W9-DHF-279

CARDIOPULMONARY BYPASS

PRINCIPLES AND PRACTICE

Second Edition

CARDIOPULMONARY BYPASS

PRINCIPLES AND PRACTICE

Second Edition
Editors

GLENN P. GRAVLEE, M.D.

Professor and Chairman
Department of Anesthesiology
College of Medicine and Public Health
Ohio State University Medical Center
Columbus, Ohio

RICHARD F. DAVIS, M.D.

Chief Clinical Executive
Portland Veterans Administration Medical Center
Professor of Anesthesiology
Oregon Health Sciences University
Portland, Oregon

MARK KURUSZ, C.C.P.

Chief Perfusionist
Division of Cardiothoracic Surgery
Assistant Professor
Department of Surgery
The University of Texas Medical Branch
Galveston, Texas

JOE R. UTLEY, M.D.

Former Chief, Cardiac Surgery Division
Spartanburg Regional Medical Center
Spartanburg, North Carolina
Former Clinical Professor, Surgery
Medical University of South Carolina
Charleston, South Carolina
University of South Carolina School of Medicine
Columbia, South Carolina

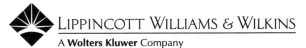

LIPPINCOTT WILLIAMS & WILKINS
A **Wolters Kluwer** Company

Philadelphia · Baltimore · New York · London
Buenos Aires · Hong Kong · Sydney · Tokyo

Acquisitions Editor: Craig Percy
Developmental Editor: Tanya Lazar
Production Editor: Kim Yi
Manufacturing Manager: Colin Warnock
Cover Designer: Christine Jenny
Compositor: Maryland Composition
Printer: Maple Press

© **2000 by LIPPINCOTT WILLIAMS & WILKINS**
530 Walnut Street
Philadelphia, PA 19106-3780 USA
LWW.com

All rights reserved. This book is protected by copyright. No part of this book may be reproduced in any form or by any means, including photocopying, or utilized by any information storage and retrieval system without written permission from the copyright owner, except for brief quotations embodied in critical articles and reviews. Materials appearing in this book prepared by individuals as part of their official duties as U.S. government employees are not covered by the above-mentioned copyright.

Printed in the USA

Library of Congress Cataloging-in-Publication Data

Cardiopulmonary bypass : principles and practice / [edited by] Glenn P. Gravlee . . . [et al.].—2nd ed.
          p. ; cm.
     Includes bibliographical references and index.
     ISBN 0-683-30476-3
        1. Cardiopulmonary bypass.   I. Gravlee, Glen P.
     [DNLM: 1. Cardiopulmonary Bypass. WG 168 C2662 2000]
RD598.C344 2000
617.4′12059–dc21

                                      99-057043

Care has been taken to confirm the accuracy of the information presented and to describe generally accepted practices. However, the authors, editors, and publisher are not responsible for errors or omissions or for any consequences from application of the information in this book and make no warranty, expressed or implied, with respect to the currency, completeness, or accuracy of the contents of the publication. Application of this information in a particular situation remains the professional responsibility of the practitioner.

The authors, editors, and publisher have exerted every effort to ensure that drug selection and dosage set forth in this text are in accordance with current recommendations and practice at the time of publication. However, in view of ongoing research, changes in government regulations, and the constant flow of information relating to drug therapy and drug reactions, the reader is urged to check the package insert for each drug for any change in indications and dosage and for added warnings and precautions. This is particularly important when the recommended agent is a new or infrequently employed drug.

Some drugs and medical devices presented in this publication have Food and Drug Administration (FDA) clearance for limited use in restricted research settings. It is the responsibility of the health care provider to ascertain the FDA status of each drug or device planned for use in their clinical practice.

10   9   8   7   6   5   4   3   2

CONTENTS

CONTRIBUTING AUTHORS

V. Simon Abraham, M.D.
Surgical Director
Children's Heart Center
St. Vincent Hospital
8333 Naab Road
Indianapolis, Indiana 46260

Scott K. Alpard, M.D.
Surgical Research Fellow
Division of Cardiothoracic Surgery
The University of Texas Medical Branch
301 University Boulevard
Galveston, Texas 77555-0528

Francisco A. Arabia, M.D.
Associate Professor of Surgery
Department of Cardiothoracic Surgery
University of Arizona
1501 North Campbell Avenue, Room 4402
Tucson, Arizona 85724

Gerard Bashein, M.D., Ph.D.
Professor of Anesthesiology
Adjunct Professor, Department of Bioengineering
University of Washington
Seattle, Washington 98195-6540

Daniel E. Berkowitz, M.B.
Associate Professor
Department of Anesthesiology and Critical Care Medicine
The Johns Hopkins Hospital
600 North Wolfe Street
Baltimore, Maryland 21287

Bruce D. Butler, Ph.D.
Professor of Anesthesiology
Director of Research, Hermann Center for Environmental,
    Aerospace and Industrial Medicine
Department of Anesthesiology
The University of Texas-Houston Medical School
6431 Fannin, MSB 5.020
Houston, Texas 77030

John F. Butterworth, M.D.
Professor and Section Head, Cardiothoracic Anesthesiology
Department of Anesthesiology
Wake Forest University School of Medicine
Medical Center Boulevard
Winston Salem, North Carolina 27157-1009

Mark E. Comunale, M.D.
Assistant Professor of Anesthesia
Harvard Medical School
Boston, Massachusetts
Associate Anesthetist-in-Chief
Beth Israel Deaconess Medical Center
Department of Anesthesia and Critical Care
330 Brookline Avenue
Boston, Massachusetts 02215

Vincent R. Conti, M.D.
Professor of Surgery
Chief, Division of Cardiothoracic Surgery
The University of Texas Medical Branch
301 University Boulevard
Galveston, Texas 77555-0528

David J. Cook, M.D.
Consultant in Anesthesiology
Mayo Foundation and Mayo Clinic
Associate Professor of Anesthesiology
Department of Anesthesiology
Mayo Medical School
200 First Street SW
Rochester, Minnesota 55905

John R. Cooper, Jr., M.D.
Associate Chief, Department of Cardiovascular
    Anesthesiology
St. Luke's Episcopal Hospital
Texas Heart Institute
P.O. Box 20345
Houston, Texas 77225-0345
Clinical Associate Professor of Anesthesiology
University of Texas Health Sciences Center
Houston, Texas 77225-0345

Jack G. Copeland, M.D.
Professor and Chief
Section of Cardiovascular and Thoracic Surgery
Michael Drummond Distinguished Professor of Surgery
University of Arizona Health Sciences Center
1501 North Campbell Avenue
Tucson, Arizona 85724

Joseph S. Coselli, M.D.
Professor, Department of Surgery
Baylor College of Medicine
6560 Fannin Street, Suite 1100
Houston, Texas 77030

Laurie K. Davies, M.D.
Associate Professor, Department of Anesthesiology
Director, Pediatric Cardiothoracic Anesthesia
University of Florida
P.O. Box 100254
Gainesville, Florida 32610

Richard F. Davis, M.D.
Chief Clinical Executive
Portland Veterans Administration Medical Center
3710 SW US Veterans Hospital Road
Professor of Anesthesiology
Oregon Health Sciences University
Portland, Oregon 97207

George J. Despotis, M.D.
Associate Professor
Department of Anesthesiology and Pathology
Washington University School of Medicine
660 South Euclid Avenue, Box 8118
St. Louis, Missouri 63110

L. Henry Edmunds, Jr., M.D.
Julian Johnson Professor of Cardiothoracic Surgery
University of Pennsylvania
5000 Ravdin Court
Hospital of the University of Pennsylvania
3400 Spruce Street
Philadelphia, Pennsylvania 19104-4382

Jane C. K. Fitch, M.D.
Associate Professor
Chief, Cardiovascular and Thoracic Anesthesiology
Department of Anesthesiology
Baylor College of Medicine
6550 Fannin, Suite 1003
Houston, TX 77030

N. Martin Giesecke, M.D.
Clinical Assistant Professor
University of Texas Health Science Center Medical School
Houston, Texas
Staff Anesthesiologist
Division of Cardiovascular Anesthesiology
St. Luke's Episcopal Hospital/Texas Heart Institute
P.O. Box 20345
Houston, Texas 77225-0345

Lawrence T. Goodnough, M.D.
Professor of Medicine and Pathology
Washington University School of Medicine
Director of Transfusion Services
Barnes-Jewish Hospital
660 South Euclid Avenue, Box 8118
St. Louis, Missouri 63110

Terry Gourlay, Ph.D.
Scientific Officer
Department of Cardiac Surgery
National Heart and Lung Institute
Imperial College School of Medicine
Hammersmith Hospital
DuCane Road
London, W12 ONN
United Kingdom

Glenn P. Gravlee, M.D.
Professor and Chairman
Department of Anesthesiology
College of Medicine and Public Health
Ohio State University Medical Center
410 West 10th Street
Columbus, Ohio 43210

Gordon R. Haddow, M.B., Ch.B., F.F.A. (S.A.)
Associate Professor of Anesthesia
Division Chief, Cardiac Anesthesia
Department of Anesthesia H3580
Stanford University Medical Center
Stanford, California 94305-5640

Richard I. Hall, M.D., F.R.C.P.C., F.C.C.P.
Professor of Anesthesiology
Associate Professor of Pharmacology and Surgery
Dalhousie University
Queen Elizabeth II Health Sciences Centre
1796 Summer Street
Halifax, Nova Scotia B3H 3A7
Canada

Eugene A. Hessel II, M.D., F.A.C.S.
Professor, Anesthesiology and Surgery (Cardio-thoracic)
Director, Cardio-thoracic Anesthesia
Department of Anesthesiology
University Hospital—Chandler Medical Center
University of Kentucky School of Medicine
800 Rose Street
Lexington, Kentucky 40536-0293

Kane M. High, M.D.
Associate Professor of Anesthesia
Pennsylvania State University College of Medicine
Co-Director Anesthesia/Surgery Intensive Care Unit
Department of Anesthesia
Hershey Medical Center
500 University Drive
Hershey, Pennsylvania 17033

Aaron G. Hill, C.C.P.
Chief Perfusionist
Inova Fairfax Hospital
3300 Gallows Road
Falls Church, Virginia 22042

Philip Hornick, B.Sc., M.B., B.Chir., F.R.C.S. (Eng)
Specialist Registrar in Cardiothoracic Surgery
Garfield Weston Senior Research Fellow and
Lecturer in Cardiothoracic Surgery
Imperial College School of Medicine at Hammersmith
 Hospital
2nd Floor Surgical Directorate
B Block
DuCane Road
London, W12 ONN
United Kingdom

Jan C. Horrow, M.D.
Clinical Professor of Anesthesiology
MCP-Hahnemann University
Philadelphia, Pennsylvania 19102
Vice-President, Clinical Development
IBEX Technologies Corporation
5 Great Valley Parkway, Suite 300
Malvern, Pennsylvania 19355

James Jaggers, M.D.
Assistant Clinical Professor, Department of General and
 Thoracic Surgery
Pediatric Cardiac Surgery
Box 3474
Duke University Medical Center
Durham, North Carolina 27710

Mark Kurusz, C.C.P.
Chief Perfusionist
Division of Cardiothoracic Surgery
Assistant Professor
Department of Surgery
The University of Texas Medical Branch
301 University Boulevard
Galveston, Texas 77555-0528

Douglas F. Larson, Ph.D., C.C.P.
Professor of Surgery
Department of Cardiothoracic Surgery
University of Arizona
1501 North Campbell Avenue, Room 4402
Tucson, Arizona 85724

Glenn W. Laub, M.D.
Chairman
Department of Cardiothoracic Surgery
Director, The Heart Hospital
St. Francis Medical Center
601 Hamilton Avenue
Trenton, New Jersey 08629-1986

Scott A. LeMaire, M.D.
Assistant Professor, Department of Surgery
Baylor College of Medicine
6560 Fannin Street, Suite 1100
Houston, Texas 77030

C. Walton Lillehei, M.D.
(deceased)

Edward Lowenstein, M.D.
Henry Isaiah Dorr Professor of Anaesthesia
Professor of Medical Ethics
Harvard Medical School
Boston, Massachusetts
Provost, Department of Anesthesia and Critical Care
Massachusetts General Hospital
32 Fruit Street
Boston, Massachusetts 02114

Christina T. Mora Mangano, M.D.
Associate Professor of Anesthesia
Stanford University
Stanford, California 94305
Ischemic Research
250 Executive Park Boulevard, Suite 3400
San Francisco, California 94134

Noel L. Mills, M.D.
Professor of Surgery
Division of Cardiothoracic Surgery
Tulane University School of Medicine
1430 Tulane Avenue
New Orleans, Louisiana 70112

Roger A. Moore, M.D.
Chair, Anesthesia Department
Deborah Heart & Lung Center
435 Camden Avenue
Moorestown, New Jersey 08057
Clinical Associate Professor of Anesthesiology
University of Medicine and Dentistry of New Jersey

Michael J. Murray, M.D., Ph.D.
Dean, Mayo School of Health Related Sciences
Professor of Anesthesiology
Mayo Clinic and Foundation
Mayo Medical Center
200 First Street SW
Rochester, Minnesota 55905

Yukihiko Nosé, M.D., Ph.D.
Professor of Surgery
Department of Surgery
Baylor College of Medicine
Texas Medical Center
One Baylor Plaza
Houston, Texas 77030

Jonathan B. Oster, M.D.
Critical Care Fellow
Department of Anesthesiology
College of Physicians and Surgeons of Columbia University
New York Presbyterian Medical Center
630 West 168th Street
New York, New York 10032

Walter E. Pae, Jr., M.D.
Professor, Department of Surgery
The Pennsylvania State University College of Medicine
P.O. Box 850
Hershey, Pennsylvania 17033

Venkat Patla, M.D., F.R.C.A.
Instructor in Anesthesia
Harvard Medical School
Boston, Massachusetts
Attending Anesthesiologist
Beth Israel Deaconess Medical Center
330 Brookline Avenue
Boston, Massachusetts 02215

Richard C. Prielipp, M.D.
Professor and Section Head
Critical Care Medicine
Department of Anesthesiology
Wake Forest University School of Medicine
Winston Salem, North Carolina 27157-1009

Steve A. Raskin, M.B.A., C.C.P.
Senior Staff Perfusionist
Baylor College of Medicine
Texas Medical Center
One Baylor Plaza
Houston, Texas 77030

Christine S. Rinder, M.D.
Associate Professor
Department of Anesthesiology and Laboratory Medicine
Yale University School of Medicine
333 Cedar Street
P.O. Box 208035
New Haven, Connecticut 06520-8035

Russell S. Ronson, M.D.
Department of Surgery
Emory University School of Medicine
550 Peachtree Street NE
Atlanta, Georgia 30322

Robert E. Shangraw, M.D., Ph.D.
Associate Professor of Anesthesiology
Department of Anesthesiology, UHS-2
Oregon Health Sciences University
3181 SW Sam Jackson Park Road
Portland, Oregon 97203-3098

Ian R. Shearer, C.C.P.
Chief Perfusionist
4291 Hospital North Box 3082
Duke University Medical Center
Durham, North Carolina 27710

Linda Shore-Lesserson, M.D.
Assistant Professor of Anesthesiology
Department of Anesthesiology
Mt. Sinai Medical Center
One Gustave L. Levy Place
Box 1010
New York, New York 10029

Harris B. Shumacker, Jr., M.D.
Department of Surgery
Uniformed Services University of the Health Sciences
4301 Jones Bridge Road
Bethesda, Maryland 20814

Robert N. Sladen, M.D., M.B., Ch.B., M.R.C.P., F.R.C.P.
Professor of Anesthesiology and Vice-Chairman
Department of Anesthesiology
Director, Cardiothoracic-Surgical Intensive Care Unit
College of Physicians and Surgeons of Columbia University
New York Presbyterian Medical Center
630 West 168th Street
New York, New York 10032

Richard G. Smith, M.S.E.E., C.C.E.
Technical Director
Artificial Heart Program
University Medical Center
University of Arizona
1501 North Campbell Avenue
Tucson, Arizona 85724

Nina Stenach, C.C.P.
Clinical Perfusionist
Clinical Programs Manager
Cardiac Surgery
Medtronic, Inc.
7000 Central Avenue NE
Minneapolis, MN 55432-3576

Benjamin C. Sun, M.D.
Director of Cardiac Transplantation
Assistant Professor of Surgery
Section of Cardiothoracic Surgery, MCH165
The Pennsylvania State University College of Medicine
P.O. Box 850
500 University Drive
Hershey, Pennsylvania 17033

Julie A. Swain, M.D.
Professor of Surgery
Gill Heart Institute
University of Kentucky College of Medicine
800 Rose Street, MN 276
Lexington, Kentucky 40536-0084

Eiki Tayama, M.D., Ph.D.
Department of Surgery
Kurume University School of Medicine
67 Asahi-machi, Kurume City
830 Japan

Kenneth M. Taylor, M.D., F.R.C.S., F.R.C.S.E., F.E.S.C.
British Heart Foundation Professor of Cardiac Surgery
Deputy Head, National Heart and Lung Institute
Imperial College School of Medicine
Cardiac Surgical Unit
Hammersmith Hospital
2nd Floor, B Block
DuCane Road
London WI2 ONN
United Kingdom

Stephen J. Thomas, M.D.
Professor and Vice Chair
Department of Anesthesiology
Weill Medical College of Cornell University
1300 York Ave
New York, New York 10021

Vinod H. Thourani, M.D.
Department of Surgery
Emory University School of Medicine
550 Peachtree Street NE
Atlanta, Georgia 30322

John M. Toomasian, M.S., C.C.P.
Staff Perfusionist
Perfusion Services
Stanford University Medical Center
300 Pasteur Drive
Stanford, California 94305

Ross M. Ungerleider, M.D.
Chief of Pediatric Cardiac Surgery
Duke University Medical Center
Box 3178
Durham, North Carolina 27710

Joe R. Utley, M.D.
Former Chief, Cardiac Surgery Division
Spartanburg Regional Medical Center
Spartanburg, North Carolina
Former Clinical Professor, Surgery
Medical University of South Carolina
Charleston, South Carolina
University of South Carolina School of Medicine
Columbia, South Carolina

Jakob Vinten-Johansen, Ph.D.
Professor of Surgery (Cardiothoracic Surgery)
Associate Professor of Physiology
Carlyle Fraser Heart Center of Crawford Long Hospital
Emory University School of Medicine
550 Peachtree Street NE
Atlanta, Georgia 30365-2225

Andrew S. Wechsler, M.D.
Professor and Chairman
Department of Cardiothoracic Surgery
Senior Associate Dean for Clinical Affairs
MCP Hahnemann University
Hahnemann University Hospital
245 North Broad Street, MS111
Philadelphia, Pennsylvania 19102-1192

Joseph B. Zwischenberger, M.D.
Professor of Surgery, Medicine, and Radiology
Director, General Thoracic Surgery Program
Director, ECMO Program
Division of Cardiothoracic Surgery
The University of Texas Medical Branch at Galveston
301 University Boulevard
Galveston, Texas 77555-0528

PREFACE TO FIRST EDITION

The rapidly expanding scope of medical knowledge threatens to overwhelm even our most diligent efforts to remain current, even within a discrete specialty arena. In a lecture reflecting on his noteworthy academic career in anesthesiology spanning over four decades, Dr. Joseph Artusio noted that there were just three English-language textbooks relevant to anesthesiology during his residency in the 1940s. He went on to say, "And now, there's a new book every week."* Amid this scenario, one might reasonably ask whether this, or any other new medical text, offers something new and worthwhile. This book was designed to provide comprehensive and scholarly discussion of cardiopulmonary bypass with a comprehensive multidisciplinary scope and a structure that differs considerably from previous texts in the field.

Current annual oxygenator utilization is estimated at 350,000 patients in the United States, and 650,000 patients worldwide, so the number of patients affected by this intervention is not insignificant. These numbers reflect continued growth in oxygenator utilization, and the complexity of disease present in patients undergoing cardiopulmonary bypass continues to escalate. Although cardiac surgical procedures account for the vast majority of oxygenators consumed, other indications for cardiopulmonary bypass are either emerging (e.g., cardiac arrest and supported angioplasty) or re-emerging (e.g., pulmonary support). In the United States, the number of hospitals offering cardiopulmonary bypass is also rapidly expanding.

The clinical management of cardiopulmonary bypass for cardiac surgery represents a team effort involving perfusionists, surgeons, and anesthesiologists. Our goal has been to provide a textbook representing the perspectives of each of those professions while addressing both practical and reference needs for practitioners and trainees. We also hope to assist cardiologists, neonatologists, and intensive care specialists who manage patients undergoing or recovering from cardiopulmonary bypass. We hope that scholarly pathophysiologic discussions will enhance the understanding and application of patient care after cardiopulmonary bypass. Like most multiauthor textbooks, some redundancy exists between individual chapters. We strove to minimize this, but elected to retain any overlap that appeared to enhance the understanding of the primary subject covered in a given chapter or represented an author's unique perspective on that particular subject. As with most medical subjects, when discussing cardiopulmonary bypass, the border between fact and opinion is often indistinct. Such is the nature of medicine as an imperfect science.

Glenn P. Gravlee, M.D.
Richard F. Davis, M.D.
Joe R. Utley, M.D.

---

* Artusio Jr JF: Rovenstine Lecture, 1991 New York Postgraduate Assembly of Anesthesiologists, New York Society of Anesthesiologists, New York, New York.

PREFACE

The goals for this edition are identical to those articulated in the Preface to the First Edition. We welcome co-editor Mark Kurusz, C.C.P., from the perfusion community, who brings a firsthand perspective. We have reorganized the sections, introduced new chapters, and added a number of new contributors. Specifically, the section titles have been simplified into the categories of History, Equipment, Physiology and Pathology, Hematology, and Clinical Applications. There are new chapters on history, blood pumps, cardiotomy suction and venting, hematologic effects, transfusion and blood conservation, and minimally invasive bypass. The subjects of blood–artificial surface interaction and oxygenators and heat exchangers have been separated into two chapters. Key Points have been included at the end of every chapter to serve as a quick overview for readers. Most changes were made in an effort to incorporate knowledge gained and techniques developed since publication of the First Edition. The second history chapter adds the perspective of another pioneer in cardiopulmonary bypass, Dr. Har-ris B. Shumacker, Jr. History was being made simultaneously in Minneapolis and in Philadelphia, and each account tells its own fascinating story. We note with sadness the passing of Dr. C. Walton Lillehei, the author of Chapter 1, and gratefully acknowledge his important contribution to this book and his enormous contributions to the development of cardiac surgery and cardiopulmonary bypass. As in the First Edition, we have striven to avoid duplication, yet have made some exceptions in order to respect the particular perspectives of different experts.

We thank the readers of the First Edition for making a Second Edition possible, and express our desire that this book be used by a diverse array of students and practitioners to enhance the care of the patients we share.

Glenn P. Gravlee, M.D.
Richard F. Davis, M.D.
Mark Kurusz, C.C.P.
Joe R. Utley, M.D.

ACKNOWLEDGMENTS

Glenn P. Gravlee thanks his wife, Joyce, and children for their support and patience during the preparation of this book. Special thanks go to Barbara Davis of the Department of Anesthesiology at Allegheny General Hospital in Pittsburgh, Pennsylvania, for her expert administrative assistance.

Richard F. Davis thanks his wife and family for their consistent support. He also gratefully acknowledges Sue Gardner and Deborah Heideman for their steadfast support with manuscript preparation, editing, correspondence, and general communication.

Mark Kurusz thanks his family and coworkers for their forbearance during the completion of this project and acknowledges H. Gibbon for manuscript processing. *Deo gratias, ad finem.*

Joe R. Utley thanks Connie Wilde for her invaluable assistance with manuscript processing, correspondence, and communication.

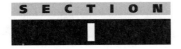

HISTORY

1

HISTORICAL DEVELOPMENT OF CARDIOPULMONARY BYPASS IN MINNESOTA

C. WALTON LILLEHEI

A physician at the bedside of a child dying of an intracardiac malformation as recently as 1952 could only pray for a recovery. Today, with the heart–lung machine, correction is routine. As a result, open heart surgery has been widely regarded as one of the most important medical advances of the 20th century. Its application is so widespread (2,000 such surgeries performed every 24 hours worldwide), performed so effortlessly, and carries such low risk at all ages that it may be difficult for the current generation of cardiologists and cardiac surgeons, much less the lay public, to appreciate that just 40 years ago the outer wall of the living human heart presented an impenetrable anatomic barrier to the surgeon's knife and to the truly incredible therapeutic accomplishments that are so commonplace today.

The keystone to this astonishing progress has been cardiopulmonary bypass (CPB) by extracorporeal circulation (ECC). These methods for ECC have allowed surgeons to empty the heart of blood, stop its beat as necessary, open any desired chamber, and safely carry out reparative procedures or even total replacement in an unhurried manner.

Beginning in 1951, a number of the developments that made the transition from the research laboratory to clinical open heart surgery possible and successful occurred in the Department of Surgery at the University of Minnesota (Table 1.1). This institution boasted two unequaled assets. One was the world's first heart hospital devoted entirely to the medical and surgical treatment of heart diseases. This 80-bed facility for pediatric and adult patients was donated to the University of Minnesota by the Variety Club of the Northwest and opened its doors to patients on July 1, 1951. The second, and perhaps even more important, advantage was the presence of Owen H. Wangensteen, a truly visionary surgeon, as Chairman of the Department of Surgery. He was not a cardiac surgeon but had made immense contributions in the field of general surgery by his innovative work in the treatment and prevention of bowel obstruction.

Over the years, beginning in 1930, he had evolved the unique "Wangensteen system" for the training of young surgeons. He placed a heavy emphasis on in-depth knowledge of the basic sciences and in research. He believed that this combination of a thorough grounding in the basic sciences and the insights gained by research gave young surgeons the confidence to disregard or abandon previously held ideas and traditions and to go forward on the basis of their own judgment and knowledge.

Proverbial also was his ability to spot talent and capabilities in his younger colleagues, whose aptitudes were not at all obvious to others—often not even to themselves. He would then proceed to develop that student using a combination of intellectual stimulation and material assistance.

THE OPEN HEART ERA IS BORN

Hypothermia

In this stimulating milieu, major accomplishments were soon forthcoming. The first of these occurred on September 2, 1952 when Dr. F. John Lewis, a medical school classmate and close personal friend, after a period of laboratory research on dogs successfully closed a secundum atrial septal defect (ASD) (1) in a 5-year-old girl under direct vision using inflow stasis and moderate total body hypothermia (Fig. 1.1).* The date has considerable historical significance because that was the world's first successful operation within the open human heart under direct vision. Dr. Lewis had been inspired by Bigelow et al.'s experimental studies (2) on general body hypothermia as a technique for open heart

---

C. W. Lillehei: *Deceased, July 1999.*

* This first patient had a normal postoperative heart catheterization. She is now the mother of two healthy children and remains entirely well, nearly 50 years after her operation.

TABLE 1.1. ORIGINAL OPEN HEART OPERATIONS AND TECHNIQUES DEVELOPED AT THE UNIVERSITY OF MINNESOTA, 1952 TO 1957

Operation/Technique	Date[a]	Technique
Atrial septal defect closure	September 2, 1952	General hypothermia
Ventricular septal defect closure	March 26, 1954	Cardiopulmonary bypass (by cross-circulation)
Atrioventricularis communis correction	August 6, 1954	Same as above
Tetralogy of Fallot intracardiac correction	August 31, 1954	Same as above
Disposable bubble oxygenator for CPB	May 13, 1955	
First use of direct cardiac stimulation by myocardial electrodes with a pacemaker for complete heart block	January 30, 1957	

[a] Dates indicate the first successful use in patients.
CPB, cardiopulmonary bypass.

repairs. Such operations became routine at the University of Minnesota Hospital, and news of these successes spread rapidly throughout the medical world. Swan et al. (3) were next to report successful direct-vision intracardiac operations in humans using general hypothermia and inflow stasis.

Hypothermia with inflow stasis proved to be an excellent method for simple atrial defects. Lewis (4) reported in 1954 that eight of nine patients had their atrial septal defects successfully closed, with only one death. Later in 1954, Lewis et al. (5) reported on closure of ASD in 11 patients,

with a mortality of only 18% (Table 1.2). By 1955, Lewis (6) reported 33 atrial septal defects closed at a 12.1% mortality rate compared with Gross' 30.2% mortality using blind techniques (atrial well). Also, the blind atrial well provided significantly fewer complete corrections (6).

Hypothermia also proved excellent for isolated congenital pulmonic or aortic stenoses (3). However, failure was uniform when this technique was applied to more complex lesions such as ostium primum, atrioventricularis communis, or ventricular septal defect (VSD). These experiences reconfirmed the oft-predicted need for a perfusion method for the more complex intracardiac lesions.

CARDIOPULMONARY BYPASS

Beginning Efforts and then Discouragement

The first attempts to use a heart–lung machine for total CPB to permit intracardiac surgery in humans were also carried out at the University of Minnesota Hospital by Dennis et al. on April 5, 1951 (7). Two patients were operated on within a month's time, but both died in the operating room. The first patient had an erroneous preoperative diagnosis despite two heart catheterizations and finger exploration of the heart's interior 5 months earlier. Instead of the

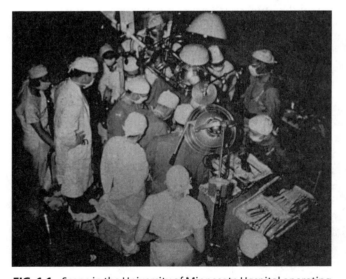

FIG. 1.1. Scene in the University of Minnesota Hospital operating room on September 2, 1952 near the end of the first successful open heart operation in medical history. On that date, Dr. F. John Lewis closed by suture an atrial secundum defect (2 cm in diameter) under direct visualization using inflow stasis and moderate total body hypothermia (26°C) in a 5-year-old girl who remains alive and well today. Postoperative heart catheterization confirmed a complete closure. She is the mother of two normal children.

TABLE 1.2. DIRECT VISION CLOSURE ATRIAL (SECUNDUM) DEFECT SYSTEMIC HYPOTHERMIA AND CAVAL OCCLUSION[a]

Patients	Defects Closed	Deaths
11[b]	10	2 (18%)

[a] Surgery performed by F. J. Lewis, M.D., at the University of Minnesota, 1952–1953 (5).
[b] One patient developed ventricular fibrillation and was not surgically repaired, but recovered.

TABLE 1.3. CLINICAL EXPERIENCE BY J. H. GIBBON, JR. WITH TOTAL CARDIOPULMONARY BYPASS USING HIS SCREEN OXYGENATOR (12,13)

Patient	Age	Date of Operation	Diagnosis Preoperatively	Postoperative Results
1	15 mo	February, 1952	ASD	Had PDA (only); died in OR
2	18 yr	May 6, 1953	ASD	Lived (long term)
3	5.5 yr	July 1953	ASD	Died in OR
4	5.5 yr	July 1953	ASD	Had also VSD, PDA; died in OR
5	Data NA	Data NA	Data NA	Died
6	Data NA	Data NA	Data NA	Died

PDA, patent ductus arteriosus; VSD, ventricular septal defect; ASD, atrial secundum defect; OR, operating room; NA, not available.

anticipated ASD, she had an unexpected partial atrioventricularis communis lesion. This pathology was baffling at the time. The second patient, operated on 2 weeks later, had an ASD repaired but died intraoperatively from massive air embolism (8).

In both operations, the failures were related to the high perfusion rates that were considered necessary. In the first patient, in addition to the unfamiliar pathology, Dennis et al. stated that they were visually handicapped by "an amazing amount of blood" lost from the coronary sinus and thebesian vein and that "adjacent tissue anteriorly was employed to attempt closure in spite of the recognition of a good deal of encroachment upon the tricuspid orifice" (7). The cardiac specimen was studied by Dr. Jesse Edwards (9), the world-renowned cardiac pathologist, who found the tricuspid orifice had been severely stenosed in the attempt to close the ostium primum defect. In the second patient, the arterial reservoir was emptied suddenly (by the high flow), resulting in air being pumped into the patient's systemic circuit (8). Later in 1951, Dr. Dennis and many of his team moved to the University of New York (Brooklyn) to continue their work.

The next milestone was reached in May 1953 by Dr. John Gibbon, Jr. (10), who had started working on a pump oxygenator in the 1930s. He had developed his apparatus and techniques to the point where 12 of 20 dogs survived the closure of a surgically created VSD for 1 week to 6 months (11). By 1952 he believed he was ready to venture into the clinical area. His first patient had died,† but the

second case, with an atrial (secundum) defect, was operated on May 6, 1953 and was a complete success (12). This success was well received in a report in the lay press 12 days later (13) but aroused surprisingly little enthusiasm or interest among cardiologists and cardiac surgeons at the time, for several reasons. First, Dr. Gibbon duplicated only once Dr. Lewis' successes beginning 8 months earlier and could not repeat or extend his one success (12,14). Second, Dr. Lewis was regularly closing ASDs under direct vision using inflow stasis and moderate hypothermia with excellent results (1,4–6). Swan and colleagues (3,15) were also duplicating these excellent results with ASD. Third, and perhaps most important, was the fact that Dr. Gibbon, not repeating his one success with ASD or achieving success with the more complex VSD, became so discouraged after five failures (Table 1.3) that he abandoned open heart surgery as a means of repair of human heart lesions. That decision by the dean of the pioneering surgeons at that time had a profound effect in the minds of many investigators on the future of open heart surgery.

From 1951 to early 1954, there were many reported—and many more unreported—attempts to use CPB for intracardiac operations (Table 1.4). In all these reported clinical attempts at open heart operations, there was a common scenario: good-to-acceptable survival in the experimental animals but universal failure when the same apparatus and techniques were applied to humans. Thus, virtually all of the most experienced investigators of that era concluded with seemingly impeccable logic that the problems were not with the perfusion techniques or the heart–lung machines but that the "sick human heart," ravaged by failure, could not possibly be expected to tolerate the magnitude of the operations required and then recover immediately, with adequate output as occurred when the same machines and techniques were applied to dogs with healthy hearts. Thus, discouragement was rampant, and pes-

---

† Similar to the experience of Dennis, Gibbon's first patient selected for intracardiac surgery to close an atrial septal defect was a 15-month-old infant with an erroneous preoperative diagnosis. At operation, no septal defect was found. Autopsy disclosed a large unrecognized patent ductus arteriosus. Patient 2 was the 18-year-old girl with the successful atrial defect closure. Patients 3 and 4 were both 5.5-year-old girls operated on in July 1953, and both died intraoperatively. Patient 3 had an ASD, and repair was attempted. Patient 4 had been diagnosed preoperatively as having an atrial septal defect but had a VSD and small patent ductus. Dr. Gibbon stated that "none of the defects could be repaired because of the flooding of the intracardiac field by blood" inside the bypassed heart (12). Kirklin (14) wrote (and also confirmed in a letter to me) that Gibbon operated on four patients

after his May 1953 success and none survived. These last two patients were never reported by Gibbon or associates, and details are not available.

TABLE 1.4. OPEN HEART SURGERY WITH TOTAL CARDIOPULMONARY BYPASS

Physician (refs)	Patients	Age	Defects	Method	Date	Result Died	Result Lived
Dennis (7,8)	2	6–8 yr	ASD, AV canal	Film oxygenator	1951	2	0
Gibbon (12–14)	6	15 mo–18 yr	PDA, ASD (2), ASD and VSD (1), NA (2)	Film oxygenator	1952–1953	5	1 (ASD)
Helmsworth (16)	1	4 yr	ASD	Bubble oxygenator	1952	1	0
Dodrill (17)	1	16 yr	Pulmonary stenosis	Autogenous lung	1953	1	0
Mustard (18)	5	10 m–11 yr	Tetralogy of Fallot	Monkey lungs	1951–1953	5	0
Clowes (19)	3	Neonate–55 yr	Lung disease, AO stenosis, left atrial myxoma	Bubble oxygenator	1953	3	0

All reported cases from 1951–1954, before cross-circulation, March 26, 1954.
ASD, atrial secundum; AV canal, atrioventricularis communis; PDA, patent ductus; VSD, ventricular septal defect; NA, not available; AO, aortic.

simism about the future of open heart surgery became widespread.

The prevalent belief was that the concept of open heart repair, however attractive, was doomed for patients with the more complex pathologic conditions who urgently required and would benefit the most from corrective procedures. What was necessary, many thought, was a means of mechanical support for the heart during its recovery period. Even today, more than three decades later, prolonged mechanical support of the failing heart during recovery still presents many unsolved problems.

A New Outlook

During some canine experiments in which the cavae were temporarily occluded to test tolerance limits of the brain and heart to ischemia (20), it was discovered that if the azygos vein was not clamped (but all other inflow to the heart was), the resulting very small cardiac output (measured at 8 to 14 mL/kg body weight/min) (21) was sufficient to sustain the vital organs safely in *every* animal for a minimum of 30 minutes at normothermia. To even mention at that time that such a low flow might be adequate for perfusions was heresy; thus, we were pleased to learn of a similar observation in 1952 in England by Andreason and Watson (22). Both studies agreed that only about 10% of the so-called basal cardiac output was needed to sustain animals unimpaired physiologically for a reasonable period of time at normothermia.

From the earliest days, the universally accepted *minimum flow* for CPB (at normothermia) was considered by the authorities at that time to be 100 to 165 mL/kg per body weight/min in animals and humans (7,12,16,19,23). Our findings of this remarkable tolerance to drastically lower flows of only 8 to 14 mL/kg/min was very surprising, but the animal (dog) results were unmistakably clear. In analyzing these findings, we described at that time (1954) at least three identifiable important physiologic adjustments that

were occurring in response to lowered blood flow (21). These compensating readjustments were additive and in their entirety at normal body temperatures accounted very well for the fact that these animals survived for 30 minutes or longer with their vital organs (brain, liver, heart, and kidneys) well protected.

At that time in our studies, we quickly found that "low flow" was a pejorative term and that advocacy of systemic flows much lower than the so-called basal cardiac output of 100 to 120 mL/kg/min was considered "totally wrong." What most clinicians and even physiologists did not appreciate was the simple fact that with the basal cardiac output, venous blood was returning with 65% to 75% of its oxygen content *unused*. There was no physiologic harm whatsoever in fully using the oxygen contained in the blood. Thus, the "azygos flow was really not low flow, but *physiologic flow* (21)."

Reducing the volume of blood necessary to be pumped had immediate and immense benefits. It has been observed repeatedly that one of the universal problems responsible in a very large part for the early failures with ECC by Dennis et al. (7), Gibbon (12), and Helmsworth et al. (16) was the enormous and unexpected blood return out of the open hearts due to well-developed systemic-to-pulmonary collaterals that made accurate vision almost impossible. Also, these unanticipated losses often made the perfusions physiologically precarious.

We immediately appreciated that the discovery of the azygos flow concept represented the sword that would eventually sever the Gordian knot of complexity that had garroted perfusion technology. I was convinced that some simple way could be found to successfully perfuse at only 20 to 25 mL/kg/min, which we set as a desirable flow rate with a comfortable safety margin. This low flow or physiologic flow quantity was only 10% to 20% of what others deemed necessary. Consequently, armed with this information in 1952, I believed that successful open heart surgery was not only possible but inevitable in the near future.

TABLE 1.5. DODRILL'S CLINICAL EXPERIENCE WITH AUTOGENOUS LUNG-PUMP BYPASS

Patient	Diagnosis	Date	Procedure	Operation	Postoperative Result
Male, 41 yr	Mitral regurgitation	7/3/52	Pump bypass of left ventricle, 50 min	Heart not opened (26); finger exploration of valve	Lived
Male, 16 yr	Pulmonary stenosis	10/21/52	Right heart bypass, 25 min	Pulmonary (27) valvuloplasty, direct vision	Lived (RV 190 mm, to 50 mm Hg, by catheter)
Unknown	Pulmonary stenosis	Before 9/16/53 (17)	Bypass both sides of heart, autogenous lungs	Pulmonary valvuloplasty	Died (fourth day)
Unknown	Mitral disease	Before 9/16/53 (17)	Pump bypass of left ventricle	Mitral valve exposed	Lived

RV, right ventricle.

Autogenous Lung for Cardiopulmonary Bypass

The low-flow principle made autogenous lung oxygenation much simpler and thus attractive. However, we found that the extra cannulas and tubing in the operative field were sensitive to even slight displacements, with the subsequent rapid onset of pulmonary edema. This rather frequent complication in our animal studies dampened our enthusiasm for potential clinical use (24). However, these venous drainage kinking problems led directly to the idea of moving these extrapulmonary cannulas completely out of the operative field by using a separate donor animal for oxygenation (cross-circulation). These experimental studies (24) convinced us that the autogenous lung was not a feasible route to pursue clinically, even with the significant advantages offered by the azygos flow concept.

The Dodrill Experience with Autogenous Lung Pump Bypass

Dodrill et al. (25), in collaboration with the General Motors Corporation engineers in Detroit, developed a blood pump for animal and clinical use as a right, left, or combined heart bypass with autogenous lung oxygenator. All their reported clinical experiences are summarized in Table 1.5. In their series of four patients, three had partial heart bypasses (two left sides, one right side). All three lived but in only one (patient 2) was a therapeutic procedure (pulmonary valvuloplasty) carried out (17). The fourth (patient 3 in Table 1.5) had bypass of both sides of the heart but did not survive pulmonary valvuloplasty.

In their patients, Dodrill et al. used high flow rates (4,500 mL/min or about 56 to 64 mL/kg body weight). Those perfusion rates led to a significant amount of collateral flow within the bypassed heart, making it difficult to open the heart without sizable blood losses, which made therapeutic maneuvers difficult or impossible. For this and various other reasons, they did not report any further clinical work.

Controlled Cross-Circulation for Cardiopulmonary Bypass

Initially, our extracorporeal perfusions using cross-circulation in dogs had been intended only as an interim method to permit some open heart experience in animals without the need for a complex conventional pump-oxygenator, which was unavailable to us at the time. The term "controlled" refers to the use of a pump to precisely control the balance of the volume of blood flowing into and out of the donor and the patient. However, as the experiments progressed, it became apparent that the dogs undergoing a 30-minute open heart interval using physiologic flow with cross-circulation not only survived at a far higher rate but recovered far more rapidly when compared with the dogs we had observed undergoing a similar period of high-flow pump-oxygenator perfusions.‡ The differences were truly astonishing, and for the first time we realized that this might be the simple and effective clinical method for intracardiac operations for which we were searching. The experimental and clinical data on cross-circulation perfusions and the reduced or physiologic perfusion flow rates based on the azygos flow studies have been documented elsewhere (27,28).

Clinical Application

Cross-circulation for clinical intracardiac operations was an immense departure from established surgical practice at the time (1954). The thought of taking a normal human being to the operating room to provide a donor circulation (with potential risks, however small), even temporarily, was con-

---

‡ In the years 1950 and 1951, Drs. C. Dennis and C.W. Lillehei had experimental laboratories next door to each other in the attic of the physiology building (Millard Hall) at the University of Minnesota Medical School.

sidered unacceptable and even "immoral" by some critics. However, we had begun to suspect massive physiologic disturbances evoked by total body perfusion and open cardiotomy about which we knew very little and that by temporarily instituting a "placental" circulation we might minimize or even correct those to permit successful operations that would have otherwise been impossible (Fig. 1.2).

The continued lack of any success in the other centers around the world that were working actively on heart–lung bypass (Table 1.4) and the widespread doubt about the feasibility of open heart surgery in humans contributed to our decision to go ahead clinically on March 26, 1954 (28) (Fig. 1.3). The cross-circulation technique was a dramatic

success in humans (28–36). In the months that followed its first use to close a VSD, a rapid succession of surgical firsts occurred for correction of congenital heart defects that previously had been inoperable (Table 1.1). Cross-circulation as the means for ECC to permit work inside the human heart was used for 45 operations (Table 1.6). There was no donor mortality and no long-lasting donor sequelae (36).

Almost overnight, the "sick human heart theory" was refuted because the patients operated on with cross-circulation, mostly infants in terminal congestive failure, could not have been worse operative risks. Thus, after 15 years in the experimental laboratory, open heart surgery moved permanently into the clinical arena.

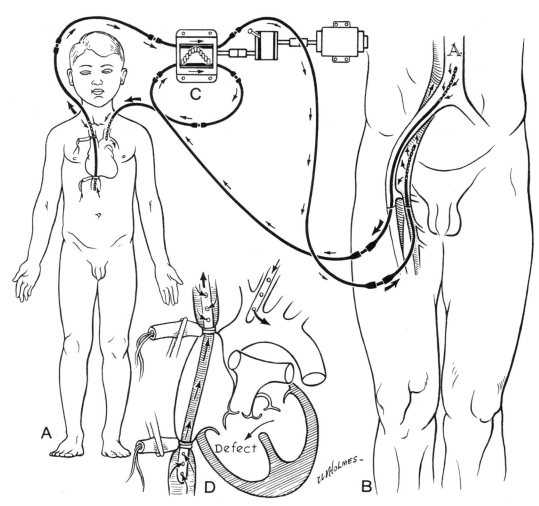

FIG. 1.2. Direct-vision intracardiac surgery using extracorporeal circulation by means of controlled cross-circulation. **A:** The patient, showing sites of arterial and venous cannulations. **B:** The donor, showing sites of arterial and venous (superficial femoral and great saphenous) cannulations. **C:** The single Sigmamotor pump controlling precisely the reciprocal exchange of blood between the patient and donor. **D:** Close-up of the patient's heart, showing the vena caval catheter positioned to draw venous blood from both the superior and inferior venae cavae during the cardiac bypass interval. The arterial blood from the donor was circulated to the patient's body through the catheter that was inserted into the left subclavian artery.

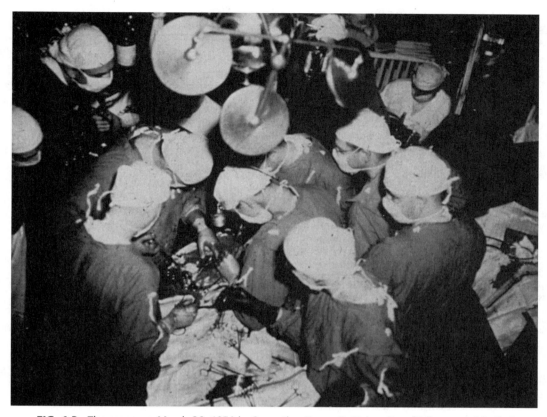

FIG. 1.3. The scene on March 26, 1954 in Operating Room B, University of Minnesota Medical Center, during the first controlled cross-circulation operation. At that time, a ventricular septal defect (VSD) was successfully visualized by ventricular cardiotomy and closed in a 12-month-old infant. The lightly anesthetized donor (the patient's father), with the groin cannulations serving as the extracorporeal oxygenator, may be seen to the far right (the patient is in the left foreground). Dr. C. W. Lillehei is immediately to the right of the scrub nurse, and opposite him is Dr. R. L. Varco. Behind Dr. Lillehei is Dr. H. E. Warden, and next to him, looking over the shoulder of the scrub nurse, is Dr. M. Cohen. Drs. Cohen and Warden are the two residents who had perfected this technique in the experimental dog laboratory. To Dr. Varco's right is Dr. J. B. Aust, an assistant resident. Behind Dr. Varco, at the left upper corner, is Dr. V. L. Gott, the surgical intern. Also, behind Dr. Varco is an observer, Dr. Norman Shumway, who was an assistant resident at the time. The VSD was closed by direct suture during a bypass interval of 19 minutes. The average flow rate was 40 mL/kg body weight/min at normothermia. The Sigmamotor pump that served to control the interchange of blood is located on Dr. Warden's right between donor and patient, but it is not visible in this photo.

A Three-Decade Follow-Up

The follow-up of a minimum of 30 years on these first patients—with VSD, atrioventricularis communis, infundibular pulmonic stenosis, and tetralogy of Fallot—to have successful intracardiac corrections has been particularly informative and impressively sanguine (36). Twenty-eight of 45 (62%) patients undergoing ECC survived their operations and were discharged from the hospital. Even more impressive was the finding that only six of these survivors had died in 30 years. Thus, 22 of 45 patients (49%) initially operated on were alive 30 years later, and all were in good health.

The 27 patients with VSDs constituted the largest category to have repair, and 17 (63%) were living and well 30

or more years later. There were only two later VSD patient deaths in all of the years after hospital discharge. Both occurred in patients with closed defects but inexorable progression of their pulmonary vascular disease. Similarly, the late follow-up on the more complex tetralogy patients has been equally rewarding (35–38).

Cross-circulation was so successful because the donor automatically corrected all the various hematologic and metabolic derangements. At that time, we had no idea what these physiologic aberrations were and thus no knowledge about measuring them, much less treating them. In 1954 to 1955, pH and blood gases were not available clinically. Even emergency plasma electrolytes took 4 to 6 hours. There was no respiratory assistance equipment for infants or children, and

TABLE 1.6. RESULTS OF DIRECT-VISION INTRACARDIAC OPERATIONS WITH CPB BY CROSS-CIRCULATION IN 45 PATIENTS FROM MARCH 26, 1954, TO JULY 9, 1955[a]

Abnormality	Corrective Operations	Patients	Mortality	
			Hospital	Late (30 yr)
VSD	Suture closure	27	8	2
PDA (with severe pulmonary hypertension)	Exploratory ventriculotomy, division of ductus	1	0	0
Tetralogy of Fallot	Closure of VSD, correction of infundibular/valvular pulmonary stenosis	10	5	3
Atrioventricularis communis	Closure of ostium primum, VSD; repair of valvular deformities	5	3	1
Isolated infundibular pulmonary stenosis	Resection of infundibulum	1	0	0
Pulmonary stenosis, ASD, anomalous pulmonary venous retum	Pulmonary valvotomy, ventricular and atrial cardiotomies, transposition of anomalous pulmonary veins, closure of septal defects	1	1	0
Total		45	17	6

[a] Cross-circulation was used exclusively from its inception through February 1955. Beginning March 1, 1955, other bypass methods (bubble oxygenator, dog-lung oxygenator, arterial reservoir) were used for lower risk patients. Cross-circulation was reserved for high-risk patients. By July 1955, the bubble oxygenator had become the sole method.
VSD, ventricular septal defect; PDA, patent ductus arteriosus; ASD, atrial (secundum) septal defect; CPB, cardiopulmonary bypass.

there were no intensive care units, much less any monitors, pacemakers, or external defibrillators. In temporarily reconstituting the placental circulation with cross-circulation, we rediscovered the world's greatest intensive care unit: the intrauterine environment. It was some years before we could duplicate these remarkable results in equally sick patients using the pump oxygenator.

PROBLEMS REQUIRING SOLUTIONS FOR SUCCESSFUL OPEN HEART SURGERY

For open intracardiac operations in humans to be regularly successful, workable solutions had to be identified for the three major obstacles that had stalled progress for so long. First, an effective method was needed for safely emptying the heart of blood for a reasonable length of time. ECC by cross-circulation fulfilled that need. Next, having gained access to the interior of the living human heart, it was soon evident that these malformations existed in a very broad spectrum and in many forms not yet described or even recognized by clinicians or pathologists. Surgical methods for dealing with these unfamiliar lesions required rapid technical development, often improvised on the spot, and sometimes with poignant failures. Moreover, given the existing state of technology, the preoperative diagnoses were often wrong or incomplete. Finally, these patients, often critically ill preoperatively, required postoperative care on a much higher level of sophistication than was known or available at the time.

Knowing now what we did not know in 1951 through 1954, it seems very probable that the only method for ECC that could possibly have succeeded so rapidly in the face of such formidable problems, in the face of such limited knowledge, and in the many high-risk infants and children with complex anatomic lesions was cross-circulation. The homeostatic mechanisms of the donor automatically corrected the untold number of mostly unknown physiologic aberrations evoked by total body perfusion.

Thirty years ago we wrote that "clinical experience with cross-circulation has made it apparent that it is unlikely that a technique for total cardiopulmonary bypass will be developed which excels this one for the patients' safety" (32). The spectacular success of clinical cross-circulation operations stimulated intensive laboratory work on alternative methods for CPB without the need for a living human donor.

Heterologous Biologic Oxygenators

Beginning on March 1, 1955, a series of clinical open heart operations was started at the University of Minnesota using a pair of canine lungs as oxygenators. Twelve patients were operated on, with 4 long-term survivors (39,40). Subsequent to those two reports, two more patients were operated on, for a total of 14, with 5 long-term survivors. In no patient was death attributable to oxygenator dysfunction. The only other attempt to use heterologous lungs at that time was the report of Mustard and associates (18,41) using

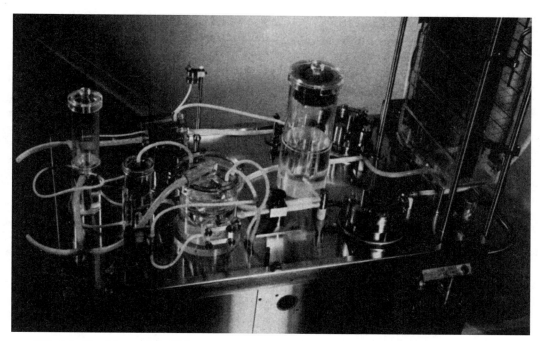

FIG. 1.4. The Mayo Clinic-Gibbon screen oxygenator. This model was used in 1955 during the first series of open heart operations performed by Dr. John Kirklin and associates at the Mayo Clinic, Rochester, MN. (Photo courtesy of J. W. Kirklin).

monkey lungs. In their series of seven patients, there were no survivors. Mustard and Thomson (18) subsequently reported on surgery using monkey lungs in 21 infants and children having ECC between 1952 and 1956; there were three survivors in this series.

Extracorporeal Circulation from a Reservoir of Oxygenated Blood

Beginning March 3, 1955, the first of a series of five patients were operated on at the University of Minnesota for intracardiac repairs of VSD or transposition of the great vessels by continuous perfusion from a reservoir of oxygenated blood (29,42,43). This very simple technique was particularly applicable to infants needing relatively simple intracardiac repairs, thereby requiring lesser blood requirements.§ The arterialized venous blood for perfusion was drawn in the blood bank a few hours preoperatively using an ordinary venipuncture in donors whose arms had been immersed in

---

§ On March 29, 1955, the patient, at age 6 months, weighing 4.7 kg, was operated on using reservoir perfusion for closure of a VSD. This patient reported on in 1955 (29,43) has now been followed for 37 years. He was recatheterized in 1964 with findings of normal pulmonary pressures and a completely closed defect. He graduated from college and was a Federal Bureau of Investigation agent for 20 years. He presently heads a private security company.

water heated to 45°C for 15 minutes before collection, which effectively oxygenated the venous blood.

THE MECHANICAL PUMP OXYGENATOR FOR CARDIOPULMONARY BYPASS—BEGINNING OF AN ERA

In two publications in 1955 from the Mayo Clinic, Jones et al. (44) and Donald et al. (45) described their experimental results using the design of the Gibbon-type pump oxygenator as originally built by IBM and modified by the Mayo Clinic (Fig. 1.4). Their first clinical application was March 22, 1955, and a report followed on their first eight patients undergoing open heart surgery (46). Two of their four survivors had VSDs, one had an atrial septal defect, and one had an atrioventricularis communis canal. The four deaths occurred in patients with VSD (two), tetralogy (one), or atrioventricularis communis canal (one) (Table 1.7). Their flow rates varied from 100 to 200 mL/kg body weight. By September 1958, 245 patients had been operated on at the Mayo Clinic by Kirklin et al. (47). In their skillful and thoughtful hands, the initial high mortality declined rapidly.

Advent of the DeWall-Lillehei Bubble Oxygenator

Before 1955, there was universal agreement among the world's authorities on ECC that the one way that blood

TABLE 1.7. MAYO CLINIC OPEN HEART EXPERIENCE[a]

Defect	No. of Patients	Lived	Hospital Deaths
Atrial (secundum)	1	1	0
Ventricular	4	2	2
AV canal	2	1	1
Tetralogy	1	0	1
Total	8	4	4 (50%)

[a] First Series (March–May 1955) with Mayo-Gibbon screen oxygenator (46).
AV canal, Atrioventricularis communis.

could *not* be arterialized for clinical CPB was by a bubble oxygenator because of potential problems with air embolism. On May 13, 1955, DeWall and Lillehei, based on their dog laboratory research, began routine clinical use of a simple disposable bubble oxygenator (Fig. 1.5A). In their first report, Lillehei et al. (48) described surgery for seven patients with closure VSD, five of whom were long-time survivors. The operations took place at normothermia with perfusion rates (using a Sigmamotor pump, SIGMA-MOTOR, INC., Middleport, NY) of 25 to 30 mL/kg body weight. All seven patients awoke postoperatively, and there was no evidence of neurologic, hepatic, or renal impairment of even a temporary nature.

In an addendum to that study (48), DeWall et al. (49) reported that 36 patients ranging in age from 16 weeks to 21 years had their hearts and lungs totally bypassed for intracardiac correction using their bubble oxygenator with similar excellent results. The congenital defects successfully corrected were VSD, tetralogy of Fallot, atrioventricularis communis canal, complete transposition, and ASDs. As the number of patients having open heart surgery by ECC increased rapidly, the bubble oxygenator was refined to increase capacity for adult patients (Figs. 1.5, B and C, and 1.6).

In the early clinical open heart operations, considerable physiologic and biochemical data (50) were collected, analyzed, and compared with the earlier animal studies (51). This information confirmed the excellence of the patients' physiologic status while undergoing perfusions from the bubble oxygenator at the lower (more physiologic) flow rates based on the azygos flow concept. Tests done by psychologists and neurologists on these patients before and after perfusion detected no significant abnormalities in cerebral function attributable to the perfusions (52).

In a 26- to 31-year follow-up of 106 patients operated on for correction of tetralogy (37), 34 (32%) had college or graduate degrees, including two MDs, two PhDs, and one lawyer (LLB). Obviously, putting people on the bubble oxygenator could not be expected to increase intelligence, but these figures were far beyond the average for a random group from the general population and at the very least confirmed the absence of any significant cerebral dysfunction.

The DeWall-Lillehei bubble oxygenator was an instant success because it had so many practical advantages. It was efficient, inexpensive, heat sterilizable, easy to assemble and check, and had no moving parts. Because it could be assembled from commercially available materials at a small material cost, it was also disposable (Figs. 1.5 and 1.6). The development of the self-contained unitized plastic sheet oxygenator (Figs. 1.5C and 1.7) in 1956 by Gott et al. (53,54) further improved this system and played an important role in the tremendous expansion of open heart surgery that occurred after 1956. The revelation that safe perfusion of the body could be maintained with several lengths of plastic tubing, a few clamps, and some oxygen had an explosive

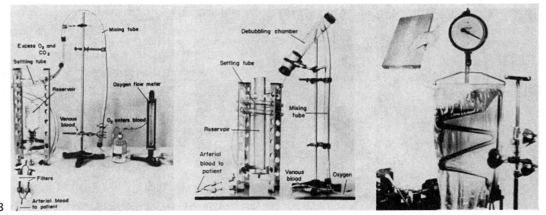

FIG. 1.5. Evolution of the simple disposable DeWall-Lillehei bubble oxygenator for open heart surgery. **A:** The first 1955 clinical model; it was successful in infants and small children. **B:** Later in 1955, helix reservoir model with adult capacity was developed. **C:** A 1956 commercially manufactured model, shipped sterile in a package (left upper inset), ready to hang up and use.

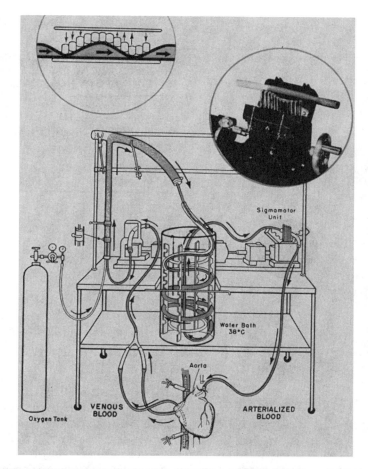

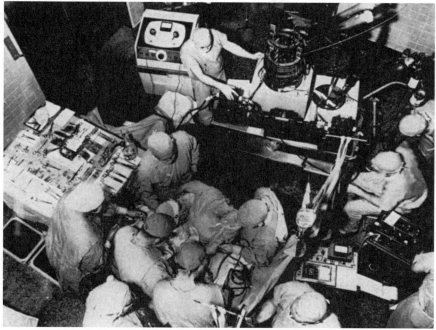

FIG. 1.6. **Top:** Diagram of the 1955 DeWall-Lillehei helix reservoir, disposable bubble oxygenator with adult capacity. The upright oxygenating column with the venous blood mixing with oxygen bubbles formed at the base, transverse debubbling chamber, and the spiral (helix) debubbling reservoir immersed in a water bath are evident. The two insets show the wavelike pattern of the Sigmamotor pump's 12 metallic "fingers" as they stroke the blood through the plastic tubing without direct contact. **Bottom:** An open heart operation in an adult patient at the University of Minnesota Hospital in 1956.

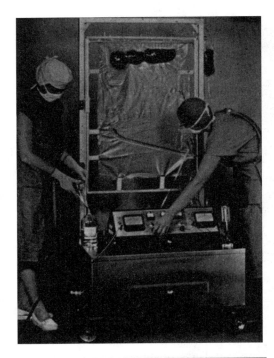

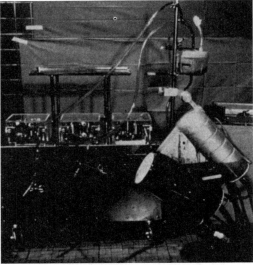

FIG. 1.7. Top: A DeWall-Lillehei unitized plastic sheet oxygenator, commercially manufactured and shipped sterile ready to hang up, prime, and use as shown here. (Courtesy of D. A. Cooley, Texas Heart Institute, Houston, TX.) **Bottom:** The Temptrol disposable bubble oxygenator with self-contained heat exchanger during a perfusion. In this unit, Dr. DeWall introduced the rigid presterilized plastic outer shell, which has been the basis of all subsequent oxygenator designs for both bubble and membrane units.

TABLE 1.8. OPEN CARDIOTOMY: SUMMARY OF THE EARLY CLINICAL EXPERIENCE AT THE UNIVERSITY OF MINNESOTA HOSPITALS (56)

Method	Period	No. of Patients
Hypothermia only	1952–1956	70
Cross-circulation	1954–1955	45
Arterial reservoir	1955	5
Dog-lung oxygenator	1955	14
Bubble oxygenator	1955–1966	2581

regularly scheduled open heart surgery by ECC: the University of Minnesota Hospital in Minneapolis (using cross-circulation). Beginning in May 1955 and well into 1956, there were only two places in the world performing these operations, the University of Minnesota in Minneapolis and the Mayo Clinic in Rochester, Minnesota, only 90 miles apart. Visitors from all parts of the world traveled to these two places to observe open heart surgery. On the one hand, there was the Mayo Clinic-Gibbon apparatus, which was very expensive, handcrafted, and very impressive in appearance but difficult to use and maintain. On the other hand, there was the unbelievably simple, disposable, heat-sterilized bubble oxygenator of DeWall and Lillehei, costing only a few dollars to assemble. It is no wonder, as Professor Naef (56) wrote, that "many surgeons left these two clinics with their minds in a totally confused state as to which method they should seek to pursue."

Dr. Denton Cooley (57), an early visitor and observer in June 1955, was to later write

> The contrast between the two institutions and the two surgeons was striking. We observed Lillehei and a team composed mostly of house staff correct a ventricular septal defect using cross-circulation. During the visit, we also saw an oxygenator developed by Richard DeWall at the University of Minnesota. The next day we observed John Kirklin and his impressive team in Rochester that was made up of physiologists, biochemists, cardiologists, and others as they performed operations using the Mayo-Gibbon apparatus. Such a device was beyond my organizational capacity and financial reach. Thus I was deeply disappointed on our return to Houston when Dr. McNamara stated that he would not permit me to operate on his patients unless I had a Mayo-Gibbon apparatus.

However, Cooley succeeded in convincing some of his cardiologists that "the era of open heart surgery had arrived" and in 1956 began to perform open heart surgery using the DeWall-Lillehei bubble oxygenator with considerable success.

Professor Naef (56) also later wrote "the homemade helix reservoir bubble oxygenator of DeWall and Lillehei, first used clinically on May 13, 1955, went on to conquer the world and helped many teams to embark on the correction of malformations inside the heart in a precise and unhurried manner. The road to open-heart surgery had been opened."

effect on the worldwide development of cardiac surgery (Fig. 1.8). The surgeon's dream of routinely performing intracardiac correction in the open heart had become a reality (55) (Table 1.8).

In 1954, there was only one place in the world doing

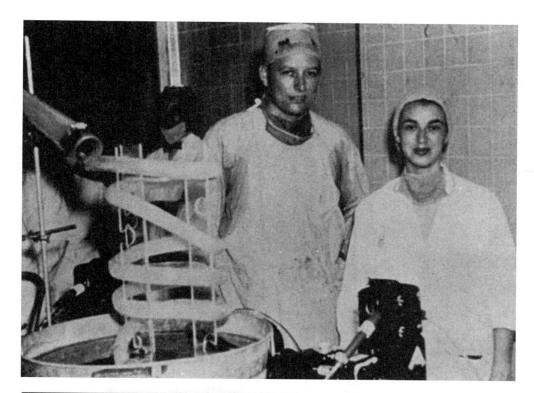

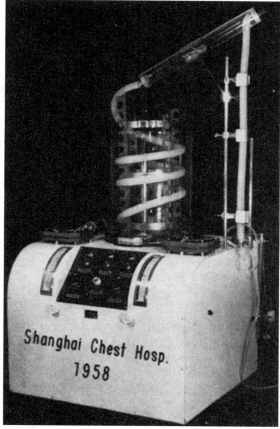

FIG. 1.8. The ready availability of the simple and effective disposable Helix Reservoir Bubble Oxygenator had an explosive effect on worldwide growth of open heart surgery. **Top:** Dr. Denton Cooley with a perfusionist after an atrial septal defect closure, September 12, 1957, in Caracas, Venezuela. **Bottom:** The equipment used by Professor Pan Chih and associates for many successful open heart operations at the Shanghai Chest Hospital in China, 1957 to 1958. The first successful cardiac operations using cardiopulmonary bypass in both China and Japan were done with the DeWall-Lillehei bubble oxygenator.

TABLE 1.9. OPEN HEART SURGERY BY EXTRACORPOREAL CIRCULATION[a]

Patient	Sex	Age (yr)	Date of Surgery	Procedure	Result
1	F	6	5/24/56	Pulmonary valvuloplasty	Died
2	F	10	1/13/57	Aortic valvuloplasty	Died
3	M	12	1/17/57	ASD closure	Lived
4	F	13	2/14/57	Pulmonary valvuloplasty	Lived
5	F	7	2/21/57	ASD closure	Lived
6	F	9	2/26/57	ASD closure	Died
7	M	8	4/2/57	Pulmonary valvuloplasty	Lived
8	F	6	4/4/57	VSD closure	Died
9	M	8	4/11/57	VSD closure	Died
10	F	3	4/18/57	VSD closure	Died
11	F	9	4/20/57	VSD closure, pulmonary valvuloplasty	Died
12	F	14	4/25/57	VSD closure	Died

[a] Early experience of R. E. Gross (62). Boston Children's Hospital. The first patient was operated on using the Harvard screen oxygenator and the remaining with the Kay-Cross rotating disc film oxygenator.
ASD, atrial septal defect; VSD, ventricular septal defect.

Rotating Disc Film Oxygenator (Kay-Cross)

After finishing his surgical training at the University of Minnesota in 1953, Dr. Frederick Cross‖ moved to Cleveland, where he developed with Earl Kay in 1956 a rotating disc oxygenator that had wide use in the later 1950s, particularly in the United States. This oxygenator, called the Kay-Cross apparatus (58,59), was based on the earlier experimental work of Bjork (60). It had multiple vertical discs placed on a horizontal axis that rotated, with the discs dipping into a pool of venous blood, creating a film on the discs in an atmosphere of oxygen. This filming unit, like the Mayo Clinic-Gibbon film oxygenator, was capable of good oxygenation, but both, being nondisposable, shared similar problems: cumbersome to use, large priming volumes, very difficult and tedious to clean and sterilize, and rapid loss of efficiency if hemodilution was attempted. However, the Kay-Cross unit became commercially available in contrast to the Mayo Clinic-Gibbon machine, which was extremely expensive to handcraft and was not available commercially in those early years. Although this oxygenator certainly accomplished its purpose, the rotating disc mechanism had clinical limitations, in addition to its cumbersome assembly and maintenance. Disc oxygenation was later supplanted everywhere by bubble oxygenation, and perfusionists no longer had to spend all day setting up for the next surgery. The blood bank personnel were equally grateful at its passing.

Robert E. Gross, who pioneered cardiac surgery in 1938 with his brilliantly conceived ligation of patent ductus, began open heart surgery with CPB at the Boston Children's Hospital in 1956 (Table 1.9). For his first patient, who died after a pulmonary valvuloplasty, he had used a screen pump oxygenator modeled after the Gibbon machine but constructed in the Harvard laboratories by an engineer, Mr. Savage. Dr. Dwight Harken, who also used this oxygenator, stated that the unit was cumbersome, not heat sterilizable, required a very large priming volume, was inefficient as an oxygenator, and was extremely noisy (61).

Gross was also disturbed by the performance of this device and instituted a moratorium on open heart surgery in his unit for almost 8 months. He restarted CPB in January 1957 using the Kay-Cross oxygenator with high flow (2.3 to 2.5 L/m²/min) at normothermia and without hemodilution. In the next 3.5 months, 11 patients had been operated on with a disastrously high mortality rate of 67% (Table 1.9). Gross persisted with the same equipment and methods, and even at the time of his Shattuck Lecture to the Massachusetts Medical Society in Boston on May 20, 1959, his operative mortality remained very high. He reported a 13% early mortality for pulmonary valvuloplasty, a 40% mortality for VSD closure, and recommended against intracardiac correction in cyanotic tetralogies (63). Looking at these results is a clear reiteration of a lesson that many pioneer cardiac surgeons had to learn, "that even consummate surgical skill could not compensate for deficiencies in perfusion physiology."

The Kay-Cross filming unit appealed to the cardiac surgeons who at that time could not or refused to believe that bubble oxygenation was more efficient, safer, ideally adapted for hemodilution, yet vastly simpler to use and less expensive than the filming units. Even the Mayo Clinic had by 1971 converted almost entirely to the use of the bubble oxygenator (64). By 1976 it was estimated that 90% of all open heart operations worldwide involved the use of a bubble oxygenator (65).

Other oxygenators for CPB that were publicly known and worthy of mention but had moderate to ephemeral

---

‖ Dr. Cross was a surgery resident at the University of Minnesota who assisted in the world's first successful open heart operation, closure of an ASD under hypothermia, on September 2, 1952 (1).

clinical applications were those of Rygg and Kyvsgaard¶ (66) (bubble), Dennis (8) (film), Clark et al. (67) (bubble), Crafoord and Senning (68) (film and bubble), Clowes et al. (19) (bubble), Clowes and Neville (69) (membrane), Melrose (70) (film), and Gerbode et al. (71) (membrane). For more information on these devices, the reader is referred to the references cited as a starting point and also to two fine review articles by DeWall et al. (72,73).

Membrane Oxygenators

Kolff et al. (74) described a disposable membrane oxygenator for experimental use in 1956. Clowes and Neville (69) described their experimental studies with membrane oxygenation and a complex apparatus they considered suitable for clinical perfusions in 1958. The belief that membrane oxygenation gives a better perfusion than the bubble or film oxygenators has been clear only with perfusions exceeding 8 hours in duration. Confusion has arisen over the innumerable comparative studies of membrane versus bubble oxygenators in shorter perfusions. With perfusions lasting 6 to 8 hours, the membrane oxygenator is associated with less reduction of platelets, less complement activation, less postoperative bleeding, and fewer microemboli. Because ECC times for most cardiac procedures are 2 to 3 hours or less, it has been difficult to prove that these changes, which are for the most part readily reversible, have any permanent side effects. Some studies have failed to show the theoretic benefits of membrane over bubble oxygenation (75–77), whereas other published data demonstrate improved hematologic tolerance of CPB with membrane oxygenators (78–80). I, with Lande et al. (81), described in 1967 the first compact, disposable, commercially manufactured membrane oxygenator for clinical use.

Further Developments in Bubble Oxygenation

In 1966, DeWall et al. (82) made a very significant advance in oxygenator design with the introduction of a hard-shell bubble oxygenator with an integrated oxygenator and omnithermic heat exchanger in a disposable, presterilized, polycarbonate unit (Fig. 1.7). The adequacy of oxygenation and acid-base balance was amply documented (83,84). The integrated hard-shell concept has been the basis of all subsequent refinements, both in the bubble and membrane oxygenators (Fig. 1.9).

In the early days of open heart surgery, postoperative cerebral dysfunction was a subject of intense interest. As the major causes were identified and resolved (52), concern

¶ The Rygg bubble oxygenator (66) was a replica of the DeWall-Lillehei technology that was manufactured in Denmark and was used particularly in countries where U.S. patents did not apply.

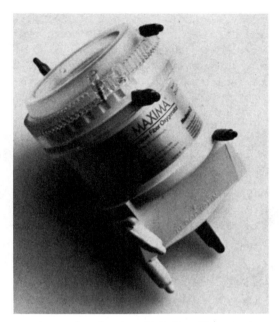

FIG. 1.9. The Maxima (Medtronic) hollow-fiber membrane oxygenator is a widely used state of the art device. This disposable unit and similar competitive devices, such as those of Cobe, Terumo, Sarns, Shiley, and Bard, have rigid outer shells with integrated heat exchangers, easily attached venous reservoirs and cardiotomy suction chambers, low priming volumes, and efficient gas transfer. Their ease of use and more competitive price differentials versus the bubblers have resulted in increasing use for routine open heart procedures.

over this matter decreased. However, there has been a resurgence of interest in the detection and prevention of more subtle changes in personality and intellect that may be associated with an otherwise successful CPB (85–88). The reality and frequency of these changes and the need for continuous electroencephalographic monitoring for immediate correction of problems are under study (89).

Hemodilution

A major technologic advance that has had an astonishing effect on the growth of ECC was the knowledge that the pump oxygenators could be primed with nonblood solutions, thereby immensely reducing the need for blood donors and at the same time improving the quality of perfusions by a reduction in viscosity and the safety by reducing foreign blood. Zuhdi et al. (90–92) developed the theory and process of hemodilution in 1961; they had trained in cardiac surgery at the University of Minnesota. DeWall et al. (93,94) confirmed the benefits of hypothermic hemodilution in ECC. Other hemodilution studies were reported from the Minnesota group that confirmed the value of low molecular weight dextran (95–97). Other comparative studies demonstrated the value of hemodilution with differing perfusates for improving renal blood flow and lessening

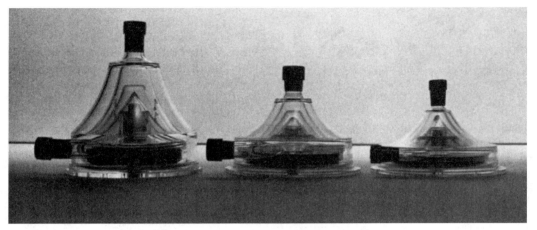

FIG. 1.10. The BioMedicus disposable centrifugal flow blood pump, with ease of use over a wide range of flows and a number of other advantages (see text), has gained steadily increasing acceptance for routine open heart operations and also for longer time circulatory support. Three sizes are available.

hemolysis (98,99). Further, the beneficial effects of hemodilution and antiadrenergic drugs on the prevention of renal ischemia during ECC were confirmed (100,101).

Progress in Pump Design

In the earliest days of ECC, the multicam-activated Sigmamotor pump was used. Then the roller pumps, because of their ease of use and reliability, gained popularity. In more recent years, the centrifugal pump described by Rafferty et al. in 1968 (102) has become commercially available as the BioMedicus Biopump (BioMedicus, Inc., division of Medtronic, Inc., Minneapolis, MN) (Fig. 1.10). Some of the advantages of this pump are reliability, ease of use over a wide range of flows, less likelihood to pump air, absence of spallation, and low hemolysis. This pump was originally developed and used for perfusions lasting hours or days. However, surgeons in growing numbers have been impressed by the centrifugal pump's performance and advantages and have begun in increasing numbers to use it for routine ECC.

As CPB became predictably reliable for a wide variety of congenital malformations, beginning in 1956 open cardiotomy was successfully applied to revolutionize the treatment of patients with acquired valvular heart disease (103,104) and subsequently to the treatment of an even larger group afflicted with coronary arteriosclerosis (105,106). By 1967, the ultimate landmark of successful human heart transplantation was reached by two surgeons, Drs. Barnard and Shumway, who had trained together in the late 1950s in my cardiac program at the University of Minnesota.

Today, the primary challenge is the need to further widen the benefits of heart replacement by both increasing the availability of donors and by an effective permanent intracorporeal mechanical heart. This latter seems a likelihood in the foreseeable future. Because of the shortage of donors, only 10% to 12% of potential recipients are being served. Short of a breakthrough with xenotransplantation (which is quite possible), the gap inevitably will have to be filled by a reliable, practical, fully implantable, total artificial heart.

SUMMARY

CPB by ECC for open heart surgery and even replacement of the heart itself were just dreams only 50 years ago. Today, after millions of total body perfusions, CPB has become a standard, widely used, low-risk procedure with immense benefits to humankind. We got where we are today by a worldwide catalytic combination of research, heterodoxy, and serendipity.

KEY POINTS

- Dr. F. John Lewis performed the first successful open heart operation (closure of ASD) using general hypothermia and inflow occlusion on September 2, 1952.
- Other than one successful case by Dr. John H. Gibbon, Jr. in 1953, early clinical experience with CPB was discouraging and had unacceptably high morality rates.
- The "azygos flow concept" led to the first clinical use of controlled cross-circulation for closure of VSD on March 26, 1954 by Dr. C. Walton Lillehei.

- Dr. John W. Kirklin and coworkers at the Mayo Clinic modified the IBM-Gibbon screen film oxygenator and used it in a large series of patients in the mid to late 1950s.
- Three major problems associated with early open heart surgery were finding an acceptable method for emptying the heart for reasonable lengths of time; unfamiliar pathology, inaccurate diagnoses, and new surgical techniques for effective repair; and lack of sophisticated postoperative care.
- Despite concerns over the potential for air embolism, the DeWall-Lillehei helix bubble oxygenator was used clinically beginning in May 1955 in a large series of patients and became the method of choice worldwide for open heart operations.
- Reasons for the success of the bubble oxygenator were its simplicity, efficiency, and low cost.
- Commercially available, prepackaged, sterile bubble oxygenators of the unitized sheet and later hard-shell design with integral heat exchanger further popularized its use.
- The rotating disc oxygenator, developed by Drs. Frederick Cross and Earl Kay, also was used widely for early open heart surgery in the United States.
- Membrane oxygenators were developed and used clinically in the 1950s through the 1970s, but lack of demonstrable benefit for short CPB times contributed to their infrequent use by most groups until microporous designs became predominant in the mid-1980s.
- Hemodilution with nonblood solutions was a major technologic advance in CPB that improved tissue perfusion, reduced hemolysis, and avoided donor blood exposure.

REFERENCES

1. Lewis FJ, Taufic M. Closure of atrial septal defects with the aid of hypothermia; experimental accomplishments and the report of one successful case. *Surgery* 1953;33:52–59.
2. Bigelow WG, Callaghan JC, Hopps JA. General hypothermia for experimental intracardiac surgery. *Ann Surg* 1950;132:531–539.
3. Swan H, Zeavin I, Blount SG Jr, et al. Surgery by direct vision in the open heart during hypothermia. *JAMA* 1953;153:1081–1085.
4. Lewis FJ. In discussion: Bigelow WG, Mustard WT, Evans JG. Some physiologic concepts of hypothermia and their applications to cardiac surgery. *J Thorac Surg* 1954;28:463–480.
5. Lewis FJ, Varco RL, Taufic M. Repair of atrial septal defects in man under direct vision with the aid of hypothermia. *Surgery* 1954;36:538–556.
6. Lewis FJ. In discussion: Watkins E, Gross RE. Experiences with surgical repair of atrial septal defects. *J Thorac Surg* 1955;30:469–491.
7. Dennis C, Spreng DS Jr, Nelson GE, et al. Development of a pump-oxygenator to replace the heart and lungs: an apparatus applicable to human patients and application to one case. *Ann Surg* 1951;134:709–721.
8. Dennis C. Perspective in review: one group's struggle with development of a pump-oxygenator. *Trans Am Soc Artif Intern Organs* 1985;31:1–11.
9. Edwards JE. Personal communication, 1951.
10. Gibbon JH Jr. Artificial maintenance of circulation during experimental occlusion of pulmonary artery. *Arch Surg* 1937;34:1105–1131.
11. Gibbon JH Jr, Miller BJ, Dobell AR, et al. The closure of interventricular septal defects in dogs during open cardiotomy with the maintenance of the cardiorespiratory functions by a pump oxygenator. *J Thorac Surg* 1954;28:235–240.
12. Gibbon JH Jr. Application of a mechanical heart and lung apparatus to cardiac surgery. *Minn Med* 1954;37:171–185.
13. Historic Operation. *Time News Magazine* 1953 May:70.
14. Kirklin JW. Open heart surgery at the Mayo Clinic—the 25th Anniversary. *Mayo Clin Proc* 1980;50:339–341.
15. Swan H. In discussion: Lewis FJ, Varco RL, Taufic M. Repair of atrial septal defects in men under direct vision with the aid of hypothermia. *Surgery* 1954;36:538–556.
16. Helmsworth JA, Clark LC Jr, Kaplan S, et al. An oxygenator pump for use in total bypass of heart and lungs. *J Thorac Surg* 1953;26:617–631.
17. Dodrill FD, Hill E, Gerisch RA, et al. Pulmonary valvuloplasty under direct vision using the mechanical heart for a complete bypass of the right heart in a patient with congenital pulmonary stenosis. *J Thorac Surg* 1953;26:584–597.
18. Mustard WT, Thomson JA. Clinical experience with the artificial heart lung preparation. *J Can Med Assoc* 1957;76:265–269.
19. Clowes GHA Jr, Neville WE, Hopkins A, et al. Factors contributing to the success of failure in the use of a pump oxygenator for complete bypass of the heart and lung, experimental and clinical. *Surgery* 1954;36:557–579.
20. Cohen M, Hammerstrom RW, Spellman MW, et al. The tolerance of the canine heart to temporary complete vena caval occlusion. *Surg Forum* 1952;3:172–177.
21. Cohen M, Lillehei CW. A quantitative study of the "azygos factor" during vena caval occlusion in the dog. *Surg Gynecol Obstet* 1954;98:225–232.
22. Andreason AT, Watson F. Experimental cardiovascular surgery. *Br J Surg* 1952;39:548–551.
23. Gibbon JH Jr. The maintenance of life during experimental occlusion of the pulmonary artery followed by survival. *Surg Gynecol Obstet* 1939;69:602–614.
24. Cohen M, Lillehei CW. Autogenous lung oxygenator with total cardiac bypass for intracardiac surgery. *Surg Forum* 1953;4:34–40.
25. Dodrill FD, Hill E, Gerish RA. Some physiologic aspects of the artificial heart problem. *J Thorac Surg* 1952;24:134–150.
26. Dodrill ARC, Hill E, Gerish A. Temporary mechanical substitute for the left ventricle in man. *JAMA* 1952;150:642–644.
27. Warden HE, Cohen M, DeWall RA, et al. Experimental closure of intraventricular septal defects and further physiologic studies on controlled cross circulation. *Surg Forum* 1954;5:22–28.
28. Warden HE, Cohen M, Read RC, et al. Controlled cross circulation for open intracardiac surgery. *J Thorac Surg* 1954;28:331.
29. Lillehei CW, Cohen M, Warden HE, et al. Direct vision intracardiac surgery: by means of controlled cross circulation or continuous arterial reservoir perfusion for correction of ventricular septal defects, atrio-ventricularis communis, isolated infundibular pulmonic stenosis, and tetralogy of Fallot. In *Proceedings of Henry Ford Hospital Symposium*. Philadelphia: W.B. Saunders, 1955:371–392.
30. Lillehei CW. Controlled cross circulation for direct vision intracardiac surgery correction of ventricular septal defects, atrioventricularis communis, and tetralogy of Fallot. *Postgrad Med* 1955;17:388–396.

31. Lillehei CW, Cohen M, Warden HEE, et al. The direct vision intracardiac correction of congenital anomalies by controlled cross circulation; results in 32 patients with ventricular septal defects, tetralogy of Fallot, and atrioventricular communis defects. *Surgery* 1955;38:11–29.

32. Lillehei CW, Cohen M, Warden HE, et al. Direct vision intracardiac surgical correction of the tetralogy of Fallot, pentalogy of Fallot, and pulmonary atresia defects: report of first ten cases. *Ann Surg* 1955;142:418–455.

33. Lillehei CW, Cohen M, Warden HE, et al. The results of direct vision closure of ventricular septal defects in eight patients by means of controlled cross circulation. *Surg Gynecol Obstet* 1955; 101:446–466.

34. Lillehei CW, Cohen M, Warden HE, et al. Complete anatomical correction of the tetralogy of Fallot defects: report of a successful surgical case. *Arch Surg* 1956;73:526–531.

35. Lillehei CW. A personalized history of extracorporeal circulation. *ASAIO J* 1982;28:5–16.

36. Lillehei CW, Varco RL, Cohen M, et al. The first open heart repairs of ventricular septal defect, atrioventricular communis, and tetralogy of Fallot using extracorporeal circulation by cross circulation: a 30-year follow-up. *Ann Thorac Surg* 1986;41: 4–21.

37. Lillehei CW, Varco RL, Cohen M, et al. The first open heart corrections of tetralogy of Fallot. A 26–31 year follow-up of 106 patients. *Ann Surg* 1986;204:490–502.

38. Gott VL. C. Walton Lillehei and total correction of tetralogy of Fallot. *Ann Thorac Surg* 1990;49:328–332.

39. Campbell GS, Crisp NW, Brown EB. Total cardiac bypass in humans utilizing a pump and heterologous lung oxygenator (dog lungs). *Surgery* 1956;40:364–371.

40. Campbell GS, Vernier R, Varco RL, et al. Traumatic ventricular septal defect. Report of two cases. *J Thorac Surg* 1959;37: 496–501.

41. Mustard WT, Chute AL, Keith JD, et al. A surgical approach to transposition of the great vessels with extracorporeal circuit. *Surgery* 1954;36:39–51.

42. Warden HE, DeWall RA, Read RC, et al. Total cardiac bypass utilizing continuous perfusion from a reservoir of oxygenated blood. *Proc Soc Exp Biol Med* 1955;90:246–250.

43. Warden HE, Read RC, DeWall RA, et al. Direct vision intracardiac surgery by means of a reservoir of "arterialized venous" blood. *J Thorac Surg* 1955;30:649–657.

44. Jones RE, Donald DE, Swan HJC, et al. Apparatus of the Gibbon type for mechanical bypass of the heart and lungs. *Proc Mayo Clin* 1955;30:105–113.

45. Donald DE, Harshbarger HG, Hetzel PS, et al. Experiences with a heart lung bypass (Gibbon type) in the experimental laboratory. *Proc Mayo Clin* 1955;30:113–115.

46. Kirklin JW, DuShane JW, Patrick RT, et al. Intracardiac surgery with the aid of a mechanical pump oxygenator system (Gibbon type): report of eight cases. *Proc Mayo Clin* 1955;30:201–206.

47. Kirklin JW, McGoon DC, Patrick RT, et al. What is adequate perfusion? In: Allen JG, ed. *Extracorporeal circulation*. Springfield, IL: Charles C Thomas, 1958:125–138.

48. Lillehei CW, DeWall RA, Read RC, et al. Direct vision intracardiac surgery in man using a simple, disposable artificial oxygenator. *Dis Chest* 1956;29:1–8.

49. DeWall RA, Warden HE, Read RC, et al. A simple, expendable, artificial oxygenator for open heart surgery. *Surg Clin North Am* 1956:1025–1034.

50. DeWall RA, Warden HE, Gott VL, et al. Total body perfusion for open cardiotomy utilizing the bubble oxygenator. *J Thorac Surg* 1956;32:591–603.

51. DeWall RA, Warden HE, Varco RL, et al. The helix reservoir pump-oxygenator. *Surg Gynecol Obstet* 1957;104:699–710.

52. Hodges PC, Sellers RD, Story JL, et al. The effects of total cardiopulmonary bypass procedures upon cerebral function evaluated by the electroencephalogram and a blood brain barrier test. In: Allen JG, ed. *Extracorporeal circulation*. Springfield, IL: Charles C Thomas, 1958:279–294.

53. Gott VL, DeWall RA, Paneth M, et al. A self-contained, disposable oxygenator of plastic sheet for intracardiac surgery. *Thorax* 1957;12:1–9.

54. Gott VL, Sellers RD, DeWall RA, et al. A disposable unitized plastic sheet oxygenator for open heart surgery. *Dis Chest* 1957; 32:615–625.

55. Lillehei CW, Varco RL, Ferlic RM, et al. Results in the first 2,500 patients undergoing open heart surgery at the University of Minnesota Medical Center. *Surgery* 1967;62:819–832.

56. Naef AP. *The story of thoracic surgery.* Toronto: Hografe and Huber, 1990:113–119.

57. Cooley DA. Recollections of early development and later trends in cardiac surgery. *J Thorac Cardiovasc Surg* 1989;98:817–822.

58. Cross FS, Berne RM, Hirose Y, et al. Description and evaluation of a rotating disc type reservoir oxygenator. *Surg Forum* 1956; 7:274–278.

59. Kay EB, Zimmerman HA, Berne RM, et al. Certain clinical aspects in the use of the pump oxygenator. *JAMA* 1956;162: 639–641.

60. Bjork VO. Brain perfusions in dogs with artificially oxygenated blood. *Acta Chir Scand* 1948;96[Suppl]:137.

61. Harken DE. Personal communication, May 1992.

62. Gross RE. Unpublished data, 1992.

63. Gross RE. Shattuck lecture. Open heart surgery for repair of congenital defects. *N Engl J Med* 1959;260:1047–1057.

64. Barnhorst DE, Moffitt EA, McGoon DC. Clinical use of the Bentley-Temptrol oxygenating system. In: Ionescu MI, Wooler GH, eds. *Current techniques in extracorporeal circulation*. London: Butterworths, 1976:91–116.

65. Bartlett RH, Harken DE. Instrumentation for cardiopulmonary bypass-past, present, and future. *Med Instrum* 1976;10: 119–124.

66. Rygg IH, Kyvsgaard E. A disposable polyethylene oxygenator system applied in a heart-lung machine. *Acta Chir Scand* 1956; 112:433–437.

67. Clark LC Jr, Gollan F, Gupta VB. The oxygenation of blood by gas dispersion. *Science* 1950;111:85–87.

68. Crafoord CA, Senning A. Utvecklingen av extra-corporeal cirkulation med hjart-lungmaskin. *Nordisk Med* 1956;56:1263.

69. Clowes GHA Jr, Neville WE. The membrane oxygenator. In: Allen JG, ed. *Extracorporeal circulation*. Springfield, IL: Charles C Thomas, 1958:81–100.

70. Melrose DM. A mechanical heart-lung for use in man. *Br Med J* 1953;2:57–66.

71. Gerbode F, Osborn JJ, Bramson ML. Experiences in the development of a membrane heart-lung machine. *Am J Surg* 1967; 114:16–23.

72. DeWall RA, Grage TB, McFee AS, et al. Theme and variations on blood oxygenators. *Surgery* 1961;50:931–940.

73. DeWall RA, Grage TB, McFee AS, et al. Theme and variations on blood oxygenators. II. Film oxygenators. *Surgery* 1962;51: 251–257.

74. Kolff WJ, Effler DB, Groves LJ, et al. Disposable membrane oxygenator (heart-lung machine) and its use in experimental surgery. *Cleve Clin Q* 1956;23:69–97.

75. Edmunds LH Jr, Ellison N, Colman RW, et al. Platelet function during cardiac operations. Comparison of membrane and bubble oxygenators. *J Thorac Cardiovasc Surg* 1982;83:805–812.

76. Sade RM, Bartles DM, Dearing JP, et al. A prospective randomized study of membrane and bubble oxygenators in children. *Ann Thorac Surg* 1980;29:502–511.

77. Trumbell HR, Howe J, Mottl K, et al. A comparison of the effects of membrane and bubble oxygenators on platelet counts and platelet size in elective cardiac operations. *Ann Thorac Surg* 1980;30:52–57.

78. van den Dungen JAM, Karlicek GF, Brenken U, et al. Clinical study of blood trauma during perfusion with membrane and bubble oxygenators. *J Thorac Cardiovasc Surg* 1982;83:108–116.

79. van Oeveren W, Kazatchkine MD, Descamps-Latscha B, et al. Deleterious effects of cardiopulmonary bypass. A prospective study of bubble versus membrane oxygenation. *J Thorac Cardiovasc Surg* 1985;89:888–899.

80. Boers M, van den Dungen JJAM, Karlicek GF, et al. Two membrane oxygenators and a bubbler. A clinical comparison. *Ann Thorac Surg* 1983;35:455–462.

81. Lande AJ, Dos SJ, Carlson RG, et al. A new membrane oxygenator-dialyzer. *Surg Clin North Am* 1967;47:1461–1470.

82. DeWall RA, Bentley DJ, Hirose M, et al. A temperature controlling (omnithermic) disposable bubble oxygenator for total body perfusion. *Dis Chest* 1966;49:207–211.

83. DeWall RA, Najafi H, Roden T. A hard shell temperature controlling disposable blood oxygenator. *JAMA* 1966;197:1065–1068.

84. Kalke BR, Castaneda A, Lillehei CW. A clinical evaluation of the new Temptrol (Bentley) disposable blood oxygenator. *J Thorac Cardiovasc Surg* 1969;57:679–687.

85. Aberg T, Kihlgren M, Jonsson L, et al. Improved cerebral protection during open-heart surgery. A psychometric investigation on 339 patients. In: Becker R, Katz J, Polonius M-J, Speidel H, eds. *Psychopathological and neurological dysfunctions following open-heart surgery.* Berlin: Springer-Verlag, 1982:343–351.

86. Aberg T, Ahlund P, Kihlgren M. Intellectual function late after open heart operation. *Ann Thorac Surg* 1983;36:680–683.

87. Henriksen L. Evidence suggestive of diffuse brain damage following cardiac operations. *Lancet* 1984;1:816–820.

88. Shaw PJ, Bates D, Carlidge NEF, et al. Early neurological complications of coronary artery bypass surgery. *Br Med J* 1985;291:1384–1387.

89. Arom KV, Cohen DE, Strobl FT. Effect of intraoperative intervention on neurological outcome based on electroencephalographic monitoring during cardiopulmonary bypass. *Ann Thorac Surg* 1989;48:476–483.

90. Zuhdi N, McCollough B, Carey J, et al. Hypothermic perfusion for open heart surgical procedures—report of the use of a heart lung machine primed with five percent dextrose in water inducing hemodilution. *J Int Coll Surg* 1961;35:319–326.

91. Zuhdi N, McCollough B, Carey J, et al. Double helical reservoir heart lung machine designed for hypothermic perfusion primed with five percent glucose in water inducing hemodilution. *Arch Surg* 1961;82:320–325.

92. Zuhdi N. Discussion of paper by Yeh TJ, Ellison LT, Ellison RG. Hemodynamic and metabolic responses of the whole body and individual organs to cardiopulmonary bypass with profound hypothermia. *J Thorac Cardiovasc Surg* 1961;42:782–792; 827–828.

93. DeWall R, Lillehei CW. Simplified total body perfusion-reduced flows, moderate hypothermia, and hemodilution. *JAMA* 1962;179:430–434.

94. DeWall R, Lillehei R, Sellers R. Hemodilution perfusions for open heart surgery. *N Engl J Med* 1962;266:1078–1084.

95. Lillehei CW. Hemodilution perfusions for open heart surgery. Use of low molecular dextran and 5 percent dextrose. *Surgery* 1962;52:30–31.

96. Cuello-Mainardi L, Bhanganada K, Mack JD, et al. Hemodilution in extracorporeal circulation: comparative study of low molecular weight dextran and 5 percent dextrose. *Surgery* 1964;56:349–354.

97. Long DM Jr, Todd DB, Indeglia RA, et al. Clinical use of dextran-40 in extracorporeal circulation—a summary of 5 years' experience. *Transfusion* 1966;6:401–403.

98. Todd DB, Indeglia RA, Simmons RL, et al. Comparative clinical study of hemolysis and renal function accompanying extracorporeal circulation utilizing hemodilution with different perfusates. *Am J Cardiol* 1965;15:149. (abst)

99. Nakib A, Lillehei CW. Assessment of different priming solutions for oxygenators by renal blood flow and metabolism. *Ann Thorac Surg* 1966;2:814–822.

100. Lillehei CW, Simmons RL, Miller ID, et al. Role of hemodilution and phenoxybenzamine (Dibenzyline) in prevention of renal ischemia during cardiopulmonary bypass. *Circulation* 1965;31[Suppl 2]:II-138. (abst)

101. Todd DB Jr, Indeglia RA, Lillehei RC, et al. An analysis of some factors influencing renal function following open heart surgery utilizing hemodilution and antiadrenergic drugs. *Am J Cardiol* 1967;19:154. (abst)

102. Rafferty EH, Kletschka HD, Wynyard M, et al. Artificial heart: application of nonpulsatile force-vortex principle. *Minn Med* 1968;51:11–16.

103. Lillehei CW, Gott VL, DeWall RA, et al. Surgical correction of pure mitral insufficiency by annuloplasty under direct vision. *Lancet* 1957;77:446–449.

104. Lillehei CW, Gott VL, DeWall RA, et al. The surgical treatment of stenotic or regurgitant lesions of the mitral and aortic valves by direct vision utilizing a pump oxygenator. *J Thorac Surg* 1958;35:154–191.

105. Favaloro RG. Saphenous vein graft in the surgical treatment of coronary artery disease, operative technique. *J Thorac Cardiovasc Surg* 1969;58:178–185.

106. Johnson WD, Flemma RS, Lepley D Jr. Direct coronary surgery utilizing multiple-vein bypass grafts. *Ann Thorac Surg* 1970;9:436–444.

2

BIRTH OF AN IDEA AND THE DEVELOPMENT OF CARDIOPULMONARY BYPASS

HARRIS B. SHUMACKER, JR.

A PATIENT IN DISTRESS

It was midafternoon on October 3, 1930 and a patient lay dying at the Massachusetts General Hospital in Boston. For 2 weeks her convalescence from an uncomplicated cholecystectomy had been uneventful. Moments before, however, returning to bed after a wheelchair trip to the toilet, she suddenly developed discomfort in her right chest, and almost immediately the discomfort gave way to sharp pain. Dr. Edward Churchill, who saw her at once in consultation, found her frightened, pale, cyanotic, cold, and moist. He believed that the diagnosis of massive pulmonary embolism was evident, and at his suggestion she was moved in her bed to the operating room where a pulmonary embolectomy could be undertaken as soon as a decision to proceed was made. John H. Gibbon, Jr. was assigned the task of watching the patient and monitoring her vital signs.

Her pulse, blood pressure, and respiration were determined and recorded at frequent intervals. Afternoon and night passed. Finally, at 8:00 a.m. the next morning, her condition worsened further, respirations ceased, a pulse could not be felt, and she lost consciousness. Within minutes, Churchill had opened the chest, made an incision in the pulmonary artery, and extracted several large clots. It was to no avail; the patient could not be revived. Gibbon told of this experience in remarks made in 1972 and published posthumously 6 years later (1):

> A correct diagnosis of massive pulmonary embolism was made and Dr. Churchill had the patient moved to the operating room where she could be continuously observed and operated upon immediately should her condition become critical.
>
> My job in the operating room was to take and record the patient's pulse and respiratory rates and blood pressure every 15 minutes. From 3:00 pm one day to 8:00 am the next day

the operating team and I were by the side of the patient. Finally at 8:00 am respirations ceased and the blood pressure could not be obtained. Within 6 minutes and 30 seconds Dr. Churchill opened the chest, incised the pulmonary artery, extracted a large pulmonary embolus, and closed the incised wound in the pulmonary artery with a lateral clamp.

The steps Churchill took were customary at the time and understandably so. Pulmonary embolectomy then was a last minute desperate undertaking. Not many operations had been undertaken during the 23 years since Friedrich Trendelenburg (2) had attempted, without success, the first procedure in Leipzig, and most efforts had ended fatally. The first success had been achieved only 6 years before by Martin Kirschner (3) in Konigsberg, and not a single operation had succeeded in the United States. Indeed, another 34 years would go by before Richard Warren and his colleagues across town at the Peter Bent Brigham Hospital would record such a result (4).

THE IDEA

The event of October 3rd marked a turning point in the history of surgery, not because of the way in which the patient was managed—it followed the standard practice—nor because of the fatal result from the pulmonary embolism—it was the usual outcome—but because it gave birth to an idea, one that would eventuate in the development of the heart–lung machine and would make contemporary cardiopulmonary bypass (CPB) and open heart surgery possible. In several publications (5–8), Gibbon told about the occasion and the idea it generated. This is how he put it in a 1970 address:

> During that long night, helplessly watching the patient struggle for life as her blood became darker and her veins more distended, the idea naturally occurred to me that if it were possible to remove continuously some of the blue blood from the patient's swollen veins, put oxygen into that blood and allow

H. B. Shumacker, Jr: Department of Surgery, Uniformed Services University of the Health Sciences, Bethesda, MD 20814.

carbon dioxide to escape from it, and then to inject continuously the now-red blood back into the patient's arteries, we might have saved her life. We would have bypassed the obstructing embolus and performed part of the work of the patient's heart and lungs outside the body.

Within a short period—Gibbon could never recall just when this happened but it was in a matter of a day or so—his original objective was enlarged substantially. Instead of building an apparatus that could take over some of the cardiorespiratory functions and make pulmonary embolectomy a safer procedure, he would attempt to build one that could perform the entire function of the heart and lungs for a period of time, a heart–lung machine that would make possible operations on the heart itself and even inside its chambers, a heart–lung machine that would make CPB a reality. He did not realize at the time that 23 years would pass before he could bring this idea to fruition. CPB was on the way, but a long bumpy road stretched ahead; an intriguing pathway nevertheless, for there were persons on the roadway who did not know just where they were going and one man who did, who traversed it, and reached his goal.

Even though Gibbon spoke of the idea in his customary modest manner as one that occurred to him "naturally," the idea was unique, and it becomes even more novel when viewed from the time it was conceived (9,10). The novelty of Gibbon's plan lay in its magnitude, building an apparatus with the oxygenating capacity necessary for use in humans, one which would permit safe total CPB in humans. Gibbon later estimated that if this objective were achieved using the rotating drum technique—a very good method for oxygenating blood—the drum would have to be as tall as a building two stories high, an estimate he still later revised to a building seven stories high!

HISTORICAL BACKGROUND

The concept of the perfusion of blood was itself not new nor was that of a mechanical device for oxygenating blood. As long ago as 1812, Cesar-Julian-Jean LeGallois (11) made the suggestion that a part of the body might be preserved by some sort of external perfusion device, a suggestion based on the observations of other investigators that some tissues and organs of apparently dead animals could be brought back temporarily to an apparent living state by restoring the flow of blood to them. Although some studies involving the perfusion of muscles and organs were carried out in the years that followed, it was not until the middle of the century that Charles Eduard Brown-Sequard (12) pointed out that the success of such perfusions depended on the use of oxygenated blood. An interesting observation he made was the temporary disappearance of the rigor mortis of muscles of guillotined criminals when they were perfused with their own blood. From Brown-Sequard's time it was evident that

supplying an adequate amount of oxygen to the blood is essential for successful perfusion and supplying the necessary amount of oxygen proved the most difficult problem in designing a mechanical CPB device.

Brown-Sequard's technique was very simple: He used syringes for perfusion and put oxygen into the dark venous blood by beating the blood vigorously, a maneuver that also defibrinated the blood. Other early investigators also used relatively simple methods for oxygenating the blood. One was that of "bubbling" the blood, a technique introduced in 1882 by Waldemar von Schroder (13) of Strasbourg. The bubbling method was based on the supposition that bubbles of a gas, such as air or oxygen passing through blood, would become surrounded by a thin layer of the blood that in turn would absorb oxygen, give off carbon dioxide, and then burst and leave the blood free of gas. The experiments that von Schroder, and subsequently others, carried out demonstrated that this method was unsatisfactory, however, because of foaming of the blood and gas embolism, difficulties that could not be overcome until antifoaming agents became available (14). A variant of the bubbling method, the "spraying" technique used by von Euler and Heymans (15) much later in 1932, only 2 years after the pulmonary embolism event in Boston, proved even more unsatisfactory, causing far too much damage to the blood to be useful. Solving the problems associated with the construction of a workable mechanism for CPB would prove to be far from simple.

It is interesting that the best technique for oxygenating the blood, the filming method, the one that would form the basis of techniques currently in use, had been proposed about 50 years previously in 1885 by Max von Frey and Max Gruber (16) of Leipzig. This method was founded on the hypothesis that a sufficiently thin film of blood exposed to oxygen would provide a good mechanism for gas exchange. Von Frey and Gruber achieved this objective by dispersing the blood as a thin film inside a rotating slanted cylinder filled with oxygen. The oxygenating capacity of their exceedingly complex apparatus was quite small, sufficient only for perfusion of isolated organs. Other investigators also used the filming method in small oxygenators of various designs. That of Richards and Drinker (17), for example, filmed the blood by having it flow down a cloth cylinder inside an oxygen chamber and that of Bayliss et al. (18) by dispersing the blood over the surface of a series of cones. Instead of cones, Daly and Thorpe's device (19) dispersed and filmed the blood on a glass cylinder down which it descended (Fig. 2.1). Thus, the basis for CPB had now been laid in the first decades of the 20th century but not for a method that would be applicable in building an apparatus for human use.

Some investigators, among them Patterson and Starling (20) and still later Hemingway (21), avoided the problem of oxygenating the blood with a mechanical device altogether by accomplishing this objective through the use of

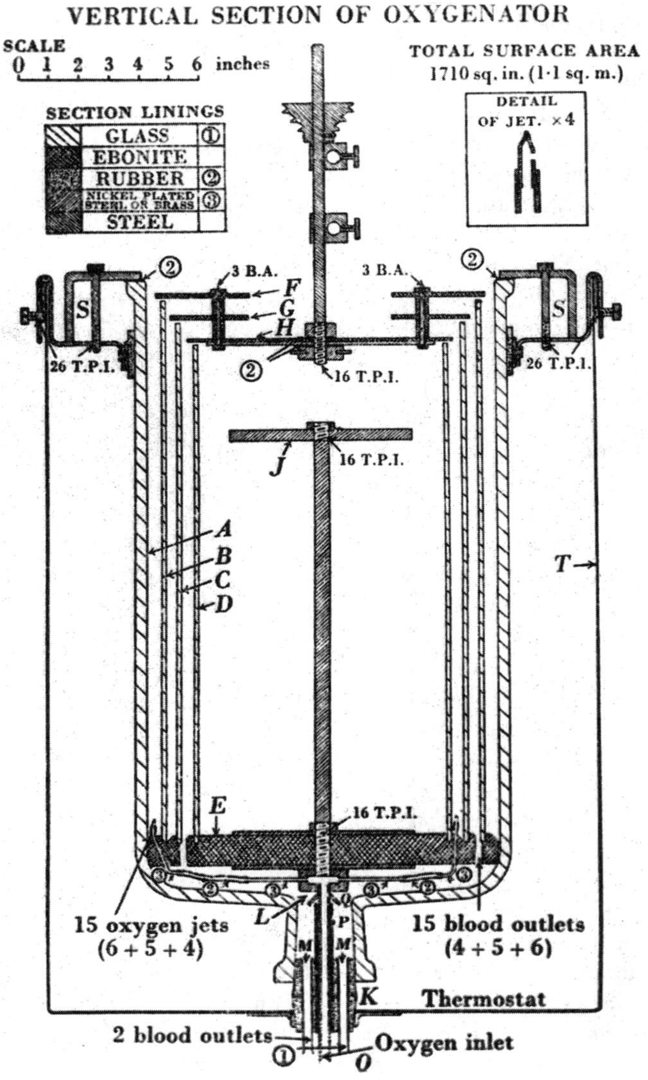

FIG. 2.1. Film oxygenator of Daly and Thorpe. This device was used for isolated dog heart preparations. Defibrinated blood was dispersed from jets onto spinning discs (*F, G, H*) where it filmed down three concentric glass cylinders (*A, B, C*). An arrangement of oxygen jets at the base provided an oxygen-rich atmosphere for gas exchange. Oxygenated blood drained through two blood outlets (*M*) to a reservoir through a filter and then into the left or right atria of the isolated heart where measurements of cardiac work and oxygen consumption were made. The surface area of the oxygenator was 1.1 m², and the system was capable of flowing 600 mL/min and handling blood volumes up to 2.5 L. The entire apparatus was immersed in a larger jar filled with water at 38°C to maintain the temperature of the circulating blood and isolated heart. Hearts continued to function for up to 6.5 hours using this device. (Reprinted from Daly IB, Thorpe WV. An isolated mammalian heart preparation capable of performing work for long periods. *J Physiol* 1933;79:202, with permission.)

the animal's own lungs. Still others used the repetitively inflated lungs of a second "donor" animal. This was the method Jacobj (22) used in his perfusion studies of isolated organs carried out during the last decade of the 19th century. His apparatus was cleverly designed but exceedingly complicated (Fig. 2.2). Later, in their experiments with kidney perfusion, Binet and Mayer (23) helped with one of the inherent problems by describing a good method for collecting the blood from the lungs of the donor animal.

The Russians Brukhonenko and Tchetchuline (24) also used the donor-lung oxygenator principle in their interesting studies that went a mammoth step beyond organ perfusion. Their experiments, described in 1929 (25), attempted to preserve temporary function of the guillotined heads of dogs (Fig. 2.3). The blood was oxygenated by passage through the repeatedly inflated lungs of a second dog before it was introduced by diaphragm-like pumps via the carotid arteries into the head of the subject animal. After achieving success in keeping the head functional for a few hours, Brukhonenko then used the same method of oxygenation in an attempt to bypass the nonfunctioning hearts of dogs. Some of these animals lived a short while after termination of the experiments but rarely was a temporary heartbeat restored. Unsuccessful as he was with these studies, Brukhonenko was optimistic about the potential of the method:

> Our conclusions, it should be understood, are of a preliminary nature. Before finishing, let us mention, in addition an idea about the methods of artificial circulation of the blood. If the method were perfected could it not be useful in the domain of medicine and especially in the case where it is essential to replace, even if it be temporary, the insufficient work of the human heart? Without going more deeply into this question, we would express the supposition based on experience with the present work that in principle the method of artificial circulation may be applicable in man (in certain cases and perhaps even for performing certain operations upon the temporarily arrested heart) but only if an adequate technique be worked out. . . .
>
> The solution of the problem of artificial circulation of the whole body opens the pathway to the question of operations upon the heart (for example upon valves).

Brukhonenko's vision was truly remarkable because it seems clear that he conceived the ultimate value of CPB and its potential use in humans. It is quite evident, however, that the method for oxygenating the blood he used in his experiments would not be acceptable for clinical application. Using the lung of a human "donor" would never be judged entirely safe and practical. It brings to mind the later short-lived cross-circulation method of C. Walton Lillehei et al. (26) (see Chap. 1).

Another person, far better known in the Western world than Brukhonenko, though in an entirely different field, also had a somewhat similar but less comprehensive vision, the building of a heart pump. Charles A. Lindbergh's *Autobiography of Values* (27) relates how the idea came to him.

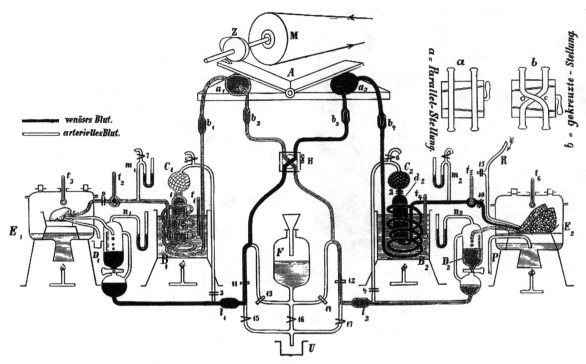

FIG. 2.2. Organ perfusion apparatus of Jacobj. This complex device relied on ventilated (*R*) donor lungs (chamber *E₂*, **right**) to provide for gas exchange. At the top center, a rotating cam (*M*) and hinged plates (*A*) arrangement alternately compressed bulbs (*a₁* and *a₂*) to pump blood to the organ to be perfused (chamber *E₁*, **left**). Note presence of open flames beneath each chamber for temperature regulation and two additional chambers (B₁, B₂) containing coiled tubing and thermometers to monitor blood temperature. (Reprinted from Jacobj C. Ein Beitrag zur Technik der kunstliechen Durchblutung ueberlebender Organe. *Arch Exp Pathol Pharmacol* 1895;36:332, with permission.)

The miracle of flying in a mechanical apparatus made him conscious of the achievements of science in general and instigated a desire to become involved in animal experimentation. He had just married Anne Morrow, and they were in the process of making plans for their home. He decided that a biologic laboratory should be put in the basement. Lindbergh was wondering what project he should undertake, what he might do "that was not already being done," when just at this time something occurred that directed his thoughts toward building a heart pump:

> My experimental interests were channeled, as so often happens, by a chance development of life—by the illness of my wife's older sister, Elisabeth. She had contracted rheumatic fever as a secondary complication of pneumonia. A lesion had developed in her heart, restricting her activities until her doctor recommended a year of complete rest in bed. Since a remedial operation of the heart was impossible, he said, her life would be limited both in activity and length. I asked him why surgery would not be effective. He said the heart could not be stopped long enough for an operation to be performed because blood had to be kept circulating through the body. I asked why a mechanical heart could not maintain the blood circulation temporarily while the heart was being operated on. He replied

that he did not know. He had never heard of a mechanical heart being used.

The same answer came from other doctors. While Lindbergh was waiting with the obstetrician and the anesthetist the night his wife was in labor with their first child, he asked the question once more. Although neither could give an answer, the anesthetist ventured the opinion that a man he knew likely could provide one. This conversation led to a meeting with Alexis Carrel, winner of the Nobel Prize and at the time director of the Rockefeller Institute for Medical Research. Lindbergh's idea was discussed thoroughly and Carrel brought up problems associated with the pumping of blood, such as clotting, infection, and hemolysis. Carrel pointed out, for example, that during a period of 20 years he had never been successful in building an infection-free organ perfusion apparatus. The result of the meeting was Lindbergh's appointment to work in Carrel's institution.

Some have assumed that Lindbergh envisioned a heart–lung machine and CPB, but a thorough search of all relevant material negates the idea that this was his dream. Instead, his dream was of a heart pump and not an extracor-

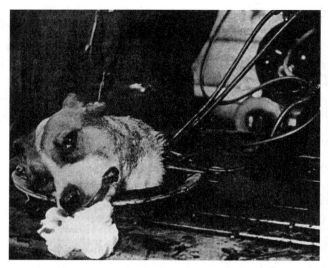

FIG. 2.3. Guillotined head of a dog in perfusion experiments of Brukhonenko and Tchetchuline. This preparation relied on gas exchange from a second donor dog's lungs. Diaphragm-like pumps pumped blood into the recipient dog's carotid arteries. Dog heads perfused in this manner remained functional for a few hours. (Reprinted from Brukhonenko S, Tchetchuline S. Experiences avec la tete isolee du chien.1.Technique et conditions des experiences. *J Physiol Pathol Gen* 1929;27:42, with permission)

poreal circuit incorporating a machine for oxygenating the blood. In this regard, Richard Bing (28), who was working at the Institute then, wrote about the research on which Lindbergh embarked:

> Charles Lindbergh's ideas immediately caught Carrel's imagination. He had always considered the concept of organ culture to be a logical extension of the concept of cell culture; but he was also aware of the considerable difficulties in designing a system for cardiorespiratory bypass, primarily because of the need to instill oxygen into the perfusate. . . . In my work with both Lindbergh and Carrel in the early 1930s, I never heard either of them refer to Lindbergh's original idea as a system for cardiopulmonary bypass. . . . Carrel convinced Lindbergh that, instead of venturing into a difficult and unexplored field, it would be wiser to attempt the culture of whole organs, which could become an immediate reality. . . .
>
> The great advantage of Lindbergh's contribution was that it permitted sterile, pulsatile perfusion at variable "pulse rates" and variable perfusion pressures. . . .
>
> Thus the perfusion system [of Lindbergh] developed into a tool that helped fulfill Carrel's wish to study the interplay between organ, blood, and lymph. An intellectual disciple of Claude Bernard's, Carrel was interested in study of the internal environment through study of the interplay between tissue fluid and organ.

In 1935, Lindbergh (29) gave details of this work with his perfusion device (Fig. 2.4), and a book on organ culture was published by Carrel and Lindbergh in 1938 (30).

Lindbergh then clearly appreciated the potential value

of a heart pump but neglected the important issue of oxygenating the blood. Brukhonenko went further, recognizing this need but providing no practical mechanism for accomplishing the task. Neither had in mind an essential component—a practical mechanical oxygenator suitable for human use. Incorporating such a mechanism into the perfusion system was indeed the primary stumbling block, and no one had tackled the problem or even conceived a suitable plan. Very shortly, however, Jack Gibbon walked onto the stage.

JOHN H. GIBBON, JR.

John H. Gibbon, Jr.* (31) was born in Philadelphia in 1903, the son of a professor of surgery and co-chairman of the surgical department at the Jefferson Medical College. Jack's early years at home in Philadelphia, on the farm in Media, and at the Penn Charter School and his young adult life at Princeton gave no indication that he would become a surgeon. Once the usual boyhood devotion to acts of physical prowess subsided, his ambition changed; he wanted to become a poet and writer. Persuaded by his father that a medical degree would do no harm and would not make him write less well, however, he entered the Jefferson Medical College.

Studying medicine was not by any means unusual in the Gibbon family. Indeed, his great-great-great-grandfather, James Lardner, was a physician in London, and five generations of Gibbons before Jack were doctors. Furthermore, there were doctors in the family of his grandmother Gibbon, two born in the colonies in 1699 and in 1731, respectively, and later three cousins. Also, the Jefferson Medical College was a logical choice for his studies. Jack's grandfather Gibbon, named Robert like his father and grandfather, studied medicine. He was the first to obtain his medical education at the Jefferson Medical College where both his son and grandson would hold surgical professorships. Not only his paternal grandfather but his uncle, his father, and his cousins as well were all graduates of Jefferson. So the would-be poet entered medical school, graduated, and became the sixth Gibbon in a direct line of descent to become a doctor.

Jack's ancestry was remarkable not only for the predilection for a medical career. Toward the close of a distinguished 43-year service in the army, his maternal grandfather, General Samuel S. B. Young, became its first chief of staff. His great uncle John Gibbon, a West Point graduate and career soldier, culminated his military service by stopping Pickett's charge at Gettysburg, during which he was wounded in

---

* A complete biography of Gibbon was recently published: Harris B. Shumacker, Jr. *A dream of the heart, the story of John H. Gibbon, Jr. and the heart surgery he revolutionized.* Santa Barbara, CA: Fithian Press, 1999.

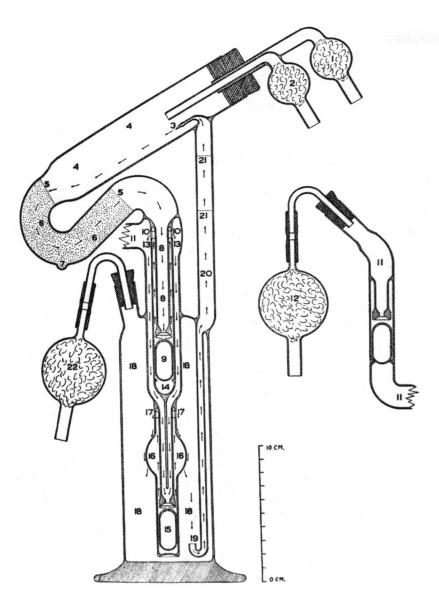

FIG. 2.4. Perfusion system of Lindbergh and Carrel. This elaborate blown-glass device provided sterile pulsatile perfusion of various organs using regulated compressed air to vary the pressure and perfusion rate. The organ chamber is the slanted portion (*4*) at the top. Cotton-filled bulb chambers (*1, 2, 12, 22*) prevented bacterial contamination of the organ and circulating fluid. Floating glass valves and other chambers provided regulation of internal and external pressures on the organ. Perfusate was filtered through a column of silica sand (*6*). Temperature of the organ and circulating fluid was maintained by placing the entire apparatus in an incubator. (Reprinted from Lindbergh CA. An apparatus for the culture of whole organs. *J Exp Med* 1935;62:415, with permission.)

close combat. Jack's great-grandfather Robert Gibbon, a doctor, became assayer of the United States mint at Charlotte, North Carolina. One of their sons, Lieutenant Lardner Gibbon, explored the Amazon with Lieutenant W. L. Herndon as a United States naval officer and wrote and illustrated the second of the two excellent published volumes that described their discoveries. Members of Jack's family, like those of other families, fought on both sides during the Civil War. With its onset, Lardner Gibbon, who had left the United States navy some years before, joined the Confederate forces and rendered excellent service as a surgeon and quartermaster in the same regiment of the Army of Northern Virginia in which his brother, Captain Nicholas Gibbon, served. Nicholas had intended to follow his father and brother into medicine, but the war inter-

rupted these plans. After it was over, he settled down in North Carolina as a farmer and was active in local and state politics, holding office as a justice of the peace and as a member of the state General Assembly.

Robert Gibbon's wife, Mary Amelia Roberts, Jack's maternal grandmother, came from a family distinguished in the ministry. Her father, Zabdiel Rogers, was a Congregational minister and spiritual leader of a church in Charleston, South Carolina but was not the first churchman in the family. John Rogers was a minister in Suffolk County, England. His second son, Reverend Nathaniel Rogers, emigrated to America in 1636.

Jack's parents then might well have anticipated that their first son would lead a useful life and likely a distinguished one, but they had no reason whatsoever to foresee that he would become a surgeon or that he would make one of the great surgical contributions of all time, that he would carry out investigations that would render human CPB feasible and in this way revolutionize surgery.

PURSUIT OF THE IDEA

When Jack returned to Philadelphia from a year in Boston working as a fellow in Churchill's laboratory, he not only brought along his haunting idea of a CPB machine but also his technical assistant and newly married wife, Maly Hopkinson, who for years would continue to work closely with him as a real partner in his investigative efforts. The time in Philadelphia provided no opportunity for starting the search for a human CPB device. Jack practiced surgery in the mornings and in the afternoons worked in the Harrison Experimental Surgical Laboratories at the University of Pennsylvania where he had obtained a staff appointment. Although he could not tackle the project, which was always on his mind, he had a profitable, indeed stimulating, time working in association with Eugene Landis, later professor of physiology at Harvard. When Jack discussed his idea of a heart–lung machine and CPB with his colleagues, he met with little or no encouragement, all too often the way new concepts are received. In general, they thought he would be wiser to investigate smaller projects, ones more certain of a successful conclusion, ones that would more likely give him an opportunity to publish his observations and thus advance his chances in the academic world. The principle of publish or perish was alive and well. Only Eugene Landis encouraged him to proceed. Jack was not dissuaded by the majority opinion, and when he was offered another fellowship year in Boston he gladly accepted it. Now he could begin to build the forerunner of his ultimate objective.

Those who work today with the relatively easily managed, small, efficient oxygenators and extracorporeal bypass circuits can hardly appreciate their humble beginnings. Fortunately, both Jack and Maly have described them. In Jack's address, published in 1978 (1) after his death, the early efforts were related:

> We. . .decided upon a vertical revolving cylinder in which the blood was introduced tangentially at the top of the cylinder in the direction of the rotation. Rotation of the cylinder kept the blood in a thin even film by centrifugal force avoiding rivulets. . . . The cylinder was tapered at the bottom to a knife-like edge, where the blood was collected in a stationary cup whose inner surface closely approximated the outer edge of the cylinder. From the cup at the bottom of the oxygenator the now red blood was returned to the animal's body through a systemic artery in a central direction.
>
> Imagine for a moment the way research was carried out in a research laboratory in the 1930s. The Federal Government was not then pouring out millions of dollars to doctors to perform research. Harvard provided my fellowship and the

Massachusetts General Hospital provided the laboratory. I bought an air pump in a second hand shop in East Boston for a few dollars, and used it to activate finger cot blood pumps. Valves were made from solid rubber corks with the small end cut transversely three quarters through to form a flap about 2 mm thick. With this flap held up, a cork borer was longitudinally passed through the center of the rubber stopper, thus creating a channel for the stream of blood. These simple valves worked well. Plastic materials were not available, so our circuit was largely rubber and glass. Heparin had just become available, but its antagonist, protamine, was not.

He gave a vivid account of the device on another occasion (7) (Fig. 2.5):

> This assemblage of metal, glass, electric motors, water baths, electrical switches, electromagnets, etc. looked for all the world like some ridiculous Rube Goldberg apparatus. Although the apparatus required infinite attention to detail it served us well and we were very proud of it. The heart–lung machines in use today bear as little resemblance to that early model as the jet plane of today bears to that magnificent conglomeration of wires, struts, and canvas that sailed into the air in 1905 from the dunes of Kitty Hawk with one of the Wright brothers at the controls.

Sometimes Jack and Maly saved money by walking about the Boston streets at night securing cats without expense. As Jack put it (5), "I can recall prowling around Beacon Hill at night with some tuna fish as bait and a gunny sack to catch any of those stray cats which swarmed over Boston in those days. To indicate the number the S.P.C.A. was killing 30,000 a year."

When the year 1934 ended in Boston and the Gibbons returned to Philadelphia, it was possible to continue work on the CPB apparatus, and in a year the machine had been improved to the point that it was satisfactory for the studies being undertaken at the time. The blood vessel cannulas were silver coated and thin walled. A piston-type air pump was being used. The oxygenated blood was delivered into the femoral artery in continuous flow with pulsatile increments. Ether was administered directly to the cats until the extracorporeal circulation took over most of the work of the heart and lungs and then was added as needed to the oxygenating device. Fortunately, no accident occurred with this potentially explosive mixture of ether and oxygen. Improved as the apparatus was, it was primitive in retrospect. So were the experiments that Maly recalled in this way (personal communication, Marly H. Gibbon, reminiscences, 1963):

> To do these experiments we had to be at the laboratory bright and early, as they often continued all that day and sometimes well into the evening. We could only manage three such experiments a week. First we had to smoke a kymograph record and get it in place on the operating table. Then, we had to bring a cat down to the laboratory from its upstairs quarters and anesthetize it. . .perform a tracheotomy and connect the animal to an artificial respirator while a "Drinker Preparation" was

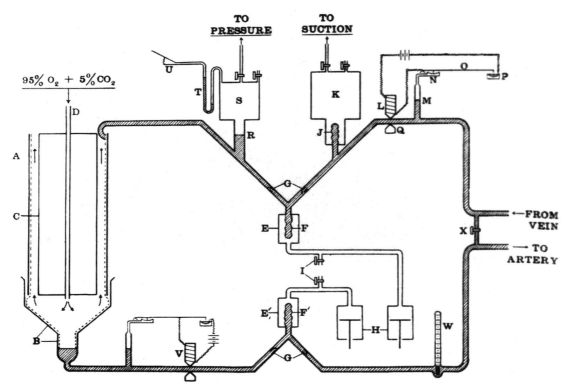

FIG. 2.5. Early extracorporeal circuit of Gibbon. Venous blood was withdrawn by a finger-cot pump (*E, F*) and transmitted to the inner wall of a vertical rotating cylinder (*A,* **left**) where it was exposed to an atmosphere of 95% oxygen and 5% carbon dioxide for gas exchange. A water manometer (*T*) measured air pressure in chamber *S* and gave an indication of total blood flow. Blood was collected in a lower chamber (*B*) and then forced back into the animal's artery by another finger-cot pump (*E', F'*). Using this apparatus, Gibbon and his wife, Maly H. Gibbon, were able to support the cardiorespiratory needs of cats for up to 68 minutes during occlusion of the pulmonary artery. (Reprinted from Gibbon JH Jr. Artificial maintenance of circulation during experimental occlusion of pulmonary artery. *Arch Surg* 1937;34:1108, with permission.)

being done, in order to expose the pulmonary artery in a (later) naturally breathing animal.... These preparations usually took four or five hours and it was midday before we were ready to start the really critical part of the experiment: gradually closing the clamp around the pulmonary artery and at the same time withdrawing blood from the jugular vein [into the apparatus]....

We would keep the clamp completely occluding the pulmonary artery for as long as we thought the cat could stand it, or nothing went wrong with the apparatus, but the things that were apt to go wrong were infinite.... [After] the period of occlusion of the pulmonary artery, [we would] remove the clamp around it, and then put the cat back on its own circulation and see if it could maintain its blood pressure at a near normal level and its respirations at a near normal rate. If it succeeded in doing this, the animal was nursed tenderly over a period of an hour or so...the kymograph record was shellacked so no diener's hand or broom should smooch our record, the instruments and general mess cleaned up, and we could go home—a long day.

A long day it was, but the Gibbons had brought CPB over a high hurdle. In 1967, Jack (6) recalled the event:

I will never forget the day when we were able to screw down the clamp all the way, completely occluding the pulmonary artery, with the extracorporeal blood circuit in operation and with no change in the animal's blood pressure! My wife and I threw our arms around each other and danced around the laboratory.

Animals were surviving a period of total CPB, and total CPB in humans was nearing reality. Jack's address was concluded with these remarks:

Although it gives me great satisfaction to know that open-heart operations are being performed daily now all over the world, nothing in my life has duplicated the joy of that dance around the laboratory of the old Bullfinch Building in the Massachusetts General Hospital 32 years ago.

When the Gibbons returned to Philadelphia it was possible to continue work with the CPB circuit and to improve

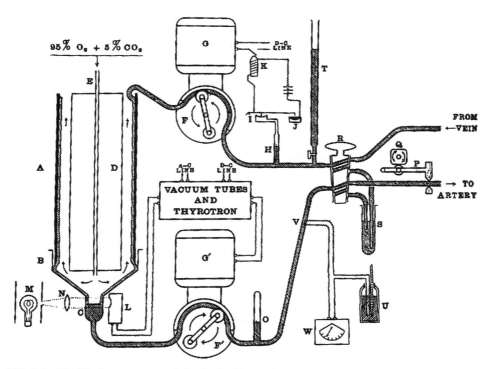

FIG. 2.6. Modified extracorporeal circuit of Gibbon. This apparatus was used in later experiments when the pulmonary arteries of cats were occluded for prolonged periods with survival (one gave birth to a litter of kittens after the experiment). Note that the apparatus is similar in design to the one described in 1937 (see Fig. 2.5), but DeBakey roller pumps are now used to withdraw and return blood to the animal's circulation, thus eliminating the need for valves. A photoelectric blood level sensor is shown (*L*) near the collection chamber (**lower left**) and was used to servoregulate the arterial pump (*F'*) and avoid air embolism. Similarly, a pressure sensor on the venous line (*H*) was used to servoregulate the venous roller pump to control the degree of suction applied to the animal's venous system. The average pump flow was approximately 250 mL/min (100 mL/kg body weight) and the maximum total flow possible was 500 mL/min. (Reprinted from Gibbon JH Jr. The maintenance of life during experimental occlusion of the pulmonary artery followed by survival. *Surg Gynecol Obstet* 1939;69:604, with permission.)

it (Fig. 2.6). After Jack reported to the 1939 meeting of the American Association for Thoracic Surgery that indefinite survival of cats in good condition had been achieved after a period of total CPB, Clarence Crafoord, widely respected head of thoracic surgery at the Karolinska Institute in Stockholm, said that a virtual pinnacle of success in surgery had been reached. Leo Eleosser, a distinguished San Francisco surgeon, remarked that Jack's work reminded him of the visions of Jules Verne, thought impossible at the time but accomplished somewhat later. These comments were unpublished but later recounted by Dr. Gibbon (8,32). CPB had surely come a long way, but its applicability in a human operation was still some years off.

INTERRUPTION AND THEN RENEWED LABORATORY WORK

The onset of World War II prompted Jack to volunteer for military service, and this necessitated deferring further work

on his project just as it had reached its most promising stage. When he took off his army uniform 4 years afterward in 1945, however, a piece of truly good luck came his way, as if in a way a reward for his patriotic service. Through a first-year Jefferson medical student who knew of his work and whose fiancee's father was a friend of Mr. Thomas Watson, chairman of the board of directors of IBM, a meeting with this far-sighted business executive was arranged. Mr. Watson had familiarized himself with Jack's work by reading reprints of his publications (33–36) and asked how he might help. Jack explained that he needed engineering assistance and added bluntly that he did not want to make any money from his idea nor did he wish IBM to do so. Watson agreed and assured Jack of the help he needed. Soon talented engineers from the corporation were working with him. No longer was this a nickel and dime operation.

A larger machine using the same rotating drum principle was soon made, each part carefully tested and constructed of the finest materials. Now the experiments yielded better results. Half the animals survived indefinitely after a period of total CPB of more than 0.5 hours. The realization that the much greater flow necessary for human use would require a drum of enormous size made it evident that the oxygenator had to undergo a drastic change. The observations of T. Lane Stokes and John Flick, Jr. (37), two young doctors working with Jack at the time, put the project on a promising path—some turbulence of flow could increase oxygenation as much as eight times. Using a screen for the oxygenator could produce the desired turbulence. One was built and worked well (Fig. 2.7). Now all the dogs survived bypass periods of up to 4 hours in good condition. A device suitable for human use was then constructed, a machine with multiple stationary vertical screen oxygenators through which the blood flowed down in an atmosphere of oxygen and carbon dioxide. Tests on large dogs went well. Indefinite survival followed prolonged exposure of the atrial septum, incision of the ventricle and bringing its septum into view, and repair of created septal defects (38). It seemed at long last that everything had been done to make certain CPB in humans was feasible, and at the May 1952 meeting of the American Association for Thoracic Surgery, Jack (39) could say "I believe that we are approaching the time when extracorporeal blood circuits of the mechanical heart lung type can be safely used in the treatment of human patients."

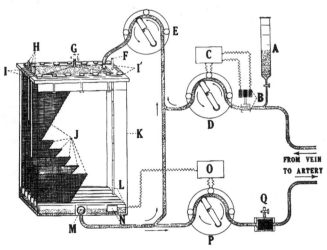

FIG. 2.7. Stationary screen extracorporeal circuit used by Gibbon in animal experiments just before clinical applications. Two roller pumps (*D and P*) are used to withdraw and reinfuse blood from the animal. A third roller pump (*E*) recirculates oxygenated blood by withdrawing it from the tubing line to the arterial pump (*P*). This maintained a constant supply of blood that was filmed down a series of screens (*J*) contained in an oxygen-rich atmosphere for gas exchange. A screen filter with stopcock (*Q*) is located in the arterial tubing line for blood filtration just before its reinfusion into the animal's artery. (Reprinted from Miller BJ, Gibbon JH Jr, Gibbon MH. Recent advances in the development of a mechanical heart and lung apparatus. *Ann Surg* 1951;134:699, with permission.)

CLINICAL APPLICATIONS: GIBBON AND OTHERS

As not infrequently happens, the first attempts were failures: a March 1951 exploration of the right atrium under partial bypass in a terminally ill patient under the erroneous diagnosis of a myxoma or large clot and a February 1952 exploration of the atrium under total CPB in a moribund infant also under the erroneous diagnosis of a septal defect. Cardiac catheterization was not a common diagnostic aid in those early days, and errors were sometimes made from ordinary clinical assessment.

Once Jack's experimental work was well under way, others attempted to design, build, and test devices for CPB. Jack welcomed these efforts, and all who were interested were free to visit his laboratory and share his experiences. Priority was not his goal. By May 1952 when Jack told those at the meeting of the American Association for Thoracic Surgery that he thought the time had come when CPB could be used in humans, it had indeed been used in three instances, although only once for an open heart procedure. In August 1951, Mario Dogliotti (40) in Turin had used his bubble oxygenator as a precautionary measure in removing a large mediastinal tumor. In the same year James Helmsworth et al. (41) in Cincinnati reported having used his in an effort to relieve severe heart failure, and in April Clarence Dennis et al. (42) used the rotating screen oxygenator he had developed at Minnesota in a fatal attempt to treat a patient thought to have an atrial septal defect but who had instead an atrioventricular canal. Not long after this effort, Dennis had another unsuccessful experience, this time due to a mistake made by the person operating the pump–oxygenator (43).

CPB had not been used successfully for an open heart procedure when 18-year-old Cecelia Bavolek became Jack's patient. Despite cardiac catheterization and angiography, the physicians at the Jefferson Hospital found the diagnosis troublesome. They concluded, however, that an atrial septal defect with a large left-to-right shunt was the correct diagnosis, and Jack agreed. Arrangements for the operation were made.

It was May 6, 1953 when Cecelia was brought to the operating room. Her heart was exposed through a bilateral fourth intercostal incision. Digital exploration of the atrium revealed a defect the size of a silver dollar. The left subclavian artery was cannulated as were the inferior vena cava through the atrial appendage and the superior cava through the atrial wall. Partial bypass was begun, a vent was placed in the left ventricle, and total bypass instituted. The defect was exposed and closed with a continuous suture reinforced with a single suture at each end. The atrial incision was closed. The extracorporeal circuit had been in place 45 minutes. The patient had been on total CPB for 26 minutes. She made an uneventful recovery. The feasibility and usefulness of CPB in humans had at long last been demonstrated. Jack had achieved success in a human (44), and his two decades of innovative and difficult work had been justified. His goal had been reached, and he was ready to leave to others the advances he knew would be made.

CPB had arrived and was here to stay.

GIBBON'S CONTRIBUTIONS TO CARDIOPULMONARY BYPASS IN CLINICAL PRACTICE

It is remarkable that John Gibbon recognized long ago so many of the essential elements of a safe and efficient apparatus for CPB and the desirable features of its secure and trustworthy use. It is doubtful that he foresaw clearly the highly trained expert professional perfusionists of today. It was consequently his desire to incorporate in the device itself every possible safeguard. He knew that major mistakes in its operation could lead to undesirable and even potentially fatal consequences. He wanted the CPB apparatus and its use to be as foolproof as possible. From 40 to 60 years ago, Gibbon used or suggested many practices currently in use with CPB. Ideally, he knew, the surface contact with blood should be inert, friendly, one might say, to the blood passing along, and this passage of blood should provide the patient with adequate circulation of undamaged properly oxygenated blood and a means for its release of carbon dioxide.

When the perfusionist Mark Kurusz looked over Gibbon's published work in 1982 (45), he listed these important contributions: the rinsing of the circuit before CPB, the use of colloids for the priming solution, and a small rather than large priming volume to reduce hemodilution. They also included the importance of measuring the oxygen saturation of the venous blood for assessing tissue perfusion and the arterial Pco_2 that he believed should be kept at a normal or slightly depressed level. Gibbon thought the systemic blood pressure should be maintained at a level of at least 50 to 65 mm Hg and that the perfusate and the blood trapped in the apparatus at the completion of CPB and the fluid collected by chest tube drainage should be salvaged and returned to the patient. He considered the heparin/protamine titration test after CPB once it became available.

His equipment included safety devices, both audible and visible, for shutting off the pump automatically in case the blood in the reservoir reached too low a level or the line pressure became too high. The inhalational anesthetic was switched to the oxygenator once CPB was established. He experimented with pulsatile flow, incorporated an in-line pH meter and a device for arterial filtration, used thin-walled stainless steel cannulas and, once it became commercially available, plastic tubing.

Dr. Gibbon demonstrated that successful operative procedures in heparinized subjects and secondary operations were possible if proper hemostatic techniques were observed. He knew that the amount of hemolysis was related to the length of CPB but that the degree of hemolysis was compatible with good outcome. He recognized that postoperative bleeding was likely to be troublesome after long periods of CPB but could be managed by administration of fresh blood and the passage of time. He knew of the danger of leaks on the negative side of the pump, described the phenomenon of heparin rebound, noted that protamine could produce hypotension, observed the differential cooling of the myocardium with hypothermic cardioplegia, and advocated the use of myocardial temperature probes.

Importantly, for the overall safety of the subject, he was aware of the immense value of an assistant who could give undivided attention to the CPB, the forerunner of the thoroughly competent perfusionist of today.

KEY POINTS

- The impetus for Dr. John H. Gibbon, Jr. to develop a heart–lung machine was the witnessing of a patient's death from pulmonary embolism and failed pulmonary embolectomy (Trendelenburg operation) in 1930.
- The concept of organ and tissue perfusion with oxygenated blood was demonstrated several times in the 1800s, beginning with the work of LeGallois in 1813.
- Early perfusion devices had limited capability to exchange gases, which limited their use to isolated organ experiments.
- Physiologists used methods such as whipping, bubbling, spraying, and filming venous blood to add oxygen and remove carbon dioxide in laboratory experiments.
- Alternative blood "oxygenators" were the native lungs of donor animals, which were also successful in preserving temporary function of perfused organs.
- In 1929, Brukhonenko speculated that artificial circulation of blood might someday be applicable for cardiac operations in humans.
- In 1935, Lindbergh and Carrel described a sophisticated pumping apparatus for organ perfusion experiments.
- Dr. Gibbon received little encouragement when he set out to develop a workable heart–lung machine in the mid-1930s.
- In 1939, Gibbon reported survival of cats in experiments that involved gradual occlusion of the pulmonary artery while gas exchange and perfusion were taken over by a rotating cylinder film oxygenator.

- In the late 1940s and early 1950s, Gibbon received engineering help from the IBM Corporation to develop a larger capacity oxygenator consisting of stationary screens, which induced mild turbulence in the blood, for potential application in humans.
- After many successful experiments in dogs in which septal defects were created and repaired, a heart–lung machine was built and used clinically by Gibbon in February 1952, but an erroneous preoperative diagnosis contributed to the death of the infant.
- Other workers who clinically used extracorporeal circulation in the early 1950s were Dogliotti, Helmsworth, Dennis, and Lillehei.
- On May 6, 1953, the Gibbon-IBM heart–lung machine was used successfully by Dr. Gibbon during closure of an atrial septal defect in an 18-year-old girl.
- Careful review of the publications of John H. Gibbon, Jr. revealed he was a meticulous investigator who solved many problems inherent with CPB and described practices still used today.

REFERENCES

1. Gibbon JH Jr. The development of the heart-lung apparatus. *Am J Surg* 1978;135:608–619.
2. Trendelenburg F. Uber die operative Behandlung der Embolie der Lungarterie. *Arch Klin Chir* 1908;86:686–700.
3. Kirschner M. Ein durch die Trendelenburgsche Operation geheilter Fall von Embolie der Art. Pulmonalis. *Arch Klin Chir* 1924;133:312–359.
4. Steenburg RW, Warren R, Wilson RE, et al. A new look at pulmonary embolectomy. *Surg Gynecol Obstet* 1958;107:214–220.
5. Gibbon JH Jr. The gestation and birth of an idea. *Philadelphia Med* 1963;Sept 13:913–916.
6. Gibbon JH Jr. The early development of an extracorporeal circulation with an artificial heart and lung. *Trans Am Soc Artif Intern Organs* 1967;13:77–79.
7. Gibbon JH Jr. Development of the artificial heart and lung extracorporeal blood circuit. *JAMA* 1968;206:1983–1986.
8. Gibbon JH Jr. The development of the heart-lung apparatus. *Rev Surg* 1970;27:231–244.
9. Romaine-Davis A. *John Gibbon and his heart-lung machine.* Philadelphia: University Pennsylvania Press, 1991.
10. Shumacker HB Jr. *John H. Gibbon, Jr., M.D. 1903–1973. A biographical memoir.* Washington, DC: National Academy Press, 1982.
11. LeGallois C-J-J. *Experiences sur le principe de la vie, notamment sur celui des mouvemens du coeur, et sur le siege de ce principe; survies du rapport fait a la premiere classe de l'Institut sur celles relatives aux mouvemens du coeur.* Paris: d'Hautel, 1812.
12. Brown-Sequard CE. Recherches experimentales sur les proprietes physiologiques et les usages du sang rouge et du sang noir et de leurs principaux elements gazeux, l'oxygene et l'acide corbonique. *J Physiol Homme* 1858;1:729–735.
13. von Schroder W. Uber die Bildungstatte des Harnstoffs. *Arch Exp Pathol Pharmacol* 1882;15:364–402.
14. Clark LC Jr, Gollan F, Gupta VB. The oxygenation of blood by gas dispersion. *Science* 1950;11:85–87.
15. von Euler E S, Heymans C. An oxygenator for perfusion experiments. *J Physiol* 1932;74:2P–3P.
16. von Frey M, Gruber M. Untersuchungen uber den Stoffwechsel isolierte Organe. Ein Respiration-Apparat fur isolierte Organe. *Virchow's Arch Physiol* 1885;9:519–532.
17. Richards AN, Drinker CK. An apparatus for perfusion of isolated organs. *J Pharmacol Exp Ther* 1915;7:467–483.
18. Bayliss LE, Fee AR, Ogden EA. Method of oxygenating blood. *J Physiol* 1928;66:443–448.
19. Daly IB, Thorpe WV. An isolated mammalian heart preparation capable of performing work for long periods. *J Physiol* 1933;79:199–217.
20. Patterson SW, Starling EH. On the mechanical features which determine the output of the ventricles. *J Physiol* 1914;48:357–379.
21. Hemingway A. Some observations on the perfusion of the isolated kidney by a pump. *J Physiol* 1913;71:201–213.
22. Jacobj C. Ein Beitrag zur Technik der kunstliechen Durchblutung ueberlebender Organe. *Arch Exp Pathol Pharmacol* 1895;36:330–348.
23. Binet L, Mayer C. Technique nouvelle de perfusion du sanguine. *Comp Rend Acad Sci* 1929;189:1330–1331.
24. Brukhonenko S, Tchetchuline S. Experiences avec la tete isolee du chien.1.Technique et conditions des experiences. *J Physiol Pathol Gen* 1929;27:31–45.
25. Brukhonenko S. Circulation artificelle du sang dans l'organisme entier d'un chien avec coeur exclus. *J Physiol Pathol Gen* 1929;27:257–272.
26. Lillehei CW, Cohen M, Warden HE, et al. The results of direct vision closure of ventricular septal defects in eight patients by means of controlled cross circulation. *Surg Gynecol Obstet* 1955;101:447–466.
27. Lindbergh CA. *Autobiography of values.* New York: Harcourt Brace Jovanovich, 1977.
28. Bing RJ. Lindbergh and the biologic sciences (a personal reminiscence). *Tex Heart Inst J* 1987;14:231–237.
29. Lindbergh CA. An apparatus for the culture of whole organs. *J Exp Med* 1935;62:409–432.
30. Carrel A, Lindbergh CA. *The culture of organs.* New York: Paul B. Hoeber, 1938.
31. Shumacker HB Jr. John H. Gibbon, Jr. (1903–1973), with a letter about his background and boyhood by Marjorie Gibbon Battles. *Indiana Med* 1985;78:916–923.
32. Gibbon JH Jr. Chairman's address: Section II, Artificial heart-lung machines. *Trans Am Soc Artif Intern Organ* 1955;1:58–62.
33. Gibbon JH Jr. Artificial maintenance of circulation during experimental occlusion of pulmonary artery. *Arch Surg* 1937;34:1105–1131.
34. Gibbon JH Jr. The maintenance of life during experimental occlusion of the pulmonary artery followed by survival. *Surg Gynecol Obstet* 1939;69:602–614.
35. Gibbon JH Jr. An oxygenator with a large surface-volume ratio. *J Lab Clin Med* 1939;24:1192–1198.
36. Gibbon JH Jr, Kraul CW. An efficient oxygenator for blood. *J Lab Clin Med* 1941;26:1803–1809.
37. Stokes TL, Flick JB Jr. An improved vertical cylinder oxygenator. *Proc Soc Exp Biol Med* 1950;73:528–529.
38. Miller BJ, Gibbon JH Jr, Greco VF, et al. The production and repair of interatrial septal defects under direct vision with the assistance of an extracorporeal pump-oxygenator circuit. *J Thorac Surg* 1953;26:598–616.
39. Gibbon JH Jr. Discussion following Helmsworth JA, Clark LC Jr, Kaplan S, Largen T. Artificial oxygenation and circulation during complete by-pass of the heart. *J Thorac Surg* 1952;24:117–133,151.

40. Dogliotti AM. Clinical use of the artificial circulation with a note on intra-arterial transfusion. *Bull Johns Hopkins Hosp* 1952;90: 131–133.

41. Helmsworth JA, Clark LC Jr, Kaplan S, et al. Clinical use of extracorporeal oxygenation with oxygenator-pump. *JAMA* 1952; 150:451–453.

42. Dennis C, Spreng DS Jr, Nelson GE, et al. Development of a pump-oxygenator to replace the heart and lungs; an apparatus applicable to human patients, and application to one case. *Ann Surg* 1951;134:709–721.

43. Dennis C. Discussion following Miller BJ, Gibbon JH Jr, Greco VF, Smith BA, Cohn CH, Allbritten FF. The production and repair of interatrial septal defects under direct vision with assistance of an extracorporeal pump-oxygenator circuit. *J Thorac Surg* 1953;26:598–616, 631.

44. Gibbon JH Jr. Application of a mechanical heart and lung apparatus to cardiac surgery. *Minn Med* 1954;37:171–180.

45. Kurusz M. Cardiopulmonary bypass during intracardiac repair of congenital defects. *Proc Am Acad Cardiovasc Perfus* 1982;3: 73–78.

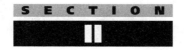

EQUIPMENT

3

BLOOD PUMPS

EIKI TAYAMA
STEVEN A. RASKIN
YUKIHIKO NOSÉ

Various types of blood pumps are available for cardiopulmonary bypass (CPB). The ideal pump for CPB should have the following characteristics:

- It must be able to pump blood at a flow rate of 7 L/min against a pressure of 500 mm Hg.
- The pumping motion should not damage the cellular or acellular components of blood.
- All parts in contact with the bloodstream should have a smooth continuous surface with no dead space to cause stagnation or turbulence, should be disposable, and should not contaminate the permanent parts of the pump.
- Calibration of pump flow should be exact and reproducible so that blood flow can be accurately monitored.
- In the event of a power failure, the pump should be manually operable.

Four types of blood pumps are currently available for CPB: roller, centrifugal, pulsatile, and nonocclusive roller.

ROLLER PUMPS

The roller pump is one type of positive displacement pump. It has been the most commonly used type for CPB for the past five decades, although its popularity has recently fallen as a result of improvements in systems using centrifugal pumps.

History

The roller pump was first patented (patent 12,753) in 1855 by Porter and Bradley (1). Potential applications listed in this patent included use as a scavenger for cleaning of privies, as a stomach pump, and as an apparatus for injection. In 1887, Allen patented a pump designed for blood transfusion. In 1934, DeBakey et al. (2) made a modification to the Porter-Bradley infusion pump to prevent creepage of the latex rubber tubing during blood transfusion (patent 2,018,998) (Fig. 3.1). This was accomplished by placing a flange on the outer circumference of the tubing that was then clamped into the pump housing. In 1959, Melrose proposed a more advanced design, in which the roller ran along the tubing held in place by a grooved backplate. The tube guides prevented lateral motion of the tubing during operation.

Structures

Roller pumps contain a length of tubing located inside a curved raceway. This raceway is placed at the travel perimeter of rollers mounted on the ends of rotating arms. These arms are arranged in such a manner that one roller is compressing the tubing at all times. By compressing a segment of the blood-filled resilient tubing, blood is pushed ahead of the moving roller, thereby producing continuous blood flow (Fig. 3.2). The output of the rotary pump is determined by the revolutions per minute (rpm) of the pump and the volume displaced with each revolution. The volume depends on the size of tubing and length of the track.

According to the number of rollers, roller pumps are classified as single, double, and multiple roller pumps. The single-roller pump consists of a circular raceway in which a 360-degree loop of tubing is inserted. Single-roller pumps were used for CPB in the 1950s and early 1960s because they produced more pulsatility than conventional double-roller pumps. The double-roller pump, which has been the most commonly used pump for CPB, consists of a 210-degree semicircular backing plate and two rollers with the rotating arms set 180 degrees apart (Fig. 3.3). When one roller ends its occlusive phase, the other has already begun its occlusive phase. Because one of the two rollers is always compressing the tubing, the double-roller pump generates

E. Tayama: Department of Surgery, Kurume University School of Medicine, Kurume City, 830 Japan.

S. A. Raskin and Y. Nosé: Department of Surgery, Baylor College of Medicine, Houston, TX 77030.

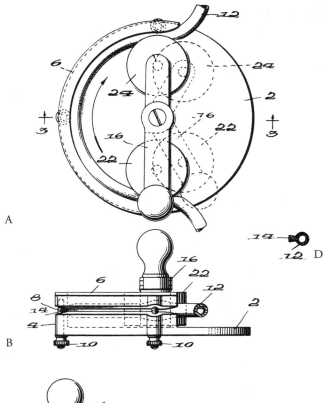

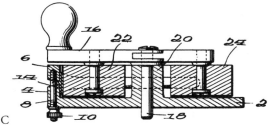

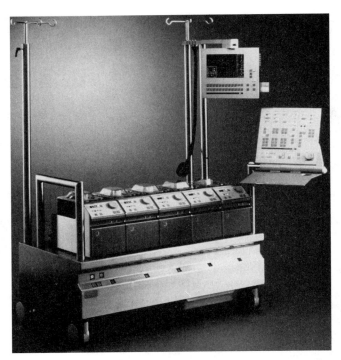

FIG. 3.1. Original DeBakey roller pump. Note dual rollers and knob for rotating roller assembly. This pump required specially edged tubing (*D*, right) for securing it between plates in the roller mechanism. **A:** Plane view of instrument. **B:** Side view. **C:** Cross-section. **D:** Cross-section of tube. (Reprinted from DeBakey ME. A simple continuous-flow blood transfusion instrument. *New Orleans Med Surg J* 1934;87:387, with permission.)

FIG. 3.2. Conventional heart–lung machine, with five roller pump modules. Typically, one roller pump is used to pump blood into the systemic circulation (usually through a membrane oxygenator) and other separate roller pumps are used for delivery of cardioplegic solutions, suction from the surgical field, and/or left ventricular venting. (Model HL-20, courtesy Jostra USA, Austin, TX.)

a relatively nonpulsatile flow. Although the multiple-roller pump has been proposed for extracorporeal blood handling, it is not clinically available because it causes more hemolysis.

Tubing

There are three basic materials currently used for tubing: silicone rubber, latex rubber, and polyvinyl chloride (PVC). These tubing materials have all been used in CPB. PVC is most widely used for roller pumps because of its durability and acceptable hemolysis rates (3,4). Latex rubber generates more hemolysis than PVC, whereas silicone rubber pro-

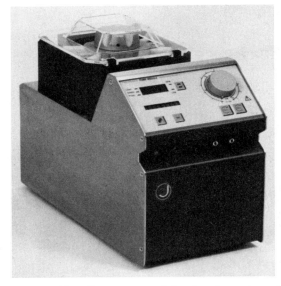

FIG. 3.3. Double-roller pump module, showing a large knob (**right**) that controls revolutions per minute, which are displayed digitally on the front of the console. (Courtesy Jostra USA, Austin, TX.)

duces less hemolysis when the pump is completely occluded (4). PVC tubing stiffens during hypothermic CPB and tends to induce spallation, which refers to the release of plastic microparticles from the inner wall of tubing as a result of roller pump compression (3–6). Silicone rubber tubing releases more particles than PVC (7).

Occlusiveness

Occlusion can be adjusted by either increasing or decreasing the compression of the tubing by the rollers. This compression appears to be critical. Excessive compression induces hemolysis and tubing wear, whereas too little occlusion may also aggravate hemolysis but, more important, compromises forward output (3). The exact output of the roller pump may vary during CPB, and it is difficult to determine the exact flow rate due to occlusion variance throughout the bypass (8). At nonocclusive settings, roller pump output can be sharply decreased, resulting in hypoperfusion (3,9). Although controversial, it is generally believed that adjusting tubing compression to be barely nonocclusive results in the least hemolysis (3,4). Rawn et al. (10) found no difference in hemolysis between a roller pump with a standard set occlusion and a centrifugal pump at a 4.5-L/min blood flow rate with an afterload of 250 mm Hg. When the occlusion is opened such that pumping at 5 rpm against occluded tubing maintains a pressure of 150 to 225 mm Hg, the roller pump induces less hemolysis than a centrifugal pump. The occlusion is set by holding the outflow line vertically so the top of the fluid is about 60 to 75 cm above the pump and then gradually decreasing occlusiveness until the fluid level falls at a rate between 1 and 12 cm/min (3,11).

Complications

Some problems arising from roller pumps include malocclusion (over- or underocclusion), miscalibration, fracture of the tubing, "runaway" pumping (12), loss of power, spallation, and the capacity to pump grossly visible air (3). If the outflow becomes occluded, pressure in the line will progressively increase until either the tubing or connectors disconnect or break. If the inflow becomes limited, the roller pumps will develop a high negative pressure producing microscopic air bubbles ("cavitation"). Roller pumps may also develop pinhole leaks, which may lead to pushing microscopic air bubbles toward the patient (3). Stoney et al. (13) attributed 92 deaths and 61 permanent injuries to arterial line embolism from roller pumps between 1972 and 1977.

CENTRIFUGAL PUMPS

Centrifugal pumps for CPB have been commercially available since 1976 (14). At many institutions, the centrifugal pump has replaced roller pumps for routine CPB for cardio-

vascular surgery. They are also used for mechanical circulatory support, including ventricular assistance, percutaneous cardiopulmonary support, and extracorporeal membrane oxygenation (15–17).

Characteristics

The basic design of a centrifugal pump consists of an impeller arranged with either vanes or a nest of smooth plastic cones inside a plastic housing. The impeller couples magnetically with an electric motor either directly or through a tether. The magnet inside the disposable pump head spins in conjunction with another magnet spinning in the drive console. This magnetic coupling means that the speed (rpm) of the driver magnet inside the console equals the rotational speed of the pump. When the impeller rotates rapidly, it generates a pressure differential causing blood flow (i.e., a negative pressure at the inlet port of the pump pulling blood into the pump housing and a positive pressure at the outlet port expelling blood). Excessive rotational speed can cause decoupling, in which the impellers or cones cannot spin as fast as the driver motor (3). The tether is driven either by a turning shaft or by an electrically powered remote magnet.

Figure 3.4 shows the relationship between the pressure differential created (pressure head) and flow rate of a centrifugal pump. In this figure, N_1, N_2, N_3, and N_4 are the arbitrary rotational pump speeds. The dotted lines indicate the pressure–flow characteristics of an ideal centrifugal pump, which can generate constant pressure regardless of flow rate, with negligible loss of pressure head inside the pump. In actual centrifugal pumps, however, the pres-

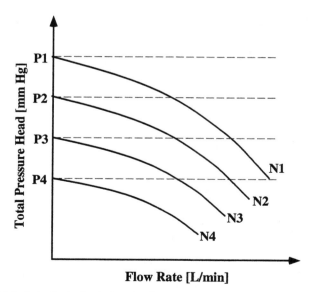

FIG. 3.4. Typical relationship between total pressure head and flow rate for a centrifugal pump. N_1 through N_4 each represent a constant level of revolutions per minute (rpm), with N_1 representing the highest rpm value and N_4 the lowest.

sure–flow relationship deviates from ideal as a result of pressure head loss in the pump head and in the inflow and outflow cannulas. As flow rate increases, pressure head loss increases. This relationship can be modeled as follows:

$$\Delta P = K_1 \times N^2 - K_2 \times Q^2$$

where N is the pump rotational speed, Q is the flow rate, and K_1 and K_2 are constants appropriate to each particular pump. The pressure head for an ideal pump can be described as $\Delta P = K_1 \times N^2$, in which the generated pressure head would be proportional to the square of the impeller rotational speed. This equation allows prediction of the pump head pressure drop from the pump rotational speed and flow.

Comparison with Roller Pumps

Table 3.1 compares advantages and disadvantages of roller pumps and centrifugal pumps. Centrifugal pumps are disposable and add approximately $150 (U.S.) or more to the cost of an individual procedure as compared with the cost of performing the procedure with a roller pump, which requires only a piece of tubing integrated into the extracorporeal circuit/oxygenator disposable kit. The most commonly used extracorporeal perfusion blood pumps (roller and centrifugal) have adverse pressure regulation properties that can lead to fatal accidents. With the standard roller pump, the most recognized hazard is overpressurization and circuit rupture if the tubing downstream from the pump (outlet side) is accidentally kinked or clamped. Additionally, if the tubing upstream from the pump (inlet side) is accidentally kinked or clamped, the roller pump will generate dangerously low negative pressures that could result in blood cavitation, hemolysis, and suction of room air through loose stopcocks or tubing connectors. Positive and negative pressure control in occlusive roller pumps is typically accomplished with additional electronic equipment such as pressure control modules or with a mechanical bladder that shuts off the pump if dangerous pressures are generated (18).

Centrifugal pumps have become popular mainly because unlike roller pumps, they cannot overpressurize. Similar to roller pumps, however, centrifugal pumps can generate very large negative pressures if the tubing upstream from the pump is restricted. Also, because they are nonocclusive, retrograde flow can occur with loss or severe reduction in forward flow from any cause. If the arterial inflow line occludes, the centrifugal pump will not generate excessive pressure (peaking at about 700 to 900 mm Hg). Likewise, if the inflow line occludes, they will not generate high negative pressures (reaching about -400 to -500 mm Hg), thereby reducing the risk of cavitation and microembolus as compared with roller pumps (3,18).

Both centrifugal and roller pumps are capable of actively sucking blood from an open venous reservoir and thus are susceptible to emptying the reservoir and pumping air to the patient. It has been claimed that centrifugal pumps hinder passage of air pulled in from an empty reservoir (18–20). This property should not be perceived as a safety feature or a method of preventing the pumping of air, however, because it has been well established that centrifugal pumps do pump air to various degrees (21).

By design, centrifugal pumps are nonocclusive, preload dependent, and afterload dependent. When the impeller is not spinning, fluid can flow through the pump head in either direction (nonocclusive). When the pump stops running for any reason, such as decoupling, blood can flow retrograde through the pump head unless the arterial line is clamped. This backflow can cause exsanguination of the patient or aspiration of air from around the purse-string sutures securing the arterial cannula (22). Therefore, when-

TABLE 3.1. COMPARISON BETWEEN ROLLER PUMPS AND CENTRIFUGAL PUMPS

	Roller Pump: Positive Displacement Pump	Centrifugal Pump: Kinetic Pump
Advantages	Reusable pump with inexpensive disposable parts Ease of sterilization Simple flow rate determination: (rpm × SV) Variable SV for different-sized patients	No possibility of disruption from excessive line pressure buildup Decreased blood trauma Less risk of massive air emboli Less cavitation Elimination of tubing wear or spallation
Disadvantages	Blood trauma Possibility of circuit disruption and termination from excessive line pressure Particulate microemboli from tubing spallation Possibility of massive air emboli Occlusion variability affecting flow rate and blood trauma Contraindicated for long-term use because of tubing wear and blood trauma	Different operator technique for initiation Flowmeter is necessary Retrograde flow when pump slows or stops More expensive non-reusable pump

rpm, pump revolutions per minute; SV; stroke volume.

ever the centrifugal pump is not running, the CPB arterial line must be clamped.

Centrifugal pumps generate increased flow when either the preload increases or the afterload decreases (preload dependent and afterload dependent). When using a roller pump, a sharp decrease in systemic vascular resistance must be accompanied by an increase in the frequency of roller head rotation if one wishes to maintain a constant arterial pressure. With centrifugal pumps, the flow rate automatically increases without a change in rotational speed when systemic vascular resistance decreases (23). Varying sensitivities to preload and afterload preclude determination of pump flow directly from rotational speed; therefore, a flow meter must be incorporated into the arterial outflow. The flow probe should be located downstream of any purge or recirculation line in the circuit to accurately measure blood flow delivered to the patient.

Electromagnetic and ultrasonic flow meters are used clinically for centrifugal pumps. Electromagnetic flow probes depend on the fact that blood flowing through an electromagnetic alters a magnetic field in a manner that can be measured continuously ("right-hand rule"). Electromagnetic flow probes require blood-contacting electrodes and are designed as connectors, which possess the disadvantages inherent to transition gaps. In contrast, ultrasonic flow probes do not contact the blood but instead wrap around the tubing. The frequency shift in the Doppler signal is related to the velocity of blood flow through the tube. Standard ultrasonic flow devices measure the maximal blood velocity and calculate the flow based on the assumption of a simple parabolic (laminar) velocity distribution (actual flow profiles are not parabolic), whereas electromagnetic devices assess mean velocity distribution. Additionally, the Doppler signal becomes very noisy at low velocities, so most ultrasonic flow probes do not measure low flows accurately (24).

A reduced risk of passing clinically significant amounts of macroscopic air into and through the arterial line to the patient has been a reported advantage of the centrifugal pump over the roller pump. If more than 32 to 52 mL of air is introduced into the circuit, the centrifugal pump becomes deprimed and stops pumping (3). Also, the centrifugal pump transmits fewer microscopic air bubbles, probably from a combination of shear force and positive pressure generation within the pump head (21).

DeBois et al. (25) prospectively compared centrifugal pumps and roller pumps in 200 patients undergoing elective coronary bypass grafting. The study demonstrated a significant reduction in length of hospital stay, a reduced 24-hour postoperative weight gain, and a net reduction in hospital cost in the centrifugal group. Clearly, both roller pumps and centrifugal pumps have advantages and disadvantages. Although clinicians may believe strongly that one or the other should be used preferentially for cardiac surgery requiring CPB, there are insufficient clinical outcome studies available as yet to reach a conclusion about the desirability of one pump type over the other for routine cases. For more prolonged applications of CPB or circulatory support, the theoretic advantages of centrifugal pumps over roller pumps become more compelling.

Complications

Centrifugal pumps are generally safe, and the overwhelming majority of cardiac operations are completed without incident. Although these pumps will not pass large quantities of gas, centrifugal pumps are nonocclusive, and therefore retrograde flow can occur whenever the pump malfunctions, stops, or when the pump slows enough so that the pressure produced is less than that needed to maintain forward flow (26). Retrograde flow can create a hemodynamic siphon that can exsanguinate the patient and can draw air into the arterial line at the cannulation site (22). *In vitro* studies demonstrated that retrograde flow could commence 540 ms after power to the pump is shut off. The reverse flow occurs even though the rotor is still spinning and can rise up to 2.5 L/min after another 470 ms (26). The only way to prevent retrograde flow is for the perfusionist to clamp the arterial line when the pump slows or stops. To sustain a pressure adequate to maintain forward flow, the perfusionist should partially occlude the arterial inflow line when low flows are requested, as when the patient is weaned from CPB. However, incidents have occurred where the perfusionist has forgotten to clamp the arterial line.

Human errors are cited as the factor believed responsible for 73.3% of perfusion accidents, compared with 19.5% for device malfunctions or failures (27). The U.S. Food and Drug Administration records about centrifugal pump malfunctions from November 1991 through October 1993 revealed that 68 pump malfunctions, 22 electrical burning smells, and 3 speed surges were reported out of 350,000 open heart operations using centrifugal pumps (failure rate, 1/3,763 cases) (28). To prevent retrograde flow associated with pump malfunction, low flow, and human errors, incorporating a one-way valve into the arterial line has been recommended (26). Although clinically available, such valves have not gained widespread use, and such issues as blood trauma, possible stasis and cavitation, the potential for valve failure, and cost effectiveness need to have further evaluation.

Specific Clinically Available Centrifugal Pumps

BioMedicus Pump

In 1976, the first centrifugal pump was used for CPB (Medtronic BioMedicus, Inc., Eden Prairie, MN). This pump was first marketed in 1978 as an alternative to the roller pumps (14). The pump head is acrylic, with inlet and outlet

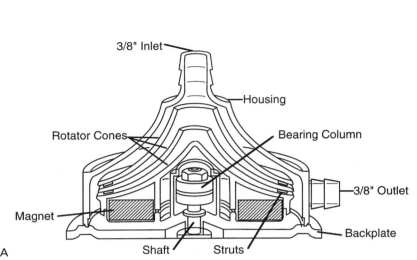

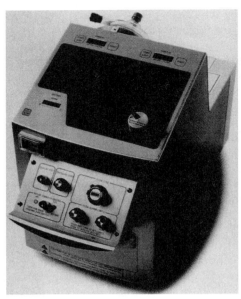

A

B

FIG. 3.5. A: Cross-sectional schematic of the BioMedicus Bio-Pump centrifugal pump. (Courtesy Medtronic BioMedicus, Inc., Eden Prairie, MN) **B:** Console that drives and regulates the BioMedicus centrifugal pump. Part of the pump is seen mounted at the top rear. Digital displays and the knob controlling the revolutions per minute are located on the console's top panel and other controls are on its front. This console is reasonably representative of those used for the centrifugal pumps of other manufacturers. (Courtesy Medtronic BioMedicus, Inc., Eden Prairie, MN.)

ports oriented at right angles to each other, and its priming volume is 80 mL (Fig. 3.5A). Pump flow rate is measured by an electromagnetic flowmeter in the CPB arterial line, which is not susceptible to inaccuracy from turbulence, hematocrit levels, temperature, and other factors. The rotor consists of a stack of parallel cones driven by magnetic coupling to the external console (Fig. 3.5B). Figure 3.6 demon-

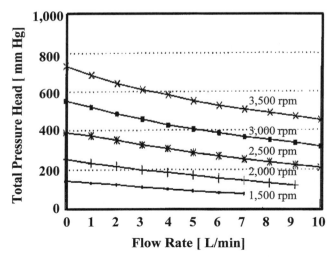

FIG. 3.6. Hydraulic performance curves for the Bio-Pump. (Courtesy Medtronic BioMedicus, Inc., Eden Prairie, MN.)

strates the pressure–flow relationship for this pump. Rotation of the parallel cones induces centrifugal force and radial flow to the blood that passes between the cones (constrained force-vortex principle). Shear rates between the cones were estimated at 100 to 400 s^{-1} at flow rates of 400 to 2,000 mL/min (29). In contrast, the shear rates between the rotating outer cone and the stationary conical pump housing vary, with a peak value of about 2.57 s^{-1}/rpm, being a function of the pump rotational speed rather than of the flow rate.

Some investigators have reported less hemolysis with the BioMedicus pump than with roller pumps (30,31), whereas others have reported the contrary (14,32) or no difference between the two (33,34). *In vitro* studies demonstrated that the BioMedicus pump induces less hemolysis at pressure-to-flow ratios below 1 mm Hg/mL/min, whereas a roller pump produces less hemolysis at the ratios above 1 mm Hg/mL/min (29). Because pressure-to-flow ratios during CPB nearly always remain well below that threshold, this distinction may have no clinical importance. Wheeldon et al. (32) compared the BioMedicus pump with the Stockert roller pump in a prospective randomized study of 16 patients undergoing coronary artery bypass grafting and found the BioMedicus pump to be associated with greater preservation of platelet numbers, less complement activation, and less microbubble transmission. In patients with CPB times over 2 hours and in those over the age of 70, perfusion with the BioMedicus pump resulted in higher postperfusion platelet counts (35). Parault and Conrad (36) found less blood damage with the BioMedicus pump than with roller pumps when CPB time exceeded 90 min. Platelet counts, plasma hemoglobin, β-thromboglobulin, and D-dimer were significantly less altered with the BioMedicus pump.

BioMedicus pumps are thought to prevent the transmission of macroscopic and microscopic air and clots better than roller pumps and other impeller pumps. These pumps are also less likely to churn air into the blood than roller pumps (14). Clots and air bubbles tend to remain in the BioMedicus pump, whereas other types of impellers may permit them to pass into the patient.

Delphin Pump

The Sarns 3M Delphin centrifugal pump (Sarns 3M, Ann Arbor, MI) has a vaned magnetically coupled impeller within an acrylic housing (Fig. 3.7). As with the BioMedicus pump, the inflow and outflow ports are oriented at right angles to each other, and the priming volume is 40 mL. Blood flow is measured by an ultrasonic flowmeter along the outlet tubing and is proportional to the rotational speed. *In vitro* comparison of the Delphin and BioMedicus pumps demonstrated that mean plasma hemoglobin levels were significantly higher with the Delphin pump at 2, 4, and 6 L/min of flow (36). Platelet counts were significantly lower with the BioMedicus pump at 2 and 4 L/min of flow, with no difference found at 6 L/min of flow.

Life Stream Pump

The Life Stream centrifugal pump (St. Jude Medical Inc., Chelmsford, MA) was introduced clinically in 1988. The

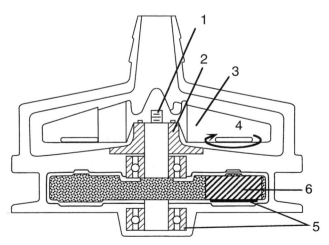

FIG. 3.7. Cross-sectional schematic of the Delphin centrifugal pump. **1:** roller shaft; **2:** sealing part; **3:** vane; **4:** absence of stagnant flow area behind the impeller; **5:** nonsealed ball bearing; **6:** magnet. (Courtesy Sarns 3M, Ann Arbor, MI.)

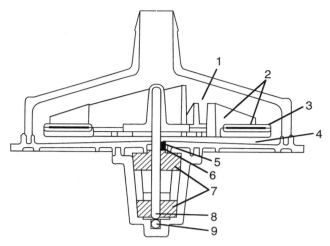

FIG. 3.8. Cross-sectional schematic of the Life Stream centrifugal pump. **1:** blood path; **2:** curved vane; **3:** thin metal drive plates; **4:** back side of vane; **5 and 6:** quad-ring double seal; **7:** sleeve bearing; **8:** stainless steel shaft; **9:** thrust bearing. (Courtesy St. Jude Medical Inc., Chelmsford, MA.)

impeller is composed of curved vanes to minimize eddies and cavitation and to optimize overall flow patterns (Fig. 3.8). The shaft, seal, and bearings have been modified to reduce the risk of blood contact and potential pump failure. The shaft is magnetically coupled to the driver console with integrated battery backup. An electromagnetic flowmeter measures blood flow. The pressure–flow relationships at various rpm are shown in Figure 3.9. An *in vitro* comparative study demonstrated similar rates of hemolysis between the BioMedicus and Life Stream pumps after 4 hours of pumping, both of which were significantly lower than that found with the Delphin pump (37). The Life Stream and Delphin pump heads were almost identical in the rotational speeds required to achieve a given flow rate and were 20% to 30% lower than those required for the same flows with the BioMedicus pump (Fig. 3.10) (37).

Capiox Pump

The Capiox centrifugal pump (Terumo Corp., Tokyo, Japan) consists of a rotor with a unique straight-path design to reduce pump rotational speed without decreasing hydraulic efficiency (38–40) (Fig. 3.11). The straight-path design with a constant cross-sectional area minimizes the change of blood flow velocity and direction. Figure 3.12 demonstrates the pump's performance, which is noteworthy for less afterload sensitivity at higher flows when compared with other centrifugal pumps. The small priming volume of approximately 46 mL may reduce stagnant flow within the rotor. *In vitro* studies revealed that the time required for blood temperature to increase from 37° to 42°C after outlet clamping was four times longer in the Capiox pump

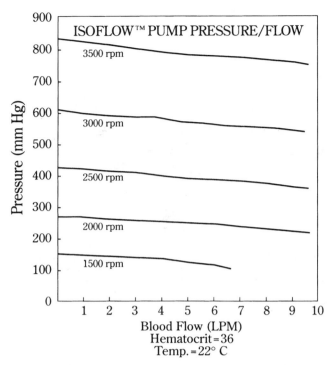

FIG. 3.9. Hydraulic performance curves for the Life Stream (Isoflow) pump. (Courtesy St. Jude Medical Inc., Chelmsford, MA.)

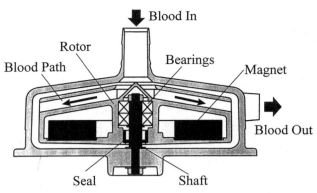

FIG. 3.11. Cross-sectional schematic of the Capiox centrifugal pump. (Courtesy Terumo Corp., Tokyo, Japan.)

caused less hemolysis than a roller pump (35) and the Bio-Medicus pump (41–43). A clinical study demonstrated less hemolysis, less platelet depletion, and lower β-thromboglobulin levels in the Capiox group than in the roller pump group (39).

Nikkiso Pump

The Nikkiso centrifugal pump (Nikkiso, Inc., Tokyo, Japan, and HIMEX Production, Inc., Houston, TX) is the smallest commercially available centrifugal pump (44–46). It has an impeller diameter of 50 mm, a priming volume of 25 mL, an outer diameter of 66 mm, a height of 58 mm, and a weight of 145 g. Figure 3.13 shows the design of the pump, which is made of polycarbonate, with a V-shape ring seal that separates the pump housing and actuator chamber. This seal, which is made of fluororubber, suppresses heat generation and prevents blood leakage (44). Six washout holes are incorporated into the impeller to generate blood

than in the Delphin pump and two times longer than in BioMedicus pump (40). These studies also demonstrated that no cavitation was observed when 0.1 mL of air was introduced into the Capiox pump under a negative pressure of 200 mm Hg. *In vitro* tests revealed that the Capiox pump

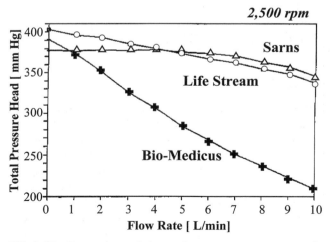

FIG. 3.10. Comparison of the performance curves among the Delphin pump, Life Stream pump, and BioMedicus pump. (Reproduced from Noon GP, Sekela ME, Glueck J, et al. Comparison of Delphin and BioMedicus pumps. *ASAIO Trans* 1990;36: M616–M619, with permission.)

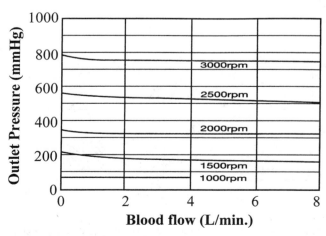

FIG. 3.12. Hydraulic performance curves of the Capiox pump. (Courtesy Terumo Corp., Tokyo, Japan.)

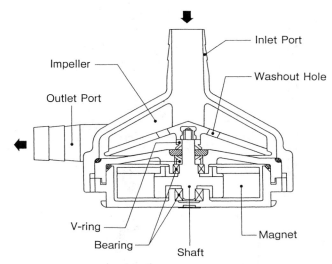

FIG. 3.13. Cross-sectional schematic of the Nikkiso centrifugal pump. (Courtesy Nikisso, Inc., Tokyo, Japan, and HIMEX Production, Inc., Houston, TX.)

flow from the back to the front surface of the impeller. These holes prevent thrombus formation in the areas behind the impeller and around the sealing part. Figure 3.14 shows the hydraulic characteristics of the Nikkiso pump. Although very small, the pump can generate 6 L/min of flow against a total pressure head of 400 mm Hg at a rotational speed of 3,500 rpm.

Because the Nikkiso pump has been marketed primarily in Japan, Japanese investigators (47–52) reported most of the clinical experience. Lower plasma free hemoglobin concentrations accompany perfusion with the Nikkiso pump than with the roller pump or the BioMedicus pump

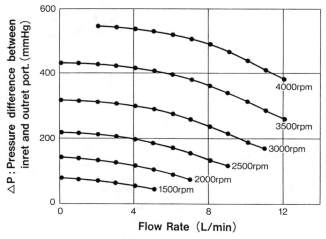

FIG. 3.14. Hydraulic performance curves for the Nikkiso pump. (Courtesy Nikisso, Inc., Tokyo, Japan, and HIMEX Production, Inc., Houston, TX.)

(48–51). It was also reported that the parameters of platelet destruction and activation (e.g., platelet factor 4 and β-thromboglobulin) increased less with the Nikkiso pump than with other pumps (52,53).

PULSATILE PUMPS

Even conventional roller pumps produce some pulsatile flow (54). However, one of the methods to generate more pulsatile blood flow during CPB is to use intraaortic balloon pumping (55). A dramatic increase in postoperative ejection fraction was observed in the pulsatile perfusion group with intraaortic balloon pumping (56). Other devices and techniques used to achieve pulsatile flow during CPB are discussed more thoroughly in Chapter 10.

NONOCCLUSIVE ROLLER PUMP

The Metaplus pump (Baxter Healthcare Corporation, Cardiovascular Group, Irvine, CA; originally Affinity model 2000, Avecor Cardiovascular, Inc., Minneapolis, MN) is a new type of blood pump that appears to incorporate some advantages of a centrifugal pump while minimizing some disadvantages of a conventional roller pump (18). This pump will not drain the venous reservoir, will not create negative pressure and cavitation, will not overpressurize, and will not allow retrograde flow.

Forward fluid flow is accomplished by a passive-filling tapered pumping chamber fabricated of two sheets of flat polyurethane tubing bonded at the edges (58). This pump chamber segment is stretched under tension over three rollers. Unlike a conventional roller pump, the Metaplus pump is considered nonocclusive because there is no backing plate against which the tubing can be compressed with rollers. The rollers are mounted on a rotor that spins to impart a peristaltic action on the fluid within the pump chamber. The priming volume is 120 mL (Fig. 3.15).

The pumping chamber shape is normally flat from being stretched over the rollers when the pump is not rotating. However, with any hydrostatic filling pressure above ambient levels, the pumping chamber expands and fills with fluid. Forward flow occurs with roller rotation, as it does with a conventional roller pump. If the tubing upstream from the pump (pump inlet) is kinked or clamped, the pump chamber will collapse into its natural flat shape. When this occurs, forward flow ceases. The pump chamber lacks the tendency to return to an inflated condition because it has no "memory." Thus, the pump cannot generate negative pressures and will not tend to damage blood and tissue or to suck air through loose tubing connectors upstream.

The pump chamber fills passively as a function of the height of the fluid column within the reservoir. Reservoir

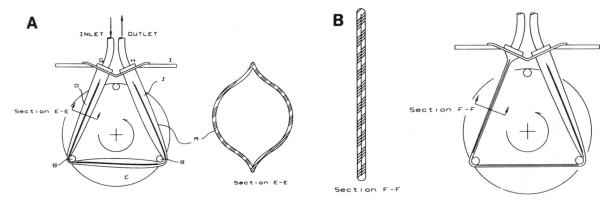

FIG. 3.15. Schematic drawing of nonocclusive roller pump. **A:** Operating principle of the triple-roller pump and pumping chamber. Polyurethane pumping chamber is stretched over the rollers, and roller rotation is counterclockwise. **E-E:** Cross-sectional view of pumping chamber distended when blood is supplied at a pressure above ambient. **B:** Pumping chamber inlet collapsed when blood is not supplied at a pressure above ambient. **F-F:** Cross-sectional view of the collapsed pumping chamber. (Reprinted from Montoya JP, Merz SI, Bartlett RH. Significant safety advantages gained with an improved pressure-regulated blood pump. *J Extra-Corp Technol* 1996;28:72–73, with permission.)

volume changes will have little effect on pump flow rate until the volume drops to a minimum level. Once that level is reached, there is insufficient hydrostatic pressure to fill the pump chamber and flow ceases, demonstrating the preload sensitivity of the pump. When venous return is reestablished, blood flow resumes gradually. As a result, air is not entrained nor does a potentially cavitating vortex form at the outlet of the CPB reservoir.

As stated earlier, the potential for retrograde flow is a key safety concern with nonocclusive pumps. With the Met-

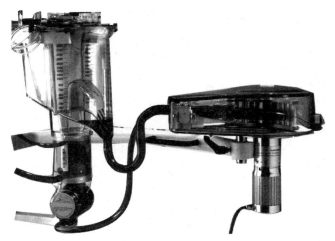

FIG. 3.16. Metaplus pump rotor and motor assembly (**right**) and membrane oxygenator (**left**). Pump position is fixed in relationship to the hard-shell venous reservoir to supply the inlet of the pump. Note requirement for large-bore, semirigid, U-shaped tubing connecting the outlet of the venous reservoir to the inlet of the pump. (Courtesy Baxter Healthcare, Cardiovascular Group, Irvine, CA.)

aplus pump, the pump chamber flattens and becomes occlusive as it wraps around the individual rollers to prevent retrograde flow from the patient. The pump is also afterload sensitive, because the pressure it generates is limited. If the arterial line occludes, the flat segment of the pump chamber becomes distended and the pump then becomes nonocclusive. This occurs at pressures lower than those required to induce failure of tubing connections. Because the system is both preload and afterload sensitive, a noninvasive electronic flow probe must be used to accurately measure blood flow, and a separate modular pump console must be used to control the pump (Fig. 3.16).

In vitro testing (57) has confirmed the inability of the pump to empty a CPB reservoir when the height of the pump inlet is placed slightly above the reservoir outlet, decreased microbubble emission when compared with conventional roller or centrifugal pumps, and lower or comparable hemolysis rates. Additional *in vitro* studies by Jaggy et al. (59) and a clinical study by Crockett et al. (60) further characterized the performance of the pump under varying preload and afterload conditions typically encountered during CPB. The cost of disposables for this new pump system are intermediate between those of the less expensive roller pump and the more expensive centrifugal pump.

KEY POINTS

- The ideal pump for CPB would be able to deliver physiologic blood flows against high resistance without damaging blood, should provide flows that are exact and easily monitored, should create no turbulence or stagnation, and should be manually operable in the event of a power failure.

- The two pumps used most commonly for CPB are roller pumps and centrifugal pumps.
- Roller pumps have the advantages of simplicity, low cost, ease and reliability of flow calculation, and the ability to pump against high resistance without reducing flow. Disadvantages include the need to assess occlusiveness, spallation of the inner tubing surface that potentially produces particulate arterial emboli, capability for pumping large volumes of air, and ability to create large positive and negative pressures.
- Compared with roller pumps, centrifugal pumps offer the advantages of lesser air pumping capabilities, lesser abilities to create large positive and negative pressures, less blood trauma, and virtually no spallation. Disadvantages include higher cost, the lack of occlusiveness (creating the possibility of accidental patient exsanguination), and afterload-dependent flow requiring constant flow measurement.
- Four commercially available centrifugal pumps demonstrate some differences in hydraulic performance, afterload sensitivity, priming volumes, ability to transmit air, and possibly blood trauma.
- A nonocclusive roller pump has been recently introduced. This pump appears to be incapable of generating dangerously high positive or negative pressures or of permitting retrograde flow. This pump is undergoing clinical evaluations to establish its appropriate clinical applications.
- In the setting of short-term CPB for cardiac surgery, it remains uncertain whether the selection of a roller pump over a centrifugal pump or of any specific centrifugal pump over another has clinical significance.

REFERENCES

1. Cooley DA. Development of the roller pump for use in the cardiopulmonary bypass circuit. *Texas Heart Inst J* 1987;14:113–118.
2. DeBakey ME. A simple continuous-flow blood transfusion instrument. *New Orleans Med Surg J* 1934;87:386–389.
3. Hessel EA. Cardiopulmonary bypass circuitry and cannulation techniques. In: Gravlee GP, Davis RF, Utley JR, eds. *Cardiopulmonary bypass, principles and practice.* Baltimore: Williams & Wilkins, 1993:55–92.
4. Bernstein EF, Gleason LR. Factors influencing hemolysis with roller pumps. *Surgery* 1967;61:432–442.
5. Hubbard LC, Kletchka HD, Olsen DA. Spallation using roller pumps and its clinical implication. *AmSECT Proc* 1975;3:27–32.
6. Kurusz M, Christman EW, Williams EH. Roller pump induced tubing wear: another argument in favor of arterial line filtration. *J Extra-Corp Technol* 1980;12:49–59.
7. Uretzky G, Landsburg G, Cohn D. Analysis of microembolic particles originating in extracorporeal circuits. *Perfusion* 1987;2:9–17.
8. Pfaender LM, Riley JB. An in vitro comparison of the effects of temperature on the stroke volume and occlusion setting of various tubing types in a roller pump. *J Extra-Corp Technol* 1979;11:78–88.
9. Noon GP, Dane LE, Feldman L, et al. Reduction of blood trauma in roller pumps for long-term perfusion. *World J Surg* 1985;9:65–71.
10. Rawn DJ, Harris HK, Riley JB, Yoda DN, Blackwell MM. An under-occluded roller pump is less hemolytic than a centrifugal pump. *J Extra-Corp Technol* 1997;29:15–18.
11. Reed CC, Stafford TB. *Cardiopulmonary bypass*, 2nd ed. Houston: Medical Press, 1985:376.
12. Kurusz M, Shaffer CW, Christman EW. Runaway pump head. *J Thorac Cardiovasc Surg* 1979;77:792–795.
13. Stoney WS, Alford WC, Burrus GR, et al. Air embolism and other accidents using pump oxygenators. *Ann Thorac Surg* 1980;29:336–340.
14. Lynch MF, Peterson D, Baker V. Centrifugal blood pumping for open-heart surgery. *Minn Med* 1978;61:536–537.
15. Curtis JJ. Centrifugal mechanical assist for postcardiotomy ventricular failure. *Semin Thorac Cardiovasc Surg* 1994;6:140–146.
16. Nishida H, Shibuya M, Kitamura M, et al. Percutaneous cardiopulmonary support as the second generation of venoarterial bypass: current status and future direction. *Artif Organs* 1993;17:906–913.
17. Black MD, Coles JG, Williams WG, et al. Determinants of success in pediatric cardiac patients undergoing extracorporeal membrane oxygenation. *Ann Thorac Surg* 1995;60:133–138.
18. University of Michigan Hospitals. *ECMO Technical Specialist Manual,* 7th edition. Ann Arbor, MI: University of Michigan Dept. of Surgery, 1984:17.
19. Anonymous. *Technical compendium. Sarns Delphin II centrifugal system.* Ann Arbor: Sarns 3M Health Care, 1993.
20. Anonymous. Medtronic BioMedicus presents more than just a pump? Eden Prairie, MN: Medtronic BioMedicus, 1991.
21. Pacheco DA, Ingram JM, Pacheco SL. A comparison of three centrifugal pumps' ability to expel micro-air under conditions of cavitation or bolus air injection. *Proc Am Acad Cardiovasc Perfus* 1992;13:73–77.
22. Kolff J, McClurken JB, Alpern JB. Beware centrifugal pumps: not a one-way street, but a dangerous siphon! [letter] *Ann Thorac Surg* 1990;50:512.
23. Berki T, Gürbüz A, Isik O, et al. Cardiopulmonary bypass using centrifugal pump. *Vasc Surg* 1992;26:123–134.
24. Schima H, Trubel W, Moritz A, et al. Noninvasive monitoring of rotary blood pumps: necessity, possibility, and limitations. *Artif Organs* 1992;16:195–202.
25. DeBois WJ, Brennan R, Wein E, et al. Centrifugal pumping: the patient outcome benefits following coronary artery bypass surgery. *J Extra-Corp Technol* 1995;27:77–80.
26. Esper E, Devineni R, Shah NS, et al. Results of the unidirectional Centri-Safe arterial valve for prevention of retrograde flow during cardiopulmonary bypass. *ASAIO J* 1994;40:M540–M546.
27. Kurusz M, Wheeldon DR. Risk containment during cardiopulmonary bypass. *Semin Thorac Cardiovasc Surg* 1990;2:400–409.
28. Kolff J, Ankney RN, Wurzel D, et al. Centrifugal pump failures. *J Extra-Corp Technol* 1996;28:118–122.
29. Tamari Y, Lee-Sensiba K, Leonard EF. The effects of pressure and flow on hemolysis caused by BioMedicus centrifugal pumps and roller pumps. *J Thorac Cardiovasc Surg* 1993;106:997–1007.
30. Jacob H, Kutshcera Y, Palzer B, et al. In-vitro assessment of centrifugal pumps for ventricular assist. *Artif Organs* 1990;14:278–283.
31. Oku T, Harasaki H, Smith W, et al. Hemolysis, a comparative study of four non-pulsatile pumps. *Trans Am Soc Artif Intern Organs* 1988;34:500–504.
32. Wheeldon DR, Bethune DW, Gill RD. Vortex pumping for routine cardiac surgery: a comparative study. *Perfusion* 1990;5:135–143.
33. Palder SB, Shaheen KW, Whittlesey GC, et al. Prolonged extra-

corporeal membrane oxygenation in sheep with a hollow-fiber oxygenator and a centrifugal pump. *ASAIO Trans* 1988;34: 820–822.

34. Kress DC, Cohen DJ, Swanson DK, et al. Pump-induced hemolysis in rabbit model of neonatal ECMO. *ASAIO Trans* 1987; 33:446–452.
35. Parault BG, Conrad SA. The effect of extracorporeal circulation time and patient age on platelet retention during cardiopulmonary bypass: a comparison of roller and centrifugal pumps. *J Extra-Corp Technol* 1991;23:34–38.
36. Jacob HG, Hafner G, Thelemann C, et al. Routine extracorporeal circulation with a centrifugal or roller pump. *ASAIO Trans* 1991; 37:M487–M489.
37. Noon GP, Sekela ME, Glueck J, et al. Comparison of Delphin and BioMedicus pumps. *ASAIO Trans* 1990;36:M616–M619.
38. Iatridis E, Chan T. An evaluation of vortex, centrifugal, and roller pump systems. In: Schima H, Thoma H, Weiselthaler G, et al. eds. *Proceedings of the International Workshop on Rotary Blood Pumps*, Baden/Vienna, Austria, 1991:123–131.
39. Kijima T, Ohsiyama H, Horiuchi K, et al. A straight path centrifugal blood pump concept in the Capiox centrifugal pump. *Artif Organs* 1993;17:593–598.
40. Nishida H, Yamaki F, Nakatani H, et al. Development of the Terumo Capiox centrifugal pump and its clinical application to open heart surgery: a comparative study with the roller pump. *Artif Organs* 1993;17:323–327.
41. Kijima T, Nojiri C, Ohsiyama H, et al. The margin of safety in the use of a straight path centrifugal blood pump. *Artif Organs* 1994;18:680–686.
42. Naito K, Suenage E, Cao ZL, et al. Comparative hemolysis study of clinically available centrifugal pumps. *Artif Organs* 1996;20: 560–563.
43. Kawahito K, Nosé Y. Hemolysis in different centrifugal pumps. *Artif Organs* 1997;21:323–326.
44. Sasaki T, Jikuya T, Aizawa T, et al. A compact centrifugal pump for cardiopulmonary bypass. *Artif Organs* 1992;16:592–598.
45. Jikuya T, Sasaki T, Aizawa T, et al. Development of an atraumatic small centrifugal pump for second-generation cardiopulmonary bypass. *Artif Organs* 1992;16:599–606.
46. Naito K, Miyazoe Y, Aizawa T, et al. Development of the Baylor-Nikkiso centrifugal pump with a purging system for circulatory support. *Artif Organs* 1993;17:614–618.
47. Orime Y, Takatani S, Sasaki T, et al. Cardiopulmonary bypass with Nikkiso and BioMedicus centrifugal pumps. *Artif Organs* 1994;18:11–16.
48. Taguchi S, Yozu R, Mori A, et al. A miniaturized centrifugal pump for assist circulation. *Artif Organs* 1994;18:664–668.
49. Ninomiya J, Shoji T, Tanaka S, et al. Clinical evaluation of a new type of centrifugal pump. *Artif Organs* 1994;18:702–705.
50. Onoda K, Kondo C, Mizumoto T, et al. Clinical experience with Nikkiso centrifugal pumps for extracorporeal circulation. *Artif Organs* 1994;18:706–710.
51. Nishinaka T, Nishida H, Endo M, et al. Less blood damage in the impeller centrifugal pump: a comparative study with the roller pump in open heart surgery. *Artif Organs* 1996;20:707–710.
52. Shomura Y, Shimono T, Onoda K, et al. Clinical experience with the Nikkiso centrifugal pump. *Artif Organs* 1996;20:711–714.
53. Ohtsubo S, Tayama E, Short D, et al. Clinical comparative study of cardiopulmonary bypass with Nikkiso and BioMedicus centrifugal pumps. *Artif Organs* 1996;20:725–730.
54. James SD, Peters J, Maresca L, et al. The roller pump does produce pulsatile flow. *J Extra-Corp Technol* 1987;19:376–383.
55. Pappas G, Winter SD, Kopriva CJ, et al. Improvement of myocardial and other vital organ functions and metabolism with a simple method of pulsatile flow (IABP) during clinical cardiopulmonary bypass. *Surgery* 1975;77:34–44.
56. Maddox G, Pappas G, Jenkins M, et al. Effect of pulsatile and nonpulsatile flow during cardiopulmonary bypass on left ventricular function early after aortocoronary bypass surgery. *Am J Cardiol* 1976;37:1000–1006.
57. Montoya JP, Merz SI, Bartlett RH. Significant safety advantages gained with an improved pressure-regulated blood pump. *J Extra-Corp Technol* 1996;28:71–78.
58. Anonymous. Technical manual. Affinity Pump System 2000. Minneapolis, MN: Avecor Cardiovascular, Inc., 1997.
59. Jaggy C, Lachat M, Leskosek B, et al. Affinity pump system: a new peristaltic pump for cardiopulmonary bypass. *Perfusion* 2000;15: 77–83.
60. Crockett G, Vocelka C, Carvalho J, et al. Predicting the blood flow rate from the Affinity model 2000 pump system. 37th International Conference of the American Society of Extra-Corporeal Technology, 8–11 April 1999, New Orleans. (abst).

PRINCIPLES OF OXYGENATOR FUNCTION: GAS EXCHANGE, HEAT TRANSFER, AND OPERATION

KANE M. HIGH
GERARD BASHEIN
MARK KURUSZ

Through common clinical usage, the term "oxygenator" has come to mean that portion of the perfusion apparatus that serves the functions of the patient's natural lungs during the period of extracorporeal circulation. More correctly, the device should be called a gas exchanger because it also transports carbon dioxide, anesthetics, and possibly other gases into and out of the circulation. In addition, all modern oxygenators have integral heat exchangers and also serve as the main reservoir and a filter for blood returned from the cardiotomy suction. Thus, the oxygenator performs all major functions of the natural lungs except for their endocrine function, which can be suspended for a short time without major ill effects.

As Chapters 1 and 2 indicated, designing a practical oxygenator constituted one of the major challenges faced by early pioneers of cardiopulmonary bypass (CPB), and it was only after disposable and relatively inexpensive oxygenators were developed that widespread practice of open heart surgery became possible. Figure 4.1 presents oxygenator use trends since 1980, showing near universal use of membrane oxygenators in the United States. An additional survey published in 1995 confirms the shift from bubble to membrane oxygenators in the United States (1). Worldwide, the annual use of disposable oxygenators has been estimated at 1.1 million, of which 80% to 90% is thought to represent membrane oxygenators (Rodger Stewart, personal communication, 1999, COBE Cardiovascular Inc., Arvada, CO). This reflects progressive improvements in both performance and cost of membrane oxygenators and a growing awareness of

the advantages over bubble oxygenators for reducing blood trauma and the risk of embolization.

Oxygenator designers strive to maximize the amount of oxygen, carbon dioxide, and other gases that can be transferred at a given blood flow rate to make gas transport easy for the perfusionist to regulate, to maximize heat-transfer efficiency, to minimize blood trauma, and to minimize the priming volume (i.e., the amount of liquid that must be added to fill the oxygenator before operation). Table 4.1 illustrates why engineers have such a formidable task in attempting to duplicate the functions of the natural lung. First, red blood cells pass through pulmonary capillaries one at a time, making the distance for O_2 diffusion much shorter than has ever been achieved in an artificial lung. The rate of oxygen transfer in natural lungs is not limited by diffusion, except in the case of severe lung disease or extreme exercise. Indeed, the difference between gas tensions measured in the natural alveoli and in the blood are mostly due to ventilation–perfusion mismatching. In contrast, in artificial lungs operating under normal conditions, a significant difference in partial pressures occurs between the gas and blood phases.

A second disadvantage to the artificial lung is a much smaller surface area over which to exchange gases (typically less than 10% of the natural lung's area). Current membrane lungs compensate for these shortcomings by increasing the blood path length (the distance that the blood travels past the gas exchange surface), thereby increasing the time available for blood exposure to the gas exchange surface (i.e., an increased dwell time). In addition, secondary flows are induced in artificial lungs to promote mixing and bring deoxygenated blood closer to the exchange surface (see Enhancing Gas Transport with Secondary Flows, below). Artificial lungs can be ventilated with 100% O_2 to maximize the driving pressure difference for O_2 diffusion, without the toxic effects that would occur in the natural lung, and the artificial lung can be ventilated with a high flow of fresh

K.M. High: Department of Anesthesia, Hershey Medical Center, Hershey, PA 17033.

G. Bashein: Department of Anesthesiology and Department of Bioengineering, University of Washington, Seattle, Washington 98195-6540

M. Kurusz: Division of Cardiothoracic Surgery, University of Texas Medical Branch at Galveston, Galveston, TX 77555-0528.

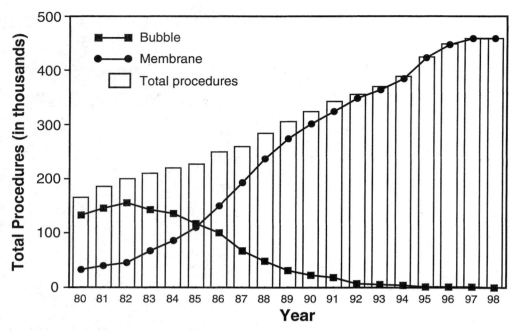

FIG. 4.1. Oxygenator use in the United States from 1980 to 1998. (Courtesy of Rodger Stewart, COBE Cardiovascular, Inc., Arvada, CO.)

gas to keep the CO_2 fraction in the gas phase low. Even the best available artificial lungs are incapable of achieving anywhere near the gas exchange of the natural lung (Table 4.1). Fortunately, hypothermia, muscle paralysis, and anesthesia all reduce the patient's metabolic requirements to the point where gas exchange requirements can ordinarily be met by one of these devices.

In what follows, we review the physical principles that determine how gas and heat transfer occur in oxygenators and how these principles are used in the design of generic bubble and membrane oxygenators. We also review studies examining interactions of blood with artificial surfaces and bubbles. Then we discuss how these considerations translate

into the performance differences of membrane and bubble oxygenators. Finally, we discuss clinical considerations in the use of bubble and membrane oxygenators and techniques for safe practice. The reader is also directed to three excellent reviews on oxygenator design (2–4).

PERTINENT PHYSICAL PRINCIPLES

Regardless of the type of oxygenator, gas transfer from the gas to the liquid phase (or the opposite direction) is driven by diffusion according to the partial pressure difference of the particular gas. Gas transfer is limited by the resistance to diffusion of the particular gas through the primary substance, whether it is a synthetic membrane, blood, or the gas phase itself. Other factors that come into play are the physical size and structure of the oxygenator and how the blood flow and gas flow affect these driving forces and resistances.

TABLE 4.1. COMPARISON OF PHYSICAL CHARACTERISTICS OF A MEMBRANE LUNG AND NATURAL LUNG

Characteristic	Membrane Lung[a]	Natural Lung[b]
Surface area (m²)	0.5–4	70
Blood path width (μm)	200	8
Blood path length (μm)	250,000	200
Membrane thickness (μm)	150	0.5
Maximum O_2 transfer (mL/min, STP)	400–600	2,000

[a] Data for a Kolobow membrane oxygenator (Avecor Cardiovascular, Minneapolis, MN).
[b] *Source:* Guyton AC. *Textbook of medical physiology.* Philadelphia: W.B. Saunders, 1976.
STP, standard temperature and pressure.

Determinants of the P_{O_2} and P_{CO_2} in Gas and Blood

The partial pressure of gases present in a mixture of gases occupying a volume acts as if each individual gas is occupying the volume independently (Dalton's law), and the sum of the individual gas partial pressures equals the total gas pressure. This applies for gases occupying a space by themselves or dissolved in solution (i.e., blood). Thus, when

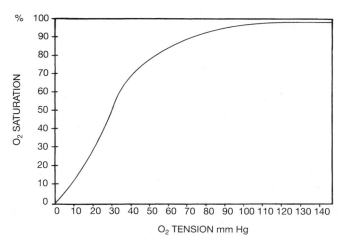

FIG. 4.2. Oxyhemoglobin dissociation curve reflecting the non-linear relationship between hemoglobin saturation and oxygen partial pressure.

blood equilibrates at atmospheric pressure, the partial pressures or gas tensions of all gases dissolved in blood must add up to 760 mm Hg at sea level. In the gas phase, the partial pressure (P), the concentration (C), and the mole fraction are equivalent.

The fact that CO_2 and O_2 blood content do not derive simply from these gases being dissolved in solution complicates analysis of gas transfer in oxygenators. The well-known oxyhemoglobin dissociation curve shown in Figure 4.2 reflects the nonlinear binding of O_2 by hemoglobin. The CO_2 in the blood combines chemically with different moieties (Fig. 4.3) to form bicarbonate, the major carrier of CO_2 in blood, and to amino groups of proteins, primarily hemoglobin, and is not linearly related to the partial pressure of CO_2. Because of the chemical combination of CO_2 and O_2

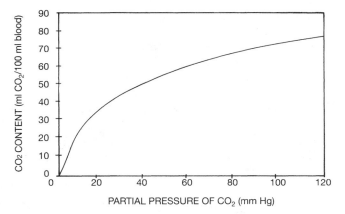

FIG. 4.3. Carbon dioxide solubility in blood is not a linear function of the partial pressure of carbon dioxide because of its chemical combination to form carbonate and its binding to hemoglobin.

to hemoglobin and the other moieties just described, both are present in much higher concentrations than would be possible simply by physical solution.

Diffusion of Gases Through Liquids and Solids

Diffusion is best considered at the molecular level. The random motion of the atoms or molecules of the diffusing gas move from regions of higher concentration to regions of lower concentration. Fick's law describes the rate at which gases diffuse through gases, liquids, and solids. This law states that the rate of diffusion is proportional to the partial pressure gradient of the gas in the direction of diffusion (i.e., the change in the partial pressure of the gas per unit distance). Mathematically, the rate of diffusion per unit area, J, at a particular location, x, along the diffusion path would be described as

$$J = -D \cdot \delta P/\delta x \qquad [1]$$

where D is the the diffusivity constant (a characteristic of the material and gas) and P is the the partial pressure of the gas at any particular location, x. The negative sign in the equation is the result of the negative value of the partial pressure difference, a result of the decreasing pressure in the direction of increasing distance, x.

Several inferences can be made from this relationship. The rate of total gas transfer can be increased by increasing the partial pressure difference (represented by δP) or the surface area available for diffusion. The rate of gas transfer can also be increased by decreasing the distance through which the gas must diffuse (represented by δx). These important concepts are discussed below in the sections on oxygenator function and design. Of course there are practical limits to how far these concepts can be taken, because they will lead to an increased oxygenator priming volume or increased pressure drop across the oxygenator as membranes are brought closer together.

The diffusivity, D, is constant for a particular gas and diffusion barrier material at a constant temperature. Kinetic theory dictates that the diffusivity is related to the molecular speed of the gas molecules and, according to Graham's law, is inversely proportional to the square root of the molecular weight of the gas. The diffusivity of a gas is related to the solubility of the gas, because increasing solubility enhances movement of the gas through a solid or liquid. This latter factor complicates the analysis of gas transfer (5,6). Gas diffusion in blood, particularly oxygen diffusion, is somewhat more complicated than predicted by Fick's law. In addition to simple diffusion through the blood plasma, the absorption of oxygen by red blood cells must be considered. Although detailed mathematical derivation of this process is beyond the scope of this book, if one assumes, as Marx et al. (5) have done, that local variations of O_2 around the red cell are small compared with the overall O_2 gradient, a

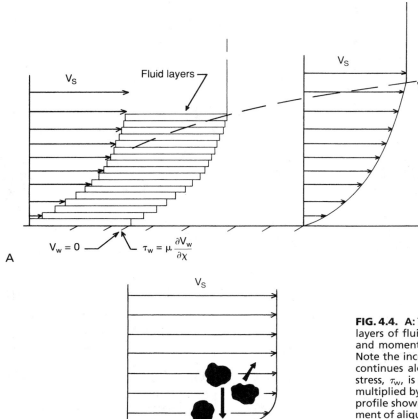

FIG. 4.4. A: The laminar velocity boundary layer of fluid showing layers of fluid dragging each other along with greater velocity and momentum as the free stream velocity, V_s, is approached. Note the increasing thickness of the boundary layer as the flow continues along the surface from left to right. The wall shear stress, τ_w, is shown as equal to the product of the viscosity, μ, multiplied by the velocity gradient, $\delta V_w / \delta x$. **B:** Turbulent velocity profile showing the steeper rise in velocity because of the movement of aliquots of fluid having a higher velocity into the boundary layer. Note that the velocity profile represents the average velocity throughout this turbulent flow.

second-order differential equation can be derived that describes diffusion of oxygen in blood as a nonlinear function of distance and time. It is not difficult to imagine that the O_2 concentration within a volume of blood will increase as the exposure time of blood to either a bubble or membrane interface increases. Thus, time (i.e., red cell dwell time within the oxygenator) becomes an important factor when considering gas transport in the blood phase. Furthermore, diffusion of O_2 within the red blood cell is not well elucidated because the shape of the cell and the packing of the hemoglobin make this analysis difficult.

Diffusion of Momentum in a Flowing Fluid and Generation of the Stagnant Boundary Layer

Blood or any other viscous fluid flowing past either a stationary surface or a bubble will have variations in velocity from zero at the interface surface to that of the free stream. The region in which this variation occurs is defined as the boundary layer. If the main stream of the fluid has a different velocity than the interface surface (a bubble could flow

within the blood flow),* a velocity gradient will be formed in which the fluid velocity varies from zero at the interface to V_s, the velocity in the main stream as shown in Figure 4.4A. This may be conceptualized as layers of fluid slipping or dragging over one another. Hence, as the distance from the wall increases, each subsequent layer has a greater velocity and momentum (momentum is the product of mass times velocity). Momentum thus varies from a maximum in the free stream to zero at the wall, which may be conceptualized as a momentum flux from the free stream through each layer to the surface. This is comparable with a flux of gas undergoing diffusion or heat transfer (see Analogues of Momentum, Mass, and Heat Transfer, below). As Figure 4.4A shows, as the flow continues along a surface, the boundary layer widens (known as the developing boundary layer). If the boundary layer widens to the point that it

---

* From a fluid mechanics viewpoint, it does not matter whether the blood is moving past the surface or the surface of a bubble past the blood. It is the relative velocity that affects the velocity boundary layer and possibly the diffusion boundary layer.

meets the growing boundary layer from the other side of the flow channel, then the flow is said to be fully developed.

The contour of the velocity boundary layer is important because it determines the overall resistance to flow or the pressure drop that occurs. At any place within the boundary layer the shear stress, τ, is proportional to the rate of change of velocity in the direction perpendicular to the main flow (the partial derivative of velocity, $\delta u/\delta x$) with the proportionality constant being the viscosity, μ, or

$$\tau = -\mu \, \delta u/\delta x \qquad [2]$$

Thus, as the velocity gradient increases, the shear stress increases.† The viscosity, μ, is constant for most fluids. Such fluids are referred to as Newtonian fluids. However, some fluids, including blood, do not have a constant viscosity (i.e., the viscosity changes depending on the nature of the flow); these are called non-Newtonian fluids. The primary determinant of blood viscosity is the concentration of red blood cells (i.e., the hematocrit), which tends to vary within boundary layers. At the wall, the shear stress, τ_w, is also related to the steepness of this velocity gradient, as shown in Figure 4.4A. The integral or summation of all the wall shear stresses over the entire wall surface is what determines the pressure drop of any viscous flow.

Velocity profiles vary with the nature of the flow stream to produce either laminar or turbulent flow. Turbulent flow generates spontaneous eddies from flow instabilities within the flow. Such a flow would have a high Reynolds‡ number (a nondimensional number used to predict the transition from laminar to turbulent flow). Turbulence can also result from an irregularity in the flow path, creating eddies within the flow (see Enhancing Gas Transport with Secondary Flows, below). Figure 4.4B shows how turbulence changes the boundary layer velocity profile by moving higher velocity fluid into the boundary layer closer to the surface, causing a steeper rise in the velocity profile (shear rate) and in shear stress.

As a fluid flows past a surface through which diffusion is occurring, a diffusion boundary is generated that is layer-similar to the velocity boundary and depends on Fick's law. For oxygen diffusion typical of a membrane lung, as shown in Figure 4.5, the oxygen partial pressure in the fluid varies from P_w, the partial pressure of oxygen at the interface with the blood, to P_s, the partial pressure within the stream not yet affected by the diffusion of gas to or from the wall. Note that in Figure 4.5 the O_2 partial pressure decreases slightly

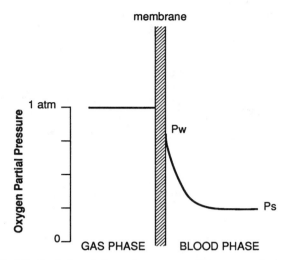

FIG. 4.5. Typical variation of oxygen partial pressure from the membrane of an artificial lung to the free stream of blood. (see text for details.)

in the membrane itself but rapidly decreases in the blood. This graphically represents the actual physical condition. In modern membrane oxygenators, most resistance to O_2 diffusion occurs in the blood (estimates are >90%) due to the low diffusivity of O_2 in blood. As the bloodstream flows along the interface, the boundary layer of O_2 grows in a manner similar to that described for the velocity boundary layer. As the width of this boundary layer increases, the diffusion distance increases and hence the rate of gas diffusion decreases because of the greater diffusion distance.

Principles of Heat Transfer

Discussion of heat transfer traditionally begins with consideration of the molecular basis of this form of energy transfer. Heat transfer represents the transfer of kinetic energy from molecules with a higher energy (higher temperature) to molecules with a lower energy (lower temperature). This transfer actually represents the transfer of kinetic energy from the higher energy source to the lower.

Heat transfer is possible in one of three forms: conduction (through solids), convection (from solids to liquids, with motion of the liquid carrying fluid away from the solid–liquid interface), and radiation (an electromagnetic mechanism). Within the CPB heat exchanger, the major forms of heat transfer are forced convection (the water and blood of the heat exchanger are actively pumped past the stainless steel interface, hence the term "forced") and conduction within the stainless steel.

The flow of energy or heat, Q, is related to the temperature difference by the thermal conductivity, K, a constitutive property of any material, such that

$$Q = -K \cdot \delta T/\delta x \qquad [3]$$

---

† Note that shear stress, τ, is a force applied to a unit area and thus has units of pressure. The force, however, is applied tangentially to or across the area, unlike pressure, in which the force is applied perpendicular to the area. Furthermore, note that the velocity gradient, $\delta u/\delta x$, is usually referred to as the shear rate.

‡ The Reynolds number is defined as the ratio of inertial to viscous forces, or Re $= \rho \cdot U \cdot d/\mu$ (ρ = density, U = velocity, d = chamber diameter, μ = viscosity)..

TABLE 4.2. COMPARISON OF MOMENTUM TRANSFER, HEAT TRANSFER, AND MASS TRANSFER (DIFFUSION)

Transfer	Driving Force	Flow	Defining Equation[a]
Momentum	Velocity gradient	Momentum	$\tau = -\mu\, {}^{\delta u}/_{\delta x}$
Heat	Temperature gradient	Heat (energy)	$Q = -K\, {}^{\delta T}/_{\delta x}$
Mass (Diffusion)	Concentration gradient	Mass (diffusing gas)	$J = -D\, {}^{\delta P}/_{\delta x}$

[a] The negative signs in these equations are the result of standard conventions used in defining positive and negative directions. See text for explanation of equations.

where T is the temperature at any point and x is the distance. This equation is the one-dimensional form of Fourier's law of heat conduction. In a similar manner to that already discussed for the other boundary layers, as blood flows past the heat exchanger surface, a thermal boundary layer is generated in which the temperature varies from the temperature of the wall to that of the free stream yet unaffected by the heat exchanger.

Analogues of Momentum, Mass, and Heat Transfer

It provides insight to consider the similarities between the various forms of mass and energy transfer that have just been discussed: diffusion, momentum transfer, and heat transfer (7). Marked similarity exists between the apparent movement of momentum in the velocity boundary layer, gas diffusion, and heat transfer in the heat exchanger. Table 4.2 summarizes these similarities. The most striking feature is the resemblance of the defining equations as shown in the right column. Although these equations are simpler than the actual equations needed to describe the physical situations, they provide insight into the nature of the equations.

Enhancing Gas Transport with Secondary Flows

The major resistance to gas diffusion occurs in the blood phase (8). Efforts to improve gas exchange have focused on reducing this diffusion barrier (9,10). As mentioned earlier, the primary methods for enhancing gas diffusion are increasing the driving gradient and dwell time or decreasing the diffusion path. Increasing the driving gradient is limited to 760 mm Hg minus the oxygen tension in the blood, because pressures above atmospheric pressure risk bulk gas transport across the membrane with resultant gas embolization. Increasing the dwell time is limited by the requirement for increased priming volume as the size of the oxygenator increases.

However, decreasing the diffusion path has been used very successfully to enhance gas transfer. First, the blood path thickness has been minimized as much as technically feasible by placing the membranes as close together as possi-

ble without causing an excessive pressure drop across the oxygenator. The major advance has been the utilization of induced eddies or secondary flows of the blood (11) from the primary stream (Fig. 4.6) into the diffusion boundary layer, thus decreasing the thickness of this layer and increasing the gas transfer. Eddies have been generated in several different ways. Some possible methods include making the surface of the membrane irregular (e.g., dimpled) (12) or positioning the elements within the flow stream to disrupt the smooth flow.

This bulk movement of venous blood into the diffusion

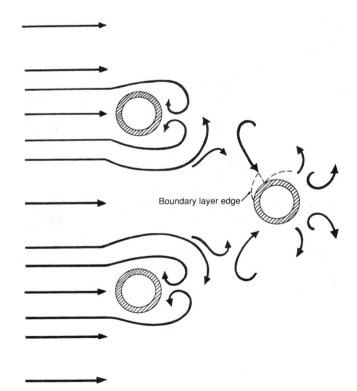

FIG. 4.6. Blood flow past hollow fibers showing the effect of an eddy on the boundary layer (cross-section) of a downstream fiber. An eddy current has an impact on the boundary layer of the fiber on the right, disrupting its development and reducing its thickness. This phenomenon occurs much more frequently and on a smaller scale than indicated here, causing continuous inhibition of the boundary layer development.

boundary layer also has an impact on the blood velocity boundary layer, thus increasing the shear stresses within the boundary layer and at the wall. This has two negative effects. First, the increased shear stress within the boundary layer can lead to increased formed element destruction, as discussed later. Furthermore, increasing wall shear stresses (membrane oxygenators) increases the blood pressure drop across the oxygenator. These factors must be balanced in the design of the blood flow pattern within a membrane oxygenator.

BUBBLE OXYGENATORS

Standard Design

Although the concepts of both bubble and membrane oxygenation were well appreciated by the early developers of CPB, the inherent simplicity of bubble oxygenation led to the earlier development of a practical device. Structurally, a typical bubble oxygenator is divided into two sections (Fig. 4.7). Venous blood first enters a mixing chamber, where fresh gas flows into the blood through a screen, which causes small bubbles to form. The blood and bubbles coalesce; sufficient time is allowed in this section for adequate gas exchange to occur before defoaming in the second section.

A major advantage of bubble oxygenators is their low

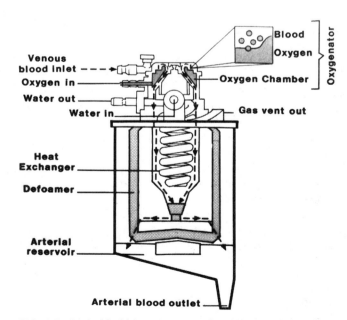

FIG. 4.7. Typical bubble oxygenator showing the mixing chamber, heat exchanger, defoamer, and arterial reservoir. Dashed line = blood path. (Reprinted from High KM, Williams DR, Kurusz M. Cardiopulmonary bypass circuits and design. In: Hensley FA, Martin DE, eds. *A practical approach to cardiac anesthesia 2nd edition.* Boston: Little, Brown & Co., 1995:471; with permission.)

pressure drop, which allows them to be placed upstream of the CPB pump where they can also act as the reservoir for the system. The flow through a bubble oxygenator is driven primarily by the hydrostatic pressure head generated in the venous perfusion tubing (which explains why CPB machines are designed to stay close to the floor). However, the mixing chamber is designed so that the blood flows through it in an upward direction, exploiting the tendency of the rising bubbles to facilitate blood flow and reduce the pressure drop. Generally, the pressure drop through a bubble oxygenator is less than 30 cm of water, in contrast to the 100 cm of water pressure drop typically found in membrane oxygenators.

The hydrostatic pressure and drag from the bubbles carry the blood over the top of a separator and into the heat exchanger, bubble remover, and reservoir. Because the heat exchanger functions similarly for both bubble and membrane oxygenators, it is described in a later section. An advantage to having the heat exchanger downstream from the bubble chamber is that gas exchange continues while heat transfer occurs. Blood is first defoamed by silicone antifoam-A, which consists of the liquid polymer dimethylpolysiloxane (96%) and particulate silica (4%). Dimethylpolysiloxane, the active defoaming agent, is mounted on the silica (which acts to disperse it in blood) (13) and destabilizes the bubbles, causing them to collapse. Bubbles are also mechanically restrained by the mesh net through which the blood and bubbles must pass.

The reservoir section has several purposes. It compensates for inevitable flow discrepancies between the passively flowing venous tubing and the pump-driven arterial tubing and it allows the perfusionist some time to react to these changes. Unlike membrane oxygenators, bubble oxygenators do not require a separate venous or arterial reservoir. Second, the reservoir also serves a debubbling function by allowing time for the blood to briefly stagnate and thus facilitate bubble elimination by allowing them to float to the top of the reservoir. Blood exits from the reservoir through the bottom, away from any bubbles floating to the top.

Bubble Considerations

Gas bubbles are eliminated from the oxygenated blood both by separation (as described above) and by absorption into the blood. The absorption of the gas in a bubble depends on the difference in partial pressures between the gas in the bubble and the liquid. In the case of oxygen bubbles coming from the oxygenator, the net pressure difference tending to drive absorption is the sum of the ambient pressure of the blood and the surface tension of the bubble minus the sum of the partial pressure of CO_2 in the bubble and the oxygen partial pressure within the blood. This difference becomes more favorable for absorption when the bubbles are compressed by the high ambient pressure of the blood present

TABLE 4.3. TOTAL BLOOD–GAS INTERFACE FOR 1 CM³ OF GAS SEPARATED INTO VARIOUS BUBBLE SIZES[a]

Bubble Diameter (μm)	Number of Bubbles (×10⁺³)	Total Surface Area (cm²)
10	238,700	3000
50	1,910	600
100	239	300
200	29.8	150
400	3.73	75

[a] Numbers calculated based on equations for volume of a sphere ($V = 4/3\pi r^3$) and surface areas of a sphere ($A - 4\pi r^2$).

in the arterial infusion tubing. Absorption of bubbles will be inhibited as the arterial P_{O_2} increases.

Bubble size also affects the rate of CO_2 and O_2 exchange. For a specified flow of oxygen into the mixing chamber, decreasing the size of the bubbles by injecting the gas through smaller holes will increase the total amount of surface area of the blood–gas interface. As Table 4.3 shows, for a given total gas volume, the total area available for gas transfer is inversely proportional to the bubble diameter (assuming all bubbles are the same diameter). Thus, as the bubble diameter decreases from 100 to 10 μm, the surface area per cubic centimeter of total gas increases 10-fold from 300 to 3,000 cm². However, as Galletti and Brecher (14) pointed out, there is a difficulty with smaller bubbles: the CO_2 tension within them will rise faster, limiting the total carbon dioxide transfer. One can imagine a limiting case where bubbles containing only a few oxygen molecules are injected, resulting in excellent blood oxygenation without any carbon dioxide diffusing into them whatsoever. Manufacturers have assessed this trade-off between oxygenation and carbon dioxide elimination and have selected bubble sizes that provide the best compromise, generally with a respiratory quotient (ratio of CO_2 elimination to O_2 uptake) of 0.8 under standard operating conditions.

Operation and Control

Control of oxygenation in bubble oxygenators is made more complicated by the interaction between oxygenation and carbon dioxide removal. This situation contrasts with natural lungs or artificial membrane lungs, where independent change in carbon dioxide elimination can be accomplished by simply changing the ventilating gas flow rate. Increasing the flow of oxygen into a bubble oxygenator will increase the number of bubbles generated and the surface available for gas transfer, resulting in increased P_{O_2} in the blood. In lieu of adding more oxygen, attempts have been made (15) to add so-called inert gases to the ventilating gas in an attempt to control the oxygenation and carbon dioxide elimi-

nation independently. The perfusionist could then adjust the ratio of the oxygen and inert gas (i.e., nitrogen or helium), thus maintaining a constant flow of oxygen while varying the total ventilating flow. However, this is dangerous because the higher total ventilating flow increases the risk of gas emboli. Furthermore, inert gases in the bubbles would absorb more slowly than the oxygen, which avidly combines with hemoglobin. Inert gases are not generally used.

One vital aspect of using a bubble oxygenator is maintaining an adequate volume of blood in the reservoir. As mentioned above, this reservoir enhances debubbling of the blood by giving the bubbles the opportunity to rise to the top of the blood pool. This volume of blood also acts as a compliance chamber for the system, giving the perfusionist time to add volume, warn surgeons of decreased venous return, and/or temporarily decrease blood pump flow rate.

MEMBRANE OXYGENATORS

Standard Design: "True" Versus Microporous Membranes

Membrane lungs attempt to achieve separation between blood and gas in a manner analogous to the natural lung. "True" membrane lungs provide a complete barrier between the gas and blood phases so that gas transfer depends totally on diffusion of gas through the membrane material. True membrane lungs are costly to manufacture and have a large priming volume, and as a result, most membrane lungs used for CPB today have micropores. The only true membrane oxygenator currently in production is the Kolobow spiral coil membrane lung (Avecor Cardiovascular, Inc., Minneapolis, MN). This lung is used primarily in extracorporeal membrane oxygenation because of its ability to maintain stable CO_2 and O_2 for long periods of time (weeks) without the decrement in gas transfer that is commonly seen with microporous membrane lungs. As depicted in Figure 4.8, the Kolobow membrane lung consists of a silicone membrane in the shape of an envelope that is coiled on itself. Blood flows through the integral heat exchanger and then past the membrane. This oxygenator is available in gas exchange surface area sizes from 0.5 to 4.5 m² to provide extracorporeal membrane oxygenation to patients ranging from neonates with congenital lung disease to adults with adult respiratory distress syndrome and conventional CPB.

Microporous membranes allow at least transient direct blood–gas interfacing at the initiation of CPB. After a short time, protein coating of the membrane and gas interface takes place, and no further direct blood and gas contact exists. Typically, the surface tension of the blood prevents large amounts of fluid from traversing the small micropores during CPB. The micropores provide conduits through the polypropylene membrane that give sufficient diffusion capa-

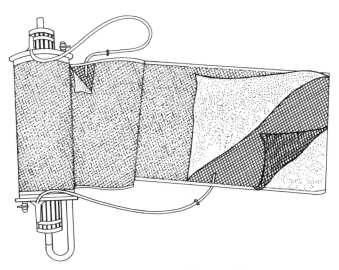

FIG. 4.8. An unfolded view of a Kolobow coiled membrane oxygenator showing the coiled silicone envelope with a mesh screen separating the membranes in the gas phase of the oxygenator. Fresh gas is supplied to the envelope by several silicone tubes (one is depicted in the figure) and removed in a similar manner. (Reproduced from Snider MT, High KM, Campbell DB, et al. Extracorporeal membrane oxygenation. In: Hensley FA, Martin DE, eds. *The practice of cardiac anesthesia.* Boston: Little, Brown & Co., 1990, with permission.)

bility to the membrane for both oxygen and carbon dioxide exchange.

However, over several hours of use, the functional capacity of micropore membrane oxygenators decreases because of evaporation and subsequent condensation of serum that leaks through the micropores (16–18). It has been suggested that this transfer may be reduced by heating the membrane lung and the gas entering it (17), the premise being that the condensation within the fibers can be minimized by maintaining the ventilating gas temperature above blood temperature to minimize condensation. Although currently unconfirmed, the initial results of this approach appear promising. Blood surface tension prevents gas leakage into the blood (provided excessive gas compartment pressures do not occur).

Membrane Configuration and the Manifolding of Gas and Blood Flow

Two primary designs of microporous membrane structure are currently being used: the hollow fiber design originally described by Bodell et al. (19) and the folded envelope design. Hollow polypropylene fibers are extruded, annealed, and stretched to produce the micropores and then heated to stabilize the structure of the polymer (20). Pore size is less than 1 μm, although the size depends on the manufacturing process used. Pores less than 1 μm are required to inhibit both gas and serum leakage across the membrane. The wide-

spread current use of membrane lungs depended on the development of the microporous membrane. Before this innovation, available materials with the necessary structural integrity (Teflon, cellulose) were incapable of sufficient gas exchange without excess surface areas. The microporous membrane provides the necessary gas transfer capability via the micropores, where there is a direct blood–gas interface with minimal resistance to diffusion.

Two basic types of hollow fiber membrane lungs have been made: those with the blood phase on the inside or outside of the fibers. Decreased oxygenator function from thrombosis within the fibers has occurred with the former design (21). However, satisfactory clinical performance continues to be achieved with both blood flow patterns. For oxygenators with blood flow outside the fiber, blood flows either perpendicular to the fiber bundle (cross-current) or in the direction of the fibers. In the latter case, blood usually flows in the opposite direction to the gas flow (counter-current). Cross-current blood flow offers the advantage of naturally induced secondary flow generation. The fibers tend to "trip" the flow, inducing eddies downstream of each fiber (Figs. 4.6 and 4.9). This flow alteration reduces the

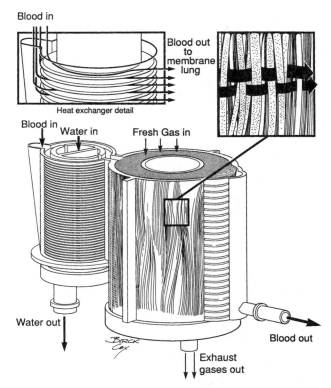

FIG. 4.9. Typical membrane lung. In this case, the heat exchanger (shown in detail in the upper left of the figure) incorporates fins that act as channels through which the blood flows. The blood first passes through the heat exchanger and then through the gas exchange portion of the membrane lung. Both the heat exchanger and gas exchanger portions contain manifolding that distributes blood flow evenly to minimize shunting within the device.

diffusion boundary layer of downstream fibers, thereby enhancing gas exchange. Another advantage to routing blood outside the hollow fibers is reduced pressure drop across the blood compartment.

Elimination of blood streamlining (direct flow through the oxygenator without gas exchange) through the oxygenator constitutes a key feature to ensuring optimal lung performance. Therefore, in hollow fiber designs where blood flows outside the fibers, adequate manifolding (the blood flow channel in and out of the oxygenator) of both the inlet and outlet blood flow is critical, as is the flow pattern within the oxygenator itself. In hollow fiber designs where blood flows inside the fibers, reducing fiber occlusions from thrombosis has been the key to successful design.

Operation and Control of Membrane Oxygenators

In contrast to bubble oxygenators, control of ventilation and oxygenation is relatively independent in membrane oxygenators. Increasing the total gas flow rate changes ventilation (CO_2 elimination) by reducing the gas phase CO_2 partial pressures and probably by decreasing the gas phase boundary layers for CO_2 transfer. Gas flow is adjusted by a flow controller upstream of the oxygenator, such that some pressurization of the gas occurs (generally only a few centimeters of water pressure).

Blood oxygenation control is accomplished simply by increasing (or decreasing) the fraction of O_2 in the gas supplied to the oxygenator. Because the membrane oxygenator separates the blood and gas phases and does not introduce gas bubbles into the blood, the addition of nitrogen to the gas flows does not increase the risk of gas emboli to the patient (as it does with bubble oxygenators). Some experts have commended the ability of membrane oxygenators to function with a reduced supply of gas oxygen fraction as an indicator of efficiency, although this capability has limited clinical relevance, except in the rare instance of a hypermetabolic patient.

QUANTIFICATION OF OXYGENATOR PERFORMANCE

Measurement of Gas Transfer

It is not common practice at this time to measure the amount of O_2 and CO_2 transferred across the artificial lung. However, situations can arise (22) in which determination of oxygenator gas exchange is critical and perhaps life saving. In the case of oxygenator dysfunction, it is vital to distinguish between primary oxygenator dysfunction and hypermetabolic states of the patient. The gas exchange of the oxygenator can rapidly be determined using either blood or gas phase measurements.

In the blood phase, gas transfer can be calculated by

application of conservation of mass (Fick's principle). This assumes that the transfer of O_2 across the membrane or bubble interface causes the difference between the oxygen content flowing into and emerging from the oxygenator. Thus, the oxygen content of the arterial and venous perfusion tubes is determined by continuous in-line monitors or blood gas determinations, and the difference is multiplied by the flow rate of blood (pump flow rate) as shown in Eq. 4:

$$V_{O_2} = Q \cdot (C_a - C_v) \qquad [4]$$

where V_{O_2} is the oxygen transport, Q is the blood flow rate, and C is the oxygen content, with a and v representing the arterial and venous values, respectively.

Gas transfer can also be determined in the gas phase, perhaps more accurately and rapidly in some cases than blood phase measurements. Using an operating room mass spectrometer or infrared gas analyzer, the gas concentrations of the gas flowing into and from the oxygenator can be sampled and gas fractions determined. The difference of O_2 in inlet and outlet gas concentrations can then be multiplied by the total gas flow rate to determine the O_2 transfer rate:

$$V_{O_2} = Q \cdot (F_iO_2 - F_eO_2) \qquad [5]$$

In this case, Q is the gas flow rate and F_iO_2 and F_{eO_2} are inlet and outlet gas oxygen fractions, respectively.

This method introduces what is usually a minor inaccuracy in the calculations. Because the rate of transfer of O_2 and CO_2 is not necessarily the same, the flow rate of the gas entering the oxygenator is slightly different than the exiting flow rate. If more accurate gas transfer rates are desired, then a dilutional gas can be added to the supply gas. Typically, a relatively inert and insoluble gas such as helium is added in a low concentration of 5% to 10%. Helium in the gas phase rapidly comes into equilibrium with blood phase helium, so that after a short time the net transmembrane helium flux is zero. Again by continuity, the helium flow into the oxygenator equals the flow out of the oxygenator. This can be rearranged so that the outflow can be calculated by:

$$Q_e = (F_{i,He}/F_{e,He}) \cdot Q_i \qquad [6]$$

where Q_i and Q_e are the total gas flow rates in and out, respectively, and $F_{i,He}$ and $F_{e,He}$ represent helium gas fractions in and out, respectively. The rate of oxygen transport can be calculated from conservation of mass by subtracting the amount of oxygen leaving the oxygenator from that entering:

$$V_{O_2} = Q_i \cdot F_iO_2 - Q_e \cdot F_eO_2 \qquad [7]$$

or by substituting Eq. 6 in Eq. 7 and rearranging terms:

$$V_{O_2} = Q_i \cdot [F_iO_2 - (F_{i,He}/F_{e,He}) \cdot F_eO_2] \qquad [8]$$

Thus, oxygen transfer within the oxygenator can be calculated by measuring only one flow and inlet and outlet gas concentrations. Similar equations can be derived for CO_2, which are usually simplified because $F_iCO_2 = O$.

Industrial Standardization of Gas Transfer and Blood Flows

The industrial method for describing oxygenator performance relates to standards outlined by the Association for the Advancement of Medical Instrumentation (AAMI; Arlington, VA), whose most recent oxygenator standard was published in 1997 (23). Bethune (24) reviewed the development of oxygenator standards. Despite widespread reliance on AAMI standards, their clinical validity has been questioned in a well-reasoned article by Fried et al. (25) and an editorial by Ueyama et al. (26). Some of the more pertinent reference conditions follow.

Carbon Dioxide Reference Blood Flow

This is the flow rate of normothermic whole blood having a hemoglobin content of 12 g/100 mL, zero base excess, and oxygen saturation of 65% that has its carbon dioxide content decreased by 38 mL carbon dioxide (standard pressure and temperature) per liter of blood flow by direct passage through the blood oxygenator.

Oxygen Reference Blood Flow

This is the flow rate of normothermic whole blood having a hemoglobin content of 12 g/100 mL, zero base excess, and oxygen saturation of 65% that has its oxygen content increased by 45 mL O_2 (standard pressure and temperature) per liter of blood flow by passage through the blood oxygenator.

REFERENCE BLOOD FLOW

This is the lowest of the following: oxygen reference blood flow, carbon dioxide reference blood flow, the manufacturer's recommended blood flow, or a blood flow of 6 L/min.

Index of Hemolysis

Quantity (in milligrams) of plasma-hemoglobin generated in the *in vitro* cellular damage test per 100 L of blood pumped through the circuit containing the oxygenator less the quantity generated in the circuit without the oxygenator.

Initial Priming Volume

Static volume of blood (in milliliters) to fill the blood phase of the device to the manufacturer's recommended minimal reservoir level. With bubble oxygenators, this is measured

with the reference oxygen flow recommended by the manufacturer for the start of perfusion.

Maximum Operating Volume

Volume of blood contained in the device at the maximum reservoir level recommended by the manufacturer at reference blood flow and reference oxygen flow.

Minimum Operating Volume

Volume contained in the device at the minimum reservoir level recommended by the manufacturer at the reference blood flow and reference oxygen flow.

HEAT TRANSFER DURING CARDIOPULMONARY BYPASS

Heat Exchangers

The design of heat exchangers for cooling and rewarming blood in the oxygenator centers around making a biologically inert surface capable of achieving the desired rate of heat exchange, without producing any localized overheating of the blood. Generally, the energy transfer into and out of the heat exchanger is provided by nonsterile water that is circulated through a heater or cooler unit, which is part of the perfusion apparatus. When cooling is desired, the water is passed through an ice bath, and when warming is desired, it is heated by electric resistance heaters. Use of water as the heat transfer fluid is simple and reliable and provides an even temperature distribution across the surface of the heat exchanger without localized hot spots, which might occur, for example, if the electric heating element were built into the oxygenator itself.

The heat transfer surface is usually made of stainless steel or aluminum. Both materials have good thermal conductivity and are readily coated with polymers to minimize blood interactions. To maximize heat efficiency of heat transfer, designers try to maximize the available surface area for heat exchange, either by making a larger heat exchanger (at the cost of increasing the priming volume) or by using fins extending into the blood. "Finning" also allows a reduced number of water channels (Fig. 4.9), which in turn simplifies construction of the heat exchanger and decreases the potential number of sites at which fluid leaks might occur. Many presently used heat exchangers consist simply of a coiled tubing, wound so that the resulting cylinder acts as the blood conduit. This design has the advantages of simplicity and a low risk of leakage. Heat exchange is also enhanced in most devices by flowing the blood and water in opposite directions (counter-current heat exchange).

Constraints on Rate of Heat Transfer

The temperature difference between the circulating water and the blood drives heat transfer. A thermal boundary layer exists in the blood flowing just beside the wall of the heat exchanger (i.e., the wall separating blood and water), an area where the temperature varies from the wall temperature to the free stream temperature (27). The exact temperature profile in the boundary layer depends on the nature of the velocity boundary layer, but a typical profile would appear similar to the curves shown earlier for gas concentrations during diffusion (Fig. 4.4). Rapid cooling is commonly used at the onset of CPB, when the circulating water is cooled to temperatures approaching 0°C by an ice bath, thus rapidly cooling the blood. Typically, the rate of cooling at the onset of CPB is limited only by this thermal boundary layer and the temperature difference between the water and the blood.

On the other hand, at the conclusion of CPB, the rate of rewarming is limited not by physical constraints but by concerns regarding blood damage due to overheating and bubble formation because of the lower gas solubility of warmer blood. In addition, concerns have emerged about exacerbating cerebral injury by creating hyperthermic central circulatory temperatures while striving to adequately rewarm more peripheral vascular beds (28,29). Blood damage, in the form of protein denaturation, limits the absolute maximum temperature (42°C) that can be safely achieved in the blood (30). In addition, the maximum difference in temperature between the water and the venous blood is limited to prevent bubble formation due to the rapidly decreasing gas solubility. It has been shown *in vitro* and in clinical CPB (31) that gaseous microemboli formation can be avoided by limiting the water and/or blood temperature difference to 10°C. Some manufacturers of membrane oxygenators have taken the additional precaution of placing the warmer upstream from the gas exchanger (where lower oxygen tensions are present). The actual advantage of this approach has not been demonstrated, and this configuration is not used by all manufacturers. Furthermore, it cannot be readily used in bubble oxygenators.

Determination of Rate of Heat Transfer

The amount of heat being transferred is readily quantifiable (32,33) by simple energy balance as defined by the first law of thermodynamics. This relationship requires that the amount of heat transferred to the blood equals the thermal energy in the blood leaving the oxygenator less the thermal energy of the blood entering the heat exchanger. The thermal energy of blood can be determined by multiplication of the specific heat of blood, C (0.90 kcal/kg/°C) (34) by the absolute temperature. Thus, the heat transfer can be calculated by

$$H = C \cdot F \cdot (T_i - T_o) \qquad [9]$$

where C is the specific heat, F is blood flow rate, and T_i

and T_o are the inlet and outlet temperatures, respectively. This provides the instantaneous heat transfer (heat/unit time usually expressed in kcal/min). If this quantity is then integrated either continuously or in a finite manner over discrete time intervals, the total amount of heat transferred into or from the patient can be determined. This may provide an alternative method of assessing the adequacy of rewarming during CPB in the future.

PERFORMANCE COMPARISON OF BUBBLE VERSUS MEMBRANE OXYGENATORS

The advantages of membrane oxygenators over bubble oxygenators have been clearly established in patients undergoing long-term extracorporeal perfusion for pulmonary insufficiency. However, in patients undergoing cardiac operations having short perfusion times, it remains a subject of debate whether the theoretic advantages of membrane oxygenators translate into a measurably improved clinical outcome.

Although the sale of oxygenators for cardiac surgery is a multimillion dollar annual business in the United States, large-scale evaluative studies of the available products are not ordinarily performed by governmental or other independent testing laboratories. Thus, it is usually left to clinicians to conduct the comparative trials of oxygenators in their practices. Because major granting agencies will seldom support evaluations of medical devices, those studies conducted are often done on very limited budgets and thus tend to evaluate only a small number of types of oxygenators with only a few performance variables.

It is important to appreciate that a complete performance assessment of an oxygenator must include numerous measures, including efficiency of gas transfer, efficiency of heat transfer, priming volume, ease of setup and debubbling, blood compatibility, clinical outcomes, and cost. Two other points should be borne in mind when comparing bubble and membrane oxygenators. First, the two types of membrane oxygenators, microporous and true membranes, may differ importantly in their performance, particularly with respect to gas exchange and blood compatibility. Second, any conclusions drawn about the performance characteristics of any particular oxygenator may not apply to other oxygenators of the same type, even when they are similar in design and come from the same manufacturer.

Early Clinical Studies

Before the early 1980s, comparative studies of oxygenators concentrated on clinical outcome assessment and common clinical laboratory measurements to evaluate differences in oxygenator performance. An early prospective randomized study found no major differences in two groups of 10 patients perfused for an average of more than 4 hours with either a bubble or membrane oxygenator (35). Clark et al. (36) performed the first large-scale randomized comparison of blood trauma in bubble versus microporous Teflon oxygenators in two prospectively selected groups of 80 patients each: those having short perfusion times (averaging 109 minutes) and those with long perfusions (averaging 188 minutes). In the short-perfusion group, the authors found no statistically significant differences in the hematologic and immunologic variables measured. However, in the long-perfusion group, the membrane patients had lower plasma hemoglobin and white cell concentrations; much smaller losses of IgG, IgM, and C3; and less bleeding and transfusion. However, the membrane oxygenator patients had a greater loss of C4, a paradoxical result that the authors suggested may have resulted from binding of C4 by the Teflon membrane.

In 1980, Hessel et al. (37) prospectively studied 32 patients, randomized to have either a bubble or microporous membrane oxygenator according to the type of operation planned. With bypass runs averaging about 2 hours, the authors found no significant differences in cardiac outcome (infarction, creatine phosphokinase-MB levels), neurologic and mental function (by time to awakening and standardized examinations), pulmonary function (duration of mechanical ventilation, alveolar-arterial oxygen tension differences), renal function (urine output, blood urea nitrogen), overall outcome (intensive care and hospital stay), and most hematologic parameters (bleeding, blood administration, plasma-free hemoglobin, gross hemoglobinuria). However, the platelet count (expressed as a fraction of the control count) was higher immediately after bypass in the patients undergoing solitary coronary artery surgery. This difference disappeared by 18 hours postoperatively. A subsequent study in dogs found increased platelet lysis with bubble oxygenators compared with the membrane oxygenator (38). However, a human study found less platelet destruction with bubble oxygenators and no difference between oxygenator types in bleeding time, tests of platelet aggregation, or postoperative blood loss (39).

Blood Cell Damage

It is well known that bubble oxygenators tend to hemolyze red blood cells to a greater extent than do membrane oxygenators, probably through the mechanism of high shear stresses induced around the bubbles (40). Studies (41–43) have confirmed the results of numerous earlier ones finding greater increases in plasma-free hemoglobin after perfusion with bubble oxygenators, suggesting that design improvements in the modern bubble oxygenators have not eliminated the hemolysis problem. A related question is whether the red cells surviving a perfusion run have a diminished lifespan. This was studied in dogs by withdrawing an aliquot of blood from each animal, tagging the red cells with a radioactive tracer, and then exposing the specimen to perfu-

sion with a bubble or membrane oxygenator or else to a control period of extracorporeal incubation (44). Red cell survival over the ensuing 30 days was found to be adversely affected by the duration of perfusion but not by the oxygenator type.

The results of early studies examining the effect of oxygenator type on platelets were contradictory. In a dog model using radiolabeled platelets, Peterson et al. (38) convincingly demonstrated a greater decrease in platelet numbers, more platelet destruction, and more deposition of platelets on the artificial surfaces of a bubble oxygenator compared with a membrane oxygenator. On the other hand, Edmunds et al. (39) found no significant differences in platelet counts, *in vitro* platelet function tests, or bleeding times between oxygenators in a clinical comparison. More clinical evaluations have tended to indicate that membrane oxygenators do preserve platelets better than bubble oxygenators, although this effect has not been accompanied by significant differences in postoperative blood loss between oxygenator types (41,45). More recent clinical studies likewise found no difference between bubble and membrane oxygenators (46,47).

White blood cell destruction during and after bypass occurs largely because of activation of the complement system; this is discussed in the next section. The general topic of blood cell activation during bypass has been extensively reviewed by Royston (48).

Complement Activation and the Inflammatory Response

The emphasis on which variables to study when comparing oxygenators appears to have shifted in the early 1980s when a group from the University of Alabama called attention to the problem of complement activation during bypass (49). The authors studied 15 patients perfused with a bubble oxygenator and found significant elevations of C3a levels, beginning within 10 minutes of starting bypass, whereas the plasma levels of C5a did not change significantly. However, after bypass they found statistically significant circulating neutrophilia and transpulmonary neutropenia, which they believed might have resulted from pulmonary sequestration of C5a-activated granulocytes. They also demonstrated that both bubble oxygenation and incubation of blood with the nylon mesh liner of the bubble oxygenators promoted complement activation. Although they did not establish a causal relationship between the actions of the anaphylatoxins and major organ dysfunction after surgery, they suggested that measurements of complement activation might be used to facilitate redesign of clinical oxygenators. All manufacturers have replaced the nylon mesh in their oxygenators with polyester or polypropylene (50).

Subsequently, this group extended their findings in a group of 116 patients undergoing CPB by relating postoperative C3a levels to postoperative cardiac dysfunction, pulmonary dysfunction, renal dysfunction, abnormal bleeding, and overall morbidity (51). They were also among the first to implicate heparin–protamine complexes as causing complement activation and potentially confounding the assessment of complement activation by oxygenators (52). The hypothesis of a "whole body inflammatory reaction of variable magnitude" to CPB evolved from these studies and earlier work. Subsequent studies in monkeys and humans suggest that membrane oxygenators activate complement predominantly by the alternative pathway, whereas bubble oxygenators activate it primarily through the classic pathway (53).

Cavarocchi et al. (54) investigated the possibility that high-dose steroid administration might compensate for the added complement activation apparently caused by bubble oxygenators. The study randomly assigned 91 patients to a silicone membrane oxygenator group or to bubble oxygenator groups, with or without pretreatment with methylprednisolone sodium succinate (30 mg/kg). The C3a activation and leukocyte sequestration in the bubble oxygenator group without methylprednisolone exceeded that in either the membrane oxygenator group or in the bubble oxygenator group with methylprednisolone. However, no clinical differences in postoperative organ function were found among the treatment groups.

In a dog model in which the surgical wound was deliberately sprayed with an aerosol of *Staphylococcus aureus*, infection developed only in the animals perfused with a bubble oxygenator (55). Host defenses were mildly impaired by use of cardiotomy suction with a membrane oxygenator and markedly impaired in the group with bubble oxygenators, whether or not cardiotomy suction was used.

An extensive study using *in vitro* circuits illustrates the complexities involved in attempting to assess the response of the complement system to CPB. In this study, fresh human blood was circulated through six different membrane and bubble oxygenators for 1 hour (56). To eliminate the effect of the gas–blood interface, no oxygen was run into the oxygenators. Complement activation was assessed by measuring levels of both C3a and the terminal complement complex (C5 to C9). The authors found a similar increase in terminal complement activation with all oxygenators. In addition, no significant C3 activation was observed in the hollow fiber membrane and soft-shell bubble oxygenators, whereas similar increases in C3 were induced by the capillary membrane, sheet membrane, nonporous membrane, and hard-shell bubble oxygenators. The authors were unable to explain the differences in C3 activation among the oxygenators, either on the basis of the types of materials used or the amount of surface area exposed to the blood. Neither the perfusion tubing nor the arterial line filter appeared to contribute significantly to complement activation. In a randomized clinical trial (57) subsequently reported by the same group, two bubble oxygenators and a nonporous silicone membrane oxygenator again produced similar eleva-

tions in terminal complement complex, although both bubblers produced greater increases in C3 activation. The authors emphasized the importance of testing for activation products at both the initial and terminal parts of the complement cascade when evaluating oxygenators. Some important issues to be considered in assessing complement activation in the setting of bypass were also discussed by Volanakis (58).

Nilsson et al. (59) studied 96 patients, randomly assigned to two bubble and two microporous membrane oxygenators, and 7 thoracotomy patients who served as control subjects. Complement activation during bypass was measured as changes in the ratio of C3d to C3, to correct for hemodilution. No significant differences were observed among the oxygenators studied. Similarly, tests of the classic and alternative pathway showed markedly decreasing complement levels during bypass, without significant differences between oxygenator groups.

The studies mentioned above (and others reviewed by Nilsson et al. [59]) are often contradictory about the degree of complement activation with bubble versus membrane oxygenators. There is a clear suggestion that the amount of complement activation depends heavily on the materials used in a particular oxygenator and its other design features and the method of testing used. Thus, it does not appear that any general conclusions can be drawn about the superiority of either oxygenator type with respect to complement activation. Furthermore, much remains to be learned about the degree to which complement activation influences patient morbidity after cardiac surgery.

Lung Injury

Possible oxygenator-type influences on postoperative lung function have been assessed in humans directly by gas exchange measurements and indirectly by measurements of pulmonary lung water and the degranulation of white cells, a process implicated in the genesis of the adult respiratory distress syndrome. In one randomized study of 30 patients (60) having perfusions of unspecified duration, extravascular lung water and pulmonary gas exchange were found to be no different between bubble oxygenator and membrane oxygenator patients for 5 hours postperfusion. However, Nilsson et al. (42) found an increased alveolar-to-arterial PO_2 gradient occurring 3 hours after bypass in patients perfused with a bubble oxygenator for more than 2 hours. In this same group of patients, two serum protein markers of white cell degranulation, lactoferrin and myeloperoxidase, were both found to be more elevated with the bubble than with the membrane oxygenators (59). Elevated lactoferrin levels have been associated with the adult respiratory distress syndrome. Because the syndrome occurs so infrequently after routine cardiac surgery today, it would be difficult to determine whether its incidence is related to the type of oxygenator used. More convincing evidence of the benefit of membrane oxygenators comes from a dog study in which bubble oxygenators produced greater pulmonary sequestration of platelets and white cells and more profound pathologic changes in the lung during reperfusion after bypass (61).

Redmond et al. (62) reported that a heparin-coated oxygenator circuit reduced pulmonary injury in pigs when compared with a standard uncoated circuit. Reeve et al. (63) compared a bubble oxygenator with a membrane oxygenator in 500 prospectively randomized patients. Extravascular lung water and atelectasis assessed by x-ray were more prevalent in the bubble oxygenator group. However, there was no difference in the duration of mechanical ventilation, mortality, or in lengths of intensive care unit or hospital stays. They concluded that neither intrapulmonary shunting nor clinical outcome were influenced by the type of oxygenator used. In 1966, Ranucci et al. (64) found that patients on whom a heparin-coated oxygenator circuit was used had better lung function postoperatively, but, like the study of Reeve et al., durations of endotracheal intubation and stay in the intensive care unit did not differ among bubble oxygenators, uncoated hollow fiber membrane oxygenators, and heparin-coated membrane oxygenators. In pediatric patients undergoing CPB, Watanabe et al. (65) reported pulmonary benefits in the immediate postoperative period. Like the earlier reports (63,64), the beneficial effects of a heparin-coated oxygenator were limited to the hours immediately after CPB.

Brain Microembolism and Injury

Although brain injury has been recognized as a complication of CPB since its inception in the middle 1950s, the exact causes, incidence, severity, and duration remain a subject of debate. Anatomic evidence of injury has been produced with a number of imaging modalities. For example, in a heterogeneous series of 64 infants and children, computed tomography demonstrated decreases in brain mass after cardiac surgery in 31% of patients in whom a bubble oxygenator and a 40-μm arterial line filter were used, whereas no such changes were found in patients perfused with either a membrane oxygenator or a bubble oxygenator with a 20-μm arterial filter (66). Although these changes suggest microembolism as the cause of the loss of brain mass, none of the patients with computed tomographic changes had clinical evidence of brain injury, and the tomographic changes disappeared after a follow-up of 6 to 11 months.

A group from the Hammersmith Hospital in London have quantitated microembolization by performing digital subtraction of an intraoperative angiogram (taken 5 minutes before weaning from CPB) and an angiogram recorded preoperatively (67). In comparing coronary bypass patients perfused with a bubble and a microporous flat-sheet membrane oxygenator, marked differences were found in the incidence of retinal embolization (100% with the bubble oxygenator

versus 44% with the membrane oxygenator), the number of ischemic lesions, and the area of retinal ischemia. Arterial filtration (40 μm) was used with both groups of patients, which may explain why most occluded vessels measured 20 μm or less in diameter. Whether the degree of retinal embolization is related to neuropsychological dysfunction after surgery is currently under investigation by this group.

Using transcranial Doppler ultrasound, Padayachee et al. (68) observed irregular signals suggestive of emboli during bypass in patients in whom a bubble oxygenator was used without arterial filtration. The rate of occurrence of these signals was related to the gas flow rate through the bubble oxygenator. On the other hand, no embolic-type signals were observed during perfusion with a membrane oxygenator and arterial line filter. Similar results were obtained independently by Pedersen et al. (69).

From the above reports, it appears clear that much less cerebral microembolization occurs with unfiltered membrane oxygenators than with unfiltered bubble oxygenators. However, it has been much more difficult to prove whether the excess of embolization that occurs with bubble oxygenators actually causes harm to patients.

Clinical Studies

The design of both membrane and bubble oxygenators has improved through continuous evolution over the years. With this in mind, one is led to give greater weight to the more recent oxygenator studies. In one study performed for the Procurement Directorate of the British National Health Service, Pearson (45) randomly assigned seven bubble and nine membrane oxygenator types to 180 patients and assessed their performance in terms of blood gas control, gaseous microemboli, and hematology. Taken as a group, it was easier for the perfusionist to achieve the targeted blood gas values with the membrane oxygenators than with the bubble oxygenators. As expected, gaseous microemboli were also far fewer in number with the membrane oxygenators, but there was a surprising degree of variability in microemboli delivery among the bubble oxygenators. It was suggested that membrane oxygenators were inherently safer than hard-shell bubble oxygenators as far as inadvertently pumping air, although the membrane oxygenators, and not the bubble oxygenators, were thought to be more likely to embolize air left over from improper priming.

With regard to platelet counts, there was generally a smaller decrement from before to after bypass with the membrane oxygenators; indeed, some membrane oxygenators actually produced a rise in the platelet count. There was also a greater rise in β-thromboglobulin, a marker of platelet activation, among patients with bubble oxygenators. However, neither the white blood count, platelet aggregation, nor postoperative blood loss were significantly different between oxygenator types. The variability in performance observed within the groups of oxygenators underscores the importance of evaluating each oxygenator design individually and of not considering the performance of a single oxygenator of each type as representative of the performance of the groups as a whole.

A further report by Nilsson et al. (41) from the study of the four oxygenators, mentioned above (42), confirms Pearson's findings of better preservation of platelet function and less release of β-thromboglobulin with membrane oxygenators. In addition, this study also found less hemolysis and less degranulation of white cells with the bubble oxygenator.

The major new development in oxygenator technology in the last decade has been applying coatings to the blood-contacting surfaces in an effort to enhance their biocompatibility. Heparin has been used most commonly, but alternative polymers are also being investigated as a means to "passivate" the extracorporeal circuit. Most studies on heparin-coated oxygenators have suggested a slight benefit by reduction of blood cellular and protein-mediated reactions. One of the earliest reports (70), however, reported no reduction in complement activation, but those authors suggested that the method used to attach heparin was important to achieving beneficial effects. Hatori et al. (71) studied two small groups of patients (seven per group) and found that systemic inflammatory reactions (i.e., platelet activation, prostaglandin production, complement activation, and activated granulocyte released substances) were reduced in those patients perfused with a Carmeda heparin-coated oxygenator (Medtronic, Inc., Minneapolis, MN). Shigemitsu et al. (72) found reduced C3a and free hemoglobin levels in a heparin-coated circuit when compared with a conventional uncoated circuit. Steinberg et al. (73) found lower levels of the inflammatory cytokines interleukin-6 and interleukin-8 when each of two types of heparin-coated circuits were compared with uncoated circuits. Moen et al. (74) found that both Duraflo II (Baxter, Inc., Irvine, CA) and Carmeda heparin-coated circuits reduced blood activation but that the Carmeda circuits exhibited lower levels of the terminal C5b-9 lytic complement complex and lesser degrees of neutrophil activation. Baksaas et al. (75) reported reduced activation of cellular and humoral inflammatory systems when blood surfaces in the CPB circuit were coated with a either a new polymer or heparin.

A secondary benefit of heparin-coated oxygenators was suggested by Palanzo et al. (76), who found that three models of uncoated hollow fiber oxygenators were more susceptible to the development of high transmembrane pressure drops during bypass. This was confirmed by Wahba et al. (77) in a retrospective study of nearly 2,000 adult cases, in which use of an uncoated circuit was associated with a higher incidence of abnormal pressure gradients across the oxygenator. Several other clinical studies (78–83) have provided additional details of the operational characteristics and acceptability of hollow fiber membrane oxygenators for routine clinical use.

In summary, a growing body of evidence favors membrane oxygenators in terms of their ability to minimize embolization and the abnormalities in laboratory indices of blood function and immune response associated with CPB. However, clear evidence has not been found for the clinical superiority of the membrane oxygenator for operations having short perfusion times. Nevertheless, because improved manufacturing techniques have reduced the cost difference between oxygenator types, there has been widespread movement toward routine use of membrane oxygenators in all cardiac surgery requiring CPB.

OXYGENATOR-RELATED CARDIOPULMONARY BYPASS ACCIDENTS

In a retrospective study of CPB accidents in approximately 573,000 patients, Kurusz et al. (84) reported that oxygenator failure was the third leading cause, following protamine reactions and hypoperfusion. Oxygenator failure occurred in 506 cases (an incidence of 1 in 13,362 cases) and caused life-threatening hypoxia in 156 patients and permanent damage or death in 42 patients. These accidents occurred with almost equal frequency with membrane and bubble oxygenators. In the 1970s, a time of predominant bubble oxygenator use, Stoney et al. (85) reported a survey of 374,000 CPB cases. Of 1,419 accidents reported, 24% involved the oxygenator, with specific problems including leakage (16%), clotting (4%), pressurization (1%), bursting (1%), contamination (1%), and chemical injury (1%).

An iatrogenic cause of oxygenator failure involves isoflurane that is spilled onto either bubble (86) or membrane (87) oxygenators while filling a vaporizer, resulting in cracks in the polycarbonate shell or venous connector. Simply avoiding the physical placement of the vaporizer over the oxygenator eliminates this risk.

SUMMARY

This chapter has delved into the principles that control the exchange of carbon dioxide and oxygen in membrane and bubble oxygenators. These principles form the basis upon which design modifications have been predicated and comparisons have been made between membrane and bubble oxygenators. Descriptions, photographs, and operating characteristics of specific oxygenators are not included because these are readily available from the manufacturers.

Although membrane oxygenators are the only type suitable for long-term perfusion, it has been difficult to demonstrate any clear-cut superiority of membrane oxygenators for a typical 2-hour perfusion time for cardiac surgery. Nevertheless, membrane oxygenators are used almost universally in North America and western Europe. In most studies, membrane oxygenators appear to lessen derangements in several hematologic variables, notably red cell damage and granulocyte and platelet activation. Similarly, most studies show less complement activation with membrane oxygenators, although the picture is clouded by different indices of complement activation measured among the various studies and by numerous other potentially confounding factors. Furthermore, although a number of deleterious effects have been associated with complement activation in humans, direct proof of its influence on morbidity in the cardiac surgery patient is lacking. In particular, the incidence of infection or lung or renal injury does not appear to be associated with the type of oxygenator used. Likewise, membrane oxygenator use reduces embolization to the cerebral circulation and brain mass reduction (by computed tomography) in children, but both of these findings were eliminated by adding an arterial filter to a the bubble oxygenator circuit.

There appears to be general agreement that benefits may be realized from using membrane oxygenators in long perfusions in adults and possibly in all perfusions in infants and small children. In adults having short perfusion times, it remains unproven whether it is worthwhile to minimize subclinical abnormalities by substituting a membrane oxygenator for a bubble oxygenator. However, because technologic advances have reduced the cost difference between membrane and bubble oxygenators, routine use of membrane oxygenators for all CPB has become the norm in most developed nations.

KEY POINTS

- The ideal extracorporeal oxygenator transfers oxygen into and carbon dioxide out of the body at physiologic blood flow rates with minimal blood trauma and a small priming volume.
- Compared with natural lungs, artificial lungs have much smaller surface areas and are limited by diffusion. Despite improved oxygenator designs that offset these differences somewhat, the maximum oxygen transfer of even the most efficient artificial lungs is less than half that of normal lungs.
- Gas transfer across an oxygenator is proportional to partial pressure difference and surface area and inversely proportional to diffusion distance.
- At the interface between gas and blood with laminar flow characteristics the velocity of blood flow incrementally increases from zero at the interface to free stream velocity at some distance from the interface. This velocity transition zone is termed the boundary layer, and gas diffusion is inversely proportional to its thickness. The thickness of this boundary layer, and thus the efficiency of the oxygenator, can be improved by creating secondary "eddy current" flows at this interface.
- Bubble oxygenators place bubbles in direct contact with the blood, with essential features that include an

optimal mix of bubble sizes, because smaller bubbles better exchange O_2 and larger ones better exchange CO_2; (2) low resistance to flow and low pressure drop across the oxygenator (compared with membrane oxygenators), such that gravity and bubble flow can "drive" gas exchange; (3) the need for a settling chamber with an antifoaming material for defoaming the blood before reinfusion; (4) O_2 and CO_2 exchange that is more interdependent than in membrane or natural lungs, with increases in gas flow simultaneously increasing P_aO_2 while decreasing P_aCO_2; and (5) maintaining an adequate reservoir volume is critical to the adequacy of both gas exchange and debubbling of the blood.
- Most membrane oxygenators actually use microporous membranes, although one device uses a true membrane. True membranes offer advantages in longer perfusions (days to weeks), because microporous membrane lungs eventually develop leaks that produce "oxygenator pulmonary edema."
- Important aspects of microporous membrane lungs include (1) absence of a direct blood–gas interface once the membrane develops a proteinaceous coating; (2) relatively high resistance to flow, such that blood must be actively pumped across the lung; and (3) independent regulation of P_aCO_2 and P_aO_2 by varying gas flow (P_aCO_2) and FiO_2 (P_aO_2).
- Standards have been developed for assessing oxygenator CO_2 and O_2 transport capacities, hemolysis indexes, priming volumes, and maximum and minimum operating volumes. Reference blood flow is defined as the lowest of the oxygen reference blood flow, carbon dioxide reference blood flow, manufacturer's reference blood flow, or a blood flow of 6 L/min.
- Heat exchangers are integrated into commercial oxygenators to permit extracorporeal cooling and warming of the bloodstream by varying the water temperature flowing into the heat exchanger. The exchange surfaces typically are made of stainless steel or aluminum and have "fins" to maximize the efficiency. Boundary layer considerations (see above) apply to this process.
- To prevent formation of gaseous microemboli, the temperature gradient between water and blood should not exceed 10°C.
- Membrane oxygenators now dominate the marketplace in the United States. Comparative studies indicate that membrane oxygenators induce less hemolysis, thrombocytopenia, and platelet activation. When perfusion times are short (less than 2 hours), clear evidence has not been found for the superiority of membrane oxygenators over bubble oxygenators. However, because technologic advances have reduced the cost differential to virtual equivalence, most centers now choose membrane oxygenators.

REFERENCES

1. Silvay G, Ammar T, Reich DL, et al. Cardiopulmonary bypass for adult patients: a survey of equipment and techniques. *J Cardiothorac Vasc Anesth* 1995;9:420–424.
2. Gaylor JDS, Hickey S, Bell G, et al. Membrane oxygenators: influence of design on performance. *Perfusion* 1994;9:173–180.
3. Voorhees ME, Brian BF III. Blood-gas exchange devices. *Int Anesthesiol Clin* 1996;34:29–45.
4. Weger JA. Oxygenator anatomy and function. *J Cardiothorac Vasc Anesth* 1997;11:275–281.
5. Marx TI, Snyder WE, St. John AD, et al. Diffusion of oxygen into a film of whole blood. *J Appl Physiol* 1960;15:1123–1129.
6. Zapol WM, Qvist J. *Artificial lungs for acute respiratory failure.* New York: Academic Press, 1976.
7. Bird RB, Stewart WE, Lightfoor EN. *Transport phenomena.* New York: John Wiley & Sons, 1960.
8. Marx TI, Baldwin BR, Miller DR. Factors influencing oxygen uptake by blood in membrane oxygenators: report of a study. *Ann Surg* 1962;156:204–213.
9. Gaylor JDS. Membrane oxygenators: current developments in design and application. *J Biomed Eng* 1988;10:541–547.
10. Bartlett RH, Kittredge D, Noyes BS Jr, et al. Development of a membrane oxygenator: overcoming blood diffusion limitation. *J Thorac Cardiovasc Surg* 1969;58:795–800.
11. Drinker PA, Bartlett RH, Bialer RM, et al. Augmentation of membrane gas transfer by induced secondary flows. *Surgery* 1969;66:775–781.
12. Dorrington KL, Gardaz J-P, Bellhouse BJ, et al. Extracorporeal oxygen and CO_2 transfer of a polypropylene dimpled membrane lung with variable secondary flows: partial bypass in the dog. *J Biomed Eng* 1986;8:36–42.
13. Smith WT. Cerebral lesions due to emboli of silicone antifoam in dogs subjected to cardiopulmonary bypass. *J Pathol Bacteriol* 1960;80:9–18.
14. Galletti PM, Brecher GH. *Heart-lung bypass: principles and techniques of extracorporeal circulation.* New York: Grune & Stratton, 1962.
15. Groom RC, Kramer M, Reed CC. Use of a sweep gas in bubble oxygenators to obtain independent control of blood carbon dioxide levels. *Proc Am Acad Cardiovasc Perfus* 1982;3:69–72.
16. Murphy W, Trudell LA, Friedman LI, et al. Laboratory and clinical experience with a microporous membrane oxygenator. *Trans Am Soc Artif Intern Organs* 1974;20A:278–285.
17. Mottaghy K, Oedekoven H, Starmans H, et al. Technical aspects of plasma leakage prevention in microporous membrane oxygenators. *Trans Am Soc Artif Intern Organs* 1989;35:640–643.
18. Gile JP, Trudell L, Snider MT, et al. Capability of the microporous membrane-lined, capillary oxygenator in hypercapnic dogs. *Trans Am Soc Artif Intern Organs* 1970;16:365–374.
19. Bodell BR, Head JM, Head LR, et al. A capillary membrane oxygenator. *J Thorac Cardiovasc Surg* 1963;46:639–649.
20. Bierenbaum HS, Isaacson RB, Druin ML, et al. Microporous polymeric films. *Ind Eng Chem Prod Res Dev* 1974;13:2–9.
21. Dutton RC, Edmunds LH Jr. Formation of platelet aggregate emboli in a prototype hollow-fiber membrane oxygenator. *J Biomed Mater Res* 1974;8:163.
22. Quinn RD, Pae WE, McGary SA, et al. Development of malignant hyperthermia during mitral valve replacement. *Ann Thorac Surg* 1992;53:1114–1116.
23. Anonymous. Cardiovascular implants and artificial organs—blood gas exchangers. American National Standard/International Organization for Standards, ISO/TC
24. Bethune DW. Standards for blood gas exchange devices. *Perfusion* 1994;9:207–209.
25. Fried DW, DeBenedetto BN, Leo JJ. Rethinking the AAMI/ISO "International standard" for oxygen transfer performance of artificial lungs. *Perfusion* 1994;9:335–342.
26. Ueyama K, Niimi Y, Nosé Y. How to test oxygenators for extracorporeal membrane oxygenation: is the Association for the Advancement of Medical Instrumentation's protocol enough? *Artif Organs* 1996;20:741–742.
27. Holman JP. *Heat transfer.* New York: McGraw-Hill, 1972.
28. Nathan HJ, Lavallee G. The management of temperature during hypothermic cardiopulmonary bypass. I. Canadian survey [comments]. *Can J Anaesth* 1995;42:663–668.
29. Cook DJ, Orszulak TA, Daly RC, et al. Cerebral hyperthermia during cardiopulmonary bypass. *J Thorac Cardiovasc Surg* 1996;111:268–269.
30. Reed CC, Stafford TB. *Cardiopulmonary bypass 2nd edition.* Houston: Medical Press, 1985:327.
31. Clark RE, Dietz DR, Miller JG. Continuous detection of microemboli during cardiopulmonary bypass in animals and man. *Circulation* 1975;54:74–78.
32. Jenkins I, Karliczek G, de Geus F, et al. Postbypass hypothermia and its relationship to the energy balance of cardiopulmonary bypass. *J Cardiothorac Vasc Anesth* 1991;5:135–138.
33. Davis FM, Parumelazhagan KN, Harris EA. Thermal balance during cardiopulmonary bypass with moderate hypothermia in man. *Br J Anaesth* 1977;49:1127–1132.
34. Mendelowitz M. The specific heat of human blood. *Science* 1948;107:97–98.
35. Chopra PS, Dufek JH, Kroncke GM, et al. Clinical comparison of the General Electric-Peirce membrane lung and bubble oxygenator for prolonged cardiopulmonary bypass. *Surgery* 1973;74:874–879.
36. Clark RE, Beauchamp RA, Magrath RA, et al. Comparison of bubble and membrane oxygenators in short and long term perfusions. *J Thorac Cardiovasc Surg* 1979;78:655–666.
37. Hessel EA II, Johnson DD, Ivey TD, et al. Membrane versus bubble oxygenator for cardiac operations. *J Thorac Cardiovasc Surg* 1980;80:111–122.
38. Peterson KA, Dewanjee MK, Kaye MP. Fate of indium 111-labeled platelets during cardiopulmonary bypass performed with membrane and bubble oxygenators. *J Thorac Cardiovasc Surg* 1982;84:39–43.
39. Edmunds LH Jr, Ellison N, Colman RW, et al. Platelet function during cardiac operation: comparison of membrane and bubble oxygenators. *J Thorac Cardiovasc Surg* 1982;83:805–812.
40. Hirayama T, Yamaguchi H, Allers M, et al. Evaluation of red cell damage during cardiopulmonary bypass. *Scand J Thorac Cardiovasc Surg* 1985;19:263–265.
41. Nilsson L, Bagge L, Nystroem SO. Blood cell trauma and postoperative bleeding: comparison of bubble and membrane oxygenators and observations on coronary suction. *Scand J Thorac Cardiovasc Surg* 1990;24:65–69.
42. Nilsson L, Tyden H, Johansson O, et al. Bubble and membrane oxygenators comparison of postoperative organ dysfunction with special reference to inflammatory activity. *Scand J Thorac Cardiovasc Surg* 1990;24:59–64.
43. Benedetti M, De Caterina R, Bionda A, et al. Blood artificial surface interactions during cardiopulmonary bypass. A comparative study of four oxygenators. *Int J Artif Organs* 1990;13:488–497.
44. Tabak C, Eugene J, Stemmer EA. Erythrocyte survival following

150/SC 2. Arlington, VA: Association for the Advancement of Medical Instrumentation, 1997.

extracorporeal circulation. A question of membrane versus bubble oxygenator. *J Thorac Cardiovasc Surg* 1981;81:30–33.

45. Pearson DT. Gas exchange: bubble and membrane oxygenators. *Semin Thorac Cardiovasc Surg* 1990;2:213–319.

46. Turri F, Della Volpe A, Leirner AA. Clinical comparison of blood oxygenators: a retrospective study. *Artif Organs* 1995;19: 263–266.

47. Martin W, McQuiston AM, Tweddel AC, et al. Quantification of extracorporeal white cell and platelet deposition in cardiopulmonary bypass; comparison of membrane and bubble oxygenators. *Nucl Med Commun* 1996;17:378–384.

48. Royston D. Blood cell activation. *Semin Thorac Cardiovasc Surg* 1990;3:341–357.

49. Chenoweth DE, Cooper SW, Hugli TE, et al. Complement activation during cardiopulmonary bypass: evidence for generation of C3a and C5a anaphylatoxins. *N Engl J Med* 1981;304:497–503.

50. Kirklin JK. Prospects for understanding and eliminating the deleterious effects of cardiopulmonary bypass [editorial]. *Ann Thorac Surg* 1991;51:529–531.

51. Kirklin JK, Westaby S, Blackstone EH, et al. Complement and the damaging effects of cardiopulmonary bypass. *J Thorac Cardiovasc Surg* 1983;86:845–857.

52. Kirklin JK, Chenoweth DE, Naftel DC, et al. Effects of protamine administration after cardiopulmonary bypass on complement, blood elements, and the hemodynamic state. *Ann Thorac Surg* 1986;41:193–199.

53. Tamiya T, Yamasaki M, Maeo Y, et al. Complement activation in cardiopulmonary bypass, with special reference to anaphylatoxin production in membrane and bubble oxygenators. *Ann Thorac Surg* 1988;46:47–57.

54. Cavarocchi NC, Pluth JR, Schaff HV, et al. Complement activation during cardiopulmonary bypass. Comparison of bubble and membrane oxygenators. *J Thorac Cardiovasc Surg* 1986;91: 252–258.

55. van Oeveren W, Dankert J, Wildevuur CR. Bubble oxygenation and cardiotomy suction impair the host defense during cardiopulmonary bypass: a study in dogs. *Ann Thorac Surg* 1987;44: 523–528.

56. Videm V, Fosse E, Mollnes TE, et al. Different oxygenators for cardiopulmonary bypass lead to varying degrees of human complement activation in vitro. *J Thorac Cardiovasc Surg* 1989; 97:764–770.

57. Videm V, Fosse E, Mollnes TE, et al. Complement activation with bubble and membrane oxygenators in aortocoronary bypass grafting. *Ann Thorac Surg* 1990;50:387–391.

58. Volanakis JE. Complement activation caused by different oxygenators [invited letter]. *J Thorac Cardiovasc Surg* 1989;98: 292–295.

59. Nilsson L, Nilsson U, Venge P, et al. Inflammatory system activation during cardiopulmonary bypass as an indicator of biocompatibility: a randomized comparison of bubble and membrane oxygenators. *Scand J Thorac Cardiovasc Surg* 1990;24:53–58.

60. Boldt J, von Bormann B, Kling D, et al. New membrane oxygenator (LPM 50): influence on extravascular lung water and pulmonary function in comparison to bubble oxygenator. *J Thorac Cardiovasc Surg* 1986;92:798–800.

61. Gu YJ, Wang YS, Chiang BY, et al. Membrane oxygenator prevents lung reperfusion injury in canine cardiopulmonary bypass. *Ann Thorac Surg* 1991;51:573–578.

62. Redmond JM, Gillinov AM, Stuart RS, et al. Heparin-coated bypass circuits reduce pulmonary injury. *Ann Thorac Surg* 1993; 56:474–478.

63. Reeve WG, Ingram SM, Smith DC. Respiratory function after

cardiopulmonary bypass; a comparison of bubble and membrane oxygenators. *J Cardiothorac Vasc Anesth* 1994;8:502–508.

64. Ranucci M, Cirri S, Conti D, et al. Beneficial effects of Duraflo II heparin-coated circuits on postperfusion lung dysfunction. *Ann Thorac Surg* 1996;61:76–81.

65. Watanabe H, Miyamura H, Hayashi J, et al. The influence of a heparin-coated oxygenator during cardiopulmonary bypass on postoperative lung oxygenation capacity in pediatric patients with congenital heart anomalies. *J Cardiol Surg* 1996;11:396–401.

66. Muraoka R, Yokota M, Aoshima M, et al. Subclinical changes in brain morphology following cardiac operations as reflected by computed tomographic scans of the brain. *J Thorac Cardiovasc Surg* 1981;81:364–369.

67. Blauth C, Smith P, Newman S, et al. Retinal microembolism and neuropsychological deficit following clinical cardiopulmonary bypass: comparison of a membrane and a bubble oxygenator. A preliminary communication. *Eur J Cardiothorac Surg* 1989;3: 135–138.

68. Padayachee TS, Parsons S, Theobold R, et al. The detection of microemboli in the middle cerebral artery during cardiopulmonary bypass: a transcranial Doppler ultrasound investigation using membrane and bubble oxygenator. *Ann Thorac Surg* 1987; 44:298–302.

69. Pedersen TH, Karlsen HM, Semb G, et al. Comparison of bubble release from various types of oxygenators. An in vivo investigation. *Scand J Thorac Cardiovasc Surg* 1987;21:73–80.

70. Svennevig JL, Geiran OR, Karlsen H, et al. Complement activation during extracorporeal circulation. In vitro comparison of Duraflo II heparin-coated and uncoated oxygenator circuits. *J Thorac Cardiovasc Surg* 1993;106:466–472.

71. Hatori N, Yoshizu H, Haga Y, et al. Biocompatibility of heparin-coated membrane oxygenator during cardiopulmonary bypass. *Artif Organs* 1994;18:904–910.

72. Shigemitsu O, Hadama T, Takasaki H, et al. Biocompatibility of a heparin-bonded membrane oxygenator (Carmeda MAXIMA) during the first 90 minutes of cardiopulmonary bypass: clinical comparison with the conventional system. *Artif Organs* 1994;18: 936–941.

73. Steinberg BM, Grossi EA, Schwartz DS, et al. Heparin bonding of bypass circuits reduces cytokine release during cardiopulmonary bypass. *Ann Thorac Surg* 1995;60:525–529.

74. Moen O, Fosse E, Brockmeier V, et al. Disparity in blood activation by two different heparin-coated cardiopulmonary bypass systems. *Ann Thorac Surg* 1995;60:1317–1323.

75. Baksaas ST, Videm V, Fosse E, et al. In vitro evaluation of new surface coatings for extracorporeal circulation. *Perfusion* 1999; 14:11–19.

76. Palanzo DA, Manley NJ, Montesano RM, et al. Potential problem when using the new lower-prime hollow-fiber membrane oxygenators with uncoated stainless steel heat exchangers. *Perfusion* 1996;11:481–485.

77. Wahba A, Philipp A, Behr R, et al. Heparin-coated equipment reduces the risk of oxygenator failure. *Ann Thorac Surg* 1998;65: 1310–1312.

78. de Somer F, De Smet D, Vanackere M, et al. Clinical evaluation of a new hollow fibre membrane oxygenator. *Perfusion* 1994;9: 57–64.

79. Stinkens D, Himpe D, Thyssen P, et al. Clinical evaluation of the oxygenation capacity and controllability of 15 commercially available membrane oxygenators during alpha-stat regulated hypothermic cardiopulmonary bypass. *Perfusion* 1996;11:471–480.

80. Fried DW. Performance evaluation of blood-gas exchange devices. *Int Anesth Clin* 1996;34:47–60.

81. Visser C, de Jong DS. Clinical evaluation of six hollow-fibre membrane oxygenators. *Perfusion* 1997;12:357–368.

82. De Vroege R, Rutten PM, Kalkman C, et al. Biocompatibility of three membrane oxygenators: effects on complement, neutrophil and monocyte activation. *Perfusion* 1997;12:369–375.

83. Stammers AH, Fristoe LW, Alonso A, et al. Clinical evaluation of a new generation membrane oxygenator: a prospective randomized study. *Perfusion* 1998;13:165–175.

84. Kurusz M, Conti VR, Arens JF, et al. Perfusion accident survey. *Proc Am Acad Cardiovasc Perfus* 1986;7:57–65.

85. Stoney WS, Alford WC, Burrus GR, et al. Air embolism and other accidents using pump oxygenators. *Ann Thorac Surg* 1980; 29:336–340.

86. Walls JT, Curtis JJ, McClatchey BJ, et al. Adverse effects of anesthetic agents on polycarbonate plastic oxygenators [Letter]. *J Thorac Cardiovasc Surg* 1988;96:667–672.

87. Cooper S, Levin R. Near catastrophic oxygenator failure [Letter]. *Anesthesiology* 1987;66:101–102.

CIRCUITRY AND CANNULATION TECHNIQUES

EUGENE A. HESSEL II
AARON G. HILL

GENERAL SURVEY OF THE CIRCUIT

The primary function of cardiopulmonary bypass (CPB) is to divert blood away from the heart (both the right and left side and usually the lungs as well) and return it to the systemic arterial system, thus allowing cardiac surgery. Therefore, it must replace the function of both the lung (gas exchange) and heart (provide energy to ensure circulation of blood). Typically, blood is drained by gravity via cannulas in the superior and inferior vena cavae (SVC, IVC) or IVC and right atrium (RA) (cavoatrial position) to the heart–lung machine where it is pumped (with a roller or centrifugal pump) through the artificial lung (most often a membrane-type "oxygenator") back into the systemic vasculature via an arterial cannula placed in the ascending aorta. In the past, when bubble oxygenators were used, the pump was placed after the oxygenator, drawing arterialized blood from a reservoir.

Because of the need to offset the cooling during the extracorporeal passage of blood and the frequent desire to intentionally cool and then rewarm the patient, a heat exchanger is included as part of the oxygenator, either before or contiguous with the gas exchange unit.

Peripheral cannulation, using the femoral or other veins and arteries, is occasionally used electively for cardiac surgery when central cannulation is not technically possible, for initiating bypass before opening the chest, for emergent situations, for aortic surgery, and for extracorporeal membrane oxygenation. Left heart bypass or proximal aorta bypass (with "venous cannulation" of the left atrium, left ventricle, or proximal aorta) and distal infusion into the distal aorta or femoral artery, incorporating only an extracorporeal pump (commonly a centrifugal pump with minimal anticoagulation), is sometimes used for aortic surgery.

Besides the major venous and arterial connections and the oxygenator, heat exchanger, and pump, there are many other components to the heart–lung machine (Fig. 5.1). An adjustable clamp or remote venous line occluder regulates the main venous drainage line and a separate tubing clamp is used on the systemic flow line whenever the patient is not on CPB to prevent backflow out of the arterial cannula, particularly when a centrifugal pump is used. The venous reservoir serves as a buffer for fluctuations in venous drainage and is a source of fluid for rapid transfusion. It usually is placed before a membrane oxygenator (before the pump but often physically attached to the membrane oxygenator housing). When a bubble oxygenator is used, it is usually incorporated as part of the oxygenator and before the pump. Various fluids, such as blood and crystalloid solutions, and drugs may be added to this reservoir. Several suction devices and systems, usually using one or more of the roller pumps, may aspirate blood and gas from the open heart chambers (hence the term "cardiotomy suction"), surgical field, aortic root (during aortic cross-clamping as a left ventricular vent and after unclamping as an air vent), and left ventricular vent. This blood is then passed into the cardiotomy reservoir, which may be incorporated in the housing of an open (hard-shell) venous reservoir or may first flow into an external cardiotomy reservoir before emptying into a separate venous reservoir or bubble oxygenator.

A cardioplegia delivery and/or coronary perfusion system is another component that typically uses one of the roller pumps for administering blood or cardioplegic solution into the coronary arteries, aortic root, or coronary sinus. This circuit usually includes a separate heat exchanger and may include a reservoir and sometimes a recirculation line from the surgical field, which is used when cardioplegic solution is not being administered into the heart, although a single-pass delivery system is more commonly used. Often, arterial blood is simultaneously mixed with crystalloid-based cardioplegic solution (usually in a 4:1 blood-to-fluid ratio) to produce blood cardioplegia (see Chap. 13).

A source of oxygen, air, and sometimes carbon dioxide,

E. A. Hessel: Department of Anesthesiology, University of Kentucky School of Medicine, Chandler Medical Center, Lexington, KY 40536.
A. G. Hill: Inova Fairfax Hospital, Falls Church, VA 22042.

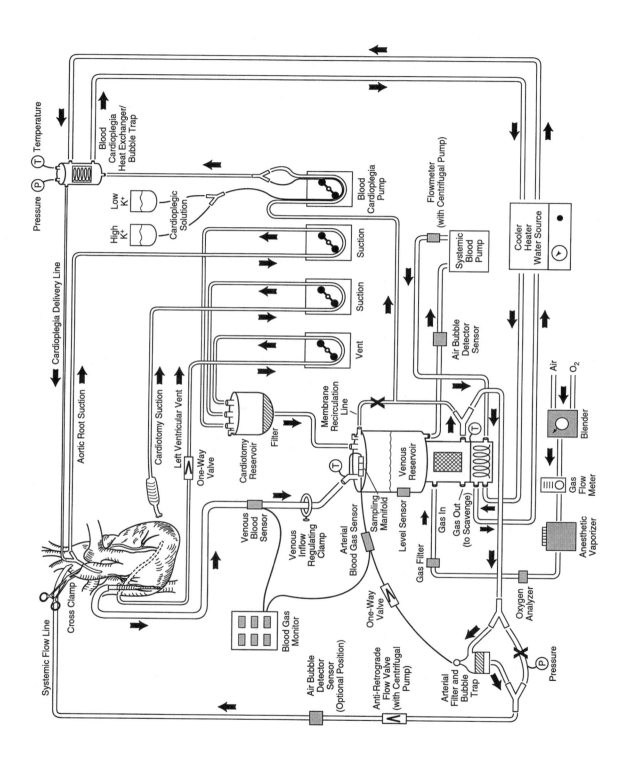

with appropriate flow meters and blenders, supplies ventilating gas to the oxygenator, usually through an in-line anesthetic vaporizer. Although at times hot and cold water is supplied from wall outlets to a mixing valve for adjusting water temperature in the heat exchangers, most commonly a dedicated stand-alone water cooler and heater is used for this purpose. A number of filters (macro or micro) are often included at various sites in the CPB circuit (e.g., cardiotomy reservoir, venous reservoir, oxygenator, and arterial line). Also included are sampling ports (pre- and postoxygenator), pressure monitoring sites such as the cardioplegia-coronary perfusion delivery line and the arterial line (after the systemic pump but before the arterial filter), and arterial and venous in-line blood-gas monitors. Temperature monitoring sites, such as water inflow and outflow for major heat exchanger, venous and arterial blood, cardioplegic solution, and water bath, are also present.

Whenever a centrifugal pump is used, a flowmeter must be included in the systemic outflow line. Various safety devices and monitors, besides those already mentioned, are frequently incorporated into the CPB circuit, including: a bubble trap on the arterial line, often incorporating a microfilter and purge line that includes a one-way valve that drains back to the venous or cardiotomy reservoir; a bypass line that goes around the arterial filter in case the latter becomes obstructed; an air bubble detector on the systemic flow line; and a low-level alarm on the venous or arterial reservoir. A hemoconcentrator is sometimes attached between the systemic flow line, or some other source of blood under pressure, and the venous or cardiotomy reservoir.

VENOUS CANNULATION AND DRAINAGE

Principles of Venous Drainage

Venous drainage is usually accomplished by gravity siphonage. However, recently there has been a renewed interest in applying suction to the venous lines, a technique that had been discarded early in the history of CPB. Siphonage places two constraints on successful venous drainage. First, the venous reservoir must be below the level of the patient and, second, the lines must be full of blood (or fluid) or else an air lock will occur and disrupt the siphon effect. The amount of venous drainage is determined by the pressure in the central veins (patient's blood volume), the difference in height of the patient and the top of the blood level in the venous reservoir or entrance of venous line into a bubble oxygenator (negative pressure exerted by gravity equals this height differential in centimeters of water), and the resistance in the venous cannulas, venous line and connectors, and venous clamp, if one is in use.

The central venous pressure is influenced by intravascular volume and venous compliance, which is influenced by medications, sympathetic tone, and anesthesia. Excessive drainage (i.e., drainage faster than blood is returning to the central veins, which may be caused by an excessive negative pressure caused by gravity) may cause the compliant vein walls to collapse around the ends of the venous cannulas (manifested by line "chattering" or "fluttering") and intermittent reduction of venous drainage. This may be ameliorated by partially occluding the clamp on the venous line, which may paradoxically increase venous drainage, or by increasing the systemic blood flow. Obviously, the ultimate limit to venous flow is the amount of blood returning to the great veins from the body.

Types and Sizes of Cannulas

Venous cannulas are either single or two stage (cavoatrial) (Fig. 5.2). The latter have a wider portion with holes in the section designed to sit in the RA and a narrower tip designed to rest in the IVC. Cannulas are usually made of a flexible plastic; most are wire reinforced to prevent kinking. They may be straight or right angled. Some of the latter are constructed of hard plastic or metal for optimal inner diameter (ID) to outer diameter (OD) ratio. The venous cannulas

FIG. 5.1. Detailed schematic diagram of arrangement of a typical cardiopulmonary bypass circuit using a membrane oxygenator with integral hard-shell venous reservoir (**lower center**) and external cardiotomy reservoir. Venous cannulation is by a cavoatrial cannula and arterial cannulation is in the ascending aorta. Some circuits do not incorporate a membrane recirculation line; in these cases the cardioplegia blood source is a separate outlet connector built-in to the oxygenator near the arterial outlet. The systemic blood pump may be either a roller or centrifugal type. The cardioplegia delivery system (**right**) is a one-pass combination blood/crystalloid type. The cooler–heater water source may be operated to supply water to both the oxygenator heat exchanger and cardioplegia delivery system. The air bubble detector sensor may be placed on the line between the venous reservoir and systemic pump, between the pump and membrane oxygenator inlet or between the oxygenator outlet and arterial filter (neither shown) or on the line after the arterial filter (optional position on drawing). One-way valves prevent retrograde flow (some circuits with a centrifugal pump also incorporate a one-way valve after the pump and within the systemic flow line). Other safety devices include an oxygen analyzer placed between the anesthetic vaporizer (if used) and the oxygenator gas inlet and a reservoir level sensor attached to the housing of the hard-shell venous reservoir (on the left). *Arrows,* directions of flow; *X,* placement of tubing clamps; *P* and *T,* pressure and temperature sensors, respectively. Hemoconcentrator (described in text) not shown.

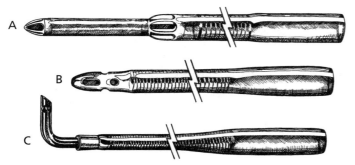

FIG. 5.2. Drawings of conventional venous cannulae. **A:** Standard, tapered, two-stage cavoatrial cannula for insertion into the right atrium (RA) and inferior vena cava (IVC). **B:** Wire-reinforced cannula for atrial or caval cannulation. **C:** Cannula with right-angled tip (usually made of metal or hard plastic because the thin wall optimizes the ratio of internal to external diameters). This type of cannula is often used for congenital or pediatric cases and may be inserted directly into the vena cava near its junction with the RA.

are typically the narrowest component of the CPB venous system and thus are a limiting factor for venous drainage. Knowing the flow characteristics of the particular catheter, which should be provided by the manufacturer or established by benchtop testing, and the required flow (about one third of total flow from SVC and two thirds of total flow from IVC), one can select the appropriate venous cannula for a patient. For example, a 1.8-m^2 patient (total estimated flow, 5.4 L/min; SVC, 1.8 L/min; IVC, 3.6 L/min) at a siphon (gravity) gradient of 40 cm would require at least a 30 French (F) SVC, a 34F IVC, or a single 38F single-stage catheter (1,2). These requirements are easily met by various 36F to 51F cavoatrial cannulas (3). Delius et al. (4) offered a new method for describing the performance of cannulas used in extracorporeal circulation called the M number. They reported the M numbers of several currently available cannulas and provided a nomogram for determining the M number and for predicting the pressure gradient across any cannula at any flow based on this number.

Although venous (and arterial) cannulas are considered disposable and are not intended for reuse, current cost-containment pressures have led to reconsideration of this practice (5).

Connection to the Patient

Usually, the venous connection for CPB is accomplished by inserting cannulas into the RA. Three basic approaches are used (Table 5.1 and Fig. 5.3): bicaval, in which separate cannulas are inserted into SVC and IVC; single atrial; and cavoatrial (i.e., the two-stage approach). The latter has a wider proximal section with holes that lie within the RA and a narrower extension with end and side holes that ex-

tends into the IVC. When bicaval cannulas are used, tapes are frequently placed around the cavae and passed through small tubes so they may be cinched down as tourniquets or snares around the cannula. This forces all the patient's venous return to pass to the extracorporeal circuit, preventing any systemic venous blood from getting into the right heart and any air (if the right heart is opened) from getting into the venous lines. This is referred to as caval occlusion, or total CPB.

Other ways of accomplishing this include the use of elastic tapes placed around the cavae and held together with vascular clips (6) and the use of specially designed external clamps that go around the cavae and their contained cannulas (7). Cuffed venous cannulas may be used, either specially designed for this purpose (e.g., model 191037, Medtronic DLP, Inc., Grand Rapids, MI) (8), or cuffed endotracheal tubes (9,10). The latter may be helpful in emergency cases and when dissection around the vena cava to place tapes could be particularly difficult or dangerous. When there is a hole in the atrium and it is not possible (or there is not enough time) to insert a purse-string suture or the suture breaks, a cuffed endotracheal tube may also be used for venous drainage (11). After insertion, the cuff is inflated and gentle traction tamponades the hole in the atrium so adequate venous drainage may be provided.

Arom et al. (12) and Bennett et al. (13) compared the efficiency of the various approaches for venous drainage (Table 5.1). Bicaval cannulation with caval occlusion is required any time the right heart is entered. This approach may provide the best caval decompression if properly positioned. However, caval cannulas cause greater interference with venous flow (and hence cardiac output) when not on CPB (i.e., after cannulation but before going on bypass and after bypass but before decannulation). When the caval tapes are tightened, no provision for decompression of the right heart (atrium and ventricle) is provided. If the right ventricle is not able to eject, then coronary sinus blood returning to the RA must be removed by opening or venting the right heart or releasing the caval tourniquets. This would be aggravated by presence of a left superior vena cava (LSVC). When the aorta is cross-clamped, coronary sinus flow is greatly reduced. However, the problem of right heart decompression recurs whenever cardioplegia or direct coronary perfusion is administered.

Bicaval cannulation without caval tourniquets is often preferred for mitral valve surgery because the retraction necessary often distorts the cavoatrial junctions, interfering with venous drainage if only a single atrial cannula is used. Right heart decompression is much better than when caval tourniquets are used but may not be as good as with atrial cannulation.

Single atrial cannulation has the advantage of being simpler, faster, and less traumatic, with one less incision, and provides fairly good drainage of both the cavae and the right heart. It interferes least with caval return when off bypass.

TABLE 5.1. COMPARISON OF VENOUS CANNULATION METHODS

	Bicaval		Single	
	With Tourniquet	**Without Tourniquet**	**Atrial**	**Cavoatrial**
Atrial incisions	2	2	1	1
Speed of cannulation	Slowest	Slow	Fast	Fast
Technical difficulty	Most difficult	Difficult	Easy	Moderately easy
Right heart exclusion	Complete	Incomplete	No	No
Coronary sinus return	Excluded	Partial	Included	Included
Right heart decompression	None	Fair	Good	Best
Right heart decompression with heart lifted up	Bad	Bad	Bad	Good
Caval drainage	Best	About as good	Good (less good for IVC)	Good (less good for SVC)
Caval drainage with heart lifted up	Good	Good	Bad	IVC adequate; SVC bad
Adequate venous drainage for all types of surgery	Yes	Yes	No	No
Potential rewarming of heart by systemic venous return	No	Yes	Yes	Yes
Myocardial preservation	Best	Good	Suboptimal	Controversial[a]

Assessments were derived from multiple sources, including Arom et al. (12), Bennett et al. (13,14), Lake (15), and Casthely and Bregman (16). *Note:* When performing bicaval cannulation, some surgeons place both catheters through a single atriotomy.
[a] See Bennett et al. (14).
SVC, superior vena cava; IVC, inferior vena cava.

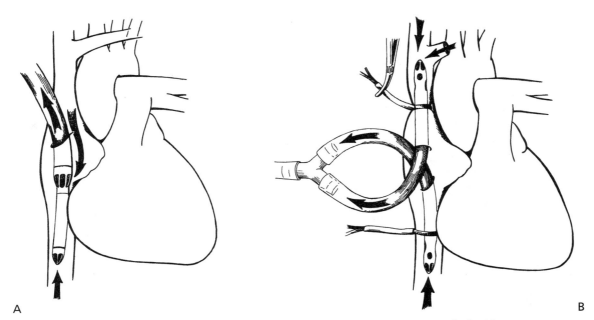

A   B

FIG. 5.3. Methods of venous cannulation. **A:** Single cannulation of right atrium (RA) with a "two-stage" cavoatrial cannula. This is typically inserted through the right atrial appendage. Note that the narrower tip of the cannula is in the inferior vena cava (IVC), where it drains this vein. The wider portion, with additional drainage holes, resides in the RA, where blood is received from the coronary sinus and superior vena cava (SVC). The SVC must drain via the RA when a cavoatrial cannula is used. **B:** Separate cannulation of the SVC and IVC. Note that there are loops placed around the cavae and venous cannulas and passed through tubing to act as tourniquets or snares. The tourniquet on the SVC has been tightened to divert all SVC flow into the SVC cannula and prevent communication with the RA.

However, the quality of its drainage of the cavae and right heart is sensitive to positioning, especially with distortion of the heart (e.g., "circumflex position" when lifting the heart to make an anastomosis to posterior branches of the circumflex coronary arteries). The cavoatrial cannula has many advantages of a single right atrial cannula but may provide superior drainage of the right heart, especially in the circumflex position, perhaps by providing some stability to the position of the atrial holes (13).

Although drainage of the IVC remains good with cavoatrial cannulation in the circumflex position, drainage of the SVC is often compromised. Proper location of the atrial holes is critical to optimal drainage by this cannula (12), and adequacy of decompression of the right heart and myocardial temperature must be monitored and appropriate adjustments made when needed. Some controversy has occurred regarding the effect of the type of venous cannulation on the adequacy of myocardial protection during aortic cross-clamping with cardioplegic arrest. The concern is that with atrial cannulation alone, relatively warm (about 25 to 30°C) blood returning from the body may bathe the right heart and interfere with myocardial protection (17).

Bennett et al. (14) studied the effects of venous drainage on myocardial preservation in a dog model and compared cavoatrial cannulation with biatrial cannulation with or without caval tourniquets. They observed the greatest myocardial cooling, the slowest rewarming (between doses of cardioplegic solution), and the least evidence of myocardial ischemia with cavoatrial cannulation, which they attributed to superior decompression of the right heart. The fact that most surgeons use a cavoatrial cannula for coronary artery bypass grafting surgery with apparent good results corroborates these observations. Specially designed swirl-tip atriocaval catheters (model VC2, Medtronic DLP, Inc.) and 45-degree two-stage cannulas (Research Medical, Inc., Midvale, UT) (18) may facilitate venous drainage, especially during limited access surgery.

Taylor and Effler (19) and Kirklin and Barratt-Boyes (2) reviewed the surgical technique of venous cannulation. Single atrial cannulas are usually inserted through the right atrial appendage after placing a purse-string suture. Bicaval cannulas are usually placed through separate incisions, although some surgeons may place both through a single incision in the atrial appendage. The SVC cannula is usually passed through the right atrial appendage. The IVC cannula is usually passed through a purse-string suture placed in the posteroinferior portion of the lateral wall of the RA near the IVC and avoiding the right coronary artery. The cavoatrial junctions may be dangerously thin. Some surgeons place purse-string sutures directly in the SVC and IVC, but this could cause narrowing when closed.

At times, venous cannulation is accomplished peripherally, usually via the femoral or iliac veins. This is used for emergency closed cardiopulmonary assist, for support of particularly ill patients before induction of anesthesia, for

prevention or management of bleeding complications during sternotomy for reoperations (20), and for certain types of aortic and thoracic surgery. The key to adequate flow rates with peripheral cannulation is use of as large a cannula as possible and advancing the catheter into the RA guided by transesophageal echocardiography (TEE), if available. Specially designed, commercially available (e.g., Medtronic BioMedicus, Inc., Eden Prairie, MN), long, ultrathin, non-kinkable, wire-reinforced catheters are available for this purpose. Insertion may be facilitated by use of an internal stylet and guidewire. Jones et al. (21) documented flows of up to 3.6 L/min (25F) to 4.0 L/min (27F and 29F) with simple gravity drainage. Using another brand of femoral venous catheter (model Femflex II, Research Medical, Inc.) and gravity drainage, Merin et al. (20) obtained flows of up to 2.5 L/min with 20F catheters and flows of 3.5 to 4.5 L/min with 28F catheters. This flow can be augmented by use of kinetic or vacuum assistance, which is discussed below.

Alternatively, venous catheters intended for percutaneous CPB may be used. Westaby (22) suggested that in cases where IVC drainage alone does not provide adequate venous return, adding a 32F cannula inserted into the SVC via a cut-down in the right internal jugular vein is effective. In contrast, Flege and Wolf (23) described using the right internal jugular vein as the sole source of venous drainage for conduct of CPB using percutaneously placed 21F 20-cm-long femoral arterial catheters (Medtronic DLP, Inc.) advanced into the RA and augmented venous drainage. Bicaval femoral venous cannulas (29F and 33F) are available (Medtronic DLP, Inc.) that allow drainage of the SVC and IVC while isolating the RA by snaring the SVC and IVC around the cannula (24).

Persistent Left Superior Vena Cava

An LSVC is present in about 0.3% to 0.5% of the general population but in 2% to 10% of patients with congenital heart disease and in up to 40% when such patients have abnormal sinus. It usually drains into the coronary sinus and then into the RA (25–28). In about 10% of cases, usually associated with other congenital heart disease, the LSVC drains into the left atrium. In some cases, there are defects in the wall between the coronary sinus and the left atrium permitting intercommunication between the left atrium and RA (e.g., coronary sinus type atrial septal defect).

The presence of an LSVC should be suspected when a large coronary sinus is noted on echocardiography (differential diagnosis includes right-sided venous hypertension, tricuspid regurgitation, and stenosis of the ostium of the coronary sinus) (29). Sometimes the LSVC itself can be seen on echocardiography posteriorly and laterally to the left atrium above the atrio-ventricular groove beside the aorta. Its presence can be confirmed by injection of agitated saline echo-contrast into a left arm vein and noting passage into the coronary sinus before its arrival into the RA. The surgeon should suspect an LSVC when the (left) innominate vein is small or absent.

The presence of an LSVC poses a number of problems during cardiac surgery. It may confuse and complicate passage of a pulmonary artery catheter or interfere with administration of retrograde cardioplegic solution (30). The latter is difficult because the coronary sinus is usually quite large in this circumstance and thus the balloon on the retrograde catheter does not seal and cardioplegic solution leaks into the RA. Furthermore, the cardioplegic solution may run off into the persistent LSVC, and the cardioplegic solution will be diluted with systemic venous blood draining down the LSVC. Patients with this anomaly may be more prone to atrial tachycardia and may have other congenital cardiac abnormalities. Finally, the presence of an LSVC poses obvious problems if the right heart is to be entered or with right heart decompression and adequacy of venous return if bicaval cannulation is used because of the flow of the additional systemic venous blood into the RA.

If the right heart is not going to be opened and a single or two-staged venous cannula is used for venous drainage and retrograde cardioplegia is not used, the presence of an LSVC poses no problems. If the right heart needs to be entered, several options are available. If an adequately sized innominate vein is present (true in about 30% of cases), the LSVC can simply be occluded during CPB. However, one must be wary of the rare possibility of the associated anomaly of atresia of the coronary sinus, in which case the LSVC provides the main outlet for cardiac venous drainage and occlusion of the LSVC could injure the myocardium (31). This condition should be suspected if the coronary sinus is not enlarged and by failure of echocontrast injected in the left arm or LSVC from entering the RA via the coronary sinus during TEE. Another obvious circumstance, in which the LSVC cannot be occluded despite the presence of an adequately sized innominate vein, is when there is associated absence of the right SVC (true in about 20% of cases).

If the innominate vein is absent (true in about 40% of cases) or small (true in about 33% of cases), occlusion of the LSVC may cause serous venous hypertension and potentially cerebral injury or ischemia and should not be done without documenting acceptable venous pressure in the LSVC cephalad to the occlusion. Otherwise, some other arrangement must be made to provide drainage of the LSVC. Use of cardiotomy suction in the coronary sinus ostium may be adequate, but cannulation, usually via a cannula passed retrograde into the LSVC through the ostium of the coronary sinus, is preferred, with a caval tape (tourniquet) placed around the LSVC. Alternatively, a cuffed caval cannula or endotracheal tube may be used (26). A caval cannula could be placed directly into the LSVC through a purse-string suture placed externally. Finally, in small infants, induction of deep hypothermia with CPB cooling

using a single venous cannula followed by circulatory arrest obviates the need for extra cannulation of the LSVC.

Augmented Venous Return

Early in the history of CPB, suction pumps (roller or finger) were used for venous drainage, but because they were difficult to control, these were discarded in favor of the more simple and effective gravity siphon method described above. Recently, there has been a renewed interest in use of regulated suction to overcome the resistance of longer and/or narrower venous cannulas used during limited (transthoracic) access or peripheral venous (e.g., jugular or femoral veins) access. With these narrower and longer venous cannulas, gravity siphon alone may not provide adequate flow for full CPB even with a maximal height differential between the patient and the venous reservoir.

Three methods to augment venous return have been described. One is to place a roller pump in the venous line between the venous cannula and the venous reservoir (32). This carries a high risk of generating excess negative pressure and collapsing the RA or great veins around the cannula tip and requires constant attention and adjustment of the roller pump flow rate. A second method substitutes a kinetic (centrifugal) pump for the roller pump in the venous line and is referred to as kinetic-assisted venous drainage (KAVD) (33). The third method involves applying a regulated vacuum to a closed hard-shell venous reservoir attached to the venous line. This method is referred to as vacuum-assisted venous drainage (34,35). This system is relatively simple and does not require regulation of a second pump. When a pump (roller or centrifugal) is used to generate the suction, some advocate placing a shunt around the pump using two Y-connectors. When a centrifugal pump is used, the shunt is clamped but is opened in the event entrained venous line air deprimes the centrifugal pump. When a roller pump is used, the shunt is only partially occluded to prevent generation of excessive negative pressures.

With all three systems, a conventional systemic pump (centrifugal or roller) then pumps blood out of the venous reservoir through the oxygenator and to the patient. Fried et al. (36) described use of a single pump for KAVD. Using their method, one centrifugal pump both aspirates venous blood and pumps it to the patient. This requires that the venous reservoir is T-ed into the venous drainage line to sequester or add blood to the system. This method reduces the problem of balancing the flow of two pumps but runs the risk of systemic air embolization (37,38).

Use of any of these systems requires careful regulation of the degree of negative pressure applied to the venous line. This is best accomplished by monitoring the pressure in the venous line about 10 cm before the inlet to the venous pump (roller or kinetic) or the hard-shell reservoir (if using a vacuum-assisted system). The negative pressure (or vacuum) measured at this site should not exceed −60 to −100 mm Hg (33). It is also desirable to observe the RA directly or via TEE. When the vacuum-assisted system is used, the degree of vacuum applied should be controlled with a vacuum regulator that can be adjusted and display low levels of suction in 10-mm Hg increments. It is important that vacuum should never be applied when there is no forward blood flow through the oxygenator to prevent air from being pulled across the microporous membrane into the blood path. The reservoir also should be open to the atmosphere when vacuum is not being applied to prevent overpressurization of the venous reservoir with reduction of venous return and risk of retrograde or antegrade air embolization. The venous reservoir should have a low positive (about +15 mm Hg) and a high negative (about −150 mm Hg) relief valve. Usually, adequate venous drainage is achieved with speeds of 1,000 to 1,200 revolutions per minute (rpm) of the kinetic pump or application of 20 to 60 mm Hg vacuum to the venous reservoir.

When a vacuum-assisted system is used with a closed reservoir, the degree of vacuum within the reservoir is influenced not only by the amount of vacuum applied to the system but also the relative flow of blood and air into the reservoir (from the venous line and cardiotomy suction and vents) and blood out of the reservoir (by the systemic pump).

There are a number of potential problems and risks associated with the use of augmented venous return methods. Excessive negative pressure may cause hemolysis because red blood cells are more easily damaged by negative than positive pressure (39,40). There also may be collapse of right atrial, tricuspid valve, or venous structures around the cannula tip resulting in impaired venous return and "chattering" in the venous line and possible damage to cardiovascular structures. Application of additional negative pressure (beyond gravity) increases the risk and amount of air aspiration from holes in walls of the RA or great veins. Air may also enter through a patent foramen ovale if the left heart is open or through any intravenous lines or introducers that may be in place (these should be closed or placed in occlusive infusion pumps during augmented venous return). Any aspirated air may cause an air lock or can deprime a centrifugal pump and stop blood flow or fill the hard-shell venous reservoir and contribute to systemic air embolization. If vacuum is applied to the closed reservoir system during a no-flow state, there is the theoretic risk of pulling air across the microporous membrane into the blood path with subsequent systemic air embolism. If the venous reservoir is not open to atmosphere when vacuum is not being applied or when KAVD is in use, the venous reservoir can become overpressurized with reduction of venous return and increase the risk of retrograde (through cardiac vents or cardioplegia line) or antegrade (systemic arterial line) air embolization. When a pump is being used to augment venous return, there also is potential for imbalance of flow between the venous drainage and the systemic flow pump, resulting in a change in intravascular volume in the patient or a risk of systemic air embolism. Thus, these methods of augmenting venous drainage require that the perfusionist must be even more attentive than when using conventional gravity siphon drainage.

Complications Associated with Achieving Venous Drainage

These include atrial dysrhythmias, laceration and bleeding of the atrium, air embolization (especially if the atrial pressure is low, which could cause systemic embolization with potential right-to-left shunts), laceration of the vena cavae (the IVC is particularly prone to this), and malposition of the tips (or atrial portion of the cavoatrial catheter), including inserting the tips into the azygos, innominate, or hepatic veins or across an atrial septal defect into the left heart. Placement of the low atrial purse-string suture for cannulation of the IVC requires retraction of the heart, which may have adverse hemodynamic consequences and sometimes is deferred until the patient is placed on bypass with a single cannula (SVC). Placing tapes around the cavae may result in lacerations of the cavae themselves or branches off the cavae or, when encircling the SVC, the right pulmonary artery. Once the venous cannulas are in place, they may interfere with venous return and cardiac output until CPB is initiated. Placing venous cannulas may displace central venous or pulmonary artery catheters inserted for hemodynamic monitoring (41). Caval tapes may occlude these lines and, conversely, their presence may prevent tight caval occlusion by the tapes. Further, these monitor lines may become caught in atrial purse-string sutures, causing malfunction and preventing their removal (42). Finally, the cavae may become obstructed when purse-string sutures placed in the cavae are closed after cannula removal (43).

Causes of Low Venous Return

Reduced venous drainage may be due to reduced venous pressure, inadequate height of the patient above the CPB reservoir, malposition of the venous cannulas (sometimes due to surgical manipulation of heart), or obstruction or excess resistance of the lines and cannulas. Inadequate venous pressure may be caused be venodilation with drugs (e.g., nitroglycerin, inhalation anesthetics) or hypovolemia. Kinks, air lock, or insertion of a pulmonary artery balloon catheter into a cannula (44) may cause obstruction, or the cannulas may be too small. During rewarming, the tendency for kinking of cannulas is potentially aggravated because of softening of the tubing and/or surgical manipulation of the heart.

ARTERIAL CANNULATION

Cannulas

Many different types of cannulas are available, made of various materials (Figs. 5.4 and 5.5). Some that are designed for insertion into the ascending aorta have right-angled tips; some are tapered; and some have flanges to aid in fixation and prevent introduction of too great a length into the aorta. The arterial cannula is usually the narrowest part of the extracorporeal circuit. High flow through narrow cannulas may lead to high pressure gradients, high velocity of flow (jets), turbulence, and cavitation with undesirable consequences, which are discussed below.

Hemodynamic evaluations of arterial cannulas have traditionally been based on measurement of the pressure drop. A useful descriptive characteristic of an arterial cannula is its performance index (pressure gradient versus OD at any given flow) (45). The narrowest portion of the catheter that enters the aorta should be as short as compatible with safety, and thereafter the cannula size should enlarge to minimize the gradient. Long catheters with a uniform narrow diameter are undesirable. The use of metal or hard plastic for the tip provides the best ID-to-OD ratio. Pressure gradients exceeding 100 mm Hg are associated with excessive hemolysis and protein denaturation (46). Thus, it is preferable to select a cannula that will provide adequate flow with no more than 100-mm Hg pressure gradient. Drews et al. (47) suggested that in small-sized cannulas, the right angle configuration (as compared with straight configuration) may aggravate hemolysis. New approaches to hemodynamic evaluation of arterial cannula include velocimetry (48) and detailed analysis of flow patterns using laser Doppler anemometry (49), color Doppler ultrasound, and high-field magnetic resonance imaging (50), but the clinical relevance of these studies is yet to be demonstrated.

The jetting effect produced by small cannulas may damage the interior aortic wall, dislodge atheroemboli and cause arterial dissections, and disturb flow into nearby vessels. Muehrcke et al. (49) described a new aortic cannula that has a closed tip and internal cone designed to reduce exit

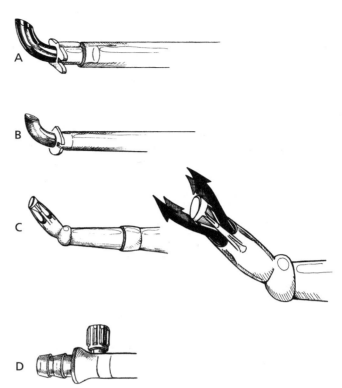

FIG. 5.5. Newer arterial cannulas. **A:** Metal-tipped right-angled cannula with plastic molded flange for securing cannula to aorta. **B:** Similar design but with a plastic right angle tip and molded flange. **C:** (Left) Diffusion-tipped angled cannula designed to direct systemic flow in four directions to avoid a "jetting effect" that may occur with conventional single-lumen arterial cannulas. An inverted cone occludes the tip. (Right) Drawing with arrows depicts flow patterns. **D:** Integral cannula connector and luer port (for de-airing) incorporated into some arterial cannulas; newer arterial cannulas may contain a self-venting cap (not shown) for removal of air during insertion.

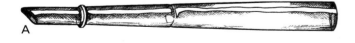

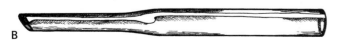

FIG. 5.4. Conventional arterial cannulas. **A:** Bevel-tipped tapered "blue line" Texas Heart Institute (THI)-type cannula with molded flange near tip. **B:** Similar cannula without a flange ("Bardic" type) that also can be used for femoral arterial cannulation.

forces and velocities to reduce these adverse jet effects (Fig. 5.5C). Hemolysis rates were similar while pressure gradients were intermediate compared with a number of other cannulas in common use.

Brodman et al. (45) evaluated 29 different types of arterial cannulas. They found that an 8-mm OD high-flow aortic arch cannula (model 15235, 3M Healthcare, Inc., Ann Arbor, MI) and an 8-mm OD aortic cannula with or without flange (models 1858 and 1860, CR Bard, Billerica, MA) were best (gradient less than 50 mm Hg at flows of 5 L/min), whereas several others were unacceptable (gradient more than 100 mm Hg at flows of 4 L/min). For cannulas not studied by them, one should refer to gradient-flow data provided by the manufacturer or conduct benchtop tests. Unfortunately, the data of Brodman et al. may underestimate clinical gradients because they used water rather than blood or a blood analogue as the fluid in their studies. Size and shape of aortic cannulas did not influence rate of transcranial Doppler-detected microemboli in one study (51).

Connection to the Patient

Ascending Aorta

In the early days of CPB, arterial inflow was via the subclavian or femoral artery (52), but currently it is usually via a cannula inserted into the ascending aorta (53). The advantages of this approach over the femoral or iliac arteries (Table 5.2) include ease, safety, and the fact that it does not require an additional incision. The surgical technique for aortic cannulation has been reviewed in detail by many others (2,19,54,55). The site for cannulation is selected based on the type of cannula to be used, the operation planned (how much of the ascending aorta must be available), and the quality of the aortic wall (56).

Atherosclerosis with or without calcification frequently involves the ascending aorta and poses problems regarding arterial cannulation and application of clamps and vascular grafts. Dislodgement of atheromatous debris either by direct mechanical disruption or from the "sand-blasting" effect of the jet coming out of the arterial cannula is thought to be a major cause of perioperative stroke (57–59). Atherosclerosis is also considered a risk factor for perioperative aortic dissection (60) and postoperative renal dysfunction (61).

Traditionally, surgeons have relied on palpation to detect these changes and select sites for cannulation, cross-clamping, and so on, and this should continue to be a component of the evaluation of the aorta (62). However, this method is much less sensitive and accurate than epivascular ultrasonic scanning (63–66). Mills and Everson (56) recommend using a 10- to 20-second period of venous inflow occlusion to reduce systemic arterial pressure to 40 to 50 mm Hg to improve the reliability of palpation of the ascending aorta. Specially designed epivascular probes, or transthoracic probes, encased in sterile sheaths with ultrasound jelly or lubricant inside and saline covering the aorta may be used for epiaortic scanning but do require some time and effort on the part of the surgeon. The use of a saline-filled glove placed between the probe and the aorta as a step-off may improve the image. Unfortunately, TEE, which is more convenient, is not sensitive enough because of limited views of the ascending aorta (65–67). However, some believe it can be used as a screening method to determine which patients need epiaortic scanning. If no significant atherosclerosis is detected in the ascending, transverse, or proximal descending aorta, it has been suggested that epiaortic imaging is not necessary (68), but others disagree (66,69).

Epiaortic and TEE should be considered complimentary (66). Beique et al. (59) suggested using epiaortic scanning in all patients who have a history of transient ischemic attacks, strokes, severe peripheral vascular disease, palpable calcification in the ascending aorta, calcified aortic knob on chest x-ray, those older than 60 years, and those with TEE findings of moderate aortic atherosclerosis. Others advocate epiaortic scanning of the ascending aorta in all patients over 50 years of age (70). If atherosclerosis is detected, then sites for insertion of cannulas, grafts, and application of vascular clamps are modified. If extensive atherosclerosis precludes arterial cannulation in the ascending aorta, then the femoral route should be considered (see below). However, in this case, the transverse and descending aorta should be evaluated by TEE to rule out extensive atheroma that might be embolized into the brain or elsewhere with retrograde flow from a femoral cannula. If such is the case, then axillary-subclavian cannulation should be considered.

If atheroma is extensive in the ascending or transverse aorta, some clinicians have suggested using a long arterial cannula that is inserted in the ascending aorta and threaded around into the proximal descending aorta to reduce the

TABLE 5.2. ARTERIAL CANNULATION

	Ascending Aorta or Arch	Femoral or Iliac
Accessibility	Easy	Difficult
Additional incision	No	Yes
Cannula size	Usually unlimited	Limited
Obstruct ascending aorta	Possible	No
Risk of malperfusion of arch vessels	Yes	No
Perfusion direction	Antegrade	Retrograde
Leg ischemia	No	Possible
Aortic dissection incidence	0.01–0.09%	0.2–1.0%
Leg wound and artery complications	0	~4%
Indications	Most cases	When aortic cannulation not feasible or desirable, peripheral cannulation under local anesthesia, bleeding complications during reentry
Contraindications	Ascending aortic aneurysms; diseased ascending aorta	When aortic cannulation feasible, occlusive disease of vessels, extensive atheroma (especially mobile) in arch and/or descending aorta

Assessments were derived from multiple sources, including Lake (15). See text for details.

"sand-blasting" effect (71). Others have advocated doing an endarterectomy under deep hypothermic circulatory arrest if severely protruding or mobile atheroma are detected (72), but in a recent study this has been associated with a higher stroke rate (35% versus 12%) and mortality (19% versus 12%) than when endarterectomy was not performed (73).

If the ascending aorta is totally calcified and rigid (so-called porcelain aorta), then entirely different strategies for cannulation and surgery must be used (74). These include no clamping of the ascending aorta, femoral or axillary-subclavian arterial cannulation, and, in selected cases, graft replacement or endarterectomy of the ascending aorta during deep hypothermic circulatory arrest (70,75). Unfortunately, graft replacement of the atherosclerotic ascending aorta may be a high-risk procedure (76). If there is no intraluminal debris, Liddicoat et al. (77) used an intraluminal balloon designed for port-access surgery that is inserted through a purse-string suture in an atherosclerotic free portion of aortic arch to occlude the aorta. Others used a Foley catheter in a similar manner (78). Studies using historical control subjects suggest improved neurologic outcome with echocardiographic-based modification of surgical techniques in handling the ascending aorta (59,64,79).

If possible, the intrapericardial aorta is chosen for aortic cannulation because this segment best resists tearing or dissection. Many surgeons insert two concentric purse-string sutures into the aortic wall. Surgeons differ as to whether these should be shallow, deep, or full-thickness bites (2,80). Most surgeons then incise and dissect away the adventitia within the purse-string suture. Most avoid using a partial occluding clamp, except in pediatric patients, to minimize clamp trauma to the aorta. Optimal arterial blood pressure during cannulation (mean arterial pressure of about 70 to 80 mm Hg, systolic pressure of about 100 to 120 mm Hg) is important: if too high, there is a greater chance of tears and dissection and blood loss and spray; if too low, the aorta tends to collapse, it is harder to make an incision and insert the cannula, and there is a greater risk of damaging the back wall of the aorta. An appropriately long full-thickness incision is then made, and the leak is controlled with a finger or by approximating the adventitia or by simultaneously inserting the cannula. Alternatively, Garcia-Rinaldi et al. (81) suggested only incising down to the intima during aortic cannulation.

Dilators are routinely or selectively used. If a right-angled tip is used, it is often initially directed toward the heart and then rotated 180 degrees to confirm intraluminal placement. Slight or vigorous back bleeding is allowed to eliminate air or atheromatous debris and to further confirm intraluminal placement, which can be additionally confirmed by noting a pulsatile pressure in the systemic flow line pressure monitor on the CPB circuit, which should approximate the radial artery pressure. Proper position of the cannula tip is critical. Most surgeons insert only 1 to 2 cm of the tip into

the aorta and direct it toward the middle of the transverse arch to avoid entering the arch vessels. Others have advocated threading a long cannula into the proximal descending aorta to reduce the velocity and turbulence in the aortic arch to reduce the "sand-blast" effect and emboli (71).

Many potential complications of aortic root cannulation exist (52,82), including: inability to introduce the cannula (interference by adventitia or plaques, too small an incision, fibrosis of wall, low arterial pressure), intramural placement, dislodgment of atheroemboli (56,64), and air embolism from the cannula or if the aortic pressure is very low, injury to the back wall of the aorta; persistent bleeding around the cannula or at the site after its removal; malposition of the tip to a retrograde position or even across the aortic valve, against the vessel wall, or into the arch vessels (52); abnormal cerebral perfusion; obstruction of the aorta in infants (83); aortic dissection; and high CPB line pressure. High systemic flow line pressure may be a clue to malposition of the tip against the vessel wall or into an arch vessel, cannula occlusion by the aortic cross-clamp, aortic dissection, a kink anywhere in the inflow system, including a line clamp still on, or use of too small a cannula for the intended CPB flow.

Inadvertent cannulation of the arch vessels or the direction of a jet into an arch vessel may cause irreversible cerebral injury and reduced systemic perfusion (52,83–88). Suggestive evidence includes: high systemic line pressure in the CPB circuit; high pressure in the radial artery if supplied by the inadvertently cannulated vessel (52) (or low pressure if not supplied by the cannulated vessel); unilateral facial blanching when initiating bypass with a clear priming solution (86); asymmetric cooling of the neck during perfusion cooling (88); and unilateral hyperemia, edema, petechia, otorrhea, or dilated pupils. Before CPB, palpation of the carotids may reveal asymmetric pulsation (reduced on cannulated side) and the opposite may be observed during pulsatile bypass (increased pulsation on cannulated side) (88). Before CPB, the radial artery catheter may reveal sudden damping if the cannula is inserted in the arch vessel supplying the monitored radial artery (89).

It has been suggested that the Coanda effect (in which a jet stream adheres to the boundary wall and hence produces a lower pressure along the opposite wall) may be associated with carotid hypoperfusion (90). This has been shown to occur experimentally and may account for some cerebral dysfunction after CPB using aortic cannulation. Salerno et al. (91) detected major electroencephalographic abnormalities due to malposition of a cannula in 3 of 84 patients undergoing arch perfusion, possibly on the basis of the Coanda effect.

Antegrade aortic dissection associated with ascending aortic cannulation has been reported to occur in between 0.01% and 0.09% of cases (Table 5.3) (54,60,80,92). Aortic dissection should be suspected when any of the following are observed: a sudden decrease in both venous return and

TABLE 5.3. ASCENDING AORTIC DISSECTION COMPLICATING CARDIAC SURGERY

	Murphy et al. (60)	Gott et al. (92)	Still et al. (80)	All
Year published	1983	1990	1992	–
Institution	Emory	Emory	MGH	–
Years covered	1971–1981	1982–1988	1982–1990	1971–1990
Total cases	6,943	11,145	14,877	32,965
Dissections[a]	24 (0.35)	27 (0.24)	24 (0.16)	75 (0.23)
Site of origin				
Aortic cannulation[a]	4 (0.06)	10 (0.09)	10 (0.07)	24 (0.07)
Partial occlusion clamp	8	3	7	18
Aortic cross clamp	1	4	8	13
Proximal SV anastamosis	4	2	1	7
Cardioplegia cannula	2	5	—	7
Vent site	—	1	—	1
Aortotomy	2	—	—	2
Unknown or other	3	2	1	6
When recognized				
Operating room	15	27	20	62
Postoperatively	9	—	4	13
Mortality				
If recognized in operating room	33%	15%	20%	—
If recognized postoperatively	78%	—	50%	—

[a] Values are number of incidents, with percentages in parentheses.
MGH, Massachusetts General Hospital; SV, saphenous vein.

arterial pressure, excessive loss of perfusate, increased CPB systemic line pressure, evidence of decreased organ perfusion (oliguria, dilated pupil, electroencephalographic changes, electrocardiographic evidence of myocardial ischemia), blue discoloration of the aortic root (because of subadventitial hematoma), and bleeding from needle or cannulation sites in the aortic root. Subadventitial hematomas tend to be less extensive and to be softer and usually resolve when incised. TEE may be useful in diagnosing aortic dissection (93). Gott et al. (92) and Still et al. (80) discussed this complication in detail.

Management usually involves prompt cessation of CPB; recannulation distal to the dissection (usually femoral but occasionally into the distal aortic arch); induction of deep hypothermia and a period of circulatory arrest while the aorta is opened and the extent of the injury analyzed and repaired either by direct closure, use of a patch, or replacement of ascending aorta with a tubular graft. Occasionally, small injuries can be repaired off bypass by closed plication (92). Survival of those recognized and treated in the operating room has ranged from 66% to 85%. When not recognized until postoperatively, survival has been 50% or less (Table 5.3). Bleeding and infected or noninfected false aneurysms are late complications of aortic cannulation (82).

Femoral Artery

Cannulation of the femoral or iliac arteries (exposed via a retroperitoneal suprainguinal approach) is indicated when there is an aneurysm of the ascending aorta or when it is otherwise unsatisfactory for cannulation (56,64). It may be indicated when there is no space available due to multiple procedures involving the ascending aorta, for peripheral cannulation under local anesthesia in unstable patients, during reoperations prophylactically (20), when bleeding complications occur during reentry, or when an antegrade dissection complicates aortic cannulation. Femoral cannulation requires a second incision and limits the size of the cannula that can be used. Hence, the adverse consequences of fluid jetting effects and high pressure gradients are more likely. Lees et al. (94) found no difference in the distribution of blood flow and vascular resistance between retrograde (femoral artery infusion) and antegrade (aortic root infusion) flow in monkeys.

Femoral cannulation is associated with many complications (20,53,91), including: trauma to the cannulated vessel, such as tears, dissection, late stenosis or thrombosis, and bleeding; lymph fistula; infection; embolization; and limb ischemia. Because the retrograde perfusion cannula usually totally occludes the blood supply to the cannulated limb, ischemic complications (acidosis, compartment syndrome, muscle necrosis, and neuropathy) may develop if cannulation exceeds 3 to 6 hours (95–97). The risk of distal ischemia can be minimized by placing a Y-connector or leur-lock port in the arterial line and attaching a smaller cannula (e.g., 8F to 14F pediatric arterial cannula) inserted distally through the same arteriotomy (96) or a 8.5F introducer catheter inserted into the distal superficial femoral artery using the Seldinger technique (98) to maintain perfusion of the leg.

Alternately, VanderSalm (99) advocated suturing a 10-mm polytetraflluoroethylene graft end-to-side on the common femoral artery into which the 24F femoral cannula is inserted. This latter technique not only prevents lower extremity ischemia but may reduce risk of arterial injury and retrograde dissection. Use of a coated Dacron graft may be associated with less bleeding (100). If distal limb perfusion is used and the ipsilateral femoral vein is also cannulated, then a method to provide better venous drainage of that limb is suggested to reduce edema. This can be minimized either by not taping the vein around the cannula (96) or placing a second (12F) venous cannula through the saphenous vein into the distal femoral vein (101). If limb ischemia does occur, Beyersdorf et al. (102) described a method of controlled limb reperfusion to improve outcome.

Femoral perfusion may lead to cerebral and coronary atheroembolism if there is extensive atheroma in the distal arch or descending aorta; ideally, this should be assessed by TEE before selecting the femoral route. If severe atherosclerosis is present, an alternate route should be used if possible. Femoral perfusion may also aggravate preexisting aortic dissections, and an alternate site for cannulation (see below) is recommended by some authors (103).

The most serious complication of femoral cannulation is retrograde arterial dissection, which may lead to retroperitoneal hemorrhage or retrograde extension all the way to the aortic root. The incidence of this complication has been reported at between 0.2% to 1.3% (104–108), although rates as high as 1 in 30 (3%) (109) and as low as 0 in 702 (91) have been reported. Kay et al. (107) noted a rate of 3% in 378 patients over 40 years old.

Femoral cannulation is being frequently used during limited access surgery and has been complicated by fatal dissection (110). Galloway et al. (111) reported a rate of about 0.8% in 1,063 patients undergoing retrograde femoral cannulation and CPB with a port-access system (HeartPort, Inc., Redwood City, CA). Retrograde arterial dissection is thought to be caused by either direct (cannula) or indirect (jet) trauma and to be more likely in the presence of atherosclerosis or cystic medial necrosis and in patients over 40 years old (53,107). Retrograde aortic dissection may present like antegrade aortic dissection already described but may be more difficult to recognize if it does not extend into the ascending aorta. In these cases it may present only by a sudden decrease in venous return and arterial pressure, excessive loss of perfusate, increased systemic line pressure, and oliguria. In this situation, TEE is extremely helpful in making the correct diagnosis.

Because of the nature of the dissection and the flap, discontinuation of retrograde perfusion and resumption of antegrade flow (via a cannula in the ascending aorta or by normal cardiac function) may resolve the problem. This may permit different management from antegrade dissections. If the dissection occurs early in the procedure, simply discontinuing CPB immediately (and hence retrograde fem-

oral perfusion) and restoring intravascular volume (which can be facilitated by attaching the arterial line to the venous cannula and infusing perfusate from the pump) and then aborting the planned operation and doing nothing to the ascending aorta, even if it is affected by the dissection, can be successful (104). If the dissection occurs later when it is not possible or desirable to come off CPB, retrograde perfusion is immediately discontinued and the arterial cannula is introduced into the true lumen in the ascending aorta (often through the false lumen). Bypass is then resumed with antegrade perfusion and the planned operation may be completed without repair of the dissection itself or the ascending aorta. Carey et al. (106) reported long-term success in six of seven patients using this approach. Others recommend graft replacement of the ascending aorta (105).

A test infusion with the systemic pump through the arterial line (regardless of location of the arterial cannula) before initiating CPB accompanied by increased line pressure may warn of possible dissection and may avoid extensive dissection.

Axillary Artery

Use of the axillary artery instead of the femoral artery when ascending aortic cannulation is not feasible or is undesirable is being increasingly advocated, either by direct cannulation or through an attached 8-mm graft (112–114). During a left thoracotomy, the intrathoracic subclavian artery may be cannulated (115). Advantages of the axillary artery over the femoral artery include: it is less likely to be involved by atherosclerosis; it has good collateral flow, decreasing the risk of ischemic complications; healing is better; and wound complications are less likely. By providing antegrade flow, it also is less likely to cause cerebral atheroembolization. Its use has also been advocated for establishing deep hypothermia before repair of type I aortic dissections because it is less likely to result in malperfusion and further expansion of the dissection as may occur with femoral perfusion (103).

Use of the right axillary artery is favored. The artery is approached through a 4- to 10-cm incision below and parallel to the lateral two thirds of the clavicle. Care must be taken to avoid traction on the brachial plexus. The axillary vein is retracted away from the artery (but may be used for venous cannulation) (113) and a purse-string suture is placed in the axillary artery and a 20F to 22F right-angled or flexible arterial cannula is inserted 2 to 3 cm. Of course, the contralateral radial or brachial artery (usually the left) must be used for intraarterial pressure monitoring. During lateral thoracotomies, the axillary artery may be approached through the axilla through a vertical incision along the lateral border of the pectoralis major (113) or the subclavian artery may be cannulated intrathoracically (115). Brachial plexus injury and axillary artery thrombosis have been reported as complications of this technique (112).

Other Sites for Arterial Cannulation

Antegrade aortic perfusion can be accomplished by cannulating through the left ventricular apex and passing the cannula (20F to 22F) across the aortic valve into the aortic root (116–118). A 10F wire-reinforced arterial cannula has been used in a similar manner in an infant (119). In this circumstance, Robicsek (118) used a special padded vascular clamp (Heinrich Ulrich Co., Ulm, Germany) that allows clamping of the ascending aorta around the perfusion cannula. Both Robicsek (118) and Norman (117) described the use of special double-lumen or double-barreled cannulas that allow for both aortic perfusion and venting of the left ventricle. Coselli and Crawford (120) described retrograde perfusion through a graft sewn onto the abdominal aorta when distal occlusive disease prevents femoral cannulation and when ascending aortic cannulation is not feasible.

TUBING AND CONNECTORS

Minimizing blood trauma, prime volume, resistance to flow, and avoiding leaks (either outward flow of blood or aspiration of air) are considerations in selection of tubing and connectors. To minimize blood trauma, one should strive to have smooth nonwettable inside walls of nontoxic materials, to avoid velocities above 100 cm/s, and to avoid exceeding a critical Reynolds' number above 1,000 (Table 5.4). The gradient necessary to propel the blood through the tubing should also be minimized (Table 5.4). The selection of large ID tubing aids in achieving these objectives. On the other hand, the larger the tubing, the greater the priming volume. Keeping tubing as short as possible will reduce prime volume, pressure gradients (resistance to flow), and blood trauma.

Desirable tubing characteristics include: transparency; resilience (reexpands after compression); flexibility; kink resistance; hardness (resists collapse); toughness (resists cracking and rupture); low spallation rate (the release of particles from the inner surface of tubing); inertness; smooth and nonwettable inner surface; toleration for heat sterilization; and blood compatibility. Medical-grade polyvinyl chloride seems to meet these standards. Silicone rubber and latex rubber tubing sometimes were used in roller pumps in the past; however, spallation and blood incompatibility are respective problems. New formulations of polyvinyl chloride are being developed for use in roller pumps to minimize spallation.

Disposable clear polycarbonate connectors with smooth nonwettable inner surfaces that make smooth junctions with plastic tubing (to minimize turbulence) are desirable. Smooth curves rather than sharp-angled bends will minimize turbulence. Connections must be tight enough to prevent leakage of blood when exposed to positive pressures (up to 500 mm Hg beyond the systemic flow pump) and aspiration of air on the venous side. The friction of fluted connectors with a larger OD than the ID of the plastic tubing or cannula into which the connector is inserted may provide sufficient tightness; otherwise, plastic bands may be applied tightly around all such connections at time of use. Most tubing and connectors are prepackaged and preassembled for convenience and safety. Heparin bonding onto the inner surface of the tubing and other components of the circuit may improve biocompatibility (see Chap. 9).

PUMPS

These are discussed in detail in Chapter 3, and only a few aspects are mentioned here. Roller pumps are used for pro-

TABLE 5.4. PRIMING VOLUME AND MAXIMUM FLOW RATES FOR VARIOUS SIZE TUBING

Tubing Size (ID)		Volume[a] (mL/M)	To Avoid All Hemolysis[b]	To Keep Pressure Gradient[b]		To Keep Reynolds' Number[b]		To Keep Velocity[c]	
Inch	mm			<5 mm Hg/m	<10 mm Hg/m	<1,000	<2,000	<100 cm/s	<200 cm/s
3/16	4.5	15	<0.1	0.1	0.2	1.8	4.0	1.0	2.0
1/4	6	30	0.11	0.5	0.9	2.1	4.5	1.7	3.4
3/8	9	65	0.35	2.0	4.0	3.7	6.5	3.9	>6
1/2	12	115	0.45	3.8	7.0	5.0	9.5	>6	—
3/4	18	255	—	—	—	—	—	—	—

In general, turbulence occurs when disrupting forces (inertial) overcome the retaining forces (viscous). This relationship is expressed by the Reynolds number [= (density × velocity × diameter) ÷ viscosity]. Empirically, turbulence has been found to occur in blood when this number exceeds 1,000, although curvature, smoothness, and inlet conditions also influence its occurrence.
[a] *Source:* Peirce EC II. *Extracorporeal circulation for open-heart surgery.* Springfield, IL: Charles C. Thomas, 1969:37, Fig. 13, with permission.
[b] *Source* Peirce EC II. *Extracorporeal circulation for open-heart surgery.* Springfield, IL: Charles C. Thomas, 1969:36, Fig. 12, with permission.
[c] Calculated by the authors.

viding flow through the systemic line back into the patient ("arterial" pump) but also for administering cardioplegia and providing suction for vents and field ("cardiotomy") suctions and augmented venous drainage. They consist of a length of tubing located inside a curved raceway at the perimeter of the travel of rollers (usually two) mounted on the ends of rotating arms (usually two, 180 degrees apart), arranged so that one roller is compressing the tubing at all times. Flow of blood is induced by compressing the tubing, thereby pushing the blood ahead of the moving roller. Flow rate depends on the size of the tubing, length of the raceway, and rpm of the rollers. For a given pump and type and size of tubing, flow is proportional to pump speed in rpm. *In vitro* calibration curves should be constructed and checked periodically. This is done by measuring the output of the pump over a measured period of time at various pump settings in a benchtop circulation, preferably using blood or blood analogue.

The degree of compression, or occlusiveness, of the tubing by the rollers can be adjusted and appears to be important. Excessive compression aggravates hemolysis and tubing wear, whereas too little occlusion may also aggravate hemolysis but, more important, may reduce forward output and invalidate flow assumptions or readings based on rpm. Although there is some disagreement, most authorities believe that the least hemolysis occurs when compression is adjusted to be barely nonocclusive (39). This is accomplished by holding the outflow line vertically so the top of the fluid (blood or asanguinous) is 60 to 75 or 100 cm (24 to 30 or 39 inches) above the pump and then gradually decreasing the occlusiveness until the fluid level falls at a rate of 1 cm every 5 seconds (39) or 1 inch/min (121) or 1 cm/min (122). Mongero et al. (123) described another method of setting occlusion. The tighter setting ensures more accurate forward flow, makes the roller pump relatively insensitive to afterload, and may not be associated with more hemolysis.

Complications associated with roller pumps include: malocclusion (with the consequences noted above), miscalibration, or miscalculation including setting the wrong tube size into the pump controller (124); fracture of the pump tubing; "run away" (125); loss of power; spallation (126–128); and pumping of large amounts of air. If the outflow becomes occluded, pressure in the line will progressively rise until the tubing in the pump ruptures or connectors and tubing separate. This can be avoided by use of a pressure-regulated shunt between the outflow and inflow lines of the roller pump (123) or use of servoregulation of the pump to arterial line pressure so that it turns off when excessive pressures are detected. If inflow becomes limited, the roller pumps will develop high negative pressures producing cavitation, microbubbles, and hemolysis.

Centrifugal pumps consist of a nest of smooth plastic cones or a vaned impeller located inside a plastic housing. When rotated rapidly (2,000 to 3,000 rpm), these pumps generate a pressure differential that causes the movement of fluid. Unlike roller pumps, they are totally nonocclusive and afterload dependent (i.e., an increase in downstream resistance or pressure decreases forward flow delivered to the patient if no adjustment is made in the rpm). This has both favorable and unfavorable consequences. Flow is not determined by rotational rate alone, and therefore a flowmeter must be incorporated in the outflow line to quantitate pump flow. Furthermore, when the pump is connected to the patient's arterial system but is not rotating, blood will flow backward through the pump and out of the patient unless the CPB systemic line is clamped. This can cause exsanguination of the patient or aspiration of air into the arterial line (e.g., from around the purse-string sutures) (129). Thus, whenever the centrifugal pump is not running, the arterial line must be clamped. Kolff et al. (129) described a check valve to prevent this problem. On the other hand, if the arterial line becomes occluded, these pumps will not generate excessive pressure (the maximum is only about 700 to 900 mm Hg) and will not rupture the systemic flow line. Likewise, they will not generate as much negative pressure and hence as much cavitation and microembolus production as a roller pump because the maximum is only about −500 mm Hg if the inflow becomes occluded.

A reputed advantage of centrifugal pumps over roller pumps is less risk of passing massive air emboli into the arterial line. This is because they will become deprimed and stop pumping if more than approximately 50 mL of air is introduced into the circuit. However, they will pass smaller but still potentially lethal quantities of smaller bubbles.

OXYGENATORS

Although numerous types of oxygenators have been used in the past, currently only two varieties are in use, the bubble and membrane oxygenators, and bubble oxygenators are rapidly disappearing from use in most parts of the world. The details concerning the function of these two types of oxygenators and the debate over whether the membrane oxygenator is superior is covered in Chapter 4. The oxygenator used does influence the configuration of the extracorporeal circuit, and often the oxygenator includes other components of the circuit (Fig. 5.6). The heat exchanger is usually an integral part of the oxygenator and usually is situated just proximal to the gas exchanging section or sometimes within the bubble chamber of a bubble oxygenator. Bubble oxygenators and some membrane oxygenators (e.g., model Capiox E, Terumo Medical, Inc., Tokyo, Japan) are positioned proximal to the pump and include an arterial reservoir, which is located distal to the oxygenating column and defoaming area and proximal to the systemic pump for which it serves as an "atrium." No additional venous reservoir is included in this circuit because the venous return

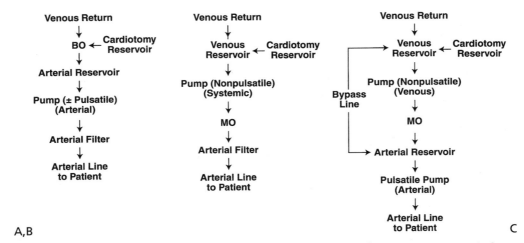

FIG. 5.6. Schematic of various arrangements of cardiopulmonary bypass components. **A:** Sequence of components when a bubble oxygenator (BO) is used. **B:** Sequence when a membrane oxygenator (MO) is used. **C:** Older arrangement for pulsatile perfusion with MO and two pumps: one removes blood from a venous reservoir and transfers it through the MO to an arterial reservoir where it can be pumped by a pulsatile pump back into the patient's arterial system. (Modified from Kirson LE, Laurnen ME, Tornbene MA. Position of oxygenators in the bypass circuit [Letter]. *J Cardiothorac Anesth* 1989;3:817–818, with permission.)

empties directly into the oxygenating column of the oxygenator, as does the cardiotomy reservoir (Fig. 5.6A).

Most membrane oxygenators are positioned after the pump because the resistance in most requires blood to be pumped through them (Fig. 5.6B). A venous reservoir receives the venous return and the drainage from the cardiotomy reservoir and serves as the atrium for the systemic pump, which pumps the blood through the oxygenator and into the patient. Some low-resistance membrane oxygenators (e.g., Capiox E) may function adequately by gravity drainage of venous blood and hence are positioned like a bubble oxygenator. For pulsatile bypass with some membrane oxygenator circuits, a second pulsatile pump is placed beyond the membrane oxygenator to avoid the damping that would occur if it were placed proximal to the membrane oxygenator (Fig. 5.6C). This requires inclusion of a second (arterial) reservoir and a bypass line to handle the excess flow of the first (venous) pump, which must run slightly faster than the arterial pump. However, pulsatile flow can be achieved with use of relatively noncompliant membrane oxygenators configured as in Figure 5.6B. If there is no arterial reservoir between the membrane oxygenator and the arterial pump, there is a risk of drawing gas bubbles across the membrane and into the CPB circuit due to pressure changes as the roller rapidly decelerates and accelerates.

Oxygenators require a gas supply system. This requires at least a source of oxygen but usually also air (via an oxygen–air blender for membrane oxygenators) and sometimes carbon dioxide, a flow regulator, and flowmeter. An oxygen analyzer should be incorporated in the gas supply line after the blender and a gas filter and moisture trap. An anesthetic

vaporizer may be incorporated in the gas supply line to the oxygenator. In this regard, one must be aware that volatile anesthetic liquids may be destructive to the plastic components of extracorporeal circuits, and hence one must consider the location of these vaporizers and use extreme care when filling them with anesthetic liquid so as not to contaminate any plastic (including tubing) component. When a vaporizer is used, a method of scavenging waste gas from the oxygenator outlet should be provided. When bubble oxygenators are used, gas flow must be initiated before the oxygenator is primed and continued thereafter to avoid back leakage of fluid through the bubble disperser plate, which may degrade its efficiency (130).

HEAT EXCHANGERS

Heat exchangers are designed to add or remove heat from the blood, thereby controlling the patient's body temperature. During its flow in the CPB circuit, the blood cools and hence heat must be added to avoid patient cooling. In addition, the patient's temperature is often deliberately lowered and then restored to normothermia before discontinuing CPB.

Although in the past separate heat exchangers were used in extracorporeal circuits, currently they are invariably included as an integral part of the disposable oxygenator. The details concerning the function and performance of blood heat exchangers are discussed in Chapter 4. They are usually located proximal to the gas exchanging section of the circuit to minimize the risk of releasing microbubbles of gas from the blood, which could occur if the blood is warmed after being saturated with gas. An additional risk of heat exchangers is water leakage into the blood path. Although this incident is rare, when it occurs it most often is manifested by the appearance of hemolysis and elevated serum potassium.

A source of hot and cold water, a regulator/blender, and temperature sensors are supplemental requirements of heat exchangers. Although hospital water supply may provide such a source, more frequently a stand-alone water cooler and heater is used. Malfunction of these cooler–heaters is one of the more common incidents during CPB (131). Separate heat exchangers are needed for administration of cardioplegic solution and/or blood for coronary perfusion.

VENOUS–ARTERIAL RESERVOIR

A reservoir is placed immediately before the systemic pump to serve as its "holding tank" or atrium and act as a buffer for fluctuation and imbalances between venous return and arterial flow. It also serves as a high capacitance (i.e., low pressure) receiving chamber for venous return and hence facilitates gravity drainage of venous blood. Additionally, it is a place to store excess blood when the heart and lungs are exsanguinated. Additional venous blood may become available from the patient when CPB is initiated and systemic venous pressure is reduced to low levels. Thus, as much as 1 to 3 L of blood may need to be translocated from the patient to the extracorporeal circuit when full CPB begins, especially in patients who have been in congestive heart failure or have long-standing valvular disease.

This reservoir may also serve as a gross bubble trap for air that enters the venous line, as the site where blood, fluids, or drugs may be added, into which the cardiotomy reservoir empties, and as a ready source of blood for transfusion into the patient. One of its most important functions, however, is to provide time for the perfusionist to act if venous drainage is sharply reduced or stopped, to avoid pumping the CPB system dry and risking massive air embolism.

When a bubble oxygenator is used, the reservoir is placed beyond the oxygenating and defoaming chambers and is usually included as an integral part of the oxygenator. This may be referred to as an "arterial reservoir" (Fig. 5.6A). In this case, venous return and cardiotomy drainage blood enter directly into the oxygenating chamber of the bubble oxygenator; hence, this inlet must be as low as possible to facilitate venous return. With membrane oxygenators, the reservoir is the first component of the extracorporeal circuit, directly receiving the venous drainage and the cardiotomy drainage (Fig. 5.6B). Blood then passes through the systemic pump and then through the membrane oxygenator. However, this reservoir (if hard-shelled and open) may be physically attached to the membrane oxygenator housing.

Reservoirs may be rigid (hard-shell) plastic canisters (referred to as "open") or soft collapsible plastic bags (referred

to as "closed"). Hard-shell reservoirs have the advantages of making it easier to measure volume, handling venous air more effectively, often having a larger capacity and being easier to prime, and permitting application of suction for vacuum-assisted venous return. Some hard-shell venous reservoirs incorporate macro- and microfilters and can also serve as the cardiotomy reservoir by directly receiving suctioned and vent blood. The soft bag reservoirs eliminate the gas–blood interface and reduce the risk of massive air embolism because they will collapse when emptied and do not permit air to enter the systemic pump. Schonberger et al. (132) observed more blood activation, blood loss, and blood administration with use of hard-shell reservoirs compared with collapsible venous reservoirs, which they attributed to additional exposure to integral filters and the blood–air interface. Another limitation of hard-shell reservoirs is that their defoaming elements are coated with silicone compounds (antifoam) that may cause systemic microembolization (133).

CARDIOTOMY RESERVOIR AND FIELD SUCTION AND VENTS

These topics are discussed in Chapter 6.

FILTERS AND BUBBLE TRAPS

Gross and microembolic material are ever present during CPB (134,135) and are fully discussed in Chapter 16. Multiple strategies have been suggested to reduce the hazards of embolization, but the most obvious is the use of micropore filters (136–138). Two types of micropore filters are available. A depth filter consists of packed fibers or porous foam. The predominant example of this is the Swank Dacron wool filter. It has no defined pore size, but presents a tortuous large wetted surface that filters by impaction and absorption. Screen filters are usually made of woven polymer thread that has a defined pore size and filters by interception, although the smallest pore screen filters (0.2 to 5.0 μm, used for prebypass filtration) are made of membranes. Screen filters vary in pore size and configuration. They not only block particulate emboli but also gross and microscopic air emboli. The latter is accomplished because the pores are filled with liquid that is maintained by surface-active forces. Excessive pressure can overcome this barrier by exceeding the so-called bubble point pressure (139).

Several studies have compared the performance of various micropore filters designed for cardiotomy (140,141) or arterial lines (142–147), and most have found the Dacron wool (depth) filter to be the most effective (140,141,144,145,147). Gourlay et al. (143–145) studied 13 commercially available arterial line filters and found all to have a similar pressure drop (24 to 34 mm Hg at a flow of 5 L/min) but to exhibit variable degrees of hemolysis and platelet loss and handling of gross and microscopic air. These findings did not appear to be related to pore size or type of material, except that again the Dacron wool (Swank) was best at removal of both microscopic and gross air. However, all filters tested were vastly superior to no filter in regards to interdiction of systemic line microemboli. Other authors expressed concern that the Dacron wool filter might cause significantly more hemolysis and thrombocytopenia and develop channeling and saturation breakthrough (136). Gourlay et al. (143) did not note excessive hemolysis, and Ware et al. (141) determined that although platelet counts were lower after the use of Dacron wool cardiotomy filters, the number of functional platelets were the same (i.e., the screen filter allowed more dysfunctional platelets to pass). Some concern has also been expressed that nylon screen filters may activate complement (136,137). Heparin-coated arterial line micropore filters have been introduced to reduce platelet aggregation and loss and facilitate debubbling and priming (148). However, studies have shown that the heparin-benzalkonium coating may leach off the screen during priming, rendering it ineffective or increasing the risk of passage of microscopic air (149).

Micropore filters may be used in several locations in the extracorporeal circuit. A survey conducted in 1993 found their frequency of use in various locations as follows: arterial line, 92%; cardiotomy reservoir, 89%; gas flow line to the oxygenator, 83%; blood product administration sets, 80%; prebypass (i.e., after priming but before connection of the circuit to the patient), 78%; and cardioplegia delivery line, 46% (150).

Most commercial cardiotomy reservoirs now contain an integrated micropore filter. Because the cardiotomy suction is a major source of microemboli (151) and because a micropore filter is more effective if placed in the cardiotomy reservoir line than arterial line (142), this would appear to be a reasonable practice. With the demonstrated presence of various foreign particulates in the disposables used for extracorporeal circuits, it also seems reasonable to use a prebypass filter during priming. The need for micropore filters on the cardioplegia delivery system has been questioned (152).

Limitations of arterial line microfilters include that they add to the cost, may obstruct, are harder to de-air (and therefore may be a source of gaseous microemboli), may generate microemboli, and cause hemolysis and platelet loss and complement activation. However, their wide use and available studies suggest little adverse effect from their use (153). Micropore arterial filters (Fig. 5.7) are excellent gross bubble traps, and on this basis alone, their routine use can probably be justified. If they are used for this purpose, however, they must have (unless they are self-venting) a continuously open purge line, which includes a one-way valve, that

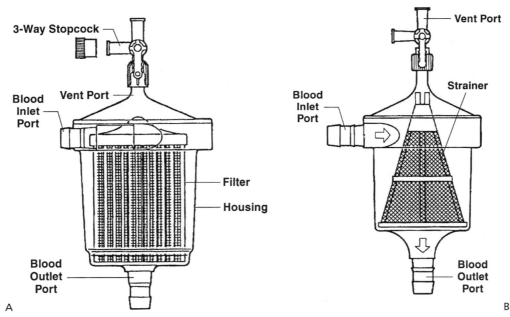

FIG. 5.7. Arterial line filters and bubble traps. **A:** Conventional adult arterial line microfilter and bubble trap. Blood enters tangentially at the top **(left),** which encourages any possibly entrained bubbles to rise to the top where they are vented out through a continuous purge line connecting the three-way stopcock to the cardiotomy or venous reservoir. Blood then passes through a screen microfilter (20- to 40-μm pore size), which also serves as a barrier to the passage of gaseous microemboli. **B:** Arterial line bubble trap. The design and flow dynamics are similar to the arterial filter, but blood only passes through a coarse screen strainer (approximately 170-μm pore size).

goes from the filter to the cardiotomy or venous reservoir to allow escape of trapped air. It is also recommended by filter manufacturers that a bypass line should be incorporated around the filter, which is clamped but can be opened in case the filter becomes obstructed.

The use of leukocyte-depleting filters is receiving much attention. Activation of leukocytes is thought to be a major contributor to the inflammatory response to CPB and postischemic injury. Active removal of leukocytes and platelets with a separate cell separator throughout CPB seems to have beneficial clinical effects (154,155). The benefits of using leukocyte-depleting filters during CPB are less clear. Animal studies have been encouraging (156), but most clinical studies have failed to document significant leukocyte depletion or clinical benefits (157,158). In contrast, Suzuki et al. (159) noted reduced cardiac enzyme levels when a leukocyte removal filter was used in the blood cardioplegia delivery circuit. Gu et al. (160) also observed clinical benefits from leukocyte filtration of residual pump blood, and Gott et al. (161) reported reduced hospital length of stay and cost savings with aggressive use of multiple leukocyte filters (arterial line, cardioplegia delivery line, autotransfused blood, and all blood product administration lines). However, this benefit was only noted in low-risk patients and despite the fact that no difference was observed in morbidity or mortality. Thus, further research is required to define the role, if any, of leukocyte filtration during CPB.

HEMOCONCENTRATORS

Hemoconcentrators (also referred to as hemofilters or ultrafiltration devices) contain semipermeable membranes (typically hollow fibers) that permit passage of water and electrolytes out of the blood. They are used in lieu of diuretics to remove excess fluid or electrolytes (e.g., potassium) and to raise the hematocrit of the perfusate. They can be connected to the CPB circuit in several different configurations. Blood may be drawn from the venous line, the arterial or venous reservoirs, or the systemic flow line, and filtered blood may be returned to the venous line or the cardiotomy or venous reservoirs. Except when blood is taken from a high pressure port or line (e.g., the systemic flow line), a pump must be used to propel blood through the device and may be used to control flow even if blood comes from the systemic flow line. Pressure is generated within the blood channels by resistance to flow through the hollow fibers or by placing a partially occluding clamp downstream. Suction may or may not be applied to the plasma water side of the membrane to facilitate filtration.

Fluid removal can be as great as 180 mL/min (at a flow of 500 mL/min) (162) but more often is in the range 30 to 50 mL/min (163). Various types of membranes are used. Molecules up to a molecular weight of 20,000 Da are re-

moved. At least some heparin is removed, and thus adequacy of heparinization must be monitored. Because of blood viscosity considerations, caution should be exercised in raising the hematocrit excessively during hypothermia.

The hemoconcentrator can be used after CPB to concentrate the pump blood before it is given back to the patient either via a bag or pumped directly into a venous line. Advantages of their use compared with centrifugal cell washers (e.g., Cell Saver) are that they conserve platelets, albumin, and coagulation factors (162) and are cheaper. However, hemoconcentrated blood still contains heparin that may need to be neutralized after infusion. Other potential adverse consequences are additional entrance into the circuit, potential for complement activation, retention of free hemoglobin and proteolytic enzymes (e.g., polymorphonuclear elastase), and loss of heparin, and excessive rise in hematocrit. However, no adverse effects were encountered by Boldt et al. (162). These authors compared six different hemofiltration devices with a conventional cell salvage device and identified some significant differences. Compared with diuretics, hemoconcentrators are more easily controlled and do not cause excessive potassium loss (164). See Chapter 7 for a further discussion of these systems.

Modified ultrafiltration (MUF) refers to a practice of withdrawing blood from the patient (usually out of the arterial cannula), after weaning from CPB, and passing it through a hemoconcentrator and pumping it back into the patient via the venous cannulas. It is primarily used in pediatric cases where, because of smaller circulating volumes, the benefits are increased (165). In a survey conducted in 1996, about 44% of pediatric cardiac surgery programs in North America used MUF (166). About 41% used it on all pediatric cases, whereas 45% based it on the patient's weight (about one-half of the respondents chose a weight of less than 10 or 15 kg). In most centers, the arteriovenous configuration is used. Venovenous MUF carries less risk of air cavitation and hemodynamic instability but may be associated with recirculation of filtered blood and does not deliver oxygenated blood to the pulmonary vasculature.

Some groups advocate use of the blood cardioplegia system as the MUF circuit, removing the crystalloid cardioplegia tubing from the cardioplegia roller head, flushing the cardioplegic solution out with CPB circuit blood, and inserting a primed hemoconcentrator distal to the blood cardioplegia pump and proximal to the blood cardioplegia system (167). The advantage of using this system is that it includes a roller pump, bubble trap, heat exchanger, and line pressure monitor and is already connected to the arterial line. It does carry the risk of accidental infusion of cardioplegic solution if not adequately flushed before MUF. Naik et al. (168) and Sutton (169) described other methods of setting up MUF circuits.

In the aforementioned survey (166), technical complications that were encountered in 84% of centers included air cavitation, patient cooling, circuit disruption, unintended infusion of cardioplegic solution, clotted circuit, and transient exsanguination. Because blood is typically aspirated from the arterial cannula by the MUF pump, air cavitation and air aspiration (from around the arterial cannulation site or through the membrane oxygenator) may occur if excessive negative pressure develops due to occlusion of the arterial cannula tip or kinking of the withdrawal line. Because of the risk of air entering the arterial circuit, antegrade flow should not be permitted once MUF has begun. For this reason, the arterial pump flow rate (which may be used to add volume from the pump oxygenator to the MUF circuit) should never exceed the MUF pump flow rate. Strategies to reduce air entry and cavitation developing in the arterial line (due to developing negative pressure) include extra vigilant monitoring of the CPB systemic line pressure, use of pressure servoregulation to stop the MUF pump if negative pressure develops in the arterial line, bypassing the arterial line filter, and having the surgeon manually maintain optimal aortic cannula position. Other safety measures include use of a bubble trap and bubble detector, inverting the hemoconcentrator so that blood enters the top, and monitoring the pressure in the MUF return line beyond the MUF pump. This topic is discussed further in Chapter 30.

MONITORING

Overall monitoring of the patient during CPB is covered in Chapter 27. This discussion focuses on ancillary devices used to monitor CPB circuit performance.

In-line Blood-gas Monitors

Noninvasive flow-through devices are available to measure blood gases and other electrolytes and the hemoglobin/hematocrit in the arterial and venous lines (170–172). The arterial monitor is similar to a pulse oximeter by providing continuous assessment of arterial oxygenation and permits more rapid and precise control of blood gases (173,174). Venous oximetry permits rapid assessment of the balance of oxygen supply and demand (175–177). Rubsamen (178), a medicolegal scholar, asserted that in-line blood-gas monitoring is a standard of care essential both from the standpoint of patient safety and prevention of devastating malpractice suits. Unfortunately, little scientific data document that this approach is superior or more safe to the visual monitoring of arterial and venous lines plus periodic discrete blood-gas sampling. Further, currently available devices are imperfect and may provide misleading information (179). For example, an apparently adequate mixed venous oxygen saturation may give a false sense of security (180). Finally, economic considerations cannot be ignored because in-line sensors add significant cost to the setup of the CPB circuit.

Another approach at more timely monitoring of blood gases and various electrolytes is the use of automated operating room analyzers (181,182), but the perfusion team or other individuals in the operating room must then accept responsibility for quality control and recognize their limitations (171,181). One must also be aware that blood drawn from the sampling port of some oxygenators may give misleading information (183). Stammers (184) summarized the clinical evaluation studies of various in-line and off-line blood-gas and electrolyte monitoring devices.

Systemic Line Pressure

The pressure in the CPB systemic flow line, measured after the pump but before the arterial line filter, should be monitored continuously to detect obstruction in the arterial line, malposition of the arterial cannula, arterial dissection, or obstruction of the filter. This pressure must be interpreted in the context of the expected pressure drop across the arterial cannula at the indicated flow rate and the patient's monitored intraarterial pressure (4). It is also a useful guide to verify proper initial arterial cannulation and as a monitor of central arterial pressure in the early postbypass period, when the radial artery pressure may be misleading. It is desirable to include an audible alarm in this systemic pressure monitoring system to alert the perfusionist if pressures are higher than expected. Many also connect this pressure site to the systemic pump so that it is servocontrolled to stop the pump if excessive pressures develop.

Systemic Line Flowmeter

A systemic line flowmeter is necessary if a centrifugal pump is being used and is a helpful adjunct to confirm proper occlusiveness and calibration when a roller pump is used. Akers et al. (185) compared four different extracorporeal blood flowmeters and the influence of changing hematocrit on measured values. The differences were small and do not appear to be clinically significant.

Oxygen Concentration

An oxygen analyzer should be placed in the gas supply line to the oxygenator. This is essential if oxygen is being diluted with another gas. The analyzer should be placed downstream from the blender (186). Monitoring gas flow into the oxygenator is also desirable. Kirson and Goldman (187) described a comprehensive system for monitoring the delivery of ventilating gas to the oxygenator.

Expired Gas

Monitoring the concentration of oxygen, carbon dioxide, and anesthetic vapors exiting the oxygenator ensures that oxygen is passing through the oxygenator and provides information regarding metabolic activity and depth of anesthesia (187). Zia et al. (188) found a fair correlation of exhaust gas CO_2 from bubble oxygenators with arterial blood CO_2 during cooling and hypothermia but a poor correlation during warming. With membrane oxygenators, another group found no correlation between exhaust gas and arterial blood CO_2 during all phases of CPB (189).

Pressure Gradient Across Membrane Oxygenators

Some manufacturers recommend monitoring the pressure gradient across membrane oxygenators because development of excessive pressure gradients has been reported to be the most frequent manifestation of oxygenator dysfunction (190,191) and may be an early indicator of possible oxygenator failure. If the gradient is not being monitored but a centrifugal systemic pump is being used, a high pressure gradient through the membrane should be suspected when systemic flow rate is unexpectedly low for the rpm setting and the CPB systemic line or patient arterial pressure.

Temperature Monitoring

Monitoring water temperature entering the heat exchangers (oxygenator and cardioplegia delivery system) ensures adequate cooling and avoids excess heating and potentially hazardous cooling and warming gradients (192). Knowledge of the temperature of the venous blood draining from the patient provides information regarding the adequacy of cooling and rewarming when inducing hypothermia and restoring normothermia, respectively. With renewed interest in the possible role of cerebral hyperthermia as a contributor to cerebral dysfunction after CPB, monitoring the temperature of the perfusate being delivered to the patient from the CPB circuit is considered by many to be essential for the safe conduct of CPB.

Low-level Sensor and Bubble Detector

A low-level sensor with alarms on the CPB reservoir and a bubble detector on the systemic flow line are considered desirable safety devices. Whether they should be connected to the systemic pump to automatically turn off the pump is the subject of debate (faster response time versus risk of false alarms). Furthermore, some reservoirs and oxygenators in current use preclude the application of the low-level alarms, emphasizing the essential role of a vigilant perfusionist.

Echocardiography

Epiaortic and TEE can be extremely helpful in conducting CPB. Besides their role in evaluating the aorta before arterial cannulation, TEE is accurate in detecting atherosclerosis in the descending aorta that might influence the use of femoral artery cannulation. It can also detect clots or tumors in the left atrium, left atrial appendage, or left ventricle and in the right-sided chambers that could influence venous cannulation and left-sided venting. Detection of a patent foramen ovale using two-dimensional images, color flow Doppler, and agitated saline echocontrast may anticipate a source of venous air if the left heart is to be opened, and detection of a patent ductus arteriosus may explain excessive return of blood to left heart during CPB (193).

Evaluations of the degree of aortic regurgitation (194) and the presence of a dilated coronary sinus (29) have impact on the administration of antegrade and retrograde cardioplegia. TEE may provide information regarding the presence of a persistent LSVC, which has an obvious impact on venous cannulation and administration of retrograde cardioplegia.

During introduction of various cannulas, TEE can evaluate positioning of peripherally introduced systemic venous cannulas, long arterial cannulas introduced into ascending aorta, retrograde coronary sinus cannulas, and left-sided venting cannulas. This is particularly helpful when the surgeon cannot directly inspect or palpate the heart due to limited access or adhesions. Use of TEE is essential to placement of various cannulas during port-access surgery and is helpful in proper placement and assessing proper function of intraaortic balloon pumps, especially when they are placed antegrade through the ascending aorta.

During bypass, TEE also can be used to assess the degree of left ventricular distension and decompression and assist with the differential diagnosis of ascending aortic hematoma and the diagnosis of aortic dissection. This is particularly important during femoral artery cannulation for systemic perfusion. During partial left heart bypass (femoral vein-to-femoral artery and left atrium-to-distal aorta or femoral artery) it can be helpful in assessing the balance of flow between the upper and lower body and blood volume regulation. Finally, it is useful in detecting intracardiac air and assessing adequacy of de-airing after cardiac surgery (195,196).

Automated Data Collection

Automatic data collection systems are available to assist with the preoperative calculations and to process and store data during CPB, which should free up the perfusionist to attend to more important tasks (197). Whether this will indeed improve outcome remains to be demonstrated (174,198).

UNUSUAL CANNULATIONS

Traditionally, CPB is conducted with the heart approached through a median sternotomy, which provides excellent exposure for venous and arterial cannulation. Approaching the heart through a right or left thoracotomy, a limited sternotomy (limited to upper portion or lower portion), or initiating CPB before exposing the heart presents special cannulation problems. These alternative approaches may be used to avoid sternotomy due to previous sternotomy, especially if complicated by prior infection or aneurysms of the ascending aorta or right ventricle and to avoid patent coronary grafts that might pass beneath the sternum (e.g., right internal mammary artery to left coronary circulation). Alternative approaches also may be appropriate for focused access to specific coronary arteries (e.g., right or circumflex) (199), for surgery involving the descending aorta, or when circulatory support is required before entering the chest (e.g., severe cardiac failure or problems encountered during attempted reentry) (20). These alternative approaches are also being used for minimal access or so-called minimally invasive cardiac surgery (Fig. 5.8).

Cannulation Through a Right Thoracotomy

This approach poses little problem with venous (atrial) cannulation but provides poor access to the ascending aorta

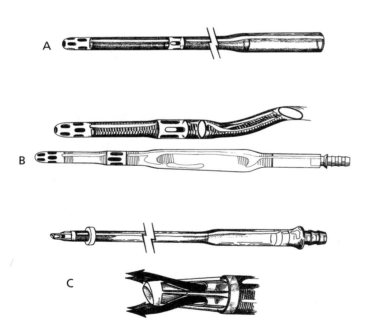

FIG. 5.8. Cannulas used for minimally invasive cardiopulmonary bypass. **A:** Smaller (typically, 29 to 29 French), nontapered, two-stage, wire-wound venous cannula that is inserted into the right atrium (RA) and inferior vena cava (IVC). **B:** Two-stage wire-wound venous cannula with a flattened section in the central portion of the cannula. This is inserted into the RA and IVC through a small chest incision. The cross-sectional area of the flattened portion of the cannula permits the same venous drainage as a round-shaped venous cannula but allows the surgeon to optimally position the cannula and avoid kinking as it exits the chest. **C:** Long, wire-wound, diffusion-tipped arterial cannula placed in the aorta. The fixation ring around the circumference near the tip is movable, and the wires in the wall allow the surgeon to position the cannula away from the surgical field.

and no access to the left ventricle. Peters et al. (24) evaluated various options for bicaval cannulation during minimal access right thoracotomies. Aortic cannulation and cross-clamping can be difficult as is de-airing the left ventricle. Arterial cannulation may be more conveniently accomplished using the femoral or axillary arteries as discussed earlier. Femoral-femoral bypass with deep hypothermia has been advocated by others (200). Placing external defibrillator pads on the left chest (front and back over the heart) may facilitate defibrillation if needed.

Cannulation Through Left Thoracotomy

One can conduct partial or complete left heart bypass and partial or complete CPB through the left chest.

Partial Left Heart Bypass

This method relies on the patient's right heart to pump blood through the lungs to the left heart and the patient's lungs to provide gas exchange. Blood is usually removed from the left heart with a large venous cannula placed directly into the left atrium. This carries a risk of systemic air embolism if one is not careful during insertion and removal of this cannula (the left heart should be well filled and ventilation momentarily interrupted during these procedures). Also, if excessive suction is applied to the venous line, especially if the atrial purse-string is not secure, air can be entrained into the left heart and venous cannula (and hence pumped into the systemic circulation). Another problem is that improper positioning or movement of the tip of the left atrial cannula can impair drainage of the left heart and flow into the left heart bypass circuit. Another way of draining blood from the left heart is by placing a cannula into the apex of the left ventricle. This may provide excellent flow of blood into the left heart circuit but adds the risks of injury to the left ventricle, bleeding, and late aneurysm formation. Arterial return may be into the descending aorta or femoral artery (usually the left, because the patient is in the right lateral decubitus position).

The extracorporeal circuit typically consists only of tubing and a centrifugal pump and does not include a reservoir, heat exchanger, or bubble trap. This minimizes the need for heparinization but precludes the ability to add or sequester fluid, adjust temperature, or prevent systemic air embolization. Some have advocated including a heat exchanger in the circuit to restore normothermia (201).

The anesthesiologist must be prepared to administer intravascular volume expanders as needed through other sites of the vascular access. Using a rapid infusion system connected to a large-bore intravenous site can facilitate volume administration.

Often this technique is used during surgery on the descending thoracic aorta. The patient's left ventricle supplies blood to the aorta proximal to the clamps and the left heart bypass circuit supplies blood to the body distal to the clamps. Typically, about two thirds of normal basal cardiac output (i.e., two thirds of 2.4 L/min/m² or about 1.6 L/min/m²) is pumped to the lower body and what is left is pumped by the left ventricle to the upper body. Arterial pressure should be measured in the proximal (right radial or brachial artery) and in the distal aorta via the right femoral artery. This will permit assessment of adequacy of flow to each part of the body, whereas the central venous and pulmonary artery diastolic or occlusion pressure will assess filling of the ventricles.

Use of TEE is particularly helpful in assessing filling and function of the left heart and left atrial cannula placement and function. If the arterial pressure is too high proximally and too low distally, the left heart bypass circuit should pump more blood. Conversely, if the arterial pressure is too low proximally and too high distally, the left heart bypass circuit should pump less blood. If both pressures are low, blood volume, and possibly a vasoconstrictor, may need to be added. If both pressures are high, more anesthesia and possibly a vasodilator should be added. O'Connor and Rothenberg (202) reviewed this topic in greater detail.

Full Left Heart Bypass

This can be accomplished with the just described cannulation technique for left-sided coronary artery surgery. If the heart fibrillates, blood can still passively pass through the right heart and lungs, but often an elevated central venous pressure is required.

Partial Cardiopulmonary Bypass

This technique is used to facilitate descending aortic surgery. The major issue is how to obtain systemic venous drainage. Several options are available: through the pulmonary artery with the cannula tip left in the main pulmonary artery or threaded retrograde into the right ventricle (203), through the right ventricular outflow tract, directly into the RA through the right atrial appendage or via the femoral vein. The problem with the latter is achieving adequate venous drainage through long small catheters, but this is usually solved by use of thin-walled cannulas threaded up into the RA with proper positioning facilitated by TEE. Augmented venous return can be used if gravity drainage is inadequate. Direct cannulation of the RA is quite difficult with risk of compression of the heart, tearing of the atrium, and bleeding. Cannulation of the pulmonary artery is somewhat easier.

The extracorporeal circuit resembles that previously described for full CPB and includes a pump, reservoir, oxygenator, heat exchanger, and bubble trap. It is important to remember that the left ventricle is still the source of blood supply to the upper part of the body, and the heart and the patient's own lungs are providing gas exchange for that

blood. Thus, the principles of relative flows to the lower part of the body and the upper part of the body described under partial left heart bypass apply. Furthermore, the adequacy of gas exchange of blood going to the upper body must be assessed separately (from samples drawn from the radial or brachial artery) from that coming out of the oxygenator and going to the lower body.

Full Cardiopulmonary Bypass

The only difference from what has just been discussed is that virtually all systemic venous return must be drained from the right heart, which accentuates the demand on venous cannulation and drainage. The CPB circuit supplies all systemic flow and gas exchange. Ascending aortic cross-clamping and administration of antegrade cardioplegia can be problematic. Sasaguri et al. (204) described a special double-lumen balloon catheter that is inserted through the left ventricular apex into the ascending aorta with TEE guidance for occlusion of the ascending aorta and administration of cardioplegic solution during thoracic aortic surgery via a left thoracotomy.

OTHER TOPICS

Heparin coating of circuits is used in an effort to improve biocompatibility and hopefully to reduce inflammatory reactions and heparinization requirements and thus improve outcome (205–207). Other surface modification methods (e.g., surface modifying additive) are being introduced (208). This topic is discussed in Chapter 9.

Circuits for CPB in children, and especially small infants, pose great challenges in terms of cannulation and miniaturization (209,210). These issues are discussed in Chapter 30.

Retrograde cerebral perfusion was first introduced as a method to treat massive air embolism (211) but is now widely used as a cerebroprotective strategy during aortic surgery and deep hypothermic circulatory arrest. This presents important issues in cannulation, monitoring, and setup of the extracorporeal circuit, which are discussed in Chapter 34.

Limited access minimally invasive surgery and, particularly, use of the HeartPort system imposes unique problems in cannulation (212). These have been covered partially in the sections on venous and arterial cannulation, augmented venous drainage, and unusual cannulation but are discussed additionally in Chapter 35. Computerized control of CPB has been described and used clinically (213).

ACKNOWLEDGMENT

We gratefully acknowledge the artwork of Norman P. Pregent, C.C.P., and Steve Schuenke.

KEY POINTS

- The primary purpose of CPB is to facilitate cardiac surgery.
- Major components include the membrane oxygenator (for gas exchange) with integral heat exchanger (for temperature regulation) and the systemic blood flow pump (roller or centrifugal type) for whole body perfusion.
- Other functions of the CPB circuit include suctioning of blood and air from the operative site and cardioplegia delivery.
- Venous drainage is most often accomplished by gravity siphonage via large-bore cannulas inserted in the RA/IVC or SVC and IVC.
- Cavoatrial cannulation is simpler and provides good drainage of both cavae and the right heart.
- Peripheral venous cannulation is facilitated by use of cannulas advanced to the RA and augmented venous assistance (kinetic or vacuum).
- Use of augmented venous drainage requires proper cannula placement and careful regulation of the degree of vacuum applied to the venous line.
- A persistent LSVC is seen infrequently but when present can negatively affect placement of a pulmonary artery catheter, delivery of cardioplegia, and right heart decompression.
- Arterial cannulas should be chosen so that the pressure drop is less than 100 mm Hg at full CPB flow.
- The risk of complications with femoral arterial cannulation is much higher than with ascending aortic cannulation.
- Use of either long or diffusion-tipped arterial cannulas can minimize the risk of dislodgment of atheroma in the ascending or transverse aorta.
- Dissection of the aorta (either retrograde or antegrade) must be promptly recognized and surgically corrected to decrease the risk of patient morbidity or mortality.
- Tubing sizes and lengths and connectors should be chosen to minimize blood velocity and priming volume.
- CPB reservoirs may be either hard-shell ("open") or soft collapsible ("closed") types, but there appears to be no advantage of one over the other unless vacuum-assisted venous return is used, which requires a hard-shell type.
- Hemoconcentrators can be used during and after CPB to remove plasma water and raise the hematocrit and are more cost effective than cell salvage and washing devices.
- Alternative thoracotomies and cannulation sites are being used for minimally invasive cardiac surgery, and newer cannulas have become available to facilitate this approach.
- TEE is a useful adjunct to CPB for assessing the aorta before cannulation, cannula placement, determining cardiac and valvular function, and evaluating the effectiveness of cardiac decompression and de-airing maneuvers.

REFERENCES

1. Peirce EC II. *Extracorporeal circulation for open-heart surgery.* Springfield, IL: Charles C Thomas, 1969.
2. Kirklin JW, Barratt-Boyes BE. *Cardiac surgery*, 2nd ed. New York: Churchill-Livingstone, 1993.
3. Riley JB, Hardin SB, Winn BA, et al. In vitro comparison of cavoatrial (dual stage) cannulae for use during cardiopulmonary bypass. *Perfusion* 1986;1:197–204.
4. Delius RF, Montoya JP, Merz SJ, et al. A new method for describing the performance of cardiac surgery cannulas. *Ann Thorac Surg* 1992;33:278–281.
5. Bloom DF, Cornhill JF, Malchesky PS, et al. Technical and economic feasibility of reusing disposable perfusion cannulas. *J Thorac Cardiovasc Surg* 1997;114:448–460.
6. Sadeghi AM, Rose EA, Michler RE, et al. A simplified method for the occlusion of the venae cavae during cardiopulmonary bypass. *Ann Thorac Surg* 1986;41:678.
7. Cooley DA. Caval occlusion clamps for temporary cardiopulmonary bypass. *J Thorac Cardiovasc Surg* 1970;59:292.
8. Al-Ebrahim KE, El-Shafei H. Cuffed venous return cannulas in minimally invasive cardiac operation [Letter]. *Ann Thorac Surg* 1998;65:1509.
9. Phillips SJ, Romanowski E. A new designed venous cannula for cardiopulmonary bypass. *J Thorac Cardiovasc Surg* 1972;63:769–770.
10. Kirsh MM, Lemer JH, Zwischenberger JB. Rapid technique of occlusion of the venae cavae for total cardiopulmonary bypass during repeat cardiac operations. *Ann Thorac Surg* 1987;43:566–567.
11. Morritt GN, Holden MP. The cuffed endotracheal tube in emergency cardiopulmonary bypass operations. *Ann Thorac Surg* 1981;31:287–288.
12. Arom KV, Ellestad C, Grover FL, et al. Objective evaluation of the efficacy of various venous cannulas. *J Thorac Cardiovasc Surg* 1981;81:464–469.
13. Bennett EV Jr, Fewel JG, Ybarra J, et al. Comparison of flow differences among venous cannulas. *Ann Thorac Surg* 1983;36:59–65.
14. Bennett EV Jr, Fewel JG, Grover FL, et al. Myocardial preservation: effect of venous drainage. *Ann Thorac Surg* 1983;36:132–142.
15. Lake CL. Controversies in the management of cardiopulmonary bypass. In: Kaplan JA, ed. *Cardiothoracic and vascular anesthesia update.* Vol. 1. Philadelphia: W.B. Saunders Co., 1990:1–21.
16. Casthely PA, Bregman D, eds. *Cardiopulmonary bypass: physiology, related complications, and pharmacology.* Mount Kisco, NY: Futura Publishing Co., 1991.
17. Rosenfeldt FL, Watson DA. Interference with local myocardial cooling by heat gain during aortic cross-clamping. *Ann Thorac Surg* 1979;27:13–16.
18. Lawrence DR, Desai JB. Forty-five degree, two-stage cannula: advantages over standard two-stage venous cannula. *Ann Thorac Surg* 1997;63:253–254.
19. Taylor PC, Effler DB. Management of cannulation for cardiopulmonary bypass in patients with adult-acquired heart disease. *Surg Clin North Am* 1975;55:1205–1215.

20. Merin O, Silberman S, Brauner R, et al. Femoro-femoral bypass for repeat open-heart surgery. *Perfusion* 1998;13:455–459.

21. Jones RE, Fitzgerald D, Cohn LH. Reoperative cardiac surgery using a new femoral venous right atrial cannula. *J Card Surg* 1990;5:170–173.

22. Westaby S. Extrathoracic cannulation for urgent cardiopulmonary bypass in cardiac tamponade: use of internal jugular vein. *J Cardiovasc Surg* 1988;29:103–105.

23. Flege JB Jr, Wolf RK. Venous drainage to the heart-lung machine via the internal jugular vein. *Ann Thorac Surg* 1997;63:861.

24. Peters WS, Stevens JH, Smith JA, et al. Minimally invasive right heart operations: techniques for bicaval occlusion and cardioplegia. *Ann Thorac Surg* 1997;64:1843–1845.

25. Choudhry AK, Conacher ID, Hilton CJ, et al. Persistent left superior vena cava. *J Cardiothorac Anesth* 1989;3:616–619.

26. Harris AM, Shawkat S, Bailey JS. The use of an endotracheal tube for cannulation of left superior vena cava via coronary sinus for repair of a sinus venosus atrial septal defect. *Br Heart J* 1987;58:676–677.

27. Horrow JC, Lingaraju N. Unexpected persistent left superior vena cava: diagnostic clues during monitoring. *J Cardiothorac Anesth* 1989;3:611–615.

28. Winter FS. Persistent left superior vena cava: survey of world literature and report of thirty additional cases. *Angiology* 1954;5:90–132.

29. Hasel R, Barash PG. Dilated coronary sinus on pre-bypass echocardiography. *J Cardiothorac Vasc Anesth* 1996;10:430–435.

30. Shahian DM. Retrograde coronary sinus cardioplegia in the presence of persistent left superior vena cava. *Ann Thorac Surg* 1992;54:1214–1215.

31. Yokota M, Kyoku I, Kitano M, et al. Atresia of the coronary sinus orifice: fatal outcome after intraoperative division of the drainage left superior vena cava. *J Thorac Cardiovasc Surg* 1989;98:30–32.

32. Babka RM. A comparison of the use of venous pumping to gravity return of blood to the oxygenator during cardioplegic arrest. *Proc Am Acad Cardiovasc Perfus* 1988;9:47–50.

33. Toomasian JM, McCarthy JP. Total extrathoracic cardiopulmonary support with kinetic assisted venous drainage: experience in 50 patients. *Perfusion* 1998;13:137–143.

34. Taketani S, Sawa Y, Massai T, et al. A novel technique for cardiopulmonary bypass using vacuum system for venous drainage with pressure relief value: an experimental study. *Artif Organs* 1998;22:337–341.

35. Darling E, Kaemmer D, Lawson S, et al. Experimental use of an ultra-low prime neonatal cardiopulmonary bypass circuit utilizing vacuum-assisted venous drainage. *J Extra-Corp Tech* 1998;30:184–189.

36. Fried DW, Zombolas TL, Weiss SJ. Single pump mechanically aspirated venous drainage (SPMAVD) for cardiac reoperation. *Perfusion* 1995;10:327–332.

37. Wallock M, Kuehn B, Hoff W. Single pump mechanically aspirated venous drainage (SPMAVD) for cardiac surgery [Letter]. *Perfusion* 1996;11:351–352.

38. Fried DW, Zombolas TL, Weiss SJ. Authors' response. *Perfusion* 1996;11:352–353.

39. Bernstein EF, Gleason LR. Factors influencing hemolysis with roller pumps. *Surgery* 1967;61:432–442.

40. Indeglia RA, Shea MA, Varco RE, et al. Mechanical and biologic considerations in erythrocyte damage. *Surgery* 1967;114:126–138.

41. Ratnaraj J, Manohar G. Pulmonary artery catheter displacement during cannulation for CPB [Letter]. *J Cardiothorac Vasc Anesth* 1991;5:648.

42. Troianos CA. Transesophageal echocardiographic diagnosis of pulmonary artery catheter entrapment and coiling. *Anesthesiology* 1993;79:602–604.

43. Ambesh SP, Singh SK, Dubey DK, et al. Inadvertent closure of the superior vena cava after decannulation: a potentially catastrophic complication after termination of bypass [Letter]. *J Cardiothorac Vasc Anesth* 1998;12:723–724.

44. Herrema IH, Winsser LJA. Flow directed pulmonary artery catheter obstructs venous drainage cannula of cardiopulmonary bypass machine [Letter]. *Anaesthesia* 1988;43:799.

45. Brodman R, Siegel H, Lesser M, et al. A comparison of flow gradients across disposable arterial perfusion cannulas. *Ann Thorac Surg* 1985;39:225–233.

46. Galletti PM, Brecher GA. *Heart-lung bypass, principles and techniques of extracorporeal circulation*. New York: Grune & Stratton, 1962:184–188.

47. Drews JA, Cleveland RJ, Nelson RJ. An approach to aortic cannulation with a caution on hemolysis associated with angled cannulas. *Rev Surg* 1974;31:57–59.

48. Groom RC, Hill AG, Kuban B, et al. Aortic cannula velocimetry. *Perfusion* 1995;10:183–188.

49. Muehrcke DD, Cornhill JF, Thomas JD, et al. Flow characteristics of aortic cannulae. *J Card Surg* 1995;10:514–519.

50. Ringgaard S, Madsen T, Pedersen EM, et al. Quantitative evaluation of flow patterns in perfusion cannulae by a new magnetic resonance imaging method. *Perfusion* 1997;12:411–416.

51. Benaroia M, Baker AJ, Mazer D, et al. Effect of aortic cannula characteristics and blood velocity on transcranial Doppler-detected microemboli during cardiopulmonary bypass. *J Cardiothorac Vasc Anesth* 1998;12:266–269.

52. Magner JB. Complications of aortic cannulation for open-heart surgery. *Thorax* 1971;26:172–173.

53. McAlpine WA, Selman MW, Kawakami T. Routine use of aortic cannulation in open heart operations. *Am J Surg* 1967;114:831–834.

54. Davidson KG. Cannulation for cardiopulmonary bypass. In: Taylor KM, ed. *Cardiopulmonary bypass: principles and management*. Baltimore: Williams & Wilkins, 1987:55–89.

55. Taylor PC, Groves LK, Loop FD, et al. Cannulation of the ascending aorta for cardiopulmonary bypass. *J Thorac Cardiovasc Surg* 1976;71:255–258.

56. Mills NL, Everson CT. Atherosclerosis of the ascending aorta and coronary artery bypass: pathology, clinical correlates, and operative management. *J Thorac Cardiovasc Surg* 1991;102:546–553.

57. Blauth CI, Cosgrove DM, Webb BW, et al. Atheroembolism from the ascending aorta. *J Thorac Cardiovasc Surg* 1992;103:1104–1112.

58. Barbut D, Grassineau D, Lis E, et al. Posterior distribution of infarcts in strokes related to cardiac operation. *Ann Thorac Surg* 1998;65:1656–1659.

59. Beique FA, Joffe D, Tousignant G, et al. Echocardiographic-based assessment and management of atherosclerotic disease of the thoracic aorta. *J Cardiothorac Vasc Anesth* 1998;12:206–220.

60. Murphy DA, Craver JM, Jones EL, et al. Recognition and management of ascending aortic dissection complicating cardiac surgical operations. *J Thorac Cardiovasc Surg* 1983;85:247–256.

61. Davila-Roman VG, Kouchoukos NT, Schechtman KB, et al. Atherosclerosis of the ascending aorta is a predictor of renal dysfunction after cardiac operations. *J Thorac Cardiovasc Surg* 1999;117:111–116.

62. Bar-El Y, Goor DA. Clamping of the atherosclerotic ascending aorta during coronary artery bypass operations. *J Thorac Cardiovasc Surg* 1992;104:469–474.

63. Ohteki H, Itoh T, Natsuaki M, et al. Intraoperative ultrasonic

imaging of the ascending aorta in ischemic heart disease. *Ann Thorac Surg* 1990;50:539–542.

64. Wareing TH, Davilla-Roman VG, Barzilai B, et al. Management of the severely atherosclerotic ascending aorta during cardiac operations: a strategy for detection and treatment. *J Thorac Cardiovasc Surg* 1992;103:453–462.

65. Sylivris S, Calafiore P, Matalanis G, et al. The intraoperative assessment of ascending aortic atheroma: epiaortic imaging is superior to both transesophageal and direct palpation. *J Cardiothorac Vasc Anesth* 1997;11:704–707.

66. Davila-Roman V, Phillips K, Davila R, et al. Intraoperative transesophageal echocardiography and epiaortic ultrasound for assessment of atherosclerosis of the thoracic aorta. *J Am Coll Cardiol* 1996;28:942–947.

67. Konstadt SN, Reich DL, Quintana C, et al. The ascending aorta: how much does transesophageal echocardiography see? *Anesth Analg* 1994;78:240–244.

68. Konstadt SN, Reich DL, Kahn R, et al. Transesophageal echocardiography can be used to screen for ascending aortic atherosclerosis. *Anesth Analg* 1995;81:225–228.

69. Guzzetta NA, Lee E, Sadel SM, et al. Does the degree of atheromatous disease in the descending aorta correlate with atheromatous disease in the ascending aorta? *Anesth Analg* 1995;80:SCA 80(abst).

70. Rokkos CF, Kouchoukos NT. Surgical management of the severely atherosclerotic ascending aorta during cardiac operations. *Semin Thorac Cardiovasc Surg* 1998;10:240–246.

71. Grossi EA, Kanchuger MS, Schwartz DS, et al. Effect of cannula length on aortic arch flow: protection of the atheromatous aortic arch. *Ann Thorac Surg* 1995;59:710–712.

72. Ribakov GH, Katz ES, Galloway AC, et al. Surgical implications of transesophageal echocardiography to grade atheromatous aortic arch. *Ann Thorac Surg* 1992;53:758–763.

73. Stern A, Tunick PA, Culliford AT, et al. Aortic arch endarterectomy increases the risk of stroke during heart surgery in patients with protruding aortic arch atheromas. *Circulation* 1997;96:I-185(abst 1024).

74. Byrne JG, Aranki SF, Cohn LH. Aortic valve operations under deep hypothermic circulatory arrest for the porcelain aorta: "no-touch" technique. *Ann Thorac Surg* 1998;65:1313–1315.

75. Svensson LG, Sun J, Cruz HA, et al. Endarterectomy for calcified porcelain aorta associated with aortic value stenosis. *Ann Thorac Surg* 1996;61:149–152.

76. King RC, Kanithanon RC, Shockley KS, et al. Replacing the atherosclerotic ascending aorta is a high-risk procedure. *Ann Thorac Surg* 1998;66:396–401.

77. Liddicoat JR, Doty JR, Stuart RS. Management of the atherosclerotic ascending aorta with endoaortic occlusion. *Ann Thorac Surg* 1998;65:1133–1135.

78. Paul D, Hartman GS. Foley balloon occlusion of the atheromatous ascending aorta: the role of transesophageal echocardiography. *J Cardiothorac Vasc Anesth* 1998;12:61–64.

79. Duda AM, Letwin LB, Sutter FP, et al. Does routine use of aortic ultrasonography decrease the stroke rate in coronary artery bypass surgery? *J Vasc Surg* 1995;21:98–107.

80. Still RJ, Hilgenberg AD, Akins CW, et al. Intraoperative aortic dissection. *Ann Thorac Surg* 1992;53:374–380.

81. Garcia-Rinaldi R, Vaughan GD III, Revuelta JM, et al. Simplified aortic cannulation. *Ann Thorac Surg* 1983;36:226–227.

82. Salama FD, Blesovsky A. Complications of cannulation of the ascending aorta for open heart surgery. *Thorax* 1970;25:604–607.

83. Parker R. Aortic cannulation. *Thorax* 1969;24:742–745.

84. Krous HF, Mansfield PB, Sauvage LR. Carotid artery hyperperfusion during open-heart surgery. *J Thorac Cardiovasc Surg* 1973;66:118–121.

85. Kulkarni MG. A complication of aortic cannulation. *J Cardiovasc Surg* 1968;9:207–208.

86. Dalal FY, Patel KD. Another sign of inadvertent carotid cannulation [Letter]. *Anesthesiology* 1981;55:487.

87. Ross WT Jr, Lake CL, Wallons HA. Cardiopulmonary bypass complicated by inadvertent carotid cannulation. *Anesthesiology* 1981;54:85–86.

88. Watson BG. Unilateral cold neck. *Anaesthesia* 1983;38:659–661.

89. McLeskey CH, Cheney FW. A correctable complication of cardiopulmonary bypass. *Anesthesiology* 1982;56:214–216.

90. Magilligan DJ Jr, Eastland MW, Lell WA, et al. Decreased carotid flow with ascending aortic cannulation. *Circulation* 1972;45[Suppl I]:I-130–I-133.

91. Salerno TA, Lince DP, White DN, et al. Arch versus femoral artery perfusion during cardiopulmonary bypass. *J Thorac Cardiovasc Surg* 1978;78:681–684.

92. Gott JP, Cohen CL, Jones EL. Management of ascending aortic dissections and aneurysms early and late following cardiac operations. *J Card Surg* 1990;5:2–13.

93. Troianos CA, Savino JS, Weiss RL. Transesophageal echocardiographic diagnosis of aortic dissection during cardiac surgery. *Anesthesiology* 1991;75:149–153.

94. Lees MH, Herr RH, Hill JD, et al. Distribution of systemic blood flow of the rhesus monkey during cardiopulmonary bypass. *J Thorac Cardiovasc Surg* 1971;61:570–586.

95. Herman BE, Wallace HW, Gadboys HL, et al. Anterior crural syndrome as a complication of cardiopulmonary bypass. *J Thorac Cardiovasc Surg* 1966;52:755–758.

96. Hendrickson SC, Glower DD. A method for perfusion of the leg during cardiopulmonary bypass via femoral cannulation. *Ann Thorac Surg* 1998;65:1807–1808.

97. Gates JD, Bichell DP, Rizzu RJ, et al. Thigh ischemia complicating femoral vessel cannulation for cardiopulmonary bypass. *Ann Thorac Surg* 1996;61:730–733.

98. Greason KL, Hemp JR, Maxwell JM, et al. Prevention of distal leg ischemia during cardiopulmonary support via femoral cannulation. *Ann Thorac Surg* 1995;60:209–210.

99. VanderSalm TJ. Prevention of lower extremity ischemia during cardiopulmonary bypass via femoral cannulation. *Ann Thorac Surg* 1997;63:251–252.

100. Sata J, Rimpilainen J, Rainio P, et al. A feasible femoral cannulation method during cardiopulmonary bypass [Letter]. *Ann Thorac Surg* 1998;65:1194.

101. Utoh J, Gotto H, Ashimura K, et al. A simple switching technique from cardiopulmonary bypass to a long-term extracorporeal life support system. *J Thorac Cardiovasc Surg* 1996;112:206–207.

102. Beyersdorf F, Mitrev Z, Ihnken K, et al. Controlled limb reperfusion in patients having cardiac operations. *J Thorac Cardiovasc Surg* 1996;111:873–881.

103. Svensson LG. Editorial comment: autopsies in acute type A aortic dissection, surgical implications. *Circulation* 1998;98:II-302–II-304.

104. Benedict JS, Buhl TL, Henney RP. Acute aortic dissection during cardiopulmonary bypass. *Arch Surg* 1974;108:810–813.

105. Bigutay AM, Garamella JJ, Danyluk M, et al. Retrograde aortic dissection occurring during cardiopulmonary bypass. *JAMA* 1976;236:465–468.

106. Carey JS, Skow JR, Scott C. Retrograde aortic dissection during cardiopulmonary bypass: "nonoperative" management. *Ann Thorac Surg* 1977;24:44–48.

107. Kay JH, Dykstra DC, Tsuji HK. Retrograde ilio-aortic dissection. A complication of common femoral artery perfusion during open-heart surgery. *Am J Surg* 1966;111:464–468.

108. Matar AF, Ross DN. Traumatic arterial dissection in open-heart surgery. *Thorax* 1967;22:82–87.

109. Jones TW, Vetto RR, Winterscheid LC, et al. Arterial complications incident to cannulation in open-heart surgery. *Ann Surg* 1960;152:969–974.

110. Reichenspurner H, Gulielmos V, Wunderlich J, et al. Port-access coronary artery bypass grafting with the use of cardiopulmonary bypass and cardioplegic arrest. *Ann Thorac Surg* 1998; 65:413–419.

111. Galloway AC, Shemin RJ, Glower DD, et al. First report of the Port-Access International Registry. *Ann Thorac Surg* 1999; 67:51–58.

112. Sabik JF, Lytle BW, McCarthy PM, et al. Axillary artery: an alternative site of arterial cannulation for patients with extensive aortic and peripheral vascular disease. *J Thorac Cardiovasc Surg* 1995;109:885–891.

113. Bichell DP, Balaguer JM, Aranki SF, et al. Axilloaxillary cardiopulmonary bypass: A practical alternative to femorofemoral bypass. *Ann Thorac Surg* 1997;64:702–705.

114. Baribeau YR, Westerbrook BM, Charlesworth DC, et al. Arterial inflow via an axillary artery graft for the severely atherosclerotic aorta. *Ann Thorac Surg* 1998;66:33–37.

115. Whitlark JD, Sutter FP. Intrathoracic subclavian artery cannulation as an alternative to femoral or axillary artery cannulation [Letter]. *Ann Thorac Surg* 1998;66:303.

116. Golding LAR. New cannulation technique for the severely calcified ascending aorta. *J Thorac Cardiovasc Surg* 1985;90: 626–627.

117. Norman JC. A single cannula for aortic perfusion and left ventricular decompression. *Chest* 1970;58:378–379.

118. Robicsek F. Apical aortic cannulation: application of an old method with new paraphernalia. *Ann Thorac Surg* 1991;51: 320–322.

119. Watanabe H, Eguchi S, Miyamura H, et al. Transapical aortic cannulation in pediatric patients. *Ann Thorac Surg* 1997;63: 1149–1150.

120. Coselli JS, Crawford ES. Femoral artery perfusion for cardiopulmonary bypass in patients with aortoiliac artery obstruction. *Ann Thorac Surg* 1987;43:437–439.

121. Stammers AH. Extracorporeal devices and related technologies. In: Kaplan JA, ed. *Cardiac anesthesia*, 4th ed. Philadelphia: W.B. Saunders, 1999:1017–1060.

122. Reed CC, Stafford TB. *Cardiopulmonary bypass*, 2nd ed. Houston: Medical Press, 1985.

123. Mongero LB, Beck JR, Orr TR, et al. Clinical evaluation of setting pump occlusion by the dynamic method: effect on flow. *Perfusion* 1998;13:360–368.

124. Tempe DK, Khanna SK. Accidental hyperperfusion during cardiopulmonary bypass: suggested safety features. *Ann Thorac Surg* 1998;65:306.

125. Kurusz M, Shaffer CW, Christman EW, et al. Runaway pump head. *J Thorac Cardiovasc Surg* 1979;77:792–795.

126. Uretzky G, Landsburg G, Cohn D, et al. Analysis of microembolic particles originating in extracorporeal circuits. *Perfusion* 1987;2:9–17.

127. Hubbard LC, Kletchka HD, Olsen DA, et al. Spallation using roller pumps and its clinical implications. *Am SECT Proc* 1975; 3:27–32.

128. Kurusz M, Christman EW, Williams EH, et al. Roller pump induced tubing wear: another argument in favor of arterial line filtration. *J Extra-Corp Technol* 1980;12:49–59.

129. Kolff J, McClurken JB, Alpern JB. Beware centrifugal pumps: not a one-way street, but a dangerous siphon! [Letter]. *Perfusion* 1990;5:225–226.

130. Dickson TA. Hypoxemia after intraluminal oxygen line obstruc-

131. tion during cardiopulmonary bypass [Letter]. *Ann Thorac Surg* 1990;49:512.

131. Jenkins OF, Morris R, Simpson JM. Australasian perfusion incident survey. *Perfusion* 1997;12:279–288.

132. Schonberger JPAM, Everts PAM, Hoffman JJ. Systemic blood activation with open and closed venous reservoirs. *Ann Thorac Surg* 1995;59:1549–1555.

133. Orenstein JM, Sato N, Arron B, et al. Microemboli observed in deaths following cardiopulmonary bypass surgery: silicone antifoam agents and polyvinyl chloride tubing as source of emboli. *Hum Pathol* 1982;13:1082–1090.

134. Pearson DT. Micro-emboli: gaseous and particulate. In: Taylor KM, ed. *Cardiopulmonary bypass: principles and management.* Baltimore: Williams & Wilkins, 1986:313–354.

135. Butler BD, Kurusz M. Gaseous microemboli: a review. *Perfusion* 1990;5:81–99.

136. Berman L, Marin F. Micropore filtration during cardiopulmonary bypass. In: Taylor KM, ed. *Cardiopulmonary bypass: principles and management.* Baltimore: Williams & Wilkins, 1986: 355–374.

137. Marshall L. Filtration in cardiopulmonary bypass: past, present and future. *Perfusion* 1988;3:135–147.

138. Joffe D, Silvay G. The use of microfilters in cardiopulmonary bypass. *J Cardiothorac Vasc Anesth* 1994;8:685–692.

139. Pascale F. Removal of gaseous microemboli from extracorporeal circulation. *Med Instrument* 1985;19:70–72.

140. Solis RT, Horak J. Evaluation of a new cardiotomy blood filter. *Ann Thorac Surg* 1979;28:487–488.

141. Ware JA, Scott MA, Horak JK, et al. Platelet aggregation during and after cardiopulmonary bypass: effect of two different cardiotomy filters. *Ann Thorac Surg* 1982;34:204–206.

142. Pearson DT, Watson BG, Waterhouse PS. An ultrasonic analysis of the comparative efficiency of various cardiotomy reservoirs and micropore blood filters. *Thorax* 1978;33:352–358.

143. Gourlay T, Gibbons M, Fleming J, et al. Evaluation of a range of arterial line filters. Part I. *Perfusion* 1987;2:297–302.

144. Gourlay T, Gibbons M, Taylor KM. Evaluation of a range of arterial line filters. Part II. *Perfusion* 1988;3:29–35.

145. Gourlay T. The role of arterial line filters in perfusion safety. *Perfusion* 1988;3:195–204.

146. Patterson RH Jr, Wasser JS, Porro RS. The effect of various filters on microembolic cerebrovascular blockade following cardiopulmonary bypass. *Ann Thorac Surg* 1974;17:464–473.

147. Pedersen T, Hatteland K, Semb BKH. Bubble extraction by various arterial filters measured in vitro with doppler ultrasound techniques. *Ultrasound Med Biol* 1982;8:71–81.

148. Hsu LC. Principles of heparin-coating techniques. *Perfusion* 1991;6:209–219.

149. Palanzo DA, Kurusz M, Butler BD. Surface tension effects of heparin coating on arterial line filters. *Perfusion* 1990;5: 277–284.

150. Silvay G, Ammar T, Reich DL, et al. Cardiopulmonary bypass for adult patients: a survey of equipment and techniques. *J Cardiothorac Vasc Anesth* 1995;9:420–424.

151. Liu J-F, Su Z-K, Ding W-X. Quantitation of particulate microemboli during cardiopulmonary bypass: experimental and clinical studies. *Ann Thorac Surg* 1992;54:1196–1202.

152. Munsch C, Rosenfeldt F, Chang V. Absence of particle-induced coronary vasoconstriction during cardioplegic infusion: is it desirable to use a microfilter in the infusion line? *J Thorac Cardiovasc Surg* 1991;101:473–480.

153. Kurusz M. Arterial line filtration during cardiopulmonary bypass: history and controversy. *Proc Am Acad Cardiovasc Perfus* 1983;4:76–86.

154. Morioka K, Muraoka R, Chiba Y, et al. Leukocyte and platelet depletion with a blood separator: effects on lung injury after

cardiac surgery with cardiopulmonary bypass. *J Thorac Cardiovasc Surg* 1996;111:45–54.

155. Chiba Y, Morioka K, Muraoka R, et al. Effect of depletion of leukocytes and platelets on cardiac dysfunction after cardiopulmonary bypass. *Ann Thorac Surg* 1998;65:107–114.

156. Lazar HL, Zhang X, Hamasaki T, et al. Role of leukocyte depletion during cardiopulmonary bypass and cardioplegic arrest. *Ann Thorac Surg* 1995;60:1745–1748.

157. Baksaas ST, Videm V, Mollnes TE, et al. Leukocyte filtration during cardiopulmonary bypass hardly changed leukocyte counts and did not influence myeloperoxidase, complement, cytokinin or platelets. *Perfusion* 1998;13:429–436.

158. Hurst T, Johnson D, Cujec B, et al. Depletion of activated neutrophils by a filter during cardiac valve surgery. *Can J Anaesth* 1997;44:131–139.

159. Suzuki I, Ogoshi N, Chiba M, et al. Clinical evaluation of a leukocyte-depleting blood cardioplegia filter (BC1B) for elective open-heart surgery. *Perfusion* 1998;13:205–210.

160. Gu YJ, deVries AJ, Boonstra PW, et al. Leukocyte depletion results in improved lung function and reduced inflammatory response after cardiac surgery. *J Thorac Cardiovasc Surg* 1996; 112:494–500.

161. Gott JP, Cooper WA, Schmidt FE, et al. Modifying risk for extracorporeal circulation: trial of four anti-inflammatory strategies. *Ann Thorac Surg* 1998;66:747–754.

162. Boldt J, Zickmann B, Fedderson B, et al. Six different hemofiltration devices for blood conservation in cardiac surgery. *Ann Thorac Surg* 1991;51:747–753.

163. Faulkner SC, Kurusz M, Manning JV Jr, et al. Clinical experience with the Amicon Diafilter during cardiopulmonary bypass. *Proc Am Acad Cardiovasc Perfus* 1987;8:66–69.

164. High KM, Williams DR, Kurusz M. Cardiopulmonary bypass circuits and design. In: Hensley FA Jr, Martin DE, eds. *A practical approach to cardiac anesthesia* 2nd edition. Boston: Little, Brown and Co, 1995:465–481.

165. Naik SK, Knight A, Elliott MJ. A successful modification of ultrafiltration for cardiopulmonary bypass in children. *Perfusion* 1991;6:41–50.

166. Darling E, Nanry K, Shearer I, et al. Techniques of paediatric modified ultrafiltration. *Perfusion* 1998;13:93–103.

167. Groom RC, Akl BF, Albus RA, et al. Alternative method of ultrafiltration after cardiopulmonary bypass. *Ann Thorac Surg* 1994;58:573–574.

168. Naik S, Elliott M. Ultrafiltration. In: Jonas RA, Elliott MJ, eds. *Cardiopulmonary bypass in neonates, infants and young children.* Boston: Butterworth-Heineman, 1994:158–172.

169. Sutton RG. Renal considerations, dialysis, and ultrafiltration during cardiopulmonary bypass. *Intern Anesth Clin* 1996;34: 165–176.

170. Alston RP, Trew A. An in vitro assessment of a monitor for continuous in-line measurement of PO_2, PCO_2 and pH during cardiopulmonary bypass. *Perfusion* 1987;2:139–147.

171. Bashein G, Pino JA, Nessly ML, et al. Clinical assessment of a flow-through fluorometric blood gas monitor. *J Clin Monit* 1988;4:195–203.

172. Pino JA, Bashein G, Kenny MA. In vitro assessment of a flow-through fluorometric blood gas monitor. *J Clin Monit* 1989;4: 186–194.

173. Pearson DT. Blood gas control during cardiopulmonary bypass. *Perfusion* 1988;3:113–133.

174. Justison GA, Parsons S. Improved quality control utilizing continuous blood gas monitoring and computerized perfusion systems. In *Proceedings of the 27th International Conference of the American Society of Extra-Corporeal Technology.* Reston, VA: American Society of Extra-Corporeal Technology, 1989:83–87.

175. Baraka A, Barody M, Harous S, et al. Continuous venous oxime-

176. Philbin DM, Inada E, Sims N, et al. Oxygen consumption and on-line blood gas determinations during rewarming on cardiopulmonary bypass. *Perfusion* 1987;2:127–129.

177. Swan H, Sanchez M, Tyndall M, et al. Quality control of perfusion: monitoring venous blood oxygen tension to prevent hypoxic acidosis. *J Thorac Cardiovasc Surg* 1990;99:868–872.

178. Rubsamen DS. Continuous blood gas monitoring during cardiopulmonary bypass: how soon will it be the standard of care [Editorial]? *J Cardiothorac Anesth* 1990;4:1–4.

179. Mark JB, Fitzgerald D, Fenton T, et al. Continuous arterial and venous blood gas monitoring during cardiopulmonary bypass. *J Thorac Cardiovasc Surg* 1991;102:431–439.

180. McDaniel LB, Zwischenberger JM, Vertrees RA, et al. Mixed venous oxygen saturation during cardiopulmonary bypass poorly predicts regional venous saturation. *Anesth Analg* 1994; 80:466–472.

181. Bashein G, Greydanus WK, Kenny MA. Evaluation of a blood gas and chemistry monitor for use during surgery. *Anesthesiology* 1989;70:123–127.

182. Nicolson SC, Jobes DR, Steven JM, et al. Evaluation of a user-operated patient-side blood gas and chemistry monitor in children undergoing cardiac surgery. *J Cardiothorac Anesth* 1989; 3:741–744.

183. Kent AP, Tarr JT, Fox MA. Where to sample during cardiopulmonary bypass [Letter]. *J Cardiothorac Anesth* 1989;3:136.

184. Stammers AH. Monitoring controversies during cardiopulmonary bypass: how far have we come? *Perfusion* 1998;13:35–43.

185. Akers T, Bolen G, Gomez J, et al. In vitro comparison of ECC blood flow measurement techniques. In *Proceedings of the 28th International Conference of the American Society of Extra-Corporeal Technology.* Reston, VA: American Society of Extra-Corporeal Technology, 1990:17–22.

186. Kurusz M, Conti VR, Arens JF. Oxygenator failure [Letter]. *Ann Thorac Surg* 1990;49:511.

187. Kirson LE, Goldman JM. A system for monitoring the delivery of ventilating gas to the oxygenator during cardiopulmonary bypass. *J Cardiothorac Vasc Anesth* 1994;8:51–57.

188. Zia M, Davies EW, Alston RP. Oxygenator exhaust capnography. A method of estimating arterial carbon dioxide tension during cardiopulmonary bypass. *J Cardiothorac Vasc Anesth* 1992;6:42–45.

189. O'Leary MJ, MacDonnell SP, Ferguson CN. Oxygenator exhaust capnography as an index of arterial carbon dioxide during cardiopulmonary bypass when using a membrane oxygenator. *J Anaesth* 1999;82:843–846.

190. Svenmarker S, Haggmark S, Jansson E, et al. The relative safety of an oxygenator. *Perfusion* 1997;12:289–292.

191. Wahba A, Philipp A, Behr R, et al. Heparin-coated equipment reduces the risk of oxygenator failure. *Ann Thorac Surg* 1998; 65:1310–1312.

192. Geissler HJ, Allen JS, Mehlhorn U, et al. Cooling gradients and formation of gaseous microemboli with cardiopulmonary bypass: an echocardiographic study. *Ann Thorac Surg* 1997;64: 100–104.

193. Amin IM, Maranets I, Barash P. Transesophageal echocardiography of the distal aortic arch. *J Cardiothorac Vasc Anesth* 1998; 12:599–560.

194. Moisa RB, Zeldis SM, Alper SA, et al. Aortic regurgitation in coronary artery bypass grafting: implication for cardioplegia administration. *Ann Thorac Surg* 1995;60:665–668.

195. Orihashi K, Matsuura Y, Hamanaka Y, et al. Retained intracardiac air in open heart operations examined by transesophageal echocardiography. *Ann Thorac Surg* 1993;55:1467–1471.

try during cardiopulmonary bypass: influence of temperature changes, perfusion flow and hematocrit level. *J Cardiothorac Anesth* 1990;4:35–38.

196. Tingleff J, Joyce FS, Pettersson G. Intraoperative echocardiographic study of air embolism during cardiac operations. *Ann Thorac Surg* 1995;60:673–677.

197. Berg E, Knudsen N. Automatic data collection for cardiopulmonary bypass. *Perfusion* 1988;3:263–270.

198. Gourlay T. Computers in perfusion practice. *Perfusion* 1987;2:79–85.

199. Uppal R, Mills NL, Wechsler AS, et al. 1993 Update: left thoracotomy for reoperative coronary artery bypass procedures. *Ann Thorac Surg* 1993;55:1575–1576.

200. Cohn LH. Update of right thoracotomy, femoro-femoral bypass, and deep hypothermia for re-replacement of mitral valve. *Ann Thorac Surg* 1997;64:578–579.

201. Ireland KW, Follette DM, Iguidbashian J, et al. Use of a heat exchanger to prevent hypothermia during thoracic and thoracoabdominal aneurysm repairs. *Ann Thorac Surg* 1993;55:534–537.

202. O'Connor CJ, Rothenberg DM. Anesthetic considerations for descending thoracic aortic surgery. Part II. *J Cardiothorac Vasc Anesth* 1995;9:734–747.

203. Westaby S, Katsumata T. Proximal aortic perfusion for complex arch and descending aortic disease. *J Thorac Cardiovasc Surg* 1998;115:162–167.

204. Sasaguri S, Fukuda T, Yamamoto T, et al. Transapical aortic occlusion for cardioplegic delivery during reconstruction of thoracoabdominal aortic aneurysm with deep hypothermic circulatory arrest. *J Thorac Cardiovasc Surg* 1999;117:186–188.

205. Aldea GS, O'Gara P, Sharpira OM, et al. Effects of anticoagulation protocol on outcome in patients undergoing CABG with heparin-bonded cardiopulmonary bypass circuits. *Ann Thorac Surg* 1998;65:425–433.

206. Mahoney CB. Heparin-bonded circuits: clinical outcome and costs. *Perfusion* 1998;13:1892–1204.

207. Shore-Lesserson L. Pro: heparin-bonded circuits represent a desirable option for cardiopulmonary bypass. *J Cardiothorac Vasc Anesth* 1998;12:705–709.

208. Gu YJ, Boonstra PW, Rijnsburger AA, et al. Cardiopulmonary bypass circuit treated with surface-modifying additives: a clinical evaluation of blood compatibility. *Ann Thorac Surg* 1998;65:1343–1347.

209. Groom RC, Akl BF, Albus R, et al. Pediatric cardiopulmonary bypass: A review of current practice. *Intern Anesth Clin* 1996;42:141–163.

210. Elliott M. Cannulation for cardiopulmonary bypass for repair of congenital heart disease. In Jonas RA, Elliott MJ eds. *Cardiopulmonary bypass in neonates, infants and young children*. Boston: Butterworth-Heineman, 1994.

211. Mills NL, Ochsner JL. Massive air embolism during cardiopulmonary bypass: causes, prevention, and management. *J Thorac Cardiovasc Surg* 1980;80:708–717.

212. Peters WS, Fann JI, Burdon TA, et al. Port-access cardiac surgery: a system analysis. *Perfusion* 1998;13:253–258.

213. Beppu T, Imai Y, Fukui Y. A computerized control system for cardiopulmonary bypass. *J Thorac Cardiovasc Surg* 1995;109:428–438.

CARDIOTOMY SUCTION AND VENTING

EUGENE A. HESSEL II
AARON G. HILL

CARDIOTOMY RESERVOIR AND FIELD SUCTION

Function

During cardiac surgery and cardiopulmonary bypass (CPB), it is necessary to aspirate variable but often large amounts of blood from the cardiac chambers and surgical field to prevent distension of cardiac chambers and air embolization and provide adequate exposure of the surgical field. It is not practical to discard the blood, and most of it is returned to the extracorporeal circuit via the cardiotomy reservoir.

Components

The cardiotomy reservoir receives blood that has been aspirated from the heart or pericardium or out of various vents. It includes a defoaming chamber containing a plastic sponge material impregnated with a substance (usually antifoam A) that lowers surface tension, a storage chamber with markings on the outer shell to measure volume, and macro- and microfilters. Blood is then returned, usually by gravity, to the venous reservoir (with membrane oxygenator systems) or into the bubble oxygenator, either intermittently or continuously by use of a tubing clamp.

When a hard-shell (rigid) venous reservoir is used in conjunction with a membrane oxygenator, this reservoir often serves as a combined or integrated venous and cardiotomy reservoir. However, the blood path of the cardiotomy section usually includes more extensive defoaming and microfiltration before this blood joins the venous return blood in the common reservoir section.

Methods

Suction is usually and most conveniently generated by use of a roller pump. The disadvantage of this system is that if the suction tip becomes occluded, a high degree of negative pressure will develop in the suction system, which can cause hemolysis of red blood cells. It also requires constant adjustment of the roller pump speed by the perfusionist and coordination with the surgeon in the event the vent or suction are not functioning. Alternatively, connecting a port on the cardiotomy reservoir to a vacuum source (e.g., wall suction) can generate suction. This avoids developing excessive negative pressure but requires an unvented cardiotomy reservoir and increases the risk of developing positive pressure in the reservoir with the risk of systemic air embolization. Another innovation is one in which the surgeon controls the degree of cardiotomy suction with a foot-controlled switch, but this is rarely used. A jet-driven aspirator has been described that removes air from the blood immediately within the suction tip and limits the degree of negative pressure to only one inch of water and reportedly reduces blood trauma (1).

Sequelae

During CPB, the cardiotomy suction and reservoir have been found to be a major source of hemolysis, particulate and gaseous microemboli (GME), fat globule formation, activation of coagulation and fibrinolysis, cellular aggregation, and platelet injury and loss (2–10). A major contributor to these adverse effects is the amount of room air that is aspirated along with the blood. Not only does this add GME to the blood, but the air–blood mixture causes turbulence and high shear stresses that can damage red blood cells and platelets.

Pearson et al. (11) analyzed the ability of various commercial cardiotomy reservoirs to remove bubbles from aspirated blood and described the following desirable features: direct injection of blood into the defoamer; avoidance of turbulence at the inlet; ensuring that all blood passes through the defoamer; avoiding free fall of blood into the reservoir; and incorporation of a micropore filter. Storing the blood in the cardiotomy reservoir for as long as possible rather than letting it continuously flow into the main extracorporeal circuit also will reduce the number of GME, as

E. A. Hessel II: Department of Anesthesiology, University of Kentucky School of Medicine, Chandler Medical Center, Lexington, KY 40536.
A. G. Hill: Inova Fairfax Hospital, Falls Church, VA 22042.

will reducing the air-to-blood ratio in the aspirated blood (11).

Edmunds et al. (2) found that the fall in platelet count was proportional to the amount of cardiotomy suction, expressed as either total amount (L per case) or as a fraction of total extracorporeal flow during CPB. de Jong et al. (12) observed a progressively greater reduction in platelet number and function and prolongation of the bleeding time with increasing amounts of air being aspirated along with blood during cardiotomy suction. Boonstra et al. (13) noted less release of β-thromboglobulin ($p < 0.05$), less depression of adenosine diphosphate-induced platelet aggregation (not significant), and less prolongation of postoperative bleeding time (not significant) when they used an automatically controlled cardiotomy suction device that prevented aspiration of air with the blood compared with conventional suction in patients undergoing coronary bypass operations. Further, there was significantly less postoperative bleeding in patients in whom controlled suction was used if large volumes (more than 65 L) with longer perfusion times (mean 3 hours) of cardiotomy suction were required. Wright and Sanderson (4) also documented the adverse effects of coaspiration of air on the platelet count and formation of microaggregates by measuring a rise in the screen filtration pressure.

Cardiotomy suction during CPB appears to be a principle source of hemolysis. This has been attributed to blood contact with the pericardium (9), (although Wright and Sanderson did not find this to be true if the pericardium had been previously washed with saline) (4), excessive negative pressure (14,15), and most important coaspiration of air (4,12). Less hemolysis has been observed when a vacuum suction pump is used rather than a roller pump (4,15). The amount of cardiotomy suction is influenced by the type of surgery and is generally greater with surgery for valvular and congenital heart disease, especially if the patient is cyanotic (4) as compared with patients undergoing coronary artery bypass surgery.

Management

The amount of blood damage can be minimized by avoiding or minimizing coaspiration of air (i.e., the suction tip should be kept below the blood level and the field not sucked "dry"), using the slowest flow rates and largest suction tips possible, and avoiding generation of high degrees of negative pressure by not occluding the sucker tip and using a controlled vacuum suction rather than a roller pump. Tobuchi et al. (8) advocated avoidance of leaving blood in the pericardium for periods of time and use of topical heparin to minimize activation of clotting.

Alternatives

An alternative method for handling blood and fluid in the surgical field is cell salvage systems (e.g., Cell Saver, Haemo-netics Corp., Braintree, MA). These aspirate the blood with a controlled vacuum, and the red cells are then automatically washed with saline and separated from the fluid by a centrifugation process. The washed red blood cells may be returned to the extracorporeal circuit or administered intravenously by anesthesia personnel (see Chap. 7). The advantage of this method is that it removes undesirable materials (microaggregates, fat, gross air, tissue debris, potassium, hormones, bioactivators, etc.) and will hemoconcentrate or raise the hematocrit of the perfusate.

The cell salvage system also can be used after CPB to process residual perfusate and recover red blood cells for transfusion. When used with a heparin-coated circuit, cell salvage and washing may provide better biocompatibility than using an uncoated cardiotomy reservoir alone (16,17). The disadvantage of cell salvage during CPB is the slow turn-around time and the loss of plasma proteins, coagulation factors, platelets, and other desirable substances in the blood. One approach is to use both a cell salvage system and conventional cardiotomy suction, choosing one or the other depending on the type of fluid (e.g., predominantly cardioplegic solution or ice melt versus predominantly blood) and source (e.g., pleural versus intracardiac). However, in recent years, cost considerations have resulted in a reduced use of cell salvage systems for routine use during CPB.

VENTING THE HEART

Venting the Right Heart

The right heart is normally drained or vented by the venous cannula(s). The relative efficiency of various types of venous lines at venting the right heart has been studied by Arom et al. (18) and Bennett et al. (19) and is summarized in Chapter 5, Circuitry and Cannulation Techniques. When bicaval cannulation with caval occlusion is used, venting of the right heart is not provided, and if the right ventricle is not able to eject, the right heart must be vented by a cannula, cardiotomy suction, or by surgically opening it to drain into the pericardial sac. The remainder of this chapter relates to venting of the left ventricle.

Purpose

The purpose of left ventricular venting is to prevent distension of the ventricle, reduce myocardial rewarming, prevent cardiac ejection of air, and to facilitate surgical exposure. Prevention of distension of the left ventricle is desirable to prevent mechanical damage to the muscle from excessive stretching. Myocardial preservation also may be improved by decreasing myocardial oxygen demand (decreased wall tension due to decreased radius of ventricle), facilitating subendocardial perfusion (subendocardial perfusion pressure equals aortic pressure minus left ventricular pressure), and preventing pulmonary venous hypertension, with possible pulmonary injury or edema and pulmonary artery hypertension.

Sources of Blood Returning to the Left Ventricle

The normal sources of blood returning to the left ventricle during CPB include bronchial and Thebesian veins and blood returning to the right heart that gets by the CPB venous cannulas and passes through the pulmonary circuit. Abnormal sources include a left superior vena cava (LSVC), patent ductus arteriosus (PDA) or a systemic-to-pulmonary artery shunt (e.g., Blalock-Taussig or Waterston), atrial or ventricular septal defects, anomalous systemic venous drainage into the left heart, and aortic regurgitation.

Even if not present to a significant degree preoperatively, aortic regurgitation commonly occurs when administering cardioplegic solution into the aortic root and from distortion of aortic root with other surgical manipulations. Even hemodynamically mild aortic regurgitation (e.g., less than 1 L/min) can become catastrophic when the heart fibrillates during CPB, yielding continuous aortic regurgitation without the ability of the left ventricle to empty itself.

Bronchial blood flow to the periphery of the lungs normally drains via the pulmonary veins. On bypass, this averages about 40 ± 182 mL/min (20), and the amount is influenced by the mean arterial pressure, which is one rationale for maintaining low perfusion pressures during CPB. Patients with chronic lung infections or inflammatory lung disease (e.g., bronchiectasis) and cyanotic congenital heart disease have exaggerated bronchial blood flow.

Coronary sinus flow into the right heart should greatly diminish with aortic cross-clamping except for noncoronary collateral flow, which averages 48 ± 74 mL/min (20), when cardioplegic solution is administered, and in the presence of an LSVC. Most coronary sinus blood should be removed if the venous cannulas are working properly, unless bicaval cannulas with caval tourniquets are used.

When excessive return of blood to the left heart is encountered, improper function or placement of the venous cannulas, an LSVC, PDA, or aortic regurgitation should be suspected. Unsuspected PDA has been discovered in about 1 in 3,500 coronary artery bypass operations (21), whereas Tunick and Kronzon (22) reported discovering five unsuspected PDAs in 8,772 adults (1/1,750) undergoing echocardiograms. PDA may be detected during intraoperative transesophageal echocardiography (TEE) (23).

Monitoring for Left Ventricular Distension

Monitoring for left ventricular distension requires the constant attention of the surgical team, which often is directing its attention elsewhere. The most common and simplest method is inspection and palpation of the heart. Particular attention should be paid to evidence of left heart distension when first establishing CPB, if the heart fibrillates, when the aorta is cross-clamped, and whenever antegrade cardioplegic solution is administered. Furthermore, moderate distension of the left ventricle may not be that easy to detect because of the posterior location of this ventricle that is often covered by blood, fluid, or ice and that, because of its thick walls, may be difficult to assess.

One definite advantage of a pulmonary artery catheter is that it can provide an indication of left atrial hypertension that accompanies left heart distension. It may be somewhat late in rising if the cause of left heart distension is aortic regurgitation and it is rendered invalid by a pulmonary artery vent. The pulmonary artery pressure reading may represent a false positive if the tip becomes wedged against a wall or is caught in the aortic cross-clamp or superior vena cava tourniquet; thus a high reading should be confirmed by examination of the pulmonary artery or left ventricle.

If a left atrial monitoring line is placed in the course of CPB, it can provide an early warning of left heart distension; however, these lines are infrequently used currently.

TEE is a powerful monitor of left heart distension during CPB. The transgastric short-axis view is optimal but can be obscured if a sponge or pad has been placed behind the left ventricle to aid exposure or to protect the phrenic nerve from ice and the heart from warming.

Indications

Venting of the left heart is indicated whenever the left ventricle is unable to handle the amount of blood that is returning to it. There is considerable debate about the need to vent the left heart during CPB, especially in the era of cold cardioplegia and for coronary artery bypass surgery (24–27). Excellent results have been reported without the use of venting in aortic (28) and coronary surgery (29). Contrary to these clinical results, experimental studies suggest that optimal myocardial recovery after an ischemic insult is best provided by full CPB and venting of the left ventricle (30). Otherwise, myocardial oxygen demand may be considerable even though the left ventricular diastolic pressure is low and the heart is not ejecting (30). Thus, left ventricular venting during reperfusion may be warranted in hearts with decreased ejection fraction or that have been incompletely revascularized or have sustained a period of severe ischemia. Olinger and Bonchek (31) found improved left ventricular performance immediately after coronary artery bypass surgery when a vent was used.

Methods

During coronary artery surgery, either no venting or venting via the cardioplegia cannula in the aortic root (32,33) is commonly practiced (Table 6.1, Fig. 6.1A). Special cardioplegia cannulas are available with a Y-arm, which allows

TABLE 6.1. METHODS OF VENTING THE LEFT HEART

Method	Advantages	Disadvantages
Ascending aortic (cardioplegia cannula)	Simple; no additional cannula. Also vents air when unclamp aorta and when LV starts to eject. Can be used to monitor aortic root infusion pressure.	Only works when aorta is cross-clamped. Does not work during administration of antegrade cardioplegia. Can cause air to be aspirated into the aortic root
Indirect LV (via stab wound in RSPV, through LA and MV)	Handles all sources of blood causing LV distension. Best for aortic regurgitation. Provides optimal decompression of LV. Avoids problems of direct LV vent.	Somewhat difficult exposure of insertion site. May be difficult to thread cannula into LV and position correctly. Risk of bleeding and tears at insertion site in RSPV. Potential for air entry into left heart. Potential problem if mechanical prosthesis in mitral valve. Potential embolism if tumor or clots in LA or LV.
Direct LV (through stab wound in apex)	Direct and simple. Avoids going across prosthetic mitral valve. Handles all sources of blood causing LV distension.	Positioning may be a problem—tip becomes easily obstructed by LV wall or MV apparatus. Risk of damage to LV and injury to coronary arteries and collaterals (myocardial ischemia) May be difficult to control bleeding from stab wound. Late LV aneurysm. Potential embolism if clots in LV. Potential for air entry into the left heart.
Direct LA (via LA appendage, roof of LA, or RSPV)	Relatively simple. Avoids going across the MV.	Does not handle AR. Potential embolism if clots in LA. Potential for air entry into the left heart.
Pulmonary artery	Simple. Reduces risk of admitting air into the left heart.	Does not handle AR. Renders use of PA pressure as a monitor of LV distension invalid. Risk of damage and bleeding from pulmonary artery.

LV, left ventricle; LA, left atrium; MV, mitral valve; PA, pulmonary artery; RSPV, right superior pulmonary vein; AR, aortic regurgitation.

one limb to be connected to suction when cardioplegic solution is not being administered through the main arm of the cannula. Other antegrade cardioplegia cannulas have a third lumen for monitoring aortic root pressure.

A limitation of aortic root venting is that it does not function during the time cardioplegic solution is being administered. If there is any aortic regurgitation or excessive blood return to the left heart, it also may be necessary to intermittently interrupt delivery of cardioplegic solution and apply suction to the vent with or without external compression of the left ventricle.

When direct venting of the left ventricle is desired, this is most commonly accomplished by inserting a catheter through a purse-string suture placed at the junction of the right superior pulmonary vein and the left atrium and advancing the catheter across the mitral valve into the left ventricle (Fig. 6.1B). One study observed less microemboli during coronary surgery when a left ventricular vent was used instead of an aortic root vent (34). This vent can be used in the left atrium at the beginning or end of surgery rather than in the left ventricle if the surgeon prefers.

Today, vents are seldom placed directly through the apex of the left ventricle (Fig. 6.1C) because of the risk of hemor-

rhage and myocardial injury. Some surgeons insert vents into the left atrium only or into the pulmonary artery (Fig. 6.2D) (25,35,36), which eliminates some risks of direct left ventricular venting but exhibit variable effectiveness. The effectiveness of pulmonary artery venting may be improved by pulmonary vein occlusion (37), but this requires careful monitoring of the adequacy of pulmonary artery venting. Pulmonary artery venting may not prevent left ventricular distension in the presence of aortic valve insufficiency and mitral valve competence (36).

All vents are then attached to suction (roller pump or siphon) and the blood is returned to the cardiotomy reservoir. When the tip of the vent is in the ventricle, the degree of suction must be constantly adjusted to avoid excessive suction (with collapse and trauma to the ventricle and the risk of aspirating air) or inadequate suction (with the risk of overdistension of the ventricle or obscuring the operative site). For this reason, some surgeons use gravity siphon drainage to vents instead of suction (38). This requires that the drainage reservoir is placed below the patient, and it may not provide adequate drainage if large volumes of blood are returning to the left heart.

Some circuits incorporate a Y-connector in the vent line

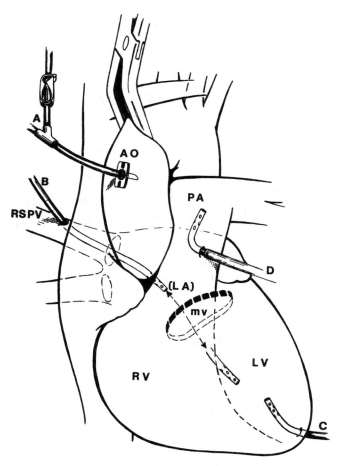

FIG. 6.1. Sites for venting the left ventricle. **A:** Aortic root cannula; one limb of the "Y" is connected to the cardioplegia administration system and the other limb to suction (siphon or roller pump) for venting left heart. **B:** Cannula inserted at the junction of the right superior pulmonary vein (RSPV) and left atrium and advanced through the left atrium and mitral valve (*mv*) into the left ventricle. **C:** Cannula is inserted directly into the apex of left ventricle. **D:** Cannula is inserted into the pulmonary artery. *AO*, aorta; *PA*, pulmonary artery; *LA*, left atrium; *RV*, right ventricle; *LV*, left ventricle. (Modified from Reed CC, Stafford TB. *Cardiopulmonary bypass*, 2nd ed. Houston: Texas Medical Press, 1985:277, with permission.)

Another method of applying suction to these vents whether they are in the left atrium, left ventricle, pulmonary artery, or aortic root is to connect them to a Y-connector or straight connector in the systemic venous drainage line. This provides automatic gravity (siphon) and/or Venturi suction of about 18 to 35 mm Hg without generating excessive suction and the need for extra pumps (40,41) but increases the risk of air entrainment in the venous line.

Complications

Left ventricular venting is not without complications, and Utley and Stephens (42) reviewed this aspect in detail. These include introduction of air into the left heart and subsequent systemic air embolism. This is most likely to occur at the time of insertion or removal of the vent if the left heart volume is low. To minimize this risk, the heart is usually allowed to fill before vent insertion, and the vents are often removed while the insertion site is covered with fluid. Excessive suction is another source of air introduction. Air may be drawn in from around purse-string sutures in the left atrium or aorta or retrograde through open coronary arteries during coronary artery surgery (43). Even pulmonary artery vents may suck air into the left heart and pulmonary veins as demonstrated by TEE. Finally, errors in function of the suction (positive pressure in reservoir, misdirection of tubing into roller pump head, reversal of roller pump) may cause air to be pumped into the ventricle. To minimize risk of this complication, some teams (44) advocate the use of a one-way valve in the left ventricular vent line. Most surgeons will test the function of the vent line at the sterile field to ensure that it aspirates fluid before implementing its use in the heart. Other risks of venting are bleeding and damage to the heart, including late left ventricular aneurysms (45). If there is a significant blood return through the left heart vent due to aortic regurgitation or bronchial blood flow, this will reduce the amount of systemic tissue perfusion. Increasing the systemic pump flow by an equivalent amount should compensate for this occurrence.

Aortic Root Air Venting

Any time the heart is opened, even simply by placing a catheter in a chamber, air may collect in the heart that, if not removed, will embolize with resumption of normal cardiac contractions. Even right heart air has the potential to pass into the left heart via septal defects or through the lungs. In addition to vigorous attempts at removal of all air before closing the left heart, the use of left heart vents, and repeated aspirations of left-sided chambers, the use of venting at the highest point of the aorta is considered the final safety maneuver against systemic air embolism (46).

Brenner et al. (47) analyzed the physiologic principles

coming from the ventricular vent so that either gravity or suction drainage can be used. Lundy et al. (39) described a combined gravity siphonage and active suction system using a roller pump and collapsible plastic bag reservoir placed between the left ventricular vent and the cardiotomy/venous reservoir and the roller pump placed between the two limbs of the reservoir bag. Using this system, the volume in the plastic reservoir bag will reflect ventricular volume. The degree of gravity suction is adjusted by the level of the reservoir bag. Active suction may be applied by clamping the outlet limb of the reservoir bag and activating the roller pump. Excessive suction is recognized by collapse of the reservoir bag.

relevant to the efficiency of aortic root air vents and studied various systems in an *in vitro* model. They found that a freely bleeding stab wound containing a nonconstricted fenestrated 10 French plastic catheter connected to suction was most efficient (97%). A freely bleeding stab wound was almost as efficient (91%), but inserting a catheter into the stab wound that was not connected to suction decreased its efficiency to 79%. Freely bleeding needles and catheter vents not connected to suction were very inefficient (20% to 36%), but efficiency was improved (to 90%) by applying suction. Marco and Barner (46) have demonstrated that the larger the vent needle area and the greater the flow out of the vent (suction), the greater its efficiency. There are obvious limits to this approach, including loss of forward flow and hemolysis.

Milsom and Mitchell (48) described a dual vent (aortic root and left ventricle via the right superior pulmonary vein) de-airing technique in which the ventricle ejects blood out the vents for a period of time before unclamping the aorta. They noted significantly fewer GME when using Doppler monitoring of the carotid artery, as compared with standard de-airing techniques. Gundry (49) described infusing blood into a left ventricular vent using the blood cardioplegia circuit to facilitate de-airing the aortic root before unclamping the aorta. Verification of the effectiveness of various de-airing techniques can be accomplished by the use of TEE.

KEY POINTS

- Cardiotomy suction and venting are intended to prevent distension of cardiac chambers and air embolism and to provide adequate surgical exposure.
- Cardiotomy reservoirs are designed to defoam, filter, and store blood before it is returned to the main CPB circuit.
- A roller pump most often is used as a source of suction, but wall suction applied to the cardiotomy reservoir also can be used.
- Major sequelae of cardiotomy suction are hemolysis, particulate and GME, fat globule formation, activation of coagulation and fibrinolysis, and platelet injury and loss.
- Careful suctioning at the surgical field and minimizing the volume of suctioned blood can decrease blood damage.
- Cell salvage and washing is an alternative sometimes used in conjunction with conventional cardiotomy suction.
- The right heart is normally drained by the CPB venous cannula and rarely needs to be vented.

- Normal sources of blood returning to the left heart include bronchial and Thebesian veins; abnormal sources include an LSVC, PDA, systemic-to-pulmonary shunt, septal defects, anomalous systemic venous drainage, and aortic regurgitation.
- The simplest method to monitor left ventricular distension is inspection and palpation of the heart by the surgeon.
- Other methods include monitoring pulmonary artery or left atrial pressure and TEE.
- Vents may be placed in the aortic root, left atrium or left ventricle via the left superior pulmonary vein, left ventricle via the apex (seldom used), or pulmonary artery.
- Venting may introduce air into the left heart and carries the risk of systemic air embolism.

REFERENCES

1. Clague CT, Blackshear PL Jr. A low-hemolysis blood aspirator conserves blood during surgery. *Biomed Inst Tech* 1995;29: 219–224.
2. Edmunds LH Jr, Saxena NC, Hillyer P, et al. Relationship between platelet count and cardiotomy suction return. *Ann Thorac Surg* 1978;25:306–310.
3. Pearson DT. Microemboli: gaseous and particulate. In: Taylor KM, ed. *Cardiopulmonary bypass: principles and management*. Baltimore: Williams & Wilkins, 1986:313–354.
4. Wright G, Sanderson JM. Cellular aggregation and trauma in cardiotomy suction systems. *Thorax* 1979;34:621–628.
5. Solis RT, Moon CP, Beall AC Jr, et al. Particulate microembolism during cardiac operations. *Ann Thorac Surg* 1974;17: 332–344.
6. Liu T-F, Su Z-K, Ding W-X. Quantitation of particulate micro emboli during cardiopulmonary bypass: experimental and clinical studies. *Ann Thorac Surg* 1992;54:1196–1202.
7. Brooker RF, Brown WR, Moody DM, et al. Cardiotomy suction: a major source of brain lipid emboli during cardiopulmonary bypass. *Ann Thorac Surg* 1998;65:1651–1655.
8. Tabuchi N, deHaan J, Boonstra PW, et al. Activation of fibrinolysis in the pericardial cavity during cardiopulmonary bypass. *J Thorac Cardiovasc Surg* 1993;106:828–833.
9. Siderys H. Pericardial fluid and hemolysis [Letter]. *Ann Thorac Surg* 1993;56:595.
10. Orenstein JKM, Soto N, Aaron B, et al. Microemboli observed in deaths following cardiopulmonary bypass surgery: silicone antifoam agents and polyvinyl chloride tubing as sources of emboli. *Hum Pathol* 1992;13:1082–1090.
11. Pearson DT, Watson BG, Waterhouse PS. An ultrasonic analysis of the comparative efficiency of various cardiotomy reservoirs and micropore blood filters. *Thorax* 1978;33:352–358.
12. de Jong JCF, ten Duis HJ, Sibinga CT. Hematologic aspects of cardiotomy suction in cardiac operations. *J Thorac Cardiovasc Surg* 1980;79:227–236.
13. Boonstra PW, van Imhoff GW, Eysman L, et al. Reduced platelet activation and improved hemostasis after controlled cardiotomy suction during clinical membrane oxygenator perfusions. *J Thorac Cardiovasc Surg* 1985;89:900–906.
14. Wielogorske JW, Cross DE, Nwadike EVO. The effects of subatmospheric pressure on the hemolysis of blood. *J Biomechan* 1975; 8:321–325.

15. Hirose T, Burman SD, O'Connor RA. Reduction of perfusion hemolysis by use of atraumatic low pressure suction. *J Thorac Cardiovasc Surg* 1964;47:242–247.

16. Borowiec JW, Rozdayi M, Jaramillo A, et al. Influence of two blood conservation techniques (cardiotomy reservoir versus cell saver) on biocompatibility of the heparin coated cardiopulmonary bypass circuit during coronary revascularization surgery. *J Card Surg* 1997;12:190–197.

17. Aldea GS, Dorsourian M, O'Gora P, et al. Heparin-bonded circuits with a reduced anticoagulation protocol in primary CABG: a prospective randomized study. *Ann Thorac Surg* 1996;62:410–418.

18. Arom KV, Ellestad C, Grover FL, et al. Objective evaluation of the efficacy of various venous cannulas. *J Thorac Cardiovasc Surg* 1981;81:464–469.

19. Bennett EV Jr, Fewel JG, Ybarra J, et al. Comparison of flow differences among venous cannulas. *Ann Thorac Surg* 1983;36:59–65.

20. Baile EM, Ling IT, Heyworth JR, et al. Bronchopulmonary anastomotic and noncoronary collateral blood flow in humans during cardiopulmonary bypass. *Chest* 1985;87:749–754.

21. Killen DA, Piehler JM, Borkon AM, et al. Occult patent ductus arteriosus encountered during coronary artery bypass procedures [Letter]. *J Thorac Cardiovasc Surg* 1994;108:588–589.

22. Tunick PA, Kronzon I. Diagnoses of patent ductus arteriosus by serendipity in the adult. *J Am Soc Echocardiogr* 1988;1:446–449.

23. Amir IM, Mardnets I, Barash P. Transesophageal echocardiography of the distal aortic arch. *J Cardiothorac Vasc Anesth* 1998;12:599–603.

24. Arom KV, Vinas JF, Fewel JE, et al. Is a left ventricular vent necessary during cardiopulmonary bypass? *Ann Thorac Surg* 1977;24:566–573.

25. Burton NA, Graeber GM, Zajtchuk R. An alternate method of ventricular venting-the pulmonary artery sump. *Chest* 1984;85:814–815.

26. Breyer RH, Meredity JW, Mills SA, et al. Is a left ventricular vent necessary for coronary artery bypass procedures performed with cardioplegic arrest? *J Thorac Cardiovasc Surg* 1983;86:338–349.

27. Buckberg GD. The importance of venting the left ventricle [Editorial]. *Ann Thorac Surg* 1975;20:488–490.

28. Najafi H, Javid H, Golding MD, et al. Aortic valve replacement without left heart decompression. *Ann Thorac Surg* 1976;21:131–133.

29. Salerno TA, Charrette EJP. Elimination of venting in coronary artery surgery. *Ann Thorac Surg* 1979;27:340–343.

30. Kanter KR, Schaff HV, Gott VL. Reduced oxygen consumption with effective left ventricular venting during postischemic reperfusion. *Circulation* 1982;66[Suppl I]:I-50–I-54.

31. Olinger GN, Bonchek LI. Ventricular venting during coronary revascularization: assessment of benefit by intraoperative ventricular function curves. *Ann Thorac Surg* 1978;26:525–534.

32. Salomon NW, Copeland JG. Single catheter technique for cardioplegia and venting during coronary artery bypass grafting. *Ann Thorac Surg* 1980;30:88–89.

33. Miller DW, Ivey TD, Bailey WW, et al. The practice of coronary artery bypass surgery in 1980. *J Thorac Cardiovasc Surg* 1981;81:423–427.

34. Hammon JW, Stump DA, Hines M, et al. Prevention of embolic events during coronary artery bypass graft surgery. *Perfusion* 1994;9:412–413(abst).

35. Little AG, Lin CY, Wernley JA, et al. Use of the pulmonary artery for left ventricular venting during cardiac operations. *J Thorac Cardiovasc Surg* 1984;87:532–538.

36. Roach GW, Bellows WH. Left ventricular distension during pulmonary artery venting in a patient undergoing coronary artery bypass surgery. *Anesthesiology* 1992;76:655–658.

37. Daily PO, Kinney T, Steinke TA. Pulmonary vein clamping during cardiopulmonary bypass: enhancement of operative field visualization and myocardial hypothermia. *Ann Thorac Surg* 1987;43:388–340.

38. Schneider B, Conti VR, Kurusz M. A cardioplegia and left heart venting technique for coronary artery bypass grafting. *Ann Thorac Surg* 1983;36:105–106.

39. Lundy EF, Gassmann CJ, Bonchek LI, et al. A simple and safe technique of left ventricular venting. *Ann Thorac Surg* 1992;53:1127–1129.

40. Casha AR. A simple method of aortic root venting for CABG [Letter]. *Ann Thorac Surg* 1998;66:608–609.

41. Victor S, Kabeer M. Venting and de-airing without a roller pump [Letter]. *Ann Thorac Surg* 1993;55:807.

42. Utley JR, Stephens DB. Venting during cardiopulmonary bypass. In: Utley JR, ed. *Pathophysiology and techniques of cardiopulmonary bypass.* Baltimore: Williams & Wilkins, 1983:115–127.

43. Robicsek F, Duncan GD. Retrograde air embolization in coronary operations. *J Thorac Cardiovasc Surg* 1987;94:110–114.

44. Hill AG, Lefrak EA. Cardiopulmonary bypass safety devices and techniques. *Proc Am Acad Cardiovasc Perfus* 1985;6:38–42.

45. Weesner KM, Byrum C, Rosenthal A. Left ventricular aneurysms associated with intraoperative venting of the cardiac apex in children. *Am Heart J* 1981;101:622–625.

46. Marco JD, Barner HB. Aortic venting: comparison of vent effectiveness. *J Thorac Cardiovasc Surg* 1977;73:287–292.

47. Brenner WI, Wallsh E, Spencer FC. Aortic vent efficiency: a quantitative evaluation. *J Thorac Cardiovasc Surg* 1971;61:258–264.

48. Milsom FP, Mitchell SJ. A dual-vent left heart deairing technique markedly reduces carotid artery micro emboli. *Ann Thorac Surg* 1998;66:785–791.

49. Gundry SR. Facile left ventricular de-airing by administration of cardioplegia into the left ventricular vent. *Ann Thorac Surg* 1998;66:2117–2118.

HEMOFILTRATION, DIALYSIS, AND BLOOD SALVAGE TECHNIQUES DURING CARDIOPULMONARY BYPASS

ROGER A. MOORE
GLENN W. LAUB

ULTRAFILTRATION

Historic Perspective

The concept of removing excess fluid from the intravascular space of patients in renal failure by the filtration of blood through an ultraporous membrane dates back to 1928 (1). However, the clinical application of ultrafiltration technology did not occur until the 1950s (2) and 1960s (3), when filtering devices were developed for the effective removal of edema fluid in overhydrated patients with renal impairment. During the 1970s, there was a refinement of ultrafiltration techniques (4,5) and the first use of this technology as part of an open heart surgical procedure (6). The use of ultrafiltration during open heart surgery was initially restricted to the severely hemodiluted patient as a method for concentrating blood remaining in the extracorporeal circuit after cardiopulmonary bypass (CPB). Ultrafiltration under these circumstances was found to be efficacious in reducing hemodilution and producing higher postoperative hemoglobins. However, by 1979 the application of ultrafiltration techniques with extracorporeal circulation was extended to use during the bypass period, though this specific application was initially limited to patients with compromised renal function (7). For these patients, ultrafiltration was chosen as an alternative to hemodialysis for managing fluid homeostasis.

In the 1980s, the use of ultrafiltration during open heart surgery spread from isolated academic centers into general clinical practice. The primary impetus that initially led to the more widespread use of ultrafiltration was the recognition that patients in renal failure could undergo open heart surgery safely. Ultrafiltration provided a simple easy method

for allowing volume control in these patients (8,9). After the initial use in patients with renal failure, ultrafiltration was secondarily recognized as an excellent method for concentrating hemodiluted blood in normal patients who had been overhydrated (10–13). Further use of ultrafiltration devices finally led to the realization that not only was volume control possible, but ultrafiltration also served as an effective method for blood conservation through the preservation of platelets and coagulation factors (14–17).

In the 1990s, the list of indications and advantages for the use of ultrafiltration continued to grow. A much greater role was assigned to ultrafiltration use in reducing post-CPB inflammatory responses and immunologic activation (8–24). The decrease in complement activation and inflammatory response with ultrafiltration was associated with improvements in postoperative pulmonary (20,25–27), cardiac (28–32), and neurologic (33) function. Ultrafiltration provided the additional benefit of moderating temperature elevations in the postoperative period due to removal of circulating pyrogens (20,34,35).

At present, ultrafiltration techniques have numerous advantageous applications, both during and after CPB. Benefits from the use of ultrafiltration can be obtained for nearly any patient undergoing extracorporeal circulation.

Basic Physiologic Principles

The primary principle governing ultrafiltration is the selective separation of plasma water and low-molecular-weight solutes from the intravascular cellular components and plasma proteins of blood, using a semipermeable membrane filter. Unlike hemodialysis, the ultrafiltration technique is simplified by eliminating the requirement for a dialysate solution. Rather than solute osmotic pressure, the driving force for ultrafiltration is provided by the hydrostatic pressure differential occurring across the ultrafiltration membrane (Fig. 7.1). The application of a negative pressure on the effluent side of the membrane or the use of an increased

R. A. Moore: Anesthesia Department, Deborah Heart & Lung Center, Moorestown, NJ 08057.

G. W. Laub: The Heart Hospital, St. Francis Medical Center, Trenton, NJ 08629–1986.

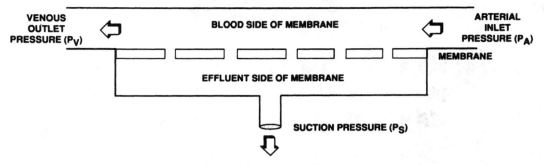

FIG. 7.1. Ultrafiltration of free water and solutes across a semipermeable membrane occurs because of a combination of the blood pressure differential across the filter—the mean of the arterial inlet pressure (P_A) and the venous outlet pressure (P_V)—and any vacuum pressure placed on the effluent side of the membrane (P_S). The combination of these pressures is equal to the transmembrane pressure, which is the primary factor determining filtration rate.

perfusion pressure applied to the blood site of the membrane results in improved solute and fluid filtration. The relationship between these pressures can be expressed by

$$\text{TMP} = \frac{P_A + P_V}{2} + P_S$$

where TMP is the transmembrane pressure gradient, which is the ultimate determinant of filtration rate; P_A is the arterial or inlet blood pressure into the ultrafilter (in mm Hg); P_V is the venous or outlet blood pressure from the ultrafiltration device (in mm Hg); and P_S is the amount of negative pressure applied to the effluent side of the ultrafiltration membrane (in mm Hg). The arterial to venous pressure difference is usually less than 100 mm Hg under normal circumstances; this fall in blood pressure is due primarily to the inherent resistance in the ultrafilter as blood flows through the filtering system. However, the arterial to venous blood pressure difference can also be affected by a variety of other variables, such as the hemoglobin, temperature, and rate of blood flow through the filter.

The range of transmembrane pressures for the normal function of any given ultrafiltration device varies, based on the manufacturer's specifications. However, transmembrane pressures in the range of 100 to 500 mm Hg are typically suggested. At equal hemoglobin levels, the resistance to blood flow through a filter is disproportionately greater when low flow is used as opposed to high flow circumstances (36). The reason for this is a basic rheologic flow dynamic principle, whereby the viscosity of blood under high shear circumstances (high flows) will be lower than in low flow conditions (37,38). Another important principle is that the cooling of blood leads to striking increases in viscosity, which in turn can increase the resistance of blood flow through the ultrafilter (Fig. 7.2) (38). Finally, the presence of high levels of serum protein is also a factor causing an increase in the arteriovenous transfilter pressure differential.

A variety of manufacturers produces ultrafiltration de-

vices and each device varies as to its efficacy in producing ultrafiltration. This efficacy can be expressed as an ultrafiltration coefficient that is intrinsic to each device. The typical ultrafiltration membrane consists of a thin membrane skin that serves as the primary microfilter placed over a thicker more porous substructure. Important characteristics in determining the ultrafiltration coefficient include the diameter of the pores in the membrane through which fluid and solutes will pass, the total number of pores on the membrane surface, and the length of the pores (membrane thickness) through which the solutes and fluids must pass. The ultrafiltration coefficient (U_C) is directly related to the efficiency of the ultrafiltration device's ability to remove fluid (Q_F):

$$Q_F = U_C \times (\text{TMP} - I_P)$$

where I_P is the protein oncotic pressure in the blood and

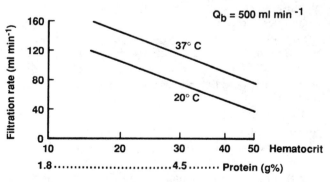

FIG. 7.2. The filtration rate of an ultrafiltration device depends on multiple factors. At a constant flow, decreases in filtration rate are observed at higher hematocrits, higher serum protein levels, and lower temperatures. Q_b, or blood flow in this representation, is kept constant at 500 mL/min. (From Wheeldon DR, Bethune DW. Blood conservation during cardiopulmonary bypass—autologous transfusion, cell saving and hemofiltration. In: Taylor KM, ed. *Cardiopulmonary bypass*. Baltimore: Williams & Wilkins, 1986:301, with permission.)

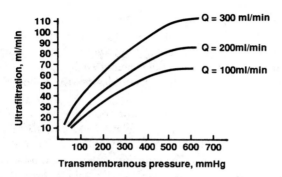

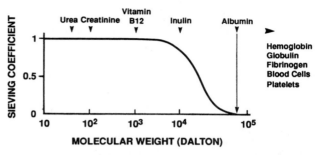

FIG. 7.3. A relatively linear relationship exists between the transmembrane pressure and the ultrafiltration rate. Note that as the blood flow increases through the filter, the slope of the ultrafiltration to transmembrane pressure relationship becomes steeper. This is a result of more rapid removal of accumulated proteins on the membrane surface. Q represents blood flow through the ultrafiltering device. (Adapted from Darup J, Bleese N, Kalmar P, et al. Hemofiltration during extracorporeal circulation. *Thorac Cardiovasc Surg* 1979;27:227, with permission.)

FIG. 7.4. The sieving coefficient is a measure of the efficiency of an ultrafiltration device to remove a soluble molecule from the blood. The sieving coefficient is directly related to molecular size. Molecules with molecular masses below 11,000 Da have a coefficient of 1, indicating that they are filtered at the same concentration as they exist in the blood. Large molecules that will not pass through the pores have a sieving coefficient of 0. (Adapted from Solem JO, Tengborn L, Steen S, et al. Cell saver versus hemofilter for concentration of oxygenator blood after cardiopulmonary bypass. *Thorac Cardiovasc Surg* 1987;35:46, with permission.)

TMP is the transmembrane pressure. The higher the serum protein concentration, the slower the filtration rate. On the other hand, the higher the transmembrane pressure, the faster the filtration rate.

Aside from differences in ultrafiltration rate due to variations in the membrane structure, the hemoglobin concentration, and the fluid temperature, fluid removal through the membrane is primarily determined by the transmembrane pressure. Absolute ultrafiltration can be increased by providing either an increase in perfusion pressure into the filter, by partially clamping the blood flow tubing from the filter thereby increasing outlet pressure, or by increasing the vacuum on the effluent side of the membrane. Typically, a relatively linear relationship exists between the transmembrane pressure and the ultrafiltration rate (Fig. 7.3). When the membrane limit is reached, a plateauing of filtration occurs. The plateau is a function of both the number of pores available for filtration and the accumulation of serum proteins on the membrane surface that occlude the ultrafiltration pores (7). By increasing the blood flow rate through the filter, the slope of the ultrafiltration curve can be increased (Fig. 7.3). The reason for this observed improvement in filtration at higher flow rates is a more rapid removal of the accumulated proteins on the membrane surface that obstruct fluid flow through the pores (7). The higher the protein content of the plasma, the greater this blood flow effect.

Membrane pore size is important for determining what soluble plasma molecules will be removed with the plasma fluid. The pore size normally ranges between 10 and 35 Å, allowing molecules up to 20,000 Da to undergo ultrafiltration. The efficiency of an ultrafiltration device to remove a soluble molecule is called the sieving coefficient and is

directly related to molecular size (Fig. 7.4) (14). The larger the molecular size of a filtered substance, the less efficient the ultrafiltration device will be in its removal. Small molecules with molecular weight below 10,000 Da, such as sodium, potassium, chloride, urea, creatinine and glucose, have a sieving coefficient of 1, meaning they are filtered at a rate equal to their concentration in the plasma. Large molecules, such as albumin (69,000 Da), hemoglobin (68,000 Da), and fibrinogen (341,000 Da) and the cellular components of blood (leukocytes, platelets, and red blood cells) are too large to traverse the pores and therefore remain within the blood. The result is a higher blood concentration of the nonfiltered elements after a period of ultrafiltration.

Of interest, the heparin molecule, which is a mucopolysaccharide between 6,000 and 25,000 Da (39,40) should be expected to be removed during ultrafiltration (41). Because of this, intensified anticoagulation monitoring has been suggested when ultrafiltration is used in conjunction with extracorporeal circulatory techniques (13). However, one investigator has found that no additional heparin supplementation is required, even when volumes as great as 15 L are removed during CPB (11). In fact, recent evidence suggests that ultrafiltration actually leads to heparin concentration within the patient rather than heparin loss (42,43). This is an unexpected observation considering the relatively small size of the heparin molecule. One hypothesis for the concentrating effect of ultrafiltration on heparin is the presence of many negative charges on the heparin molecule that promote interaction of the heparin molecule with serum proteins (42,44). The binding of the heparin molecule to proteins may inhibit its ability to be filtered. Because the effect of ultrafiltration on heparin concentration is not totally predictable, a possible concentrating effect must be anticipated when reinfusing blood that has undergone ultrafiltration from the CPB circuit (42).

Ultrafiltration may also reduce serum levels of anesthetic agents (20,45). Specifically, midazolam and alfentanil concentrations in the plasma have been noted to decrease when zero-balance ultrafiltration (when total volume is kept constant by adding fluids to compensate for ultrafiltered volume) is used (46). However, the decrease in anesthetic levels observed were not in a range that was clinically significant. Maintenance of the anesthetic concentrations within the therapeutic range may be due to protein binding of these drugs, which impedes the filtration process (46). Further determination of ultrafiltration effects on a variety of hypnotic, analgesic, and paralytic agents is necessary. Of equal concern is the effect of ultrafiltration on the medications the patient is being provided for other therapeutic purposes. For instance, the aprotinin molecule has been shown to be removed with ultrafiltration (44). Pharmacologic agents with low molecular weights, which the patient requires for physiologic stability, may have increased clearance from the plasma and therefore may require supplementation when ultrafiltration is used.

Technical Concerns

Historically, ultrafiltration devices have either been developed as parallel membrane sheets, requiring a bulky mechanical framework for their support, or as hollow membrane fibers that are internally supported. The hollow-fiber construction, because of its less bulky nature, simplicity of use, and requirement for smaller priming volume, has be-

come the most practical and widely used type of device for ultrafiltration. Hollow-fiber filters are composed of thousands of hollow polysulfone, polyacrylonitrite, or cellulose acetate fibers, with each fiber having an internal diameter of approximately 200 μm. Examples of two hollow-fiber devices are shown in Figure 7.5.

The placement of the ultrafiltration device within the extracorporeal circuit will partially depend on whether the decision to use ultrafiltration is made before or after the institution of CPB and whether a membrane or bubble oxygenator is to be used in the extracorporeal circuitry. In the event that the use of ultrafiltration is decided on before the initiation of CPB, the inlet tubing leading to the ultrafiltering device can be placed as a branch connection from the arterial line filter with both membrane and bubble oxygenators (Fig. 7.6). The outflow from the ultrafiltering device is returned to the cardiotomy reservoir with both oxygenators. A separate graduated collection container is attached to the effluent side of the filter for collection of ultrafiltration fluids and solutes for eventual measurement and disposal. The collection container for the fluids and solutes is placed on a variable pressure vacuum line allowing the adjustment of suction pressure. The advantage of this approach is that a single arterial pump head is used to perfuse the patient and the filter. The primary disadvantage of using a single pump head is that when blood flow to the patient is varied, the blood flow to the ultrafiltering device is varied. Also, pump head flow rates should be increased to compensate for flow that is diverted from the patient

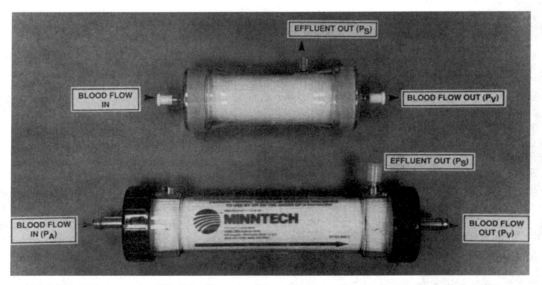

FIG. 7.5. Two examples of hollow-fiber ultrafilters. The upper filter is the Diafilter-20 Hemofilter (Amicon), which has a overall unit length of 17.5 cm, a membrane area of 0.25 m², a priming blood volume of 20 mL, and a hemoconcentrating rate of 10 to 110 mL/min. The lower ultrafilter is the Hemocor Plus 950 Hemoconcentrator (Minntech). This unit's overall length is 21.5 cm, the membrane area is 0.95 m², the priming volume is 70 mL, the hemoconcentrating rate is 30 to 113 mL/min, and the molecular mass cutoff is 17,000 Da.

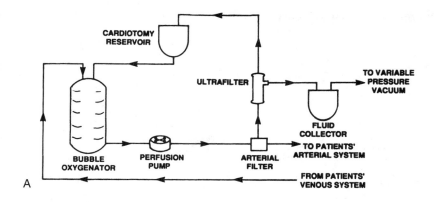

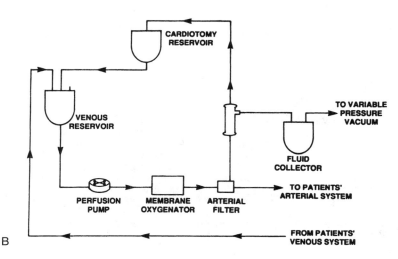

FIG. 7.6. If the use of an ultrafilter is decided on before the initiation of cardiopulmonary bypass and a bubble oxygenator is used, a branch connector from the arterial line filter is the easiest method for establishing ultrafiltration **(A)**. With the use of a membrane oxygenator, a branch connection from the arterial line filter can also be used effectively, with return of the filtered blood to the cardiotomy reservoir **(B)**. The effluent outlet in both cases is connected to a variable pressure vacuum.

to the ultrafilter. The postbypass concentration of residual pump blood can be accomplished by clamping the arterial tubing distal to the side branch of the arterial filter leading to the patient and simply recirculating blood through the ultrafilter device (10). A simplification of a CPB circuit containing a membrane oxygenator with hemofiltration function has been developed (47). A silicone-coated hollow-fiber membrane allows gas exchange at a 312-mL/min oxygen transfer rate using a blood flow of 6 L/min. The membrane is also able to provide an ultrafiltration rate of 3.5 L/hr at a blood flow rate of 4 L/min (47). Continued modification and improvements in oxygenators may in the future allow inexpensive use of dual oxygenation and ultrafiltration functions for all CPB circuits.

If use of the ultrafilter is decided on after the institution of CPB and a bubble oxygenator is being used, an acceptable alternative for providing blood flow to the ultrafilter is to run tubing through an extra pump head from the coronary arterial port of the bubble oxygenator directly to the ultrafilter. In this situation, the separate dedicated pump head provides the needed blood flow through the ultrafilter (Fig.

7.7A). Ultrafiltered blood will be returned to the pump oxygenator via the cardiotomy reservoir. In the case of a membrane oxygenator, when an ultrafilter is decided on after the initiation of bypass, the simplest method is to establish a branch from the recirculation tubing directly to the ultrafilter (Fig. 7.7B). Because the same pump head is being used both for patient perfusion and ultrafilter perfusion, the pump speed should be increased to compensate for lost patient perfusion through the ultrafilter. With all these approaches, ultrafiltration can be increased with partial cross-clamping of the ultrafilter venous outlet or with the initiation of suction on the effluent side of the ultrafilter membrane (48,49).

Ultrafiltration methodology is increasingly being categorized by the timing and technique used in the ultrafiltration process. *Modified ultrafiltration* refers to the use of ultrafiltration after separation from CPB when blood is pumped retrograde from the aortic cannula through the hemoconcentrator and returned to the right atrium (23). *Conventional ultrafiltration* is performed on CPB, usually during the rewarming phase, and the volume removed is based on

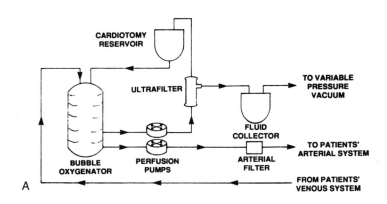

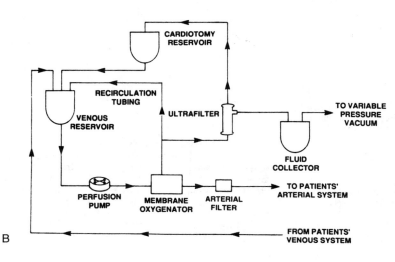

FIG. 7.7. If the use of an ultrafilter is decided on after the institution of cardiopulmonary bypass and a bubble oxygenator is used, a separate dedicated pump head can be used to direct blood from the coronary arterial port of the oxygenator into the ultrafilter **(A)**. In the case of a membrane oxygenator **(B)**, blood flow to the ultrafilter can be established by using a branch connector from the recirculation tubing. In this situation, the perfusion pump flow should be increased to compensate for perfusion that is redirected from the patient into the ultrafilter.

the volume within the CPB circuit (23). *High volume zero-balance ultrafiltration* is a modification of conventional ultrafiltration during which the ultrafiltration volume removed is replaced with an equal volume of crystalloid. Further modification of these techniques will continue to expand the ultrafiltration nomenclature.

Indications for Use of Ultrafiltration During Open Heart Surgery

Ultrafiltration has a growing list of acceptable therapeutic uses and clinical indications for patients undergoing CPB.

Free Water Removal in Patients with Compromised Renal Function Undergoing Open Heart Surgery

From its inception, hemofiltration has been recognized as a rapid and efficient method for managing fluid overload in patients with renal failure (48,50,51). The first clinical report of ultrafiltration use during open heart surgery for volume management occurred in 1979 by Darup et al. (7). Effective control of excess fluid during CPB in the 10 pa-

tients studied resulted in minimal postoperative weight gain. After their initial report, the efficacy of hemofiltration in the management of volume and electrolytes, in both pediatric (9) and adult (8,11,13,17) patients having open heart surgery and presenting with renal failure, has been substantiated. Because the patient in renal failure undergoing CPB is unable to concentrate hemodiluted intravascular volume through renal mechanisms, ultrafiltration serves as a useful method for reducing hemodilution secondary to excess pump prime, unscavenged cardioplegic solution, and preexisting volume overload. Ultrafiltration also has minimal adverse effects on hemostasis (15,52) and red blood cell integrity in these patients (11,53). These advantages become particularly important when long-term hemofiltration (continuous slow ultrafiltration) is performed after open heart surgery in pediatric (9) and adult patients (54) treated for acute renal failure.

Free Water Removal in Patients with Normal Renal Function Undergoing Open Heart Surgery

Extensive hemodilution can occur in any patient during CPB due to a combination of pump prime dilution, crystalloid cardioplegia return into the pump, and prebypass fluid loading. Hemodilution during CPB has been related to postoperative increases in the extravascular water of the lungs (12) and other organs. The use of hemofiltration during CPB to remove free water from the intravascular space has been found to be efficacious in reducing extravascular water accumulation (10,12,55). The reduction of extravascular water is due to a combination of excess intravascular free water removal and an increase in intravascular colloid osmotic pressure (49,56). Hemofiltration has repeatedly been shown to be an effective adjunct to CPB, as a mechanism for oxygenator volume control (41,57,58). At present, recommendations for the use of ultrafiltration extend from limiting this modality to only those patients with prolonged periods on bypass (longer than 2 hours) or preoperative evidence of excessive body water (edema) (10) all the way up to routinely using ultrafiltration during any open heart surgical procedure (17,52).

Preservation of Hemostasis

An important indication for hemofiltration is providing a means of hemoconcentration while preserving intravascular coagulation factors and platelets. Whether ultrafiltration is used during or after extracorporeal circulation is not of importance, because preservation of hemostasis (14–16) and reduction in blood product requirements (14) occur in either case. In one study of 100 patients undergoing ultrafiltration after CPB, platelet counts rose by 57%, fibrinogen by 102%, hemoglobin by 85%, and albumin by 91% (49). Other studies support the observation that ultrafiltration leads to significant increases in hemoglobin and hematocrit (42,59–61) and many hemostatic-promoting factors. The concentration of hemostatic-promoting factors translates clinically into less postoperative blood loss (19–21,59, 62–64). However, the relationship between reduced postoperative blood loss and the use of ultrafiltration is not simply due to a concentration of procoagulant factors (20). Rather it is a complex interplay between the concentration of hemostatic factors, the lowering of cytokine levels, and the alterations in both the hemostatic promoting processes (65,66) and fibrinolysis (67). More intuitive, the ability of ultrafiltration to concentrate and preserve both platelets and clotting factors provides for better postoperative hemostasis than techniques of cell washing, where platelets and coagulation factors are discarded (14–16,52,68).

Alteration of Immune Function

CPB is a strong mediator for inducing the inflammatory cascade. Dysfunction in the immune system is expressed in the postbypass period by significant alterations and compromise of end-organ function (8). The kidneys, brain, lungs, and the heart are all adversely affected by the exaggerated inflammatory response that characterizes the post-CPB period. Complement activation and the release of cytokine and chemokines during CPB lead to significant increases in serum concentrations of neutrophils, endotoxins, and elastases (18,20,23).

Ultrafiltration with the removal of proinflammatory mediators might be expected to have a positive clinical effect (20). In fact, ultrafiltration has been found to immediately reduce serum concentrations of tissue necrosis factor, complement fragment 3a, and myeloperoxidase. By 24 hours after ultrafiltration, the proinflammatory cytokines, interleukin-1 and interleukin-6 and the neutrophil chemoattractant called interleukin-8, the neutrophil counts, and the myeloperoxidase levels (a marker of neutrophil degranulation) are all decreased compared with patients who did not receive ultrafiltration (20). However, hemofiltration by itself can also be an inducer of the inflammatory reaction, but polyacrylonitrile filters induce less complement activation than cuprophane filters (69,70).

The removal of activated complement fragment 3a with ultrafiltration is not unexpected because it is a hydrophilic low-molecular-weight molecule. However, interleukin-8 is not cleared as well because of significant red blood cell binding (19,21,22). Bradykinin levels are also decreased using ultrafiltration (24). The bypass circuit leads to the generation of large amounts of bradykinin through consumption of factor XII, prekallikrein, and high-molecular-weight kininogen. Decreasing bradykinin levels might have a beneficial clinical effect by reducing the potent vasodilation and microvascular permeability induced by bradykinin (24).

Postoperative fever after CPB is most likely the result of endogenous pyrogen release from increased cytokine levels. Endogenous pyrogens, such as interleukin-1, interleukin-6, and interleukin-8 (34,35) are lowered with ultrafiltration. Improvements in postoperative temperature management in patients receiving ultrafiltration may simply be a function of endogenous pyrogen removal (20).

Serum elastase levels, along with other serum proteins, are elevated after hemofiltration (15). Elastase, which is released from activated polymorphonuclear leukocytes during extracorporeal circulation, may have a role in producing postoperative pulmonary dysfunction (71). However, the increase in elastase levels observed after open heart surgery, when hemofiltration is used, is transient. Within 5 hours after CPB, the elastase levels are undistinguishable from patients not receiving ultrafiltration (15).

A potentially adverse effect of ultrafiltration on the immune system is the removal of interleukin-10. Interleukin-10 serves to inhibit the release of tissue necrosis factor and interleukin-8, which are inducers of the inflammatory response (18,20). Therefore, ultrafiltration may serve to not only remove adverse circulating proinflammatory agents from the serum but also protective agents. The modulation of both positive and negative actions on the immunologic response with use of ultrafiltration points out the complex nature of attempts in quantitating the exact immunologic outcome when ultrafiltration is used.

End-Organ Effects

Although directly related to the immunologic response, ultrafiltration can provide significant improvements in end-organ integrity.

Pulmonary

Neutrophil adhesion to pulmonary vascular endothelium and neutrophil sequestration are augmented in the presence of complement fragment 3a deposits (19). The removal of C3a with ultrafiltration during operations on congenital heart patients produces a reduction in postoperative pulmonary vascular resistance and reduces the need for intensive postoperative ventilatory support (20,72). Improved clinical outcomes with ultrafiltration include faster extubation times and improved postoperative arterial-alveolar oxygen differences (20). In addition, ultrafiltration may have a beneficial effect on pulmonary function unrelated to moderating the inflammatory response. In particular, lung water reduction with ultrafiltration leads to an increase in postbypass dynamic pulmonary compliance (27,73). A decrease in mean airway pressure and improvements in total pulmonary status are the result.

Cardiac

Use of ultrafiltration has been related to improved post-CPB hemodynamic function, including lower heart rate, increased systolic pressure, higher cardiac index, and reduced pulmonary vascular resistance (28,31). Improvements in diastolic compliance can also be realized by a decreased myocardial cross-sectional area, an increase in end-diastolic length, and a decrease in end-diastolic pressure (29,30). The improved hemodynamics may be directly related to a decrease in the myocardial inflammatory response, leading to a decrease in myocardial edema and improved left ventricular compliance (73).

Renal

The vascular endothelium of the renal tissue reacts in a manner similar to pulmonary tissue to proinflammatory agents (19). Interleukin-1, tissue necrosis factor, and interleukin-8 are proinflammatory agents that induce leukocyte adhesion to endothelial cells, thereby obstructing intravascular blood flow and initiating the inflammatory sequence. In one study, evaluating patients with severe heart failure refractory to inotropic support and with associated reduced renal function, early institution of continuous hemofiltration before institution of CPB led to a significant reversal of cardiac dysfunction and restoration of renal function (72). The improvements were considered to be the result of removing toxic metabolites, although the specific toxic metabolites were not identified.

Brain

Use of modified ultrafiltration after deep hypothermic circulatory arrest has been related to improved postoperative brain function (73). Ultrafiltration leads to a decrease in cerebral edema, which may be a reflection of the decreased total body water, which in turn improves the cerebral oxygen delivery and the cerebral metabolic rate of oxygen consumption (33). Of course, removal of immunologically related mediators of leukocyte activation may also play a role (23).

Contraindications

At present, no absolute contraindication exists for the use of ultrafiltration during or after open heart surgery. Theoretically, the passage of blood through a filtering system might lead to an increase in red blood cell damage. However, significant increases in the serum free hemoglobin concentration in patients undergoing ultrafiltration have not been observed (52,53). As indicated previously, another potential concern is the activation of complement and the sequestration of leukocytes in the pulmonary circuit (71). Significant immunologic reactivity has been described when the material used in the ultrafilter construction includes cuprophane or cellulose acetate, whereas membranes made from polyacrylonitrite or polysulfone seem to have less immunologic reactivity. Despite this potential for reactivity with the immunologic system, the occurrence of hypersensitivity reactions during or after ultrafiltration is extremely rare and the use of ultrafiltration in association with CPB seems to have a more beneficial than damaging effect on the immune response of the body (12). Ultrafiltration is also a valuable method for removing excess plasma water during CPB and may well lead to an improvement in the general postoperative state of the patient. The primary consideration arguing against the use of ultrafiltration would be the extra cost in providing this intervention (74). The use of ultrafiltration is safe, and the slight theoretic concerns associated with its use are heavily outweighed by its proven value in reducing intravascular volume, preserving postoperative hemostasis, and improving postoperative end-organ function.

HEMODIALYSIS

Historical Perspective

The first apparatus used for hemodialysis (described as "vividiffusion") was constructed in 1913 and used to treat uremic animals (75). It was composed of parallel rows of semipermeable celloidin tubes through which blood flowed, whereas a saline solution was infused outside the tubes for removal of diffusible impurities. Anticoagulation was imperfectly provided using hirudin. The clinical application of hemodialysis was delayed until the 1940s, when effective anticoagulation and more efficient dialysis membranes became available. In 1944, with the use of heparin for anticoagulation and cellophane semipermeable membrane tubes, the first clinical use of hemodialysis in a patient was described (76). The patient had end-stage nephritis, and the use of dialysis provided periodic improvement during her 12-day hospital stay. On the 12th day, the inability to provide dialysis due to arterial access difficulties led to the patient succumbing to her disease process. Over the next 15 years, continued improvement occurred in the design and materials used in dialyzing units (77–79). The primary objective was to develop a dialyzer that was disposable, had a small blood volume capacity (low blood priming volume), showed high dialysis efficiency, was simple to set up, was safe to use, and was economic in both the personnel needed to run the dialyzer and the equipment needed to provide dialysis.

In 1970, an animal experiment was performed, predating clinical consideration of the intraoperative use of hemodialysis, using a dialyzer in conjunction with extracorporeal cardiac and pulmonary support. This experiment showed that dialysis in conjunction with extracorporeal circulation could be used efficaciously (80). Also during the 1970s, the concept of offering open heart surgery to patients in chronic renal failure began to develop. Patients on hemodialysis were known to be at increased risk for developing advanced atherosclerotic heart disease (81–83). Mortality rates from heart disease in the hemodialysis patient were five times greater than in patients having hypertension without known renal disease (82). The causes for the accelerated atherosclerosis in these patients were believed to be related to multiple factors, including a high incidence of hypertensive disease, comparatively greater sustained cardiac output due to anemia, hypertriglyceridemia, abnormal carbohydrate metabolism, and increased vascular calcification (81,84).

The primary circumstance that eventually brought patients with chronic renal failure into the operating room for open heart surgery was the limited ability to provide hemodialysis to a subset of these patients, secondary to severe anginal symptoms during the dialysis process. In 1974, the first report of coronary artery bypass grafting performed on a patient in chronic renal failure appeared in the literature (85). Soon after this report, numerous descriptions of the successful performance of open heart surgery, despite chronic renal failure, appeared in the literature (84,86–91). The primary point these reports transmitted was that patients in chronic renal failure could have marked improvement in their New York Heart Association functional classification (84,86,91–93) while sustaining acceptably low operative mortality (91–95). Of interest, the long-term risk of death from coronary artery disease did not change for dialysis patients who had undergone coronary artery bypass grafting, when compared with a similar cohort of patients without open heart surgery (93,94,96). Despite actuarial mortality rates being similar, the primary difference remained that patients having undergone open heart surgery had substantial improvement in lifestyle and functional status. It was for this reason that operative intervention for

these patients was considered to be justified. Though operative mortality was low, these patients did have increased postoperative morbidity, as shown by relatively longer periods of intubation and hemodynamic support, and longer stays in the intensive care unit and hospital (95).

The preoperative medical management of patients on chronic hemodialysis undergoing open heart surgery typically included preoperative red blood cell transfusion to hematocrits greater than 30% (83,96) and the provision of hemodialysis for stabilization of electrolytes within 24 hours before the planned surgical procedure (88–90,96). After the operative procedure, hemodialysis was reinstituted either within 24 hours (88,91,97) or within the first few days immediately after surgery, based on the potassium, blood urea nitrogen, and volume status (84,96,98). The primary concern for the early postoperative use of hemodialysis was an increased risk of bleeding because of the requirement for heparinization during the dialysis process. Regional heparinization, which entailed the addition of heparin to blood flowing into the dialyzer and protamine reversal of blood leaving the dialyzer, was one method used to alleviate this problem (96,99). One way of delaying immediate postoperative hemodialysis was the provision of dialysis during CPB (100,101). In 1979, the first intraoperative use of hemodialysis during open heart surgery was successfully performed on a patient with severe aortic regurgitation, congestive heart failure, and volume overload unresponsive to daily hemodialysis (100). The use of hemodialysis during CPB in this patient allowed postoperative hemodialysis to be delayed for 3 days. Since this report, other investigators have successfully used hemodialysis during extracorporeal circulation (11,101–103) and during prolonged circulatory support with a left ventricular assist device (104).

Basic Physiologic Principles

Hemodialysis is similar to ultrafiltration in that a semipermeable membrane allows the differential passage of fluid and soluble molecules through pores of about 50 Å. Sodium, calcium, urea, creatinine, and glucose and indoles, phenols, and guanidines that accumulate in uremic patients are able to diffuse through the membrane. Unlike ultrafiltration, which depends solely on differential hydrostatic pressures to provide the driving force for removal of fluid and soluble molecules, hemodialysis also depends on the concentration gradient for solutes existing between the blood and the dialysate. The clearance of a substance from the blood during dialysis is described by

$$CS = \frac{S_A - S_V}{S_A} \times Q_F$$

where CS is the clearance of a substance from blood, S_A is the substance concentration entering the filter, S_V is the substance concentration leaving the filter, and Q_F is the rate of blood flow through the filter.

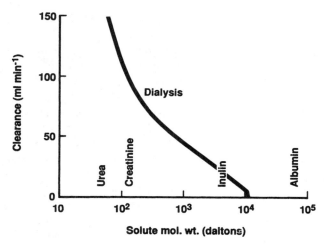

FIG. 7.8. The clearance rate of a solute during dialysis decreases as the molecular weight of the soluble molecule increases. Note the high clearance rate of the small molecule, urea, compared with the poor clearance for the larger molecule, albumin. (Adapted from Hakim M, Wheeldon DW, Bethune BB, et al. Haemodialysis and haemofiltration on cardiopulmonary bypass. *Thorax* 1985;40:101–106, with permission.)

As blood flow through the filter increases, clearance of the substance also increases. Also, as the serum concentration increases, the concentration gradient is greater, allowing better clearance (4). Obviously, clearance presupposes that the molecule being cleared is small enough to pass through the semipermeable membrane. Clearance rates also increase as the molecular weight of the substances decrease (Fig. 7.8) (11,38).

Hemodialysis requires the use of a dialysate, which carries the fluids and solutes removed from the blood away from the semipermeable membrane (Fig. 7.9). The choice of the components constituting the dialysate will, in part, be determined by the concentration of the undesirable substances in the patient's serum. If the patient has an abnormally high serum potassium, a dialysate formula lacking potassium is chosen to maximize potassium clearance. In a similar respect, if fluid overload in the patient exists, the choice of a dialysate with a higher osmotic pressure can be made to maximize free water removal (76). The best use of the concentration difference in the dialyzing apparatus is provided through the use of a countercurrent flow mechanism (Fig. 7.9), where blood flow across the membrane occurs in one direction and dialysate flow occurs in the opposite direction. The concentration of the diffusible substance progressively decreases in the blood as it flows through the filter and encounters dialysate fluid with a progressively lower concentration of the substance. The countercurrent mechanism allows a consistently higher relative diffusion gradient to be maintained throughout the filtering process and is similar to the loop of Henle in the glomerulus (105). Within a certain range, the faster the rate of dialysate flow through the filter, the more effective the solute removal (Fig. 7.10) (79,106).

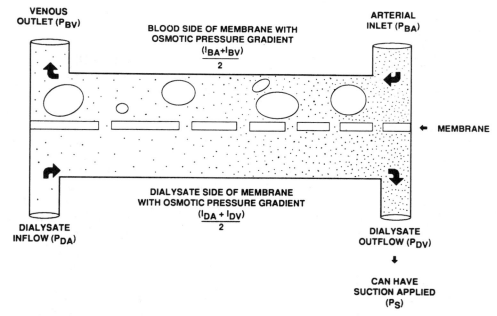

FIG. 7.9. Hemodialysis occurs across a semipermeable membrane. Solutes and fluids leave the blood into the dialysate, as the blood travels from the arterial inlet to the venous outlet. The dialysate carries the solute away and the countercurrent flow of blood and dialysate, as they travel by the semipermeable membrane, serves to increase total solute removal.

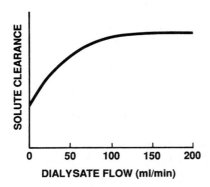

FIG. 7.10. Within the specifications of the membrane, solute clearance is a direct function of dialysate flow. Plateauing of solute clearance with an increase in dialysate flow is related to the membrane coefficient, which is determined by the number, size, and depth of the membrane pores.

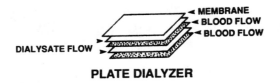

PLATE DIALYZER

COIL DIALYZER

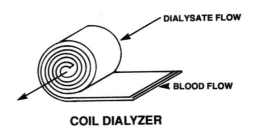

HOLLOW FIBER DIALYZER

FIG. 7.11. Dialyzers have been developed with the objective of providing the greatest blood to dialysate interface across the semipermeable membrane. Three methods for increasing the interface include using layers of parallel plates in the plate dialyzer, coiling the blood—dialysate interface in the coil dialyzer, and multiple small hollow fibers in the hollow-fiber dialyzer.

The semipermeable membrane used in various dialyzers is made from a variety of substances, including cellophane, cellulose acetate, polyacrylonitrite, and polysulfone. These membranes allow high permeability to molecules below 300 Da, and, to a lesser extent, molecules up to 10,000 Da, and high free water movement. The primary determinant for the removal of free water is the hydrostatic and osmotic pressure differentials that exist between the plasma and dialysate compartments of the filter, expressed by

$$TMP = \left(\frac{P_{BA} + P_{BV}}{2}\right) - \left(\frac{P_{DA} + P_{DV}}{2}\right)$$
$$+ \left(\frac{I_{DA} + I_{DV}}{2}\right) - \left(\frac{I_{BA} + I_{BV}}{2}\right) + P_S$$

where TMP is the transmembrane pressure for fluid removal, P_{BA} is the blood pressure at the inlet of the filter, P_{BV} is the blood pressure at the outlet of the filter, P_{DA} is the dialysate inlet pressure, P_{DV} is the dialysate outlet pressure, I_{DA} is the dialysate inlet osmotic pressure, I_{DV} is the dialysate outlet osmotic pressure, I_{BA} is the serum osmotic pressure at the inlet of the filter, I_{BV} is the serum oncotic pressure at the outlet of the filter, and P_s is negative pressure at the dialysate side of the membrane.

Technical Concerns

The membranes of dialyzing devices are typically arranged in one of three basic orientations: parallel plates, coils, or hollow fibers (Fig. 7.11). The objective in each of these designs is to provide the blood flowing through the dialyzer with the greatest possible surface area. Resistance to blood flow is greatest in coil dialyzers, whereas the hollow-fiber dialyzers present the lowest resistance to blood flow because of the short path for blood flow and the thousands of fibers through which the blood can flow. Despite the small cross-sectional internal diameter of each individual hollow fiber

of only 200 μm, which would be expected to have high resistance to blood flow, the 10,000 or more fibers within each filter ensure an overall low resistance to blood flow. The small size, simplicity of use, and high efficiency of hollow-fiber dialyzers make them readily adaptable for intraoperative use during open heart surgery and for continuous arteriovenous hemodialysis postoperatively (104–108). An example of a hollow filter dialyzer is shown in Figure 7.12.

Placement of the dialyzer in the extracorporeal bypass circuitry is similar to the positioning of an ultrafiltration device. A side branch of the arterial line filter, the coronary perfusion port of the oxygenator, or the recirculation line can each serve as adequate access ports for dialyzer attachment. Blood from the dialyzer is returned in each case to the cardiotomy reservoir. Perfusion of the dialyzer with dialysate is usually provided with a separate pump head, though gravitational flow of dialysate can be used with some filters. Dialysate, which has traversed the filter, is collected in a graduated container for measurement of volume before discarding or recirculating through the filter (Fig. 7.13).

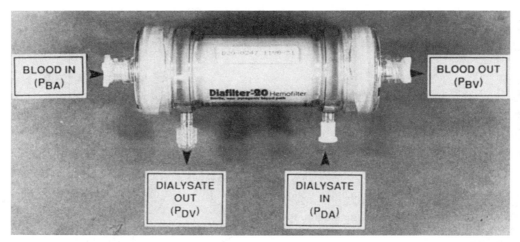

FIG. 7.12. An example of a hollow-fiber dialyzer that shows the countercurrent flow of blood and dialysate is the Diafilter-20 Hemofilter (Amicon). This device can also function as an ultrafilter by eliminating the dialysate and providing effluent removal through the dialysate inlet.

Many patients who have been on chronic hemodialysis will have a surgically placed arteriovenous fistula present in an extremity. Extreme caution must be taken with these patients to protect this shunt from reduced blood flow or pressure occlusion. A blood pressure cuff should not be placed on the arm containing an arteriovenous fistula (97), and that arm should be avoided during the placement of either intravenous or arterial catheters. In fact, avoiding the use of either arm in patients with chronic renal disease has

been suggested to save the arm vessels as future access sites for hemodialysis (90). Of interest, the presence of an arteriovenous fistula has not been related to a decreased venous oxygen saturation in patients undergoing hypothermic CPB at flow rates of 2.2 L/min/m^2 (109). Theoretically, shunting of blood through the fistula could have an adverse effect on systemic oxygenation.

Concern about maintaining adequate heparinization and other drug levels in patients undergoing hemodialysis exists

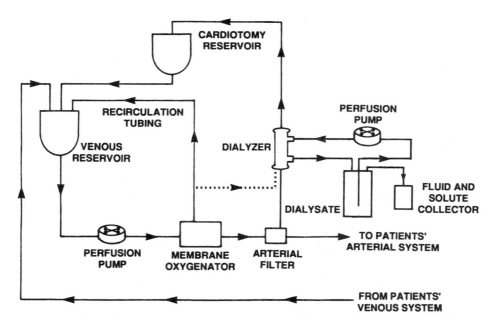

FIG. 7.13. Placement of the dialyzer in the extracorporeal circuit when a membrane oxygenator is used can be accomplished with a side branch from the arterial line filter or from the recirculation tubing. Dialysate flow is provided to the dialyzer with a separate perfusion pump or by gravitational flow.

because of the increased drug clearance occurring during the hemodialysis process. However, these concerns are no greater with hemodialysis than with ultrafiltration techniques (11,13,49).

Indications

Chronic Renal Failure

Some 180,000 patients in the United States receive some form of chronic hemodialysis. Considering the accelerated atherosclerotic disease that occurs in these patients (81–83), it would not be unreasonable to expect that a fairly large percentage might require coronary artery bypass graft surgery at some point in their lives. Normally, the preoperative care of these patients can be adequately managed by providing hemodialysis the day before surgery, followed by postoperative hemodialysis at some point governed by the laboratory findings and the volume status of the patient (88,91,96). However, limitations in the ability to provide adequate preoperative dialysis due to severe anginal symptoms (93,103) or the unexpected intraoperative exposure of the patient to a potassium overload from a massive blood transfusion (103) or poor retrieval of cardioplegic solution (110) may necessitate the intraoperative use of hemodialysis. Simple volume overload is more easily handled with ultrafiltration. However, a more frequent use of intraoperative hemodialysis is advocated by some as a method for avoiding hemodialysis in the 2- to 3-day period after open heart surgery (101). Anticoagulation for hemodialysis soon after surgery may increase the risk for postoperative bleeding. However, excellent control of electrolytes, urea, creatinine, and fluids can be realized (111).

Acute Renal Failure

Renal compromise after the use of extracorporeal circulatory techniques is not uncommon, occurring with a reported incidence of between 1.5% (112) and 5.3% (113,114). Preoperative left ventricular dysfunction (114), preoperative renal compromise (112,114,115), and duration of the surgical procedure (115) have all been related to the development of postoperative acute renal failure. Though the use of pulsatile flow (116,117) and the early institution of low-dose dopamine infusions intraoperatively (118) may reduce the occurrence of postoperative acute renal failure in some patients, these modalities alone are unable to ensure postoperative renal integrity. Patients who develop acute renal failure during extracorporeal circulation can be immediately placed on continuous arteriovenous hemodialysis (104,108). This intervention can be initiated intraoperatively and continued during the patient's intensive care unit stay. Continuous arteriovenous hemodialysis provides more efficient urea and creatinine clearance and the removal of other toxic metabolites compared with ultrafiltration techniques (108). The

early institution of hemodialysis in patients with acute renal failure may have beneficial effects on long-term survival and return of normal renal function.

INTRAOPERATIVE BLOOD SALVAGE TECHNIQUES

Cardiac surgical procedures are a major source of the total amount of blood used for transfusion purposes in the United States (119–122). The propensity for major blood loss during open heart surgical procedures is due to a combination of the extensive intervention involving major vascular structures and the inherent derangement of hemostasis that accompanies the use of extracorporeal circulatory techniques (123–127). The destruction of both red blood cells and coagulation factors during CPB results in an increased need for blood and blood products with these procedures. However, increasing pressure to reduce or eliminate the exposure of patients to blood and blood products exists because of the widespread recognition of the multiple dangers associated with homologous blood transfusion (Table 7.1). These dangers mandate that alternative strategies are used to circumvent the need for homologous blood transfusion.

Two intraoperative strategies developed for reducing homologous blood usage are autologous donation with reinfusion and scavenging of shed blood with reinfusion. The use of these techniques not only reduces the burden that open

TABLE 1. DISADVANTAGES ASSOCIATED WITH HOMOLOGOUS BLOOD USE

Infection transmission
  Human immunodeficiency viruses
  Hepatitis viruses
  Cytomegalovirus
  Syphilis
  Malaria
  African trypanosomiasis
  American filariasis
  Leishmaniasis
  Toxoplasmosis
  Babesiosis
  Bacterial contamination
Incompatibility reactions
  Hemolytic Rh reactions
  Hemolytic ABO reactions
  Graft-versus-host reactions
Febrile reactions
  Leukocyte reaction
  Heat-stable pyrogens
Deficiencies
  2,3-Diphosphoglycerate
  Platelets
  Polymorphonucleocytes (loss of phagocytosis after 48 hr)
  Factors V and VIII (decrease 10–20% in 24 hr)
Limited blood supply

heart surgical procedures place on the limited blood supply but also eliminates the many risks associated with homologous blood transfusion. Intraoperative autologous blood donation during the early phases of the surgical procedure and the intraoperative scavenging of shed blood during surgery both play an important role in reducing homologous blood transfusion requirements.

Autologous Blood Donation

Historical Perspective

Preoperative autologous blood donation for postoperative reinfusion was first successfully reported in 1921 (128) but was not adopted for routine use because of the advances in techniques for homologous blood collection. With the development of cardiovascular surgery and the attendant substantial increases in the demand for homologous blood transfusion, interest in autologous blood donation reappeared. The use of 8 to 12 units of blood during each open heart surgical procedure was not uncommon (121,129). In the early 1970s, as coronary bypass surgery became an accepted surgical intervention, there was concern that the nation's entire blood supply might be consumed by cardiac surgery alone (130). In addition, the complications and risks associated with homologous blood transfusion served as a further stimulus to find alternative methods for avoiding homologous blood transfusions (120,130,131). Early recognition that the best donor for a blood transfusion was the patient gave primary impetus for the development of autologous blood transfusion techniques (132,133). It was known that normal healthy volunteers could be phlebotomized for three to five units of whole blood each week for as many as 23 weeks with maintenance of a stable hemoglobin, as long as iron supplementation was provided (134). Debilitated patients also could tolerate preoperative phlebotomy of up to four units of blood during the 10 days before the planned surgical procedure with maintenance of hemoglobins over 10 g/dL, with supplemental iron (135).

A boost to the concept of preoperative autologous blood collection was provided with the finding that patients readily tolerated hemodilution during CPB without long-term sequelae. From these observations an immediate interest developed for collecting autologous blood preoperatively whenever major intraoperative blood losses could be predicted (136–138). It was not long thereafter that the collection of autologous blood intraoperatively during the planned surgical procedure, using hemodilution techniques, was recommended for reducing homologous blood usage (136,137,139–143).

Intraoperative autologous blood donation not only avoided the risks of homologous blood exposure but, when reinfused, provided the patient with fresh blood that was richer in 2,3-diphosphoglycerate, platelets, and clotting factors than bank blood (144). By the reinfusion of the freshly collected autologous blood, a reduction in total operative blood requirements could be realized (136,137,143,144). The primary method advocated for the intraoperative collection of autologous blood during open heart surgery was its removal before the initiation of CPB through hemodilution (136,137,144,145).

Basic Physiologic Principles

Autologous blood transfusion can be conceptually differentiated into several categories depending on the method and timing of blood collection. If the blood is removed before the operative procedure, it is termed predonation (134,135). The preoperative donation of autologous blood is especially useful for patients with unusual serum antibodies for which a shortage of homologous blood exists. Much more common is the intraoperative collection of autologous blood, either before the institution of CPB or during the very early phases of the bypass process. The donated blood volume is usually replaced with isotonic intravenous fluid, resulting in hemodilution (136,137,144).

Intraoperative autologous blood donation for open heart surgery involves withdrawing several hundred milliliters of blood from the patient and storing it, before exposing the patient's blood to the deleterious effects of the heart—lung machine. Reinfused after termination of CPB, this fresh autologous blood is an excellent oxygen-carrying volume expander, containing a full complement of coagulation factors and platelets. Most cardiac surgical patients are candidates for intraoperative blood donation as long as they meet two important criteria: The patients must be hemodynamically stable and must have sufficient red blood cell mass to maintain adequate oxygen-carrying capacity once hemodilution has occurred. Although the lowest acceptable hematocrit during CPB remains controversial, for most patients a hematocrit of 20% is safe (129,130,146–148). The reduced hemoglobin is offset by the decreased viscosity of the blood, which in turn decreases myocardial work and improves the coronary microcirculation (148–152).

To ensure adequate hemoglobin during bypass, it is essential to calculate what the patient's hemoglobin will be after the dilution occurring with prebypass donation and the dilution from the pump prime in the extracorporeal circuit. The hemoglobin after intraoperative donation can be estimated by

$$Hb_d = Hb_i \left[\frac{V_b - V_d}{V_b} \right]$$

where Hb_d is the hemoglobin after donation, Hb_i is the initial predonation hemoglobin, V_b is the total blood volume, and V_d is volume of blood donated. Typically, the patient's blood volume can be approximated to be between 6% and 8% of the kilogram body weight depending on the age, size, gender, and clinical status of the patient (153–155).

A patient's hemoglobin on bypass (Hb_b) after further dilution with the extracorporeal prime will equal the post-donation hemoglobin (Hb_d), from Eq. 5, multiplied by the proportion of the total blood volume (V_b) to the combined total blood volume and bypass prime volume (V_e):

$$Hb_b = Hb_d \left[\frac{V_b}{(V_b + V_e)} \right]$$

Combining the hemoglobin-reducing effects of blood donation and hemodilution from pump prime, the maximum volume of blood that can be donated ($V_{d,max}$) to maintain the hemoglobin above a predetermined minimal level ($Hb_{e,min}$) can be calculated by

$$V_{d,max} = V_b - (V_b + V_e) \left[\frac{Hb_{e,min}}{Hb_i} \right]$$

The extracorporeal circuit prime volume (V_e), the estimated blood volume of the patient (V_b), and the initial hemoglobin (Hb_i) serve as the variable factors. In most cases it is possible to safely remove autologous blood equal to at least 10% of the patient's blood volume before bypass (130,136,137,140). Harvesting smaller amounts of autologous blood will decrease the quantity of hemostatic elements available with reinfusion and decrease the impact on total red blood cell mass.

Technical Concerns

The objective of intraoperative predonation is the removal of the maximum quantity of blood possible, maintenance of that blood in satisfactory condition throughout the period of CPB, and reinfusion of the blood at the end of CPB. During donation, the blood must be removed in such a way as to maintain the patient's hemodynamic stability while preserving the hemoglobin at a clinically acceptable level. Electrocardiographic and hemodynamic monitoring are essential during the donation process. It is important to obtain the blood isovolumetrically to prevent hemodynamic instability. Support of the intravascular volume with administration of crystalloid or colloid solutions during the process of autologous blood removal is required. The blood's oxygen-carrying capacity must also be maintained at a sufficient level to prevent hypoxia.

Several techniques can be used for collecting blood intraoperatively. For each, blood is donated before or immediately after the initiation of CPB. This minimizes the contact of blood and blood elements with the artificial surfaces of the extracorporeal circuit. After initiation of CPB, not only is the blood diluted with the prime but coagulation factors and platelets are exposed to the artificial surfaces, reducing the value of the blood for later hemostatic control (142,156–158). Numerous techniques have been proposed for obtaining blood, but the most widely accepted access routes are through a central venous catheter, an arterial catheter, or the venous tubing of the heart—lung machine (159). Whichever technique is used, maintenance of hemodynamic stability is essential throughout the donation process.

If blood is to be collected from a central venous catheter, the catheter is connected by a short segment of sterile intravenous tubing to a blood collection bag that contains an anticoagulant. The blood collection bag is placed below the level of the patient's right atrium, and the blood is allowed to collect into the bag by gravity (Fig. 7.14A). Simultaneously, the patient's blood volume is replaced with crystalloid solution through a peripheral intravenous line. After the blood has been collected, it is labeled and usually left connected to the patient for later reinfusion. This technique is attractive for several reasons: it requires no complex equip-

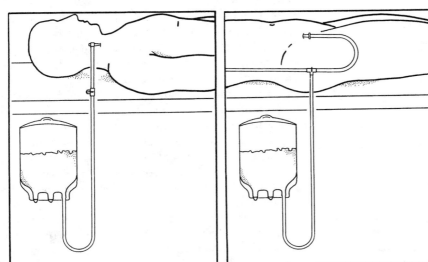

FIG. 7.14. A: Intraoperative collection of autologous blood from a central venous catheter. The blood is collected in a anticoagulated blood collection bag placed below the level of the patient to allow gravity flow. **B:** Intraoperative collection of autologous blood from a femoral arterial catheter. The arterial pressures serve as the driving force, allowing the filling of the anticoagulated blood collection bag.

ment or training to accomplish; the blood loss is gradual and can be easily compensated for by intravenous fluid replacement; and the quantity of anticoagulant in the blood storage bag is usually small, causing a minimal effect on coagulation when the blood is reinfused. The major limitation of this technique is that it is relatively slow. In many operating room environments, time is of the essence, and the period from the start of anesthesia to the initiation of CPB may be relatively short. In addition, another disadvantage of this technique is that the anesthesiologist's attention may be diverted from the patient during the collection process, which may increase the potential for an adverse event.

Another method of blood collection is through an arterial cannula (Fig. 7.14B). An advantage for blood collection through this route is that donation can be accomplished fairly rapidly. Of course, there is an increased risk for transient hypovolemia and hypotension during the donation process. In addition, monitoring the blood pressure may be problematic if only one arterial line is in place.

Alternatively, the blood can be collected immediately before the initiation of CPB through a Y-connector placed in the venous tubing, proximal to the venous reservoir of the extracorporeal circuit (Fig. 7.15). This connector allows blood either to pass unimpeded into the venous reservoir or to be diverted into a separate circuit draining into a blood collection bag. Immediately before the initiation of CPB, the limb of the Y-connector leading to the collection bag is clamped and the pump prime is allowed to drain into the reservoir until venous blood begins entering the reservoir. At that point, the venous return to the reservoir is clamped and blood is diverted into the collection bag. Simultaneously, pump prime is transfused through the arterial cannula

to replace the volume loss. After a calculated quantity of blood has been harvested, the drainage tubing to the collection bag is clamped and the venous return is diverted back into the reservoir. With this technique, the blood collection bag does not have to be anticoagulated because of the patient's full heparinization. The bagged blood is labeled and can be reinfused into the extracorporeal circuit by the perfusionist if the hemoglobin on bypass becomes unacceptably low. If the blood is not returned during CPB, the anesthesiologist can reinfuse it later during the surgical procedure.

Immediate prebypass collection of blood is attractive because of the ability to rapidly sequester large volumes before the initiation of CPB. Also, it is relatively simple to institute because complex preparation is not required. Hypovolemia can easily be avoided by the rapid administration of volume through the heart—lung machine. One disadvantage of this technique is that sequestered blood contains a significant level of heparin, which requires neutralization with protamine, when the blood is eventually reinfused. However, the preservation of platelets and coagulation factors by using this technique is excellent (159).

Indications

Although some early studies failed to demonstrate that reinfusion of autologous blood during open heart surgical procedures had any value in reducing blood bank requirements (160,161), numerous subsequent studies have confirmed the benefit of this technique. In fact, most studies have found that intraoperative autologous blood donation with reinfusion decreases total homologous blood requirements by at least 20% to 50% (129,136,137,143,146,159, 162–169). In addition, a decrease in the requirement for fresh frozen plasma, needed for control of postoperative coagulopathies, can be realized (163–165,169). Reinfusion of fresh autologous blood that is obtained before exposure of the blood to the deleterious effects of the heart—lung machine has several advantages for maintaining hemostasis. Several studies have demonstrated an improvement in both the quantitative (143,159,170) and qualitative (171) platelet availability when compared with patients not having undergone predonation and reinfusion. In addition, postoperative coagulation factor defects are less extensive in patients receiving the reinfusion of fresh autologous blood (159), and significant improvements in coagulation and lytic parameters have been demonstrated immediately after the infusion of autologous blood (164). The improvements in coagulation status may be directly responsible for a reduction in postoperative blood loss seen in some studies (165,167), but not all investigations have observed such improvements (166).

The safety of autologous blood donation has been demonstrated repeatedly (130,136,137,140,159,166,167,172). Although transient hypotension during donation has been reported (137,140), serious complications have not oc-

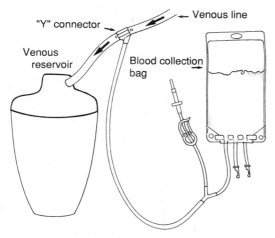

FIG. 7.15. The technique for the intraoperative collection of autologous blood from the venous line of the extracorporeal circuit is depicted. During cardiopulmonary bypass, a side branch or Y-connector allows the diversion of blood from the venous line into a blood collection bag. Because the blood is already heparinized, anticoagulant is not needed in the collection bag.

curred when the procedure is performed properly. The use of intraoperative donation of autologous blood before CPB might well be indicated for any patient whose preoperative hemoglobin would allow the necessary hemodilution associated with this technique.

Intraoperative autologous donation is highly attractive as a blood conservation technique for most patients undergoing cardiac surgery. It is an inexpensive simple method for providing fresh blood that is essentially free of risk from transmission of disease, allergic reaction, alloimmunization, and blood banking mishaps. Additionally, autotransfusion does do not pose a burden on the limited blood supply. Intraoperative autologous donation appears to yield the ideal blood product for reinfusion after CPB because it not only yields red blood cells but also fresh coagulation factors, platelets, and other essential serum components. Because the results are favorable and the risks are low, intraoperative autologous blood donation and reinfusion should be considered in all patients undergoing open heart surgical procedures.

Intraoperative Blood Scavenging

Historical Perspective

One method for minimizing homologous blood usage is the intraoperative salvage of shed blood from the operative field and, after processing, reinfusion of the red blood cells. This approach is particularly advantageous during operative procedures, such as open heart surgery, where surgical blood losses constitute a significant portion of the transfusion requirement. The salvage, processing, and reinfusion of blood that is lost during a surgical procedure is called autotransfusion.

The first recorded application of autotransfusion occurred in 1818 and is credited to John Blundell (173), who reinfused shed blood in 10 patients with severe postpartum hemorrhage. William Highmore (174) published the first scientific article in 1874 advocating the value of intraoperative autotransfusion, and subsequently in 1886, John Duncan (175) reported a case of reinfusion of shed operative blood during a leg amputation. In the early 1900s, the development of techniques for blood storage and blood banking began to change the emphasis from autotransfusion to homologous blood usage (131,176,177). This was further extended during World War II when increased awareness by the public of the value of donating blood, in combination with the cumbersome nature of the techniques required for the collection of shed blood, led to a reduction in the enthusiasm for autologous blood salvage.

However, interest in autotransfusion reemerged during the 1960s with the advent of the Vietnam War. Vietnam War casualties required massive transfusions, which placed an inordinate drain on the homologous blood supply. In response, Bentley Laboratories developed a device specifi-

cally for the rapid intraoperative autotransfusion of lost blood. Shed blood was aspirated from the surgical field and collected in a reservoir. The processing of the blood entailed defoaming and filtering before immediate reinfusion (132,178,179). As much as 40 L of blood could be reinfused during an operative procedure using this technique. Although the Bentley system was useful, its disadvantages included the need to anticoagulate either the patient or the salvaged blood, the reinfusion of activated clotting factors resulting in a coagulopathy, renal failure from reinfusion of large amounts of free hemoglobin present in the filtered blood, and high risk for inadvertent but fatal air embolization during the reinfusion process.

In the 1970s, the number of cardiac surgical procedures increased exponentially, which placed a tremendous burden on blood banks, because the average open heart procedure required between 8 and 12 units of blood (119,121, 129,136,161). More recently, concerns about disease transmission associated with homologous blood transfusion, especially human immunodeficiency virus, served as an additional impetus for adopting autotransfusion techniques (119,177).

Because of the difficulties associated with the Bentley system, an alternative approach for intraoperative salvage was sought. The result was the development of red blood cell washing and reinfusing devices (178). The advantages of a red cell washing system were the removal of activated coagulation factors, free hemoglobin, and other blood cell debris and the virtual elimination of the risk for inadvertent air embolization. Unfortunately, the washing procedure also entailed the removal of normal clotting factors and pharmacologic agents existing in the serum, including heparin (131,180,181). Early cell washing systems also had the disadvantage of requiring a long interval between the time the blood was collected and the time the cells could be reinfused.

Over the past decade, the primary improvement in intraoperative salvage of blood has been in the design of the cell washing—reinfusion equipment. At present, commercially available devices from several manufacturers have reduced red blood cell processing time to as little as 3 minutes. Other improvements in equipment design include easier operation, greater reliability, and additional safety features. Present systems nearly fulfill the requirements set forth by Gilcher and Orr (182) in 1975 for the ideal autotransfusion system.

Technical Concerns

During open heart surgical procedures when the patient is fully heparinized, most shed blood can be returned to the patient through the cardiotomy suction of the heart—lung machine. However, before heparinization and after neutralization of the heparin with protamine, the use of the cardiotomy suction is not possible because of the risk for clot

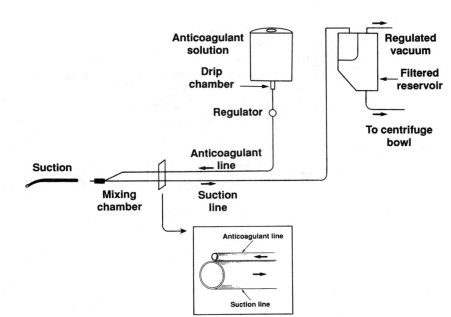

FIG. 7.16. The typical blood collection system includes a suction apparatus that aspirates blood into a filtered reservoir. As blood is drawn from the surgical field, it enters a small mixing chamber to which an anticoagulant solution is added. After mixing, the anticoagulated blood is carried to a reservoir where it is filtered and stored until centrifugation is desired. A close-up of the double-lumen suction tubing shows a small tube providing the anticoagulant solution to the mixing chamber and a large tube serving to transport the aspirated blood.

formation within the extracorporeal circulatory device. To prevent the irretrievable loss of this shed blood, other strategies had to be developed.

Autotransfusion techniques are divided into two approaches: blood is recovered and filtered before reinfusion and blood is recovered, filtered, and washed before reinfusion. In the simplest autotransfusion system, the blood is collected from the operative field using a suction-based aspiration device that anticoagulates the blood as it is collected. The collected blood is filtered and stored for reinfusion. The technique is extremely simple and inexpensive. However, simply filtering the blood does not remove serum factors that can potentiate or worsen the coagulation deficits commonly seen after CPB. Because of this, simple blood retrieval and reinfusing systems during open heart surgery have been supplanted by the more advanced blood-processing technique of cell washing (131,180).

Cell washing techniques incorporate four basic steps: blood harvesting from the operative site, processing of the shed blood with removal of the serum, storage of the red blood cells that are harvested, and reinfusion of the red blood cell mass. Harvesting the shed blood is accomplished using double-lumen suction tubing. The larger lumen provides the suction uptake of blood and the smaller lumen carries heparinized saline to the suction catheter tip (Fig. 7.16). Typically, between 10,000 and 100,000 units of heparin are added to 1 L of normal saline and allowed to drip into a mixing chamber at the suction catheter's tip (183–185). The mixing chamber allows immediate anticoagulation of any blood aspirated from the surgical field. The anticoagulated blood is then transported to a disposable reservoir where clots and other debris are filtered out before

further processing. The flow rate of the heparinized saline into the mixing chamber is controlled by the amount of vacuum applied by the suction apparatus and by the infusion rate set on the anticoagulant drip bag.

The filtered anticoagulated blood is processed in a centrifuge bowl, which is typically composed of two subassemblies. The inner subassembly is stationary and contains an inlet and outlet port through which fluid is able to enter or leave the processing chamber. The inner subassembly is positioned over an outer subassembly that rotates and contains the primary processing chamber. Blood components are separated in the outer spinning centrifuge bowl based on the differential densities of the components. The heavier more dense blood components are centrifuged outward, toward the bowl's perimeter. The lighter lower density components float inward, toward the bowl's center (Fig. 7.17).

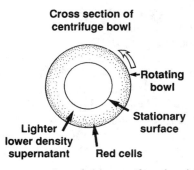

FIG. 7.17. A cross-section of the centrifuge bowl is shown. As the bowl rotates, the higher density cells migrate to the outer wall while the lighter density supernatant remains more central.

As blood is pumped into the spinning bowl, the lighter supernatants are displaced from the bowl through the outlet and discarded. After the bowl is filled with red blood cells, normal saline wash solution is pumped into the bowl and circulated through the red cell layer. The result is displacement of debris, plasma, free hemoglobin, and any anticoagulants by the wash solution through the outlet into a waste bag. After the wash cycle, the remaining red blood cells are aspirated from the inlet port into a collection bag (Fig. 7.18). The final blood collected with this system can have a hematocrit as high as 70% (180,185–187).

Control of the processing in all currently available devices is provided by a microprocessor, controlled by internal air detectors and solenoid valves (Fig. 7.19). The valves ensure the exact control of the fluid paths and the identification of status conditions and end points in the processing sequence. Most commonly available blood salvage systems have standard disposable equipment that includes a centrifuge bowl, reinfusion bag, and waste bag. The list price of the disposable separator, bowl, and tubing is typically in the range of $100 to $400. Other disposable materials, including the reservoir, suction assembly tubing, and anticoagulant solution, typically cost an additional $25 to $50. The hardware cost is in the range of $18,000 to $40,000. Although the microprocessor control simplifies the operation of the equipment, qualified personnel are still necessary to set up and operate the device. Typically, during open heart surgery, the equipment can be run by a perfusionist.

Indications

Intraoperative salvaging and washing of shed blood during an operative procedure has emerged as an important technique for blood conservation during cardiac surgery. The aim of intraoperative red blood cell salvage and reinfusion is a reduction in homologous blood transfusion requirements. Most studies (186–194) have demonstrated that the use of this technique is safe and effective in reducing homologous blood transfusion during open heart surgery by as much as 32% to 62%. Initially, there was some concern that reinfusion of a platelet and coagulation factor-depleted blood product would exacerbate the extracorporeal circulatory-induced coagulation defects, but a dilutional coagulopathy has not been demonstrated with the use of routine blood salvage techniques (186–188). However, a comparison between the red blood cell salvaging, washing, and reinfusing technique and the ultrafiltration technique for concentrating blood remaining in the CPB circuitry after an open heart operation did indicate better postoperative hemostasis with the use of an ultrafiltration approach (15). Although red cell washing techniques may be a less desirable method for salvaging and concentrating red blood cell mass in the extracorporeal circuit after bypass, reinfusion of blood salvaged and washed from the pump circuit remains a well-accepted technique. In addition, bleeding as a result of reinfusing the salvaged blood has not been demonstrated to be a clinically important problem.

Another concern associated with the transfusion of red blood cells recovered from the operative field was that the processing might alter the cell membrane's stability and viability. However, when autologous red cell viability was compared with donor blood (185), autologous red cells were found to be more resistant to osmotic stress than the homologous blood. Red blood cells that had been collected, processed, and reinfused also had similar survival times when compared with autologous red blood cells obtained by venous puncture (186,195,196). There is additional concern that salvaged blood may contain plasma, residual heparin,

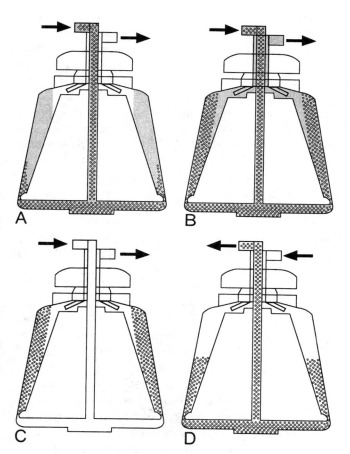

FIG. 7.18. The cell saving and washing process occurs sequentially. **A:** Blood collected in a reservoir from the surgical field is pumped through the inlet port of the centrifuge bowl, causing displacement of saline from the bowl out of the outlet. **B:** With centrifugation, the heavier more dense red blood cells are spun to the periphery of the bowl and the waste plasma overflows into a waste collection bag. **C:** After the centrifuge bowl has been filled with red blood cells, the flow of blood from the reservoir is stopped and a saline wash solution is started. The saline is pumped through the layers of red blood cells, removing free hemoglobin, coagulation factors, debris, and other plasma components. **D:** After washing of the red blood cells, the centrifuge is stopped. The washed red blood cells are aspirated from the inlet port and placed into a reinfusion bag.

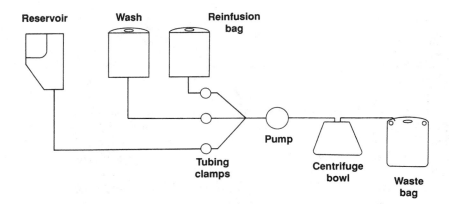

FIG. 7.19. Schematic drawing of typical cell separator showing the reservoir bag into which aspirated anticoagulated blood is accumulated. Other portions of the apparatus include a reservoir for saline wash solution, a bag for collecting the washed blood, serial tubing clamps that are operated by a microprocessor, a pump head that allows flow in either direction (depending on which tubing clamps are open or shut), a centrifuge bowl for cell separation, and a waste bag for discarding supernatant during the washing process.

cellular debris, and free hemoglobin from damaged cells. However, the intraoperatively scavenged and washed blood generally yields a safe product (197).

Although not universally confirmed (198), most studies have found autologous red blood cell salvage and reinfusion to be cost effective (187,189,191,192,199). In most evaluations of cost, the immediate cost of processing the shed blood was compared with the cost savings associated with avoidance of homologous blood usage. The cost of using blood salvage techniques was more than offset by the decreased use of blood and blood products. However, the need for trained personnel and the initial capital expense and the cost of maintaining and running the equipment must be considered.

Contraindications

The risks of using red cell salvaging systems can be subdivided into three areas: equipment malfunction, operator error, and blood contamination. Advances in design and microprocessor control have greatly reduced the chance that a device malfunction will result in harm to a patient. In addition, increased user experience and refinements in the design of the equipment contributed to significant reductions in operator error. However, a persistent concern is the danger associated with the use of blood that has been contaminated on the surgical field. Although current autotransfusion devices are very effective in removing damaged red blood cells and other particulate matter, they do not completely remove bacteria, malignant cells, and certain medications (132,200,201). The centrifugation and washing process removes a large proportion of any bacterial contamination, but unacceptable numbers of bacteria may remain within the red cell mass (202). Therefore, salvaging blood from an infected surgical site should be avoided. However, in the setting of massive hemorrhage, cell salvage from a contaminated site should not be withheld, because several studies have shown no increase in infectious complications in this situation (203,204). It has also been recom-

mended that blood collected from an area of malignancy should not be reinfused because malignant cells within the processed blood could, theoretically, cause diffuse metastases (205). Interestingly, there are little clinical data on this subject. One study of patients with bladder cancer failed to demonstrate any evidence for increased dissemination of tumor caused by autotransfusion after a mean follow-up of 24 months (206). Because of the short duration and nonrandomized poorly controlled nature of these studies, generalization of the results is not justified. Therefore, avoidance of autotransfusion in malignancy continues to be a reasonable approach (205, 207).

It must also be realized that blood collected from the surgical field can be contaminated with agents placed there by the operating surgical team (208). Certain agents used to irrigate the operative site and bound to the red blood cell membrane are not removed by the device and are potentially toxic if infused intravenously. Theoretically, drugs carried in the plasma are eliminated by the cell washing process, such as topical bacitracin and neomycin (209). However, in general it is not advisable to salvage blood from an area contaminated with an antibiotic or other agent, which would be toxic if infused intravenously (210). For example, a frequently encountered surgical situation of potential concern occurs with the use of topical hemostatic agents that might be dangerous if given intravenously. Microfibrillar collagen hemostat is not removed during the wash cycle in scavenged blood (211). Although blood exposed to thrombin from the incision is probably acceptable for salvage (212), blood exposed to Avitene (Alcon, Inc., Puerto Rico) and Surgicel (Johnson and Johnson, Arlington, TX) can potentially induce a coagulopathy if reinfused (211).

Red blood cell salvage is an important blood conservation technique during cardiac surgery. Although cost benefit and other concerns associated with the use of salvage devices must be considered, there remains a strong incentive for the use of any technique that can reasonably reduce homologous transfusion requirements.

KEY POINTS

- Ultrafiltration during CPB allows safe and effective removal of free water, solutes (electrolytes, urea, creatinine, and glucose), and pharmacologic agents (analgesia drugs, hypnotic drugs, paralytic agents, and aprotinin).
- Heparin appears to be (somewhat paradoxically) concentrated on the blood side of the filter.
- Ultrafiltration is efficacious in patients with abnormal and normal renal function.
- Ultrafiltration may improve coagulation function and decrease the inflammatory response after CPB.
- Beneficial effects of ultrafiltration have been clinically shown for pulmonary, renal, cardiac, and brain function after CPB.
- Hemodialysis during CPB decreases the need for early postoperative dialysis when the patient may be unstable and difficult to manage.
- Autologous (preoperative) blood donation and intraoperative blood removal before CPB with hemodilution decrease banked blood usage.
- Appropriate collection methods include preoperative phlebotomy and intraoperative collection using a central venous catheter and gravity drainage, an arterial catheter, and a Y-connector in the CPB venous circuit to divert blood into a collection bag at the start of CPB.
- Intraoperative autologous blood collection decreases the use of banked blood by 20% to 50%.
- Intraoperative blood salvage decreases homologous blood requirements
- Red blood cell viability after cell salvage techniques is not different from banked blood.
- Few cost-effectiveness data compare ultrafiltration, autologous collection, and shed blood salvage techniques.

REFERENCES

1. Brull L. Realization de l' ultrafiltration in vivo. *C R Soc Biol (Paris)* 1928;99:1605–1608.
2. Lunderquist A, Alwall N, Tornberg A. On the artificial kidney. XXI. The efficacy of the dialyzer ultrafilter intended for human use. Including a preliminary report on treatment of oedemic patients by means of ultrafiltration. *Acta Med Scand* 1952;143:307.
3. Nakamoto S. Removal of edema fluid by ultrafiltration with the disposable twin-coil artificial kidney. *Cleve Clin Q* 1961;28:10–15.
4. Kobayashi K, Shibata M, Kato K. Studies on the development of a new method of controlling the amount and contents of body fluids (extracorporeal ultrafiltration method.ECUM) and the application of this method for patients receiving long-term hemodialysis. *Jpn J Nephrol* 1972;14:1.
5. Henderson LW. Pre vs. post dilution hemofiltration. *Clin Nephrol* 1979;11:120.
6. Romagnoli A, Hacker J, Keats AS, et al. External hemoconcentration after deliberate hemodilution. Annual meeting of the American Society of Anesthesiologists, extracts of scientific papers, San Francisco, October 1976, p. 269.
7. Darup J, Bleese N, Kalmar P, et al. Hemofiltration during extracorporeal circulation (ECC). *Thorac Cardiovasc Surg* 1979;27:227–230.
8. Intonti F, Alquati P, Schiavello R, et al. Ultrafiltration during open heart-surgery in chronic renal failure. *Scand J Thorac Cardiovasc Surg* 1981;15:217–220.
9. Heiss KF, Pettit B, Hirschl RB, et al. Renal insufficiency and volume overload in neonatal ECMO managed by continuous ultrafiltration. *Trans Am Soc Artif Intern Organs* 1987;33:557–560.
10. Magilligan DJ. Indications for ultrafiltration in the cardiac surgical patient. *J Thorac Cardiovasc Surg* 1985;89:183–189.
11. Hakim M, Wheeldon D, Bethune DW, et al. Haemodialysis and haemofiltration on cardiopulmonary bypass. *Thorax* 1985;40:101–106.
12. Magilligan DJ, Oyama C. Ultrafiltration during cardiopulmonary bypass: laboratory evaluation and initial clinical experience. *Ann Thorac Surg* 1984;37:33–39.
13. Klineberg PL, Kam CA, Johnson DC, et al. Hematocrit and blood volume control during cardiopulmonary bypass with the use of hemofiltration. *Anesthesiology* 1984;60:478–480.
14. Solem JO, Tengborn L, Steen S, et al. Cell saver versus hemofilter for concentration of oxygenator blood after cardiopulmonary bypass. *Thorac Cardiovasc Surg* 1987;35:42–47.
15. Boldt J, Kling D, Bormann B, et al. Blood conservation in cardiac operations. *J Thorac Cardiovasc Surg* 1989;97:832–840.
16. Boldt J, Zickmann B, Czeke A, et al. Blood conservation techniques and platelet function in cardiac surgery. *Anesthesiology* 1991;75:426–432.
17. Osipov VP, Lurie GO, Khodas M, et al. Hemoconcentration during open heart operations. *Thorac Cardiovasc Surg* 1985;33:81–85.
18. Herskowitz A, Mangano D. Inflammatory cascade. Editorial views. *Anesthesiology* 1996;85:957–960.
19. Journois D, Pouard P, Greeley WJ, et al. Hemofiltration during cardiopulmonary bypass in pediatric cardiac surgery. Effects on hemostasis, cytokines and complement components. *Anesthesiology* 1994;81:1181–1189.
20. Journois D, Israel-Biet D, Pouard P, et al. High-volume, zero-balanced hemofiltration to reduce delayed inflammatory response to cardiopulmonary bypass in children. *Anesthesiology* 1996;85:965–976.
21. Millar AB, Armstrong L, van der Linden J, et al. Cytokine production and hemofiltration in children undergoing cardiopulmonary bypass. *Ann Thorac Surg* 1993;56:1499–1502.
22. Neote K, Darbonne W, Ogez J, et al. Identification of a promiscuous inflammatory peptide receptor on the surface of red blood cells. *J Biol Chem* 1993;268:12247.
23. Ramamoorthy C, Lynn AM. Con: the use of modified ultrafiltration during pediatric cardiovascular surgery is not a benefit. *J Cardiothorac Vasc Anesth* 1998;12:483–485.
24. Sakurai H, Maeda M, Murase M, et al. Hemofiltration removes bradykinin generated in the priming blood in cardiopulmonary bypass during circulation. *Ann Thorac Cardiovasc Surg* 1998;4:59–63.
25. Stein B, Pfenninger E, Grunert A, et al. The consequences of continuous haemofiltration on lung mechanics and extravascular lung water in a porcine endotoxic shock model. *Intensive Care Med* 1991;17:293–298
26. Gillinov AM, Redmond JM, Winkelstein JA, et al. Complement and neutrophil activation during cardiopulmonary bypass: a

study in the complement-deficient dog. *Ann Thorac Surg* 1994; 57:345–352.

27. Meliones JN, Gaynor JW, Wilson BG, et al. Modified ultrafiltration reduces airway pressures and improves lung compliance after congenital heart surgery. *J Am Coll Cardiol* 1995;25:217A.

28. Naik S, Balaji S, Elliott M. Modified ultrafiltration improves hemodynamics after cardiopulmonary bypass in children. *J Am Coll Cardiol* 1992;19:37A.

29. Gaynor JW, Tulloh RMR, Owen CH, et al. Modified ultrafiltration reduces myocardial edema and reverses hemodilution following cardiopulmonary bypass in children. *J Am Coll Cardiol* 1995;25:200A.

30. Davies MJ, Nguyen K, Gaynor JW, et al. Modified ultrafiltration improves left ventricular systolic function in infants after cardiopulmonary bypass. *J Thorac Cardiovasc Surg* 1998;115:361–370.

31. Ad N, Snir E, Katz J, et al. Use of the modified technique of ultrafiltration in pediatric open-heart surgery: a prospective study. *Isr J Med Sci* 1996;32:1326–1331.

32. Coraim FI, Wlner E. Continuous hemofiltration for the failing heart. *New Horizons* 1995;30:725–731.

33. Skaryak LA, Kirshbom PM, DiBernardo LR, et al. Modified ultrafiltration improves cerebral metabolic recovery after circulatory arrest. *J Thorac Cardiovasc Surg* 1995;109:744–752.

34. Dinarello CA. Interleukin-1 and tumor necrosis factor and their naturally occurring antagonists during hemodialysis. *Kidney Int* 1992;38[Suppl]:S68–S77.

35. Strijbos PJ, Hardwick AJ, Relton JK, et al. Inhibition of central actions of cytokines on fever and thermogenesis by lipocortin-1 involves CRF. *Am J Physiol* 1992;263:E632–E636.

36. Lister G, Hellenbrand WE, Kleinman CS, et al. Physiologic effects of increasing hemoglobin concentration in left-to-right shunting in infants with ventricular septal defects. *N Engl J Med* 1982;306:502–506.

37. Kontras S, Bodenbender J, Craenen J, et al. Hyperviscosity in congenital heart disease. *J Pediatr* 1970;76:214–220.

38. Wheeldon DR, Bethune DW. Blood conservation during cardiopulmonary bypass—autologous transfusion, cell saving and haemofiltration. In: Taylor KM, ed. *Cardiopulmonary bypass—principles and management.* Baltimore: Williams & Wilkins, 1986:289–311.

39. Salzman EW. Low-molecular-weight heparin. Is small beautiful? *N Engl J Med* 1986;315:957–959.

40. Rosenberg RD, Lam L. Correlation between structure and function of heparin. *Proc Natl Acad Sci USA* 1979;76:1218–1222.

41. Holt DW, Landis GH, Dumond DA, et al. Hemofiltration as an adjunct to cardiopulmonary bypass for total oxygenator volume control. *J Extra-Corp Technol* 1982;14:373–377.

42. Williams GD, Ramamoorthy C, Totzek FR, et al. Comparison of the effects of red cell separation and ultrafiltration on Heparin concentration during pediatric cardiac surgery. *J Cardiothorac Vasc Anesth* 1997;11:840–844.

43. Despotis GJ, Levine V, Filos KS, et al. Hemofiltration during cardiopulmonary bypass: the effect on anti-Xa and anti-IIa heparin activity. *Anesth Analg* 1997;84:479–483.

44. Pouard P, Journois D, Greeley WJ. Hemofiltration and pediatric cardiac surgery. In: Greeley WJ, ed. *Perioperative management of the patient with congenital heart disease.* Baltimore: Williams & Wilkins, 1996:121–132.

45. den Hollander JM, Hennis PJ, Burm AG, et al. Pharmacokinetics of alfentanil before and after cardiopulmonary bypass in pediatric patients undergoing cardiac surgery. Part I. *J Cardiothorac Vasc Anesth* 1992;6:308–312.

46. Hynynen M, Hynninen M, Soini H, et al. Plasma concentration and protein binding of alfentanil during high-dose infusion for cardiac surgery. *Br J Anaesth* 1994;72:571–576.

47. Nishida H, Suzuki S, Endo M, et al. An oxygenator with a built-in hemoconcentrator. In vitro performance and pre clinical in vivo assessment of the final prototype. *ASAIO J* 1996;42:M593–597.

48. Ing TS, Ashbach DL, Kanter A. Fluid removal with negative-pressure hydrostatic ultrafiltration using a partial vacuum. *Nephron* 1975;14:451–455.

49. Nelson RL, Tamari Y, Tortolani AJ, et al. Ultrafiltration for concentration and salvage of pump blood. In: Utley JR, ed. *Pathophysiology and technique of cardiopulmonary bypass.* Vol. 2. Baltimore: Williams & Wilkins, 1983:229–241.

50. Silverstein ME, Ford CA, Lysaght MJ, et al. Treatment of severe fluid overload by ultrafiltration. *N Engl J Med* 1974;291:747–751.

51. Henderson LW, Ford CN, Colton CK, et al. Uremic blood cleaning by diafiltration using hollow-fiber ultrafilter. *Trans Am Soc Artif Intern Organs* 1970;16:107–114.

52. Nakamura Y, Masuda M, Toshima Y, et al. Comparative study of cell saver and ultrafiltration nontransfusion in cardiac surgery. *Ann Thorac Surg* 1990;49:973–978.

53. Karliczek GF, Tigchelaar I, Dijck L, et al. How much additional blood trauma is caused by haemofiltration during cardiopulmonary bypass? *Life Support Syst* 1986;4[Suppl 1]:167–173.

54. Paganini EA, Nakamoto SI. Continous slow ultrafiltration in oliguric acute renal failure. *Tran Am Soc Artif Intern Organs* 1980;26:201–204.

55. Boldt T, Kling D, Bormann B, et al. Extravascular lung water and hemofiltration during complicated cardiac surgery. *Thorac Cardiovasc Surg* 1987;35:161–165.

56. Osipov VP, Lure GO, Marochnik SL, et al. Experience in hemoconcentration by ultrafiltration in operations using artificial circulation at the all-union scientific center of surgery of the USSR Academy of Medical Sciences. *Grud Serdechnososudistaia Khir* 1990;7:3–6.

57. Tamari YR, Nelson R, Levy R, et al. Concentration of blood in the extracorporeal circuit using ultrafiltration. *J Extracorp Technol* 1983;15:133–142.

58. Hopeck JM, Lane RS, Schroeder JW. Oxygenator volume control by parallel ultrafiltration to remove plasma water. *J Extra-Corp Technol* 1981;13:267–271.

59. Draaisma AM, Hazekamp MG, Frank M, et al. Modified ultrafiltration after cardiopulmonary bypass in pediatric cardiac surgery. *Ann Thorac Surg* 1997;115:521–525.

60. Friesen RH, Campbell DN, Clarke DR, et al. Modified ultrafiltration attenuates dilutional coagulopathy in pediatric open heart operations. *Ann Thorac Surg* 1997;64:1787–1789.

61. Gurbuz AT, Novick WM, Pierce CA, et al. Impact of ultrafiltration on blood use for atrial septal defect closure in infants and children. *Ann Thorac Surg* 1998;65:1105–1109.

62. Casey WF, Hauser GJ, Hannallah RS, et al. Circulating endotoxin and tumor necrosis factor during pediatric cardiac surgery. *Crit Care Med* 1992;20:1090–1096.

63. Casey LC. Role of cytokines in the pathogenesis of cardiopulmonary-induced multisystem organ failure. *Ann Thorac Surg* 1993;56:92–96.

64. Naik SK, Knight A, Elliott M. A prospective randomized study of a modified technique of ultrafiltration during pediatric open-heart surgery. *Circulation* 1991;84:422–431.

65. Hashimoto Y, Hirohata S, Kashiwado T, et al. Cytokine regulation of hemostatic property and IL-6 production of human endothelial cells. *Inflammation* 1992;16:613–621.

66. van der Poll T, Levi M, Hack CE, et al. Elimination of interleukin-6 attenuates coagulation activation in experimental endotoxemia in chimpanzees. *J Exp Med* 1994;179:1253–1259.

67. Levi M, ten Cate H, Bauer KA, et al. Inhibition of endotoxin-induced activation of coagulation and fibrinolysis by pentoxifyl-

line or by a monoclonal anti-tissue factor antibody in chimpanzees. *J Clin Invest* 1994;93:114–120.

68. Page PA. Ultrafiltration versus cell washing for blood concentration. *J Extra-Corp Technol* 1990;22:142–150.

69. Pascual M, Schifferli JA. Adsorption of complement factor D by polyacrylonitrile dialysis membranes. *Kidney Int* 1993;43: 903–911.

70. Mulvihill J, Cazenave JP, Mazzucotelli JP, et al. Minimodule dialyser for quantitative ex vivo evaluation of membrane hemocompatibility in humans: comparison of acrylonitrile copolymer, cuprophan and polysulphone hollow fibres. *Biomaterials* 1992;13:527–536.

71. Craddock PR, Fehr J, Brigham KL. Complement and leukocyte mediated pulmonary dysfunction in hemodialysis. *N Engl J Med* 1977;296:769–774.

72. Bando K, Vijay P, Turrentine MW, et al. Dilutional and modified ultrafiltration reduces pulmonary hypertension after operations for congenital heart disease: a prospective randomized study. *J Thorac Cardiovasc Surg* 1998;115:517–527.

73. Montenegro LM, Greeley WJ. Pro: the use of modified ultrafiltration during pediatric cardiac surgery is a benefit. *J Cardiothorac Vasc Anesth* 1998;12:480–482.

74. Sutton RG. Renal considerations, dialysis, and ultrafiltration during cardiopulmonary bypass. *Int Anesthesiol Clin* 1996;34: 165–176.

75. Abel JJ, Rowntree LG, Turner BB. On removal of diffusable substances from the circulating blood in living animals by dialysis. *J Pharmacol Exp Ther* 1914;5:275–316.

76. Kolff WJ, Berk HT. The artificial kidney: a dialyzer with a great area. *Acta Med Scand* 1944;117:121–134.

77. Alwall N. On the artificial kidney. I. Apparatus for dialysis of blood in vivo. *Acta Med Scand* 1947;128:317–326.

78. Kolff WJ, Watschinger B, Vertes V. Results in patients treated with coil kidney (disposable dialyzing unit). *JAMA* 1956;161: 1433–1437.

79. MacNeill AE, Doyle JE, Anthone R, et al. Technic with parallel flow, straight tube blood dialyzer. *NY State J Med* 1959: 4137–4149.

80. Awad JA, Brassard A, Binet J, et al. Pulmonary and cardiac assistance during hemodialysis. An experimental method for the oxygenation of the blood and the support of the heart during extracorporeal dialysis. *J Urol* 1970;103:388–392.

81. Lazarus JM, Lowrie KG, Hampers CL. Cardiovascular disease in uremic patients on hemodialysis. *Kidney Int* 1975;2[Suppl]: 167.

82. Lindner A, Charra B, Sherrana DJ, et al. Accelerated atherosclerosis in prolonged maintenance hemodialysis. *N Engl J Med* 1974;290:697–701.

83. Hellerstedt WL, Johnson WJ, Ascher N, et al. Survival rates of 2,728 patients with end-stage renal disease. *Mayo Clin Proc* 1984;59:776–783.

84. Byrd LH, Sullivan JF. Successful coronary artery bypass in hemodialysis patients. *J Dialysis* 1978;2:33–42.

85. Menzoian JO, Davis RC, Idelson BA, et al. Coronary bypass surgery and renal transplantation: a case report. *Ann Surg* 1974; 179:63–64.

86. Laws KH, Merrill WH, Hannon JW, et al. Cardiac surgery in patients with chronic renal disease. *Ann Thorac Surg* 1986;42: 152–157.

87. Francis GS, Sharma B, Collins AJ, et al. Coronary artery surgery in patients with end-stage renal disease. *Ann Intern Med* 1980; 92:499–503.

88. Sakurai H, Ackad A, Friedman HS, et al. Aorto-coronary bypass graft surgery in a patient on home hemodialysis. *Clin Neprol* 1974;2:208–210.

89. Lamberti JJ, Cohn LH, Collins JJ. Cardiac surgery in patients

undergoing renal dialysis or transplantation. *Ann Thorac Surg* 1975;19:135–141.

90. Posner MA, Reves JG, Lell WA. Aortic valve replacement in a hemodialysis-dependent patient: anesthetic consideration—a case report. *Anesth Analg* 1975;54:24–28.

91. Chawla R, Gailiunas P, Lazarus JM, et al. Cardiopulmonary bypass surgery in chronic hemodialysis and transplant patients. *Trans Am Soc Artif Intern Organs* 1977;23:694–697.

92. Zamora JL, Burdine JT, Karlberg H, et al. Cardiac surgery in patients with end-stage renal disease. *Ann Thorac Surg* 1986; 42:113–117.

93. Opsahl JA, Husebye DG, Helseth HK, et al. Coronary artery bypass surgery in patients on maintenance dialysis: long-term survival. *Am J Kidney Dis* 1988;12:271–274.

94. Marshall WG, Rossi NP, Meng RL, et al. Coronary artery bypass grafting in dialysis patients. *Ann Thorac Surg* 1986; 42[Suppl]:S12–S15.

95. Deutsch E, Bernstein RC, Addonizio VP, et al. Coronary artery bypass surgery in patients on chronic hemodialysis. *Ann Intern Med* 1989;10:369–372.

96. Francis GS, Compty CM, Sharma B, et al. Myocardial revascularization in chronic renal disease patients. In: Love J, ed. *Cardiac surgery in patients with chronic renal disease.* New York: Futura, 1982:115–132.

97. Van Devanter SH, Cohn LH, Koster TK, et al. Cardiac valve replacement in chronic renal disease patients. In: Love J, ed. *Cardiac surgery in patients with chronic renal disease.* New York: Futura, 1982:151–165.

98. Monson BK, Wickstrom PH, Haglin JJ, et al. Cardiac operation and end stage renal disease. *Ann Thorac Surg* 1980;30:267–272.

99. Gordon LA, Simon ER, Rukes M, et al. Studies in regional heparinization. *N Engl J Med* 1956;255:1063–1066.

100. Soffer O, MacDonell RC, Finlayson DC, et al. Intraoperative hemodialysis during cardiopulmonary bypass in chronic renal failure. *J Thorac Cardiovasc Surg* 1979;77:789–791.

101. Zawada ET, Stinson JB, Done G. New perspectives on coronary artery disease in hemodialysis patients. *South Med J* 1982;75: 694–696.

102. Goebel TK, Stote RM, Dubb JW, et al. Intraoperative dialysis techniques. *ANNA J* 1987;14:121–124.

103. Murkin JM, Murphy DA, Finlayson DC, et al. Hemodialysis during cardiopulmonary bypass: report of twelve cases. *Anesth Analg* 1987;66:899–901.

104. Paganini EP, Suhoza K, Swann S, et al. Continuous renal replacement therapy in patients with acute renal dysfunction undergoing intraaortic balloon pump and/or left ventricular device support. *Trans Am Soc Artif Intern Organs* 1986;32: 414–417.

105. Goudsouzian N. The kidneys. In: Goudsouzian N, Karamanian AA, eds. *Physiology for the anesthesiologist.* Norwalk, CT: Appleton Century Crofts, 1984:429–454.

106. Lunderquist A. On the artificial kidney for human use. Including a preliminary report on treatment of oedemic patients by means of ultrafiltration. *Acta Med Scand* 1952;143:307–314.

107. Lamer C, Valleaux T, Plaisance P, et al. Continuous arteriovenous hemodialysis for acute renal failure after cardiac operations. *J Thorac Cardiovasc Surg* 1990;99:175–176.

108. Geronemus R, Schneider N. Continuous arteriovenous hemodialysis: a new modality for treatment of acute renal failure. *Trans Am Soc Artif Intern Organs* 1984;30:610–613.

109. Karzai W, Priebe HJ. Oxygen consumption in hemodialysis patients undergoing cardiopulmonary bypass. *J Cardiothorac Vasc Anesth* 1998;12:415–417.

110. Kopman EA. Scavenging of potassium cardioplegic solution to prevent hyperkalemia in hemodialysis-dependent patients. *Anesth Analg* 1983;62:780–782.

111. Kubota T, Miyata A, Maeda A, et al. Continuous haemodiafiltration during and after cardiopulmonary bypass in renal failure patients. *Can J Anaesth* 1997;44:1182–1186.

112. Gailiunas P, Chawla R, Lazarus JM, et al. Acute renal failure following cardiac operations. *J Thorac Cardiovas Surg* 1980;79:241–243.

113. Rigden SPA, Barratt TM, Dillon MJ, et al. Acute renal failure complicating cardiopulmonary bypass surgery. *Arch Dis Child* 1982;57:425–430.

114. Hilberman M, Myers BD, Carrie BJ, et al. Acute renal failure following cardiac surgery. *J Thorac Cardiovasc Surg* 1979;77:880–888.

115. Abel RM, Buckley MT, Austem WG, et al. Incidence and prognosis of renal failure following cardiac operations. Result of a prospective analysis of 500 consecutive patients. *J Thorac Cardiovasc Surg* 1976;71:323–333.

116. Olinger GN, Hutchinson LD, Bonchek LI. Pulsatile cardiopulmonary bypass for patients with renal insufficiency. *Thorax* 1983;38:543–550.

117. Matsuda H, Hirose H, Nakano S, et al. Results of open heart surgery in patients with impaired renal function as creatinine clearance below 30 ml/min. *J Cardiovasc Surg* 1986;27:595–599.

118. Davis RF, Lappas DG, Kirklin JK, et al. Acute oliguria after cardiopulmonary bypass: renal functional improvement with low-dose dopamine infusion. *Crit Care Med* 1982;10:852–856.

119. Tyson GS, Slanden RN, Spainhour V, et al. Blood conservation in cardiac surgery: preliminary results with an institutional commitment. *Ann Surg* 1989;209:736–742.

120. Utley JR, Moores WY, Stephens DB. Blood conservation techniques. *Ann Thorac Surg* 1981;31:482–490.

121. Roche JK, Stengle JM. Open-heart surgery and the demand for blood. *JAMA* 1973;225:1516–1521.

122. Goodnough LT, Johnston MFM, Toy PT, et al. The variability of transfusion practice in coronary artery bypass surgery. *JAMA* 1991;265:86–90.

123. Milam JD. Blood transfusion in heart surgery. *Clin Lab Med* 1982;1:65–85.

124. Cosgrove DM, Loop FD, Lytle BW, et al. Determinants of blood utilization during myocardial revascularization. *Ann Thorac Surg* 1985;40:380–384.

125. Campbell FW, Addonizio VP Jr. Platelet function alterations during cardiac surgery. In: Ellison N, Jobes DR, eds. *Effective hemostasis in cardiac surgery*. Philadelphia: W.B. Saunders, 1988:85–109.

126. Edmunds LH, Addonizio VP Jr. Platelet physiology during cardiopulmonary bypass. In: Utley JR, ed. *Pathophysiology and techniques of cardiopulmonary bypass*. Baltimore: Williams & Wilkins, 1982:106–119.

127. Gravlee GP, Hopkins MB. Blood plasma products. In: Ellison N, Jobes DR, eds. *Effective hemostasis in cardiac surgery*. Philadelphia: W.B. Saunders, 1988:69–83.

128. Grant FC. Autotransfusion. *Ann Surg* 1921;74:253–254.

129. Cohn LH, Fosberg AM, Anderson RP, et al. The effects of phlebotomy, hemodilution and autologous transfusion on systemic oxygenation and whole blood utilization in open heart surgery. *Chest* 1975;68:283–287.

130. Tector AJ, Gabriel RP, Mateicka WE, et al. Reduction of blood usage in open heart surgery. *Chest* 1976;4:454–457.

131. Brzica SM, Pineda AA, Taswell HF. Autologous blood transfusion. *Mayo Clin Proc* 1976;51:723–737.

132. Council on Scientific Affairs. Autologous blood transfusions. *JAMA* 1986;256:2378–2380.

133. Yomtovian RA. Autologous blood transfusion: past performance and current concerns. *Minn Med* 1986;69:353–356.

134. Hamstra RD, Block MH. Erythropoiesis in response to blood loss in man. *J Appl Physiol* 1969;27:503–507.

135. Newmann MM, Hamstra R, Block M. Use of banked autologous blood in elective surgery. *JAMA* 1971;218:861–863.

136. Hallowell P, Bland JHL, Chir B, et al. Transfusion of fresh autologous blood in open-heart surgery. *J Thorac Cardiovasc Surg* 1972;64:941–948.

137. Ochsner JL, Mills NL, Leonard GL, et al. Fresh autologous blood transfusions with extracorporeal circulation. *Ann Surg* 1973;177:811–817.

138. Barbier-Bohm G, Desmonts JM, Couder E, et al. Comparative effects of induced hypotension and normovolaemic haemodilution on blood loss in total hip arthroplasty. *Br J Anaesth* 1980;52:1039–1043.

139. Cuello L, Vazquez E, Rios R, et al. Autologous blood transfusion in thoracic and cardiovascular surgery. *Surgery* 1967;62:4814–4818.

140. Hardesty RL, Bayer WL, Bahnson HT. A technique for the use of autologous fresh blood during open-heart surgery. *J Thorac Cardiovasc Surg* 1968;5:683–688.

141. Newman MM, Hamstra R, Block M. The use of banked autologous blood in elective surgery. *JAMA* 1971;218:861–863.

142. Dobell ARC, Mitri M, Galva R. Biologic evaluation of blood after prolonged recirculation through film and membrane oxygenators. *Ann Surg* 1965;4:617–622.

143. Wagstaffe JG, Clarke AD, Jackson PW. Reduction of blood loss by restoration of platelet levels using fresh autologous blood after cardiopulmonary bypass. *Thorax* 1972;27:410–414.

144. Kramer AH, Hertzer NR, Beven KG. Intraoperative hemodilution during elective vascular reconstruction. *Surg Gynecol Obstet* 1979;149:831–836.

145. Jobes DR, Gallagher J. Acute normovolemic hemodilution. *Int Anesthesiol Clin* 1982;20:77–95.

146. Lawson NW, Ochsner JL, Mills NL, et al. The use of hemodilution and fresh autologous blood in open-heart surgery. *Anesth Analg* 1974;53:672–683.

147. Buckley MJ, Austen WG, Goldblatt A, et al. Severe hemodilution and autotransfusion for surgery of congenital heart disease. *Surg Forum* 1971;22:160–162.

148. Seager OA, Nesmith MA, Begelman KA, et al. Massive acute hemodilution for incompatible blood reaction. *JAMA* 1974;229:790–792.

149. Nahas RA, Mundth ED, Buckley MJ, et al. Effect of hemodilution on left ventricular function with regional ischemia of the heart. *Surg Forum* 1972;23:149–150.

150. Yoshikawa H, Powell WJ, Bland JHL, et al. Effect of acute anemia on experimental myocardial ischemia. *Am J Cardiol* 1973;32:670–678.

151. Pavek K, Carey JS. Hemodynamics and oxygen availability during isovolemic hemodilution. *Am J Physiol* 1974;226:1172–1177.

152. Messmer K, Sunder-Plasmann L, Jesch L, et al. Oxygen supply to the tissues during limited normovolemic hemodilution. *Res Exp Med* 1973;159:152.

153. Albert SN. *Blood volume*. Springfield, IL: Charles C Thomas, 1963:26.

154. Miller D. Normal values and examination of the blood: perinatal period, infancy, childhood and adolescence. In: Miller DR, Baechner RL, McMillan CW, et al., eds. *Blood diseases of infancy and childhood*. St. Louis: CV Mosby, 1984:21–22.

155. Shoemaker WC. Fluids and electrolytes in the acutely ill adult. In: Shoemaker WC, Ayres S, Grevik A, et al., eds. *Textbook of critical care*, 2nd ed. Philadelphia: W.B. Saunders, 1989:1130–1150.

156. Bick RL. Alterations of hemostasis associated with cardiopulmo-

nary bypass, pathophysiology, prevention, diagnosis and management. *Semin Thromb Hemost* 1976;3:59–82.

157. de Leval MR, Hill JD, Mielke CH Jr, et al. Blood platelets and extracorporeal circulation. Kinetic studies on dogs on cardiopulmonary bypass. *J Thorac Cardiovasc Surg* 1975;69:144–151.

158. Fong SW, Burns NE, Williams C, et al. Changes in coagulation and platelet function during prolonged extracorporeal circulation (ECC) in sheep and man. *Trans Am Soc Artif Intern Organs* 1974;20:239–247.

159. Kaplan JA, Cannarella C, Jones EL, et al. Autologous blood transfusion during cardiac surgery: a re-evaluation of three methods. *J Thorac Cardiovasc Surg* 1977;74:4–10.

160. Pliam MB, McGoon DC, Tarhan S. Failure of transfusion of autologous whole blood to reduce banked-blood requirements in open-heart surgical patients. *J Thorac Cardiovasc Surg* 1975;70:338–343.

161. Sherman MM, Dobnik DB, Dennis RC, et al. Autologous blood transfusion during cardiopulmonary bypass. *Chest* 1976;70:592–595.

162. Silver H. Banked and fresh autologous blood in cardiopulmonary bypass surgery. *Transfusion* 1975;15:600–603.

163. Lilleaasen P, Froysaker T. Fresh autologous blood in open heart surgery. Influence on blood requirements, bleeding and platelets counts. *Scand J Thor Cardiovasc Surg* 1979;13:41–46.

164. Whitten CW, Allison PM, Latson TW, et al. Evaluation of laboratory coagulation and lytic parameters resulting from autologous whole blood transfusion during primary aortocoronary artery bypass grafting. *J Clin Anesth* 1996;8:229–235.

165. Kochamba GS, Pfeffer TA, Sintek CF, et al. Intraoperative autotransfusion reduces blood loss after cardiopulmonary bypass. *Ann Thorac Surg* 1996;61:900–903.

166. Helm RE, Klemperer JD, Rosengart TK, et al. Intraoperative autologous blood donation preserves red cell mass but does not decrease postoperative bleeding. *Ann Thorac Surg* 1996;62:1431–1441.

167. Khan R, Siddiqui A, Natrajan KM. Blood conservation and autotransfusion in cardiac surgery. *J Card Surg* 1993;8:25–31.

168. Lee J, Ikeda S, Johnston MF. Efficacy of intraoperative blood salvage during coronary artery bypass grafting. *Min Cardioangiol* 1997;45:395–400.

169. Petry AF, Jost T, Sievers H, et al. Reduction of homologous blood requirements by blood-pooling at the onset of cardiopulmonary bypass. *J Cardiothorac Surg* 1994;5:1210–1214.

170. Iyer VS, Russell WJ. Fresh autologous blood transfusion and platelet counts after cardiopulmonary bypass surgery. *Anaesth Intens Care* 1982;10:348–352.

171. Dale J, Lilleaasen P, Erikssen J. Hemostasis after open-heart surgery with extreme or moderate hemodilution. *Eur Surg Res* 1987;19:339–347.

172. Zubiate P, Kay JH, Mendez AM, et al. Coronary artery surgery: a new technique with use of little blood, if any. *J Thorac Cardiovasc Surg* 1974;68:263–267.

173. Blundell J. Experiments on the transfusion of blood by the syringe. *Med Chir Trans* 1818;9:56–92.

174. Highmore W. Practical remarks: overlooked source of blood-supply for transfusion in postpartum haemorrhage. *Lancet* 1874;1:891.

175. Duncan J. Reinfusion of blood in primary and other amputations. *Br Med J* 1886;1:192–193.

176. Wilson JD, Taswell HF. Autotransfusion historical review and preliminary report on a new method. *Mayo Clin Proc* 1968;43:26–35.

177. Yomtovian RA. Autologous blood transfusion past performance and current concerns. *Minn Med* 1986;69:353–356.

178. Rosenblatt R, Dennis P, Draper LD. A new method for massive fluid resuscitation in the trauma patient. *Anesth Analg* 1983;62:613–616.

179. Stehling LC, Zauder HL, Rogers W. Intraoperative autotransfusion. *Anesthesiology* 1975;43:337–345.

180. Orr MD. Autotransfusion: intraoperative scavenging. *Anesthesiol Clin* 1982;24:97–117.

181. Umlas J, O'Neill TP. Heparin removal in an autotransfusion device. *Transfusion* 1981;21:70–73.

182. Gilcher RO, Orr M. Intra-operative autotransfusion. *Transfusion* 1975;15:520.

183. Messick KD, Gibbons GA, Fosburg RG, et al. Intraoperative use of the haemonetics cell saver. Proceedings of the Blood Conservation Institute, Haemonetics, Braintree, MA, 1978.

184. Haemonetics. *Cell saver plus autologous blood recovery system owner's operating and maintenance manual.* Braintree, MA: Haemonetic Corporation, 1986:1–68.

185. Orr MD, Blenko JW. Autotransfusion of concentrated, selected washed red cells from the surgical field: a biochemical and physiological comparison with homologous cell transfusion. *Proceedings of the Haemonetics Blood Conservation Institute*, 1978.

186. Cordell AR, Lavender SW. An appraisal of blood salvage techniques in vascular and cardiac operations. *Ann Thorac Surg* 1981;31:421–425.

187. Keeling MM, Gray LA, Brink MA, et al. Intraoperative autotransfusion. Experience in 725 consecutive cases. *Ann Surg* 1983;197:536–541.

188. Mayer ED, Welsch M, Tanzeem A, et al. Reduction of postoperative donor blood requirement by use of the cell separator. *Scan J Thorac Cardiovasc Surg* 1985;19:167–171.

189. Laub GW, Murali D, Riebman JB, et al. The impact of intraoperative autotransfusion on cardiac surgery. *Chest* 1993;104:686–689.

190. Breyer RH, Engelman RM, Rousou JA, et al. Blood conservation for myocardial revascularization. *J Thorac Cardiovasc Surg* 1987;93:512–522.

191. Parrot D, Lancon JP, Merle JP, et al. Blood salvage in cardiac surgery. *J Cardiothorac Vasc Anesth* 1991;5:454–456.

192. Pelley WB. Cost-effectiveness of blood conservation. *J Extra-Corp Technol* 1980;12:148–151.

193. Vertrees RA, Auvil J, Rohrer C, et al. Intra-operative blood conservation during cardiac surgery. *J Extra-Corp Technol* 1980;12:60–62.

194. Cosgrove DM, Thurer RL, Lytle BW, et al. Blood conservation during myocardial revascularization. *Ann Thorac Surg* 1979;28:184–188.

195. Giordano GF, Goldman DS, Mammana B, et al. Intraoperative autotransfusion in cardiac operation. Effect on introperative and postoperative transfusion requirements. *J Thorac Cardiovasc Surg* 1988;3:382–386.

196. Ansell J, Parrilla N, King M, et al. Survival of autotransfused red blood cells recovered from the surgical field during cardiovascular operations. *J Thorac Cardiovasc Surg* 1982;84:387–391.

197. Spain DA, Miller FB, Bergamini TM, et al. Quality assessment of intraoperative blood salvage and autotransfusion. *Am Surg* 1997;63:1059–1063.

198. Ray JM, Flynn JC, Bierman AH. Erythrocyte survival following intraoperative autotransfusion in spinal surgery: an in vivo comparative study and 5-year update. *Spine* 1986;11:879–882.

199. Winton TL, Charrette EJP, Salerno TA. The cell saver during cardiac surgery: does it save? *Ann Thorac Surg* 1982;33:379–381.

200. Cutler BS. Avoidance of homologous transfusion in aortic operations: the role of autotransfusion, hemodilution, and surgical technique. *Surgery* 1984;95:717–722.

201. Yaw PB, Sentary M, Link WJ, et al. Tumor cells carried through

autotransfusion: contraindication to intraoperative blood recovery? *JAMA* 1975;231:490–491.

202. Klebanoff G, Phillips J, Evans W. Use of disposable autotransfusion unit under varying conditions of contamination. *Am J Surg* 1970;120:351–354.

203. Ozmen V, McSwain NE, Nichols RL, et al. Autotransfusion of potentially culture-positive blood (CPB) in abdominal trauma: preliminary data from a prospective study. *J Trauma* 1992;32:36–39.

204. Timberlake GA, McSwain NE. Autotransfusion of blood contaminated by enteric contents: a potentially life-saving measure in the massively hemorrhaging trauma patient. *J Trauma* 1988;28:855–857.

205. Desmond MJ, Thomas MJ, Gillon J, et al. Consensus Conference on Autologous Transfusion. Perioperative red cell salvage. *Transfusion* 1996;36:644–651.

206. Kimberg I, Sirois R, Wajsman Z, et al. Intraoperative autotransfusion in urologic oncology. *Arch Surg* 1986;121:1326–1329.

207. Fujimoto J, Okamoto E, Yamanaka N, et al. Efficacy of autotransfusion in hepatectomy for hepatocellular carcinoma. *Arch Surg* 1993;128:1065–1069.

208. Yawn DH. Ensuring quality during intraoperative blood salvage. *Lab Med* 1994;25:626–631.

209. Boudreaux, Bornside GH, Cohn I. Emergency autotransfusion: partial cleansing of bacteria laden blood by cell washing. *Trauma* 1983;23:31–35.

210. Paravicini D, Thys J, Hein H. Rinsing the operative field with neomycin-bacitracin solution with intraoperative autotransfusion in orthopedic surgery. In: Lawin P, ed. *Clinic of anesthesiology and operative intensive medicine*. Munster: Westphalian Wilhelm University, 1983:1–12.

211. Robicsek F, Duncan GD, Born GVR, et al. Inherent dangers of simultaneous application of microfibrillar collagen hemostat and bloodsaving devices. *J Thorac Cardiovasc Surg* 1986;92:766–770.

212. Blood conservation update. Electromedics, Inc. Englewood, CO: 1989;3:2.

8

CIRCULATORY ASSIST DEVICES: APPLICATIONS FOR VENTRICULAR RECOVERY OR BRIDGE TO TRANSPLANT

FRANCISCO A. ARABIA
JACK G. COPELAND
DOUGLAS F. LARSON
RICHARD G. SMITH

CLINICAL APPLICATIONS AND MANAGEMENT

At the present time, orthotopic heart transplantation is acknowledged as the best therapy for end-stage congestive heart failure. It is estimated that 164,000 people in the United States die each year as a result of end-stage heart disease. About 20% to 40% of potential cardiac recipients die while waiting for a heart transplant (1). Approximately 1,600 to 2,000 heart transplants are performed every year under the current procurement system (2,3). The discrepancy between the possible recipients and the available donors generates a realistic need for circulatory systems for cardiac support and replacement.

The first indication for the use of mechanical circulatory assistance was in the treatment of postcardiotomy cardiogenic shock (4–7). This category encompasses approximately 2,000 patients who cannot be weaned from cardiopulmonary bypass (CPB) (8). Some circulatory devices were designed for this purpose, "pending recovery of the natural heart." Some of these systems, and others, are currently used for a second indication: temporary cardiac support until a donor heart becomes available for transplantation, or "bridge to transplantation" (9–13). As progress continues to be made in the medical and engineering sciences, there is no doubt that permanent assist devices or devices that can totally replace the heart will eventually become available.

The spectrum of devices discussed in this chapter ranges from the intraaortic balloon pump (IABP) to the total artificial heart (TAH). Each system is described in detail.

Patient Selection, Initiation of Support, Outcome

Patients with severe cardiac failure are at once diverse, each having a unique medical history and pattern of organ dysfunction, and homogeneous, all sharing many aspects of congestive heart failure, low-output syndrome, and cardiogenic shock. They frequently have been treated with maximal medical inotropic and afterload reduction therapy and also often have had treatment with an IABP. For those who continue to decompensate, a number of possible solutions are available.

Patient selection is the most important factor in determining survival with mechanical circulatory assistance (6,14,15). The younger the patient, the better the survival. The experience with the use of postcardiotomy devices for cardiac recovery has shown that patients younger than 60 years have a survival rate of 21% to 31%, whereas patients older than 60 years have a survival of 12%. The survival rate for patients over 70 years is 6%. Other factors that contribute to the success of these devices include the performance and selection of the device, and the skill, experience, and judgment of the surgeon who is using the devices (16).

Various criteria have been applied in the past as guidelines for the placement of ventricular assistance (Table 8.1). Considered together, these criteria function as a definition of cardiogenic shock (17). They are presented as basic guidelines. They do not exclude such other parameters as a requirement for high-dose catecholamine support with or without adjuvant drugs, such as phosphodiesterase III inhibitors, systemic hypotension (mean arterial pressure <60 mm Hg, systolic <80 mm Hg), respiratory distress, waxing and waning state of consciousness, failure to separate from bypass, and metabolic acidosis. Common to all these patients is a global picture indicating inadequate perfusion of organs and tissues as a result of cardiac failure. Prompt

F. A. Arabia, J. G. Copeland, D. F. Larson, and R. G. Smith: Department of Cardiothoracic Surgery, University of Arizona, Tucson, Arizona 85724.

TABLE 8.1. CRITERIA FOR PLACEMENT OF VENTRICULAR ASSIST DEVICES

Cardiac index <2.0 L/min/m^2
Systemic vascular resistance >2,100 dyn-sec/cm^{-5}
Atrial pressure >20 mm Hg
Urine output <20 mL/h with
   Optimal preload
   Maximal drug therapy
   Corrected metabolism
   Intraaortic balloon pump

Adapted from Pennington DG, Joyce LD, Pae Jr WE, et al. Circulatory support symposium 1988; patient selection. *Ann Thorac Surg* 1989;47:77–81, with permission.

institution of mechanical circulatory assistance is of great importance. Prolonged hypotension (>12 hours) is associated with multisystem failure and poor recovery (16). To assess simultaneously the physiologic need for and the results of circulatory support, the cardiac output and direct atrial pressures should be measured. In this context, direct left atrial pressure is preferable to pulmonary capillary wedge pressure as an index of left ventricular failure, as the latter may be less accurate in cases of pulmonary edema. The need for univentricular or biventricular support should also be addressed very early in the process of determining the degree of support. Patients who are awaiting transplantation often require biventricular support. Patients who have a low right atrial pressure, normal or slightly elevated pulmonary vascular resistance, and no ventricular dysrhythmias may benefit from left ventricular support only. Approximately 20% of patients who receive left ventricular support ultimately require right ventricular support also (18–20). A large number of patients require inotropic agents for right ventricular support during the first 48 hours after implantation of a left ventricular device. The current criteria most often used to differentiate between the need for univentricular or biventricular support are summarized in Table 8.2.

The merits of paracorporeal biventricular support versus left ventricular support may be disputed, but once the decision to provide support is made, little technically separates the two approaches. The only requirements for biventricular support are two extra cannulas and a few extra minutes of operating time. Biventricular support is not associated with a higher incidence of thrombotic, infectious, cannulation, and mechanical problems in comparison with univentricular assistance (21). It appears that mortality is higher in patients receiving biventricular support; however, whether this is a consequence of the degree of preexisting myocardial damage that dictates biventricular rather than univentricular support or of the extent of support *per se* has not been established. The need for univentricular versus biventricular support should be individualized for each patient, (Table 8.2).

Another factor that has to be taken into consideration once the need for support has been established is whether a continuous-flow or pulsatile device should be used. The use of prolonged continuous flow has been associated with end-organ dysfunction (14). The use of an IABP in addition to a continuous-flow device (centrifugal pump) appears to improve end-organ function (22). If a device that provides pulsatile flow is chosen, then a selection must be made between synchronous or asynchronous contractions of the device with the native heart. Synchronous counterpulsatile flow has been postulated to improve myocardial recovery when reversible damage is suspected and a need to augment blood flow to the endocardium is desired. Asynchronous pulsatile flow may be used when irreversible myocardial damage is present and maximal blood flow is required to maintain end-organ function. Other considerations may also be important, such as the inability to track the electrocardiogram in tachyarrythmias and chaotic rhythms and the desirability of controlling rate to optimize device filling or to decrease the amount of device-related hemolysis. The mode of device filling may dictate a counterpulsating pumping mode. Each device has its own peculiarities in this area.

Availability of Devices

In 1976, an amendment to the Food, Drug and Cosmetics Act gave the Food and Drug Administration (FDA) the responsibility to oversee clinical trials. Inherent in this regulation is the requirement that the FDA must ensure that anticipated benefits to the individual patient, and to society

TABLE 8.2. CRITERIA OF SUPPORT

Right ventricular failure: right VAD and IABP
   Left atrial pressure <15 mm Hg
   Right atrial pressure >20 mm Hg
   Few or no dysrhythmias
   Near-normal left ventricle function by echocardiogram, ventriculogram, or MUGA
Left ventricular failure: left VAD only
   Left atrial pressure >20 mm Hg
   Right atrial pressure <15 mm Hg
   Few or no dysrhythmias
   Near-normal pulmonary vascular resistance
   Normal right ventricle function by echocardiogram, ventriculogram, or MUGA
Biventricular failure: right VAD plus left VAD ± IABP
   Right and left atrial pressure ≥20 mm Hg
   Ventricular tachycardia or fibrillation
   Severely impaired right and left ventricular function by echocardiogram, ventriculogram, or MUGA

VAD, ventricular assist device; IABP, intraaortic balloon pump; MUGA, multigated acquisition scan.
Adapted from Pennington DG, Reedy JE, Swartz MT, et al. Univentricular versus biventricular assist device support. *J Heart Lung Transplant* 1991;10:258–263, with permission.

at large, outweigh the risks involved in subjecting patients to an unproven device. Before any clinical trials begin, the FDA reviews an application (Investigational Device Exemption, or IDE), submitted by the sponsor of the proposed study. The IDE application includes a description of the device, details of materials and manufacturing, a description of any bench and animal testing, results of and conclusions derived from these tests, and a protocol of the proposed clinical trial, including indications, criteria for patient selection, methods proposed to evaluate results, and a patient informed-consent document (23). A local institutional review board oversees each clinical study. The institutional review board is expected "to apply local community attitudes and ethical standards in making a judgment that the benefits to subjects and the knowledge to be gained outweigh the risks" (24).

Because devices that existed before 1976 did not require an IDE application, any device that could show "substantial equivalence" to a preamendment device could be exempted from the IDE requirement by filing a request for exemption (510k). Importantly, the device categories of balloon pumps, centrifugal pumps, and resuscitative systems do not require an IDE application because similar technology existed before 1976. Although centrifugal pump technology existed before the amendment was created, its use for ventricular assistance did not. Because of the absence of a rigorous clinical study with these exempted devices, issues involving patient selection, complications, and informed consent are unclear (25). Once the IDE study is concluded, the accumulated data are submitted to the FDA for premarketing approval. The FDA staff and a panel of non-FDA experts review all data presented by the IDE sponsor. Approval at this point is the prerequisite to marketing any new device.

Complications of Circulatory Support Systems

Bleeding

Bleeding can be quite significant at the time an intrathoracic device is placed, especially if CPB has taken more than $2\frac{1}{2}$ hours. Activation of platelets and the coagulation system during exposure of the blood to artificial surfaces and turbulent flow patterns of the heart–lung machine may lead to a severe coagulopathy characterized by platelet dysfunction (26). Once surgical bleeding has been controlled, control of bleeding from suture lines, conduits, and raw surfaces as a result of deficiencies in the coagulation system become the next major clinical undertaking. Clear professional communication between the surgeon, anesthesiologist, hematologist, and blood bank may prove to be life-saving if persistent bleeding continues. Prompt control of bleeding is necessary to decrease the incidence of end-organ dysfunction as a result of transfusions.

The bleeding time becomes greater than 30 minutes after 2 hours of CPB (27). It appears that platelets become dysfunctional when they interact with the oxygenator surfaces, either bubble or membrane. Normalization of platelet function appears to begin 30 minutes after termination of CPB. A platelet count above $100,000/\mu L$, with normally functioning platelets, should provide clinically adequate hemostasis. A platelet count below this level at the completion of CPB will most often require exogenous platelet administration. A prolonged bleeding time with a platelet count above $100,000/\mu L$ indicates platelet dysfunction, and exogenous administration of platelets may be required. Desmopressin, a synthetic analog of the hormone arginine vasopressin, has been very useful in augmenting platelet function to improve hemostatic plug formation (28–30). Its mode of action is mediated by factor VIII complex; therefore, adequate levels of factor VIII are required. It is administered intravenously at a dose of 0.3 μg/kg over 10 minutes. A response, a decrease in bleeding time, may be measured 30 to 90 minutes after administration.

Dilution of the coagulation factors to less than one-half of normal concentration as a result of the nonblood prime appears not to affect hemostasis adversely. However, the persistent dilution by more than 50% coupled with the consumption that is encountered during prolonged operations requires the administration of coagulation factors, either in fresh-frozen plasma or cryoprecipitate. The use of cell-salvage devices helps to return red cells from the operative field back to the circulation, but it contributes to hemodilution and platelet dysfunction in that any procoagulant factors and platelets are lost in the washing process.

In the postoperative period, brisk bleeding or tamponade can decrease cardiac filling and thus prevent filling of any circulatory assist device. The same criteria for reoperation used for routine operations should be applied when devices are implanted. Evidence of tamponade in the face of rapid bleeding, a sudden decrease in chest tube drainage, and ongoing bleeding of more than 200 mL/h for longer than 3 to 4 hours are commonly accepted criteria for reoperation.

Bleeding may also become a significant problem at the time of removal of assist devices. Dense, immature adhesions between the device and intrathoracic organs tend to cause diffuse hemorrhage.

Thromboembolism

Protocols for anticoagulation differ among institutions using mechanical assist devices, mainly because no single regimen seems to be more effective than the others. Many agents have been used at different times after implantation and in varying combinations. These agents include low-molecular-weight heparin, warfarin, aspirin, dipyridamole, and ticlopidine.

A typical regimen may start with continuous intravenous infusion of heparin to maintain the partial thromboplastin time (PTT) at 50 to 60 seconds. Dipyridamole may be started simultaneously with heparin. The patient is maintained on heparin and dipyridamole unless a relatively long implant time is anticipated. In this case, warfarin is favored over heparin, with maintenance of the prothrombin time (PT) at approximately 18 to 22 seconds (international normalized ratio, or INR, of 2.5 to 3.5.) Aspirin is also started very early to decrease platelet adhesion.

More recently, for patients implanted with a TAH, our regimen has been modified to include the use of other agents, such as 250 mg of ticlopidine every other day and 1,200 mg of pentoxifylline per day, in combination with heparin, warfarin, aspirin, and dipyridamole to stabilize platelet function and balance the different coagulation pathways (31). To monitor the effectiveness of anticoagulation therapy, in addition to the usual measurement of PT and PTT, we examine factor X, fibrinogen, fibrin degradation products, platelet count, bleeding time, and *in vitro* platelet aggregability in response to four different stimulators (adenosine, adrenaline, collagen, and arachidonic acid). Antithrombin III in plasma and serum is used to calculate the antithrombotic potential index relating the amount of antithrombin III available to interact against thrombin. The use of thromboelastography, probably the best available indicator of overall coagulation mechanisms, and calculation of the thrombodynamic potential index provide a measurement of the coagulability of blood by examining the rapid phase of clot formation.

With most types of devices, specific internal sites are relatively more prone to the formation of thrombus. In the case of centrifugal pumps, thrombus tends to form at the cones (18). We know from our own experience that in the Novacor (Division of Baxter Healthcare, Oakland, California) left ventricular assist device, clots may form around the inflow valve. If the inflow site for the Novacor is the left ventricular apex, thrombus can form within the ventricle and then embolize in and out of the device. Examination of the Jarvik 7 TAH revealed deposits of platelets in the groove formed by the graft–valve housing and at the junction of the diaphragm with the device housing (32,33).

Other factors that appear to be involved in the development of thrombus within devices are a low or reduced blood flow and infection. The low-flow state and the contact of blood with an artificial surface may accelerate thrombus formation. Infection can lead to a hypercoagulable state, with activation of inflammatory cells and mediators leading to the formation of thrombus. Infection within a device on valves or adherent thrombus is more likely to be seen after prolonged periods of support. The risk for this complication in "nonpermanent" implants appears to be low.

The brain is by far the most sensitive organ to thromboembolism and therefore is the organ most often affected by thromboembolism. Fortunately, irreversible neurologic damage has not been a common clinical observation during the use of circulatory assist devices. Transient ischemic attacks have been among the more frequently reported events. Embolism to the kidneys, ophthalmic artery, lung, and heart via the coronary arteries has also been documented. Embolism to other organs, such as the liver, should be expected to be more difficult to document. Based on current experience, thrombosis, thromboembolism, and infections are increasingly common beyond 30 days and may be interrelated (34).

Infection

Patients who need circulatory assistance are at risk for the development of infection, not only because of the presence of a large foreign body but also because of their often debilitated and malnourished state. Improvement of the nutritional status of the patient should be considered of great importance. Prophylactic antibiotics should be routinely used during the perioperative period. A common practice is to begin administering a combination of vancomycin and gentamicin before surgery and continue the drugs until the chest tubes are removed.

The rate of infection is directly related to the duration of circulatory support. It appears that pneumonia and mediastinitis are the most prevalent infections encountered. In one series, in which the Thoratec (Pleasanton, California) ventricular assist device was used, the most common infection was sepsis resulting from nosocomial pneumonia caused by gram-negative bacilli (35). In another common infectious complication, infection involves not only the support device and inflow and outflow conduits but also the drive lines. These infections require systemic antibiotics and surgical debridement. Fungal infections, with *Candida* and *Aspergillus* organisms, have been reported in immunosuppressed patients who required circulatory support (18,32). Infection in these patients increases the rates of morbidity and mortality (2.5% to 31%). However, many of these patients can be successfully treated with antibiotics and become good candidates for cardiac transplantation. Prior immunosuppression should be a relative contraindication for the use of a TAH because sepsis resulting from mediastinitis and pneumonia appears to be a common infectious cause of death in patients with a TAH (36,37).

Hemolysis

Hemolysis is commonly observed during extended bypass. Chronic hemolysis can be associated with anemia and a requirement for transfusions, which may sensitize a potential transplant patient to tissue antigens and thereby create a less compatible potential recipient. Chronic hemolysis can also be associated with chronic renal failure. None of the currently approved investigational devices, when used as recommended, produce excessive hemolysis (free hemoglobin >10 mg/dL). Most clinical hemolysis is related to patient-specific, not device-specific, parameters (18). In the bridge to transplant setting, drive parameters of devices should be set to minimize blood trauma while accepting a blood flow index of 2.5 L/min/m² body surface area. Blood transfusions should not be given unless the hematocrit falls below 20%, and then blood that has been in storage for less than 1 week should be used and administered with a white blood cell filter.

Multiple Organ Failure

Multiple organ failure is multifactorial. Many "device patients" are in some degree of cardiogenic shock preoperatively. This may persist if the device fails to produce the desired increase in cardiac output. Many of these patients have clinically significant bleeding during placement of the device and require large amounts of blood products. Postoperatively, many will require inotropic support for the first 24 to 48 hours to maintain an adequate output. The presence of sepsis compounds multiple organ failure. Infection and multiple organ failure are the two most common causes of mortality in patients who undergo placement of a TAH (36).

Renal failure in this patient population is associated with mild azotemia and abnormal clearance of free water. Its onset is associated with a high mortality. The onset of acute renal failure in patients who had received the Thoratec device was associated with a mortality rate above 90% (38). The management of renal failure by hemodialysis, ultrafiltration, peritoneal dialysis, or a combination of these did not affect the outcome. Massive transfusions may be associated with adult respiratory distress syndrome. Hypoxemia is usually one of the first manifestations of pulmonary failure. Increased intrapulmonary shunt and decreased compliance are common clinical accompaniments. Jaundice is the most common evidence of liver failure. Although an elevated bilirubin level may represent hemolysis, elevations in the levels of liver enzymes may help make the diagnosis of liver failure. Gastrointestinal failure presents as bleeding from the gastrointestinal tract. Also, we have occasionally seen prolonged ileus. The outcome of patients with multiple organ failure is well-known. The more organs involved in failure, the higher the mortality.

Weaning and Bridging

The goal with all these devices is that the patient will be successfully weaned from mechanical support or that a heart transplant will be performed. When these devices are used as a bridge to transplantation, the potential recipient should meet all the usual transplant selection criteria before elective cardiac transplantation is undertaken. It appears that 35% to 70% of patients who receive a mechanical support device are either successfully weaned or receive a heart transplant (33,37).

CIRCULATORY ASSIST DEVICES

Intraaortic Balloon Pump

The IABP is at present the simplest and most frequently used circulatory assist device (1). It was first introduced by Moulopoulos et al. (39) in 1962 and then described clinically by Kantrowitz et al. (40) in 1968. It offers the least complicated means of circulatory assistance. Operation of the balloon is timed with the electrocardiogram or aortic pressure waveform. It inflates during diastole (counterpulsation), which propels blood into the coronary arteries and the periphery. The effects of the IABP on the circulation (Fig. 8.1) include augmentation of diastolic pressure, a decrease in afterload, and a decrease in myocardial oxygen consumption (41). Use of the IABP improves cardiac function, augmenting cardiac output by approximately 10% or 500 to 800 mL/min. It is generally used in combination with inotropic agents, which are usually at near-maximal levels at the time of IABP insertion.

The IABP has many therapeutic uses in modern medicine. It is widely used in left ventricular failure following CPB for revascularization or valve replacement. It is also used in cases of cardiogenic shock in patients on maximal inotropic support while awaiting cardiac transplantation (42), cardiogenic shock following myocardial infarction, or intractable angina. Other limited uses include left main coronary disease, ventricular dysrhythmias, right ventricular failure (43), septic shock, and pulmonary embolus. In cases of right ventricular failure, the IABP can be placed in the pulmonary artery. This is performed in the operating room with the heart and great vessels exposed (43).

Contraindications for the use of the IABP include aortic valve insufficiency, aortic aneurysm, and severe aortoiliac or femoral disease precluding insertion of the balloon. Augmentation of the diastolic pressure will cause an increase in regurgitant flow across an incompetent aortic valve, resulting in left ventricular distension. The same augmentation or passage of the balloon may perforate the aortic wall in patients with an aortic aneurysm.

The IABP is usually inserted percutaneously in one of the femoral arteries by the Seldinger technique (44) and advanced into the descending aorta just distal to the origin of the left subclavian artery (Fig. 8.2). If the femoral artery pulse is not palpable, especially after bypass, insertion may require a femoral artery cutdown. In cases of severe obstruction of the iliac and femoral vessels, the IABP may be placed in the operating room directly into the ascending aorta and advanced into the descending aorta.

The advantages of the IABP are that (a) it is a non-IDE device, (b) it is inexpensive ($35,000 per console and $650 to $750 per balloon), (c) it is easy to insert and use, (d) there is a large experience and minimal surveillance is required (physicians, perfusionist, nurses), and (e) anticoagulation not absolutely necessary (recommended during weaning). The disadvantages are (a) a complication rate of 20%, (b)

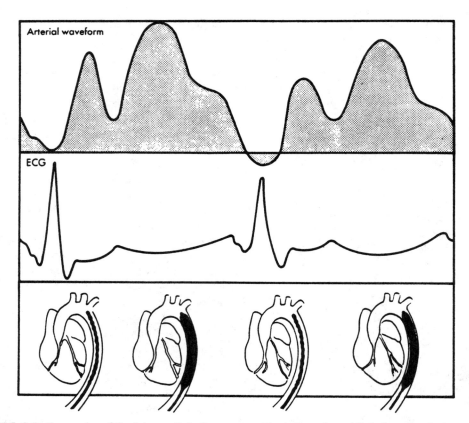

FIG. 8.1. Two cycles of the intraaortic balloon pump. The balloon is rapidly inflated at the beginning of diastole, just after aortic valve closes. Rapid deflation follows before next systole. (From Quaal SJ. Balloon's effect on a failing heart. In: Norwitz BE, ed. *Comprehensive intra-aortic balloon pumping.* St. Louis: Mosby, 1984:81, with permission.)

a limited increase in cardiac output, (c) no effective preload reduction, and (d) a limited effectiveness in cases of tachycardia, dysrhythmias, and right ventricular failure (25).

Complications related to the IABP occur during insertion, pumping, and removal, or shortly thereafter. These include dissection of the aorta, perforation, compromised blood flow to the lower extremity (when placed in the femoral artery) leading to ischemia, bleeding, thrombosis, embolism, thrombocytopenia, and infection. Peripheral pulses should be monitored frequently and on a regular schedule to document adequate blood flow to the extremity where the IABP has been placed. Monitoring of the arterial pressure is required to verify maximal augmentation of diastolic pressure. This will result in a decrease in the afterload and myocardial oxygen consumption.

Axial Flow Pump

The Hemopump or Nimbus pump (Johnson and Johnson, Rancho Cordova, California) is a device that can provide nonpulsatile flow rates of up to 3.5 L/min. It shares some of the simplicity of the IABP. The device is actually a minia-

ture axial flow pump at the end of a catheter. The pump is inserted through a 12-mm woven graft that is sutured to a femoral or iliac artery. The cannula is advanced into the aorta and across the aortic valve, and the tip is positioned at the apex of the left ventricle under fluoroscopic guidance (Fig. 8.3). The axial pump actually sits in the descending aorta in a cylindrical housing at the end of a 20-cm-long flexible inflow cannula (45). It aspirates blood from the left ventricle and pumps it directly into the descending aorta. The pump generates 3 L/min when rotating at a speed of 24,500 rpm, discharging into an output load of 100 mm Hg of pressure (46). Stationary blades provide directional flow of the blood as it exits the axial pump. The Hemopump is a disposable device intended for one-time use. The average time for insertion has been approximately 20 minutes.

Indications for placement are similar to those for the IABP. These include the presence of cardiogenic shock despite maximal medical support, a pulmonary capillary wedge pressure above 18 mm Hg, and a cardiac index below 2 L/min per square meter. The Hemopump has been used in patients with refractory cardiogenic shock after coronary artery bypass grafting, acute myocardial infarction, ischemic

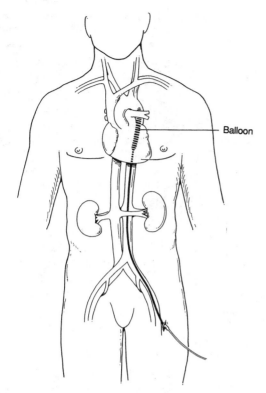

FIG. 8.2. The intraaortic balloon pump is usually inserted via the femoral arteries. The tip of the balloon should be placed just distal to the origin of the left subclavian artery.

cardiomyopathy, postpartum cardiomyopathy, and rejection of a transplanted heart (47,48). A contraindication for use of the Hemopump is severe aortoiliac disease that will prevent introduction of the inflow cannula and pump into the aorta. Advantages of the Hemopump are that it is (a) inserted without sternotomy, (b) less invasive, (c) comparable in cost with the IABP, and (d) small in size. Disadvantages are that (a) it cannot provide right ventricular support; (b) it can be used only for short periods of time; (c) an IDE is required at present; (d) complications are associated with insertion, including injury to the aortic valve, hemolysis, bleeding, and ischemic injury to the extremity used for placement; and (d) it requires an artery with a 7- to 10-mm lumen, which may in turn require a retroperitoneal approach to the iliac artery. The time range for its use has been 13 to 120 hours.

Internal Ventricular Assist Devices

The Novacor ventricular assist device and TCI ventricular assist device (Thermo Cardiosystems, Woburn, Massachusetts) represent prototypes of implantable devices for cardiac assistance that required more than 20 years of research and development, which was funded by the National Institutes

of Health. These devices work in a similar fashion, and both provide pulsatile assistance to a failing left ventricle. They represent a family of univentricular assist devices that are used in profound cardiogenic shock unresponsive to maximal inotropic support and IABP.

The Novacor left ventricular assist system is an electrically driven pump that energizes a solenoid that moves a dual-pusher plate to propel blood into the aorta. It was initially described in 1983 to provide long-term assistance, and it may well become the first totally implantable "permanent" left ventricular assist device (49). It has been used to support patients in profound cardiogenic shock after cardiac surgery, but its main application has been as a bridge to heart transplantation (50). The device is implanted in the left upper quadrant of the abdomen, anterior to the fascia of the rectus abdominis muscle (Fig. 8.4). It weighs approximately 3.3 kg and occupies a volume of about 400 mL. The inflow to the device comes via a low-porosity Dacron conduit that is anastomosed to a hole cored in the apex of the left ventricle. The outflow is also via a similar Dacron conduit that usually leads to the ascending aorta but may also be anastomosed to the abdominal aorta. Bioprosthetic inflow and outflow valves maintain unidirectional flow. The blood pump is made of a seamless, smooth-surfaced polyurethane sac. The power line and a vent travel subcutaneously and exit the patient in the right lower quadrant of

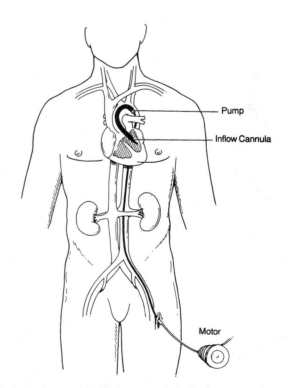

FIG. 8.3. The Hemopump is inserted via the femoral arteries. The inflow to the pump sits in the left ventricle and the outflow in the proximal descending aorta.

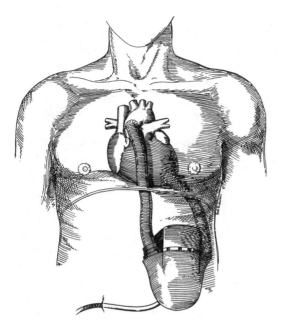

FIG. 8.4. The Novacor left ventricular assist device (electromechanical).

the abdomen. A series of sensors are attached to the pump mechanism and exit the body in the same line. These connect to a console with two controllers, one serving as a backup. Information about filling and stroke volumes, pump rate, and energy use are displayed on the console for analysis. This device can provide flows of up to 8 L/min (51). The Novacor ventricular assist device can be triggered in three different settings: (a) at a fixed rate independent of the intrinsic cardiac activity, (b) following the native QRS complex of the electrocardiogram, or (c) following changes in the rate of pump filling. It is most widely used in the latter setting. This allows filling of the ventricular assist device during ventricular systole, which triggers device ejection. However, the device has been used in patients who are in ventricular fibrillation. In this case, filling of the device occurs by a pressure gradient; 10 mm Hg is the minimum required. According to a current protocol, patients are sent home with a Novacor device while they wait for heart transplantation (27). The surgical implantation of the Novacor left ventricular assist system requires cardiopulmonary bypass.

The TCI ventricular assist device is a totally implantable, pneumatically driven dual-chamber pump in a rigid titanium housing. A flexible polyurethane diaphragm sits between the air and blood chambers (Fig. 8.5). The remainder of the blood chamber is made of sintered titanium microspheres. This surface promotes coating of the lining with the patient's own blood while minimizing clot formation (52). The device, which has been used since 1985 (53), is positioned in the left upper quadrant of the abdomen. The

inlet low-porosity Dacron conduit is anastomosed to a hole cored in the apex of the left ventricle. A longer outlet Dacron conduit goes to the aorta. Porcine valves sit at the inlet and outlet of the device and provide unidirectional flow. The pneumatic drive line travels subcutaneously and exits the skin at a distance from the device; it then connects to the console. An electric vented ventricular assist device is also available that allow patients to be discharged home. This device can generate blood flows of up to 8 L/min.

Indications for placement of the Novacor or TCI ventricular assist device are similar. The following criteria must be met: (a) approved transplant candidate; (b) systolic blood pressure below 80 mm Hg or mean blood pressure below 60 mm Hg with a pulmonary capillary wedge pressure of 20 mm Hg or more and a cardiac index of less than 2.0 L/min per square meter; (c) maximal inotropic support; and (d) IABP support. Clinical criteria that contraindicate the use of these devices include the following: body weight of less than 50 kg, body surface area of less than 1.5 m^2, age below 65 years, chronic renal insufficiency requiring hemodialysis within 1 month before surgery, unresolved pulmonary infarction secondary to pulmonary embolism, severely depressed right ventricular function with estimated ejection fraction below 10%, fixed pulmonary hypertension with pulmonary vascular resistance above 6 Wood units after a trial of prostaglandin E_1 or inhalation oxygen therapy, severe hepatic failure with either total bilirubin above 10 mg/dL or biopsy-proven cirrhosis, unresolved malignancy, severe blood dyscrasia, severe cerebrovascular or peripheral vascular disease, prior cerebrovascular accident or transient ischemic attack, acute systemic infection, and positive result on HIV antibody test.

The advantages of implantable ventricular assist devices are pulsatile flow, mobilization of patients, possible support

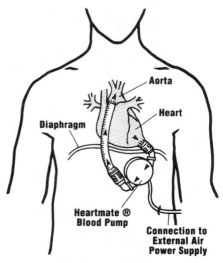

FIG. 8.5. TCI Heartmate.

for long periods, and high cardiac output capability. The disadvantages are that (a) they require a median sternotomy with extension into the upper abdominal wall or abdominal cavity; (b) fit problems are possible in smaller patients; (c) they cannot support the right ventricle; (d) anticoagulation is required; (e) they are expensive ($100,000 per console and $50,000 per pump); and (f) complications of bleeding, infection, or thromboembolism can occur.

Management of the Novacor Ventricular Assist Device after Implantation

Frequent monitoring of the cardiovascular, respiratory, hepatic, and renal systems is performed according to established protocols required of each institution. Bleeding from drainage tubes and coagulation profiles are serially determined to establish the requirement for blood products. Stroke volume and cardiac output are displayed on the left ventricular assist device monitor; inotropic support is given as needed to support the right ventricle. Of great concern is the development of right ventricular failure, manifested by low device output, peripheral edema, hepatic congestion, a high central venous pressure, and a decrease in the pulmonary capillary wedge pressure. In this case, a centrifugal right ventricular assist device may be necessary. A euvolemic state should be maintained for proper functioning of the ventricular assist device.

Heparin is usually started shortly after implant. Dipyridamole in a dosage of 100 mg every 6 hours is given via a nasogastric tube in the immediate postoperative period and is continued for the duration of the implant. Chest tubes are removed as soon as minimal drainage is observed. Ventilatory support is weaned, following by extubation and early mobilization of the patient. Prophylactic broad-spectrum intravenous antibiotics are recommended for the first 24 to 48 hours. If evidence of sepsis or acute infection is noted, cultures from all body fluids, including fluids in chest tubes, are obtained and appropriate antibiotics are started. All central, monitoring, and peripheral lines are removed as soon as possible.

Early nutritional support, which is of extreme importance, is initiated, preferably via the gastrointestinal route, with tube feedings or by mouth. Frequent calorie counts may be required. All wounds, especially the cable exit site, are examined for early detection of infection. To avoid the formation of cytotoxic antibodies, strategies that minimize giving the patient blood products are used. Blood is drawn by "microtechnique" (with small tubes such as are used in neonates), only single-donor platelets are given, and white blood cell filters are utilized. The hematocrit is allowed to fall to 18% to 20% before blood is replaced. Iron supplements and erythropoietin are utilized when appropriate. When blood is required, the freshest (<7 days old) possible units are administered to minimize hemolysis associated with these devices (38). The recommended long-term anti-

coagulation with the Thermo Cardiosystems left ventricular assist device consists of aspirin alone.

Univentricular or Biventricular Devices

Centrifugal Pumps

This family of pumps utilizes centrifugal force to generate a nonpulsatile flow. The flow rate depends on the rotational speed of the pump. Blood enters the pump at the apex and is accelerated outward. Currently, this type of pump is manufactured by Medtronic-BioMedicus (Eden Prairie, Minnesota); Sarns (Ann Arbor, Michigan); and Aries Medical (Chelmsford, Massachusetts). These pumps can be used to assist either the left or right ventricle, or both (54). The inflow cannula to the pump originates from the left or right atrium, and the outflow goes to the aorta or pulmonary artery. The centrifugal pump is extracorporeal, with the inflow and outflow cannulas passing through the chest wall (Fig. 8.6). The pump is electromagnetically coupled to a motor that connects to the control console (55). In this way, the pump console is completely sealed from blood contacting surfaces in the "pump head."

Flows ranging from 2 to 5 L/min are obtained with these devices. The current adult centrifugal pumps should not be run below outputs of 0.5 L/min. It is recommended that the activated clotting time be maintained at 1.5 times normal with continuous heparin infusions. During weaning of these devices, the dosage of heparin should be increased to decrease the potential for thrombus formation (56).

Indications for the use of the centrifugal pumps are similar to those described above. They have been used in cases of cardiogenic shock (57), as a bridge for transplantation

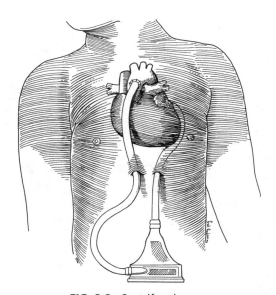

FIG. 8.6. Centrifugal pump.

(58,59), to support a failing heart after transplantation (60), and in patients who could not be weaned from bypass (61).

The advantages of centrifugal pumps are as follows: (a) They are non-IDE devices; (b) they are comparatively inexpensive ($11,000 per console and $150 per disposable pump head); (c) they can be used for left or right ventricular support, or for both simultaneously; (d) the console size is small; (e) the flow probe provides feedback on the pump flow. The disadvantages are the following: (a) Intensive monitoring is required, so that a perfusionist must generally be present at all times; (b) full anticoagulation is needed; (c) patients must be immobilized; (d) support is limited to a few days, so use as a bridge to transplant is limited; (e) hemolysis, bleeding, infection, and thromboembolism are potential complications; and (f) the pump head requires changing every 24 to 48 hours.

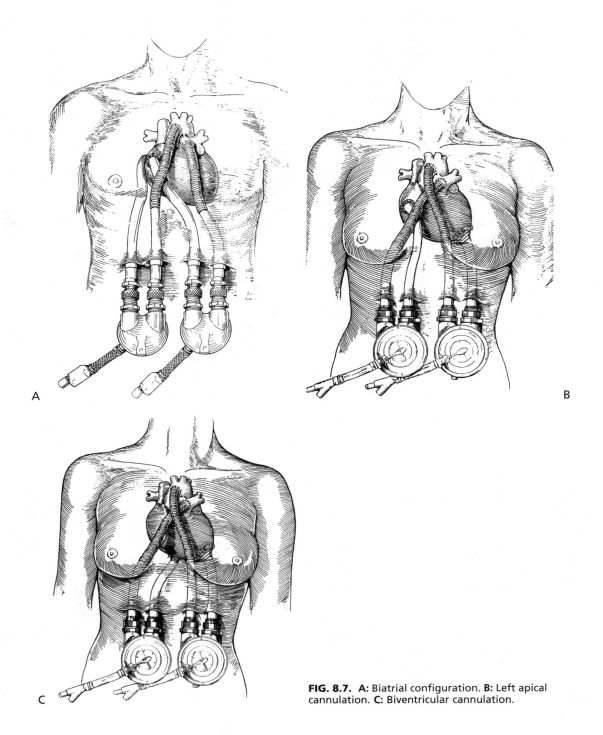

FIG. 8.7. A: Biatrial configuration. **B:** Left apical cannulation. **C:** Biventricular cannulation.

Pulsatile Paracorporeal Pumps

The family of paracorporeal pumps provides univentricular or biventricular pulsatile flow. A system of two or four cannulas provides inflow and outflow to the blood pumps (Fig. 8.7).

The Thoratec ventricular assist device is a pneumatically driven paracorporeal prosthetic ventricle. This system has been very successful when used as a bridge for cardiac transplantation (62) (Fig. 8.7). Better device filling is obtained if the pump inflow cannula comes from the patient's left and right ventricles (63). Bjork-Shiley valves sit at the inlet and outlet of each ventricle and provide unidirectional flow. A polyurethane sac divides the blood chamber from the air chamber within the prosthetic ventricle. When the device is used as a bridge to transplantation and sacrifice of a sizable portion of left ventricular apex will thus have no long-term consequence, the inflow to the left ventricular device may be anastomosed to an apical left ventriculotomy. The stroke volume from each paracorporeal ventricle is about 65 mL. The pneumatic drive lines connect to a console a few feet from the patient. This system can be triggered in a similar fashion to the one described above. A similar anticoagulation regimen is recommended.

The Abiomed BVS 5000 system is also a paracorporeal, pulsatile pneumatic device that can provide biventricular support (Fig. 8.8). Each blood pump, for right- or left-sided heart support, consists of two polyurethane chambers. Each chamber is separated from the other with trileaflet polyurethane valves. Blood flows continuously in both systole and diastole by gravity from the atrium to the first chamber within the blood pump. From there, it flows passively across an inlet valve into the active ventricle-like chamber, where it is pneumatically propelled into the great vessel composite cannula with a distal Dacron conduit. The pumps are operated by a console that determines the pulsatile rate and the systole-to-diastole ratio based on the compressed air flow into and out of the chambers. The system maintains a stroke volume of 82 mL (64). It was designed as a support for hearts that have sustained reversible damage, particularly in failed attempts at weaning in CPB situations. Patients must be kept at bed rest with this pump, which can be used for univentricular or biventricular support. In this instance, anticoagulation was maintained with intravenous heparin during the full duration of assist, with the activated coagulation time kept at 150 to 200 seconds (65).

The advantages of the paracorporeal systems are the following: (a) right, left, or biventricular support; (b) pulsatile flow; (c) patient mobilization (patients cannot be mobilized with the Abiomed system); (d) versatility for bridge to transplant; (e) useful in smaller patients; (f) long periods of support possible; (g) feedback and control of device cardiac output; (h) easier implantation; (i) commercial availability. The disadvantages of these systems include the following: (a) Cannulas limit flow to 4 to 6 L/min; (b) hemolysis, thromboembolism, bleeding, and infection are associated complications; (c) anticoagulation is required.

Total Artificial Heart

The TAH provides complete support of the circulation, but removal of the native heart is required. This device has been used to provide permanent support; however, its most important role is to serve as a bridge to cardiac transplantation. The first implantable experimental design was introduced in 1958 (66,67). An artificial heart was first used clinically in 1969 by Cooley et al. (68), who implanted the Liotta heart to supporting a patient for 64 hours until a donor heart became available. The use of the TAH as a permanent device was initiated by Jarvik et al. (69). In 1982, the Jarvik 7 was implanted in Dr. Barney Clark (70), who survived for 112 days. The Jarvik TAH was first used successfully as a bridge to cardiac transplantation by Copeland et al. (71) in 1985, in a 25-year-old man with idiopathic cardiomyopathy (72,73). The TAH was also used by the same group in patients with viral and ischemic cardiomyopathies, and in adults with congenital heart disease (72,74,75). TAHs are currently manufactured by CardioWest and Hershey Medical Center (Hershey, Pennsylvania).

The CardioWest C-70 is a pneumatically driven biventricular device (Fig. 8.9). Placement of a TAH requires a median sternotomy. Blood is withdrawn before heparinization for preclotting of the Dacron outflow grafts. Following

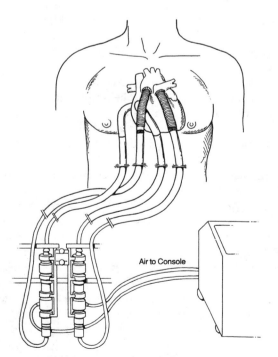

FIG. 8.8. The Abiomed circulatory support system with inflow and outflow cannulae, prosthetic ventricles, and console.

Air to Console

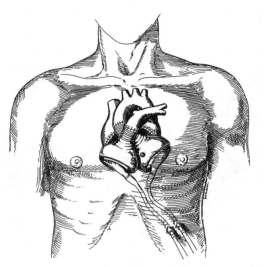

FIG. 8.9. Total artificial heart (pneumatic).

heparinization, double atrial and single ascending aortic cannulations are performed. Cardiopulmonary bypass is established and fibrillation is induced electrically. The ascending aorta is cross-clamped and a cardiectomy is performed at the atrioventricular level. The great vessels are transected just superior to the commissures of the semilunar valves. The polyurethane/Dacron atrial cuffs are then sutured in place with 3-0 polypropylene. The aortic graft anastomosis and pulmonary artery anastomoses are also performed with 3-0 polypropylene. The drive lines are tunneled subcutaneously. The left ventricle is then prefilled with saline solution and snapped to the atrial and aortic connection. Air is then removed from the ventricle. The technique of implanting the right ventricle is identical to that for the left (73,76).

The prosthetic ventricles are made of polyurethane. Mechanical heart valves (Medtronic-Hall, Minneapolis, Minnesota) sit at the inlet and outlet of the ventricles to provide unidirectional flow. A four-layered segmented polyurethane diaphragm separates blood and air. This diaphragm retracts during diastole and is displaced forward by compressed air during systole, which propels blood out of the prosthetic ventricle.

Each console has both primary and backup controllers, as well as pressurized air tanks for backup and patient transport (77). The controller provides adjustment of the heart rate, systolic duration, and drive line pressures for each of the ventricles. A personal computer monitors the mechanical function of the TAH. It displays the stroke volume and cardiac output for each of the ventricles. The CardioWest C-70 is set for incomplete filling but complete emptying with each stroke. The atrial pressure on each side determines ventricular filling. As atrial pressure increases, a higher stroke volume and cardiac output are obtained. An atrial pressure of 5 mm Hg provides a cardiac output of 4 to 5

L/min; an atrial pressure of 10 to 15 mm Hg may result in a cardiac output as high as 12 L/min at the same heart rate.

The Penn State (Hershey, Pennsylvania) heart is a pneumatically driven device that also requires removal of the native ventricles. It consists of two prosthetic ventricles that are anastomosed to the respective atria and great vessels. Each ventricle contains two chambers, one where the blood enters and is pressurized. The other chamber is filled with compressed carbon dioxide. A polyurethane diaphragm separates the two chambers within the prosthetic ventricle. The stroke volume is about 70 mL. Mechanical valves at the inlet and outlet provide unidirectional flow. The left system is set to maintain a given aortic pressure by increasing or decreasing the rate of contraction. The right system is set to maintain a given left atrial pressure, also by changing the rate of contraction.

CONSIDERATIONS IN CHOOSING A DEVICE

Circulatory assist devices have become more common and more accessible in the last few years. At the same time, a larger number of devices with overlapping purposes have become available. The considerations presented here should serve only as guidelines. It is expected that newer and more complicated devices will be developed within the coming years.

The Novacor left ventricular assist device requires implantation in the subcutaneous or intramuscular planes of the abdomen. The device should fit between the costal margin and the superior iliac spine on the left side. The patient should probably weigh a minimum of 50 kg to avoid size incompatibility. The possible problem of right ventricular failure, or an increase in pulmonary vascular resistance, must be considered before such a device is implanted. The necessity for right ventricular support should be anticipated. The Novacor should be used as a device for bridging to transplant in view of the obligatory excision and ischemia (from sutures) of the left ventricular apex. At the present time, the Novacor is recommended for transplantable patients over 50 kg and under the age of 45. The patient should also have normal pulmonary vascular resistance and probably no right ventricular failure.

The Thoratec and Abiomed ventricular assist devices are clearly the devices of choice when the cardiac pathology is felt to be reversible. Implantation of these devices may not require bypass. They can be used as the next step after IABP. The maximal cardiac output with these devices appears to be approximately 5 L/min. Thus, to provide an adequate blood flow index (>2.5 L/min per square meter), the patient should weigh less than 80 kg.

The TAH should be used when global cardiac decompensation that is not likely to be reversible is present. The best candidate for a TAH is a patient who weighs over 75 kg, is under the age of 45, and rapidly decompensates while waiting for a transplant. Implantation should be performed in a setting in which the wait for a donor is not extended (preferably, transplantation can be expected within the first 3 to 4 weeks after implantation) (37).

RESULTS WITH DEVICES USED AS A BRIDGE TO TRANSPLANTATION

For more than a decade, multiple types of circulatory devices have been utilized worldwide as bridges to heart transplantation. From 1984 through February 1996, a total of 1,286 devices were implanted worldwide, with the intent of bridging terminal patients in severe congestive heart failure to heart transplantation. Throughout the world, an additional 234 patients were bridged with nine different types of TAHs between 1969 and 1996.

Demographics among the four different manufacturers have been difficult to obtain because of proprietary data. The male-to-female ratio was 6.8 (n = 382). The most common etiology among the 1,286 patients requiring a bridge was idiopathic cardiomyopathy (n = 363), followed by ischemic cardiomyopathy (n = 226); the etiology was unclear in 697 patients. The mean age range was 42 to 47 years (n = 678). A total of 776 (60%) reached heart transplantation, and 687 were eventually discharged home. The overall success rate of discharging a patient home after heart transplantation reached was 88.5%. The similarity of the individual success rates of the bridge devices (range, 81% to 94%) demonstrates their efficacy in bridging a patient to heart transplantation. The fact that the rates are similar should serve to improve the selection criteria for use of the devices. Patient needs may one day dictate what device should be utilized (37).

FUTURE DIRECTIONS

Congestive heart failure affects approximately 4 million people in the United States. Approximately 3% to 10% of these patients will die each year as a result of the complications of congestive heart failure. It is estimated that $3.1 billion per year would be required to support every patient needing a circulatory support system. It is thought that treatment of patients with circulatory assist devices may enable them to return to the work force and contribute to society an income greater in value than the total investment (77,78). Many new models of assist devices will appear during the next few years. TAHs with electrical motors are under study (79,80). The concept of xenotransplantation, or the use of a donor heart from another species to be used in a human recipient, continues to be controversial and biologically impossible. However, this alternative continues to be explored (81). The technology that has been developed and the knowledge that has been acquired with all types of circulatory assist devices represent one of humankind's great achievements. The quest for new materials, new power supplies, and better devices will undoubtedly open new frontiers to change human life as we know it.

KEY POINTS

- Appropriate patient selection and early initiation of support are key to the successful utilization of circulatory support devices.
- Major complications of circulatory support device use include bleeding, thromboembolization, infection, hemolysis, and multiple organ system failure.
- Between 35% and 70% of patients receiving circulatory support device therapy will recover to be weaned successfully from support or to the point of transplantation. Approximately 60% of patients who received mechanical support with the intent of bridging to transplantation actually received an allograft organ, and of these, 88.5% were subsequently discharged home.
- Device categories include intraaortic, internal ventricular assist (single or dual ventricular), external ventricular assist (also single or dual ventricular) devices, and the total artificial heart.
  - Intraaortic devices are the intraaortic balloon counterpulsation pump and the axial pump.
  - Internal assist devices may be univentricular or biventricular, and they may have atrial or ventricular supply sites with corresponding outflow vessel discharge sites. Power supply may be compressed gas or electrical.
  - External devices include centrifugal pumps and two paracorporeal pulsatile pumps (Thoratec ventricular assist device and Abiomed ventricular assist device).
  - Current total artificial hearts are pneumatically driven biventricular devices that require excision of the native ventricles.
- Indications for support device use are keyed to patient criteria and therapeutic targets.
  - Intraaortic devices may be the first line but are largely limited to short-term support.
  - External devices provide longer-term support but may limit patient mobility (except for the Thoratec device). In general, these are best suited for situations in which myocardial recovery is anticipated.
  - The internal devices appear to be the current choice when transplantation is the target therapy and a bridging interval is required, provided patient characteristics meet device criteria.

■ The total artificial heart necessitates that the native ventricles are excised with device implantation, so that only permanent device dependence (not currently feasible) and transplantation are left as therapeutic alternatives.

REFERENCES

1. Levinson MM, Copeland JG. The artificial heart and mechanical assistance prior to heart transplantation. In: Cerrilli CJ, ed. *Organ transplantation and replacement.* Philadelphia: JB Lippincott Co, 1987:661–679.

2. Iglehart JK. Transplantation: the problem of limited resources. *N Engl J Med* 1983;309:123–128.

3. Evans RW, Manninen DL, Garrison LP Jr, et al. Donor availability as the primary determinant of the future of heart transplantation. *JAMA* 1986;255:1892–1898.

4. Pierce WS, Parr GVS, Myers JL, et al. Ventricular-assist pumping in patients with cardiogenic shock after cardiac operations. *N Engl J Med* 1981;305:1006–1010.

5. Pae WE, Pierce WS, Pennock JL, et al. Long-term results of ventricular assist pumping in postcardiotomy cardiogenic shock. *J Thorac Cardiovasc Surg* 1987;93:434–441.

6. Pennington DG, McBride LR, Schwartz MT, et al. Use of the Pierce-Donachy ventricular assist device in patients with cardiogenic shock after cardiac operations. *Ann Thorac Surg* 1989;47:130–135.

7. Rose DM, Conolly M, Cunningham JN, et al. Technique and results with a roller pump left and right heart assist device. *Ann Thorac Surg* 1989;47:124–129.

8. DePaulis R, Riebman JB, Delenze P, et al. The total artificial heart: indications and preliminary results. *J Card Surg* 1987;2:275.

9. Pennock JL, Pierce WS, Campbell DB, et al. Mechanical support of the circulation followed by cardiac transplantation. *J Thorac Cardiovasc Surg* 1986;92:994–1004.

10. Carpentier A, Perier P, Brugger JP, et al. Heterotopic artificial heart as a bridge to cardiac transplantation. *Lancet* 1986;2:97–98.

11. Hill JD, Farrar DJ, Hershon JJ, et al. Use of a prosthetic ventricle as a bridge to cardiac transplantation for postinfarction cardiogenic shock. *N Engl J Med* 1986;314:626–628.

12. Farrar DJ, Hill JD, Gray LA, et al. Heterotopic prosthetic ventricles as a bridge to cardiac transplantation. A multicenter study in 29 patients. *N Engl J Med* 1988;318:333–340.

13. Pennington DG, Codd JE, Merjavy JP, et al. The expanded use of ventricular bypass systems for severe cardiac failure and as a bridge to cardiac transplantation. *J Heart Transplant* 1984;3:170–175.

14. Ott RA, Mills TC, Eugene J, et al. Clinical choices for circulatory assist devices. *ASAIO Trans* 1990;36:792–798.

15. Hill JD. Bridging to cardiac transplantation. *Ann Thorac Surg* 1989;47:167–171.

16. Hill JD, Hardesty RL, Baumgartner WA, et al. Intraoperative management. *Ann Thorac Surg* 1989;47:82–87.

17. Pennington DG, Swartz LD, Pae WE, et al. Circulatory support symposium 1988: patient selection. *Ann Thorac Surg* 1989;47:77–81.

18. Pierce WS, Gray LA, McBride LR, et al. Other postoperative complications: circulatory support. *Ann Thorac Surg* 1989;47:96–101.

19. Portner PM, Oyer PE, Pennington DG, et al. Implantable electrical left ventricular assist system: bridge to transplantation and the future. *Ann Thorac Surg* 1989;47:142–150.

20. Kormos RL, Borovetz HS, Gasior T, et al. Experience with univentricular support in mortally ill cardiac transplant candidates. *Ann Thorac Surg* 1990;49:261–272.

21. Pennington DG, Reedy JE, Swartz MT, et al. Univentricular versus biventricular assist device support. *J Heart Lung Transplant* 1991;10:258–263.

22. Ott RA, Joyce L, Emery RW. Current status of mechanical circulatory assistance. *Bull Minn Heart Inst Found* 1988;6:13–18.

23. Acharya A. Development of PMA guidance for ventricular assist devices and total artificial heart. *IEEE Eng Med Biol* 1988;7:90–91.

24. *Federal Register* 1985 Jan 18:45:3732–3747.

25. Smith RG, Cleavinger M. Current perspectives on the use of circulatory assist devices. *AACN Clin Issues Crit Care Nurs* 1991;3:488–499.

26. Joist JH, Pennington DG. Platelet reactions with artificial surfaces. *ASAIO Trans* 1987;33:341–343.

27. Copeland JG, Harker LA, Joist JH, et al. Bleeding and anticoagulation. *Ann Thorac Surg* 1989;47:88–95.

28. Czer LS, Bateman TM, Gray RJ, et al. Treatment of severe platelet dysfunction and hemorrhage after cardiopulmonary bypass: reduction in blood product usage with desmopressin. *J Am Coll Cardiol* 1987;9:1139–1147.

29. Seear MD, Wadsworth LD, Rogers PC, et al. The effect of desmopressin acetate (DDAVP) on postoperative blood loss after cardiac operations in children. *J Thorac Cardiovasc Surg* 1989;98:217–219.

30. Salzman EW, Weinstein MJ, Weintraub RM, et al. Treatment with desmopressin acetate to reduce blood loss after cardiac surgery: a double-blind randomized trial. *N Engl J Med* 1986;314:1402–1406.

31. Icenogle TB, Smith RG, Cleavinger M, et al. Thromboembolic complications of the Symbion AVAD system. *Artif Organs* 1989;13:532–538.

32. Levinson MM, Smith RG, Cork RC, et al. Thromboembolic complications of the Jarvik-7 total artificial heart: case report. *Artif Organs* 1986;10:236–244.

33. Griffith BP. Interim use of the Jarvik-7 artificial heart: lessons learned at Presbyterian-University Hospital of Pittsburgh. *Ann Thorac Surg* 1989;47:158–166.

34. Didisheim P, Olsen DB, Farrar DJ, et al. Infections and thromboembolism with implantable cardiovascular devices. *ASAIO Trans* 1989;35:54–70.

35. McBride LR, Ruzevich SA, Pennington DG, et al. Infectious complications associated with ventricular assist device support. *ASAIO Trans* 1987;33:201–202.

36. Muneretto C, Solis E, Pavie A, et al. Total artificial heart: survival and complications. *Ann Thorac Surg* 1989;47:151–157.

37. Copeland JG, Smith RG, Cleavinger MR, et al. Bridge to transplantation indications for Symbion TAH, Symbion AVAD and Novacor LVAS. In: Akutsu T, ed. Artificial heart 3. *Proceedings of the 3rd International Symposium on Artificial Heart and Assist Device.* Tokyo: Springer-Verlag, 1991:303–308.

38. Kanter KR, Swartz MT, Pennington DG, et al. Renal failure in patients with ventricular assist devices. *ASAIO Trans* 1987;33:426–428.

39. Moulopoulos SD, Topaz S, Kolff W. Diastolic balloon pumping (with carbon dioxide) in the aorta—a mechanical assistance to the failing circulation. *Am Heart J* 1962;63:669.

40. Kantrowitz A, Tjonneland S, Freed PS, et al. Initial clinical experience with intra-aortic balloon pumping in cardiogenic shock. *JAMA* 1968;203:113–118.

41. Quaal SJ. Balloon's effect on a failing heart. In: Norwitz BE, ed. *Comprehensive intra-aortic balloon pumping.* St. Louis: Mosby, 1984:84–94.

42. Hardy MA, Dobelle W, Bregman D, et al. Cardiac transplanta-

tion following mechanical circulatory support. *Am Soc Artif Intern Organs* 1979;25:182–185.

43. Park SB, Lieblet GA, Burkholder JA, et al. Mechanical support of the failing heart. *Ann Thorac Surg* 1986;42:627–631.
44. Seldinger SI. Catheter replacement of the needle in percutaneous arteriography: a new technique. *Acta Radiol* 1953;39:368–376.
45. Roundtree WD. The hemopump temporary cardiac assist device. *AACN Clin Issues Crit Care Nurs* 1991;3:562–574.
46. Butler KC, Moise JC, Wampler RK. The Hemopump—a new cardiac prosthesis device. *IEEE Trans Biomed Eng* 1990;37: 193–196.
47. Phillips SJ, Barker L, Balentine J, et al. Hemopump support for the failing heart. *ASAIO Trans* 1990;36:M629–M632.
48. Deeb GM, Bolling J, Nicklas RS, et al. Clinical experience with the Nimbus pump. *ASAIO Trans* 1990;36:M632–M636.
49. Portner PM, Oyer PE, Jassawalla JS, et al. An alternative in end-stage heart disease: long-term ventricular assistance. *J Heart Transplant* 1983;3:47–59.
50. Portner PM, Oyer PE, Pennington DG, et al. Implantable electrical left ventricular assist system: bridge to transplantation and the future. *Ann Thorac Surg* 1989;47:142–150.
51. Shinn JA. Novacor left ventricular assist system. *AACN Clin Issues Crit Care Nurs* 1991;3:575–586.
52. Abou-Awdi NL. Thermo Cardiosystems left ventricular assist device as a bridge to cardiac transplant. *AACN Clin Issues Crit Care Nurs* 1991;3:545–551.
53. Bernhard WF, Clay W, Gernes D, et al. Temporary and permanent left ventricular bypass: laboratory and clinical observations. *World J Surg* 1985;9:54–64.
54. Drinkwater DC, Laks H. Clinical experience with centrifugal pump ventricular support at UCLA Medical Center. *ASAIO Trans* 1988;34:505–508.
55. Quaal SJ. Centrifugal ventricular assist devices. *AACN Clin Issues Crit Care Nurs* 1991;3:515–526.
56. Magovern GJ, Golding LAR, Oyer PE, et al. Weaning and bridging. *Ann Thorac Surg* 1989;47:102–107.
57. Park SB. Mechanical support of the failing heart. *Ann Thorac Surg* 1986;42:627–631.
58. Golding LAR, Stewart RW, Sinkenwich M, et al. Nonpulsatile ventricular assist bridging to transplantation. *ASAIO Trans* 1988; 34:476–479.
59. Bolman RM, Cox JL, Marshall W, et al. Circulatory support with a centrifugal pump as a bridge to cardiac transplantation. *Ann Thorac Surg* 1989;47:108–112.
60. Hooper TL, Odom NJ, Fetherston GJ, et al. Successful use of the left ventricular assist device for primary graft failure after heart transplantation. *J Heart Transplant* 1988;7:385–387.
61. Joyce LD, Kiser JC, Eales F, et al. Experience with the Sarns centrifugal pump as a ventricular assist device. *ASAIO Trans* 1990;36:M619–M623.
62. Farrar DJ, Lawson JH, Litwak P, et al. Thoratec VAD system as a bridge to heart transplantation. *J Heart Transplant* 1990;9: 415–423.
63. Arabia FA, Paramesh V, Toporoff B, et al. Biventricular cannulation for the Thoratec ventricular assist device. *Ann Thorac Surg* 1998;66:2119–2120.
64. Dixon JF, Farris CD. The Abiomed BVS 5000 system. *AACN Clin Issues Crit Care Nurs* 1991;3:552–561.
65. Champsaur G, Ninet J, Vigneron M, et al. Use of the Abiomed BVS 5000 as a bridge to cardiac transplantation. *J Thorac Cardiovasc Surg* 1990;100:122–128.
66. Akutsu T, Kolff WJ. Permanent substitutes for valves and hearts. *Trans ASAIO* 1958;4:230–235.
67. Akutsu T, Houston CS, Kolff WJ. Artificial hearts inside the chest, using small electric motors. *Am Soc Artif Intern Organs* 1960;6:299.
68. Cooley DA, Liotta D, Hallman GL, et al. First human implantation of cardiac prosthesis for staged total replacement of the heart. *Trans ASAIO* 1969;15:252–263.
69. Jarvik RK, Smith LM, Lawson JH, et al. Comparison of pneumatic and electrically powered total artificial heart *in vivo*. *Am Soc Artif Intern Organs* 1978;24:593–599.
70. DeVries WL, Anderson JL, Joyce LD, et al. Initial human application of the Utah total artificial heart. *N Engl J Med* 1984;310: 273–278.
71. Copeland JG, Levinson MM, Smith R, et al. The total artificial heart as a bridge to transplantation. *JAMA* 1986;256: 2991–2995.
72. Levinson MM, Smith RG, Cork RC, et al. Three recent cases of the total artificial heart before transplantation. *J Heart Transplant* 1986;5:215–228.
73. Levinson MM, Copeland JG. Technical aspects of the total artificial heart: implantation and temporary applications. *J Card Surg* 1987;2:3–19.
74. Copeland JG, Smith RG, Icenogle T, et al. Orthotopic total artificial heart bridge to transplantation: preliminary results. *J Heart Transplant* 1989;8:124–138.
75. Copeland JG, Smith RG, Icenogle TB, et al. Early experience with the total artificial heart as a bridge to cardiac transplantation. *Proceedings of the 2nd International Symposium on Artificial Heart and Assist Device*, 1987:217–223.
76. DeVries WC, Joyce LD. The artificial heart. *Clin Symp* 1983; 35:1–32.
77. Barker LE. The total artificial heart. *AACN Clin Issues Crit Care Nurs* 1991;3:587–597.
78. Poirier VL. Can our society afford mechanical hearts? *ASAIO Trans* 1991;37:540–544.
79. Davis PK, Rosenberg G, Snyder AJ, et al. Current status of permanent total artificial hearts. *Ann Thorac Surg* 1989;47:172–178.
80. Poirier VL. The quest for the permanent LVAD. We must continue. We must push forward. *ASAIO Trans* 1990;36:787–788.
81. Bailey LL. Biologic versus bionic heart substitutes. Will xenotransplantation play a role? *ASAIO Trans* 1987;33:51–53.

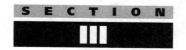

SECTION

III

PHYSIOLOGY AND PATHOLOGY

9

BLOOD–SURFACE INTERFACE

L. HENRY EDMUNDS, JR.
NINA STENACH

Extracorporeal circulation and open heart surgery (OHS) expose the entire blood mass to biomaterials in the perfusion circuit and nonendothelial cells in the wound. Normally, blood cells and proteins interface only with endothelium, which is designed to maintain the fluidity of blood and the integrity of the vascular system simultaneously. Endothelial cells accomplish this dual purpose by producing both anticoagulants and procoagulants to maintain a fragile balance between the fluid and gel forms of blood. Contact with nonendothelial surfaces, whether biomaterial, basement membrane, cell membrane, or matrix, tips the balance toward thrombosis. Contact of the blood with foreign surfaces during cardiopulmonary bypass (CPB) and OHS triggers a defense reaction so explosive that essentially every cell within the body is affected.

Extracorporeal circulation is not possible without anticoagulation (1). Although other anticoagulants have been used successfully in special situations (2–4), CPB for OHS requires high concentrations of heparin during perfusion to maintain the fluidity of blood. Heparin has both advantages and disadvantages; the most notable advantages are immediate onset of action and reversibility with protamine or recombinant platelet factor 4 (5). Heparin does not directly inhibit coagulation; rather, it acts indirectly by accelerating the actions of the natural protease inhibitor antithrombin (6). Antithrombin primarily binds thrombin; its actions on factors Xa and IXa are much slower and, during CPB, inconsequential. Thus, heparin inhibits coagulation at the end of the cascade after most coagulation proteins have been converted to active enzymes. Because antithrombin is a large molecule (58 kDa), heparin does not inhibit thrombin trapped within clots (7). Heparin also activates several blood constituents: platelets (8–10), factor XII (11), complement, neutrophils, and monocytes (12–14). Heparin concentrations are difficult to monitor in the operating room, so crude, indirect methods are used (15,16). Heparin is associ-

ated with an allergic response; heparin-induced thrombocytopenia occurs in 2% to 4% of patients, and the devastating complication of heparin-induced thrombocytopenia and thrombosis affects 0.1% to 0.2% (17). And perhaps worst of all, heparin only partially suppresses thrombin formation during CPB (18,19). Despite the administration of doses two to three times those used for other indications, thrombin is steadily generated and circulated during CPB. Thus, heparin is far from an ideal anticoagulant, but in practical terms, it is the only one we have.

When heparinized blood comes in contact with a biomaterial, plasma proteins are instantly (<1 sec) adsorbed onto the surface to form a *monolayer* of selected proteins (20–22). For a given protein, the amount adsorbed depends on its bulk concentration in plasma and the intrinsic surface activity of the protein for each biomaterial. The *intrinsic surface activity* differs between plasma proteins and also between biomaterial surfaces. The physical and chemical composition of the *biomaterial surface* determines the intrinsic surface activity of the biomaterial. Thus, concentrations of plasma proteins on a given biomaterial differ from concentrations in bulk plasma. Similarly, concentrations of surface-adsorbed proteins from the same plasma differ for different biomaterials. The composition of the protein monolayer is specific for the biomaterial and for various concentrations of proteins in the plasma, but it is not certain that the topography of the adsorbed protein layer is uniform across the surface of the biomaterial (23). On most biomaterial surfaces, fibrinogen is selectively adsorbed, but the adsorbed concentration of fibrinogen and other proteins can change over time (22). Adsorbed proteins "compete" for space on the biomaterial surface and are tightly packed, irreversibly bound, and immobile. Calculations indicate that the density of surface-adsorbed proteins is two to three orders of magnitude greater than the density of the proteins in bulk plasma (23). The complexity of blood–biomaterial interactions is further compounded by the fact that adsorbed proteins often undergo limited conformational changes (24,25) that may expose "receptor" amino acid groups recognized by specific blood cells or plasma proteins such as factor XII, complement protein 3, or platelets (23). For a given ad-

L. H. Edmunds, Jr.: Department of Surgery, Hospital of the University of Pennsylvania, Philadelphia, Pennsylvania 19104.

N. Stenach: Medtronic, Inc., Minneapolis, Minnesota.

sorbed protein, these conformational changes can vary between biomaterial surfaces, and thus change the reactivity of the adsorbed protein with cells and blood proteins in the bulk phase.

Thus, the interface between heparinized blood and the wound and perfusion circuit is an aggregate of many separate reactions between circulating blood constituents and exposed tissues and an undefined monolayer of adsorbed proteins. This infinite number of small reactions changes the composition of the circulating blood, which in turn triggers responses from normal endothelial cells lining the heart and blood vessels. A host of blood proteins are converted to active enzymes, and all blood cells are stimulated to express receptors, release granule contents, and synthesize new enzymes and chemicals. These reactions during CPB and OHS are described as the "whole body inflammatory response" (26), which temporarily transforms homeostasis into chaos.

BLOOD PROTEINS AND CELLS

Because blood circulates and reaches every cell, the enzymatic stew produced by CPB and OHS mediates the thrombotic, bleeding, and inflammatory reactions and the temporary organ dysfunction associated with CPB and OHS. A detailed explanation of these events is beyond the knowledge of these authors; only a simplified approach beginning with the major blood elements involved can be offered. The thrombotic, bleeding, and inflammatory responses to CPB and cardiac surgery primarily involve *five blood protein systems* (the contact, intrinsic coagulation, extrinsic coagulation, fibrinolytic, and complement protein systems) and *five types of blood cells* (platelets, endothelial cells, neutrophils, monocytes, and lymphocytes). Basophils and eosinophils are also involved in the inflammatory response, but their numbers and probable impact are small. Lymphocytes are definitely activated during CPB and cardiac surgery and these changes affect immunity and resistance to infection, but they have little impact on thrombosis and inflammation.

Contact System

The contact system consists of four proteins: factor XII, prekallikrein, high-molecular-weight kininogen (HMWK), and factor XI (27). Adsorption of factor XII (Hageman factor) onto a foreign surface in the presence of prekallikrein and HMWK changes the three-dimensional geometry of the protein to produce active proteases, factors XIIa and XIIf (23). In a feedback loop, factor XIIa cleaves prekallikrein to produce kallikrein and HMWK to produce bradykinin, a short-acting vasodilator (27). Factor XIIa in the presence of kallikrein and HMWK also activates factor XI to factor XIa. Factor XIa activates the intrinsic coagulation cascade, which proceeds through factor IX to activate factor X and form thrombin. Kallikrein is a major agonist for neutrophils; factor XIIa is a weak agonist.

The contact proteins are activated during *in vitro* recirculation of heparinized blood in a perfusion circuit and during CPB and OHS (12). The intensity of activation of these proteins may vary with surface composition, but this hypothesis has not yet been quantified.

Intrinsic Coagulation Pathway

Figure 9.1 diagrams the intrinsic coagulation pathway, which eventually produces the tenase complex composed of activated factors VIII and IX, calcium, and a phospholipid surface (28,29). This complex binds factor X and produces factor Xa, which is the gateway protein of the common coagulation pathway. Factor Xa slowly cleaves prothrombin to α-thrombin, the active enzyme, and a fragment, F1.2, but the reaction is 300,000 times faster if catalyzed by the *prothrombinase complex* (30–33). The prothrombinase complex is produced when factor Xa, in the presence of Ca^{2+}, is anchored by factor Va onto a phospholipid surface provided by platelets, monocytes, or endothelial cells (30–33). Either factor Xa or thrombin activates factor V to factor Va (34). The prothrombinase complex cleaves prothrombin to thrombin and a fragment, F1.2, and is the major pathway producing thrombin (35). F1.2 is a useful marker of the reaction. Thrombin, a powerful protease with multiple reactions, is neutralized when it forms an irreversible complex with antithrombin.

Although the extrinsic coagulation pathway is more important than the intrinsic pathway during clinical CPB and OHS (36), there is direct evidence that the intrinsic pathway is activated and that thrombin is produced in the extracorporeal perfusion circuit (37).

Extrinsic Coagulation Pathway

Tissue factor is a membrane-bound protein that is constitutively expressed by most tissue cells, including vascular adventitia, fat, muscle, and epicardium, but not by pericardium or hepatocytes (38–40). Stimulated monocytes and endothelial cells also express tissue factor (41,42). Tissue factor initiates the extrinsic coagulation pathway by activating factor VII to factor VIIa. This enzyme in turn combines with factor Va, calcium, and a phospholipid surface to convert factor X to factor Xa (29–31). Thus, factor Xa is produced by both the intrinsic and extrinsic coagulation pathways during CPB and OHS. The intrinsic pathway is primarily activated in the perfusion circuit; the extrinsic pathway predominates in the wound (39). During CPB, thrombin is steadily produced and circulates (18,19). Thrombin, which is a powerful protease with multiple reactions, is neutralized when it forms an irreversible complex with the native protease inhibitor antithrombin.

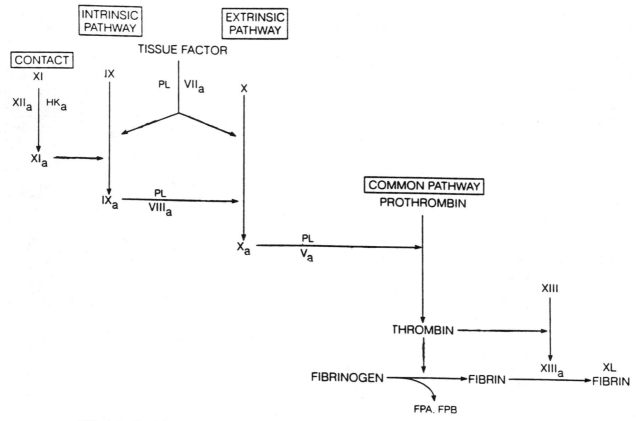

FIG. 9.1. Simplified diagram of the clotting cascade. The central precipitating event involves tissue factor (*TF*), which under physiologic conditions is not exposed to blood. With vascular or endothelial cell injury, TF acts in concert with activated factor VIIa and phospholipid (*PL*) to convert factor IX to IXa and factor X to Xa. The "intrinsic pathway" includes "contact" activation of factor XI by the XIIa/activated high-molecular-weight kininogen (*HMWKa*) complex. Factor XIa converts factor IX to IXa, and factor IXa in turn converts factor X to Xa, in concert with factors VIIIa and PL. However factor Xa is formed, it is the active catalytic ingredient of the prothrombinase complex, which includes factor Va and PL and converts prothrombin to thrombin. Thrombin cleaves fibrinopeptides (*FPA, FPB*) from fibrinogen to allow the resultant fibrin monomers to polymerize, and converts factor XIII to XIIIa, which cross-links (*XL*) the fibrin clot. (From Colman RW, Marder VJ, Salzman EW, et al. Overview of hemostasis. In: Colman RW, Hirsch J, Marder VJ, et al., eds. *Hemostasis and thrombosis: basic principles and clinical practice,* 3rd ed. Philadelphia: JB Lippincott Co, 1994:9, with permission.)

Fibrinolysis

The fourth protein system activated during CPB and OHS is the fibrinolytic system (43,44). Circulating thrombin activates endothelial cells to produce tissue plasminogen activator (t-PA), which binds avidly to fibrin (45,46). Kallikrein, produced by the contact system, cleaves prourokinase to urokinase; however, this enzyme is less important during CPB and OHS because urokinase binds poorly to fibrin (46). The combination of t-PA, fibrin, and plasminogen cleaves plasminogen to plasmin; plasmin cleaves fibrin. The reaction produces a useful marker protein fragment, D-dimer. Fibrinolysis is controlled by native protease inhibitors: α_2-antiplasmin, α_2-macroglobulin, and plasminogen activator inhibitor-1. Plasminogen activator inhibitor-1,

produced by endothelial cells, directly inhibits t-PA and urokinase, but little is produced during CPB; peak concentration occurs the day after operation (47). α_2-antiplasmin rapidly inhibits unbound plasmin and prevents the enzyme from circulating, but it poorly inhibits plasmin bound to fibrin. α_2-macroglobulin is a slow inhibitor of plasmin.

Complement

Complement is activated by both the classic and alternative pathways during CPB and OHS (12,48,49). Surface contact in the perfusion system activates the classic pathway via C1, C2, and C4 to form C3 convertase to cleave C3 into C3a and C3b (12). The alternative pathway, involving factors

B and D and C3b, also forms C3 convertase, and because it is amplified by the production of C3b, it is the predominant pathway during CPB and OHS (49). At the end of CPB, the classic pathway is activated a second time when heparin is neutralized by protamine; the heparin–protamine complex strongly activates complement via the classic pathway (12,49).

C3b is the active enzyme that cleaves C5 to C5a and C5b. C5b initiates the formation of the terminal complement complex (TCC) by sequentially binding C6, C7, C8, and finally several molecules of C9 (50). Hydrophobic domains of the TCC interact with fatty acid chains of cellular membrane phospholipids to form transmembrane channels that eventually lyse the cell. C3a, C4a, and C5a are anaphylatoxins with vasoactive properties. C5a is a major agonist for neutrophils (51,52). The TCC accelerates thrombin formation via its action on the prothrombinase complex (53). Blockade of C5a and TCC generation inhibits neutrophil and platelet activation during CPB (54).

Platelets

Although technically not cells, platelets are activated during CPB and OHS by surface contact, heparin, circulating thrombin, and platelet-activating factor (PAF) formed by a variety of cells. Heparin increases the sensitivity of platelets to soluble agonists (8), inhibits binding to von Willebrand's factor (10), and modestly increases template bleeding times (8,9). Initially, platelets are most likely activated by circulating thrombin, which is a powerful agonist and binds with a specific thrombin receptor (55). As CPB continues, activated complement (C5b–9) (53), plasmin (56–58), hypothermia (58,59), PAF, interleukin-6 (IL-6) (60), cathepsin G, serotonin, epinephrine, and other agonists also activate platelets and contribute to their loss and dysfunction.

Platelets immediately undergo shape change and express pseudopods and surface receptors. Activated platelets express glycoprotein (GP) IIb/IIIa and GPIb receptors (61,62) and secrete soluble and bound P-selectin receptors from α-granules (63). GPIIb/IIIa receptors nearly instantaneously bind platelets to exposed binding sites on the a- and y-chains on surface-adsorbed fibrinogen (64–66). Expressed GPIIb/IIIa receptors bind platelets to other platelets using fibrinogen as a bridge. By using P-selectin, platelets bind monocytes and neutrophils to form aggregates (63,67). In the wound, platelets use expressed GPIb receptors and von Willebrand's cofactor to adhere to exposed basement membranes (68). As CPB continues, some adherent platelets detach to produce platelet microparticles and partially fragmented platelets (61,66,69,70). Platelet adhesion and aggregate formation reduce the circulating platelet count, which has already been reduced by dilution with pump priming solutions.

A small percentage of activated platelets synthesize and release a variety of chemicals and proteins from granules,

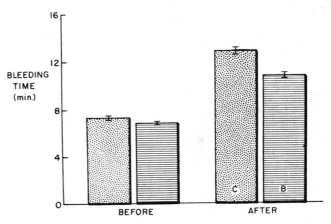

FIG. 9.2. Template bleeding times with standard errors of the mean before and 1 hour after protamine in patients undergoing clinical cardiopulmonary bypass (*CPB*) and open heart surgery (*OHS*) with bubble (*stippled*; n = 12) or membrane (*hatched*; n = 22) oxygenators. *C*, p<0.005 vs. before; *B*, p<0.01 vs. before. (From Edmunds LH Jr, Ellison N, Colman RW, et al. Platelet function during open heart surgery: comparison of the membrane and bubble oxygenators. *J Thorac Cardiovasc Surg* 1982;83:805–812, with permission.)

including thromboxane A$_2$ (71), platelet factor 4, β-thromboglobulin (72), P-selectin (63), serotonin, adenosine diphosphate, adenosine triphosphate, calcium, mitogens, acid hydrolases (73), and neutral proteases.

At the end of CPB, the circulating platelet population is a heterogeneous mixture that probably varies between patients and perfusion systems. Hemodilution, adhesion, aggregation, release, and destruction reduce platelet numbers by 30% to 50% (74,75). Some platelets are intact and discoid, whereas others show pseudopod formation (75). Some larger platelets recently arrived from the bone marrow are present (76), in addition to partially and completely degranulated platelets, platelet membrane fragments, resealed platelets, and platelet microparticles (66). Most of these platelets appear morphologically normal (75). Overall, function of the platelet mass is reduced, and bleeding times are prolonged to approximately twice normal values for several hours (74) (Fig. 9.2).

Endothelial Cells

Endothelial cells are activated during CPB and OHS by a variety of agonists, including thrombin, C5a (77), and various cytokines [e.g., IL-1, tumor necrosis factor (TNF)] (45,78). Endothelial cells produce: prostacyclin (PGI$_2$); heparan sulfate; thrombomodulin and protease nexin-1 (both of which remove thrombin); protein S, which accelerates the natural anticoagulant protein C; tissue factor pathway inhibitor, which regulates the extrinsic coagulation pathway; and t-PA. Endothelial cells produce vasoactive substances, such as nitric oxide, PGI$_2$, endothelin-1 (79,80), and PAF, and inactivate others, such as histamine, norepinephrine, and bradykinin (81). Prostacyclin concentrations increase rapidly at the beginning of CPB and then begin to decrease (82). Endothelin-1 peaks several hours after CPB ends (83).

Activation of endothelial cells during CPB stimulates expression of protein and cellular receptors, including tissue factor and both P- and E-selectin. Tissue factor is procoagulant; P- and E-selectin mediate rolling adhesion of neutrophils and monocytes to facilitate arrest and eventually transmigration to the extravascular space. VCAM-1 (vascular cell adhesion molecule-1) and ICAM-1 (intercellular adhesion molecule-1) are endothelial cell-expressed immunoglobulins that serve as ligands for Mac-1 (CD11b/CD18) and $\alpha_4\beta_1$ receptors on neutrophils and monocytes. Experimentally, ICAM-1 is upregulated during CPB in pulmonary vessels (84). There is evidence that P- and E- selectin are upregulated during CPB and in myocardial ischemia–reperfusion sequences; the roles of ICAM-1 and VCAM-1 are not clearly defined.

Neutrophils

Neutrophils are strongly activated during cardiopulmonary bypass. The principal agonists are kallikrein and C5a, which are produced by the contact and complement systems, respectively (27,52,85). Other agonists during CPB include factor XIIa, heparin, leukotriene B_4, IL-1β, IL-8, and TNF (86). Neutrophil granules contain a "smorgasbord" of cytotoxic enzymes, oxidants, and chemicals (Table 9.1). During CPB and OHS, neutrophils release neutral proteases (e.g. elastase) (87), lysosomal enzymes, myeloperoxidase, hydrogen peroxide, hydroxyl radicals, hypochlorous acid, hypobromous acid, acid hydrolases, and collagenases. During CPB, neutrophils express the Mac-1 (CD11b/CD18) receptor and CD11c/CD18, which binds to fibrinogen and a complement fragment (78). Mac-1 is an important receptor for binding neutrophils to endothelial cells and collagen. Mac-1 also binds factor X and fibrinogen and thus facilitates thrombin formation (88). Activated neutrophils express L-selectin, a receptor for P-selectin expressed by endothelial

TABLE 9.1. CONTENT OF NEUTROPHILIC GRANULES

Azurophilic Granules	Specific Granules	Respiratory Burst
Elastase	Lysozyme	Hydrogen peroxide
Cathepsin G	Lactoferrin	Hydroxyl radicals
Lysozyme	Collagenase	Hypobromous acid
Myeloperoxidase		Hypochlorous acid
Defensins		
Acid hydrolases		
Bacterial permeability agent		

cells and platelets, and $\alpha_4\beta_1$ receptors, which are involved in cellular adhesion. Neutrophils play a major role in ischemia–reperfusion injuries and are responsible for much of the inflammatory response associated with CPB and OHS.

Monocytes

Monocytes are activated to express tissue factor, both in the wound and the perfusion circuit (39), but activation in the perfusion circuit is delayed for several hours (89). Blood in contact with the surgical field contains higher concentrations of factor VIIa, F1.2, and monocytes expressing tissue factor than do simultaneous samples taken from the perfusion circuit during CPB and OHS (39). Addition of this blood to the perfusate increases monocyte tissue factor expression in the circulating perfusate (39); however, if the amount of field blood added to the perfusate is small, the increase in percentage of circulating monocytes expressing tissue factor is modest (90). In another study, no increase in monocyte tissue factor was observed at the end of CPB and OHS (91), but other monocyte cellular receptors [Mac-1, monocyte chemotactic protein-1 (MCP-1)] were upregulated at the end of CPB, and tissue factor was strongly expressed 20 hours after operation (91). This study correlated suppression of monocyte tissue factor at the end of CPB with high concentrations of the antiinflammatory cytokine IL-10. Although the process is not completely clear, it appears that monocyte tissue factor is generated in the wound and by adherent monocytes in the perfusion circuit. The status of circulating monocytes at the end of CPB is undecided and may be affected by the balance between antiinflammatory and inflammatory cytokines (91). A delayed increase in monocyte tissue factor expression occurs 20 hours after CPB ends (91).

Monocytes also express Mac-1, L-selectin, and MCP-1 during CPB and OHS (78,92) and form aggregates with platelets (63). MCP-1 is a powerful monocyte agonist (92) that is produced by monocytes and several other cells. Other agonists include C5a (85), immune complexes, endotoxin, and IL-1 1β. The number of circulating monocytes does not change during CPB and OHS, but it increases afterward, peaking at 20 hours (93–95). Monocyte expression of CD14 is downregulated during CPB and OHS (93)

Monocytes produce various cytokines involved in the inflammatory response to CPB and OHS, notably IL-β, IL-6, and TNF-α (86,93,95). Production of these cytokines by macrophages is stimulated during CPB and OHS, but peak concentrations occur several hours after CPB ends (95–98).

Lymphocytes

The numbers of B and T cells and the responsiveness of lymphocytes to mitogens and other agonists are reduced during the first week after CPB and OHS (99–102). The decrease involves B, CD4+ (helper/inducer), and CD8+ (cytotoxic/suppressor) cells in some studies (103,104); in others, the number of CD8+ cells and the ratio of CD8+ to CD4+ cells increase (94,102). Production of IL-2 and interferon-α decreases (94,104); IL-2 receptor expression also decreases (99). These changes are independent of blood transfusions (103) and indicate depression of the immune response.

SURFACES

Surfaces, not the bulk, interface between biomaterials and surrounding tissues (e.g., blood). Although bulk properties of biomaterials are very important with respect to manufacture, mechanical properties, durability, and function, physical and chemical characteristics determine the intrinsic surface activity of any material in contact with blood (see above). Surfaces of solids differ from the bulk, are very reactive and often mobile, and are easily contaminated (105). These characteristics, summed by the term *intrinsic surface activity*, can be partially described by sophisticated physical and chemical measurements (Table 9.2). Unfortunately, very few general correlations can be made between a measurement and the ability or inability of the biomaterial to activate various blood elements. For example, surface "roughness" increases platelet adhesion on hydrophobic surfaces in comparison with hydrophilic surfaces (106), and it is generally accepted that a "hydrophilic environment at the blood–polymer interface is beneficial in reducing platelet adhesion and thrombus formation" (107). In a baboon arteriovenous shunt model, platelet adhesion correlates inversely with the fraction of hydrocarbon-type groups in the ESCA C1s spectra of polyurethanes (108). Essentially all

TABLE 9.2. PHYSICAL PROPERTIES OF BIOMATERIAL SURFACES THAT MAY CORRELATE WITH BIOREACTIVITY

Wettability	Subsurface features
Hydrophilic/hydrophobic ratio	Distribution of functional
Polar/dispersive character	receptor sites
Surface chemistry	Elastic modulus
Specific functional groups	Hydrogel (swelling)
Surface electrical properties	character
Roughness/porosity	Mobility
Domains of surface chemicals	Adventitious
	contamination
	Trace quantities of
	groups

Reproduced from Ratner BD. Correlation of material surface properties with biological responses. In: Ratner BD, Hoffinan AS, Schoen FJ, et al., eds. *Biomaterials science. An introduction to materials in medicine.* San Diego: Academic Press, 1996:447, with permission.

the correlations between physical and chemical properties of biomaterials and activation of blood elements are made retrospectively; to date, it is not possible to predict blood reactivity on the basis of the physical and chemical properties of a "new" biomaterial. Thus, development of new blood-compatible biomaterials is a process of trial and error.

Many methods have been developed to modify surfaces of biomaterials to increase their biocompatibility with heparinized blood. (*Biocompatibility* can be defined as minimal activation of blood elements; the term is obviously imprecise.) Physicochemical means to modify surfaces include attachment or deposition of octadecyl groups, silicone-containing block copolymers, plasma fluoropolymers, plasma siloxane polymers, radiation-grafted hydrogels, and chemically modified polystyrene (109). Polyethylene oxide is a particularly useful nonionic hydrogel that can be immobilized on hydrophobic surfaces to increase water solubility, provide a large excluded volume to repel proteins and cells, increase surface mobility, and provide side chains for attachment of other molecules (107). Drugs, antibodies, and enzymes immobilized within or on biomaterial surfaces are also described (110). Examples include surfaces coated with albumin (111), a nitric oxide donor (112), and heparin (107).

MEDIATORS

The interaction between blood, the wound, and biomaterial surfaces of the perfusion circuit produces an angry brew that is circulated without normal reflex vasomotor controls by a separated extracorporeal pump. Cardioplegia and reperfusion washout of the heart, part of nearly every operation, add more activated blood elements and cell-signaling proteins to the mixture (113,114). During and after CPB, the perfusate contains a host of vasoactive substances, enzymes, cell-signaling proteins, and cytotoxins. Vasoactive substances are defined as substances that cause endothelial or vascular smooth-muscle cells to contract or relax or that alter myocyte contractility (79). Reports describing blood or perfusate concentrations of some substances, particularly complement fragments and cytokines, during CPB and OHS often vary with respect to the time of peak concentration or whether the vasoactive material is altered at all (79,115–117). Substances that cause vasodilation of vascular smooth muscle or contraction of endothelial cells, or that are chemotactic for neutrophils or monocytes, are proinflammatory; other substances, such as IL-10 and IL-13, are antiinflammatory. Endotoxin, thought to be absorbed from the gut during CPB, is proinflammatory, but it is not always detected during CPB (118). An ever-growing but undoubtedly incomplete list of cell-signaling substances reported to be altered during CPB and OHS appears in Table 9.3. The list includes hormones, autocoids, electrolytes, ana-

TABLE 9.3. CELL SIGNALING SUBSTANCES ALTERED BY CARDIOPULMONARY BYPASS AND OPEN HEART SURGERY

Epinephrine	Glucagon	Platelet-Activating Factor	Platelet Microparticles
Norepinephrine	Thyroxine	Nitric oxide	P-selectin
Dopamine	Triiodothyronine	Endothelin-1	Leukotriene B_4
Renin	Complement 3a, 4a, 5a	Interleukin-1–interleukin-13	MCP-1
Angiotensin II	Ca++, K+, Mg++	Interleukin-6	
Vasopressin	Serotonin	Interleukin-8	
Aldosterone	Histamine	Tumor necrosis factor-α	
Bradykinin	Prostacyclin	Interleukin-10	
Atrial natriuretic factor	Prostaglandin E_2	Interleukin-13	
Corticosteroids	Thromboxane A_2	Interferon-γ	

Cell signaling substances include hormones, autocoids, cytokines, electrolytes, anaphylatoxins, and paracrines, which are soluble agents that act on cells. They do not include cytotoxic substances such as C5b–9, free radicals, proteases, hydrolases, and lysozmes.
MCP-1, monocyte chemotactic protein-1.

phylatoxins, cytokines, soluble cell receptors, eicosanoids, and paracrines—all soluble substances that act on cells. Many are vasoactive; none is considered cytotoxic, although cytotoxins also circulate (117). Many of these substances are designed for local activity and not intended for distribution to the entire body. At present, contradictory reports and undefined variables preempt a clear and quantitative understanding of the complex interrelationships between circulating mediators and target cells during CPB and OHS.

In addition to these soluble substances, circulating cells express numerous receptors for interaction with circulating enzymes and other blood cells (Table 9.4). Most cells stay within the vascular system, but a few neutrophils and macrophages migrate to the extravascular space along with various cell-signaling proteins and enzymes. These activated, circulating blood cells and cell-signaling substances mediate much of the inflammatory response to CPB and OHS (119). Microemboli account for most of the remainder.

TABLE 9.4. BLOOD CELLULAR RECEPTORS THAT ARE UPREGULATED DURING CARDIOPULMONARY BYPASS

Platelets	**Neutrophils**
GPIIb/IIIA; GPIb	Mac-1 (CD11b/CD18)
P-selectin	CD11c/CD18
Thrombin receptor	L-selectin
Endothelial cells	$\alpha_4\beta_1$
ICAM-1; VCAM-1	**Monocytes**
E- and P-selectins	Mac-1
Tissue factor	Tissue factor
Lymphocytes	L-selectin
L-selectin	Monocyte chemotactic protein-1
HLA-DR	

GP, glycoprotein; CD, cluster of differentiation; ICAM, intercellular adhesion molecule; VCAM, vascular cell adhesion molecule.

CONSEQUENCES

The complications of bleeding associated with CPB and OHS are related to preexisting coagulation deficiencies, heparin, platelets, and fibrinolysis. Preexisting coagulation deficiencies are detected and treated preoperatively. CPB dilutes soluble coagulation factors and reduces factors V and VIII to concentrations below those expected from dilution (120), but bleeding rarely, if ever, is caused by these factors. Inadequate or unsustained neutralization of heparin with protamine commonly causes bleeding after extracorporeal circulation. Heparin "rebound" describes an increase in bleeding 1 to 3 hours after operation that results from the release of heparin bound to endothelial cells and macrophages after protamine has been cleared from the circulation (121). Heparin-induced thrombocytopenia is an allergic reaction involving heparin-induced immunoglobulin G (IgG) antibodies and platelets (17). This phenomenon, which occurs approximately 5 days after operation (or sooner if it has been previously experienced) and is manifested by an unexpected decrease in the platelet count, is related to heparin-induced thrombocytopenia and thrombosis, which is a major catastrophe. Causes of bleeding related to platelets and fibrinolysis are described above.

Discovery of clot within the wound or perfusion circuit during CPB and OHS is a cause for alarm and an indication for immediate administration of more heparin. Better to treat heparin overdose than to circulate thrombus or abruptly lose the heart–lung machine with the heart open or arrested.

Cardiopulmonary bypass produces a variety of large and small emboli that are reduced but not totally prevented by filtration (122) (Table 9.5). A depth filter or a 40-μm (pore size) arterial line screen filter removes most but not all emboli larger than 40 μm. Screen filters with smaller pore sizes increase the pressure difference across the filter, interfere

TABLE 9.5. EMBOLIC MATERIAL PRODUCED DURING CARDIOPULMONARY BYPASS AND OPEN HEART SURGERY

Fibrin
Fat (free fat, denatured lipoproteins, chylomicrons)
Denatured protein
Platelet aggregates
Leukocyte aggregates
Red cell debris
Gas (nitrogen, oxygen)
Foreign material (calcium, tissue debris, suture material)
Spallated material (primarily roller pumps)

with pump flow, and are not generally used. During CPB, arterioles, precapillaries, and capillaries are bombarded with microemboli (<40 μm), but cell death is diffusely distributed and involves relatively few cells in any one location. For the most part, microemboli are not detected during CPB but can be documented by special studies (123–125).

Blood activation and surgery itself produce fibrin emboli, macroaggregates of denatured proteins and lipoproteins, fat globules, and platelet and leukocyte aggregates (122,123). The embolic load is directly proportional to the duration of CPB. Foreign material may enter the perfusion system. Homologous blood contains platelet and leukocyte aggregates, fibrin, lipid precipitates, and red cell debris and should be filtered before it is added to the perfusate (122).

Crystalloid solutions may contain inorganic debris, and dust may remain on the inside of commercially produced tubing. Roller pumps cause spallation of bits of compressed tubing (122). Bubble oxygenators produce microbubbles of oxygen (123).

Most particulate emboli are aspirated from the wound by cardiotomy suckers; they include fibrin, fat, calcium, cellular debris, suture material, and other foreign matter (122). Aspiration of large quantities of air produces nitrogen microbubbles, which are poorly soluble in plasma. Because of poor blood solubility, these microbubbles are more dangerous than those of oxygen or carbon dioxide.

The surgical procedure itself is the most important source of macroemboli and microemboli, which produce lasting damage to the central nervous system (125–128). Cannulation and manipulation of the ascending aorta cause atheromatous macroemboli to form, particularly in patients with soft, atheromatous material in the aorta (126,129). Microemboli also are produced during cardiac surgery and cause postoperative neuropsychologic deficits in proportion to their numbers (125–126). Surgical steps, particularly aortic cannulation and manipulation of either the heart or the aorta, correlate with the production of microemboli (126) (See Chap. 16).

Interstitial fluid increases as capillary permeability increases (130) in response to circulating vasoactive substances that cause endothelial cells to contract (Fig. 9.3). There is little or no evidence that intracellular fluid increases. The

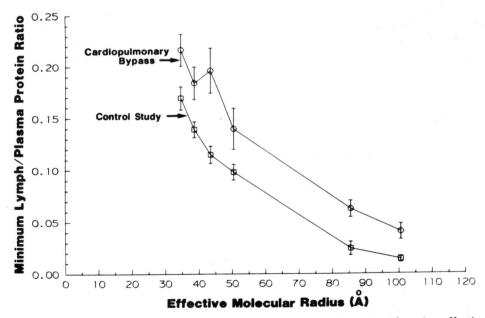

FIG. 9.3. Average minimum lymph/plasma concentration ratios of proteins of varying effective molecular radius after cardiopulmonary bypass or sham procedure (control study), as determined by gel electrophoresis. The *vertical bars* represent one standard error. (From Smith EEJ, Naftel DC, Blackstone EH, et al. Microvascular permeability after cardiopulmonary bypass. *J Thorac Cardiovasc Surg* 1987;94:225, with permission.)

accumulation of extravascular water is directly proportional to the duration of CPB and can be massive (e.g., 20 L) in patients with complicated operations. This fluid is removed by diuresis during the early postoperative period.

The combination of circulating cell-signaling and cytotoxic substances and microemboli together with excess interstitial fluid produces dysfunction of essentially every organ in the immediate postoperative period. Organ dysfunction is temporary or at least not detectable beyond the immediate postoperative period except in the brain. In up to 30% of patients, subtle neuropsychologic changes are demonstrable 1 year after operation (128); most of these changes probably derive from the presence of microemboli, but other causes cannot be excluded. During the immediate postoperative period, heart, lung, and kidney function are most important for survival and must be sufficient to provide an adequate, stable circulation, diuresis of excess interstitial fluid, and weaning from the ventilator. Other chapters in this book describe in detail the impact of CPB on various organ systems.

CONTROL OF THE BLOOD–SURFACE INTERFACE

There are two logical approaches to controlling the blood–surface interface and the bleeding, thrombotic, and inflammatory complications associated with CPB and OHS (131). The most desirable approach is to develop biomaterials with surface properties similar to those of endothelial cells. Because active metabolic processes in endothelial cells maintain the fluidity of blood and integrity of the vascular system, this goal is still far distant and probably not achievable except through tissue engineering and populating endothelial cells on synthetic scaffolds. The goal is worthwhile, however, because success in attaining it would overcome the major barrier to the development of artificial organs that could process blood, as is normally done in lung, liver, kidney, and other organs (132). An alternative approach is to prevent the activation of blood elements during the period in which blood is exposed to the wound and biomaterials of the perfusion circuit. Although this goal is more readily achievable, it applies only to extracorporeal perfusion systems.

A review of past and current investigative attempts to produce "nonthrombogenic" or "thromboresistant" biomaterial surfaces is well beyond the scope of this chapter. However, two surface modifications that are used clinically and claim to improve "biocompatibility" deserve discussion. These modifications are surface-bound heparin and surface-modifying additives. Clinical experience with promising new materials, such as nitric oxide-releasing coatings, is either lacking or too limited for complete evaluation.

Surface-bound Heparin

Heparin can be bound to certain biomaterials by either ionic or covalent bonds (107,133). The commercial Duraflo II heparin coating (Baxter Healthcare Corporation, Irvine, California) binds heparin ionically by means of a proprietary process to retard heparin leaching (134). The Carmeda heparinized surface (Medtronic, Minneapolis, Minnesota) covalently binds partially degraded heparin attached to "spacer arms" to laminated biomaterial surfaces (135). Although occasional studies report minor advantages of one coating over the other, these are inconsistent and not associated with any important clinical differences between the two coatings (136,137). Proponents of surface-bound heparin perfusion circuits allege that their use suppresses thrombin formation, reduces blood loss and transfusion requirements, attenuates the inflammatory response, and decreases platelet activation, and that clinical indicators of CPB and OHS morbidity are less than in operations in which uncoated perfusion circuits are used.

An enormous literature reports an extensive clinical experience with heparin-bonded versus uncoated perfusion circuits (138). However, with few exceptions, other variables are simultaneously introduced into most comparisons. The three most important additional variables relate to *patient selection, exclusion or washing of blood aspirated from the surgical field,* and *reducing the dose of systemic heparin.* Most comparative studies have been made in patients undergoing first-time myocardial revascularization (139–154); for the most part, these are relatively short-term perfusions with minimal return of unwashed field blood to the perfusate. Fewer studies report experience in patients with complex procedures or reoperations (155–160). Only a few reports compare the intensity of blood activation in the wound with that in the perfusion circuit (36,29,161). However, available studies show that thrombin formation (39), fibrinolysis (162), monocyte activation (39), and platelet expression of GPIb receptors (163) are greater in the wound than in the circuit; these findings suggest that other markers of inflammation may also be higher in the wound. Thus, the amount of unwashed field blood added to the perfusate during CPB and OHS has a profound influence on the markers of thrombosis, bleeding, and inflammation measured in the perfusate.

The third confounding variable is the dose of heparin. Abundant evidence indicates that heparin is an agonist for directly activating several blood zymogens and cells (8–14); therefore, although little dose-response, quantitative information is available, reducing systemic heparin may reduce activation of these blood elements. Several studies show that when a reduced dose rather than a full dose of systemic heparin is administered to patients in whom heparin-coated circuits are used, neutrophil activation is reduced (164–166). Finally, it must be recognized that clinical studies of the efficacy of heparin-bonded perfusion circuits are severely constrained by the absolute necessity of administering some heparin and by our inability to measure circulating thrombin concentrations continuously in real time. No one knows the amount of thrombin that can be safely circulated in patients during CPB and OHS; furthermore, it is highly likely that "safe" concentrations of circulating thrombin vary between patients. Because macroscopic clotting within the perfusion circuit is a major disaster and microscopic clotting is undesirable, the authors strongly recommend erring on the side of too much heparin rather than too little.

Neither ionic nor covalent bound heparin-coated perfusion circuits convincingly reduce the rate of thrombin formation, although the coating binds antithrombin onto the surface (156). Although some studies indicate reduced rates of rise of F1.2 and TAT (thrombin–antithrombin complex) during CPB and OHS (145), most studies show no difference in these markers of thrombin formation and accumulation between heparin-coated and uncoated perfusion circuits (139,146,151,156–158,165,167–171). When these circuits are used for life support without systemic heparin, the incidence of visible thrombus within the ventricle or pump head is 27% (172). Clotting has occurred in other circumstances when heparin-coated circuits were used with reduced systemic heparin (169,173) or no heparin (174).

Reports are mixed regarding whether heparin-coated perfusion circuits reduce postoperative blood losses and transfusion requirements. Several investigators report decreases in postoperative mediastinal drainage of between 4.5% to 24% (in comparison with control groups) (139,140,153, 164,165,169,175,176); others report no reduction in blood loss (142,144–146,152,154,156,158,177–179).

Findings in the voluminous literature are mixed regarding whether markers of inflammation (i.e., complement activation, neutrophil release, cytokine production) are attenuated by heparin-bonded perfusion circuits. Most studies combined heparin-coated circuits with reduced systemic heparin in first-time revascularization patients in whom field aspirated blood is minimal. Under these conditions, most studies show reduced generation of complement fragments (136,142,160,164,171,176,180,181). A few studies do not (141,145). When using heparin-bonded circuits and reduced systemic heparin in patients undergoing more complex procedures, Videm et al. (160) noted a decrease in complement fragments, but with full-dose systemic heparin, Gorman et al. did not (156). Nearly all studies except one (179) show reduced concentrations of C5b–9, the TCC (136,140–142,148,150,160,165,180,182).

The literature is more mixed regarding activation of neutrophils and other leukocytes. Some reports found reduced plasma concentrations of neutrophil elastase (164,171, 176,182), lactoferrin (136,140,142,164), TNF-α (183), and myeloperoxidase (140,142,153) (Fig. 9.4) when heparin-bonded circuits were used. Others failed to find significant changes in plasma elastase (145,150,156,184), lactofer-

rin (148,180) or myeloperoxidase (136,148,180) (Fig. 9.4). Two observers found a reduction in markers of eosinophil activation (143,185). Moen and colleagues (148) noted an upregulation of neutrophil CR3 receptors but no change in CR1, CR4, and L-selectin. Garred and Mollnes (186) found reduced Mac-1 and CD45 expression but no change in CDI4 and CDI6.

Reports are also mixed with respect to changes in circulating cytokines. In patients perfused with heparin-bonded circuits, IL-6 is unchanged (182) or reduced (149,155,171), IL-8 is increased (149,155) or not (182,183), TNF is reduced (149,183) or unchanged (155,182), IL-1 is unchanged (155), and kallikrein–C1 inhibitor complex is reduced (168).

Boonstra and colleagues (152) reported no change in bleeding times in first-time myocardial revascularization patients perfused with heparin-bonded circuits and full systemic heparin. Two studies reported less platelet adhesion with heparin-bonded circuits (156,176), and four indicated no significant change (139,146,152,171). Most reports show no significant change in release of β-thromboglobulin (139,146,152,156,158); a few show small reductions (176,179). Boonstra et al. (152) found no change in thromboxane B$_2$ concentrations; Muehrcke et al. (158) found no change in soluble P-selectin.

Clinical benefits are difficult to document. In the largest clinical study, involving 11 centers and 805 patients, no clinical benefits from the use of heparin-bonded perfusion circuits with full systemic concentrations of heparin were discovered (144). Results of other studies are mixed. Clinical benefits, such as reduced length of stay, quicker extubation, and less temperature elevation, are reported in some studies (150,154,165,172,179,182), but not in others (144,159, 160,178,187,188). The weight of evidence indicates that heparin-bonded perfusion circuits are associated with reduced formation of the TCC, but in a large study, this reduction was not associated with clinical benefit (187).

Perhaps it is now appropriate to conclude that heparin-bonded perfusion circuits offer little benefit to low-risk patients unless the systemic dose of heparin is substantially reduced and unwashed field blood is not added to the perfusate (189). However, even under these conditions, the benefits in terms of reduced bleeding, reduced transfusions, reduced inflammatory response, and quicker recovery are at best controversial (190). Considering that circulating thrombin cannot be measured continuously in real time, is the benefit of reducing systemic heparin and using heparin-bonded circuits worth the risk and extra cost?

Surface-modifying Additives

Surface-modifying additives are chemicals used in low concentrations to reduce interfacial energy. They are added to mobile bulk biomaterials during fabrication. These additives spontaneously migrate to the surface and dominate

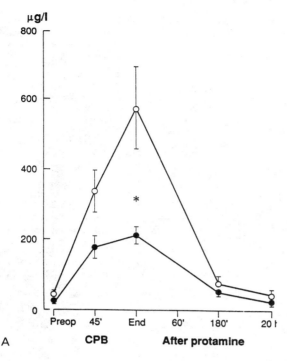

A

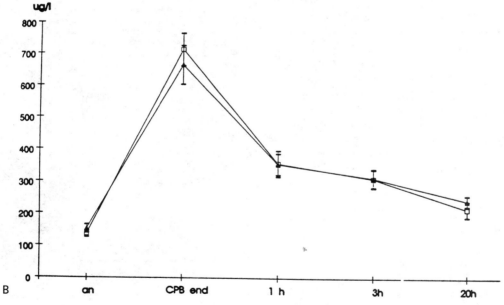

B

FIG. 9.4. A: Myeloperoxidase in plasma during and after clinical cardiopulmonary bypass (means ± SEM). *Solid circles,* heparin-coated circuits; *open circles,* uncoated circuits. *p <0.05. (From Borowiec J, Thelin S, Bagge L, et al. Heparin-coated circuits reduce activation of granulocytes during cardiopulmonary bypass. *J Thorac Cardiovasc Surg* 1992;104:644, with permission.) **B:** Myeloperoxidase in plasma before, during, and after clinical cardiopulmonary bypass and open heart surgery (means ± SEM). *Solid triangles,* heparin-coated circuits; *open squares,* uncoated circuits. (From Borowiec J, Thelin S, Bagge L, et al. Decreased blood loss after cardiopulmonary bypass using heparin-coated circuit and 50% reduction of heparin dose. *Scand J Thorac Cardiovasc Surg* 1992;26:177–185, with permission.)

surface molecules. One commercially available surface-modifying additive uses a triblock copolymer containing polar and nonpolar polymer chains of polycaprolactone-polydimethylsiloxanepolycaprolactone (COBE Cardiovascular, Arvada, Colorado) (191). Other formulations with different intrinsic surface activities remain under investigation (192,193). In a clinical investigation of first-time myocardial revascularization patients, the available surface-modifying additive product significantly reduced platelet activation, adhesion, and release; reduced thrombin genera-

tion; and reduced t-PA production. No differences in postoperative blood loss were noted (194).

Blood Modification

Preoperative administration of corticosteroids attenuates complement activation and may attenuate cytokine production during CPB and OHS (195); hypothermia may or may not attenuate cytokine production (196,197). A number of promising inhibitors of specific serine proteases and activated blood cells are in the investigative pipeline, and a few are in phase I clinical trials. Some of these inhibitors are reversible and others are not. Three are discussed, more as examples of this approach to the problem than as final answers.

Aprotinin and two ω-aminocarboxylic acids, tranexamic acid and ϵ-aminocaproic acid, are antifibrinolytic agents that reduce postoperative blood loss by 40% to 50% after reoperative cardiac surgery and OHS in patients taking aspirin (198). Aprotinin, a protease inhibitor derived from bovine lungs, inhibits plasmin directly (199); the ω-aminocarboxylic acids inhibit cleavage of plasminogen to plasmin. Although there are differences between these drugs, all are effective and relatively safe. In high doses, aprotinin partially inhibits kallikrein and has a platelet-sparing effect (200).

"Platelet anesthesia" describes a strategy of reversibly inhibiting platelets during CPB and OHS and reversing the inhibition at the end of CPB when protamine is given and wound hemostasis is needed. The goal is a normal bleeding time at the time protamine is given. Primate experiments *in vivo*, in which either tirofiban or eptifibatide with or without nitric oxide was used in the oxygenator sweep gas, achieved this goal and demonstrated successful preservation of platelets (201–203). Use of nitric oxide alone in patients demonstrated partial protection (204).

Nafamostat mesilate (FUT-175) is a synthetic, broad-spectrum protease inhibitor active against thrombin, kallikrein, activated factors X and XII, plasmin, and complement C1r and C1s. Several clinical studies from Japan indicate that the drug attenuates complement activation and fibrinolysis and reduces postoperative blood loss. Perhaps because of the dosage and other variables, significant inhibition of other markers of blood activation did not reach statistical significance (205,206).

CONCLUSION

Interaction at the blood–nonendothelial cell interface during CPB and OHS triggers a massive defense response that is responsible for bleeding, thromboembolic, and inflammatory reactions associated with CPB. Although some microemboli are not composed of blood elements, the combination of "angry blood" and microemboli causes temporary dysfunction of every organ during the early postoperative period. Control of this interface is a prerequisite for extending applications of extracorporeal perfusion technology. In the short term, selective inhibition of specific blood constituents that mediate the defense reaction by the use of cellular and protease inhibitors may be the easiest way to achieve this goal. In the long term, development of biomaterials coated with endothelial cells or that replicate many of the attributes of endothelial cells is the foundation necessary for the successful implantation of artificial organs.

KEY POINTS

- When blood contacts nonendothelial cell surfaces, plasma proteins are instantly adsorbed onto the surface to form a monolayer of *selected* proteins on the surface. The composition of the protein monolayer is specific for different biomaterials and for different concentrations of each adsorbed protein in the bulk plasma. The adsorbed protein layer is densely packed, immobile, and irreversibly bound, but some proteins can undergo conformational change to express receptors to circulating blook proteins and cells.
- Contact between heparinized blood and biomaterials and the wound during cardiopulmonary bypass (CPB) activate at least five plasma protein systems and five blood cells and initiate what is termed a "whole body inflammatory response." This response produces the unique bleeding, thrombotic, embolic complications of CPB and OHS, the accumulation of interstitial fluid, and the temporary organ dysfunction observed in nearly every organ after operation.
  - Activation of the *contact protein system* initiates coagulation by the *intrinsic coagulation pathway* and generates kallikrein and bradykinin.
  - Blood contact with cell bound tissue factor in the wound initiates the *extrinsic coagulation pathway*. Both coagulation pathways generate thrombin, a powerful protease that cleaves fibrinogen to form fibrin and clot. Thrombin generation during CPB produces the thrombotic and part of the embolic and bleeding complications of CPB.
  - Circulating thrombin stimulates endothelial cells to produce t-PA and *fibrinolysis*.
  - The *complement system* is activated by blood contact with biomaterial surfaces and by the heparin–protamine complex at the end of CPB.
  - Circulating thrombin also activates *platelets* to adhere to nonendothelial surfaces, aggregate, and release granular contents. The resulting loss of platelet numbers and function increase postoperative bleeding times.
  - *Neutrophils* and *monocytes* are also activated to express reactive cellular receptors, release vasoactive and cytotoxic substances and produce cytokines. Activated complement proteins and products from neutrophils and monocytes mediate much of the inflammatory response to CPB and OHS. The number and responsiveness of *lymphocytes* are reduced.
  - The reactions above and other factors combine to activate *endothelial cells* within the body, which release a further variety of inflammatory, vasoactive, procoagulant (and anticoagulant) mediators. This

process exposes endothelial cell surface receptors that attract neutrophils and monocytes, which may then spread the inflammatory response by migrating extravascularly.

- Efforts to control this "whole body inflammatory response" include modification of biomaterial surfaces and administration of selective inhibitors of important blood reactions.
- Heparin coated biomaterial surfaces have been widely studied. This vast literature is difficult to analyze because many studies often include other variables that affect outcome markers. The most important confounding variables involve patient selection, exclusion of field aspirated blood from the perfusate, and reduction of heparin dose. Available data support the following conclusions.
  - Heparin coated surfaces do not suppress thrombin generation.
  - Heparin coated surfaces may or may not reduce postoperative bleeding; other variables are usually more relevant.
  - Heparin coated surfaces reduce concentrations of the complement terminal attack complex.
  - Several, but not all, clinical studies document reduction in some clinical markers of the "whole body inflammatory response" when heparin coated surfaces are used with exclusion of unwashed field aspirated blood from the perfusate.
- Since thrombin cannot be measured continuously in real time, strategies to reduce "the whole body inflammatory response" by reducing the systemic dose of heparin during CPB using heparin coated surfaces assume the risk of producing potentially catastrophic thrombotic complications.

REFERENCES

1. Gravlee GP. Anticoagulation for cardiopulmonary bypass. In: Gravlee G, Davis RF, Utley JR, eds. *Cardiopulmonary bypass, principles and practice.* Baltimore: Williams & Wilkins, 1993: 340.
2. Riess F-C, Lower C, Seelig C, et al. Recombinant hirudin as a new anticoagulant during cardiac operations instead of heparin: successful aortic valve replacement in man. *J Thorac Cardiovasc Surg* 1995;110:265–267.
3. Wilhelm MJ, Schmid C, Kececioglu D, et al. Cardiopulmonary bypass in patients with heparin-induced thrombocytopenia using Org 10172. *Ann Thorac Surg* 1996;61:920–924.
4. Gillis S, Merin G, Zahger D, et al. Danaparoid for cardiopulmonary bypass in patients with previous heparin-induced thrombocytopenia. *Br J Haematol* 1997;98:657–659.
5. Bernabei AF, Gikakis N, Maione T, et al. Reversal of heparin anticoagulation by recombinant platelet factor 4 and protamine sulfate in baboons during cardiopulmonary bypass. *J Thorac Cardiovasc Surg* 1995;109:765–771.
6. Rosenberg RD, Bauer KA. The heparin-antithrombin system: a natural anticoagulant mechanism. In: Colman RW, Hirsh J,

Marder VJ, et al., eds. *Hemostasis and thrombosis: basic principles and clinical practice.* Philadelphia: JB Lippincott Co, 1994:837.
7. Weitz JI, Hudoba M, Massel D, et al. Clot-bound thrombin is protected from inhibition by heparin antithrombin III-independent inhibitors. *J Clin Invest* 1990;86:385.
8. Euison N, Edmunds LH Jr, Colman RW. Platelet aggregation following heparin and protamine administration. *Anesthesiology* 1978;48:65–68.
9. Khuri S, Valeri CR, Loscalzo J, et al. Heparin causes platelet dysfunction and increases fibrinolysis before the institution of cardiopulmonary bypass. *Ann Thorac Surg* 1995;60: 1008–1014.
10. Sobel M, McNeill PM, Carlson PL, et al. Heparin inhibition of von Willebrand factor-dependent platelet function *in vitro* and *in vivo. J Clin Invest* 1991;87:1878–1893.
11. Pixley RA, Cassello A, De La Cadena RA, et al. Effect of heparin on the activation of factor XII and the contact system in plasma. *Thromb Haemost* 1991;66:540.
12. Wachtfogel YT, Harpel PC, Edmunds LH Jr, et al. Formation of Cis-Ci-inhibitor, kallikrien-C1-inhibitor and plasmin-alpha 2-plasmin inhibitor complexes during cardiopulmonary bypass. *Blood* 1989;73:468–471.
13. Cavarocchi NC, Schaff HY, Orszulak TA, et al. Evidence for complement activation by protamine-heparin interaction after CPB. *Surgery* 1985;98:525–530.
14. Kirklin JK, Chenoweth DE, Naftel DC, et al. Effects of protamine administration after cardiopulmonary bypass on complement, blood elements, and the hemodynamic state. *Ann Thorac Surg* 1986;41:193–199.
15. Despotis GJ, Summerfield MD, Joist JH, et al. Comparison of activated coagulation time and whole blood heparin measurements with laboratory plasma anti-Xa heparin concentration in patients having cardiac operations. *J Thorac Cardiovasc Surg* 1994;108:1076.
16. Hardy J-F, Belisle S, Robitaille D, et al. Measurement of heparin concentration in whole blood with the Hepcon/HMS device does not agree with laboratory determination of plasma heparin concentration using a chromogenic substrate for activated factor X. *J Thorac Cardiovasc Surg* 1996;112:154–161.
17. Warkentin TE, Levine MN, Hirsch J, et al. Heparin-induced thrombocytopenia in patients treated with low-molecular-weight heparin or unfractionated heparin. *N Engl J Med* 1995; 332:1330.
18. Brister SJ, Ofosu FA, Buchanan MR. Thrombin generation during cardiac surgery: is heparin the ideal anticoagulant? *Thromb Haemost* 1993;70:259.
19. Boisclair MD, Lane DA, Philippou H, et al. Thrombin production, inactivation and expression during open heart surgery measured by assays for activation fragments including a new ELISA for prothrombin fragment F1 + 2. *Thromb Haemost* 1993;70: 253.
20. Uniyal S, Brash JL. Patterns of adsorption of proteins from human plasma onto foreign surfaces. *Thromb Haemost* 1982; 47:285.
21. Ziats NP, Pankowsky DA, Tierney BP, et al. Adsorption of Hageman factor (factor XII) and other plasma proteins to biomedical polymers. *J Lab Clin Med* 1990;116:687.
22. Horbett TA. Principles underlying the role of adsorbed plasma proteins in blood interactions with foreign materials. *Cardiovasc Pathol* 1993;2:137S–148S.
23. Horbett TA. Proteins: structure, properties, and adsorption to surfaces. In: Ratner BD, Hoffman AS, Schoen FJ, et al., eds. *Biomaterials science. An introduction to materials in medicine.* San Diego: Academic Press, 1996:133–141.
24. Brash JL, Scott CF, ten Hove P, et al. Mechanism of transient

adsorption of fibrinogen from plasma to solid surfaces: role of the contact and fibrinolytic systems. *Blood* 1988;71:932.

25. Lindon JN, McManama G, Kushner L, et al. Does the conformation of adsorbed fibrinogen dictate platelet interactions with artificial surfaces? *Blood* 1986;68:355.

26. Blackstone EH, Kirklin JW, Stewart RW, et al. The damaging effects of cardiopulmonary bypass. In: Wu KK, Roxy EC, eds. *Prostaglandins in clinical medicine: cardiovascular and thrombotic disorders.* Chicago: Year Book, 1982:355.

27. Colman RW. Surface-mediated defense reactions. The plasma contact activation system. *J Clin Invest* 1984;73:1249.

28. Bauer KA, Kass BL, ten Cate H, et al. Factor IX is activated *in vivo* by the tissue factor mechanism. *Blood* 1990;76:731.

29. Limentani SA, Furie BC, Furie B. The biochemistry of factor IX. In: Colman RW, Hirsh J, Marder VJ, et al., eds. *Hemostasis and thrombosis: basic principles and clinical practice*, 3rd ed. Philadelphia: JB Lippincott Co, 1994:94–108.

30. Nesheim MC, Taswell JB, Mann KG. The contribution of bovine factor V and factor Va to the activity of prothrombinase. *J Biol Chem* 1979;254:10952.

31. Tracy PB, Rohrbach MS, Mann KG. Functional prothrombinase complex assembly on isolated monocytes and lymphocytes. *J Biol Chem* 1983;258:7264.

32. Tracy PB, Eide LL, Mann KG. Human prothrombinase complex assembly and function on isolated peripheral blood cell populations. *J Biol Chem* 1985;260:2119.

33. Scandura JM, Walsh PN. Factor X bound to the surface of activated human platelets is preferentially activated by platelet-bound factor IXa. *Biochemistry* 1996;35:8890–8901.

34. Hoyer LW, Wyshock EG, Colman RW. Coagulation cofactors: factors V and VIII. In: Colman RW, Hirsch J, Marder VJ, et al., eds. *Hemostasis and thrombosis: basic principles and clinical practice*, 3rd ed. Philadelphia: JB Lippincott Co, 1994:109–133.

35. Mann KG. Prothrombin and thrombin. In: Colman RW, Hirsch J, Marder VJ, et al., eds. *Hemostasis and thrombosis: basic principles and clinical practice*, 3rd ed. Philadelphia: JB Lippincott Co, 1994:184–199.

36. Boisclair MD, Lane DA, Phillippou H, et al. Mechanisms of thrombin generation during surgery and CPB. *Blood* 1993;82:3350–3357.

37. Gilcakis N, Khan MMH, Hiramatsu Y, et al. Effect of factor Xa inhibitors on thrombin formation and complement and neutrophil activation during *in vitro* extracorporeal circulation. *Circulation* 1996;94[Suppl II]:341–346.

38. Banner EW. The factor VIIa/tissue factor complex. *Thromb Haemost* 1997;78:512–515.

39. Chung JH, Gikakis N, Rao AK, et al. Pericardial blood activates the extrinsic coagulation pathway during clinical cardiopulmonary bypass. *Circulation* 1996;93:2014.

40. Drake TA, Morrissey JH, Edgington TS. Selective cellular expression of tissue factor in human tissues. *Am J Pathol* 1989;134:1087–1096.

41. Drake TA, Ruf W, Morrissey JH, et al. Functional tissue factor is entirely cell surface expressed on lipopolysaccharide-stimulated human blood monocytes and a constitutively tissue factor-producing neoplastic cell line. *J Cell Biol* 1989;109:389.

42. Grabowski EF, Rodriguez M, Nemerson Y, et al. Flow limits factor Xa production by monolayers of fibroblasts and endothelial cells. *Blood* 1990;76[Suppl 1]422(abst).

43. Stibbe J, Kluft C, Brommer EJP, et al. Enhanced fibrinolytic activity during cardiopulmonary bypass in open-heart surgery in man is caused by extrinsic (tissue-type) plasminogen activator. *Eur J Clin Invest* 1984;14:375.

44. Gram J, Janetzko T, Jespersen J, et al. Enhanced effective fibrinolysis following the neutralization of heparin in open heart

surgery increases the risk of post-surgical bleeding. *Thromb Haemost* 1990;63:241.

45. Francis CW, Marder VJ. Physiologic regulation and pathologic disorders of fibrinolysis. In: Colman RW, Hirsch J, Marder VJ, et al. *Hemostasis and thrombosis: basic principles and clinical practice*, 3rd ed. Philadelphia: JB Lippincott Co, 1994:1076–1103.

46. Levin EG, Marzec U, Anderson J, et al. Thrombin stimulates tissue plasminogen activator release from cultured human endothelial cells. *J Clin Invest* 1984;74:1988.

47. Lu H, Du-Bruit C, Soria J, et al. Postoperative hemostasis and fibrinolysis in patients undergoing cardiopulmonary bypass with or without aprotinin therapy. *Thromb Haemost* 1994;72:438.

48. Chenoweth DE, Cooper SW, Hugli TE, et al. Complement activation during cardiopulmonary bypass: evidence for generation of C3a and C5a anaphylatoxins. *N Engl J Med* 1981;304:497.

49. Kirklin JK, Chenoweth CE, Naftel DC, et al. Effects of protamine administration after cardiopulmonary bypass on complement, blood elements, and the hemodynamic state. *Ann Thorac Surg* 1986;41:193–199.

50. Volanakis JE. Overview of the complement system. In: Volanakis JE, Frank MM, eds. *The human complement system in health and disease.* New York: Marcel Dekker Inc, 1998:9–32.

51. Berger M. Complement-mediated phagocytosis. In: Volanakis JE, Frank MM, eds. *The human complement system in health and disease.* New York: Marcel Dekker Inc, 1998:285–308.

52. Chenoweth DE, Hugli TE. Demonstration of specific C5a receptor on intact human polymorphonuclear leukocytes. *Proc Natl Acad Sci U S A* 1978;75:3943.

53. Wiedmer T, Esmon CT, Sims PJ. Complement proteins C5b–9 stimulate procoagulant activity through the platelet prothrombinase. *Blood* 1986;68:875–880.

54. Rinder CA, Rinder HM, Smith BR, et al. Blockade of C5a and C5b–9 generation inhibits leukocyte and platelet activation during extracorporeal circulation. *J Clin Invest* 1995;96:1564–1572.

55. Coughlin SR, Vu T-K H, Hung DT, et al. Characterization of a functional thrombin receptor. *J Clin Invest* 1992;89:351.

56. Niewiarowski S, Senui AF, Gillies P. Plasmin-induced platelet aggregation and platelet release reaction. *J Clin Invest* 1973;51:1647.

57. Cramer EM, Lu H, Caen JP, et al. Differential redistribution of platelet glycoproteins Ib and IIb–IIIa after plasmin stimulation. *Blood* 1991;77:894.

58. Lu H, Soria C, Cramer EM, et al. Temperature dependence of plasmin-induced activation or inhibition of human platelets. *Blood* 1991;77:996.

59. Michelson AD, MacGregor H, Barnard MR, et al. Reversible inhibition of human platelet activation by hypothermia *in vivo* and *in vitro*. *Thromb Haemost* 1994;71:633–640.

60. Weerasinghe A, Taylor KM. The platelet in cardiopulmonary bypass. *Ann Thorac Surg* 1998;66:2145–2152.

61. Abrams CS, Ellison N, Budzynski AZ, et al. Direct detection of activated platelets and platelet-derived microparticles in humans. *Blood* 1990;75:128–138.

62. Lefkovits J, Plow EF, Topol EJ. Platelet glycoprotein Iib/IIIa receptors in cardiovascular medicine. *N Engl J Med* 1995;332:1553–1559.

63. Rinder CS, Bonnert J, Rinder HM, et al. Platelet activation and aggregation during cardiopulmonary bypass. *Anesthesiology* 1991;74:388–393.

64. Gluszko P, Rucinski B, Musial J, et al. Fibrinogen receptors in platelet adhesion to surfaces of extracorporeal circuit. *Am J Physiol* 1987;252:H615–H621.

65. Shepeck RA, Bentz M, Dickson C, et al. Examination of the

roles of glycoprotein Ib and glycoprotein IIb/IIIa in platelet deposition on an artificial surface using clinical antiplatelet agents and monoclonal antibody blockade. *Blood* 1991;78:673.

66. Wenger RK, Lukasiewicz H, Mikuta BS, et al. Loss of platelet fibrinogen receptors during clinical cardiopulmonary bypass. *J Thorac Cardiovasc Surg* 1989;97:235–239.

67. Rinder HM, Bonan JL, Rinder CS, et al. Activated and unactivated platelet adhesion to monocytes and neutrophils. *Blood* 1991;78:1760–1769.

68. Saehnan EUM, Niewenhuis HK, Hese KM, et al. Platelet adhesion to collagen types I through VIII under conditions of stasis and flow is mediated by GPIa/IIa. *Blood* 1994;83:1244–1250.

69. George JN, Pickett EB, Saucerman S, et al. Platelet surface glycoproteins; studies on resting and activated platelets and platelet membrane microparticles in normal subjects, and observations in patients during adult respiratory distress syndrome and cardiac surgery. *J Clin Invest* 1986;78:340–348.

70. Miyamoto S, Marcinkiewicz C, Edmunds LH Jr, et al. Measurement of platelet microparticles during cardiopulmonary bypass by means of captured ELISA for GPIIb/IIIa. *Thromb Haemost* 1998;80:225–230.

71. Addonizio VP Jr, Smith JB, Strauss JF III, et al. Thromboxane synthesis and platelet secretion during cardiopulmonary bypass with bubble oxygenator. *J Thorac Cardiovasc Surg* 1980;79:91–96.

72. Hennessy VL Jr, Hicks RE, Niewiarowski S, et al. Effects of surface area and composition on the function of human platelets during extracorporeal circulation. *Am J Physiol* 1977;232:H622–H628.

73. Addonizio VP Jr, Strauss JF III, Li-Feng C, et al. Release of lysosomal hydrolases during extracorporeal circulation. *J Thorac Cardiovasc Surg* 1982;84:28–34.

74. Edmunds LH Jr, Ellison N, Colman RW, et al. Platelet function during open heart surgery: comparison of the membrane and bubble oxygenators. *J Thorac Cardiovasc Surg* 1982;83:805–812.

75. Zilla P, Fasol R, Groscurth P, et al. Blood platelets in cardiopulmonary bypass operations. *J Thorac Cardiovasc Surg* 1989;97:379–388.

76. Laufer N, Merin G, Grover NB, et al. The influence of cardiopulmonary bypass on the size of human platelets. *J Thorac Cardiovasc Surg* 1975;70:727–731.

77. Saadi 5, Plait JL. Endothelial cell responses to complement activation. In: Volanakis JE, Frank MM, eds. *The human complement system in health and disease.* New York: Marcel Dekker Inc, 1998:335–353.

78. Asimakopoulos G, Taylor KM. Effects of cardiopulmonary bypass on leukocyte and endothelial adhesion molecules. *Ann Thorac Surg* 1998;66:2135–2144.

79. Downing SW, Edmunds LH Jr. Release of vasoactive substances during cardioplumonary bypass. *Ann Thorac Surg* 1992;54:1236.

80. Vane JR, Anggard EE, Betting RM. Regulatory functions of the vascular endothelium. *N Engl J Med* 1990;323:27.

81. Jaffe EA. Endothelial cell structure and function. In: Hoffman R, Benz EJ Jr, Shattil SI, et al., eds. *Hematology.* New York: Churchill Livingstone, 1991:1198.

82. Faymonville ME, Deby-Dupont G, Larbuisson R, et al. Prostaglandin E$_2$, prostacyclin, and thromboxane changes during nonpulsatile cardiopulmonary bypass in humans. *J Thorac Cardiovasc Surg* 1986;91:858.

83. Hashimoto K, Horikoshi H, Miyamoto H, et al. Mechanisms of organ failure following cardiopulmonary bypass: the role of elastase and vasoactive mediators. *J Thorac Cardiovasc Surg* 1992;104:666.

84. Dreyer WJ, Bums AR, Phillips SC, et al. Intercellular adhesion molecule-1 regulation in the canine lung after cardiopulmonary bypass. *J Thorac Cardiovasc Surg* 1998;115:689–699.

85. Ember JA, Jagels MA, Hugli TE. Characterization of complement anaphylatoxins and their biological responses. In: Volanakis JE, Frank MM, eds. *The human complement system in health and disease.* New York: Marcel Dekker Inc, 1998:241–244.

86. Insel PA. Analgesic-antipyretic and antiinflammatory agents and drugs employed in the treatment of gout. In: Hardman IG, Limbird LE, eds. *Goodman and Gilman's pharmacological basis of therapeutics.* New York: McGraw-Hill, 1996:618–619.

87. Wachtfogel YT, Kucich U, Greenplate J, et al. Human neutrophil degranulation during extracorporeal circulation. *Blood* 1987;69:324–330.

88. Kappelmeyer J, BernabeiA, Gikakis N, et al. Upregulation of Mac-1 surface expression on neutrophils during simulated extracorporeal circulation. *J Lab Clin Med* 1993;121:118–126.

89. Kappelmayer J, Berrnabei A, Edmunds LH Jr, et al. Tissue factor is expressed on monocytes during simulated extracorporeal circulation. *Circ Res* 1993;72:1075–1081.

90. Barstad RM, Ovrum E, Ringdal M-AL, et al. Induction of monocyte tissue factor procoagulant activity during coronary artery bypass surgery is reduced with heparin-coated extracorporeal circuit. *Br J Haematol* 1996;94:517–525.

91. Enofsson M, Thelin S, Siegbahn A. Monocyte tissue factor expression, cell activation, and thrombin formation during cardiopulmonary bypass: a clinical study. *J Thorac Cardiovasc Surg* 1997;113:576–584.

92. Enofsson M, Siegbahn A. Platelet-derived growth factor-BB and monocyte chemotactic protein-1 induce human peripheral blood monocytes to express tissue factor. *Thromb Res* 1996;83:307–320.

93. Fingerle-Rowson G, Auers J, Kreuzer E, et al. Down-regulation of surface monocyte lipopolysaccharide-receptor CD14 in patients on cardiopulmonary bypass undergoing aorta-coronary bypass operation. *J Thorac Cardiovasc Surg* 1998;115:1172–1178.

94. Markewitz A, Faist E, Lang S, et al. Successful restoration of cell-mediated immune response after cardiopulmonary bypass by immunomodulation. *J Thorac Cardiovasc Surg* 1993;105:15–24.

95. Haeffner-Cavaillon N, Roussellier N, Ponzio O, et al. Induction of interleukin-1 production in patients undergoing cardiopulmonary bypass. *J Thorac Cardiovasc Surg* 1989;98:1100–1106.

96. Steinberg JB, Kapelanski DP, Olson JD, et al. Cytokine and complement levels in patients undergoing cardiopulmonary bypass. *J Thorac Cardiovasc Surg* 1993;106:1008–1016.

97. Frering B, Philip I, Dehoux M, et al. Circulating cytokines in patients undergoing normothermic cardiopulmonary bypass. *J Thorac Cardiovasc Surg* 1994;108:636–641.

98. Kawahito K, Kawakami M, Fujiwara T, et al. Interleukin-8 and monocyte chemotactic activating factor responses to cardiopulmonary bypass. *J Thorac Cardiovasc Surg* 1995;110:99–102.

99. Roth JA, Golub SH, Cukingnan RA, et al. Cell-mediated immunity is depressed following cardiopulmonary bypass. *Ann Thorac Surg* 1981;31:350–356.

100. Ide H, Kakiuchi T, Furuta N, et al. The effect of cardiopulmonary bypass on T cells and their subpopulations. *Ann Thorac Surg* 1987;44:277–282.

101. Hisatomi K, Kobayashi A, Moriyama Y, et al. Combined suppressive effect of cardiopulmonary bypass and aging on cell-mediated immunity. *J Thorac Cardiovasc Surg* 1997;114:140–141.

102. Nguyen DM, Mulder DS, Shennib H. Effect of cardiopulmonary bypass on circulating lymphocyte function. *Ann Thorac Surg* 1992;53:611–616.

103. DePalma L, Yu M, McIntosh CL, et al. Changes in lymphocyte subpopulations as a result of cardiopulmonary bypass. *J Thorac Cardiovasc Surg* 1991;10l:240–244.

104. Hisatomi K, Isomura T, Kawara T, et al. Changes in lymphocyte subsets, mitogen responsiveness, and interleukin-2 production after cardiac operations. *J Thorac Cardiovasc Surg* 1989; 98:580–591.

105. Ratner BD. Surface properties of materials. Characterization of biomaterial surfaces. In: Ratner BD, Hoffman AS, Schoen FJ, et al., eds. *Biomaterials science. An introduction to materials in medicine.* San Diego: Academic Press, 1996:21–35.

106. Zingg W, Neumann AW, Strong AB, et al. Effect of surface roughness on platelet adhesion under static and under flow conditions. *Can J Surg* 1982;25:16–19.

107. Kim SW. Nonthrombogenic treatments and strategies. In: Ratner BD, Hoffman AS, Schoen FJ, et al., eds. *Biomaterials science. An introduction to materials in medicine.* San Diego: Academic Press, 1996:297–308.

108. Hanson SR, Harker LA, Ratner BD, et al. Evaluation of artificial surfaces using baboon arteriovenous shunt model. In: Winter GD, Gibbons DF, Plenk H Jr. *Biomaterials, advances in biomaterials.* Chichester, UK: John Wiley and Sons, 1982:519–530 (vol 3).

109. Ratner BD, Hoffman AS. Thin films, grafts and coatings. In: Ratner BD, Hoffman AS, Schoen FJ, et al., eds. *Biomaterials science. An introduction to materials in medicine.* San Diego: Academic Press, 1996:105–118.

110. Hoffman AS. Biologically functional materials. In: Ratner BD, Hoffman AS, Schoen FJ, et al., eds. *Biomaterials science. An introduction to materials in medicine.* San Diego: Academic Press, 1996:124–130.

111. Munro MS. Quattrone AJ, Ellworth SR, et al. Alkyl substituted polymers with enhanced albumin affinity. *ASAIO Trans* 1981; 27:499–503.

112. Annich GM, Meinhardt JP, Mowery KA, et al. Reduced platelet activation and thrombosis in extracorporeal circuits coated with nitric oxide release polymers. *J Thorac Cardiovasc Surg* (in press).

113. Wan S, DeSmet J-M, Barvais L, et al. Myocardium is a major source of proinflammatory cytokines in patients undergoing cardiopulmonary bypass. *J Thorac Cardiovasc Surg* 1996;112: 806–811.

114. Hennein HA, Ebba H, Rodriquez IL, et al. Relationship of the proinflammatory cytokines to myocardial ischemia and dysfunction after uncomplicated coronary revascularization. *J Thorac Cardiovasc Surg* 1994;108:626–635.

115. Wan S, LeClerc J-L, Vincent J-L. Cytokine responses to cardiopulmonary bypass: lessons learned from cardiac transplantation. *Ann Thorac Surg* 1997:63:269–276.

116. Butler J, Chong GL, Baigrie RJ, et al. Cytokine responses to cardiopulmonary bypass with membrane and bubble oxygenation. *Ann Thorac Surg* 1992;53:833–838.

117. Toivonen HJ, Ahotupa M. Free radical reaction products and antioxidant capacity in arterial plasma during coronary artery bypass grafting. *J Thorac Cardiovasc Surg* 1994;108:140–147.

118. Edmunds LH Jr. Extracorporeal perfusion. In: Edmunds LH Jr, ed. *Cardiac surgery in the adult.* New York: McGraw-Hill, 1997:281.

119. Kirklin JK, Westaby S, Blackstone EH, et al. Complement and the damaging effects of cardiopulmonary bypass. *J Thorac Cardiovasc Surg* 1983;86:845.

120. Harker LA, Malpass TW, Branson HE, et al. Mechanism of abnormal bleeding in patients undergoing cardiopulmonary bypass: acquired transient platelet dysfunction associated with selective alpha granule release. *Blood* 1980;56:824.

121. Pifarre R, Babka R, Sullivan HJ, et al. Management of postoperative heparin rebound following cardiopulmonary bypass. *J Thorac Cardiovasc Surg* 1981;81:378.

122. Blauth CI, Smith PL, Arnold JV, et al. Influence of oxygenator type on the prevalence and extent of microembolic retinal ischemia during cardiopulmonary bypass. *J Thorac Cardiovasc Surg* 1990;99:61.

123. Clark RE, Magraf HW, Beauchamp RA. Fat and solid filtration in clinical perfusion. *Surgery* 1975;77:216.

124. Blauth CI. Macroemboli and microemboli during cardiopulmonary bypass. *Ann Thorac Surg* 1995;59:1300.

125. Clark RE, Brillman J, Davis DA, et al. Microemboli during coronary artery bypass grafting. *J Thorac Cardiovasc Surg* 1995; 109:249.

126. Pugsley W, Klinger L, Paschalis C, et al. The impact of microemboli during cardiopulmonary bypass on neuropsychological functioning. *Stroke* 1994;25:1393.

127. Blauth CI, Cosgrove DM, Webb BW, et al. Atheroembolism from the ascending aorta. An emerging problem in cardiac surgery. *J Thorac Cardiovasc Surg* 1992;103:1104.

128. Hammon JW, Stump DA, Kon ND, et al. Risk factors and solutions for the development of neurobehavioral changes after coronary artery bypass grafting. *Ann Thorac Surg* 1997;63: 1613–1618.

129. Wareing TH, Davila-Roman VG, Barzilai B, et al. Management of the severely atherosclerotic ascending aorta during cardiac operations: a strategy for detection and treatment. *J Thorac Cardiovasc Surg* 1992;103:453.

130. Smith EEJ, Naftel DC, Blackstone EH, et al. Microvascular permeability after cardiopulmonary bypass. *J Thorac Cardiovasc Surg* 1987;94:225.

131. Edmunds LH Jr. The sangreal. *J Thorac Cardiovasc Surg* 1985; 90:1–6.

132. Edmunds LH Jr. Breaking the blood–biomaterial barrier (Hasting Lecture). *ASAIO J* 1995;41:824–830.

133. Gott VL, Whiffen JD, Dutton RC. Heparin bonding on colloidal graphite surfaces. *Science* 1963;142:1297–1298.

134. Hsu L-C. Principles of heparin-coating techniques. *Perfusion* 1991;6:209–219.

135. Larm O, Larsson R, Olsson P. A new non-thrombogenic surface prepared by selective covalent binding of heparin via a modified reducing terminal residue. *Biomat Med Dev Artif Org* 1983;11: 161.

136. Ovrum E, Mollnes TE, Fosse E, et al. Complement and granulocyte activation in two different types of heparinized extracorporeal circuits. *J Thorac Cardiovasc Surg* 1995;110:1623–1632.

137. Moen O, Fosse E, Brockmeier V, et al. Disparity in blood activation by two different heparin-coated cardiopulmonary bypass systems. *Ann Thorac Surg* 1995;60:1317–1323.

138. Gravlee GP. Heparin-coated cardiopulmonary bypass circuits. *J Cardiothorac Vasc Anesth* 1994;8:213–222.

139. Ovrum E, Am Holen E, Tangen G, et al. Completely heparinized cardiopulmonary bypass and reduced systemic heparin: clinical and hemostatic effects. *Ann Thorac Surg* 1995;60: 365–371.

140. Moen O, Fosse E, Brockmeier V, et al. Disparity in blood activation by two different heparin-coated cardiopulmonary bypass systems. *Ann Thorac Surg* 1995;60:1317.

141. Pekna M, Hagman L, Halden E, et al. Complement activation during cardiopulmonary bypass: effect of immobilized heparin. *Ann Thorac Surg* 1994;58:421–424.

142. Fosse E, Moen O, Johnson E, et al. Reduced complement and granulocyte activation with heparin-coated cardiopulmonary bypass. *Ann Thorac Surg* 1994;58:472–477.

143. Nilsson L, Peterson C, Venge P, et al. Eosinophil granule proteins in cardiopulmonry bypass with and without heparin coating. *Ann Thorac Surg* 1995;59:713–716.

144. The European Working Group on Heparin-Coated Extracorporeal Circulation Circuits. Clinical evaluation of Duraflo II heparin-treated extracorporeal circulation circuits (2nd version). *Eur J Cardiothorac Surg* 1997;11:616–623.

145. Pradhan MJ, Fleming JS, Nkere UU, et al. Clinical experience with heparin-coated cardiopulmonary bypass circuits. *Perfusion* 1991;6:235–242.

146. Wagner WR, Johnson PC, Thompson KA, et al. Heparin-coated cardiopulmonary bypass circuits: hemostatic alterations and postoperative blood loss. *Ann Thorac Surg* 1994;58:734.

147. Boroweic J, Bagge L, Saldeen T, et al. Biocompatibility reflected by haemostasis variables during cardiopulmonary bypass using heparin-coated circuits. *Thorac Cardiovasc Surg* 1997;45:163–167.

148. Moen O, Hogasen K, Fosse E, et al. Attenuation of changes in leukocyte surface markers and complement activation with heparin-coated cardiopulmonary bypass. *Ann Thorac Surg* 1997;63:105–111.

149. Weerwind PW, Maessen JG, van Tits LJH, et al. Influence of Duraflo II heparin-treated extracorporeal circuits on the systemic inflammatory response in patients having coronary bypass. *J Thorac Cardiovasc Surg* 1995;110:1633–1641.

150. Jansen PGM, te Velthuis H, Huybregts RAJM, et al. Reduced complement activation and improved postoperative performance after cardiopulmonary bypass with heparin-coated circuits. *J Thorac Cardiovasc Surg* 1995;110:829–834.

151. Ovrum E, Brosstad F, Am Holen E, et al. Complete heparin-coated (CBAS) cardiopulmonary bypass and reduced systemic heparin dose; effects on coagulation and fibrinolysis. *Eur J Cardiothorac Surg* 1996;1O:449–455.

152. Boonstra PW, Gu YJ, Akkerman C, et al. Heparin coating of an extracorporeal circuit partly improves hemostasis after cardiopulmonary bypass. *J Thorac Cardiovasc Surg* 1994;107:289–292.

153. Boroweic J, Thelin S, Bagge L, et al. Decreased blood loss after cardiopulmonary bypass using heparin-coated circuit and 50% reduction of heparin dose. *Scand J Thorac Cardiovasc Surg* 1992;26:177–185.

154. Baufreton C, Le Besnerais P, Jansen P, et al. Clinical outcome after coronary surgery with heparin-coated extracorporeal circuits for cardiopulmonary bypass. *Perfusion* 1996;11:437–443.

155. Steinberg BM, Grossi EA, Schwartz DS, et al. Heparin bonding of bypass circuits reduces cytokine release during cardiopulmonary bypass. *Ann Thorac Surg* 1995;60:525–529.

156. Gorman RC, Ziats NP, Gikakis N, et al. Surface-bound heparin fails to reduce thrombin formation during clinical cardiopulmonary bypass. *J Thorac Cardiovasc Surg* 1996;111:1–12.

157. Enofsson M, Thelin S, Siegbahn A. Thrombin generation during cardiopulmonary bypass using heparin-coated or standard circuits. *Scand J Thorac Cardiovasc Surg* 1995;29:157–165.

158. Muehrcke DD, McCarthy PM, Kotte-Marchant K, et al. Biocompatibility of heparin-coated extracorporeal bypass circuits: a randomized, masked clinical trial. *J Thorac Cardiovasc Surg* 1996;112:472–483.

159. Watanabe H, Miyamura H, Hayashi J, et al. The influence of a heparin-coated oxygenator during cardiopulmonary bypass on postoperative lung oxygenation capacity in pediatric patients with congenital heart anomalies. *J Card Surg* 1996;11:396–401.

160. Videm V, Mollnes TE, Bergh K, et al. Heparin-coated cardiopulmonary bypass. II. Mechanisms for reduced complement activation *in vivo. J Thorac Cardiovasc Surg* 1999;117:803–809.

161. Spanier TB, Chen JM, Oz MC, et al. Selective anticoagulation with active site-blocked factor IXa suggests separate roles for intrinsic and extrinsic coagulation pathways in cardiopulmonary bypass. *J Thorac Cardiovasc Surg* 1998;116:860–869.

162. Tabuchi N, Haan J, Boonstra PW, et al. Activation of fibrinolysis in the pericardial cavity during cardiopulmonary bypass. *J Thorac Cardiovasc Surg* 1993;106:828.

163. Maquelin KN, Berckmans RJ, Nieuwland R, et al. Disappearance of glycoprotein Ib from the platelet surface in pericardial blood during cardiopulmonary bypass. *J Thorac Cardiovasc Surg* 1998;115:1160–1165.

164. Ovrum E, Mollnes TE, Fosse E, et al. High and low heparin dose with heparin-coated cardiopulmonary bypass: activation of complement and granulocytes. *Ann Thorac Surg* 1995;60:1755.

165. Aldea GS, O'Gara P, Shapira OM, et al. Effect of anticoagulation protocol on outcome in patients undergoing CABG with heparin-bonded cardiopulmonary bypass circuits. *Ann Thorac Surg* 1998;65:425–433.

166. Videm V. Heparin in clinical doses "primes" granulocytes to subsequent activation as measured by myeloperoxidase release. *Scand J Immunol* 1996;43:385–390.

167. Ovrum E, Brosstad F, Am Holen E, et al. Effects on coagulation and fibrinolysis with reduced versus full systemic heparinization and heparin-coated cardiopulmonary bypass. *Circulation* 1995;92:2579–2584.

168. Te Velthuis H, Baufreton C, Jansen PGM, et al. Heparin coating of extracorporeal circuits inhibits contact activation during cardiac operations. *J Thorac Cardiovasc Surg* 1997;114:117–122.

169. Kuitunen AH, Heikkila LJ, Salmenpera MT. Cardiopulmonary bypass with heparin-coated circuits and reduced systemic anticoagulation. *Ann Thorac Surg* 1997;63:438–444.

170. Bannan S, Danby A, Cowan D, et al. Low heparinization with heparin-bonded bypass circuits: is it a safe strategy? *Ann Thorac Surg* 1997;63:663–668.

171. Kagisaki K, Masai T, Kadoba K, et al. Biocompatibility of heparin-coated circuits in pediatric cardiopulmonary bypass. *Artif Org* 1997;21:836–840.

172. Muehrcke DD, McCarthy PM, Stewart RW, et al. Complications of extracorporeal life support systems using heparin-bound surfaces. *J Thorac Cardiovasc Surg* 1995;110:843.

173. Cheung AT, Levin SK, Weiss SJ, et al. Intracardiac thrombus: a risk of incomplete anticoagulation for cardiac operations. *Ann Thorac Surg* 1994;58:541–542.

174. Van Dyck MJ, Lavenne-Pardonge E, Azerad MA, et al. Case 5—1996. Thrombosis after the use of a heparin-coated cardiopulmonary bypass circuit in a patient with heparin-induced thrombocytopenia. *J Cardiothorac Vasc Anesth* 1996;10:809–815.

175. von Segesser LK, Weiss BM, Garcia E, et al. Risk and benefit of low systemic heparinization during open heart surgery. *Ann Thorac Surg* 1994;58:391.

176. Fuktomi M, Kobayshi S, Niwaya K, et al. Changes in platelet, granulocyte and complement activation during cardiopulmonary bypass using heparin-coated equipment. *Artif Org* 1996;20:767–776.

177. Ladowski JS, Schatzlein MH, Peterson AC, et al. Clinical heparin-coated cardiopulmonary bypass: reduction of systemic heparin requirements for redo cardiac surgery. *ASAIO J* 1996;42:34–36.

178. Ovrum E, Am Holen E, Tangen G, et al. Heparinized cardiopulmonary bypass and full heparin dose marginally improve clinical performance. *Ann Thorac Surg* 1996;62:1128–1132.

179. Schreurs HH, Wijers MJ, Gu YJ, et al. Heparin-coated bypass circuits: effects on inflammatory response in pediatric cardiac operations. *Ann Thorac Surg* 1998;66:166–171.

180. Fosse E, Thelin S, Svennevig JL, et al. Duraflo II coating of cardiopulmonary bypass circuits reduces complement activation, but does not affect the release of granulocyte enzymes: a

European multicenter study. *Eur J Cardiothorac Surg* 1997;11: 320–327.

181. Videm V, Mollnes TE, Garred P, et al. Biocompatibility of extracorporeal circulation. *J Thorac Cardiovasc Surg* 1991;10l: 654–660.

182. Moen O, Fosse E, Dregelid E, et al. Centrifugal pump and heparin coating improve cardiopulmonary bypass biocompatibility. *Ann Thorac Surg* 1996;62:1134–1140.

183. Yamada H, Kudoh I, Hirose Y, et al. Heparin-coated circuits reduce the formation of TNF-alpha during cardiopulmonary bypass. *Acta Anaesthesiol Scand* 1996;40:311–317.

184. Ashraf S, Tian Y, Cowan D, et al. Release of proinflammatory cytokines during pediatric cardiopulmonary bypass: heparin-bonded versus nonbonded oxygenators. *Ann Thorac Surg* 1997; 64:1790–1794.

185. Ovrum E. Eosinophil granulocyte activation and heparin-coated cardiopulmonary bypass. *Ann Thorac Surg* 1996;61:1038.

186. Garred P, Mollnes TE. Immobilized heparin inhibits the increase in leukocyte surface expression of adhesion molecules. *Artif Org* 1997;21:293–299.

187. Videm V, Mollnes TE, Fosse E, et al. Heparin-coated cardiopulmonary bypass: I. Biocompatibility markers and development of complications in a high-risk population. *J Thorac Cardiovasc Surg* 1999;117:794–802.

188. Ranucci, Cirri S, Conti D, et al. Beneficial effects of Duraflo II heparin-coated circuits on postperfusion lung dysfunction. *Ann Thorac Surg* 1996;61:76–81.

189. DeHaan J, Boonstra PW, Tabuchi N, et al. Retransfusion of thoracic wound blood during heart surgery obscures biocompatibility of the extracorporeal circuit. *J Thorac Cardiovasc Surg* 1996;111:272–275.

190. Levy M, Hartman AR. Heparin-coated bypass circuits in cardiopulmonary bypass: improved biocompatibility or not? *Int Cardiol J* l996;53:S81–S87.

191. Gu YJ, Boonstra PW, Rijnsburger AA, et al. Cardiopulmonary bypass circuit treated with surface-modifying additives: a clinical evaluation of blood compatibility. *Ann Thorac Surg* 1998;65: 1342–1347.

192. Kawahito K, Tasai K, Murata S, et al. Evaluation of the anti-thrombogenicity of a new microdomain structured copolymer. *Artif Org* 1995;19:857–863.

193. Tsai C-C, Deppisch RM, Forrestal LJ, et al. Surface-modifying additives for improved device–blood compatibility. *ASAIO J* 1994;40:M619–M624.

194. Rubens FD, Labow RS, Lavallee GR, et al. Hematologic evaluation of cardiopulmonary bypass circuits prepared with a novel block copolymer. *Ann Thorac Surg* 1999;67:689–696.

195. Wan S, LeClerc J-L, Vincent J-L. Cytokine responses to cardiopulmonary bypass; lessons learned from cardiac transplantation. *Ann Thorac Surg* 1997;63:269–276.

196. Menasche P, Haydar S, Pernet J, et al. A potential mechanism of vasodilation after warm heart surgery: the temperature-dependent release of cytokines. *J Thorac Cardiovasc Surg* 1994; 107:293–299.

197. Frering B, Philip I, Dehoux M, et al. Circulating cytokines in patients undergoing normothermic cardiapulmonary bypass. *J Thorac Cardiovasc Surg* 1994;108:636–641.

198. Royston D. Coagulation in cardiac surgery. *Adv Card Surg* 1996;8:19–45.

199. Royston D. Aprotinin versus lysine analogues: the debate continues. *Ann Thorac Surg* 1998;65:S9–S19.

200. Wachtfogel YT, Kucich U, Hack CE, et al. Aprotinin inhibits the contact, neutrophil and platelet activation systems during simulated extracorporeal perfusion. *J Thorac Cardiovasc Surg* 1993;106:1–10.

201. Hiramatsu Y, Gikakis N, Anderson HL, et al. Tirofiban provides "platelet anesthesia" during cardiopulmonary bypass in baboons. *J Thorac Cardiovasc Surg* 1996;113:182–193.

202. Suzuki Y, Hillyer P, Miyamoto S, et al. Integrilin prevents prolonged bleeding times after cardiopulmonary bypass. *Ann Thorac Surg* 1998;66:373–381.

203. Suzuki Y, Malekan R, Hansen CW III, et al. Platelet anesthesia with nitric oxide with or without eptifibatide during cardiopulmonary bypass in baboons. *J Thorac Cardiovasc Surg* 1999;117: 987–993.

204. Mellgren K, Mellgren G, Lundin S, et al. Effect of nitric oxide gas on platelets during open heart operations. *Ann Thorac Surg* 1998;65:1335–1341.

205. Sato T, Tanaka K, Kondo C, et al. Nafamostat mesilate administration during cardiopulmonary bypass decreases postoperative bleeding after cardiac surgery. *ASAIO Trans* 1991;37: M194–M195.

206. Usui A, Hiroura M, Kawamura M, et al. Nafamostat mesilate reduces blood–foreign surface reactions similar to biocompatible materials. *Ann Thorac Surg* 1996;62:1404–1411.

10

PULSATILE CARDIOPULMONARY BYPASS

TERRY GOURLAY
KENNETH M. TAYLOR

Interest in the pulsatile nature of blood flow and the physiologic importance of this flow modality is not new. This area of research predates the clinical application of cardiopulmonary bypass (CPB) by a considerable time. Indeed, the very earliest physicians expressed an interest in the pulse and the pulsatile motion of the blood vessels. Aristotle (384–322 B.C.) noted, "The blood in animals throbs within their veins," and with particular reference to the heart, "The veins pulsate as a whole synchronously and successively inasmuch as they depend on the heart. It keeps moving and so do they." These apparently simple and logical conclusions, made without the aid of modern instruments, demonstrate that the pulsatile nature of the circulation did not go unnoticed by these early observers. However, it was not until much later that its significance could be thoroughly investigated.

Many early investigations of the significance of the pulsatile nature of blood flow were carried out by using isolated organ preparations. Hamel (1) demonstrated that pulsatile flow was of considerable importance to renal function. These findings were confirmed by Gesell (2), who suggested that this maintenance of function was the consequence of improved gas exchange at the capillary level, together with freer flow of lymph. Using a depulsed isolated organ preparation, Kohlstaedt and Page (3) further confirmed the importance of pulse pressure to kidney function, and in particular demonstrated that renin secretion is affected by the flow modality employed. Renal function and blood flow were the focus of many of the early flow studies. However, other factors were also studied in an effort to confirm the importance of the pulsatile nature of blood flow. McMaster and Parsons (4) demonstrated that lymph flow is greatly reduced during periods of nonpulsatile blood flow. The pulsatile nature of blood flow was studied intensely during the period leading up to the development of clinical CPB, and the results, although not universally accepted, offer considerable evidence supporting the importance of pulsatile blood flow, rather than simply bulk blood flow, in the maintenance of normal physiologic organ function.

These studies were of greater academic interest than practical importance until the development of clinical CPB. With the development and application of clinical CPB, it became necessary to support the total circulation to enable heart surgery to be performed. The early heart–lung machine of Gibbon (5) utilized a nonpulsatile pumping mechanism of the type designed by DeBakey (6) for this purpose. Despite the fact that this type of mechanism appeared to work well during CPB, interest still existed in examining the application of pulsatile blood flow during CPB. Mindful of the early results of the study of pulsatile blood flow in isolated organ preparations, the pioneers of CPB and cardiac surgery investigated the possibility of utilizing a pulsatile blood flow regime during CPB. Several attempts were made to produce pulsatile blood pumps for clinical CPB, but clinical acceptance was hampered by clinicians' fears of the complexity of such devices and of the potential for damage to formed blood elements. These fears persisted until a reliable commercial pulsatile blood pump (Fig. 10.1) was made available in the late 1970s, more than 20 years after the first clinical application of CPB.

The availability of this relatively simple modified roller pump system spurred a number of investigators to readdress the issue of pulsatile blood flow in the context of CPB. This area of research persists to this day and has led to some degree of understanding of the importance of pulsatile blood flow in the maintenance of normal physiologic response patterns during CPB. Nonetheless, the issue of pulsatile blood flow during CPB remains controversial (7).

During the years since the introduction of clinical CPB, research into the significance of pulsatile blood flow has focused mainly on two areas—metabolic effects and hemodynamic effects. In addition to these areas of research, the development of technology to generate pulsatile blood flow

T. Gourlay and K. M. Taylor: Department of Cardiac Surgery, National Heart and Lung Institute, Imperial College, Hammersmith Hospital, London W12 ONN, United Kingdom.

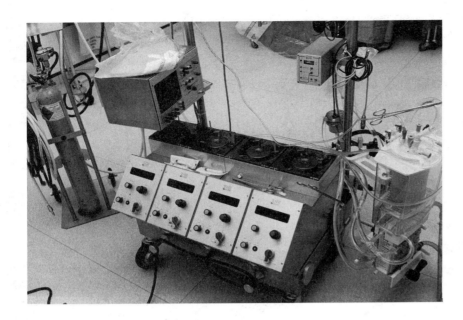

FIG. 10.1. Stockert pulsatile roller pump system (Stockert, Munich, Germany). This system is seen in a modern console- based configuration, but the pump modules and control system do not differ significantly from those in the first pump of this type produced.

that is compatible with other components of the CPB circuit continues.

PRINCIPLES OF PULSATILE BLOOD FLOW

Before considering the benefits attributed to pulsatile blood flow during CPB, one should consider the principles underlying these benefits. The two fundamental differences between pulsatile and nonpulsatile flow relate to flow–pressure architecture (shape of the flow–pressure complex) and energy delivery.

Blood Flow–Pressure Architecture

In pulsatile blood flow or pressure, a specific shape or architecture characterizes the pulse. The architecture is determined by the mechanism generating the blood flow and its interaction with the environment in which it operates. Some characteristics of pressure wave shape that can be used to describe the architecture of a pulse waveform (Fig. 10.2) include frequency, amplitude, rise time, decay time, and mean pressure or flow.

All these parameters have been employed to describe pulsatile blood flow during clinical and experimental CPB (8–10), and they represent the descriptive parameters most accessible to the clinician. In the absence of more advanced measurement and monitoring techniques, the arterial blood pressure waveform is commonly used to indicate "how pulsatile" a perfusion is during clinical practice. Although this constitutes a reasonably useful indicator capable of discriminating between pulsatile and nonpulsatile perfusion, it is not sufficient to describe fully the pulsatile properties of a particular flow modality.

Since the introduction of the pulsatile roller pump, most clinical investigations of pulsatile blood flow have employed the pulse pressure simply as a marker to confirm whether some form of pulse is present. Our group has employed a standard pulsatile pump control during more than two decades of clinical and experimental CPB in animals (11). The settings used have been based on safety considerations and represent the midrange of control options available to the clinician without claiming to offer optimum or physiologic pulsatility. The arterial pulse waveform generated with this configuration is not physiologic insofar as it does not resemble that of the native heart (Fig. 10.3).

Roller pump-generated pulsatile flow has been described as "ripple flow" (12). Nonetheless, this suboptimal flow modality has been associated in many investigations with significant clinical advantages, ranging from maintenance of relatively normal hemodynamics to reduced patient morbidity and mortality (13–16).

It is conceivable that the benefits attributed to roller pump-generated pulsatile flow would be further enhanced if the pulse output were made more physiologic. This would seem logical, and some *in vitro* and clinical experiments have assessed the degree to which the roller pump mechanism generates physiologic pulse pressure–flow architecture. Our experiments, in which an *in vitro* model of the human systemic circulatory system was used (17,18), suggest that although the roller pump offers a range of control for almost every aspect of pressure architecture, it is not capable of generating truly physiologic pulsatility. In our experience, when the maximum pulsatile control configurations are em-

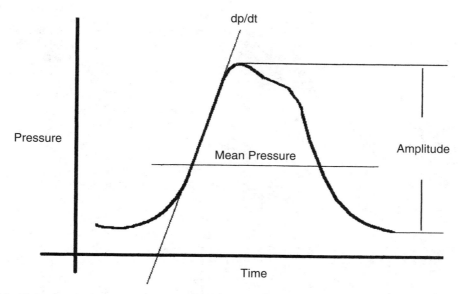

FIG. 10.2. Some of the factors that can be employed to describe the architecture of a pulse pressure waveform.

ployed clinically, the pressure architecture differs little from the conventional configuration (18), and both configurations produce unphysiologic waveforms. As it exists today, the roller pump mechanism may not therefore be the best one for delivering physiologic pulsatile blood flow architecture. This apparent limitation makes it difficult to understand the clinical benefits that have been demonstrated with this system. Optimizing the output profile within the performance envelope of this mechanism does not appear to enhance the situation significantly.

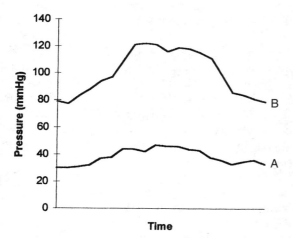

FIG. 10.3. Graph showing typical roller pump (A) and heart-generated (B) pulsatile blood pressure taken from the radial artery of a patient undergoing open heart surgery.

Delivery of Energy

The perfusion pump, whether the heart itself or some mechanical system, does no more than deliver mechanical energy to the circulation. This energy accrues in the form of blood flow and intravascular pressure. The rate at which the energy is delivered is defined as hydraulic power (19). The overall delivery of hydraulic power consists of both pulsatile and nonpulsatile, or mean, components, and these can be measured and used to characterize the flow delivery of the system. Separation of hydraulic power into its mean and pulsatile components is a complex matter involving phase shifting and Fourier analysis of the pressure and flow complexes. Total hydraulic power is the sum of mean power (product of mean pressure and flow) and pulsatile hydraulic power (derived from the sum of a number of pressure and flow harmonics). Computing total hydraulic power is not a simple matter, as it ideally requires that both blood flow and pressure be measured invasively at a common site. Although some investigators have managed to perform these measurements clinically (18,20), such an approach is not always possible or advisable in the operating theater, and the assessment of hydraulic power is generally reserved for research environments. However, extensive studies of this parameter have been carried out, and it has been established in both *in vitro* and animal models as a useful tool to assess the pulsatile blood flow-generating capabilities of several pumping systems. Studies by Gourlay (18) and Wright (19) demonstrate the limited pulsatile hydraulic power-generating capability of the standard pulsatile roller pump in comparison with that of a pulsatile ventricular system (Fig. 10.4).

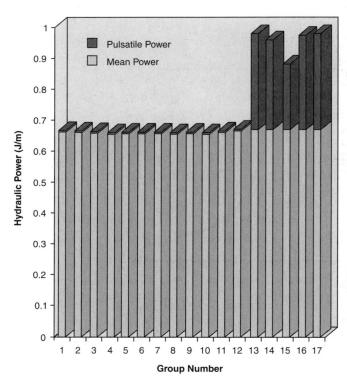

FIG. 10.4. Graph showing the pulsatile and nonpulsatile hydraulic power components of pulsatile blood flow generated by a roller and a ventricular pump. The ventricular pump groups are numbers 13 through 17 and are clearly associated with significantly more hydraulic power in the pulsatile domain. The mean pulsatile power remains similar between the two pump types. It can be seen that the roller pump is associated with very little hydraulic power in the pulsatile domain. These results are taken from an *in vitro* study of two pump systems.

For a number of reasons, particularly expense, pulsatile pumps of the ventricular type are not generally available for routine clinical use; therefore, the true clinical benefits of using this type of pumping mechanism during clinical CPB have not, as yet, been fully determined. However, the importance of energy transfer associated with pulsatile blood flow has been the focus of considerable research effort (21–23), and it is generally believed that it is of considerable importance. Shepard et al. (24) concluded that at the same mean blood pressure and flow rate, a pulsatile perfusion regime delivered up to 3.4 times as much energy to the circulation, and that this improved energy delivery might be responsible for maintaining normal peripheral blood flow distribution under pulsatile blood flow conditions. This factor may be responsible for many of the observed and perceived advantages associated with pulsatile CPB. Pulsatile flow is a complex issue that remains the focus of much study, and clearly the roller pump pulsatile flow system is not the ideal one from a fluid dynamic or hydraulic standpoint. Ventricular systems appear to offer more control of the pulse architecture and enhanced energy delivery, but use

of such systems is confounded by expense and technologic complexity. In the meantime, the roller pump system is the only clinically available option, and its use, despite suboptimal output characteristics, has been associated with reduced patient mortality and morbidity (7,25,26). The reasons for this are clearly open to some degree of speculation, but many investigations indicate that energy transfer and pulse shape are involved.

HEMODYNAMIC EFFECTS OF PULSATILE CARDIOPULMONARY BYPASS

In a recent review of pulsatile perfusion, Hornick and Taylor (7) observed that progressive systemic arterial vasoconstriction is the inevitable consequence of nonpulsatile CPB. This vasoconstriction may ultimately lead to reduced visceral perfusion. At separation from CPB, afterload might be increased at a time when the left ventricle is already functionally compromised from the insult of the operative procedure, which predisposes to a low cardiac output syndrome and potential visceral organ damage. This sequence of events, familiar to most clinicians, had been described by Taylor et al. (27) as a vicious cycle that is generally controlled by a "cocktail" of vasodilator and inotropic drugs in the immediate postperfusion period. Taylor and colleagues also showed that the use of pulsatile perfusion during CPB appears to be associated with a reduction in the vasoconstriction commonly present at the termination of bypass. When combined with the improved myocardial contractility resulting from modern myocardial preservation techniques, this improved post-CPB hemodynamic state should hasten the return to normal myocardial performance. Common approaches to increased systemic vascular resistance in the period after bypass (e.g., sodium nitroprusside) do improve cardiac performance (28,29). Pulsatile flow during the CPB period can potentially offer a similar benefit by avoiding the development of increased systemic vascular resistance in the first place.

The mechanisms underlying the hemodynamic effects of pulsatile and nonpulsatile blood flow during CPB are complex and as yet not fully understood; however, a number of mechanisms have been proposed. Mechanisms purportedly involved in the development of postperfusion vasoconstriction consequent to nonpulsatile blood flow include activation of the renin–angiotensin system and the release of catecholamines, vasopressin, and local tissue vasoconstrictors.

Renin secretion increases under nonpulsatile blood flow conditions (30,31). This may ultimately increase plasma concentrations of angiotensin II, one of the most potent endogenous vasoconstrictors. Taylor et al. (32) associated the use of an angiotensin I- and angiotensin II-specific converting-enzyme inhibitor during CPB with significant and rapid reduction in systemic vascular resistance during CPB and an increase in cardiac index immediately following CPB. Plasma vasopressin levels are also elevated during nonpulsatile CPB (33); however, the importance of this finding to the development of postoperative vasoconstriction is unresolved. Similarly, many reports demonstrate that catecholamines are secreted during CPB and that this secretion may be attenuated by the use of pulsatile flow (34,35).

The hemodynamic response to nonpulsatile CPB and the mechanisms involved are varied and complex. However, a substantial body of evidence suggests that many of the undesirable postoperative sequelae of nonpulsatile flow can be prevented by using pulsatile blood flow during CPB. This may reduce the need for pharmacologic interventions in the critical post-CPB period. Clinical studies have demonstrated that pulsatile CPB reduces the requirement for inotropic agents and intraaortic balloon pump support after CPB (25,26,36). In addition, these studies demonstrate a reduction in hemodynamically related mortality in patients receiving pulsatile perfusion in comparison with those exposed to nonpulsatile CPB.

METABOLIC EFFECTS OF PULSATILE CARDIOPULMONARY BYPASS

The metabolic effects of pulsatile and nonpulsatile CPB can be characterized at the cellular level and at the vital organ level. The effects of pulsatile and nonpulsatile blood flow on most vital organs have been studied. The cellular metabolic effects of pulsatile flow continue to be studied, particularly as new metabolic assays become available.

Pulsatile Blood Flow and Cell Metabolism

Nonpulsatile CPB has been associated with the development of metabolic acidosis and reduced tissue oxygen consumption (37–40), whereas pulsatile flow during CPB has been associated with a higher rate of oxygen consumption and a reduction in the level of metabolic acidosis (41).

The mechanisms underlying the maintenance of relatively normal cell metabolism during pulsatile bypass have not been clearly ascertained. However, it has been postulated that the enhanced energy associated with a pulsatile regimen may be responsible for maintaining the patency of the microcirculation, thereby improving the delivery of nutrients (42,43).

Pulsatile Blood Flow and Organ Function

The effect of pulsatile CPB on organ function has been studied in a wide variety of experimental models and in a number of target organs. Many of the earliest animal studies are now being repeated as the technology for evaluating the effects of flow modality on organ function evolve into tools that can be utilized clinically, although many of the effects of pulsatile and nonpulsatile blood flow on major organ function during CPB have been well described.

Pulsatile Blood Flow and the Kidney

As early as 1889, Hamel (1) determined that the pulse has an important influence on kidney function. His conclusions were confirmed by Gesell (2), who postulated that improved kidney function is the result of better gas exchange at the capillary level together with the maintenance of normal lymph flow. Kohlstaedt and Page (3), by performing a series of experiments on isolated kidneys, confirmed the importance of pulse pressure to kidney function and in particular to the secretion of renin. During these experiments, blood flow to the kidney was depulsed. They found that renin secretion is much higher in the group exposed to nonpulsatile blood flow. In all these experiments, the mean pressure was similar in both the pulsatile and nonpulsatile groups.

Mavroudis (36), in his excellent 1978 review, pointed out that some investigators contested these early findings. Ritter (44), Goodyer and Glenn (45), Oelert and Eufe (46), and Selkurt (47) all found that renal function is not affected by the presence or absence of a pulse in an isolated preparation, provided that the mean blood pressure is maintained. Mavroudis observed, however, that the blood flow architecture varied widely in the pulsatile flow groups involved in these experiments, an issue that is of considerable concern to this day. The pulse pressure profiles employed by the latter investigators were quite different from those used by Hooker in 1910 (48) in experiments in which normal pressure architecture was maintained in isolated tissue preparations, which leads to the conclusion that pulsatile blood flow enhances kidney function.

In common with most other investigators, Many et al. (30) confirmed the importance of pulsatility to kidney function in a series of experiments in which they found that animals undergoing nonpulsatile perfusion experience increased renin levels, along with attendant fluid and electrolyte imbalances. Many investigators considered improved distribution of blood flow to be the prime reason for the enhancement of renal function associated with pulsatile blood flow. Boucher et al. (49), using radioactively labeled microspheres, found renal blood flow to be preserved under pulsatile flow conditions. Nakayama et al. (50) had already reported that renal venous return is preserved under pulsatile blood flow conditions.

Earlier, Fintersbusch et al. (51) demonstrated a loss in normal renal artery configuration associated with nonpulsatile blood flow in a perfused dog model. Barger and Herd (52), using the same model, associated this finding with a shift in intrarenal blood flow that results in decreased sodium excretion. Mori et al. (53) discovered that after a period of hypothermic circulatory arrest, renal blood flow is substantially higher and the kidneys recover function more fully and rapidly in dogs exposed to pulsatile blood flow during the reperfusion period. Studies of renal function in open heart surgical patients by German et al. (54) confirmed that nonpulsatile blood flow is associated with a more rapid onset of renal hypoxia and acidosis than is pulsatile flow, despite an adequate systemic rate of blood flow and oxygen extraction. Paquet (55) had already described a similar phenomenon in an isolated porcine kidney model. Mukherjee (56) et al. demonstrated decreased tissue oxygen pressure in the renal medulla, together with increased local lactate levels and decreased oxygen uptake, when blood flow is nonpulsatile. Landymore et al. (15), working with essentially the same model, found that urine output is enhanced with pulsatile flow and once again that plasma renin levels are higher with nonpulsatile flow.

Clinical studies have tended to confirm the results of animal investigations. Williams et al. (57), in a study of infants undergoing open heart surgery during profound hypothermia, found urine output, used as an indicator of renal function, to be 100% greater in the pulsatile flow group than in the nonpulsatile group. Many clinical investigators have had difficulty in discerning any particular advantage directly attributable to the pulsatile nature of blood flow. This may be a consequence of many factors, including variations in clinical management during cardiac surgical procedures. Indeed, Louagie et al. (58) concluded that pulsatile blood flow is associated with reduced urine output in patients undergoing open heart surgery. Although these findings are at odds with those in most of the scientific literature, they may be an indication of how critical the clinical model is in establishing the beneficial effects of flow modality.

The effects of pulsatile flow on renal function may be most apparent and significant under the most challenging conditions. A number of clinical studies have focused on the importance of pulsatile flow in patients undergoing cardiac surgery who have renal insufficiency preoperatively. On the basis of a substantial clinical trial, Matsuda et al. (59) recommended that pulsatile blood flow be employed in this group of patients, having established that renal function is best preserved in these patients under pulsatile flow conditions.

The effect of pulsatility on kidneys being preserved for transplantation has also been studied. Belzer et al. (60) demonstrated that isolated kidneys subjected to nonpulsatile perfusion show a gradual but clearly defined rise in vascular resistance that is not present with pulsatile perfusion. This appears to confirm the development of rising vascular resistance with nonpulsatile flow, even in an isolated organ preparation. They further demonstrated that once transplanted, kidneys perfused in a pulsatile manner return to normal function more quickly than those perfused with nonpulsatile flow. This confirms the enhanced preservation associated, they surmised, with improved tissue perfusion. This is perhaps one area in which the frequently reported association between pulsatile blood flow and improved tissue perfusion may still be of considerable practical benefit.

Pulsatile Blood Flow and the Brain

The brain, although protected by autoregulation, is still susceptible to injury during cardiac surgery. Taylor et al. (61) showed that the autoregulatory mechanisms can be modified by several factors, including temperature, pattern of blood flow, viscosity, oxygen and carbon dioxide tension, and various pharmacologic agents. Simpson (62) determined that certain brain tissues require substantially higher blood flow rates than others. He further suggested that these may be compromised by the breakdown of autoregulatory mechanisms and flow disruption associated with CPB. As early as 1969, Hill et al. (63) described significant neuropathologic manifestations associated with cardiac surgery. These findings included histologic evidence of focal brain lesions resulting from extracorporeal circulation. Sanderson et al. (64), employing a canine model, demonstrated that the diffuse brain cell damage associated with nonpulsatile perfusion can be prevented by pulsatile flow. Taylor et al. (61), using a similar canine perfusion model, demonstrated that the level of creatine phosphokinase BB isoenzyme in the cerebrospinal fluid, a sensitive marker of cerebral injury, is significantly higher in animals exposed to nonpulsatile blood flow than in those receiving pulsatile blood flow. These findings may be related to those of DePaepe et al. (65), who described significantly smaller cerebral capillary diameters with nonpulsatile than with pulsatile flow, which suggests the possibility of reduced cerebral blood flow under nonpulsatile conditions. Taylor and colleagues (66,67) found markedly different hypothalamic–pituitary axis responses to surgical stress with pulsatile and nonpulsatile blood flow conditions. They found that the anterior pituitary gland fails to respond to thyrotropin-releasing hormone under nonpulsatile conditions, in contrast to the normal profile exhibited during major surgery not utilizing CPB. The secretion of cortisol was also found to be significantly reduced under nonpulsatile flow conditions. In all cases, they noted a return of normal responses within 1 hour of cessation of nonpulsatile bypass. Taylor et al. (68) further demonstrated that the pituitary–adrenal axis responds normally under pulsatile perfusion conditions. Philbin et al. (69) demonstrated a similar response pattern of vasopressin secretion during nonpulsatile CPB.

All these findings demonstrate differences in the cerebral metabolic response to different CPB perfusion modalities. Several investigations have compared the adequacy of brain blood flow with pulsatile and nonpulsatile flow. Briceno and Runge (70) showed that pulsatile flow prevents the cerebral acidosis often observed during the early phase of nonpulsatile CPB. This may be a consequence of better preservation of regional cerebral blood flow. In comparison with nonpulsatile perfusion in patients, Kono et al. (71) found that pulsatile flow reduces cerebral vascular resistance by as much as 25%. This highly significant difference and the proposed improvement in regional blood flow distribution may be responsible for the reduced cerebral lactate production demonstrated by Mori et al. (72). They suggested that regional blood flow is maintained and anaerobic metabolism is suppressed with the application of pulsatile blood flow, particularly during the critical cooling and rewarming phases of the operative procedure. In a canine stroke model, Tranmer et al. (73) used computerized mapping to demonstrate that pulsatile perfusion better maintains cerebral blood flow in ischemic regions. In another canine CPB study, Onoe et al. (74) found that pulsatile blood flow preserves cerebral circulation, even during profound hypothermia, which suggests a cerebral protective effect of pulsatile blood flow.

A number of studies focusing on the brain contest the evidence supporting pulsatile blood flow. Invariably, these studies do not offer nonpulsatile blood flow as a superior mode of perfusion, but rather indicate that pulsatile blood flow provides little or no advantage over nonpulsatile flow. In particular, two studies showed no differences in neurologic or neuropsychological outcomes between pulsatile and nonpulsatile flow (75,76), but Murkin et al. (77) did find a reduction in cardiovascular morbidity in their pulsatile flow group. Hindman et al. (78), in a 1995 study focusing on cerebral blood flow and cerebral oxygen consumption in a rabbit model, found no difference between pulsatile and nonpulsatile flow regimes. In comparing roller pump-generated pulsatile and nonpulsatile blood flow, Chow et al. (79) found no differences in a number of cerebral metabolic markers. Despite this conflicting evidence, considerable evidence favors pulsatile blood flow for the maintenance of normal cerebral function, metabolism, and blood flow distribution during CPB.

Pulsatile Blood Flow and the Liver and Pancreas

Interest in the effects of CPB on pancreatic function was stimulated by sporadic findings pointing to increased plasma levels of amylase after nonpulsatile bypass. Feiner (80) reported a 16% incidence of ischemic pancreatitis in patients who had undergone CPB. Baca et al. (81), using a canine model, found that post-CPB pancreatic function was significantly better immediately and 48 hours after bypass in dogs exposed to pulsatile CPB than in those that underwent nonpulsatile CPB. Saggau et al. (82), monitoring insulin, glucose, glucagon, and growth hormone levels in human and animal studies, concluded that pulsatile CPB preserves pancreatic function better than nonpulsatile CPB. They found "normal function" of the pancreatic β-cells in the pulsatile blood flow group and reduced function in the nonpulsatile group. Using a clinical model, Murray et al. (83) were able to demonstrate improved pancreatic function associated with a reduced incidence of elevated amylase levels in patients undergoing CPB with pulsatile flow. Mori et al. (72) concluded that pancreatic function is preserved in dogs perfused under both hypothermia and normother-

mia in the presence of pulsatile blood flow. In contrast, they found pancreatic function to be reduced in dogs exposed to a nonpulsatile regimen. Further evidence supporting the role of pulsatile flow in the maintenance of normal hepatic function was provided by Pappas et al. (84), who, employing serum glutamic oxaloacetic transaminase (SGOT) as a marker of hepatic injury, concluded that pulsatile blood flow preserves hepatic tissues and function. Mathie and colleagues (85) found similar results in a canine CPB model. This was echoed in the results of a series of clinical studies carried out by Chiu et al. (86), who found that hepatic function is preserved with pulsatile blood flow during CPB, as reflected in postoperative SGOT levels. They demonstrated that hepatic blood flow shows a typical vasoconstrictive response to nonpulsatile CPB, coupled with a reduction in hepatic oxygen consumption.

Pulsatile Blood Flow and the Gut

Abdominal complications associated with CPB have become increasingly recognized as a significant component of operative morbidity and mortality. In one study, Gauss et al. (87) reported that 1.8% of 500 patients who underwent cardiac surgery had some type of abdominal complication. The mortality rate was 44% in this group. From his own retrospective study of 5,924 patients and two other reports, Baue (88) noted that postoperative gastrointestinal morbidity occurs in 0.29% to 2% of patients undergoing CPB, with an associated mortality of 23.5% to 44%. He suggested that the primary cause of these complications is mesenteric hypoperfusion leading to ischemia and subsequent gut-related morbidity or mortality. Bowles et al. (89) reported that CPB is associated with endotoxemia in some patients and that mesenteric ischemia may be an important contributor to this problem. Endotoxemia associated with CPB in children has been the focus of study for some years. Anderson and Baek (90) postulated that the high levels of endotoxin found in children after CPB may derive from ischemia-induced increases in gut permeability. The incidence of this undesirable post-CPB endotoxemia remains undetermined.

However, there have been reports of substantially elevated endotoxin levels in patients with no apparent preoperative infection (91). Two studies (92,93) highlighted the period immediately following removal of the aortic cross-clamp as a critical time in the development of endotoxemia. In a canine CPB model, Ohri et al. (94) demonstrated a disparity between mesenteric oxygen consumption and oxygen delivery during the rewarming phase of CPB. Further studies using the same model confirmed an increase in gut permeability during this period. Tao et al. (95) demonstrated in pigs that gut mucosa becomes ischemic during CPB, apparently from blood flow redistribution and shifting tissue oxygen demand.

Riddington et al. (96) confirmed these findings in the clinical model. They found that patients undergoing CPB exhibit increased gut mucosal ischemia and gut permeability, and endotoxin was detectable in the plasma of 42% of these patients. They further found that an elevated intestinal pH did not return to normal until the nonpulsatile flow regimen was terminated and the heart took over the circulation. Quigley et al. (97) established that perfusion pressure is one important factor in preventing endotoxemia. When the perfusion pressure was maintained in excess of 60 mm Hg throughout the perfusion period, there was no measurable endotoxemia in either the pulsatile or nonpulsatile groups. A number of preventive measures have been proposed to modify and reduce the impact of this potentially injurious course of events. Fiddian-Green (98) suggested that pulsatile blood flow results in improved blood flow to the gut, reducing mucosal ischemia and increasing oxygen delivery. He further suggested the application of preoperative gut lavage and parenteral antibiotics. Reilly and Bulkey (99) proposed that the vasoactive gut response to circulatory shock is mediated by activation of the renin–angiotensin system, which increases gut permeability. Pulsatile blood flow, therefore, may offer a simple but significant method for avoiding the potentially injurious results of impaired gut perfusion. There is little to suggest any harmful effects of pulsatile blood flow on the gut, although a 1998 case report (100) attributes a case of bowel necrosis to pulsatile blood flow dislodging plaque during CPB. The authors claim that this is a risk with pulsatile blood flow, but they provide no substantiation other than this perhaps coincidental complication.

FACTORS INFLUENCING PULSATILE BLOOD FLOW ARCHITECTURE DURING CARDIOPULMONARY BYPASS

At the beginning of this chapter, we described the current state of clinical pulsatile blood flow as suboptimal in terms of pulse architecture. This derives from a combination of factors, including the interaction between the pump and other circuit components and the ever-changing hemodynamic status of patients undergoing cardiac surgery. The hemodynamics change considerably during CPB as a result of hemodilution, pharmacologic interventions, and changes in perfusion flow and temperature. All these factors may importantly influence the quality of the perfusion delivered by a pulsatile pump system. However, the quality of the system employed and its inherent pulse-generating capability are critical to the architectural integrity of pulsatile flow delivery. Many systems claiming to have some degree of pulsatile blood flow capability have evolved, some of which have been tested and characterized. However, the roller

pump remains the most commonly used system for this purpose.

BLOOD PUMPS AND SYSTEMS FOR DELIVERING PULSATILE BLOOD FLOW

A number of pumping systems are available to clinicians involved in CPB practice. The degree to which each of these systems is capable of delivering pulsatile blood flow varies greatly and has been the focus of much study.

Roller Blood Pump

The roller pump mechanism is simple and reliable, features that are extremely important for a clinical support mechanism. These pumps were used for circulatory support for some time before extracorporeal circulation and oxygenation were added. DeBakey (101) and Wesolowski (102) both reported the early use of a roller pump mechanism in total circulatory support in animals. The roller pump mechanism, which works on the principle of two or more diametrically opposed rollers "milking" a constrained piece of tubing (Fig. 10.5), offers the advantages of simplicity and predictability.

The occlusive nature of the mechanism induces negative pressures at the inlet side, rendering this type of mechanism appropriate for both arterial blood pumping systems and suction pumping (103). This inherent flexibility led to the

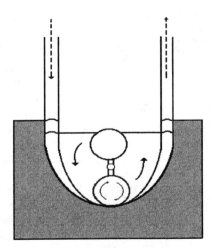

FIG. 10.5. Typical roller pump head arrangement. The *broken arrows* show the direction of blood flow, and the *solid arrows* show the direction of rotation of the head components. In this case, two rollers are shown on a common axle. Each roller is capable of independent rotation in either a clockwise or counterclockwise direction. By rotating the roller mechanism over a constrained piece of tubing, a positive displacement of the perfusate contained within the tube is achieved by a "milking" process; each roller operates as a one-way valve when in contact with the tubing.

mechanism being adopted as the pump of choice for heart–lung machines from a very early point in the evolution of CPB. Initially, commercially available roller pumps did not offer a pulsatile flow option. However, interest in the investigation of pulsatile flow as a modality for clinical CPB led to the development of modified systems. Ogata et al. (104) reported the modification of a roller pump to generate pulsatile blood flow. This study was followed by those of Nonoyama (105) and Nakayama et al. (106), who each employed essentially the same roller pump system with limited mechanical success but with reported clinical benefit. These systems were associated with poor mechanical reliability, possibly resulting from the effects of inertia of the heavy pump heads.

In the 1970s, a pulsatile roller pump for clinical use was made available for the first time by the Stockert company (Stockert Instruments, Munich, Germany). This innovation was made possible by the development of a pump head with low inertia made of aluminum and stainless steel and the incorporation of a "stepping" motor mechanism. The principal design requirement for this pumping system was that it be capable of generating some degree of pulsatile blood flow during CPB. The combination of a light pump head and the stepping motor permitted the pump head to be controlled precisely during the rapid acceleration and deceleration phases of the pulse cycle. The manufacturers also recognized the need for control of flow architecture and offered, in a limited way, some degree of user determination of output profile. While using the pump control module, it is possible to adjust the output frequency, pulse duration, and baseline flow rate in addition to total flow rate. A common fear among potential users was that the rapid acceleration and deceleration of the pump head during pulsatile flow might lead to an increase in hemolysis as the result of an increase in shear rate occurring under pulsatile blood flow conditions (107). However *in vitro* (108) and *ex vivo* studies (109,110) showed this not to be the case.

A number of clinical and laboratory experiments in which the Stockert pulsatile flow system was used have been carried out with considerable success during almost two decades. Demand for these systems has been such that several other manufacturers of blood pumps now offer a pulsatile blood flow option on roller-type blood pumps. However, Wright (19) has indicated that the roller pump may not be the most efficient mechanism for generating pulsatile flow. There is some question regarding whether the output generated by a roller pump in the pulsatile mode can truly be described as pulsatile in the physiologic sense. At best, the roller pump may be capable of generating only a "ripple" flow pattern. Subsequent studies (18) using a model of the systemic circulation and circuitry that mimics the typical perfusion add weight to this assertion. It has been established that the roller pump is not capable of matching the hydraulic power output of the human heart (20), but there is clear evidence that, even though the output of such sys-

tems is less than optimal, clinical benefits are derived from its use.

Ventricular Blood Pumps

These devices are probably the most physiologic method for generating pulsatile blood flow in that they operate in a similar manner to the ventricle of the heart. In simple terms, ventricular systems consist of compressible sac and two one-way valves permitting blood to flow into and out of the ventricle in only one direction. There are many configurations of ventricular mechanisms, one of which is shown in Fig. 10.6.

Typically, these systems are driven by either hydraulic or pneumatic means. Hydraulic systems generally employ a noncompressible fluid, such as distilled water, as the drive medium. The total blood flow generated by ventricular systems depends on frequency and stroke volume. Any alteration in stroke volume or frequency (e.g., when the system is synchronized with a patient's electrocardiogram) will affect the total output of the system. This problem can be solved by ensuring that total blood flow is maintained independently of all other control demands by some form of compensating software. This requires a substantial reserve capacity within the system to enable adjustments of output.

Ventricular systems have been associated with architecturally physiologic pulse pressure–flow profiles during experimental procedures. Pumps of this type have been employed in clinical practice with some success (111). However, widespread use of such systems has been hampered by their considerable cost, in terms of both mechanical and disposable components. It is possible that as the interest in physiologic pulsatile blood flow increases (112), interest in ventricular pumps will also increase and more systems will find their way into clinical practice.

Compression Plate Pumps

The principle of the compression plate pumping system is simple and not dissimilar to that of the ventricular models. Like ventricular pumps, compression plate pumps can produce only pulsatile flow. Simply put, a length of tubing of known diameter is placed on a rigid back plate and compressed by a moving plate that descends for a preselected stroke length, thereby ejecting a volume of perfusate from the tube (Fig. 10.7). The direction of blood flow is ensured by valves positioned at the inlet and outlet of the ventricle or sac.

The pulse rise time can be controlled by the rate of compression of the tube, and the flow rate by altering either the frequency or the length of travel of the compression plate. These systems offer significant control of pulse wave architecture. The filling aspect of the pumping cycle, like that of the ventricular mechanisms, can be either passive or active. Passive filling systems depend on a head of pressure

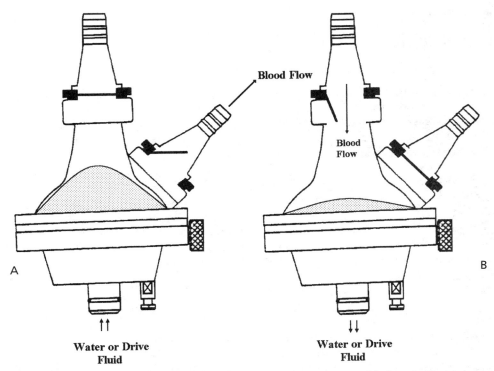

FIG. 10.6. Ventricular pumping mechanism, mode of action. The ventricle is typically driven by either water or air. The driving medium fills a sac within the blood chamber, thereby displacing a volume of blood (*A*). The blood flow is directed by one-way inlet and outlet valves. During the fill cycle, the driving medium is drawn out of the sac and is replaced by blood in the blood chamber (*B*). The driving force for the displacement of blood is the displacement of the driving medium.

at the inlet side of the device to fill the ventricle after the ejection cycle has been completed. Such systems employ ventricles with little or no elastic memory; therefore, the filling is entirely passive, limiting the application of such pumps. Active filling systems do not entirely depend on a head of pressure at the inlet side to effect a filling cycle. In these systems, the material employed in constructing the ventricle has an elastic memory that effects filling by generating a negative pressure. This condition augments the positive pressure at the inlet side of the device. A similar outcome can be achieved by connecting the ventricle to both the constraining and compression plates, whereby the return of the compression plate to the neutral position will effect the filling of the ventricle by generating a negative pressure within the ventricle. Active filling systems are the only compression plate systems that can be considered for routine CPB applications as stand-alone systems. Passive filling systems commonly require an additional or "priming" pump

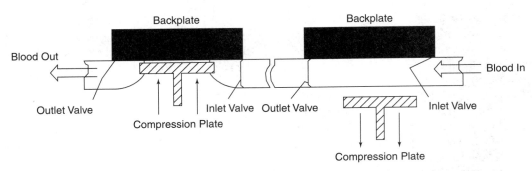

FIG. 10.7. Typical compression plate mechanism. This diagram shows both the fill and ejection cycles. The valves that ensure flow direction can be either pressure-driven or cam-driven.

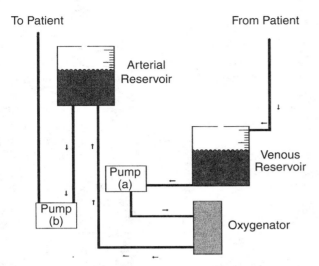

FIG. 10.8. Circuit diagram of the feeder reservoir system for employing a passive-filling ventricle pump system. Venous blood flows into the venous reservoir in the normal manner and is pumped from there by a roller pump (*a*) through the membrane oxygenator. Rather than passing directly to the patient, the blood is held in a second reservoir (arterial reservoir). The arterial reservoir is the most elevated aspect of the perfusion circuit and fills the pump head (*b*) by gravity flow. Such a system permits passive-filling ventricles to be used for routine cardiopulmonary bypass.

if the system is to operate without being affected by position within the perfusion circuitry (Fig. 10.8). The passive filling system has attractive attributes; notably, negative pressures are not generated within the system, and it can pump only the volume of blood supplied by the inlet conditions, matching output with inlet flow. Active filling ventricles powered by the elastic memory of the ventricular material have been the basis of several systems in the past (18,113) and have proved adequate for CPB, although their flow capabilities are somewhat limiting. The valves employed in ventricular pumping systems have produced significant problems. Internal valves have proved prohibitively expensive through the years, which has led to many promising systems being shelved on economic grounds before clinical use. One possible solution to this issue is to position the valves on the outside of the tubing or ventricle. This arrangement, used in the University of Texas preload-responsive pump (114), has proved to be both economical and efficient. The use of mechanical, externally positioned valves may require another compromise. The tubing employed in the pump head must be soft enough to allow the passively operated valves to compress it to the point of closure. This removes to a great extent the strong elastic memory required to power an active fill cycle, and the system reverts to being a passive filling system.

Ventricular pumps are pulsatile and capable of generating pulsatile flow of physiologic proportions. As research into the beneficial effects of pulsatile blood flow continues,

it is conceivable that interest in ventricular pumps will expand with the realization that this pump is uniquely capable of generating nearly physiologic pulse architecture.

Centrifugal Blood Pumps

Centrifugal blood pumps are a relatively recent innovation in pumping technology for routine CPB applications. Leschinski et al. (115) described them as pumps in which the working elements rotate a drive shaft; they can be axial, nutational, or rotary in nature. The drive for these pumps is invariably provided by an electric motor coupled to the drive shaft. The coupling of the motor to the drive shaft offers a complex design problem. The drive components must be sealed so that sterility of the blood path can be ensured. The accepted solution to this problem is to couple the drive motor to the drive shaft magnetically (Fig. 10.9). Pennington (116) determined that centrifugal pumps are afterload-dependent, as the output is related to pump speed and pressure gradient. It is, therefore, necessary to measure the pump output with a flow probe during use.

There are as many pump head designs as there are pump types, but in general, designs fall into one of three categories—vaned pump mechanisms, concentric disk pump mechanisms, or combinations of both.

Centrifugal pumps have been used for a considerable time with success. These pumps may be susceptible to the generation of stagnant zones and high vortex areas, which can result in hemolysis and the formation of thrombi on the working parts of the pump mechanism. Centrifugal

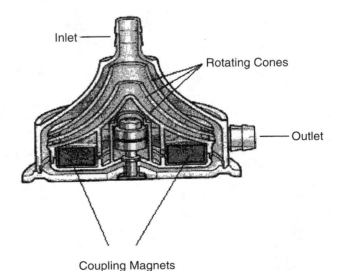

FIG. 10.9. Schematic diagram of a centrifugal pump head (Bio-Medicus pump, Medtronic, Minneapolis, Minnesota) showing the rotating cone arrangement, inlet and outlet orientation, and drive magnets. The rotating components are held in place by a bearing assembly.

pumps have been extensively studied in the long-term assist arena, where they have been found to offer significant advantages over roller pumps (117). Increasingly, however, centrifugal pumps are being employed for short-term, routine CPB procedures. Interest in the use of centrifugal pumps for routine clinical practice has been fired by the safety features associated with these systems, particularly a reduced risk for air embolism. Centrifugal pumps, particularly those of the disk type, have been associated with reduced hemolysis in clinical use. Berki et al. (118) noted a reduction in operative hemolysis with the disk centrifugal pump, and also an improvement in postoperative hemostasis and preservation of the platelet count, in comparison with the roller pump. They further noted a reduced microembolic load with the centrifugal pump, which they thought was probably a consequence of the elimination of tubing spallation traditionally associated with the roller pump. These findings confirmed those of Mandl (119) and Noon et al. (120), who noted that centrifugal pumps, particularly constrained vortex pumps, are associated with a lower particulate and gaseous embolic load than are roller pumps. Improved blood handling with the centrifugal pump during routine clinical use was confirmed by Matsukura (121), who noted improved platelet preservation in comparison with the roller mechanism. Maas et al. (122) confirmed this, observing reduced hemolysis and improved postoperative platelet counts.

Because fluid displacement in such systems depends on centrifugal impulsion, which requires a very high rotational speed to produce blood velocity, a pulsatile output is difficult to achieve. To do so, the impeller would have to accelerate very rapidly to an extremely high rotational speed. Attempts to achieve this have been made with varying degrees of success; however, pulsatile blood flow with centrifugal systems has been slow to develop. Recent studies by Nishida et al. (123) with the Terumo Capiox (Terumo Corporation, Kanagawa, Japan) centrifugal pump in the pulsatile mode confirmed that physiologic arterial wave profiles are difficult to achieve clinically. Use of a rapidly accelerating rotor head achieved a radial artery pressure of only 10 mm Hg, which is no greater than the ripple pressure amplitude seen with roller pump mechanisms in a nonpulsatile mode. Gobel et al. (124) described a new centrifugal pump that they determined to be capable of generating pulsatile flow of physiologic proportions. In a comparative study, they further noted that pumps without vanes are incapable of generating pulsatile flow at all because energy is transferred to the perfusate by friction only in such systems. Vaned pumps could produce varying degrees of pulsatility during testing but tended to "decouple" under the increased strain, potentially resulting in unacceptably low blood flows. Komada et al. (125) found that pulsatile blood flow generated by a centrifugal blood pump is not associated with the normally observed reduced peripheral vascular resistance and that the pressure profiles observed are damped. They found, however, that the centrifugal system does offer other advantages normally associated with roller pump-generated pulsatile blood flow, such as reduced angiotensin levels and a reduction in the need for postoperative inotropic agents. Ninomiya and colleagues (126) recognized the limitations of the centrifugal pump in generating pulsatile blood flow and employed a centrifugal pump in conjunction with a pulsatile assist device to generate pulsatile flow. They concluded that under these complex conditions, the centrifugal pump can produce sufficient pulsatile blood flow. In comparison with a nonpulsatile centrifugal pump, Dreissen et al. (127) observed reduced complement activation with a pulsatile centrifugal pump. They further found a higher incidence of postoperative respiratory tract infection in the nonpulsatile group, and the classic whole body inflammatory response (i.e., complement activation) appeared to be reduced when a pulse was added to centrifugal blood flow.

Centrifugal pump-generated pulsatile flow has not been well accepted, probably because generating physiologic pulsatility is not possible with currently available mechanisms. This belief appears to have been borne out in clinical practice. However, this area of research continues to attract much attention.

Pulsatile Assist Device

The pulsatile assist device is an intermittent occlusive device that employs an intraaortic balloon pump apparatus to produce pulsatile blood flow in the arterial line of the CPB circuit (Fig. 10.10). The pulse is generated by occluding the arterial line of the circuit under flowing conditions, thereby creating a large pressure and volume delay within the arterial side of the circuit. On deflation of the balloon in the arterial line, the pressure and blood volume are released into the aorta of the patient as a "pulse." Bregman and colleagues (128) described using this system during CPB to produce pulsatile blood flow at the beginning of as well as before and after CPB to produce arterial counterpulsation. The control module of the balloon pump permits control of the balloon inflation and deflation times, together with the rate of inflation and volume of gas infused into the balloon. The level of control offered by such a system is significant, and clinical studies involving this technology have been promising. Maddoux et al. (129) and Philbin et al. (130) were both impressed by the versatility of the system. However, there have been some concerns regarding its use, particularly regarding the possibility of balloon rupture (131) and generation of hemolysis (132). The pulsatile assist device chamber is positioned in the arterial line of the circuit and, in the event of a balloon rupture, the contents of the balloon can be discharged into the arterial line and from there into the aorta, with potentially disastrous consequences. However, the most convincing argument against this technology from the clinical standpoint is that it adds complexity to a traditional roller pump mechanism. Despite

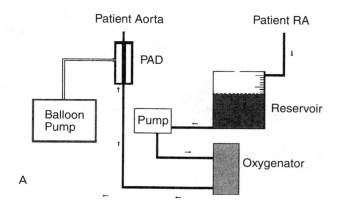

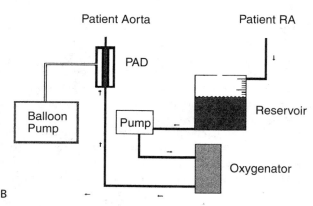

FIG. 10.10. Diagram of mode of operation of pulsatile assist device (PAD). Blood from the roller pump passes through the device when the balloon is deflated (*A*). When the balloon is inflated, the blood flow is prevented from passing through the device (*B*). This process is repeated at the desired pulse frequency, and a considerable degree of pulsatility can be achieved. Timing of the mechanism is critical, and extremely high circuit arterial "line" pressures are normal. RA, right atrium.

filter, and aortic cannula. In addition to these devices, the tubing connecting the patient to the heart–lung machine has energy-adsorbing properties that can affect energy delivery. Wright (133) noted that the tubing should be as short and rigid as possible with the minimum number of connectors if energy delivery is to be maximized. When tubing is long and unrestrained between pump and patient, it can often be seen swinging under pulsatile flow conditions, with the energy utilized in producing this pendular motion originating at the arterial pump. Highly flexible tubing can be seen to expand and contract under pulsatile flow conditions. Some of the pulsatile energy will be lost as a result of these processes, which then will impair the ability of the system to deliver physiologic pulsatility to the patient. Most recently, Inzoli et al. (134) found that the arterial tubing has a much greater overall damping effect on pulsatile structure and energy delivery than does the membrane oxygenator. Studies of the effects of tubing type and configuration on pulsatile flow delivery are few; however, many more studies have concentrated on the effects of membrane oxygenators on this important factor. Two studies (17,133) showed that the inclusion of a membrane oxygenator between the pump and the patient reduces hydraulic power delivery and alters pressure architecture. Specifically, Gourlay (18) showed that the membrane reduces hydraulic power only in the pulsatile domain when measured in a model of the human systemic circulation (Fig. 10.11). However, because the proportional

excellent clinical results with these devices, the increase in circuit complexity together with the fear of balloon rupture have led to its relative disuse.

Compatibility of Pulsatile Blood Flow with Perfusion Circuit Components

There are a number of ways in which perfusion circuit components other than the blood pump can influence the quality of pulsatile blood flow delivery to patients undergoing CPB. Of particular interest, because of their apparent involvement in the beneficial effects of pulsatile blood flow, are the energy adsorption characteristics of devices positioned in the arterial line of the perfusion circuit. The three devices commonly positioned between the arterial blood pump and the patient are the membrane oxygenator, arterial

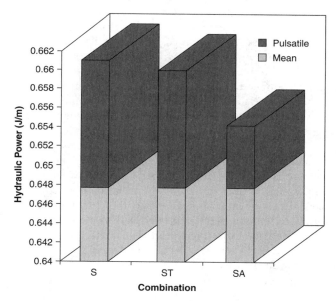

FIG. 10.11. The effects of including a membrane oxygenator on total hydraulic power. Group S has no oxygenator in line, group ST has an oxygenator positioned in the venous line, and group SA has the membrane in the arterial line. Clearly, energy absorption is greatest when the oxygenator is positioned in the arterial line. It is interesting to note that power in the mean domain is unaffected.

contribution to total hydraulic power arising from the pulsatile domain is small with a roller pump system, the resultant reduction in hydraulic power may not be clinically significant (135). In the same series of experiments, the effect of an arterial line filter on energy delivery was evaluated, and no significant effect was found.

The third circuit component between the pump and the patient, the aortic cannula, is critical to the transmission of pulsatile blood flow. Runge et al. (136) stated that it may be impossible for truly physiologic pulsatile flow to be achieved with current aortic cannulas. They further suggested that the excellent results achieved with pulsatile flow in animal studies cannot be repeated in the clinical environment without radically altering cannulation techniques. Clearly, the optimally sized aortic cannula for pulsatile blood flow transmission has an internal diameter that is the same as that of the arterial infusion tubing. Not surprisingly, it might be difficult to find a cardiac surgeon willing to insert such a large "pipe" into a patient's aorta.

Special attention must be paid to sheer stress and velocity associated with catheter size and tip geometry under pulsatile blood flow conditions. Kayser (137) stated that the high velocity of blood passing through aortic cannulas under pulsatile blood flow conditions may increase hemolysis. Wright (107) determined that the degree to which blood undergoes hemolysis in an arterial cannula depends on several factors—shear rate, velocity profile, and dimensions of the cannula. Most importantly, however, this depends on whether the flow within the cannula becomes turbulent or not. Wright determined by experimentation that hemolysis can be expected to occur when a shear rate of 200 Nm^{-2} is exceeded (107). Taylor et al. (67) measured the shear stress under pulsatile blood flow conditions at varying flow rates with two commonly used aortic cannulas and showed that not all cannulas are compatible with roller pump-generated pulsatile blood flow. One of these cannula types, although both were largely similar in design, was associated with high levels of hemolysis under the test conditions.

Aortic cannulas are generally considered benign in relation to perfusion. This may well be the case, but only if attention is paid to velocity profile, shear rate, and pressure drop during use. Runge et al. (136) summed up the importance of aortic cannulas to pulsatile blood flow by saying simply that cannula size should be maximized to optimize transmission of pulsatility. In effect, the only approach to aortic cannulation that can deliver physiologic pulsatile architecture is one that preserves the diameter of the aortic return line all the way into the patient's aorta. Clearly, without a radical change in cannulation technique and approach, this will not be achievable.

PULSATILE BLOOD FLOW: SAFETY CONSIDERATIONS

Generating pulsatile flow with roller pump technology is relatively simple. However, there are several safety consider-

ations that must be carried out. In a previous section, we described interactions that take place between the pump and other circuit components that adsorb hydraulic energy. Other interactions between these devices can, under some circumstances, induce considerably more hazardous consequences. In particular, the interaction between the pulsatile flow modality and the membrane oxygenator can generate gaseous microemboli (17,138).

Interaction between Pulsatile Flow and Membrane Oxygenators

Membrane oxygenators are generally microporous in nature and rely on a positive pressure gradient between the blood and gas phases to maintain integrity. It is possible for oxygenating gas to enter the blood phase in the form of microbubbles if the pressure gradient is, even momentarily, positive in favor of the gas phase (138). Pearson (139) described this phenomenon and the presence of microbubbles in the arterial tubing of the perfusion circuit in association with large transient negative pressure "spikes" generated by pulsatile roller pumps. In our own series of experiments (18), we found a relationship between the flow configuration and the number of microbubbles present in the arterial line of the circuit (Fig. 10.12.).

The gaseous microembolic activity associated with the combination of pulsatile blood flow and a membrane oxygenator is significant, but it can be dealt with quite adequately by including a screen filter downstream from the membrane oxygenator. The generation of microbubbles associated with this combination of technologies must be considered when pulsatile flow is used in the clinical setting; in particular, the fact that the number of microbubbles present increases with increasing pulsatility and blood flow (18) must be borne in mind during any decision regarding which pulsatile flow configuration to use.

Although increased microbubble production and energy adsorption are disadvantages to combining pulsatile flow technology with membrane oxygenators, there may be advantages. Pulsatile blood flow can enhance gas exchange within the membrane by generating secondary flows at the membrane–blood interface, and by breaking down boundary layers (see Chap. 4). This may not be immediately apparent in routine clinical practice, during which the membrane oxygenator's reserve capacity is not challenged. However, if the device is stressed by an increase in oxygen demand, pulsatile flow within the membrane compartment can assist in meeting this challenge (140).

The effect of pulsatile blood flow on the other main function of the modern blood oxygenator, heat exchange, has also been the focus of study. Sheperd (141) determined that pulsatile blood flow enhances the performance of the heat exchanger of one commercially available membrane oxygenator. He reasoned that under pulsatile blood flow conditions, the boundary layer effect within the heat exchanger is broken down, leading to improved heat transmission. This factor is

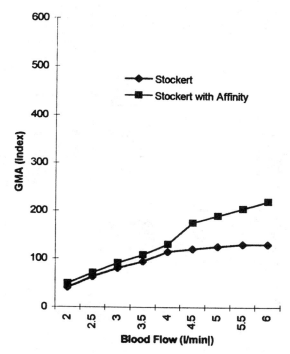

FIG. 10.12. Graph showing free circulating gaseous microembolic activity (GMA) in an *in vitro* circuit running at the clinical range of blood flow rates with normal clinical pulsatile control configuration (Stockert roller pump mechanism, Stockert, Munich, Germany). In this case, the pump was used with and without an Affinity membrane oxygenator (Avecor Cardiovascular Inc., Minneapolis, MN) in the arterial line. It can be seen that inclusion of the membrane is associated with an increase in activity across the flow range, but a particularly high response can be seen at the higher levels of blood flow.

potentially important because the reduced systemic vascular resistance encountered during pulsatile CPB may place greater demand on the heat exchanger, particularly during the rewarming phase of the procedure.

Overall, the combination of pulsatile blood flow and membrane oxygenation has advantages and disadvantages. It is particularly important that all these be understood fully before the pulsatile flow route is undertaken. The combination is safe and effective provided that adequate safety measures are taken to ensure that the optimum combination of devices and control configuration are employed.

CONCLUSIONS

The clinical use of pulsatile flow during CPB has a considerable history; however, evolving technologies require that the issue be continually readdressed. Pulsatile CPB remains a controversial issue (7). Studies of pulsatile blood flow during CPB have focused on a broad spectrum of factors, ranging from cellular metabolism to organ function and including both hemodynamic and metabolic responses. However,

most of this work, particularly the clinical studies, has been carried out without a truly physiologic pulsatile blood flow having been achieved. This results from the lack of a device capable of delivering such a flow pattern during routine CPB. Despite evidence in its favor, pulsatile CPB still remains controversial; however, it is conceivable that production of a pulsatile blood pump capable of generating physiologic pulsatile flow during routine CPB will resolve the controversy. This leaves considerable opportunity for future investigation. Despite the safety issues raised in the latter half of this chapter, it seems logical that a flow modality closely resembling the natural state will deliver the best result. It remains to be seen whether this can be safely achieved within the size constraints imposed by arterial cannulas. With advancing technologic development, it may not be long before this controversy is resolved.

KEY POINTS

- It has long been recognized that pulsatile flow is of physiologic importance and that reproducing pulsatility during cardiopulmonary bypass may be beneficial, but the safe delivery of pulsatile blood flow during cardiopulmonary bypass presents some formidable technologic obstacles.
- Simply generating a normal pulse pressure may not be sufficient to sustain normal circulatory physiology during cardiopulmonary bypass; rather, reproducing a normal pulsatile "architecture" should be the goal.
- Nonpulsatile cardiopulmonary bypass induces a progressive increase in systemic vascular resistance, potentially compromising organ perfusion during cardiopulmonary bypass and setting the stage for increased myocardial oxygen demand after bypass. Mechanisms involved in the increase of systemic vascular resistance include an increase in circulating catecholamines and vasopressin and activation of the renin–angiotensin system.
- Investigations in animals have generally found that urine output and renal blood flow are better preserved with pulsatile than with nonpulsatile bypass, yet clinical studies most often have not noted improved renal outcomes with pulsatile bypass, perhaps because the pulsatile flow has not been sufficiently physiologic.
- Pulsatile cardiopulmonary bypass has been shown experimentally to reduce both cerebral acidosis and markers of brain injury and neurohumoral dysfunction, but again, clinical studies have not demonstrated improved outcomes.
- Investigations suggest that hepatic, pancreatic, and gut function are better preserved during pulsatile cardiopulmonary bypass, quite possibly because of a reduction in the development of mucosal ischemia, which can induce endotoxemia. The clinical implications of these findings remain unclear.

- Several different types of systems can be used to deliver pulsatile cardiopulmonary bypass. These are briefly highlighted as follows:
  - Rhythmically varying the speed of a traditional roller pump head is the most widely available mechanism, but the architectural form and hydraulic power generated by these pumps have been suboptimal. Nevertheless, studies have shown some improvement in process variables such as systemic vascular resistance and stress hormone release, although improved clinical outcomes remain elusive.
  - Ventricular pumps use a compressible sac and one-way valves to generate pulsatility that is more architecturally physiologic than that obtained with other devices. Clinical trials show promise, but high cost remains a limiting factor.
  - Compression plate pumps and pulsatile assist devices compress the extracorporeal arterial flow between the oxygenator and the arterial inflow cannula to produce pulsatility. For various reasons, these devices have not become widely used.
  - Pulsatility can be produced with centrifugal pumps under ideal conditions, but their dependence on afterload renders them unreliable for this purpose.
- Obstacles to transmitting pulsatile flow into the patient include distensibility of the arterial tubing and resistance and damping imposed by membrane oxygenators, arterial filters, and arterial infusion cannulas that intervene between the source of pulsatility and the patient's arterial circulation. The small size of the aortic cannula in relation to the arterial tubing creates the extracorporeal equivalent of severe aortic stenosis, resulting in loss of pulsatility and possible hemolysis when sufficient energy is transmitted across the cannula to induce architecturally physiologic intraarterial pulsatility.

REFERENCES

1. Hamel G. Dei Bedeutung des pulses fur den blutstrom. *Z Biol NSF* 1889;474–497.
2. Gesell RA. On relation of pulse pressure to renal function. *Am J Physiol* 1913;32:70.
3. Kohlstaedt LA, Page IH. The liberation of renin by perfusion of kidneys following reduction of pulse pressure. *J Exp Med* 1940;72:201–211.
4. McMaster PD, Parsons RJ. The effect of the pulse on the spread of substances through tissues. *J Exp Med* 1938;68:377–400.
5. Gibbon JH Jr. Application of a mechanical heart and lung apparatus to cardiac surgery. *Minn Med* 1954;37:171–185.
6. DeBakey ME. A simple continuous flow blood instrument. *New Orleans Med Surg J* 1934;87:387–389.
7. Hornick P, Taylor KM. Pulsatile and nonpulsatile perfusion: the continuing controversy. *J Cardiothorac Vasc Anesth* 1997;11:310–315.
8. Gourlay T, Gibbons M, Taylor KM. Pulsatile flow compatibility of a group of membrane oxygenators. *Perfusion* 1987;2:115–126.
9. Hutcheson IR, Griffith TM. Release of endothelium-derived relaxing factor is modulated both by frequency and amplitude of pulsatile flow. *Am J Physiol* 1991;261:H257–H262.
10. Runge TM, Cohen DJ, Hantler CB, et al. Achievement of physiologic pulsatile flow on cardiopulmonary bypass with a 24 French cannula. *J ASAIO* 1992;38:M726–M729.
11. Taylor KM, Bain WH, Maxted KJ, et al. Comparative studies of pulsatile and nonpulsatile flow during cardiopulmonary bypass. I. Pulsatile system employed and its hematologic effects. *J Thorac Cardiovasc Surg* 1978;75:569–573.
12. Wright G, Furness A. What is pulsatile flow? *Ann Thorac Surg* 1985;39:401–402.
13. Gourlay T, Taylor KM, Russell M, et al. Comparative retrospective study of pulsatile and non-pulsatile flow in 380 consecutive cardiac patients. *Proceedings of the First World Congress on Extracorporeal Circulation*, Brighton, England, 1983.
14. Taylor KM, Bain WH, Davidson KG, et al. Comparative clinical study of pulsatile and non-pulsatile perfusion in 350 consecutive patients. *Thorax* 1982;37:324–330.
15. Landymore RW, Murphy DA, Kinley CE, et al. Does pulsatile flow influence the incidence of postoperative hypertension? *Ann Thorac Surg* 1979;28:261–268.
16. Kono M, Orita H, Shimanuki T, et al. A clinical study of cerebral perfusion during pulsatile and non-pulsatile cardiopulmonary bypass. *Nippon Geka Gakkai Zasshi* 1990;91:1016–1022.
17. Gourlay T, Taylor KM. Pulsatile flow and membrane oxygentors. *Perfusion* 1994;9:189–196.
18. Gourlay T. Controlled pulsatile architecture in cardiopulmonary bypass: *in vitro* and clinical studies [Thesis]. Strathclyde University, 1997.
19. Wright G. The hydraulic power outputs of pulsatile and non-pulsatile cardiopulmonary bypass pumps. *Perfusion* 1988;3:251–262.
20. Wright G, Ping J, Campbell C, et al. Computation of haemodynamic power and input impedance in the ascending aorta of patients undergoing open heart surgery. *Cardiovasc Res* 1988;22:179–184.
21. Wilcox BR, Coulter NA, Peters RM, et al. Power dissipation in the systemic and pulmonary vasculature of dogs. *Surgery* 1967;62:25.
22. Westerhof N, Elzinga G, Sipkema P. An artificial arterial system for pumping hearts. *J Appl Physiol* 1971;31:776–781.
23. Wright G. Hemodynamic analysis could resolve the pulsatile blood flow controversy. *Ann Thorac Surg* 1994;58:1199–1204.
24. Shepard RB, Simpson DS, Sharp JF. Energy equivalent pressure. *Arch Surg* 1966;93:730–740.
25. Gourlay T, Taylor KM, Russell M, et al. Comparative retrospective study of pulsatile and non-pulsatile flow in 380 consecutive cardiac patients. *Proceedings of the First World Congress on Extracorporeal Circulation*, Brighton, England, 1983.
26. Taylor KM, Bain WH, Davidson KG, et al. Comparative clinical study of pulsatile and non-pulsatile perfusion in 350 consecutive patients. *Thorax* 1982;37:324–330.
27. Taylor KM, Bain WH, Morton JJ. The role of angiotensin II in the development of peripheral vasoconstriction during open heart surgery. *Am Heart J* 1980;100:935–937.
28. Stinson EB, Holloway EL, Derby GC, et al. Control of myocardial performance early after open heart operations by vasodilator treatment. *J Thorac Cardiovasc Surg* 1977;73:523–530.
29. Taylor KM, Bain WH, Russell M, et al. Peripheral vascular resistance and angiotensin II levels during pulsatile and non-pulsatile cardiopulmonary bypass. *Thorax* 1979;34:594–598.

30. Many M, Soroff HS, Birtwell WC, et al. The physiologic role of pulsatile and nonpulsatile blood flow. II. Effects on renal function. *Arch Surg* 1968;95:762–767.

31. Kohlstaedt LA, Page IH. The liberation of renin by perfusion of kidneys following reduction of pulse pressure. *J Exp Med* 1940;72:201–211.

32. Taylor KM, Casals J, Morton JJ. The haemodynamic effect of angiotensin blockage after cardiopulmonary bypass. *Br Heart J* 1979;41:380–385.

33. Levine FH, Philbin DM, Kono K, et al. Plasma vasopressin levels and urinary sodium excretion during cardiopulmonary bypass with and without pulsatile flow. *Ann Thorac Surg* 1981;32:63–67.

34. Minami K, Korner M, Vyska K. Effects of pulsatile perfusion on plasma catecholamine levels and haemodynamics during and after cardiac operations with cardiopulmonary bypass. *J Thorac Cardiovasc Surg* 1990;99:82–91.

35. Taylor KM. Pulsatile perfusion. In: Taylor KM, ed. *Cardiopulmonary bypass—principles and management*. London: Chapman and Hall, 1986.

36. Mavroudis C. To pulse or not to pulse. *Ann Thorac Surg* 1978:25:259–271.

37. Jacobs LA, Klopp EH, Seamone W, et al. Improved organ function during cardiac bypass with a roller pump modified to deliver pulsatile flow. *J Thorac Cardiovasc Surg* 1969;58:703–712.

38. Dunn J, Kirsh MM, Harness J, et al. Hemodynamic, metabolic and hematologic effects of pulsatile cardiopulmonary bypass. *J Thorac Cardiovasc Surg* 1974;68: 138–147.

39. Steed D, Follette D, Foglia R. Effects of pulsatile and nonpulsatile perfusion on subendocardial perfusion during cardiopulmonary bypass. *Ann Thorac Surg* 1978;26:133–141.

40. Shepard RB, Kirklin JW. Relation of pulsatile flow to oxygen consumption and other variables during cardiopulmonary bypass. *J Thorac Cardiovasc Surg* 1969;58:694–702.

41. Ogata T, Ida Y, Takeda J, et al. A comparative study of the effectiveness of pulsatile and nonpulsatile blood flow in extracorporeal circulation. *Arch Jpn Chir* 1960;29:59–65.

42. Prior FGR, Moorcroft V, Gourlay T, et al. Further testing of pulse reverse osmosis. A new theory of the maintenance and control of blood pressure. *Int J Artif Organs* 1995;18: 469–473.

43. Prior FGR, Moorecroft V, Gourlay T, et al. The therapeutic significance of pulse reverse osmosis. *Int J Artif Organs* 1996; 19:487–492.

44. Ritter ER. Pressure-flow relations in kidney: alleged effects of pulse pressure. *Am J Physiol* 1952;168:480–489.

45. Goodyer AVN, Glenn WL. Relation of arterial pulse pressure to renal function. *Am J Physiol* 1951;167:689–697.

46. Oelert H, Eufe R. Dog kidney function during total left heart bypass with pulsatile and non-pulsatile flow. *J Cardiovasc Surg (Torino)* 1974;15:674–678.

47. Selkurt EE. Effects of pulse pressure and mean arterial pressure modification on renal haemodynamics and electrolyte and water excretion. *Circulation* 1951;4:541–546.

48. Hooker DR. A study of the isolated kidney: the influence of pulse pressure upon renal function. *Am J Physiol* 1910;27: 24–44.

49. Boucher JK, Rudy LW, Edmunds LH. Organ blood flow during pulsatile cardiopulmonary bypass. *J Appl Physiol* 1974;36: 86–90.

50. Nakayama K, Tamiya T, Yamamoto K, et al. High-amplitude pulsatile pump in extracorporeal circulation with particular reference to hemodynamics. *Surgery* 1963;54:798–805.

51. Fintersbusch W, Long DM, Sellers RD. Renal arteriography during extracorporeal circulation in dogs with preliminary report upon effects of low-molecular-weight dextran. *J Thorac Cardiovasc Surg* 1961;41:252–260.

52. Barger AC, Herd JA. Study of renal circulation in the unanaesthetized dog with inert gases (Proceedings of the Third International Congress of Nephrology). *Nephrology* 1966;1:174.

53. Mori A, Watanabe K, Onoe M, et al. Regional blood flow in the liver, pancreas and kidney during pulsatile and nonpulsatile perfusion under profound hypothermia. *Jpn Circ J* 1988;52: 219–227.

54. German JC, Chalmers GS, Hirai J, et al. Comparison of nonpulsatile and pulsatile extracorporeal circulation on renal tissue perfusion. *Chest* 1972;61:65–69.

55. Paquet KJ. Hemodynamic studies on normothermic perfusion of the isolated pig kidney with pulsatile and nonpulsatile flows. *J Cardiovasc Surg (Torino)* 1969;10: 45–53.

56. Mukherjee ND, Beran AV, Hirai J. *In vivo* determination of renal tissue oxygenation during pulsatile and non-pulsatile left heart bypass. *Ann Thorac Surg* 1973;15:334–363.

57. Williams GD, Seifen AB, Lawson NW, et al. Pulsatile perfusion versus conventional high-flow non-pulsatile perfusion for rapid core cooling and rewarming of infants for circulatory arrest in cardiac operation. *J Thorac Cardiovasc Surg* 1979;78:667–677.

58. Louagie YA, Gonzalez M, Collard E, et al. Does flow character of cardiopulmonary bypass make a difference? *J Thorac Cardiovasc Surg* 1992;104:1628–1638.

59. Matsuda H, Hirose H, Nakano S, et al. Results of open heart surgery in patients with impaired renal function as creatinine clearance below 30 mL/min. The effects of pulsatile perfusion. *J Cardiovasc Surg (Torino)* 1986;27: 595–599.

60. Belzer FO, Ashby BS, Huang JS. Etiology of rising perfusion pressure in isolated organ perfusion. *Ann Surg* 1968;168: 382–391.

61. Taylor KM, Devlin BJ, Mittra S, et al. Assessment of cerebral damage during open heart surgery. A new experimental model. *Scand J Thorac Cardiovasc Surg* 1980;14:197–203.

62. Simpson JC. Cerebral perfusion during cardiac surgery using cardiac bypass. In: Longmore E, ed. *Towards safer cardiac surgery*. MTP, Lancaster, 1981.

63. Hill JD, Aguilar KJ, Baranco A, et al. Neuropathological manifestations of cardiac surgery. *Ann Thorac Surg* 1969;7:409–419.

64. Sanderson JM, Wright G, Sims FW. Brain damage in dogs immediately following pulsatile and non-pulsatile blood flows in extracorporeal circulation. *Thorax* 1972;27:275–286.

65. DePaepe J, Pomerantzeff PMA, Nakiri K, et al. Observations of the microcirculation of the cerebral cortex of dogs subjected to pulsatile and non-pulsatile flow during extracorporeal circulation. In: *A Propos du Débit Pulse*. Belgium: Cobe Laboratories, 1979.

66. Taylor KM, Wright GS, Reid JS, et al. Comparative studies of pulsatile and non-pulsatile flow during cardiopulmonary bypass. II. The effects on adrenal secretion of cortisol. *J Thorac Cardiovasc Surg* 1978;75:574–578.

67. Taylor KM. Pulsatile perfusion. In: Taylor KM, ed. *Cardiopulmonary bypass—principles and management*. London: Chapman and Hall, 1986.

68. Taylor KM, Wright GS, Bain WH, et al. Comparative studies of pulsatile and non-pulsatile flow during cardiopulmonary bypass. III. Anterior pituitary response to thyrotrophin-releasing hormone. *J Thorac Cardiovasc Surg* 1979;75:579–584.

69. Philbin DM, Coggins CH, Emerson CW, et al. Plasma vasopressin levels and urinary sodium excretion during cardiopulmonary bypass: a comparison of halothane and morphine anesthesia. *J Thorac Cardiovasc Surg* 1979;77:582–585.

70. Briceno JC, Runge TM. Monitoring of blood gases during prolonged cardiopulmonary bypass and their relationship to brain pH, P_{O_2} and P_{CO_2}. *J ASAIO* 1994;40:M344–M350.

71. Kono M, Orita H, Shimanuki T, et al. A clinical study of cerebral perfusion during pulsatile and non-pulsatile cardiopul-

monary bypass. *Nippon Geka Gakkai Zasshi* 1990;91: 1016–1022.

72. Mori A, Watanabe K, Onoe M, et al. Regional blood flow in the liver, pancreas and kidney during pulsatile and nonpulsatile perfusion under profound hypothermia. *Jpn Circ J* 1988:52: 219–227.

73. Tranmer BI, Gross CE, Kindt GW, et al. Pulsatile versus non-pulsatile blood flow in the treatment of acute cerebral ischemia. *Neurosurgery* 1986;19:724–731.

74. Onoe M, Mori A, Watarid S, et al. The effect of pulsatile perfusion on cerebral blood flow during profound hypothermia with total circulatory arrest. *J Thorac Cardiovasc Surg* 1994;108: 119–125.

75. Henze T, Stephan H, Sonntag H. Cerebral dysfunction following extracorporeal circulation for aortocoronary bypass surgery: no differences in neuropsychological outcome after pulsatile versus nonpulsatile flow. *Thorac Cardiovasc Surg* 1990;38:65–68.

76. Murkin JM, Martzke JS, Buchan AM, et al. A randomized study of the influence of perfusion technique and pH management strategy in 316 patients undergoing coronary artery bypass surgery: II. Neurological and cognitive outcomes. *J Thorac Cardiovasc Surg* 1995;110:349–362.

77. Murkin JM, Martzke JS, Buchan AM, et al. A randomized study of the influence of perfusion technique and pH management strategy in 316 patients undergoing coronary artery bypass surgery: I. Mortality and cardiovascular morbidity. *J Thorac Cardiovasc Surg* 1995;110:340–348.

78. Hindman BJ, Dexter F, Smith T, et al. Pulsatile versus nonpulsatile flow. No difference in cerebral blood flow or metabolism during normothermic cardiopulmonary bypass in rabbits. *Anesthesiology* 1995;82:241–250.

79. Chow G, Roberts IG, Harris D, et al. Stockert roller pump generated pulsatile flow: cerebral metabolic changes in adult cardiopulmonary bypass. *Perfusion* 1997;12:113–119.

80. Feiner H. Pancreatitis after cardiac surgery. *Am J Surg* 1976; 131:684–688.

81. Baca I, Beiger W, Mittmann U, et al. Comparative studies of pulsatile and continuous flow during extracorporeal circulation. Effects on liver function and endocrine pancreas secretion. *Chir Forum Exp Klin Fortschr* 1979;49–53.

82. Saggau W, Baca I, Ros E, et al. Clinical and experimental studies on pulsatile and continuous flow during extracorporeal circulation. *Herz* 1980;5:42–50.

83. Murray WR, Mittra S, Mittra D, et al. The amylase creatinine clearance ratio following cardiopulmonary bypass. *J Thorac Cardiovasc Surg* 1982;82:248–253.

84. Pappas G, Winter SD, Kopriva CJ, et al. Improvement of myocardial and other vital organ functions and metabolism with a simple method of pulsatile flow (IAPB) during clinical cardiopulmonary bypass. *Surgery* 1975;77:34–44.

85. Mathie R, Desai J, Taylor KM. Hepatic blood flow and metabolism during pulsatile and non-pulsatile cardiopulmonary bypass. *Life Support Systems* 1984;2:303–305.

86. Chiu IS, Chu SH, Hung CR. Pulsatile flow during routine cardiopulmonary bypass. *J Cardiovasc Surg (Torino)* 1984;25: 530–536.

87. Gauss A, Druck A, Hemmer W, et al. Abdominal complications following heart surgery. *Anaesthesiol Intensivmed Notfallmed Schmerzther* 1994;29:23–29.

88. Baue AE. The role of the gut in the development of multiple organ dysfunction in cardiothoracic patients. *Ann Thorac Surg* 1993;55:822–829.

89. Bowles CT, Ohri SK, Nongchana K, et al. Endotoxaemia detected during cardiopulmonary bypass with a modified Limulus amoebocyte lysate asay. *Perfusion* 1995;10:219–228.

90. Andersen LW, Baek L. Transient endotoxaemia during cardiac surgery. *Perfusion* 1992;7:53–58.

91. Andersen LW, Baek L, Degen H, et al. Presence of circulating endotoxins during cardiac operations. *J Thorac Cardiovasc Surg* 1987;93:115–119.

92. Rocke DA, Gaffin SL, Wells MT, et al. Endotoxaemia associated with cardiopulmonary bypass. *J Thorac Cardiovasc Surg* 1987;93:832–837.

93. Jansen NJ, van Oeveren W, Gu YJ, et al. Endotoxin release and tumor necrosis factor formation during cardiopulmonary bypass. *Ann Thorac Surg* 1992;54:744–747.

94. Ohri SK, Bowles CT, Siddiqui A, et al. The effect of cardiopulmonary bypass on gastric and colonic mucosal perfusion. A tonometric assessment. *Perfusion* 1994;9:101–108.

95. Tao W, Zwischenberger JB, Nguyen TT, et al. Gut mucosal ischemia during normothermic cardiopulmonary bypass results from blood flow redistribution and increased oxygen demand. *J Thorac Cardiovasc Surg* 1995;110:819–828.

96. Riddington DW, Venkatesh B, Boivin CM, et al. Intestinal permeability, gastric intramucosal pH, and systemic endotoxemia in patients undergoing cardiopulmonary bypass. *JAMA* 1996;275:1007–1012.

97. Quigley RL, Caplain MS, Perkins JA, et al. Cardiopulmonary bypass with adequate flow and perfusion pressure prevents endotoxaemia and pathologic cytokine production. *Perfusion* 1995; 10:27–33.

98. Fiddian-Green RG. Gut mucosal ischemia during cardiac surgery. *Semin Thorac Cardiovasc Surg* 1990;4:389–399.

99. Reilly PM, Bulkey GB. Vasoactive mediators and splanchnic perfusion. *Crit Care Med* 1993;21:S55–S68.

100. Ogino H, Miki S, Ueda Y, et al. A case of bowel necrosis due to acute mesenteric ischemia following pulsatile cardiopulmonary bypass. *Ann Thorac Cardiovasc Surg* 1998;4:34–36.

101. DeBakey ME. A simple continuous flow blood instrument. *New Orleans Med Surg J* 1934;87:387–389.

102. Wesolowski SA, Miller HH, Halkett AE. Experimental replacement of the heart by a mechanical extracorporeal pump. *Bull N Engl Med Center* 1950;12:41–50.

103. Gourlay T, Taylor KM. Perfusion pumps. In: Jones RA, Elliott MJ, eds. *Cardiopulmonary bypass in neonates and young children.* London: Butterworth–Heineman, 1994.

104. Ogata T, Ida Y, Takeda J. Experimental studies on the extracorporeal circulation by use of our pulsatile arterial pump. *Lung* 1959;6:381–383.

105. Nonoyama A. Haemodynamic studies on extracorporeal circulation with pulsatile and non-pulsatile blood flows. *Arch Jpn Chir* 1960;29:381–406.

106. Nakayama K, Tamiya T, Yamamoto K, et al. High-amplitude pulsatile pump in extracorporeal circulation with particular reference to hemodynamics. *Surgery* 1963;54:798–803.

107. Wright G. Blood cell trauma. In: Taylor KM, ed. *Cardiopulmonary bypass.* London: Chapman and Hall, 1986:249–276.

108. Gourlay T, Taylor KM. Pulsatile flow and membrane oxygenators. *Perfusion* 1994;9:189–196.

109. Taylor KM, Bain WH, Maxted KJ, et al. Comparative studies of pulsatile and nonpulsatile flow during cardiopulmonary bypass. I. Pulsatile system employed and its hematologic effects. *J Thorac Cardiovasc Surg* 1978;75: 569–573.

110. Adams S, Fleming J, Gourlay T, et al. Clinical experience with the Sarns pulsatile pump during open heart surgery. *Perfusion* 1986;1:53–56.

111. Rottenberg D, Sondak E, Rahats S, et al. Early experience with a true pulsatile pump for heart surgery. *Perfusion* 1995;10: 171–175.

112. Mutch WA, Lefevre GR, Theissen DB, et al. Computer-con-

trolled cardiopulmonary bypass increases jugular venous oxygen saturation during rewarming. *Ann Thorac Surg* 1998;65:59–65.

113. Sanderson JM, Morton PG, Tolloczko TS, et al. The Morton-Keele pump—a hydraulically activated pulsatile pump for use in extracorporeal circulation. *Med Biol Eng* 1973;Mar,11(2): 182–190.

114. Runge TM, Grover FL, Cohen DJ, et al. Preload-responsive, pulsatile flow, externally valved pump: cardiovascular bypass. *J Invest Surg* 1989;2:269–279.

115. Leschinski BM, Itkin GP, Zimin NK. Centrifugal blood pumps—a brief analysis: development of new changes. *Perfusion* 1991;6:115–123.

116. Pennington DG, Merjavy JP, Swartz MT, et al. Clinical experience with centrifugal pump ventricular assist devices. *Trans Am Soc Artif Intern Organs* 1982;28:93–99.

117. Nose Y. Nonpulsatile mode of blood flow required for cardiopulmonary bypass and total body perfusion. *Artif Organs* 1993; 17:92–102.

118. Berki T, Gurbuz A, Isik O, et al. Cardiopulmonary bypass using a centrifugal pump. *Vasc Surg* 1992;26:123–134.

119. Mandl JP. Comparison of emboli production between a constrained vortex pump and a roller pump. *Proceedings AmSECT*, 1977.

120. Noon GP, Sekela ME, Glueck, et al. Comparison of *in vitro* blood trauma and spallation produced by the Bio-medicus and roller pump during hypothermia. International Workshop on Rotary Blood Pumps, Baylor College, 1988.

121. Matsukura H. An experimental study of the preservation of platelet during extracorporeal circulation. *Jpn J Thorac Surg* 1983;36:11.

122. Maas C, Kok R, Segers P. Comparison between a centrifugal and a roller pump. Abstract of presentation at Pathophysiology and Techniques of Cardiopulmonary Bypass, San Diego, California, February, 1993.

123. Nishida H, Uesugi H, Nishinaka T, et al. Clinical evaluation of pulsatile flow mode of Terumo Capiox centrifugal pump. *Artif Organs* 1997;21:816–821.

124. Gobel C, Eilers R, Reul H, et al. A new blood pump for cardiopulmonary bypass: the HiFlow centrifugal pump. *Artif Organs* 1997;21:841–845.

125. Komada T, Maet H, Imawaki S, et al. Haematologic and endocrinologic effects of pulsatile cardiopulmonary bypass using a centrifugal pump. *Nippon Kyobu Geka Zasshi* 1992;40: 901–911.

126. Ninomiya J, Shoji T, Tanaka IS, et al. Clinical evaluation of a new type of centrifugal pump. *Artif Organs* 1994;18:702–705.

127. Dreissen JJ, Dhaese H, Fransen G, et al. Pulsatile compared with nonpulsatile perfusion using a centrifugal pump for cardiopulmonary bypass during coronary artery bypass grafting. Effects on systemic haemodynamics, oxygenation and inflammatory response parameters. *Perfusion* 1995;10:3–12.

128. Bregman D, Bowman FO Jr, Parodi EN, et al. An improved method of myocardial protection with pulsation during cardiopulmonary bypass. *Circulation* 1977;56[Suppl 2]:157–160.

129. Maddoux G, Pappas G, Jenkins M, et al. Effect of pulsatile and nonpulsatile flow during cardiopulmonary bypass on left ventricular ejection fraction early after aortocoronary bypass surgery. *Am J Cardiol* 1976;37:1000–1006.

130. Philbin DM, Levine FH, Emerson CW, et al. Plasma vasopressin levels and urinary flow during cardiopulmonary bypass in patients with valvular heart disease: effects of pulsatile flow. *J Thorac Cardiovasc Surg* 1979;78:779–783.

131. Tomatis L, Nemiroff M, Raihi M, et al. Massive arterial air embolism due to rupture of pulsatile assist device. Successful treatment in the hyperbaric chamber. *Ann Thorac Surg* 1981; 32:604–608.

132. Zumbro GL, Shearer G, Fishback ME, et al. A prospective evaluation of the pulsatile assist device. *Ann Thorac Surg* 1979; 28:269–273.

133. Wright G. Factors affecting the pulsatile hydraulic power output of the Stockert roller pump. *Perfusion* 1989;4:187–195.

134. Inzoli F, Pennati G, Mastrantonio F, et al. Influence of membrane oxygentors on the pulsatile flow in extracorporeal circuits: an experimental analysis. *Int J Artif Organs* 1997;20:455–462.

135. Gourlay T, Taylor KM. Pulsatile flow and membrane oxygenators. *Perfusion* 1994;9:189–196.

136. Runge TM, Cohen DJ, Hantler CB, et al. Achievement of physiologic pulsatile flow on cardiopulmonary bypass with a 24 French cannula. *J ASAIO* 1992;38:M726–M729.

137. Kayser KL. Pulsatile perfusion problems. *Ann Thorac Surg* 1979; 27:284–285.

138. Karichev Z, Muler A, Vishnevsky M. Unusual oxygen transfer in microporous blood oxygenator. *Int J Artif Organs* 1997;21: 522.

139. Pearson DT. Microemboli. In: Taylor KM, ed. *Cardiopulmonary bypass—principles and management.* London: Chapman and Hall, 1986.

140. Bellhouse BJ. Design of the Oxford membrane oxygenator and its performance during prolonged support of newborn lambs. In: Zapol WM, ed. *Membrane lungs for acute respiratory failure.* New York: Academic Press, 1976.

141. Shepherd S, Pierce JMT. Pulsatile flow during cardiopulmonary bypass speeds thermal energy transfer: a possible explanation for the reduced afterdrop. *Perfusion* 1995;10:111–114.

11

HEMODILUTION AND PRIMING SOLUTIONS

JOHN R. COOPER, JR.
N. MARTIN GIESECKE

HISTORICAL PERSPECTIVE

Historical perspective is particularly important in assessing the progression of techniques for hemodilution and how they affect the physiology of extracorporeal circulation and the development of related complications. John Gibbon (1), who developed the first heart–lung machine and performed the first successful operation using cardiopulmonary bypass (CPB), envisioned a perfusion technique employing a prime of normal composition (i.e., blood) with "normal" flow rates (70 to 80 mL/kg per minute) and normal blood pressure. When Gibbon withdrew from this area of research, his original methods were continued by Kirklin and colleagues (2). Lillehei and his associates, first in their procedures with controlled cross-circulation (3) and then with CPB (4), employed significantly lower flow rates (30 to 35 mL/kg per minute) than did Gibbon. This modification (based on the "azygos flow principle") (5) was derived from the observation that dogs could survive when both the superior and inferior venae cavae were occluded. In this situation, the azygos venous drainage of dogs, unlike that of humans, still returns to the heart because of a more central entry, and this amount of flow (10% of normal cardiac output) proved adequate for survival for up to 1 hour. This observation was rapidly accepted and applied to CPB by many who perceived the harm to blood elements by high flows and excessive suctioning. Hypothermia was added to many high flow rate and most low flow rate techniques to "protect" various organs, even though Lillehei's original cross-circulation procedures were carried out at normothermia (3). Despite lower flows, the priming solution for the extracorporeal circuit with oxygenator remained the same—whole blood, either freshly drawn and heparinized, or collected into citrated bags, but as fresh as possible.

Spurred by animal research and the occasional emergent clinical experience with asanguineous prime, surgeons,

around 1960, began electively using crystalloid solutions or plasma-expanding colloids to reduce or eliminate blood from the prime (Table 11.1). Hypothermia was now increasingly applied to protect organs from the "adverse effects" of not only low flow, but also hemodilution. Nevertheless, the technique of hemodilution gained increasing popularity, and presently it is used almost universally. It should be noted that the following discussion pertains to short-duration clinical CPB as used for cardiac surgery. Applicability of hemodilution to longer CPB support is discussed elsewhere.

IMMEDIATE BENEFITS OF HEMODILUTION

A major reason for employing asanguineous primes was to reduce the severe strain placed on hospital blood banks by the use of whole blood for priming CPB circuits. The need for at least two units of whole blood, and possibly as many as five or six, just for prime in each patient often caused severe logistical problems for physicians trying to run an active cardiac surgical service. Many cases were postponed for lack of the correct type or amount of blood. Crystalloid primes also improved access to CPB as an emergency procedure by reducing the time and resources required to have a usable circuit available (Table 11.1).

Another immediate, but unforeseen, clinical benefit of crystalloid primes was improved oxygenation during CPB. Bubble oxygenators of that period, the type most widely used, produced a high proportion of relatively large bubbles in comparison with modern devices. Compared with the smaller, more numerous bubbles produced by later oxygenators, these larger bubbles were relatively inefficient for the transfer of oxygen because of the smaller surface area of the oxygen bubbles relative to the number of red cells. Hemodilution, especially in patients with polycythemia, produced an absolute reduction in the number of red cells and increased the likelihood of exposure to oxygen. Arterial oxygen tension on CPB was generally higher, and additional crystalloid was given to maintain hemodilution if oxygen tension started to fall with diuresis.

J. R. Cooper, Jr. and N. M. Giesecke: Department of Cardiovascular Anesthesiology, St. Luke's Episcopal Hospital, Texas Heart Institute, Houston, Texas 77225.

TABLE 11.1. HISTORICAL PERSPECTIVE OF PRIMING SOLUTIONS AND USE OF HEMODILUTION DURING CARDIOPULMONARY BYPASS

Surgeon	Priming Solution	Technique
Gibbon (1)	Whole blood	High flow
Kirklin (2)	Whole blood	High flow
Lillehei (3)	Whole blood	Low flow
DeWall and Lillihei (4)	5% Dextrose	Hemodilution and hypothermia
Zuhdi (6)	5% Dextrose	Hemodilution and hypothermia
Panico (7)	Saline solution	Hemodilution
Long (8)	Dextran and 5% albumin	Hemodilution and hypothermia
Cooley (9)	5% Dextrose	Hemodilution and normothermia

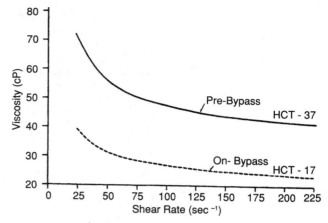

FIG. 11.1. Viscosity change (in centipoise) plotted against shear rate (in sec^{-1}) in a patient whose hematocrit fell from 37% to 17% after hemodilution at the initiation of cardiopulmonary bypass. (Modified from Gordon RJ, Ravin M, Rawitscher RE, et al. Changes in arterial pressure, viscosity and resistance during cardiopulmonary bypass. *J Thorac Cardiovasc Surg* 1975;69:552–561, with permission.)

A special impetus to the development of nonhemic prime techniques was provided by members of the Jehovah's Witness faith, who totally refused to accept transfusions of blood or blood products, although they would allow their own blood to circulate outside their body as long as fluid continuity was constantly maintained in the CPB circuit. The use of nonhemic prime has permitted cardiac operations to be performed in more than 1,000 Jehovah's Witnesses at the Texas Heart Institute alone (10). These patients constitute a unique "control" group for comparison of other techniques of blood conservation.

PHYSIOLOGIC CONSEQUENCES OF HEMODILUTION

Rheology of Blood

A detailed review of the rheologic properties of blood is beyond the scope of this chapter. However, some basic definitions and concepts are required, as changes in blood rheology are central to any discussion of hemodilution physiology. An exhaustive review can be found in the text by Gordon et al. (11). A force applied to an area of a liquid confined between two plates, sufficient to set the liquid in motion, is known as the *shear stress*. The velocity at which the liquid moves in proportion to the separation of the plates is known as the *velocity gradient* or *shear rate*. The shear stress is proportional to the shear rate, and the coefficient of proportionality is the fluid viscosity (Eq. 1).

$$\text{Shear Stress} = \text{Viscosity} \times \text{Shear Rate} \qquad [1]$$

For most uniform fluids, such as water, viscosity is constant; these are known as *newtonian fluids*. The viscosity of blood is not constant; rather, it depends on the shear rate

when flowing (Fig. 11.1); thus, blood is a non-newtonian fluid. Lower shear rates are associated with higher viscosity, as the cellular elements and plasma proteins tend to aggregate, form rouleaux, and resist flow. This aggregation at low shear rates primarily results from intracellular bridging by fibrinogen; as flow rates increase, these bridges disintegrate.

Non-newtonian behavior of blood is also influenced by the effective cell volume (12). When solid particles (cells) are added to a fluid, they influence viscosity not only by their absolute presence, but also by their effect on the surrounding fluid. The effective cell volume is the cell volume plus the surrounding fluid that behaves as though it were a part of the cell, much like the earth and its atmosphere. Red cells are deformable, and as shear rates increase, they tend to form ellipsoid shapes with the major axis aligned with the direction of flow. This latter effect, combined with the disaggregation of red cells, causes blood to behave in a more newtonian fashion at higher velocity gradients.

One further concept about behavior of fluids is important. The amount of shear stress that must be applied to a stationary newtonian liquid to begin its movement is at or near zero. For non-newtonian blood, because of cellular geometry and aggregation, a force known as the *yield stress* is required to induce flow. At low shear rates, the yield stress represents part of the viscous resistance and depends on both fibrinogen and hematocrit (13).

Circulatory Effects

Both organ blood flow and total cardiac output are directly proportional to perfusion pressure and inversely related to total peripheral resistance (Eq. 2A). This resistance to flow is proportional to vascular resistance and viscosity of the perfusate (Eq. 2B).

$$\text{Flow (Cardiac Output)} \propto \frac{\text{Perfusion Pressure}}{\text{Total Peripheral Resistance}} \quad [2A]$$

$$\text{Flow} \propto \frac{\text{Perfusion Pressure}}{\text{Vascular Resistance} \times \text{Viscosity}} \quad [2B]$$

These relationships are often specifically expressed in the Hagen-Poiseuille equation:

$$Q = \frac{\pi \, (P_1 \, dP_2) \, R^4}{8\mu L} \quad [3]$$

where Q equals flow, $(P_1 \, dP_2)$ equals pressure drop along a tube of radius R and length L, and μ equals viscosity. Application of this equation to blood flow is limited because it is accurate only for the laminar flow of newtonian liquids in long tubes with rigid walls. It does serve to further emphasize, however, the influence of viscosity and vascular geometry on flow. In humans, the aorta and larger vessels provide little impedance to blood flow; most of the vascular resistance comes from the smaller vessels: arterioles, capillaries, and venules. As vessel diameter decreases, shear rate decreases, and because blood viscosity is inversely related to shear rate, viscosity rises as flow falls. As a result, peripheral resistance also rises. Flow is lowest and viscosity highest in the postcapillary venules (14).

These physiologic effects are potentially quite harmful if CPB is performed without considering viscosity. In most centers, modern CPB involves the use of flow rates that are somewhat lower than those of "normal" blood: 50 mL/kg per minute or 2.0 L/m² per minute. Frequently, hypothermia is also used if flow rates are further reduced to provide a bloodless operative field or, more commonly, to augment myocardial protection. Reductions in both flow rate and perfusion pressure would tend to increase viscosity and thus peripheral resistance; this in turn would decrease tissue perfusion. Hemodilution works to limit the adverse effects of CPB by significantly reducing blood viscosity during bypass. There is a direct relationship between viscosity and hematocrit (15) (Fig. 11.1). Therefore, reducing hematocrit produces a marked decrease in total resistance and results in an increase in tissue perfusion (Eq. 2B). For example, in canine experiments, a decrease in hematocrit from 42% to 25% produces a 50% increase in flow at the same pressure (14). Extremes of hemodilution (hematocrit <10%) permit blood to act as a newtonian fluid (16).

Clinically, the most noticeable effect of hemodilution is a marked drop in perfusion pressure at initiation of CPB. Gordon et al. (15) showed that when hemodilution is used to decrease hematocrit and flow rate on CPB is held constant, perfusion pressure falls in direct proportion to the

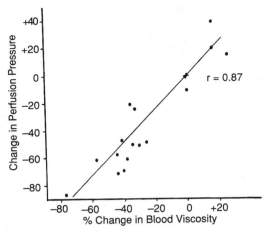

FIG. 11.2. Change in perfusion pressure versus change in viscosity in a series of patients on cardiopulmonary bypass at constant flow rates. (Modified from Gordon RJ, Ravin M, Rawitscher RE, et al. Changes in arterial pressure, viscosity and resistance during cardiopulmonary bypass. *J Thorac Cardiovasc Surg* 1975;69: 552–561, with permission.)

change in viscosity (Fig. 11.2). Additionally, Guyton and Richardson (17) found that hemodilution passively increases venous return in dogs, which is probably attributable to the marked increase in flow in small vessels, especially the postcapillary venules (Fig. 11.3). This same phenomenon was noted during CPB in humans by Cooley et al. (9).

The addition of induced hypothermia to CPB further influences the rheologic behavior of blood. Temperature reduction decreases flow by inducing direct vasoconstriction and increasing viscosity (18) (Fig. 11.4). The relationship is not, however, as direct as that of hematocrit and viscosity. For example, a decrease of 10°C in temperature causes about a 20% to 25% increase in viscosity. Of course, this adverse effect of hypothermia is partially or completely offset by the planned reduction in oxygen consumption.

Organ blood flow during hemodilution reflects the interplay of all these concepts. In animals, with progressive normovolemic hemodilution to a hematocrit of 19%, oxygen tension has been shown to increase in skeletal muscle, liver, pancreas, small intestine, and kidney (14). Cerebral blood flow during hemodilution has also been shown to increase 50% to 300% in comparison with pre-bypass levels (19,20). Decreases in hematocrit correlate with increases in cerebral blood flow velocity by transcranial Doppler (21). However, because cerebral flow is also significantly influenced by local autoregulation, changes in carbon dioxide tension, and extremes of perfusion pressure (22), absolute statements about the regional benefits of hemodilution are difficult to make, although hemodilution in general appears to have a salutary effect.

An exceedingly important consequence of hemodilution during CPB is an "uncoupling" of the normal relationship

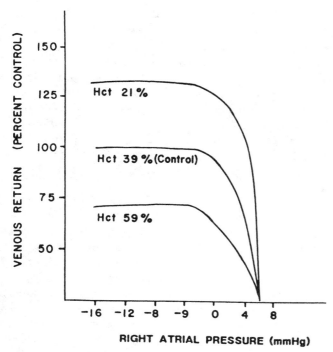

FIG. 11.3. Decreasing viscosity leads to increasing venous return (at a constant right atrial pressure). (From Guyton AC, Richardson TQ. Effect of hematocrit on venous return. *Circ Res* 1961;9: 157–163, with permission.)

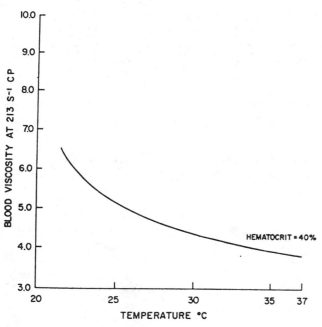

FIG. 11.4. Relationship between blood viscosity (in centipoise at a constant shear rate of 213 sec^{-1}) and temperature. (From Rand PW, Lacombe E, Hunt HE, et al. Viscosity of normal human blood under normothermic and hypothermic conditions. *J Appl Physiol* 1964;19:117–122, as modified by Gordon RJ, Ravin MB, Daicroff GR. Blood rheology. In: *Cardiovascular physiology for anesthesiologists.* Springfield, IL: Charles C. Thomas Publisher, 1979:27–71, with permission.)

between perfusion pressure and blood flow. Thus, perfusion pressure cannot serve as the marker of adequacy of flow because pressure is a function of two variables: flow and viscosity. This pivotal concept bears directly on the incidence and causes of complications associated with the use of CPB, as will be discussed below.

Hemodilution, Anesthetic Agents, and Adjuvants

Anesthetic agents and vasoactive adjuvant drugs can influence vascular geometry during CPB and thereby alter vascular resistance; these effects are independent of those related to hemodilution. Hemodilution can also alter the pharmacokinetics and pharmacodynamics of drugs, principally by dilution and decreased protein binding. Although total drug concentration is usually decreased during CPB because of dilution, the amount of free active drug probably changes little because of decreased protein binding (23). During CPB, drug kinetics are also influenced by temperature, pH, oncotic pressure, and sometimes sequestration in the CPB circuit or excluded vascular beds (i.e., the pulmonary vascular bed). These multiple factors make study of drug activity during CPB interesting but exceedingly difficult (24).

Considerations in Oxygen Transport

Hemoglobin Physiology

Oxygen transport is the movement of molecular oxygen from the atmosphere to the cellular mitochondria. This movement depends on the availability of oxygen, cardiac output, hemoglobin, tissue perfusion, and the ability of the tissues to extract oxygen. Hemoglobin provides a tremendous physiologic advantage to the process of oxygen transport in that relatively larger volumes of oxygen can be brought to the tissues bound to the hemoglobin molecule than could be transported in simple solution in the plasma.

Reduction of hemoglobin concentrations to below normal still permits adequate oxygen transfer. In fact, when oxygen transport is expressed as the product of cardiac output and oxygen-carrying capacity and plotted against changes in hematocrit (Fig. 11.5), maximal delivery occurs at a hematocrit of approximately 30%; more importantly, delivery falls only about 10% below normal between hematocrits of 20% to 50% (25). This preservation of oxygen delivery obviously depends on a compensatory increase in cardiac output at lower hematocrit ranges. Hemoglobin concentrations are reduced as a normal consequence of CPB with hemodilution. Without an increase in cardiac output, such a reduction will decrease oxygen delivery, but this is usually well tolerated clinically. The lower limit to which hemoglobin can be reduced under any circumstance and not compromise a patient's safety is not known. A hemoglobin concentration of 10 g/dL was traditionally accepted (and

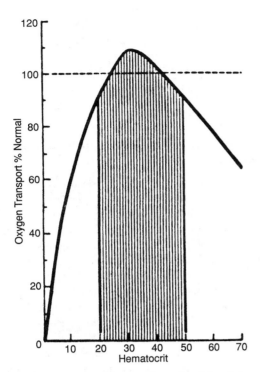

FIG. 11.5. Oxygen transport versus hematocrit level showing an approximate 10% change in oxygen transport (cardiac output times oxygen-carrying capacity) between hematocrits of 20% and 50%. (From LeVeen HH, Ip M, Ahmed N, et al. Lowering blood viscosity to overcome vascular resistance. *Surg Gynecol Obstet* 1980;150:139–149, with permission.)

institutionalized) as adequate for patients undergoing noncardiac surgery based on the above oxygen transport concepts, although a level of 8 g/dL has now been shown not to increase the frequency of adverse occurrences (26).

Environmental Effects

The oxygen-carrying capacity of hemoglobin is influenced by pH, P_{CO_2}, temperature, concentration of 2,3-diphosphoglycerate (2,3-DPG), and the specific type of hemoglobin. These factors may shift the oxygen–hemoglobin dissociation curve to the right (easier dissociation of oxygen from hemoglobin—higher P_{50}) or to the left (more firmly attached oxygen—lower P_{50}). Metabolic acidosis, hypercarbia, hyperthermia, increased levels of 2,3-DPG, and anemia shift the curve to the right, whereas metabolic alkalosis, hypocarbia, decreased 2,3-DPG, and hypothermia shift it to the left. Abnormal forms of hemoglobin may have a normal, increased, or decreased affinity for oxygen. The absolute clinical significance of each of these influences is not known.

Physiology of Chronic Anemia

Chronic anemia, or reduction in the volume of circulating red blood cells, tends to develop gradually and permit com-

pensation. These mechanisms include an increase in plasma volume to maintain a euvolemic or even hypervolemic state, an increase in heart rate and stroke volume, and a passive (but real) increase in cardiac output as a result of decreased viscosity. In the intact human, this occurs with little or no increase in myocardial oxygen extraction (14). Another compensatory mechanism is an increased oxygen extraction by the tissues, often associated with a decreased affinity of hemoglobin for oxygen (produced by an increase in the 2,3-DPG level in red blood cells). This mechanism is not usually operative at hemoglobin levels continuously above 7 g/dL (14).

Reduction in physical activity with a subsequent decrease in oxygen consumption is an important additional mechanism. The chronically anemic patient who is well compensated may be compromised if metabolic demands are increased (e.g., by enhanced physical activity, fever, or an inability to increase cardiac output secondary to intrinsic or acquired heart disease). In this context, an anesthetized patient will demonstrate improved tolerance to anemia because of a reduced total body oxygen consumption (overall, about 15%) and especially a reduced myocardial oxygen demand (27). Hypothermia is an important physiologic method for reducing oxygen utilization by tissues and plays a greater or lesser role, depending on the clinical circumstances. Again, anesthesia has a significant role because normal compensatory mechanisms maintaining normothermia, such as shivering, which markedly increases oxygen consumption, are blocked by anesthesia and muscle relaxation.

The acute anemia produced by hemodilution, coupled with lower than normal flow rates at the institution of CPB, must also be associated with operative compensatory mechanisms to permit adequate oxygen delivery. These include general anesthesia and muscle relaxation, normovolemia, improved microcirculatory perfusion as a consequence of decreased viscosity, and sometimes induced hypothermia.

Hemodilution and Complications of Cardiopulmonary Bypass

Despite the early success of open heart operations in which CPB was used, a high rate of complications was common. Specifically, CPB was associated with postoperative neurologic, pulmonary, and renal dysfunction, and these were seen with both high and low flow rate techniques. Each was attributed to a variety of physiologic or clinical factors.

Neurologic dysfunction was thought to be associated with low perfusion pressures. Stockard et al. (28) mathematically related an increased incidence of neurologic complications to degree and duration of hypotension. Pulmonary complications (postperfusion pulmonary insufficiency, "pump lung") were attributed to parenchymal hypoxia, pulmonary venous distension, the oxygenator itself, or other mechanical factors (29). Renal failure was related to low perfusion pressure and, secondarily, to low urine output during CPB (30). When Cooley et al. (9) reported their first 100 cases in which hemodilution with dextrose and water prime was used, they anecdotally noted a reduction of postoperative cerebral, pulmonary, and renal complications. Hemodilution may have been instrumental in the reduction of morbidity associated with CPB for each of these organ systems.

The uncoupling of flow and pressure with hemodilution, as discussed above, modifies the relation between perfusion pressure and neurologic complications. The patients described by Stockard et al. (28) all had a blood prime for CPB. The relationship between perfusion pressure and an incidence of neurologic complications has disappeared since hemodilution has been universally adopted (31,32). Subsequent reports by Govier et al. (33) and Prough et al. (34) have also demonstrated the maintenance of cerebral autoregulation in patients undergoing hemodilution at varying levels of flow, temperature, and P_{CO_2}.

Similar differences in reports of renal dysfunction with and without blood priming are also revealing. Bhat et al. (30) found bypass time, low perfusion pressure, volume of urine formed during CPB, and hemoglobinemia to be factors for postoperative dysfunction when blood priming was employed. In the same year, Abel et al. (35) found none of these factors to be predictive when hemodilution was used. It now appears that in the absence of low cardiac output before or after CPB or excessive perioperative transfusion, preoperative renal dysfunction is the only predictor of postoperative dysfunction (32). Postperfusion respiratory failure still occurs for multiple reasons, but these are often related to extrapulmonary factors (36). The "pump lung" of the 1960s has markedly decreased in incidence, and this is at least partly because of hemodilution techniques (9,37).

Another problem, referred to as the "homologous blood syndrome," was blamed for both intraoperative and postoperative bleeding diatheses and also for contributing to postoperative cerebral, pulmonary, and renal dysfunction (38). The syndrome was sometimes thought to result from incompatibility or cross-reactions between the patient and one or more of the multiple units of donor blood used in the prime. More likely, with correct donor–patient crossmatching, it represented a reaction occurring between units of homologous blood from different donors when mixed together in the CPB circuit before bypass. Whatever the exact mechanism, it also disappeared with the introduction of crystalloid priming.

Hemodilution alone is not solely responsible for the reduction in complications associated with CPB. Other factors, such as more accurate initial diagnoses, improved anesthetic methods, better CPB equipment, and quicker recognition and treatment of ventricular failure, have all contributed. Specifically, filtering of blood has helped to decrease pulmonary complications (39), and a reduction in hemolysis through a reduced need to suction large amounts of fluid from the surgical field has helped to decrease renal dysfunction.

PRIMING SOLUTIONS

Crystalloid Primes

The use of a crystalloid priming solution is the norm in the present-day management of CPB. There is probably as much institutional variation in specific primes and components as there is in cardioplegic solutions, as they both developed in empiric fashion. In general, modern priming solutions are similar in electrolyte content to plasma and have a similar osmolarity. Balanced salt solutions such as lactated Ringer's solution, with or without glucose, are common basic priming solutions. The addition of colloid may be justified in perfusion procedures of long duration to prevent the development of excessive edema. In addition to institutional variations in types of priming fluids used, differences in the volumes of priming solutions also are common, as a consequence of the differences in priming requirements for the variety of oxygenators, connecting tubing, and arterial filters employed. Some institutions have a "standard" prime volume that is used for all adult patients, whereas others vary the volume depending on the patient's weight or body surface area. Each specific oxygenator–tubing system will obviously have a minimum "safe" priming volume—that is, one that will allow the initiation of CPB without undue risk for air embolism and permit adequate flow rates.

The degree of hemodilution can be predicted based on the patient's weight and hematocrit, the amount of intravenous fluids administered before CPB, and the oxygenator's priming volume. The blood volume can be calculated by multiplying the weight in kilograms by 7% (female patients) to 7.5% (male patients) (Table 11.2). If use of the intended prime volume will cause unacceptable hemodilution, then packed red blood cells can be added to the CPB circuit to compensate.

Children, and especially infants, present a special problem, as most pediatric CPB circuits have a minimum prim-

---

TABLE 11.2. PREDICTION OF INITIAL HEMATOCRIT DURING CARDIOPULMONARY BYPASS

$$\text{Predicted Hct during CPB} = \frac{\text{Patient's Red Blood Cell Volume before CPB}}{\text{Patient's Estimated Blood Volume} + \text{CPB Prime Volume} + \text{Pre-CPB Intravenous Fluid Volume}}$$

Estimated blood volume is equal to the patient's weight times 0.08 to 0.085 for infants, times 0.075 for children and male adults, and times 0.07 for female adults.
One unit of packed red blood cells or whole blood equals approximately 150 mL of red blood cell volume.

ing volume of 700 to 800 mL. Because this priming volume is often larger than the infant's blood volume, blood must usually be added empirically to the prime to achieve appropriate hemodilution by most institutional protocols. The acceptable range for the hematocrit is essentially the same for children and adults.

Allowable Hemodilution

The degree of allowable hemodilution is an important consideration in the composition of the initial prime. There are also large institutional variations in the range of "acceptable" hemodilution. In general, because hemodilution has a salutary effect on perfusion and there is a theoretical decrease in microcirculatory flow with hematocrits above 30% (14), most centers try to achieve hematocrits below 30% during CPB. With priming volumes in the range of 1,400 to 2,000 mL, this is easily achieved in most adults. Patients with large blood volumes, high hematocrits, or both may require pre-pump phlebotomy or additional dilution while on CPB (Table 11.2).

Hypothermia also influences the acceptable range of hematocrits, but guidelines are again institutional. Because of the viscosity–flow relationship and the influence of hypothermia, it is appropriate to target a hematocrit of less than 30% if the temperature is lowered to 30°C, and lower hematocrits, generally below 25%, are preferred if temperatures are to be reduced below 25°C. Experimental evidence suggests that hematocrits below 20% may be associated with an abnormal distribution of flow to organs (40,41). However, hematocrits below this level appear to be well tolerated clinically, with values in the range of 15% to 18% commonly seen during the initial stages of CPB. Physiologic compensatory mechanisms may be operative in addition to the benefits of anesthesia and hypothermia. Even extreme hemodilution to hematocrits below 15%, used for hypothermic circulatory arrest or sometimes in patients who are Jehovah's Witnesses (10), appear to be clinically well tolerated (42).

Another consideration in allowable hemodilution is an acceptable hematocrit for separation from bypass. Here, too, there is much institutional variation and few hard data. Because maldistribution of coronary flow away from the subendocardium occurs experimentally with hematocrits at or below 15% (40,43), especially if the coronary circulation is compromised, it would seem prudent to separate from bypass at hematocrits above this level. Evidence of myocardial ischemia would be further cause to add blood. An argument against maintenance of higher hematocrits (≥34%) is that the higher hematocrits have been shown to be associated postoperatively with a greater risk for Q-wave myocardial infarction, worsened left ventricular function, and mortality after coronary bypass grafting (44).

The safety of hemodilution, especially with crystalloid solutions, was initially questioned because of fear of increased postoperative bleeding secondary to dilutional coagulopathy. These fears proved unfounded in general, even

with extreme hemodilution (45). In polycythemic patients with congenital heart disease, adequate hemodilution (hematocrit <30%) has been associated with a decreased incidence of postoperative coagulopathies (46).

Use of Glucose

Recently, there has been considerable debate over intraoperative glucose management (47) and intraoperative use of glucose-containing fluids in general because of an association of worsened neurologic outcome with hyperglycemia in a series of noncardiac surgical cases (48). These data theoretically affect the management of CPB prime because the use of glucose-containing fluids remains a common practice, and without appropriate control, blood glucose concentrations on bypass can reach unacceptable values (e.g., 500 to 800 mg/dL). Metz and Keats (49) have shown that the addition of glucose to priming solutions, by raising the osmotic pressure of the prime, significantly reduces perioperative fluid requirements and postoperative fluid retention. The seeming lack of complications of the use of glucose during CPB may relate to the putative mechanism, as both animal and human data suggest that central nervous system damage associated with hyperglycemia occurs when either global or focal injury is followed by immediate reperfusion of the ischemic area (50). Cerebral injury after CPB, in the absence of low cardiac output, is almost always embolic in origin, and areas affected would not be expected to be reperfused immediately.

Based on this line of reasoning and the demonstrable beneficial effects in regard to fluid requirements, dextrose (5%) in lactated Ringer's solution is used as the crystalloid prime for CPB at many institutions. Some centers do not use glucose in patients who may be subject to a global central nervous system ischemia followed by reperfusion, such as those undergoing aortic arch aneurysm repair requiring circulatory arrest or descending thoracic aorta aneurysm repair. Other centers, equally without documented support, have taken a completely opposite approach and have removed all glucose from CPB circuits.

However, evidence is mounting that perioperative hyperglycemia in diabetic patients is associated with an increased risk for wound infections, and that postoperative control of glucose may be an important factor in decreasing the incidence of these infections (51,52). With this in mind, one can still advocate the benefits of a glucose-containing prime in diabetic patients so long as appropriate postoperative glucose control is emphasized.

Colloidal Primes

A consequence of hemodilution in CPB is a fall in the plasma colloidal oncotic pressure secondary to dilution of the circulating plasma proteins. This may result, especially in the absence of glucose, in increased movement of fluid out of the vascular space into the interstitial and intracellular spaces, which can lead to postoperative edema and be associated with dysfunction of the lung and possibly other organs. In an effort to attenuate these changes, the addition of colloidal particles to a crystalloid prime, or even the use of a colloidal solution as the principal priming fluid, has been advocated. Solutions used include 5% and 25% albumin, dextran 40 and dextran 70, 5% plasma protein fraction, 6% hydroxyethyl starch, and human plasma. These solutions have been compared in various combinations with a crystalloid prime alone or with each other. Differences in lung water or total body water are reported between groups, most notably immediately after bypass, but these differences tend to diminish quickly in the immediate postoperative period (53,54). The relative importance of colloid in short-term CPB is therefore hard to judge, and individual decisions can be made on the basis of availability and cost. No significant harm is associated with synthetic or heat-treated colloid. However, human plasma should not be used without a specific indication, usually a clinically apparent and laboratory-documented bleeding diathesis.

Other Additives

Additional components that have been used in primes for varying reasons are listed in Table 11.3, with the rationale for each. Much institutional variation exists here also.

Experimental Priming Solutions

The use of oxygen-carrying solutions in CPB has paralleled their experimental use as blood substitutes in noncardiac

TABLE 11.3. ADDITIONAL COMPONENTS FOR CARDIOPULMONARY BYPASS PRIMING SOLUTIONS

Component	Amount	Rationale
Heparin	10–25 mg (1,000–2,500 U)/L of priming volume	Additional safety factor if systemic heparinization is not adequate.
Calcium	200 mg/L of priming volume	Prevents chelation of circulating calcium if citrated blood is added to the prime; may be especially important in pediatric patients because of frequent use of blood in the prime.
Mannitol	25–50 g	To prevent tissue edema and to induce an osmotic diuresis.
Corticosteroids	Various	Prevention or attenuation of activation of inflammatory processes by cardiopulmonary bypass.

surgery and has been confined to two types: perfluorocarbons (55) and stroma-free hemoglobin (56). The evaluation of these liquids, which can carry relatively large amounts of dissolved oxygen in comparison with untreated human plasma, has progressed for several years. Their benefit is the ability to permit oxygen delivery even in the face of profound native anemia.

As they are insoluble in blood, perfluorocarbons (also known as fluorocarbons) must be emulsified before use. They are nearly chemically inert substances with a high natural solubility for oxygen. The oxygen solubility of perfluorocarbons is linear, unlike that of hemoglobin, and because of this, they are able to release oxygen in very low PO_2 environments (57). The release of oxygen by perfluorocarbons is not related to pH or temperature (58). Perfluorocarbon particles are small (0.118 μm), and their viscosity is roughly one-half that of blood; these characteristics allow them to bypass stiffened red blood cells readily and perfuse distal capillary beds (57). However, when perfluorocarbons were used in patients of the Jehovah's Witness faith who were profoundly anemic, survival was not increased (59). These solutions are currently undergoing clinical efficacy trials.

The substitution of hemoglobin for the transfusion of red blood cells would seem ideal because of the natural oxygen-carrying capacity and osmotic activity of hemoglobin. Hemoglobin solutions have a number of benefits over banked blood (60). They are readily available, with a long shelf-life, and they do not require blood typing or cross-matching. They were thought to be free of infectious contamination, but this has been questioned (61). They do not cause immunosuppression, as blood can. The viscosity of hemoglobin-based substitutes, like that of perfluorocarbons, is low. Bovine hemoglobin, chemically cross-linked to prevent its filtration by the kidneys, has a low oxygen affinity, similar to that of human hemoglobin in erythrocytes (62). Preclinical testing and early clinical safety trials of both human- and bovine-based hemoglobin solutions have been completed. The number of different hemoglobin products and the potential variation between batches of a single manufacturer's product make evaluation and comparison of efficacy a daunting task in further clinical studies (63). Clinical trials during CPB of hemoglobin solutions produced by chemical modification of human hemoglobin or synthesis of hemoglobin by recombinant technology have been conducted, but the results to date remain proprietary information. Perhaps the eventual availability of recombinant human hemoglobin will provide a safer alternative.

ASSESSING ADEQUACY OF PERFUSION WITH HEMODILUTION

The most notable effect of the use of modern asanguineous priming solutions, as noted above, is a marked fall in perfusion pressure on institution of bypass. In almost all instances, this is secondary to the resulting hemodilution and corresponding fall in viscosity, not to dilution of circulating catecholamines or vasodilation (Fig. 11.2). Because hemodilution results in an uncoupling of the relationship between perfusion pressure and blood flow, the adequacy of perfusion must be assessed by other means. Standard flow rates of 50 mL/kg per minute or 2 L/m^2 per minute are a tested reference, athough they may be modified by age, weight, or temperature.

Monitoring of organ perfusion is probably the most reliable method of determining perfusion adequacy during CPB with hemodilution; however, clinical methods of monitoring organ perfusion are most often indirect and inadequate. Global cerebral function can be followed by electroencephalographic means, but whether such monitoring confers the ability to detect and modify an impending central nervous system adverse event is open to question. The obvious parameter of renal function, urinary output, is easily and virtually uniformly measured, but clinical studies have shown that the volume of urine produced during CPB has little or no bearing on postoperative renal function. Measurement of arterial blood gases will monitor oxygenator function, and measurement of mixed venous oxygen tension may detect inadequate perfusion. However, a normal mixed venous oxygen tension does not ensure adequate regional perfusion because it may not reflect local organ conditions.

SUMMARY

In summary, hemodilution probably represents the most significant advance in CPB technique after the development of the pump oxygenator itself. It permits the maintenance of organ homeostasis under what would otherwise be often inadequate circumstances, with a resultant decrease in complications and conservation of blood resources.

KEY POINTS

- Hemodilution
- Advantages of hemodilution include the following:
  - Decreased blood viscosity
  - Improved regional blood flow
  - Improved oxygen delivery to tissues
  - Decreased exposure to homologous blood products
  - Improved blood flow at lower perfusion pressure (lower shear stress), especially during hypothermic perfusion
- Hemodilution affects the pharmacokinetic and pharmacodynamic properties of drugs used during cardiopulmonary bypass, predominantly by changing protein binding through dilution of plasma proteins.
- Hemodilution decreases bypass-related complications (neurologic, renal, and pulmonary).

- Cardiopulmonary bypass priming solutions
- Crystalloid priming solutions are the norm in the present-day practice of cardiopulmonary bypass.
  - Most commonly used solutions are "balanced salt or physiologic saline" solutions.
  - The use of 5% dextrose is common, but it complicates the control of blood glucose concentration during cardiopulmonary bypass.
  - Hyperglycemia during and after cardiopulmonary bypass may predispose the patient to neurologic damage and infectious complications.
  - Colloid solutions (e.g., albumin, hydroxyethyl starch) are widely used empirically as priming components.
  - In the near term, oxygen-carrying colloidal solutions of perfluorocarbons or hemoglobin will be available for use during cardiopulmonary bypass.

REFERENCES

1. Gibbon JH. Application of a mechanical heart and lung apparatus to cardiac surgery. *Minn Med* 1954;37:171–180.
2. Kirklin JW, Donald DE, Harshbarger HG, et al. Studies in extracorporeal circulation. I. Applicability of Gibbon-type pump-oxygenator to human intracardiac surgery: 40 cases. *Ann Surg* 1956;144:2–8.
3. Lillehei CW, Cohen M, Warden HE, et al. The results of direct vision closure of ventricular septal defects in eight patients by means of controlled cross-circulation. *Surg Gynecol Obstet* 1955;101:447–466.
4. DeWall RA, Lillehei RC, Sellers RD. Hemodilution perfusions for open-heart surgery. *N Engl J Med* 1962;266:1078–1084.
5. Cohen M, Lillehei CW. A quantitative study of the "azygos factor" during vena caval occlusion in the dog. *Surg Gynecol Obstet* 1954;98:225–232.
6. Green AE, Carey JM, Zuhdi N. Hemodilution principle of hypothermic perfusion. A concept of obviating blood priming. *J Thorac Cardiovasc Surg* 1962;43:640–648.
7. Panico FG, Neptune WB. A mechanism to eliminate the donor blood prime from the pump-oxygenator. *Surg Forum* 1959;10:605–609.
8. Long DM, Sanchez L, Varco RL, et al. The use of low molecular weight dextran and serum albumin as plasma expanders in extracorporeal circulation. *Surgery* 1961;50:12–28.
9. Cooley DA, Beall AC, Grondin P. Open-heart operations with disposable oxygenators, 5 per cent dextrose prime, and normothermia. *Surgery* 1962;52:713–719.
10. Cooper JR. Perioperative considerations in Jehovah's Witnesses. *Int Anesthesiol Clin* 1990;28:210–215.
11. Gordon RJ, Ravin MB, Daicoff GR. Blood rheology. In: *Cardiovascular physiology for anesthesiologists*. Springfield, IL: Charles C. Thomas Publisher, 1979:27–71.
12. Chien S. Present state of blood rheology. In: Messmer K, Schmid-Schoenbein H, eds. *Hemodilution. Theoretical basis and clinical application*. Basel: Karger, 1972:1–45.
13. Priebe H. Hemodilution and oxygenation. *Int Anesthesiol Clin* 1981;190:237–255.
14. Messmer K. Hemodilution. *Surg Clin North Am* 1975;55:659–678.
15. Gordon RJ, Ravin M, Rawitscher RE, et al. Changes in arterial

pressure, viscosity and resistance during cardiopulmonary bypass. *J Thorac Cardiovasc Surg* 1975;69:552–561.

16. Laver MB, Buckley MJ. Extreme hemodilution in the surgical patient. In: Messmer K, Schmid-Schoenbein H, eds. *Hemodilution. Theoretical basis and clinical application.* Basel: Karger, 1972: 215–222.

17. Guyton AC, Richardson TQ. Effect of hematocrit on venous return. *Circ Res* 1961;9:157–163.

18. Rand PW, Lacombe E, Hunt HE, et al. Viscosity of normal human blood under normothermic and hypothermic conditions. *J Appl Physiol* 1964;19:117–122.

19. Lundar T, Froysaker T, Lindegaard K, et al. Some observations or cerebral perfusion during cardiopulmonary bypass. *Ann Thorac Surg* 1985;39:381–423.

20. Lundar T, Lindegaard K, Froysaker T, et al. Cerebral perfusion during nonpulsatile cardiopulmonary bypass. *Ann Thorac Surg* 1985;40:144–150.

21. Brass LM, Pavlakis SG, DeVivo D, et al. Transcranial Doppler measurements of the middle cerebral artery. Effect of hematocrit. *Stroke* 1988;19:1466–1469.

22. Reves JG, Greely WJ. Cerebral blood flow during cardiopulmonary bypass: some new answers to old questions. *Ann Thorac Surg* 1989;48:752–754.

23. Levy JH, Hug CC. Use of cardiopulmonary bypass in studies of the circulation. *Br J Anaesth* 1988;60:35S–37S.

24. Okutani R, Philbin DM, Rosow CE, et al. Effect of hypothermic hemodilutional cardiopulmonary bypass on plasma sufentanil and catecholamine concentrations in humans. *Anesth Analg* 1988; 67:667–670.

25. LeVeen HH, Ip M, Ahmed N, et al. Lowering blood viscosity to overcome vascular resistance. *Surg Gynecol Obstet* 1980;150: 139–149.

26. Carson JL, Poses RM, Spence RK, et al. Severity of anaemia and operative mortality and morbidity. *Lancet* 1988;1:727–729.

27. Theye RA, Michenfelder JD. Individual organ contributions to the decrease in whole-body V_{O_2} with isoflurane. *Anesthesiology* 1975;42:35–40.

28. Stockard JJ, Bickford RG, Schauble JF. Pressure-dependent cerebral ischemia during cardiopulmonary bypass. *Neurology* 1973; 23:521–529.

29. Tilney NL, Hester WJ. Physiologic and histologic changes in the lungs of patients dying after prolonged cardiopulmonary bypass: an inquiry into the nature of post-perfusion lung. *Ann Surg* 1967; 166:759–766.

30. Bhat JG, Gluck MC, Lowenstein J, et al. Renal failure after open heart surgery. *Ann Intern Med* 1976;84:677–682.

31. Slogoff S, Girgis KZ, Keats AS. Etiologic factors in neuropsychiatric complications associated with cardiopulmonary bypass. *Anesth Analg* 1982;61:903–911.

32. Slogoff S, Reul GJ, Keats AS, et al. Role of perfusion pressure and flow in major organ dysfunction after cardiopulmonary bypass. *Ann Thorac Surg* 1990;50:911–918.

33. Govier AV, Reves JG, McKay RD, et al. Factors and their influence on regional cerebral blood flow during nonpulsatile cardiopulmonary bypass. *Ann Thorac Surg* 1984;38:592–600.

34. Prough DS, Stump DA, Roy RC, et al. Response of cerebral blood flow to changes in carbon dioxide tension during hypothermic cardiopulmonary bypass. *Anesthesiology* 1986;64:576–581.

35. Abel RM, Buckley MJ, Austen WG, et al. Acute postoperative renal failure in cardiac surgical patients. *Surg Res* 1976;20: 341–348.

36. Matthay MA, Wiener-Kronish JP. Respiratory management after cardiac surgery. *Chest* 1989;95:424–434.

37. Hepps SA, Roe BB, Wright RR, et al. Amelioration of the pulmonary postperfusion syndrome with hemodilution and low molecular weight dextran. *Surgery* 1963;54:232–243.

38. Gadboys HL, Slonim R, Litwak RS. Homologous blood syndrome: I. Preliminary observations on its relationship to clinical cardiopulmonary bypass. *Ann Surg* 1962;156:793–804.

39. Solis RT, Gibbs MB. Filtration of the microaggregates in stored blood. *Transfusion* 1972;12:245–250.

40. Race D, Dedichen H, Schenk WG. Regional blood flow during dextran-induced normovolemic hemodilution in the dog. *J Thorac Cardiovasc Surg* 1967;53:578–585.

41. Brazier J, Cooper N, Maloney JV, et al. The adequacy of myocardial oxygen delivery in acute normovolemic anemia. *Surgery* 1974;75:508–516.

42. Laver MB, Buckley MJ, Austen WG. Extreme hemodilution with profound hypothermia and circulatory arrest. *Bibl Haematol* 1975;41:225–238.

43. Hagl S, Heimisch W, Meisner H, et al. The effect of hemodilution on regional myocardial function in the presence of coronary stenosis. *Basic Res Cardiol* 1977;72:344–364.

44. Spiess BD, Ley C, Body SC, et al. Hematocrit value on intensive care unit entry influences the frequency of Q-wave myocardial infarction after coronary artery bypass grafting. The institutions of the Multicenter Study of Perioperative Ischemia (McSPI) Research Group. *J Thorac Cardiovasc Surg* 1998;116:460–467.

45. Niinikoski J, Laato M, Laaksonen V, et al. Effects of extreme haemodilution on the immediate post-operative course of coronary artery bypass patients. *Eur Surg Res* 1983;15:1–10.

46. Milam JD, Austin SF, Nihill MR, et al. Use of sufficient hemodilution to prevent coagulopathies following surgical correction of cyanotic heart disease. *J Thorac Cardiovasc Surg* 1985;89: 623–629.

47. Sieber FE, Smith DS, Traystman RJ, et al. Glucose: a reevaluation of its intraoperative use. *Anesthesiology* 1987;67:72–81.

48. Pulsinelli WA, Levy DE, Sigsbee B, et al. Increased damage after ischemic stroke in patients with hyperglycemia with or without established diabetes mellitus. *Am J Med* 1983;74:540–544.

49. Metz S, Keats AS. Benefits of a glucose-containing priming solution for cardiopulmonary bypass. *Anesth Analg* 1991;72: 428–434.

50. Lanier WL, Stangland KJ, Scheithauer BW, et al. The effects of dextrose infusion and head position on neurological outcome after complete cerebral ischemia in primates: examination of a model. *Anesthesiology* 1987;66:39–48.

51. Pomposelli JJ, Baxter JK, Babaineau TJ, et al. Early postoperative glucose control predicts nosocomial infection rate in diabetic patients. *J Parenteral Enteral Nutr* 1998;22:77–81.

52. Zerr KJ, Furnary AP, Grunkemeier GL, et al. Glucose control lowers the risk of wound infection in diabetics after open heart operations. *Ann Thorac Surg* 1997;63:356–361.

53. Lumb PD. A comparison between 25% albumin and 6% hydroxyethyl starch solutions on lung water accumulation during and immediately after cardiopulmonary bypass. *Ann Surg* 1987;206: 210–213.

54. Marelli D, Paul A, Samson R, et al. Does the addition of albumin to the prime solution in cardiopulmonary bypass affect clinical outcome? *J Thorac Cardiovasc Surg* 1989;98:751–756.

55. Stone JJ, Piccione W, Berrizbeitia LD, et al. Hemodynamic, metabolic and morphological effects of cardiopulmonary bypass with a fluorocarbon priming solution. *Ann Thorac Surg* 1986; 41:419–424.

56. Gould SA, Sehgal LR, Rosen AL, et al. The efficacy of polymerized pyridoxylated hemoglobin solution as an O_2 carrier. *Ann Surg* 1990;211:394–398.

57. Fennema M, Erdmann W, Faithful NS. Myocardial oxygen supply under critical conditions, the effects of hemodilution and fluorocarbons. In: Erdmann W, Bruley DF, eds. *Oxygen transport to tissue XIV.* New York: Plenum Publishing, 1992:527–544.

58. Holman WL, Spruell RD, Ferguson ER, et al. Tissue oxygenation with graded dissolved oxygen delivery during cardiopulmonary bypass. *J Thorac Cardiovasc Surg* 1995;110:1–85.

59. Gould SA, Rosen AL, Sehgal LR, et al. Fluosol-DA as a red-cell substitute in acute anemia. *N Engl J Med* 1986;314:1653–1656.

60. Cohn SM. The current status of haemoglobin-based blood substitutes. *Ann Med* 1997;29:371–376.

61. Dietz NM, Joyner MJ, Warner MA. Blood substitutes: fluids, drugs, or miracle solutions? *Anesth Analg* 1996;82:390–405.

62. Bunn HF. The role of hemoglobin-based blood substitutes in transfusion medicine. *Transfus Clin Biol* 1995;2:433–439.

63. Ogden JE, Parry ES. The development of hemoglobin solutions as red cell substitutes. *Int Anesthesiol Clin* 1995;33:115–129.

HYPOTHERMIA: PHYSIOLOGY AND CLINICAL USE

LAURIE K. DAVIES

The use of hypothermia as an adjunct to the treatment of a wide variety of disorders has been advocated for centuries. Lowered body temperature has been employed to combat cancer, infection, trauma, and central nervous system disease, and as a regional method to produce anesthesia for amputation (1,2). However, it was not until 1950 that Bigelow et al. (3) demonstrated longer tolerance to inflow occlusion in hypothermic animals than in their normothermic counterparts. This work led to the first clinical application of hypothermia in cardiac surgery. Lewis and Taufic (4) used surface cooling to 28°C with 5.5 minutes of inflow occlusion to facilitate successful closure of an atrial septal defect in a 5-year-old child. In 1952, Gibbon (5) introduced the pump oxygenator to clinical practice, and in 1958, Sealy et al. (6) used hypothermia in conjunction with the cardiopulmonary bypass (CPB) circuit for intracardiac repairs. The use of the pump oxygenator and hypothermia has allowed cardiac surgery to flourish. Complex lesions are repaired routinely with remarkably low mortality. A better understanding of the principles of hypothermia will maximize the advantages and safe application of this technology.

PHYSIOLOGY OF HYPOTHERMIA

One of the main difficulties in devising a reasonable strategy for the application of hypothermia in humans is the fact that they are naturally homeothermic beings. Humans and other homeothermic species have very effective homeostatic systems, which ensure that body temperature remains consistently near 37°C regardless of changes in environmental temperatures. This tight regulation of temperature is accomplished by multiple mechanisms. Thermoreceptors in the skin sense cold, which then causes the hypothalamus to trigger a strong sympathetic nervous system response. Vasoconstriction of skin vessels, which decreases convective heat loss, occurs simultaneously with vasodilation of the skeletal muscle vascular beds, which augments muscular activity to produce heat by tensing and shivering. The endocrine system is activated, oxygen consumption is increased, and heart rate, cardiac output, and blood pressure are elevated. Because of the complexity of these interactions, one can appreciate the difficulty in understanding the physiologically appropriate response to the unnatural state of induced hypothermia in humans. One must extrapolate from animal studies, biochemical equations, accidental hypothermia survivors, and normal organ temperature gradients to maximize the beneficial effects and minimize the complications of hypothermia.

Rationale for the Use of Hypothermia

Why is hypothermia often employed during CPB? The obvious purpose of using hypothermia is to provide a degree of organ (and organism) protection and safety margin during CPB. Hypothermia exerts its protective effect by multiple mechanisms. The most obvious mechanism is a reduction in metabolic rate and oxygen consumption (7) (Fig. 12.1). This metabolic suppression may not explain all the protective effects observed. Hypothermia also helps to preserve high-energy phosphate stores and reduces excitatory neurotransmitter release, which is especially important to central nervous system protection (8,9). Normally, ischemic neuronal cells rapidly release neuroexcitatory amines, especially glutamate (10). The accumulation of these excitotoxic amines causes the opening of calcium channels and activation of multiple destructive enzymatic systems. Hypothermia attenuates this excitotoxic cascade, helping to prevent calcium entry into the cell and restricting membrane permeability (11) (Fig. 12.2).

Alteration of temperature causes a change in the reaction rate of all biochemical processes, especially enzymatic reactions. This temperature dependence of reaction rates has been described by the concept of Q_{10}, which is defined as the increase or decrease in reaction rates or metabolic processes in relation to a temperature change of 10°C. For

L. K. Davies: Department of Anesthesiology, University of Florida, Gainesville, Florida 32610.

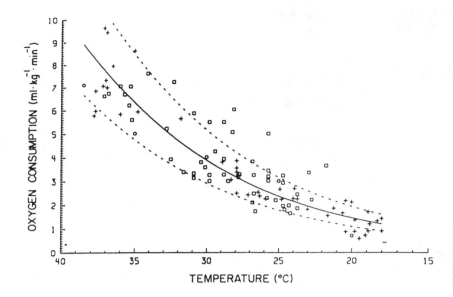

FIG. 12.1. Whole body oxygen consumption as a function of body temperature in dogs made hypothermic by surface cooling. (From Kirklin JW. *Cardiac surgery.* New York: Churchill Livingstone, 1993:61–127, with permission.)

instance, the reaction rate of a process with a Q_{10} of 2 will double with a 10°C increase in temperature or be halved with a drop of 10°C. Most reactions, including total body oxygen consumption, have a Q_{10} of 2 to 3 (7).

Some biochemical processes, especially those localized to cell membranes, show an abrupt change in reaction rates at certain critical temperatures. This has been termed a *phase*

transition and is thought to be a result of a change in the cell membrane from a fluid to a gel (12). In mammalian tissues, phase transitions often occur at about 25° to 28°C and may disturb cell homeostasis. Biophysical processes such as osmosis and water diffusion are also affected by temperature. Typically, a linear change of about 3%/10°C is seen. Thus, this effect is minimal at clinical levels of hypo-

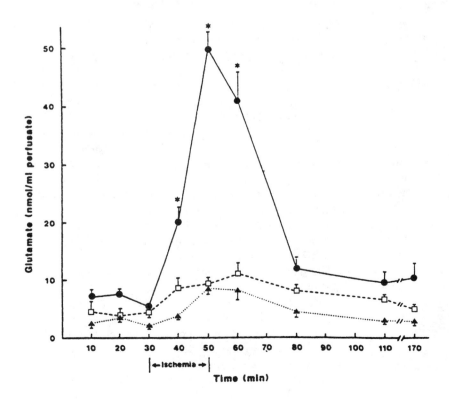

FIG. 12.2. Line plot of the time course of changes in the perfusate concentration of glutamate (in nmol/mL) in animals with ischemic brain temperature maintained at 36°C, 33°C, and 30°C. (From Busto R, Blobus MY-T, Dietrich WD, et al. Effect of mild hypothermia on ischemia-induced release of neurotransmitters and free fatty acids in rat brain. *Stroke* 1989;20:904–910, with permission.)

thermia. However, if the freezing point of water is approached, ice is formed in the tissue, a condition that is not tolerated. The solutes concentrate in a hyperosmolar fashion in the residual nonfrozen water, causing marked fluid shifts and membrane disruption. Mammalian tissue does not regain function on thawing from a frozen state. For this reason, there is a limit to the beneficial effects of hypothermia.

In cardiac surgery, CPB in conjunction with systemic hypothermia allows lower pump flows, better myocardial protection, less blood trauma, and better organ protection than does normothermic perfusion (13). Oxygen needs predictably fall with lowered temperature. It was recognized early that lowered bypass flows could be employed in this setting and still provide adequate perfusion as assessed by mixed venous oxygen tension and return of organ function following bypass. Relating oxygen consumption (Vo_2) to perfusion flow rate at various temperatures also can be valuable in assessing adequacy of tissue perfusion (Fig. 12.3). At a given temperature, a fall in Vo_2 with a decrease in flow rate implies a flow-limited Vo_2, indicating that oxygen delivery is not adequate. Hickey and Hoar (14) have shown in humans that a reduction in flow rate from 2.1 to 1.2 L/min per square meter body surface area at 25°C does not alter Vo_2 or tissue perfusion. Slogoff and colleagues (15) were unable to correlate low flows (<40 mL/kg per minute) or pressures (<50 mm Hg) during bypass in which moderate hypothermia and hemodilution were used with postoperative renal or central nervous system dysfunction. Lower perfusion flow rates allow better visualization by the surgeon. Venous return from the bronchial, pulmonary, and noncoronary collateral vessels is also decreased. Because this returning blood is at systemic temperature, it can inappropriately warm the heart and jeopardize myocardial protec-

tion. Blood trauma is minimized because of both the lower pump flows and the hemodilution employed during bypass. Because the etiology of most central nervous system damage on bypass is embolic in origin (16), lower bypass flows can minimize these focal insults. Systemic hypothermia also provides some margin of safety for organ protection if equipment failure occurs or circulatory arrest must be employed.

Acid–Base Alteration with Temperature Change

One of the more often discussed aspects of clinical hypothermia is the appropriate acid–base management strategy during hypothermia. To understand acid–base regulation during hypothermia, it is helpful to consider several example conditions. "Normal" values for pH and Pco_2 are usually thought of as 7.40 pH units and 40 mm Hg, respectively. However, it must be kept in mind that these values are appropriate only at 37°C in blood. There is a temperature-dependent spectrum of "normal" values depending on the temperature of the specific site in the body. For example, arterial blood leaves the heart at 37°C with a pH of 7.40 and a Pco_2 of 40 mm Hg. When that same blood perfuses working skeletal muscle, where the ambient temperature may be 40°C, it will have a pH of approximately 7.35 and a somewhat higher Pco_2, despite a constant CO_2 content before any respiratory exchange with the muscle. In contrast, the same arterial blood perfusing exposed skin, where temperature may be 20°C in cool weather, will have a pH of 7.65 and a proportionately lower Pco_2, again with no change in CO_2 content. Stated another way, a sample of arterial blood held in a gas-tight syringe will have a Pco_2 that varies directly with temperature, and a pH that varies inversely with temperature, despite constant CO_2 content.

This change in Pco_2 with temperature is a consequence of the change in solubility of gases in liquids with temperature change. As a general rule, decreasing the temperature of a solution increases the solubility of a given gas in that solution and therefore decreases the partial pressure of that gas while the overall content of the gas in the fluid remains constant. Increasing the temperature of a solution increases the kinetic energy of the molecules in the solution, which both increases the tendency of dissolved gas molecules to leave the solution (decreased solubility) and increases the relative pressure caused by those remaining in solution (increased partial pressure). This concept is intuitive to anyone who has opened a container of warm carbonated beverage and observed that its tendency to "fizz" (CO_2 bubbling out of solution) is much greater than that of a cold beverage.

The relationship of pH to temperature is somewhat more complex than the Pco_2 change with temperature. There is clearly a direct relationship between the concentration of H^+ [H^+] in a water solution and the CO_2 content of that solution. The higher the CO_2, the more H^+ in solution, hence the lower the pH. This is largely caused by the ten-

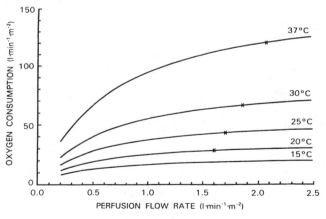

FIG. 12.3. Nomogram of an equation expressing the relation of oxygen consumption to perfusion flow rate at different temperatures in animals. The x represents the perfusion flow rates used clinically at these temperatures. (From Kirklin JW. Hypothermia, circulatory arrest, and cardiopulmonary bypass. In: Kirklin JW, Barratt-Boyes BG, eds. *Cardiac surgery.* New York: Churchill Livingstone, 1993:61–127, with permission.)

dency of CO_2 to combine chemically with water to produce carbonic acid, which then dissociates in solution to yield H^+. Accordingly, one might expect that the change in pH of blood with temperature is caused by the changes in P_{CO_2} with temperature discussed above. It is true that cooling an anaerobic blood sample decreases both the P_{CO_2} and the $[H^+]$. But, and very importantly, the change in $[H^+]$ and pH that occurs with temperature change *is independent of a change in CO_2 content and therefore does not depend on the change in CO_2 solubility with temperature change.*

All acids and bases, including water, exist in solution in equilibrium between the undissociated form and the ionized components of the parent molecule. The dissociation constant (K) is the equilibrium ratio of the product of the concentrations of the ionized components to the un-ionized component. For water at 25°C, the equilibrium dissociation equation is as follows:

$$K_{(H_2O, 25°C)} = \frac{[H^+] \times [OH^-]}{[H_2O]} = 1.08 \times 10^{-14}$$

Because at equilibrium in water $[H^+]$ equals $[OH^-]$, and because the concentration of H_2O is essentially 1, $[H^+]$ equals $[OH^-]$ equals $\sqrt{10^{-14}}$, or 10^{-7}. Because the definition of pH is the negative $\log_{10}$ of $[H^+]$, the pH of pure water at equilibrium at 25°C is 7. This pH value has come to be called the *neutral pH*, or *pN*, of water. Temperature change has a significant effect on the tendency of molecules in solution to dissociate. In thermodynamic terms, the increased kinetic energy associated with increased temperature promotes dissociation, whereas decreased temperature has the opposite effect. For example, within the temperature range seen in clinical CPB (approximately 15°C to 40°C), the dissociation constant of water increases from 0.451×10^{-14} to 2.919×10^{-14}. These values of K_{H_2O} relate to a change in $[H^+]$ from approximately 67 nmol/L at 15°C to 170 nmol/L at 40°C. This nearly threefold change in $[H^+]$ is *solely a consequence of the effects of temperature change on dissociation.* Pure water may be considered the simplest weak acid–base solution. The major importance of these concepts is that water is the fundamental solvent of all biologic systems, and the dissociation of virtually all weak acids and bases in biologic solutions follows the same pattern as that described for water.

The behavior of body fluids (intracellular and extracellular, intravascular and extravascular) is far more complex than the simple scenario described above for water, but biologic fluids behave much like water in terms of the intrinsic temperature-related changes in the dissociation constants of the many weak acids and weak bases of which they are composed. The amino acids in proteins, the simple sugars in polysaccharides, the fatty acids in lipids, and the major buffer systems all follow this same basic pattern. As temperature decreases the tendency to dissociate decreases, and the concentrations of the ionized components (H^+ and R^-) all decrease.

At normal body temperature (37°C), blood and tissue fluids are alkaline (lower $[H^+]$ and correspondingly higher pH) relative to water at the same temperature. A number of buffer systems create and maintain this relative alkalinity so that the ratio of $[OH^-]$ to $[H^+]$ remains constant at approximately 16:1 despite temperature variation. As temperature changes, the intrinsic dissociation of these buffer systems also changes to maintain the ratio of $[OH^-]$ to $[H^+]$ constant. Thus, the intrinsic pH shift of blood and tissue fluid parallels the pN_{H2O} as temperature changes, and this relative alkalinity remains constant in comparison with water (17) (Fig. 12.4).

A major buffering system responsible for this constant relationship of blood and tissue fluid pH to pN with temperature change is the imidazole moiety of the amino acid histidine, which is commonly found in body proteins. The pK_a of this component of histidine is close to 7.0 at body temperature, a property that confers potent buffering capacity for maintaining a constant ratio of $[H^+]$ to $[OH^-]$ despite significant changes in the absolute concentration of each as temperature varies. These considerations are applicable to the previous example of arterial blood with a constant CO_2 content perfusing tissues with different temperatures. The observed pH shift with cooling follows the pN_{H2O}, and the buffering capacity of the imidazole moiety of histidine preserves the constant relative alkalinity and ratio of $[OH^-]$ to $[H^+]$ in the blood (Fig. 12.5). In cold-blooded vertebrates, the blood pH–temperature curve also runs parallel to the pH of neutral water. Intracellular pH has also been measured in various animals and shows changes with temperature identical to those that have been described for pN_{H2O} (18) (Fig. 12.6). The intracellular pH parallels the pN and blood pH slopes with temperature changes and differs from the extracellular pH by a constant but species-specific factor of about -0.6 to -0.8 pH units. Thus, at 37°C, intracellular pH is about 6.8 to 6.9 and so the $[H^+]$

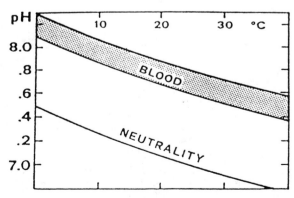

FIG. 12.4. Blood pH of various ectothermic species and the pH of neutral water as a function of body temperature. (From Rahn H. Body temperature and acid-base regulation [Review Article]. *Pneumonologie* 1974;151:87–94, with permission.)

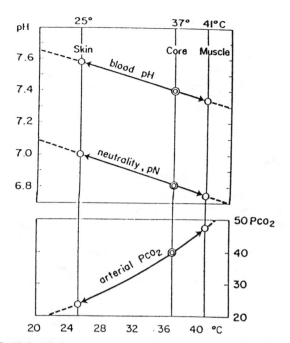

FIG. 12.5. Changes in arterial pH and P_{CO_2} as blood at 37°C arrives at skin and exercising muscle at temperatures of 25° and 41°C, respectively. Neutrality of water (pN) changes in parallel with changes in blood pH. Thus, the relative alkalinity of the blood or the ratio between [OH^-] and [H^+] ions remains constant. (From Rahn H. Body temperature and acid–base regulation [Review Article]. *Pneumonologie* 1974;151:87–94, with permission.)

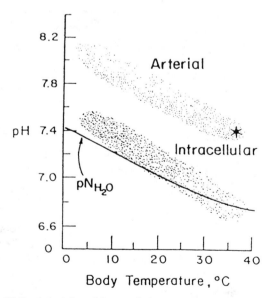

FIG. 12.6. Arterial and intracellular pH as a function of body temperature in ectothermic animals. Intracellular pH closely follows the neutral pH of water; relative arterial alkalinity is maintained at all temperatures. (From White FN, Weinstein Y. Carbon dioxide transport and acid–base regulation during hypothermia. In: Utley JR, ed. *Pathophysiology and techniques of cardiopulmonary bypass*, vol II. Baltimore: Williams & Wilkins, 1983:40–48, with permission.)

is somewhat higher. In a fashion similar to the observed change in blood pH with temperature, the reaction kinetics of numerous respiratory enzyme systems [lactate dehydrogenase, Na^+-K^+-ATPase (sodium–potassium adenosine triphosphatase), acetyl CoA carboxlyase, fatty acid synthetase, NADH (reduced nicotinamide adenine dinucleotide) cytochrome *c* reductase, and succinate cytochrome *c* reductase] all show optimal catalytic function with temperature change when the pH of the reaction medium parallels the temperature-mediated pN_{H_2O} change (18A).

This constant internal milieu is accomplished, as has been mentioned, predominantly by the buffering capacity of the imidazole group of the amino acid histidine. As temperature changes, the imidazole groups in protein change pK_a in parallel with the pN of water. The ratio of the unprotonated histidine imidazole groups to H^+, a value known in the chemistry world as *alpha*, remains constant; total CO_2 remains constant; and pH changes as temperature changes. The term *alpha-stat* has come to indicate an acid–base management strategy in which the net charge (dissociation) of proteins remains constant as temperature changes. Typically during CPB, this is managed by keeping total CO_2 stores constant and allowing pH and $PaCO_2$ to follow their thermodynamically mediated dissociation changes with temperature change.

The alternative method of acid–base strategy is termed *pH-stat*. With this method, pH is the value that is maintained constant at varying temperatures. Obviously, if the pH-stat strategy is used as blood is cooled, CO_2 must be added to maintain a $PaCO_2$ of 40 and a pH of 7.40. Extracellular and intracellular ratios of [OH^-] to [H^+] are altered and total CO_2 stores are elevated.

Why might one strategy be chosen over another? During the first two decades of hypothermic CPB, pH-stat management with the addition of 5% CO_2 to the oxygenator gas flow was used almost exclusively. An understanding of the expected changes in pH with temperature seemed to be lacking, and CO_2 was thought to be beneficial for cerebral vasodilation and maintenance of cerebral blood flow (CBF). In the past 15 to 20 years, this practice has been questioned, and many institutions have shifted toward an alpha-stat management protocol. It is only recently that sufficient data have accumulated to enable a rational decision to be made to employ one strategy rather than the other in a given situation.

On a theoretical basis, alpha-stat management may be preferable in certain situations. Maintenance of constant intracellular electrochemical neutrality appears to be essential for normal cellular function (19). Intracellular metabolic intermediates of high-energy phosphates can be depleted if the intracellular pH changes and these metabolites lose their charged state. These substrates are then free to diffuse across lipid membranes. Most enzymes depend on optimal pH for their function. Electrochemical neutrality is also important in maintaining the Donnan equilibrium across cellular membranes to allow normal intracellular anion concentrations and water content (20).

Poikilothermic animals, whose tissues must function optimally despite wide variations in temperature, follow an alpha-stat acid–base strategy. On the other hand, hibernating mammals appear to maintain a pH-stat strategy, with constant (temperature-corrected) blood pH_a and P_{CO_2} (19). These animals hypoventilate as they hibernate, the tissue CO_2 stores increase, and intracellular pH becomes acidotic in most tissues. This acidotic state causes a further depression of metabolism that teleologically may be useful by further decreasing the energy consumption of nonfunctioning tissues, such as skeletal muscle, gastrointestinal tract, and higher brain centers. In contrast, active tissues such as heart and liver adopt a different strategy by actively extruding H^+ across their cell membranes to maintain intracellular pH at or near the values predicted by alpha-stat methodology. Thus, hibernating mammals are able to vary their intracellular-to-extracellular pH gradient differently in different tissues, depending on the state of metabolic activity of the tissue. This functionally provides a different type of acid–base regulation in different tissues, depending on the metabolic activity of the tissue. The first noticeable change associated with arousal from hibernation is hyperventilation. This depletes CO_2 stores, raises intracellular pH, and increases the metabolic rate. The animal reverts to an overall alpha-stat pH control pattern during awakening, which allows tissues to regain optimal function. Thus, in hibernating mammals, the issue of acid–base maintenance is not clearly defined because intracellular acid–base regulation can be independent of blood regulation both within and among different tissues in the same animal.

Despite the preceding discussion, the practical question of how acid–base status should be regulated during hypothermic bypass in humans remains open. Some animal studies suggest that alpha-stat acid–base management is beneficial in terms of myocardial protection. McConnell et al. (21) evaluated alpha-stat regulation during hypothermia in dogs and demonstrated that significant elevations in coronary blood flow, left ventricular oxygen consumption, and lactate utilization occurred with maintenance of a pH of 7.7 at 28°C (alpha-stat) in comparison with a pH of 7.4 (pH-stat). There was also a significant increase in peak ventricular pressure when a standard preload was applied. Poole-Wilson and Langer (22) demonstrated a greater contractility in hypothermic perfused papillary muscle when the pH of the perfusate was more alkaline than 7.4. They also demonstrated a rapid fall in myocardial tension in addition to changes in Ca^{2+} flux when the perfusate Pa_{CO_2} was increased (23). On the other hand, Sinet et al. (24) found no effect of pH on isolated rat heart performance. The myocardium is often not perfused but is purposely made ischemic to facilitate cardiac surgery. In this setting, alkalinization of the blood before ischemia has been shown to decrease the development of acidosis in coronary sinus

blood and improve contractility on reperfusion (25). It also appears that the pH of the blood reperfusing the heart may be critical to recovery of ventricular performance. Becker et al. (26) studied the myocardial effects of an acid–base strategy in which alkalinization greater than that of alpha-stat was used. They found myocardial performance after 1 hour of circulatory arrest and cardioplegia was improved with moderate alkalinization in comparison with alpha-stat. Acid–base management also appears to be important in cardiac electrophysiology. Swain et al. (27) showed the electrical stability of the heart to be increased, with less spontaneous ventricular fibrillation, when alpha-stat blood regulation was compared with pH-stat. Kroncke et al. (28) found a 40% incidence of ventricular fibrillation in patients cooled to 24°C during pH-stat management and a 20% incidence in those managed with alpha-stat.

The appropriate acid–base management for optimal cerebral perfusion has also been questioned. Clearly, CBF decreases significantly with hypothermia. Cerebral metabolic rate also decreases during hypothermic bypass. The response of the cerebral circulation to changes in Pa_{CO_2} is preserved, at least during moderate hypothermia (29); thus, alpha-stat management will result in lower cerebral flows than those seen with pH-stat management. However, because of the lowered metabolic demands, a lower CBF may be appropriate and indicative of a maintained coupling of blood flow and metabolic demand. Govier et al. (30) demonstrated intact autoregulation in humans following alpha-stat strategy at temperatures from 21° to 29°C. Murkin et al. (31) showed coupling of CBF and metabolism that was independent of cerebral perfusion pressure within the range of 20 to 100 mm Hg when alpha-stat management was employed. In contrast, cerebral autoregulation was abolished and CBF varied with perfusion pressure when pH-stat strategy was used (Fig. 12.7). It has been argued that the CBF during pH-stat hypothermia actually represents excessive blood flow and may be detrimental. Unnecessarily high blood flows may put the brain at risk for damage by microemboli or high intracranial pressure. With deep hypothermia (i.e., temperatures <20°C), the normal vascular responses are lost and CBF becomes pressure-dependent (32,33). At deep hypothermic temperatures, coupling of cerebral flow and metabolism is also lost. It is important to note, though, that the responses of CBF and CMR_{O_2} (cerebral metabolic rate of oxygen) are quantitatively different at deep hypothermic conditions. CBF decreases linearly with the decrease in temperature, whereas CMR_{O_2} drops exponentially. The net result is that CBF becomes more luxuriant at deep hypothermic temperatures. At normothermia, the mean ratio of CBF to CMR_{O_2} is 20:1, and at deep hypothermia, the ratio increases to 75:1 (34). This situation is important in the context of low-flow CPB. At very low temperatures, data indicate that pump flow rates may be reduced to as little as 10 mL/kg per minute before flow becomes inadequate for cerebral metabolic requirements (35).

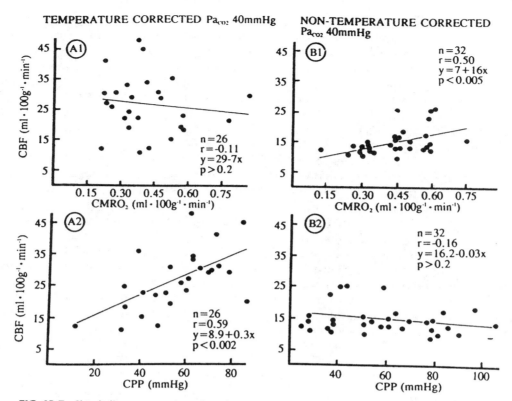

FIG. 12.7. Simple linear regression of cerebral blood flow (*CBF*) versus cerebral perfusion pressure (*CPP*) or cerebral oxygen consumption (*CMRo₂*) for temperature-corrected and temperature-uncorrected groups. **Upper panel:** There is no significant correlation between CBF and CMRo₂ in the temperature-corrected group (*A1*), whereas CBF significantly correlates with CMRo₂ in the temperature-uncorrected group (*B1*). **Lower panel:** CBF is significantly correlated with CPP in the temperature-corrected group (*A2*), whereas CBF is independent of CPP in the temperature-uncorrected group (*B2*). (From Murkin JM, Farrar JK, Tweed WA, et al. Cerebral autoregulation and flow/metabolism coupling during cardiopulmonary bypass: the influence of Paco₂. *Anesth Analg* 1987;66:825–832, with permission.)

On a microcirculatory level, some evidence suggests that alpha-stat management may be beneficial to the brain. Norwood et al. (36) studied the brains of hypothermic dogs perfused with anoxic blood and found a decrease in extent and magnitude of lesions when the perfusate had a higher pH. Acidic perfusate enhanced the extent of the lesions.

Theoretically, hypocarbia (and increased pH) result in a leftward shift of the oxyhemoglobin dissociation curve, which causes oxygen to be less readily available to the tissues. However, more oxygen is dissolved in the plasma during hypothermia, so that these two effects tend to cancel each other out. The relatively low CBF during alpha-stat management has been shown still to be in excess of cerebral metabolic needs (31).

In adults, the preponderance of evidence suggests either that CO_2 management on CPB does not matter or that an alpha-stat strategy is advantageous. Bashein and colleagues (37) examined the influence of pH management in 86 adults in whom mild hypothermia was utilized (about 30°C). They found no difference in cardiac or neuropsycho-

logical outcome regardless of acid–base management. It is important to realize, however, that it would have been unlikely for them to be able to demonstrate a difference in this study under their conditions. The differences in P_{CO_2} between the two groups amounted only to about 6 to 7 mm Hg, and the degree of hypothermia was not very profound. Contrast their scenario to that of a patient in deep hypothermia, for whom the difference in P_{CO_2} between the two strategies approaches 80 mm Hg! Also, their analysis looked for differences in mean group performances rather than changes of individual patient performance, a methodology that may have decreased the sensitivity of the study to detect any existing difference. Three recent randomized prospective studies of moderate hypothermia in adults have demonstrated that postoperative neurologic or neuropsychological outcome is slightly, but consistently, better with alpha-stat management (38–40).

Although acid–base management is probably not as important when moderate hypothermic temperatures are used, it may be critical in the setting of deep hypothermia. Proponents of the alpha-stat method suggest that the unnecessarily high blood flows (with pH-stat management) may put the brain at risk for damage from microemboli, cerebral edema, or high intracranial pressure, or may actually predispose to an adverse redistribution of blood flow ("steal") away from marginally perfused areas in patients with cerebrovascular disease. On the other hand, proponents of the pH-stat strategy suggest that enhanced CBF may be helpful in improving cerebral cooling before the initiation of circulatory arrest. In fact, total CBF is increased, global cerebral cooling is enhanced, and brain blood flow is redistributed during pH-stat management. An increased proportion of CBF is distributed to deep brain structures (thalamus, brainstem, and cerebellum) when pH-stat management is used (41) (Figs. 12.8 and 12.9). However, other data suggest that cerebral metabolic recovery after circulatory arrest may be better with the alpha-stat method than with the pH-stat mode. This variation in results has led some authors to advocate a crossover strategy in which a pH-stat approach is used during the first 10 minutes of cooling to provide maximal cerebral metabolic suppression, followed by an alpha-stat strategy to remove the severe acidosis that accumulates dur-

ing profound hypothermia during pH-stat. This approach appears to offer maximal metabolic recovery in animals (42) (Fig. 12.10). The choice of acid–base management may be particularly important in the subgroup of patients with aortopulmonary collaterals, for whom cerebral cooling is problematic. It appears that the addition of CO_2 during cooling enhances cerebral perfusion and improves cerebral metabolic recovery (43). Kurth and colleagues (44) demonstrated in a piglet model two mechanisms by which pH-stat management may be beneficial to the brain. They showed that pH-stat increases the rate of brain cooling and that the rate of depletion of brain oxygen during deep hypothermia and circulatory arrest (DHCA) is considerably slower with pH-stat management than with alpha-stat management (Fig. 12.11). A recent randomized single-center trial in human infants less than 9 months of age found that infants managed with a pH-stat strategy generally had better outcomes than those in the alpha-stat group (45). The pH-stat infants had a significantly shorter recovery time to first electroencephalographic activity and a tendency to fewer electroencephalographically manifested seizures. In this study, within the subset of infants with transposition of the

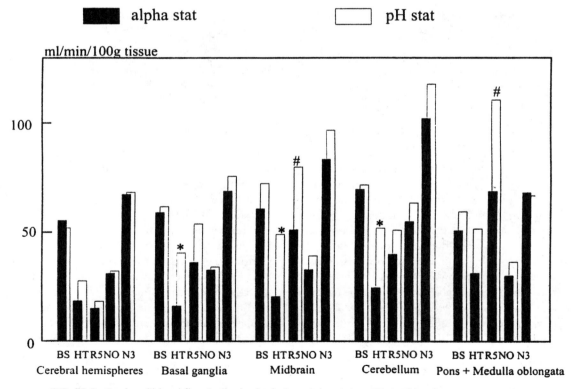

FIG. 12.8. Regional blood flow in the brain during alpha-stat or pH-stat blood gas management. *BS*, baseline on normothermic cerebral blood pressure (*CBP*); *HT*, at the end of 30 minutes of hypothermic CPB; *R5*, 5 minutes after initiation of reperfusion and rewarming after 1 hour of circulatory arrest; *N0*, after 45 minutes of rewarming, when normothermia was achieved; *N3*, after 3 hours of reperfusion at normothermia. *p <0.01, #p <0.05 for group difference. (From Aoki M, Nomura F, Stromski ME, et al. Effects of pH on brain energetics after hypothermic circulatory arrest. *Ann Thorac Surg* 1993;55:1093–1103, with permission.)

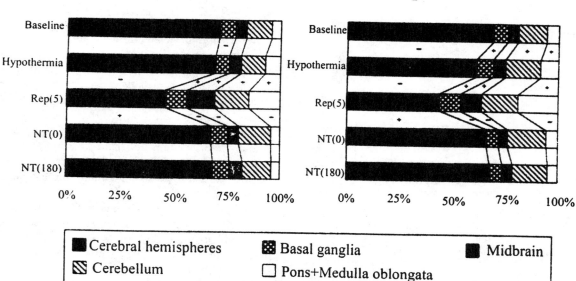

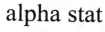

FIG. 12.9. Intracerebral distribution of blood flow: alpha-stat vs. pH-stat. *Rep(5),* 5 minutes after initiation of reperfusion and rewarming after 1 hour of circulatory arrest; *NT(0),* after 45 minutes of rewarming, when normothermia was achieved; *NT(180),* after 180 minutes of reperfusion at normothermia. $+p <0.05$ for the within-group increase by paired t test; $-p <0.05$ for the within-group decrease by paired t test. (From Aoki M, Nomura F, Stromski ME, et al. Effects of pH on brain energetics after hypothermic circulatory arrest. *Ann Thorac Surg* 1993;55:1093–1103, with permission.)

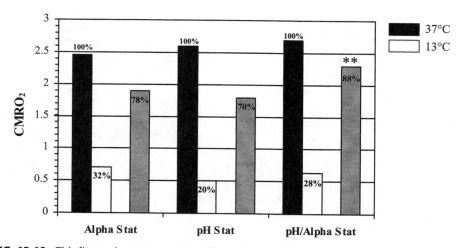

FIG. 12.10. This figure demonstrates the effects of three different cooling strategies (alpha-stat, pH-stat, and a crossover of pH-stat followed by alpha-stat) on cerebral metabolic suppression before deep hypothermic circulatory arrest (*DHCA*) and the recovery of cerebral metabolism after DHCA. The addition of CO_2 (i.e., the pH-stat strategy) provides better cerebral metabolic suppression before DHCA, but cerebral metabolic recovery after DHCA is poor. Initial cooling with a pH-stat strategy followed by conversion to alpha-stat before DHCA results in the greatest cerebral metabolic recovery. (From Kern FH, Greeley WJ. pH-stat management of blood gases is not preferable to alpha-stat in patients undergoing brain cooling for cardiac surgery. *J Cardiothorac Vasc Anesth* 1995;9:215–218, with permission.)

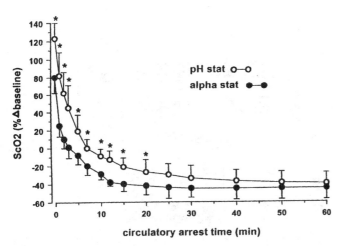

FIG. 12.11. Cortical oxygen saturation (Sco_2) during deep hypothermic circulatory arrest in the pH-stat and alpha-stat groups. Mean ± SD, eight animals per group. *p <0.05 between groups. The Sco_2 half-life during arrest was significantly greater in the pH-stat than in the alpha-stat group. (From Kurth CD, O'Rourke MM, O'Hara IB. Comparison of pH-stat and alpha-stat cardiopulmonary bypass on cerebral oxygenation and blood flow in relation to hypothermic circulatory arrest in piglets. *Anesthesiology* 1998;89:110–118, with permission.)

great vessels, those assigned to pH-stat tended to have a higher cardiac index despite a lower requirement for inotropic agents, less frequent acidosis and hypotension, and a shorter duration of mechanical ventilation and intensive care unit stay. Although the numbers of infants studied in this investigation were small, the study challenges the concept that alpha-stat management is more physiologic and protective during deep hypothermia in infants. The data suggest that pH-stat management may actually enhance systemic and cerebral protection in this group of patients.

Why the apparent difference in outcome between adults and children relative to pH management? It may relate to differences in the mechanism of brain injury on CPB. In adults, emboli appear to play a prominent role in adverse neurologic outcome (46). It is thus postulated that the lesser CBF associated with alpha-stat management may be protective by limiting the formation of cerebral microemboli. On the other hand, the mechanism of injury in children may relate more to hypoperfusion or activation of excitotoxic pathways (47). If a pH-stat strategy is employed, the increase in CBF may be beneficial in ensuring complete brain cooling and slowing oxygen consumption, thus increasing the tolerance of the brain for DHCA.

Alterations in Organ Function

Hypothermia causes a decrease in blood flow to all organs of the body. However, some areas experience greater declines than others. Skeletal muscle and the extremities have the greatest reduction in flow, followed by the kidneys,

splanchnic bed, heart, and brain. Despite these decreases in flow, differences in arteriovenous oxygen content either decrease or are not changed, which implies that oxygen supply is adequate to meet the metabolic requirements.

With cooling, heart rate decreases but contractility remains stable or may actually increase. Dysrhythmias become more frequent as temperature decreases and may include nodal, premature ventricular beats, atrioventricular block, atrial and ventricular fibrillation, and asystole. The mechanism of this dysrhythmogenic effect is unknown but may involve electrolyte disturbances, uneven cooling, and autonomic nervous system imbalance. Because coronary blood flow is well-preserved during hypothermia, it is unlikely that myocardial hypoxia plays a role in the genesis of these dysrhythmias.

The pulmonary system is characterized by a progressive decrease in ventilation as the temperature is lowered. Physiologic and anatomic dead space increases during dilation of the bronchi by cold. Gas exchange is largely unaffected.

The kidneys show the largest proportional decrease in blood flow of all the organs. Hypothermia increases renal vascular resistance, with diminished outer and inner cortex blood flow and oxygen delivery. Tubular transport of sodium, water, and chloride are decreased, and concentrating ability becomes impaired. Tubular reabsorption is decreased. Urine flow may be increased with hypothermia, but this effect can be masked by the stress-induced release of arginine vasopressin and antidiuretic hormone. The ability of the hypothermic kidney to handle glucose is impaired, and glucose often appears in the urine. Hemodilution in combination with hypothermic CPB improves renal blood flow and protects the integrity of the renal tubules postoperatively.

In general, significant hepatic injury with hypothermic CPB is rare. Hepatic arterial blood flow is reduced in proportion to the fall in cardiac output. The most significant effect of hypothermia is the decrease in metabolic and excretory function of the liver. Obviously, drug actions and requirements will be modified by this change in liver function. With rewarming, hepatic efficiency reverts to normal.

Marked hyperglycemia is often a feature of hypothermic CPB. Endogenous insulin production is decreased; glycogenolysis and gluconeogenesis may be increased because of increases in catecholamines. Even if exogenous insulin is administered, its efficacy is reduced during hypothermia, and hyperglycemia may develop.

It is difficult to separate the effects of hypothermia from those of hemodilution and CPB. Tissue water content is increased during hypothermic bypass, primarily as a consequence of hemodilution (48). Cell swelling and edema occur, which may be related to an accumulation of sodium and chloride within cells secondary to a decrease in reaction rates of membrane Na^+-K^+-ATPase (13). Hypothermia decreases free water clearance and causes a decrease in plasma potassium and an increase in osmolarity.

Hypothermia cas marked changes in the peripheral circulation. Systen and pulmonary vascular resistance typically rise with ing below 26°C (49). This increase in vascular resistan elates to increases in blood viscosity and catecholamines moconcentration, cell swelling, and perhaps active vaso strictor substances in the lung. In addition, arteriovenc shunts appear at low temperatures (50) and may cause arther diminution in tissue oxygen delivery. The increas blood viscosity occurs because of fluid shifts, with loss plasma volume from capillary leak and cell swelling. Th d blood cell volume remains unchanged even though e hematocrit rises. Red blood cell aggregation and roulx formation can occur, further impeding blood flow. ese changes can be somewhat attenuated by adequate a thesia, hemodilution, heparinization, and the use of va dilators. Hypothermia also causes thrombocytopenia by a versible sequestration of platelets in the portal circulatior

The hormonal respo to hypothermia depends on the level of anesthesia. Non esthetized subjects demonstrate a marked sympathetic res nse to cold. This response can be almost ablated if deep ar thesia is used. After deep hypothermia and total circulat y arrest, a massive release of catecholamines occurs (51), ich may contribute to the impaired cerebral perfusion und by Greeley and colleagues (52). Corticosteroid relea is suppressed with long-term hypothermia below 28°C lt appears to be normal during short periods of hypotherm (53). Complement activation occurs during CPB and is as ciated with neutrophil activation. Respiratory complicatic s correlate with the degree of complement activation (54). Iypothermia, hemodilution, and heparin reduce complem nt activation and subsequent neutrophil response and may potect patients from harmful sequelae. Circulating bradykin increases during hypothermia and CPB and may contribue to altered vascular permeability and circulatory instabili (55).

CLINICAL USE OF HYPOTHERMIA

Currently, hypothermia is used most commonly in cardiac surgery, although its use has also been described for major vascular procedures, intracranial surgery, and removal of hepatic and renal tumors. In most cardiac procedures, mild to moderate systemic hypothermia (>25°C) is used for its protective effects, previously described. More profound selective myocardial hypothermia is also often used during aortic cross-clamping to aid in the preservation of ischemic myocardium. Myocardial hypothermia is typically obtained in two ways: by coronary perfusion with cold cardioplegic solution, and by topical application of an ice slush or cold pericardial lavage. The optimal temperature for myocardial protection is controversial; however, most studies have demonstrated superior protection down to 2 to 4°C, as long as freezing temperatures are avoided, alkalosis is present, and the heart is promptly arrested during cooling (56).

Deep Hypothermic Circulatory Arrest

The most dramatic application demonstrating the protective effects of hypothermia is in DHCA. Systemic temperatures of 20° to 22°C or less are used to allow cessation of the circulation for periods up to 40 to 60 minutes, often without detectable organ injury (7). DHCA can be used in a variety of situations. In pediatric cardiac surgical patients (particularly those weighing <8 to 10 kg), the repair of complex congenital cardiac lesions is often facilitated by the asanguineous surgical field provided with circulatory arrest. It is often used in procedures requiring occlusion of multiple cerebral vessels, particularly repair of aortic arch aneurysms. It may be used to enhance surgical exposure and speed in procedures that could lead to uncontrollable hemorrhage.

Central Nervous System Effects of Deep Hypothermic Circulatory Arrest

The brain is the organ at greatest risk for injury, which limits the duration of "safe" arrest time. Cerebral metabolic activity is decreased with temperature but never ceases altogether, even at temperatures approaching 0°C. As mentioned earlier, the protective effect of hypothermia may involve more than just a reduction in cerebral metabolic rate. A Q_{10} of 2.7 would predict a "safe" arrest time of only about 15 minutes at 20°C. Clinical and experimental evidence indicate, however, that 30 to 45 minutes is typically tolerated, so there appears to be a disproportionate cerebral protective effect to profound levels of hypothermia. Other factors, such as extracellular pH, may play a role. Swain and colleagues (57) showed that hypothermia significantly increases the tissue energy state and intracellular pH in both heart and brain. This increase in high-energy phosphate levels may partially explain the beneficial effects of hypothermia on organ tolerance to ischemia. On the other hand, it may be that cerebral oxygen consumption decreases in a nonlinear fashion and more precipitously with profound hypothermia than was previously thought. Michenfelder and Milde (58) showed a change in Q_{10} from 2.23 between 37° and 27°C to 4.53 between 27° and 14°C. They postulated that this marked drop in oxygen consumption at lower temperatures could be explained by a primary effect of hypothermia on integrated neuronal function (as shown by suppression of the electroencephalogram).

The rate of cooling also appears to be important in the production of brain injury. Wide gradients between body and perfusate temperature in dogs correlated with brain cell necrosis and death (59). The optimal site for temperature monitoring is controversial, but it must be remembered that gradients exist among the different regions (60) (Fig. 12.12). Monitoring multiple sites to ensure uniform cooling

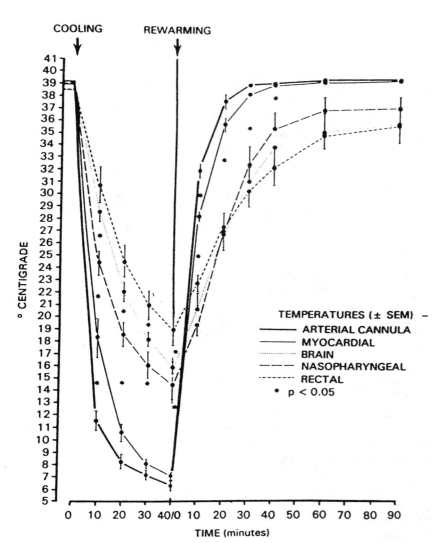

FIG. 12.12. Average temperature (± SEM) of arterial cannula, myocardium, cerebral cortex, nasopharynx, and rectum during 40 minutes of cooling and 90 minutes of rewarming under cardiopulmonary bypass in pigs. (From Stefaniszyn HJ, Novick RJ, Keith FM, et al. Is the brain adequately cooled during deep hypothermic cardiopulmonary bypass? *Curr Sur* 1983;40:294–297, with permission.)

before arrest is advisable. Coselli et al. (61) suggested using electroencephalographic monitoring to determine the ideal depth of cooling for safe circulatory arrest. They advocated using electroencephalographic silence as the appropriate end-point in cooling, but found that no peripheral body temperature consistently predicts this level of hypothermia. There was a wide variation in temperature among body sites when electroencephalographic silence occurred.

A consequence of ischemia and anoxia is the "no-reflow" phenomenon. The cerebral microcirculation can shut down multifocally, causing incomplete reperfusion when flow is resumed. The etiology of this problem is not completely understood but may involve increased blood viscosity, vascular smooth-muscle contraction resulting from increased extracellular potassium, and precapillary shunting (62). It can occur with or without total circulatory arrest and can be prevented by hypothermia (36). Microscopic cellular damage in the brain occurs to some degree following hypo-

thermia to 18°C, regardless of whether pulsatile or nonpulsatile perfusion or total circulatory arrest is employed (63).

The main concern with the use of DHCA is the potential harmful effects on the organ most at risk, the brain. As mortality decreases with improvements in technique, the question of an effect on later intellectual development after hypothermic bypass with or without circulatory arrest becomes critical. Several studies have shown evidence of a decreased intelligence quotient and developmental capacity related to the duration of circulatory arrest (64–66). However, other studies have not been able to demonstrate an adverse effect on intellectual capacity and development when circulatory arrest times are less than 60 minutes at nasopharyngeal temperatures of about 20°C (67–69). It is difficult to interpret many of these studies because of the difficulty in defining an appropriate control group. Blackwood and colleagues (70) used each child as his or her own control and found no difference between preoperative and postoperative scores with arrest intervals as long as 74 minutes. In 1993 (71), Newburger and colleagues reported a greater neurologic risk to neonates and infants with DHCA than with continuous low-flow bypass. They reported modest but statistically significant reductions in psychomotor developmental performance in those children in the circulatory arrest group (72). Many investigators have tried to determine a "safe" duration of DHCA, but the answer is still not known. Extensive clinical experience suggests that periods of DHCA as long as 60 minutes are often well tolerated. Although patients vary widely, the data of Newburger et al. data suggest minimal adverse effects on psychomotor test results with circulatory arrest times of about 35 minutes at 18°C.

Choreoathetosis

Choreoathetosis has been reported in 1% to 20% of children undergoing DHCA (73–74). Choreoathetosis usually appears 2 to 6 days postoperatively and generally lessens in severity with time. However, in severe cases, choreoathetoid movements or generalized hypotonia may persist indefinitely. Choreoathetosis has also been occasionally observed following continuous CPB, especially with profound hypothermia (10° to 12°C) (75). Numerous etiologies have been proposed, including hyperglycemia (76), uneven cooling (71), the no-reflow phenomenon (77,78), dopaminergic neurotransmitter alterations (79), and cerebral excitatory amino acid neurotoxicity (80). It is generally thought that this hyperkinetic movement disorder is a result of injury to basal ganglia, although often the pathology is not detectable by conventional cranial computed tomography (CT) or magnetic resonance imaging (MRI). It appears that there may also be an age-related phenomenon with regard to choreoathetosis. Data from Boston Children's Hospital suggest that the most vulnerable period starts at 6 to 9 months and ends after 5 to 6 years (81). A mild, transient form of the condition was observed to develop in younger children, whereas older children manifested a severe, persistent disorder with a high mortality. The Boston group also noted that choreoathetosis is most likely to occur in children with significant systemic–pulmonary collateral vessels. Perhaps the phenomenon of "steal" from the cerebral circulation to the pulmonary arteries, particularly in the setting of inadequate brain cooling, contributes to this problem.

Seizures

Seizures following CPB in neonates are much more common than in adults. Seizures occur clinically in approximately 20% of neonates following CPB (82,83). Seizures detected by electroencephalogram occur even more commonly than clinically observed seizures, a fact to be kept in mind if pharmacologic paralysis becomes necessary in the postoperative period. The seizures are generally self-limited

and can occur whether or not circulatory arrest has been used. Some series have reported no long-term adverse sequelae, whereas others have suggested a decrement in psychomotor developmental performance in addition to neurologic and MRI abnormalities (84–86). The long-term prognosis for these children is still unclear. The question also arises of whether seizures themselves actually add to the damage or are just a reflection of severe underlying brain pathology. At present, the answer is unknown, with further research necessary in this important area. Also, the relative involvement of hypothermia or other elements of CPB has not been determined.

Thus, the question of a "safe" circulatory arrest time is complex and cannot be answered with certainty. Hypothermia can delay but not prevent the appearance of metabolic and structural changes during ischemia that lead to functional neurologic impairment. A nomogram has been devised that, although not rigorously defined, provides a best estimate of safe circulatory arrest times at three temperatures (7) (Fig. 12.13). Although patients vary widely, the data of Newburger et al. in children suggest minimal adverse effects on psychomotor testing with circulatory arrest times of about 35 minutes at 18°C (71).

Central Nervous System Cooling

Because deep hypothermia and very low flow rates or circulatory arrest will most likely remain important tools in cardiac surgery, especially in congenital heart surgery and aortic arch repair, much effort has been expended in trying to understand better the physiology involved. Newer monitoring and protective strategies are evolving in an attempt to improve cerebral outcome in these patients. One of the areas of focus has been cooling methods before circulatory arrest. The rate of cooling and the efficiency of brain cooling are important factors in neurologic protection. Marked variability in cerebral cooling occurs, and sufficient time must be allotted before circulatory arrest to ensure uniform brain cooling. One group of investigators reported slower brain cooling in one third of neonates studied by jugular venous saturation monitoring (87). It appears that cooling periods of less than 20 to 25 minutes before the initiation of circulatory arrest with alpha-stat regulation are associated with a lower developmental quotient in neonates undergoing DHCA (88) (Fig. 12.14). Uniform cerebral cooling may also be problematic in certain groups of patients. Cyanotic patients with aortopulmonary collaterals appear to be at increased risk for neurologic injury during CPB (89). A reduction in total and regional measures of CBF occurs in these patients, resulting in less efficient cerebral cooling. Because the brain is acidotic and a tremendous metabolic debt develops during DHCA, the method of reestablishing CPB and rewarming may also be critically important. Some intriguing data suggest that a period of cold reperfusion with delayed rewarming after reestablishment of CPB may

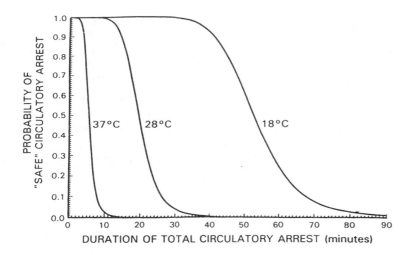

FIG. 12.13. Nomogram of an estimate (not rigorously derived) of the probability of "safe" total circulatory arrest (absence of structural or functional damage) according to the arrest time at nasopharyngeal temperatures of 37°C, 28°C, and 18°C. (From Kirklin JW. *Cardiac surgery.* New York: Churchill Livingstone, 1993:61–127, with permission.)

be beneficial (90). These authors demonstrated an improvement in CBF velocity in the group of infants in whom rewarming was delayed by 10 minutes. It is also becoming clear that too aggressive rewarming with hyperthermic overshoot is deleterious to neurologic outcome and should be avoided. Martin et al. (91) and Mora and colleagues (92) reported an increased risk for neurologic injury in adult patients actively warmed to 37°C with a CPB circuit water bath maintained at 39° to 40°C in comparison with patients allowed to "drift" to systemic temperatures of 33° to 36°C in a more tepid approach to warm heart bypass. They suggested that many if not all of their "normothermic" patients experienced cerebral hyperthermia (>37°C), which may potentiate ischemic pathologic processes in the brain during cardiac operations. Animal data have demonstrated that even small (2°C) increases in brain temperature can exacerbate neuronal injury, with changes in blood–brain permeability, increases in postischemic release of glutamate, and increased mortality (93,94).

Cardiac surgery has advanced remarkably during the last 30 years. Hypothermia has contributed substantially toward improving patient outcome. Current efforts must be directed toward defining methods of maximizing cerebral protection and refining critical techniques.

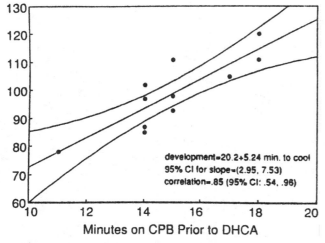

FIG. 12.14. Scatter plot of duration of core cooling (minutes of cardiopulmonary bypass before deep hypothermic circulatory arrest) and developmental index for infants with "short" periods of core cooling (<20 minutes). The best-fit regression line and its 95% confidence interval (*CI*) are shown. (From Bellinger DC, Wernovsky G, Rappaport LA, et al. Cognitive development of children following repair of transposition of the great arteries using deep hypothermic circulatory arrest. *Pediatrics* 1991;87:701–707, with permission.)

KEY POINTS

- Acid–base balance is significantly affected by hypothermia.
  - Biologic fluids are water solutions of weak acids and weak bases.
  - Hypothermia decreases the tendency for weak acids and bases to dissociate in solution.
  - Blood pH is maintained at moderately alkaline values (0.4 pH units) relative to water.
  - Maintenance of a constant ratio of $[OH^-]$ to $[H^+]$ (16:1) as temperature decreases
  - Allows optimum function of many respiratory enzymes.
  - Requires an alkaline pH shift with cooling.
  - Alpha-stat regulation preserves the ratio of $[OH^-]$ to $[H^+]$ with temperature change and produces an alkaline shift with cooling.
  - pH-stat regulation maintains absolute a constant $[H^+]$ regardless of temperature and requires added H^+, usually as CO_2, with cooling.

- The solubility of gases in biologic fluids increases with hypothermia.
  - At a constant CO_2 content, $Paco_2$ decreases as temperature falls.
- Protection of the brain during deep hypothermia (temperature $<20°C$) may be best accomplished with a mixed acid–base strategy:
  - pH-stat during the initial cooling phase.
  - Alpha-stat during reperfusion, rewarming, and termination of cardiopulmonary bypass.
- Hypothermia causes a decrease in blood flow to all vascular beds in proportion to the reduced metabolic demands.
  - The most profound effects occur in skeletal muscle and the extremities, followed by the kidneys, splanchnic bed, heart, and brain.

REFERENCES

1. Fay T. Observations on prolonged human refrigeration. *N Y State J Med* 1940;40:1351–1354.
2. Crossman LW, Ruggiero WF, Hurley V, et al. Reduced temperatures in surgery. II. Amputations for peripheral vascular disease. *Arch Surg* 1942;44:139–156.
3. Bigelow WG, Callaghan JC, Hopps JA. General hypothermia for experimental intra-cardiac surgery. *Ann Surg* 1950;132:531–539.
4. Lewis FJ, Taufic M. Closure of atrial septal defects with the aid of hypothermia; experimental accomplishments and the report of one successful case. *Surgery* 1953;33:52–59.
5. Gibbon JH. Application of a mechanical heart and lung apparatus to cardiac surgery. *Minn Med* 1954;37:171–180.
6. Sealy WC, Brown IW Jr, Young WG Jr. A report on the use of both extracorporeal circulation and hypothermia for open heart surgery. *Ann Surg* 1958;147:603–613.
7. Kirklin JW, Barratt-Boyes BG. Hypothermia, circulatory arrest, and cardiopulmonary bypass. *Cardiac surgery*, 2nd ed. New York: Churchill Livingstone, 1993:61–127.
8. Swain JA, McDonald TJ, Griffith PK, et al. Low-flow hypothermic cardiopulmonary bypass protects the brain. *J Thorac Cardiovasc Surg* 1991;102:76–84.
9. Michenfelder JD. The hypothermic brain. In: Michenfelder JD, ed. *Anesthesia and the brain*. New York: Churchill Livingstone, 1988:23–34.
10. Rothman SM, Olney JW. Glutamate and the pathophysiology of hypoxic-ischemic brain damage. *Ann Neurol* 1986;19:105–111.
11. Busto R, Globus MY-T, Dietrich WD, et al. Effect of mild hypothermia on ischemia-induced release of neurotransmitters and free fatty acids in rat brain. *Stroke* 1989;20:904–910.
12. Hearse DJ, Braimbridge MV, Jynge P. *Protection of the ischemic myocardium: cardioplegia*. New York: Raven Press, 1981.
13. Cameron DE, Gardner TJ. Principles of clinical hypothermia. *Cardiac surgery: state of the art reviews* 1988;2:13–25.
14. Hickey RF, Hoar PF. Whole body oxygen consumption during low-flow hypothermic cardiopulmonary bypass. *J Thorac Cardiovasc Surg* 1983;86:903–906.
15. Slogoff S, Reul GJ, Keats AS, et al. Role of perfusion pressure and flow in major organ dysfunction after cardiopulmonary bypass. *Ann Thorac Surg* 1990;50:911–918.
16. Nussmeier NA, Arlund C, Slogoff S. Neuropsychiatric complications after cardiopulmonary bypass: cerebral protection by a barbiturate. *Anesthesiology* 1986;64:165–170.
17. Rahn H. Body temperature and acid-base regulation [Review Article]. *Pneumonologie* 1974;151:87–94.
18. Malan A, Wilson TL, Reeves RB. Intracellular pH in cold-blooded vertebrates as a function of body temperature. *Respir Physiol* 1976;28:29–47.
18A. Hazel JR, Garlick WS, Sellner PA. The effects of assay temperature upon the pH optima of enzymes from poikilotherms: a test of imidazole alphastat hypothesis. *J Comp Physiol* 1978;123:97–102.
19. Hickey PR, Hansen DD. Temperature and blood gases: the clinical dilemma of acid-base management for hypothermic cardiopulmonary bypass. In: Tinker JH, ed. *Cardiopulmonary bypass: current concepts and controversies*. Philadelphia: WB Saunders, 1989:1–20.
20. Reeves RB. Temperature-induced changes in blood acid-base status: Donnan r_{Cl} and red cell volume. *J Appl Physiol* 1976;40:762–767.
21. McConnell DH, White F, Nelson RL, et al. Importance of alkalosis in maintenance of "ideal" blood pH during hypothermia. *Surg Forum* 1975;26:263–265.
22. Poole-Wilson PA, Langer GA. Effect of pH on ionic exchange and function in rat and rabbit myocardium. *Am J Physiol* 1975;229:570–581.
23. Poole-Wilson PA, Langer GA. Effects of acidosis on mechanical function and Ca^{2+} exchange in rabbit myocardium. *Am J Physiol* 1979;236:H525–H533.
24. Sinet M, Muffat-Joly M, Bendaace T, et al. Maintaining blood pH at 7.4 during hypothermia has no significant effect on work of the isolated rat heart. *Anesthesiology* 1985;62:582–587.
25. Austen WG. Experimental studies on the effects of acidosis and alkalosis on myocardial function after aortic occlusion. *J Surg Res* 1965;5:191–194.
26. Becker H, Vinten-Johansen J, Buckberg G, et al. Myocardial damage caused by keeping pH 7.40 during systemic deep hypothermia. *J Thorac Cardiovasc Surg* 1981;82:810–820.
27. Swain JA, White FN, Peters RM. The effect of pH on the hypothermic ventricular fibrillation threshold. *J Thorac Cardiovasc Surg* 1984;87:445–451.
28. Kroncke GM, Nichols RD, Mendenhall JT, et al. Ectothermic philosophy of acid-base balance to prevent fibrillation during hypothermia. *Arch Surg* 1986;121:303–304.
29. Prough DS, Stump DA, Roy RC, et al. Response of cerebral blood flow to changes in carbon dioxide during hypothermic cardiopulmonary bypass. *Anesthesiology* 1986;64:576–581.
30. Govier AV, Reves JG, McKay RD, et al. Factors and their influence on regional cerebral blood flow during nonpulsatile cardiopulmonary bypass. *Ann Thorac Surg* 1984;38:592–600.
31. Murkin JM, Farrar JK, Tweed WA, et al. Cerebral autoregulation and flow/metabolism coupling during cardiopulmonary bypass: the influence of $Paco_2$. *Anesth Analg* 1987;66:825–832.
32. Greeley WJ, Kern FH, Ungerleider RM, et al. The effect of hypothermic cardiopulmonary bypass and total circulatory arrest on cerebral metabolism in neonates, infants and children. *J Thorac Cardiovasc Surg* 1991;101:783–794.
33. Greeley WJ, Ungerleider RM, Kern FH, et al. Effects of cardiopulmonary bypass on cerebral blood flow in neonates, infants and children. *Circulation* 1989;80[suppl I]:I209–I215.
34. Swain JA. Acid-base status, hypothermia and cardiac surgery. *Perfusion* 1986;1:231–238.
35. Kern FH, Ungerleider RM, Reves JG, et al. The effect of altering pump flow rate on cerebral blood flow and metabolism in neonates, infants and children. *Ann Thorac Surg* 1993;56:1366–1372.
36. Norwood WI, Norwood CR, Castaneda AR. Cerebral anoxia: effect of deep hypothermia and pH. *Surgery* 1979;86:203–209.
37. Bashein G, Townes BD, Nessly ML, et al. A randomized study

of carbon dioxide management during hypothermic cardiopulmonary bypass. *Anesthesiology* 1990;72:7–15.

38. Stephan H, Weyland A, Kazmaier S, et al. Acid-base management during hypothermic cardiopulmonary bypass does not affect cerebral metabolism but does affect blood flow and neurological outcome. *Br J Anaesth* 1992;69:51–57.

39. Patel RL, Turtle MR, Chambers DJ, et al. Alpha-stat acid-base regulation during cardiopulmonary bypass improves neuropsychologic outcome in patients undergoing coronary artery bypass grafting. *J Thorac Cardiovasc Surg* 1996;111:1267–1279.

40. Murkin JM, Martzke JS, Buchan AM, et al. A randomized study of the influence of perfusion technique and pH management strategy in 316 patients undergoing coronary artery bypass surgery. II. Neurologic and cognitive outcomes. *J Thorac Cardiovasc Surg* 1995;110:349–362.

41. Aoki M, Nomura F, Stromski ME, et al. Effects of pH on brain energetics after hypothermic circulatory arrest. *Ann Thorac Surg* 1993;55:1093–1103.

42. Skaryak LA, Chai PJ, Kern FH, et al. Blood gas management and degree of cooling: effects on cerebral metabolism before and after circulatory arrest. *J Thorac Cardiovasc Surg* 1995;110:1649–1657.

43. Kirshbom PM, Skaryak LA, DiBernardo LR, et al. pH-stat cooling improves cerebral metabolic recovery after circulatory arrest in a piglet model of aorto-pulmonary collaterals. *J Thorac Cardiovasc Surg* 1996;111:147–157.

44. Kurth CD, O'Rourke MM, O'Hara IB. Comparison of pH-stat and alpha-stat cardiopulmonary bypass on cerebral oxygenation and blood flow in relation to hypothermic circulatory arrest in piglets. *Anesthesiology* 1998;89:110–118.

45. DuPlessis AJ, Jonas RA, Wypij D, et al. Perioperative effects of alpha-stat versus pH-stat strategies for deep hypothermic cardiopulmonary bypass in infants. *J Thorac Cardiovasc Surg* 1997;114:990–1001.

46. Hammon JW, Stump DA, Kon ND, et al. Risk factors and solutions for the development of neurobehavioral changes after coronary artery bypass grafting. *Ann Thorac Surg* 1997;63:1613–1618.

47. Vannucci RC. Mechanisms of perinatal ischemic brain damage. In: Jonas RA, Newburger JW, Volpe JJ, eds. *Brain injury and pediatric cardiac surgery*. Boston: Butterworth–Heineman, 1996:201–214.

48. Utley JR, Wachtel C, Cain RB, et al. Effects of hypothermia, hemodilution, and pump oxygenation on organ water content, blood flow and oxygen delivery, and renal function. *Ann Thorac Surg* 1981;31:121–133.

49. Cooper KE. The circulation in hypothermia. *Br Med Bull* 1961;17:48–51.

50. Suzuki M, Penn I. A reappraisal of the microcirculation during general hypothermia. *Surgery* 1965;58:1049–1060.

51. Wood M, Shand DG, Wood AJJ. The sympathetic response to profound hypothermia and circulatory arrest in infants. *Can Anaesth Soc J* 1980;27:125–132.

52. Greeley WJ, Ungerleider RM, Smith LR, et al. The effects of deep hypothermic cardiopulmonary bypass and total circulatory arrest on cerebral blood flow in infants and children. *J Thorac Cardiovasc Surg* 1989;97:737–745.

53. Blair E. *Clinical hypothermia*. New York: McGraw-Hill, 1964.

54. Moore FD Jr, Warner KG, Assousa S, et al. The effects of complement activation during cardiopulmonary bypass: attenuation by hypothermia, heparin, and hemodilution. *Ann Surg* 1988;208:95–103.

55. Pang LM, Stalcup SA, Lipset JS, et al. Increased circulating bradykinin during hypothermia and cardiopulmonary bypass in children. *Circulation* 1979;60:1503–1507.

56. Swanson DK, Dufek JH, Kahn DR. Improved myocardial preservation at 4°C. *Ann Thorac Surg* 1980;30:519–526.

57. Swain JA, McDonald TJ Jr, Balaban RS, et al. Metabolism of the heart and brain during hypothermic cardiopulmonary bypass. *Ann Thorac Surg* 1991;51:105–109.

58. Michenfelder JD, Milde JH. The relationship among canine brain temperature, metabolism, and function during hypothermia. *Anesthesiology* 1991;75:130–136.

59. Almond CH, Jones JC, Snyder HM, et al. Cooling gradients and brain damage with deep hypothermia. *J Thorac Cardiovasc Surg* 1964;48:890–897.

60. Stefaniszyn HJ, Novick RJ, Keith FM, et al. Is the brain adequately cooled during deep hypothermic cardiopulmonary bypass? *Curr Surg* 1983;40:294–297.

61. Coselli JS, Crawford ES, Beall AC Jr, et al. Determination of brain temperatures for safe circulatory arrest during cardiovascular operation. *Ann Thorac Surg* 1988;45:638–642.

62. Mavroudis C, Greene MA. Cardiopulmonary bypass and hypothermic circulatory arrest in infants. In: Jacobs ML, Norwood WI, eds. *Pediatric cardiac surgery: current issues*. Boston: Butterworth–Heineman, 1992.

63. Molina JE, Einzig S, Mastri AR, et al. Brain damage in profound hypothermia: perfusion versus circulatory arrest. *J Thorac Cardiovasc Surg* 1984;87:596–604.

64. Wells FC, Coghill S, Caplan HL, et al. Duration of circulatory arrest does influence the psychological development of children after cardiac operation in early life. *J Thorac Cardiovasc Surg* 1983;86:823–831.

65. Wright JS, Hicks RG, Newman DC. Deep hypothermic arrest: observations on later development in children. *J Thorac Cardiovasc Surg* 1979;77:466–468.

66. Settergren G. Öhqvist G, Lundberg S, et al. Cerebral blood flow and cerebral metabolism in children following cardiac surgery with deep hypothermia and circulatory arrest. Clinical course and follow-up of psychomotor development. *Scand J Thorac Cardiovasc Surg* 1982;16:209–215.

67. Dickinson DF, Sambrooks JE. Intellectual performance in children after circulatory arrest with profound hypothermia in infancy. *Arch Dis Child* 1979;54:1–6.

68. Clarkson PM, MacArthur BA, Barratt-Boyes BG, et al. Developmental progress after cardiac surgery in infancy using hypothermia and circulatory arrest. *Circulation* 1980;62:855–861.

69. Messmer BJ, Schallberger U, Gattiker R, et al. Psychomotor and intellectual development after deep hypothermia and circulatory arrest in early infancy. *J Thorac Cardiovasc Surg* 1976;72:495–502.

70. Blackwood MJA, Haka-Ikse K, Steward DJ. Developmental outcome in children undergoing surgery with profound hypothermia. *Anesthesiology* 1986;65:437–440.

71. Newburger JW, Jonas RA, Wernovsky G, et al. A comparison of the perioperative neurologic effects of hypothermic circulatory arrest versus low-flow cardiopulmonary bypass in infant heart surgery. *N Engl J Med* 1993;329:1057–1064.

72. Bellinger DC, Jonas RA, Rappaport LA, et al. Developmental and neurologic status of children after heart surgery with hypothermic circulatory arrest or low-flow cardiopulmonary bypass. *N Engl J Med* 1995;332:549–555.

73. Clarkson PM, MacArthur BA, Barratt-Boyes BG, et al. Developmental progress after cardiac surgery in infancy using profound hypothermia and circulatory arrest. *Circulation* 1980;62:855–861.

74. Brunberg JA, Reilly EL, Doty DB. Central nervous system consequences in infants of cardiac surgery using deep hypothermia and circulatory arrest. *Circulation* 1974;50[Suppl II]:II60–II68.

75. Egerton N, Egerton WS, Kay JH. Neurologic changes following profound hypothermia. *Ann Surg* 1963;157:366–374.

76. Brunberg JA, Doty DB, Reilly EL. Choreoathetosis in infants following cardiac surgery with deep hypothermia and circulatory arrest. *J Pediatr* 1974;84:232–235.

77. Ames A III, Wright RL, Kowada M, et al. Cerebral ischemia. II. The no-reflow phenomenon. *Am J Pathol* 1968;52:437–453.

78. Norwood WI, Norwood CR, Castaneda AR. Cerebral anoxia: effect of deep hypothermia and pH. *Surgery* 1979;86:203–209.

79. Robinson RO, Samuels M, Pohl KR. Choreic syndrome after cardiac surgery. *Arch Dis Child* 1988;63:1466–1469.

80. Wical BS, Tomasi LG. A distinctive neurologic syndrome after induced profound hypothermia. *Pediatr Neurol* 1990;6: 202–205.

81. Wessel DL, duPlessis AJ. Choreoathetosis. In: Jonas RA, Newburger JW, Volpe JJ, eds. *Brain injury and pediatric cardiac surgery.* Boston: Butterworth–Heineman, 1996:353–362.

82. Tharion J, Johnson DC, Celermajer JM, et al. Profound hypothermia with circulatory arrest: nine years' clinical experience. *J Thoracic Cardiovasc Surg* 1982;84:66–72.

83. Coles JG, Taylor JM, Pearce JM, et al. Cerebral monitoring of somatosensory evoked potentials during profoundly hypothermic circulatory arrest. *Circulation* 1984;70[Suppl I]:I96–I102.

84. Ehyai A, Fenichel GM, Bender HW Jr. Incidence and prognosis of seizures in infants after cardiac surgery with profound hypothermia and circulatory arrest. *JAMA* 1984;252:3165–3167.

85. O'Dougherty M, Wright FS, Garmezy N, et al. Later competence and adaptation in infants who survive severe heart defects. *Child Dev* 1983;54:1129–1142.

86. Rappaport LA, Wypij D, Bellinger DC, et al. Relation of seizures after cardiac surgery in early infancy to neurodevelopmental outcome. Boston Circulatory Arrest Study Group. *Circulation* 1998; 97:773–779.

87. Kern FH, Greeley WJ. Con: Monitoring of nasopharyngeal and rectal temperatures is not an adequate guide of brain cooling before deep hypothermic circulatory arrest [Editorial Pro-Con]. *J Cardiothorac Vasc Anesth* 1994;8:363–365.

88. Bellinger DC, Wernovsky G, Rappaport LA, et al. Cognitive development of children following repair of transposition of the great arteries using deep hypothermic circulatory arrest. *Pediatrics* 1991;87:701–707.

89. Kirshbom PM, Skaryak LA, DiBernardo LR, et al. Effects of aortopulmonary collaterals on cerebral cooling and cerebral metabolic recovery after circulatory arrest. *Circulation* 1995;92[Suppl II]:II490–II494.

90. Rodriguez RA, Austin EH III, Audenaert SM. Postbypass effects of delayed rewarming on cerebral blood flow velocities in infants after total circulatory arrest. *J Thorac Cardiovasc Surg* 1995;110: 1686–1691.

91. Martin TC, Craver JM, Gott JP, et al. Prospective, randomized trial of retrograde warm-blood cardioplegia: myocardial benefit and neurologic threat. *Ann Thorac Surg* 1994;57:298–304.

92. Mora CT, Henson MB, Weintraub WS, et al. The effect of temperature management during cardiopulmonary bypass on neurologic and neuropsychological outcomes in coronary revascularization patients. *J Thorac Cardiovasc Surg* 1996;112: 514–522.

93. Dietrich WD, Busto R, Valdes I, et al. Effects of normothermic versus mild hyperthermic forebrain ischemia in rats. *Stroke* 1990; 21:1318–1325.

94. Mitani A, Kataoka K. Critical levels of extracellular glutamate mediating gerbil hippocampal delayed neuronal death during hypothermia: brain microdialysis study. *Neuroscience* 1991;32: 661–670.

13

SURGICAL MYOCARDIAL PROTECTION

**JAKOB VINTEN-JOHANSEN
RUSSELL S. RONSON
VINOD H. THOURANI
ANDREW S. WECHSLER**

The need to protect the myocardium from intraoperative damage predates the availability of cardiopulmonary bypass (CPB). The introduction of inflow occlusion techniques permitted the repair of simple intracardiac defects, and in many cases the occlusion time could be increased by adding moderate systemic hypothermia (30°C) (1). After the development of clinical CPB, the recognition that simple hypothermia could protect the myocardium against ischemic injury induced by aortic cross-clamping led to the use of profound systemic hypothermia for the protection of the heart and other body organs. The development of hypothermia for organ preservation permitted longer periods of ischemic cardiac arrest for the repair of more complicated lesions.

Myocardial protection during cardiac surgery has evolved during many years (Fig. 13.1). The development of extracorporeal circulation techniques allowed cardiac procedures to proceed without threat of hemodynamic collapse. However, performing complicated procedures on the heart was made difficult by its continuous motion. Ischemia was known ultimately to achieve cardiac arrest through the depletion of high-energy phosphate stores, on which cardiac contraction depends. However, myocardial ischemia led to necrosis and a hypocontractile, "stone" heart on reperfusion (2–4), from which recovery was impossible. Once the limitations of ischemic (anoxic) arrest were recognized, attempts were made to arrest the heart chemically, in theory to preserve high-energy phosphate stores lost during ischemia. Chemical arresting agents were first used by Melrose and associates in 1955 (5) and 1957 (6) to induce asystole during CPB. [Parenthetically, the Melrose formulation may represent the primordial blood cardioplegia solution, as a 2.5%

potassium citrate solution was drawn up into a blood-filled syringe, which was then infused into the aortic root proximal to the aortic cross-clamp by way of a syringe. Hence, the Melrose blood solution predates the blood cardioplegia formulation of Follette et al. (7) by some 23 years.] This arresting solution, later called "cardioplegia" solution by Lam et al. (8,9), was based on potassium citrate at concentrations sufficient to initiate immediate cardiac standstill. Other contemporaries of Melrose used alternative arresting agents, such as acetylcholine alone (8,9) or in combination with other drugs (10). Although cardioplegia was indeed achieved with the Melrose potassium citrate solution, the concept of elective cardiac arrest was soon abandoned in the United States following reports of high morbidity and pathologic complications in chemically arrested hearts (11). In other parts of the world, however, Bretschneider et al. (12) and Kirsch et al. (13) used intracellular crystalloid formulations clinically.

Before the popular use of chemical cardioplegia, efforts were made to minimize damage during surgical ischemia. Topical cardiac hypothermia was introduced by Shumway and Lower (14) and others (15,16) in 1959. Using CPB and hypothermia, these groups achieved a marked reduction in operative mortality. In the late 1960s, reports described scattered myocardial or subendocardial necrosis in patients who had died after cardiac surgical operations, suggesting that current techniques of myocardial protection were inadequate (17). Laboratory studies demonstrated that topical hypothermia protected inadequately against intraoperative injury, which resulted in postoperative myocardial subendocardial necrosis and metabolic and postischemic functional depression (18–20).

The use of chemical cardioplegia as a concept was revived in the United States by Gay and Ebert (21) and Tyers et al. (22,23), who found that the constituents in the Melrose formulation were inappropriate rather than that the concept of chemical cardioplegia itself was ineffective. These reports popularized the use of potassium-based cardioplegia to

J. Vinten-Johansen: Departments of Surgery and Physiology, Emory University School of Medicine, Atlanta, Georgia 30365.

R. S. Ronson and V. H. Thourani: Department of Surgery, Emory University School of Medicine, Atlanta, Georgia 30322.

A. S. Wechsler: Department of Cardiothoracic Surgery, Hahnemann University, Philadelphia, Pennsylvania 19102.

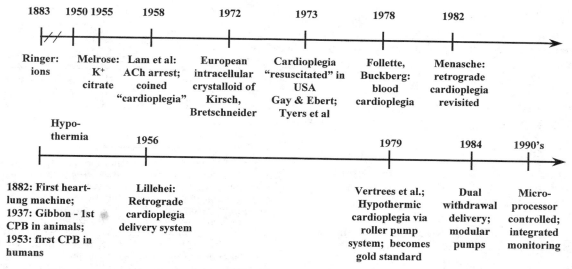

FIG. 13.1. Some highlights in the development of myocardial protection techniques. The *upper line* reports concepts of myocardial protection, and the *lower line* reports technologic advances in the delivery of myocardial protection. Dual-withdrawal delivery refers to the technique of diluting crystalloid cardioplegia solution with blood from the venous reservoir, with the modular aspect referring to a separate roller head dedicated to cardioplegia infusion. Microprocessor: Integrated refers to computerized monitoring of such parameters as cardioplegia infusion pressure with automatic negative feedback.

achieve electromechanical arrest. Today, a variety of both crystalloid and blood cardioplegia solutions are used clinically worldwide to achieve elective cardiac arrest and a bloodless field. Hearse and associates (24) at St. Thomas' Hospital in London developed an extracellular solution based on a more scientific understanding of the determinants of ischemic injury. With specific components such as potassium designed to initiate cardiac arrest and maintain a soft, flaccid myocardium, their solution has become popular internationally, and it represents a major advance in the area of myocardial protection. In the late 1970s and early 1980s, Follette and colleagues (7,25,26) introduced the concept of cold hyperkalemic blood cardioplegia. The physiologic attributes of blood, including its superior buffering capacity, endogenous oxygen radical scavengers, detoxifying substances, and superior oxygen-transport capacity, has established this concept of cardioplegia as a popular strategy with excellent clinical results (27–32).

This chapter reviews the new, emerging concepts of myocardial protection, in addition to some now conventional strategies used during open heart surgery and CPB that have evolved and developed during the past 25 years. Since the first writing of this chapter (33), the concepts of myoprotective strategies have changed significantly as our understanding of the pathophysiologic determinants of ischemia, and particularly the exquisitely complex mechanisms involved in reperfusion, have expanded. Early empiric observations have given way to complex biochemical and molecular interactions, which in some cases have reinforced physiologic

intuition and in other cases have provided a scientific underpinning to a more molecular approach in developing target-specific strategies of myocardial protection. The function of the endothelium and its critical importance in the pathophysiology of ischemia–reperfusion injury, atherosclerosis, and CPB have been identified. The role of neutrophils, proinflammatory mediators, and adhesion molecules in initiating cell–cell interactions that result in coronary vascular endothelial dysfunction (34–39), with consequences of cellular and tissue injury, has come to the forefront. Out of the explosion of research on the vascular biology of CPB and ischemia–reperfusion have come new therapeutic approaches to myocardial protection, such as inhibition of neutrophil function and endothelial activation with nitric oxide (NO), adenosine, monoclonal antibodies to adhesion molecules, and genetic alterations in adhesion molecule expression. It is the new understandings of pathophysiology of ischemia–reperfusion that form the future (and present) biologic rationale for myocardial protection. With attention diverted to the use of cardioplegia as a primary vector of delivering protection (hypothermia, arrest, cardioprotective drugs), off-pump surgery, without the comforts and convenience of extracorporeal techniques and the ability to deliver cardioplegia, has obviated the use of conventional techniques for the delivery of extracorporeally based myocardial protection, including chemical cardioplegia, and has therefore challenged scientists and surgeons alike to create new approaches to myocardial protection. The efforts of basic science in understanding the complex web of surgical ischemia–reperfusion injury under circumstances incorporating or excluding extracorporeal techniques will, it is hoped, reap dividends of clinically applicable strategies for protecting the heart.

PATHOPHYSIOLOGY OF SURGICAL ISCHEMIA–REPERFUSION INJURY

Because a complex array of forces affect the postoperative outcome of hearts with various and complex preoperative pathophysiologic features, developing strategies that adequately protect all hearts during cardiac surgery is often problematic. The heart under consideration may present a complex picture of preoperative disease, myocardial and cellular dysfunction, global or regional ischemia, differing vulnerabilities to ischemic and reperfusion injury, and various impediments to the distribution of the cardioprotective solution of choice. However, rational myocardial protection must be based on a sound scientific underpinning. Obviously, a single cardioprotective strategy may be inadequate to suit all preferences and target all mechanisms determining postischemic contractile function and cell viability. Hence, the surgical team must often mold the composition of the cardioplegic solution or its modality of delivery to meet the requirements of the pathologic scenario at hand, as well as the choice of on- or off-pump approaches. The measures taken to protect the heart during elective cardiac arrest should represent a balance struck between the requirements of the heart during aortic cross-clamp or reperfusion, with appropriate adjustments made for special considerations (hypertrophy, diffuse coronary disease) and the convenience of the anesthesia and surgical teams.

Myocardial injury sustained in the surgical setting can be divided into three phases: (a) antecedent ischemia (which includes preoperative disease status) precipitated before the institution of CPB or the delivery of cardioplegia solution (i.e., "unprotected" ischemia); (b) "protected" ischemia initiated electively by chemical cardioplegia; and (c) reperfusion injury sustained during intermittent infusions of the cardioplegic solution, after removal of the aortic cross-clamp, or after discontinuation of CPB. Reperfusion injury itself can be divided into an early phase (<4 hours) and a later phase (>4 to 6 hours). This division is based on early neutrophil- and adhesion molecule-dependent interactions (40,41) and later extension of injury by as yet unknown mediators (42). The stages in surgical operations in which ischemic and reperfusion injury can be inflicted are diagrammed in Fig. 13.2.

Unprotected ischemia: Ischemic injury can result from severe hypotension (e.g., ventricular fibrillation, cardiogenic shock) or coronary artery spasm before CPB; reperfusion injury can potentially occur when these conditions resolve before effective cardioprotective measures are implemented.

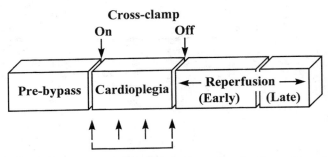

FIG. 13.2. A schematic diagram representing the chronology of a cardiac surgical procedure in which extracorporeal circulation and intermittent cardioplegia are used. Injury from ischemia can occur (a) before cardiopulmonary bypass is initiated, as a result of coronary artery disease or other disease processes, hypotension, or ventricular fibrillation; (b) during intermittent cardioplegia between infusions of solution, or when cardioplegia is poorly distributed because of coronary lesions present before revascularization or obstructions in the grafts; (c) during the reperfusion period, which can be divided into early and late components. In reality, the potential for reperfusion injury exists at each of these intervals when (a) resolution of pre-bypass hypotension or dysrhythmias restores blood flow; (b) cardioplegia solution is infused at high delivery pressures ("perfusion" injury) or has an inappropriate composition; and (c) coronary blood flow with unmodified systemic blood is restored after removal of the cross-clamp, especially if a terminal "reperfusion" dose of cardioplegia is not given. Systemic hypotension and physical or embolic obstructions to coronary blood flow can also induce injury during this period.

Protected ischemia: Ischemia can occur during maldistribution of cardioplegia solution distal to occluded coronary arteries, between intermittent infusions of cardioplegia solution, or during unintentional interruption of continuous cardioplegia; the potential for reperfusion injury exists even during this time of theoretically complete protection.

Reperfusion: Ischemia can occur with kinking of the bypass graft, during embolization (air or particulate), during performance of the proximal aortic anastomosis when a partially occluding aortic clamp is applied, during infusion of the terminal cardioplegia (pressure-induced, compositionally related, or from air embolization at the cold–warm interface), or after release of the aortic cross-clamp.

Understanding the pathophysiologic mechanisms of myocardial injury occurring at these intervals and appreciating the principles of myocardial protection will help avoid injury induced by the very techniques intended to preserve the myocardium. Unlike the cardiologist, the surgical team has the opportunity to intervene directly to control many facets of elective ischemic and reperfusion injury and to limit at some point the mechanisms causing injury, thereby more favorably directing the outcome of the postischemic heart. The pathophysiology of ischemia and reperfusion is described in the following sections. Interventions targeting these various pathologic processes are discussed under Myocardial Protection Therapy.

Determinants of Ischemic Injury

Optimal cardiac function is conventionally determined by the imbalance between myocardial oxygen demand and supply. However, there must also be sufficient blood flow to wash out metabolites of aerobic and anaerobic metabolism, which can be injurious if they accumulate in myocardial tissue. An expanded definition of ischemia, therefore, is "inadequate tissue perfusion to sustain steady-state oxidative metabolism at a given level of cardiac performance." The conventional definition of ischemic injury has been modified in two important ways: (a) acknowledgment that the accumulation of tissue metabolites (lactate, carbon dioxide, and hydrogen ions) may contribute to ischemic dysfunction and metabolic abnormalities, and (b) recognition that the coronary vasculature may not regulate the levels of perfusion appropriately in response to metabolic needs imposed by increased cardiac work, even in the absence of coronary lesions. An important advancement in the past few years has been the understanding that a delicate balance exists between endothelium-derived vasoactive substances, such as the vasodilators NO and adenosine, and the vasoconstrictors endothelin and the thromboxanes. These autacoids contribute to coronary artery autoregulation of myocardial blood flow, which may be threatened by the neutrophil-mediated inflammatory response characteristic of ischemia–reperfusion injury and CPB.

Our understanding of the pathophysiologic determinants of ischemic injury by the above definition has changed little in the past few years. The duration of ischemia, collateral blood flow available to offset primary vessel occlusion, ambient oxygen demands of the myocardium, and baseline health of the tissue are the major factors determining the extent of ischemic injury. There is an important distinction to be made between global and regional myocardial ischemia. The onset time of irreversible ischemic injury varies with the type (regional or global) and severity of ischemia and so becomes more than an academic examination of a Gordian knot. The strategy employed to correct ischemia may ideally be predicated on the severity and type of ischemic injury. For example, global ischemia under profound hypothermia induced by cardioplegia poses a different picture from that of chronic ischemic heart disease or normothermic ischemia in hearts with left ventricular hypertrophy. Therefore, the potential nature of the ischemia presented by the patient's preoperative or pre-CPB pathophysiology requires a well-conceived and executed plan by the surgical team.

Severity and Duration of Ischemia

The potential for myocardial injury is related, in part, to the duration of warm ischemia. The time to onset of irreversible ischemic injury will depend on many factors, including the severity of ischemia, myocardial temperature, energy demands, and collateral blood flow, but irreversible injury can become apparent after as little as 30 minutes of coronary occlusion in the working myocardium. However, shorter durations of global ischemia can result in mild to severe systolic and diastolic dysfunction without irreversible tissue necrosis (the so-called "stunning" model). Therefore, the duration of warm ischemia, both preceding CPB and intraoperatively after application of the cross-clamp, has often been used as a predictor of postoperative myocardial injury. Because the surgical team often does not have control over the duration of warm ischemia (particularly antecedent ischemia caused by coronary occlusive disease), other factors are more often targeted for modification to reduce the severity of postischemic injury. Therefore, strategies such as (a) initiating rapid arrest (asystole), (b) venting the left ventricle to reduce the higher oxygen requirements of passive wall stress and the morphologic consequences of overdistension, and (c) imposing cardiac hypothermia all specifically target the reduction of myocardial energy demands, thereby reducing the progression of ischemia and consequentially increasing the limits of "safe" ischemic time during aortic cross-clamping. With these cardioprotective strategies in place, the duration of aortic clamping that can be safely imposed can be increased from as little as 15 to 45 minutes to as much as 4 hours with intermittent hypothermic cardioplegia (Fig. 13.3).

The physiologic basis underlying the greater severity and accelerated progression of injury associated with regional ischemia in comparison with global ischemia may be related principally to differences in oxygen demand of the ischemic myocardium between the two types of ischemia. Oxygen demand in regionally ischemic myocardium is 70% that in nonischemic working myocardium and exceeds that of globally ischemic myocardium by a factor of 4 (10.2 mL O_2/min per 100 g of tissue vs. 2.6 mL O_2/min per 100 g of tissue) (43,44). Hence, the regionally ischemic myocardium has a greater mismatch between energy supply and demand than does its globally ischemic counterpart when blood flow is reduced, and consequently it has a more severe ischemic insult per unit time. For example, 45 minutes of global ischemia followed by unmodified reperfusion reduces systolic function by 50% to 60% without evidence of necrosis (45,46). A similar period of regional ischemia results in substantial subendocardial infarction with significant contractile dysfunction in the ischemic segment (47,48). This difference in the vulnerability and chronology of ischemic injury is important in off-pump surgery, in which regional ischemia is imposed routinely, with consequences to such phenotypic expressions of injury as regional contractile function, endothelial function, regional myocardial blood flow, neutrophil accumulation in the area at risk, and the appearance of apoptosis (49–52).

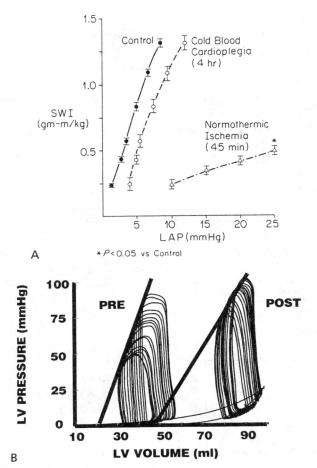

FIG. 13.3. Left ventricular performance measured by *in situ* Starling curves (**A**) or pressure–volume relations (**B**) after 45 minutes of unprotected ischemia and reperfusion. The ischemic time can be significantly extended (i.e., to 4 hours) by appropriate use of myocardial protection with intermittent hypothermic potassium blood cardioplegia (panel A). *SWI*, stroke work index; *LAP*, left atrial pressure. (Panel A data adapted from Rosenkranz ER, Buckberg GD. Myocardial protection during surgical coronary reperfusion. *J Am Coll Cardiol* 1983;1:1235–1246, with permission.)

Myocardial Oxygen Demand

Myocardial oxygen demand is determined by the work of the chamber of interest (e.g., stroke volume, aortic pressure, or wall stress for the left ventricle), heart rate, inotropic state, and minor factors, including basal metabolism, ionic homeostasis after electromechanical activity, and oxidative energy diverted to myocyte repair (in the postischemic heart). More recently, the pressure–volume relations as determinants of cardiac work have been used to describe oxygen requirements of the heart (53,54). Total CPB and diastolic arrest substantially reduce cardiac work by 50% or more, and oxygen demand is further reduced by hypothermia to minimize basal energy requirements. Ventricular decompression with venting the cardiac chamber further reduces the oxygen supply–demand mismatch in both

regional and global ischemia, thereby slowing the course of injury. In the specific case of acute coronary occlusion, reducing myocardial oxygen demands by CPB and venting can substantially delay the development of necrosis or other manifestations of injury, as wall stress from bulging imposes high energy demands on the myocardium at risk. These reductions in oxygen supply–demand mismatch and possible delays in the development of injury with techniques such as venting or hypothermia are not available in off-pump surgical techniques. Therefore, in the setting of coronary occlusive disease, substantial delays in revascularization may have a greater impact in off-pump procedures.

DETERMINANTS OF REPERFUSION INJURY

Although reperfusion of the myocardium is the ultimate goal of both surgical and nonsurgical revascularization, reperfusion carries with it the potential for extending postischemic injury to myocytes, coronary vascular endothelium, and the microvasculature. For the present discussion, we can define reperfusion injury as pathology that is extended or accelerated or that develops separately from that observed during ischemia, as a consequence of events occurring after restoration of blood flow. This definition is rather broad in that it takes into consideration the fact that the *rate* of injury in addition to the final long-term *extent* of injury may well be altered by reperfusion or reperfusion therapy. Deceleration of the rate of reperfusion injury in the early postoperative period may be important in counteracting myocardial "stunning," which is defined as postischemic contractile dysfunction in the absence of morphologic injury or necrosis. Although debate has often been spirited regarding whether reperfusion injury even exists (55–58), a consensus is developing that reperfusion is indeed an important component of postischemic myocardial injury in animals and humans (59,60). The concept of reperfusion injury is relatively new. In the years between 1966 and 1975, there was no mention of "reperfusion injury" in the literature; between 1976 and 1984, two articles mentioned reperfusion injury (both citations related to the kidney), and in the years between 1985 and 1989, there were 244 citations. During the last decade, however, there has been an explosion of research on the subject of reperfusion injury, with a total of 3,683 citations between 1990 and the writing of this chapter. The major players in reperfusion injury in addition to the therapeutic targets are being identified. Among the more important mechanisms in the pathophysiology of myocardial ischemia–reperfusion injury are (a) calcium influx and loss of normal intracellular calcium homeostasis, (b) neutrophils and neutrophil-derived products, (c) oxygen radicals generated not only by neutrophils but also by myocytes and vascular endothelium, and (d) edema. These mechanisms of injury do not operate independently, nor are they mutually exclusive. However, reperfusion injury is a malleable process that can be attenuated by utilizing a number of possible therapies targeting these various perpetrators of injury. In cardiac surgery in which extracorporeal circulation techniques are employed, therapeutic agents can be administered intravenously or by using cardioplegia as a vector for delivering agents. Extracorporeally supported cardioplegia techniques offer a unique opportunity to modify the *conditions* of reperfusion (hydrodynamics, temperature, route) and the *composition* of the solution (pH, metabolic substrates, hypocalcemia, oxygen, pharmaceuticals) that target the pathophysiologic mechanisms of injury. However, the recent interest in off-pump cardiac surgery imposes a formidable challenge to both surgical precision and myocardial protection in that most of the opportunities available with extracorporeal technology (i.e., cardioplegia solution, reducing the cardiac work load, hypothermia) are not available in the off-pump surgical armamentarium. Consequently, the current cardioprotective strategies designed during the past 25 years to attenuate reperfusion injury are somewhat disarmed or must be significantly revised. Mechanical or pharmacologic alternatives to restrict cardiac motion during off-pump procedures through bradycardia, temporary asystole (50), or stabilization devices are under investigation.

Calcium as a Mediator of Reperfusion Injury

Calcium dyshomeostasis during reperfusion is a significant factor contributing to postischemic myocardial injury and functional impairment (61,62). Under basal conditions, intracellular calcium concentrations are maintained at low levels (<200 nmol) against a 5,000-fold transsarcolemmal concentration gradient by voltage-gated calcium channels that remain closed until electrophysiologic activation (62). Increases in intracellular calcium occur primarily during reperfusion and are only minimally increased during relatively brief periods of ischemia (63,64). Rapid rises in cytosolic calcium during reperfusion result from uncontrolled calcium influx from both the extracellular space through L-type channels and via release from calcium stores in the sarcoplasmic reticulum (63,64). The physiologic consequences of calcium accumulation in the cytosol include depletion of high-energy phosphate stores required for adenosine triphosphate (ATP) production; activation of catalytic enzymes, leading to cellular injury; and alteration of calcium-related excitation–contraction coupling of the actin–myosin–troponin system, potentially leading to myocardial contracture and the phenomenon known as "stone heart."

The mechanisms for reperfusion-induced intracellular calcium overload are numerous and complex. Influx of calcium across the plasma membrane is normally controlled by both active and passive processes (Fig. 13.4). These balanced calcium transport systems are potentially injured by exposure to oxygen radicals, cytokines, and activated complement during reperfusion, which leads to calcium influx through multiple pathways: (a) diffusion through overt membrane disruptions or opened calcium channels, fueled by the differential concentration gradient of calcium; (b)

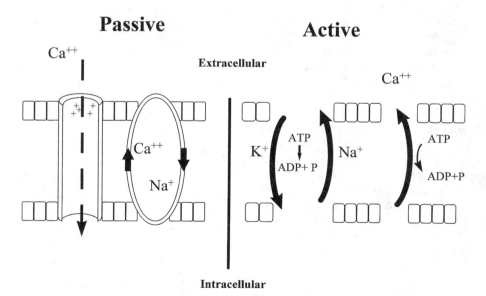

FIG. 13.4. Mechanisms of Ca^{2+} regulation involving transmembrane (plasmalemma) Ca^{2+} channels and Na$^+$-Ca^{2+} symporter (passive) and active exchange systems. The Na$^+$-K$^+$ exchange pump will, in part, regulate intracellular Na$^+$ and hence the movement of Ca^{2+} by the Na$^+$-Ca^{2+} exchange symporter. Active Ca^{2+} exchange by the expenditure of adenosine triphosphate also influences intracellular Ca^{2+} to some extent but drains energy.

facilitation of entry via α-adrenoreceptor activation and cyclic adenosine monophosphate (AMP)-dependent processes, which increase during postischemic catecholamine release; and (c) reversal or inhibition of the sodium–calcium exchanger driven by the intracellular accumulation of sodium.

Under normal physiologic conditions, uptake of cytosolic calcium into the sarcoplasmic reticulum (and to some extent into mitochondria) is a primary means of limiting intracellular calcium buildup. This calcium sequestration requires ATP. During both unprotected and cardioplegia-protected ischemia, sequestration of calcium into the sarcoplasmic reticulum competes for a limited amount of ATP. This paradox creates a cycle whereby a high intracellular calcium level binds high-energy phosphates to limit ATP availability, which then attenuates the ability of the sarcoplasmic reticulum to remove the calcium actively from the cytoplasm, resulting in a further increase in cytosolic calcium. Attenuating intracellular calcium accumulation during reperfusion is important to myocardial protection; strategies include reducing available extracellular calcium and altering ionic balances (K^+, Na^+, Mg^{2+}, Ca^{2+}) to favor the extracellular transport of calcium (65). Techniques to maximize the beneficial effects of hypocalcemia are summarized in the section on Strategies for Myocardial Protection.

Oxygen Radicals and Oxygen Radical-Mediated Injury

Molecular oxygen is relatively inert by virtue of the shared electron pair in the outer molecular shell. However, oxygen-derived free radicals, defined as molecules in which one unpaired electron is added to the outer shell of oxygen, are highly reactive with a broad range of biologic substrates including sugars, amino acids, phospholipids, and DNA (66). With such a large catalogue of biologic targets, oxygen-derived free radicals and their metabolites are potentially toxic to cells, and at the same time they are critical in the host defense mechanism and bactericidal activities of neutrophils and phagocytes (67). In the ischemic–reperfused myocardium, oxygen-derived free radical-induced injury includes peroxidation of lipid components of myocellular membranes (leading to damage to mitochondria and sarcoplasmic reticulum) (68,69) and impairment of vascular endothelial function through production of vasoactive and antiinflammatory autacoids such as adenosine (70,71) and NO (72). These injury mechanisms contribute significantly to postischemic dysfunction (73), dysrhythmias (74), morphologic injury (66), and necrosis (67).

Sources of Oxygen Radicals

Both enzymatic and nonenzymatic reactions produce oxygen radicals. Some of these reactions are listed in Table

13.1. The superoxide radical reacts robustly with biologic components and is produced by a number of sources, including mitochondria, the vascular endothelium, and activated neutrophils.

Mitochondria: The sequential univalent reduction of oxygen to H_2O (Table 13.1, Eq. 1) normally occurs in the electron transport chain at very low rates but is greatly accelerated during both ischemia and reperfusion (75).

Vascular endothelium: Superoxide anion is produced by the conversion of hypoxanthine to xanthine and uric acid by the enzyme xanthine oxidase (Table 13.1, Eq. 2). Normally, this enzyme exists mostly in the dehydrogenase form and uses nicotinamide adenine dinucleotide (NAD) as an electron acceptor (Table 13.1, Eq. 2A). During ischemia, however, two events favor the xanthine oxidase reaction: (a) hypoxanthine accumulates as a result of the sequential catabolism of purine high-energy phosphates (ATP, ADP, AMP) and deamination of adenosine, and (b) the dehydrogenase form of the enzyme is converted to the superoxide-producing oxidase form by a protease activated by increased levels of intracellular calcium (76). The biologic significance of this reaction in human endothelium remains controversial (77,78). A more important source of superoxide radicals originating from the vascular endothelium may be the NAD(P)H (reduced nicotinamide adenine dinucleotide phosphate) oxidase system. This enzyme is a membrane-bound, flavin-containing NADH/NADPH-dependent oxidase present in endothelial and vascular smooth-muscle cells. The molecular structure, function, and regulation are somewhat similar to those of the neutrophil enzyme system, requiring assembly of cytosolic components onto the membrane components before superoxide generation can occur. The NAD(P)H system is partially controlled by angiotensin II-mediated and also by nitrate-mediated activation of the renin–angiotensin system (79,80). However, superoxide anion production in the vicinity of NO production may favor the biradical neutralization and elimination of NO and the formation of peroxynitrite. The elimination of NO impairs not only vascular relaxation and autoregulatory control of postischemic myocardial perfusion, but also neutrophil-mediated postischemic inflammatory responses.

Neutrophils: Activated neutrophils represent the major source of oxygen-derived free radicals in the heart, including superoxide anion, hydrogen peroxide, and hypochlorous acid. Neutrophils are activated by various chemotactic factors stimulated by either CPB or ischemia–reperfusion [C3a and C5a anaphylatoxins, f-Met-Leu-Phe, interleukin-8 (IL-8), and platelet-activating factor], which triggers a "respiratory burst" with an increase in oxygen consumption and activation of the hexose monophosphate shunt. CPB (independently of ischemia) activates the complement cascade (81,82), with the subsequent activation of neutrophils (83) and their adherence-triggered release of cytotoxic products, all of which contribute to tissue injury in the ischemic–re-

TABLE 13.1. BIOCHEMICAL REACTIONS INVOLVED IN PRODUCTION OF OXYGEN FREE RADICALS

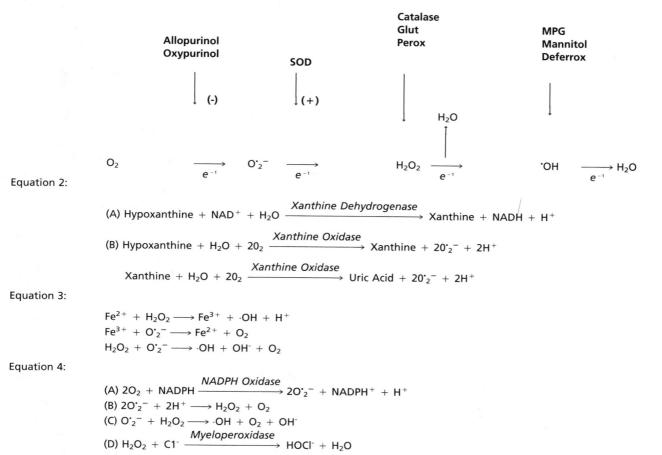

Equation 1:

Equation 2:

(A) Hypoxanthine $+ NAD^+ + H_2O \xrightarrow{\text{Xanthine Dehydrogenase}}$ Xanthine $+ NADH + H^+$

(B) Hypoxanthine $+ H_2O + 2O_2 \xrightarrow{\text{Xanthine Oxidase}}$ Xanthine $+ 2O_2^{\cdot-} + 2H^+$

Xanthine $+ H_2O + 2O_2 \xrightarrow{\text{Xanthine Oxidase}}$ Uric Acid $+ 2O_2^{\cdot-} + 2H^+$

Equation 3:

$Fe^{2+} + H_2O_2 \longrightarrow Fe^{3+} + \cdot OH + H^+$
$Fe^{3+} + O_2^{\cdot-} \longrightarrow Fe^{2+} + O_2$
$H_2O_2 + O_2^{\cdot-} \longrightarrow \cdot OH + OH^- + O_2$

Equation 4:

(A) $2O_2 + NADPH \xrightarrow{\text{NADPH Oxidase}} 2O_2^{\cdot-} + NADPH^+ + H^+$
(B) $2O_2^{\cdot-} + 2H^+ \longrightarrow H_2O_2 + O_2$
(C) $O_2^{\cdot-} + H_2O_2 \longrightarrow \cdot OH + O_2 + OH^-$
(D) $H_2O_2 + Cl^- \xrightarrow{\text{Myeloperoxidase}} HOCl^- + H_2O$

Equation 5:

$LH + R\cdot \longrightarrow L\cdot + RH$ — Initiation Phase (i.e., peroxidation by $\cdot OH$)

$L\cdot + O_2 \longrightarrow LO_2^{\cdot}$
$LH + LO_2^{\cdot} \rightarrow LOOH + L\cdot$ — Propagation Phase

$L\cdot + L\cdot \rightarrow LL$
$LO_2^{\cdot} + LO_2^{\cdot} \rightarrow LOOL + O_2$
$L_2^{\cdot} + L\cdot \rightarrow LOOL$ — Termination Phase

L, lipid; Glut Perox, glutathione peroxidase; SOD, copper-zinc superoxide dismutase; R, radical; Deferrox, deferroxamine; MPG, mercaptopropanyl glycine.

perfused myocardium (83,84). During the respiratory burst that occurs seconds after stimulation by cytokines or ischemia–reperfusion, the superoxide anion in the neutrophil is produced by a membrane-associated NADP oxidase, which transfers an electron to molecular oxygen (Table 13.1, Eq. 4A). Production of hydrogen peroxide (Table 13.1, Eq. 4B) by neutrophils or reduction of superoxide to hydrogen peroxide by superoxide dismutase (SOD) pro-

vides substrate for hydroxyl radical (Table 13.1, Eq. 4C) or the oxidant hypochlorous acid by myeloperoxidase (Table 13.1, Eq. 4D). Hypochlorous acid reacts with low-molecular-weight amines to give rise to lipophilic chloramines, which can promote membrane lipid peroxidation.

Other sources of oxygen-derived free radicals include the oxidation of catecholamines, metabolism of arachidonic acid to peroxy compounds and hydroxyl radicals by the cyclooxygenase and lipoxygenase pathways, and by the metal-catalyzed Haber-Weiss reactions. The latter series of reactions (Table 13.1, Eq. 3) may be important in the setting of CPB because they can be recruited by neutrophil activation during CPB (85). In addition, iron-containing products released by hemolysis may facilitate this reaction.

When Are Oxygen Radicals Generated?

Myocardial ischemia, whether induced globally by aortic cross-clamping or regionally by coronary artery occlusion, favors the generation of oxygen free radicals. In addition, tissue concentrations of the endogenous antioxidants superoxide dismutase, catalase, glutathione, and glutathione peroxidase are depleted during ischemia, thereby attenuating the natural defense mechanisms of the heart (86–88). Therefore, ischemia creates the biochemical setting for oxyradical production and tissue vulnerability to oxygen radical-mediated damage. However, the primary substrate, oxygen, is in scant supply during ischemia and is not readily available until reperfusion. The appearance of a "burst" of oxygen radicals on reperfusion is supported by both direct and indirect evidence. Direct evidence of oxygen radical production *in vivo* has been obtained by electron spin resonance spectroscopy (89). These studies show that oxygen radicals are produced to some extent during ischemia, but a more significant respiratory burst occurs during the early phase of reperfusion followed by decreased production for several hours thereafter (89–91). Indirect evidence to support this reperfusion oxidative burst comes from a wealth of data in which inhibitors or scavengers of oxygen radicals, or antineutrophil agents, demonstrated beneficial effects when administered during reperfusion (92–99).

In the surgical setting, the myocardium may be vulnerable to oxygen radical-induced injury at several points when oxygen is introduced into the myocardium: (a) initial induction delivery of cardioplegia into the heart with antecedent unprotected ischemia, or initial delivery of oxygenated cardioplegia to a newly revascularized myocardial segment; (b) intermittent reinfusions of cardioplegia if a multidose strategy is being used; and (c) release of the aortic cross-clamp to initiate normothermic reperfusion. The quantity of oxygen radicals generated during cardiac surgery depends on the severity of ischemic injury, activation and recruitment of neutrophils to the myocardium, the level of oxygen in cardioplegic (or blood) solutions, and the status of endogenous scavengers and inhibitors (depleted during ischemia). Blood cardioplegia theoretically provides a greater oxygen substrate for oxygen radical production than do crystalloid solutions. However, plasma-dissolved oxygen may be the pool from which oxygen is drawn for the generation of oxygen radicals, and the oxygen content in this compartment may not differ dramatically between blood and crystalloid solutions. The oxygen in blood cardioplegia used as substrate for oxygen radical production may be reduced

with "normoxic" blood cardioplegia (100,101). In addition, blood cardioplegia may offer the advantage of endogenous antioxidants (superoxide dismutase, catalase, glutathione, albumin) that are not present in crystalloid cardioplegia solutions.

Neutrophils and Neutrophil-Mediated Injury

Neutrophils play a critical role in the pathogenesis of myocardial reperfusion injury (34,102–104). The inflammatory component of reperfusion injury requires an interaction between activated neutrophils and vascular endothelium during the early moments of reperfusion, which is prerequisite to activation of the full inflammatory cascade. A well-orchestrated sequence of events mediates the interaction between adhesion molecules on neutrophils and endothelium (Fig. 13.5). These adhesion molecules are categorized into three families.

I. The selectins (P-selectin, L-selectin, E-selectin) are glycoproteins involved in the interactions between neutrophils and the endothelium in the early moments of reperfusion (0 to 15 minutes) (105–109). P-selectin is stored in endothelial cells, and its surface expression is triggered by proinflammatory mediators such as oxygen radicals (110), thrombin (111), complement components, histamine, and hydrogen peroxide released during ischemia–reperfusion and CPB (112,113). In addition, IL-8 (released from hypoxic endothelial cells following ischemia or CPB) also increases the adhesiveness of endothelial cells for neutrophils (114–116). P-selectin surface expression peaks after 10 to 20 minutes of reperfusion, and P-selectin is subsequently shed to soluble fragments in blood. In contrast to P-selectin, L-selectin is constitutively expressed on the surface of neutrophils and may be the counterligand for P-selectin during early reperfusion (117). Loose adherence and "rolling" of neutrophils on endothelium (Fig. 13.5) may involve interaction with a glycoprotein sialyl Lewis^x or a high-affinity glycoprotein ligand termed P-selectin glycoprotein ligand-1 (PSGL-1) (118). The third member of the selectin family, E-selectin, is expressed on the surface of endothelial cells. It is expressed later in reperfusion (4 to 6 hours) and may therefore be involved in later events, such as infarct extension.

II. The β_2-integrins (CD11/CD18 complex) are a family of glycoproteins located on external membranes of neutrophils. There are three distinct α-chains (CD11a, CD11b, CD11c) and a common β-subunit. Surface expression of perhaps the major complex CD11b/CD18 is triggered by a number of proinflammatory mediators, including circulating and endothelium-derived (acylated) platelet-activating factor. After initial tethering of neutrophils by endothelial P-selectin, firm adherence is mediated by interaction with CD11b/CD18 and its counterligand ICAM-1 on the endothelium (Fig. 13.5).

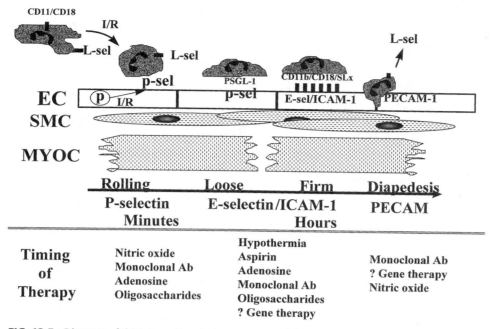

FIG. 13.5. Diagram of the interactions between neutrophils and endothelium (*EC*) with reference to the adhesion molecules on both cell types mediating the interactions during early (minutes) and later (hours, days) reperfusion events. Neutrophils can be recruited toward the endothelium by proinflammatory mediators such as platelet-activating factor, complement products released by blood–extracorporeal surface interactions, or ischemia–reperfusion (*IR*). In addition, the endothelium is activated by proinflammatory mediators such as thrombin, histamine, and superoxide anions, which increase the surface expression of P-selectin (*p, p-sel*). The early response of rolling involves selectin-mediated [P-selectin, L-selectin (*L-sel*)] loose adherence, whereas later firm adherence and diapedesis (transendothelial neutrophil migration) are mediated by E-selectin (*E-sel*), intercellular adhesion molecule-1 (*ICAM-1*) and platelet–endothelial cell adhesion molecule-1 (*PECAM-1*) receptors on endothelium, and CD11b/CD18/SL^x (sialyl Lewis^x) on neutrophils. Timing of therapy: Agents that attenuate neutrophil–endothelial cell interactions are listed below the mechanism inhibited. For example, nitric oxide inhibits P-selectin-mediated rolling and diapedesis. *MYOC*, myocytes; *SMC*, smooth-muscle cells; *Ab*, antibodies.

III. The third family of adhesion molecules is the immunoglobulin superfamily, including ICAM-1 (intercellular adhesion molecule-1), VCAM-1 (vascular cell adhesion molecule-1), and PECAM-1 (platelet–endothelial cell adhesion molecule-1). ICAM-1, the counterligand for CD11/CD18 on neutrophils, is constitutively expressed on endothelial cells and is upregulated by cytokines 2 to 4 hours after myocardial ischemia–reperfusion (119,120), coincidentally with the upregulation of CD11/CD18. Subsequently, a high-affinity bond between the neutrophil and endothelial cell occurs via integrins (CD11/CD18) on neutrophils and ICAM-1 and ICAM-2 on endothelial cells. Once the neutrophil has firmly attached to the endothelial surface, it migrates through the endothelial cell junctions to the myocardium, partly mediated by IL-8 (121). The shedding of L-selectin from the neutrophil and the presence of PECAM on the endothelium may be required for neutrophil transendothelial migration. The prerequisite nature of this interaction mediated by adhesion molecules for the propagation of inflammatory response makes antineutrophil and antiadhesion therapy a new and potentially very effective strategy, as these agents intervene at proximal points in the cascade (discussed below). Figure 13.5 lists some of these potential strategies.

Evidence supporting the rapid accumulation of neutrophils within ischemic–reperfused myocardium following the neutrophil–endothelial cell interactions was appreciated not only by our laboratory, but also by Sommers and Jennings (122). We (123–125) and others (126–128) have demonstrated an association between the extent of postischemic injury and neutrophil accumulation within ischemic–reperfused myocardium as well as a reduction of postischemic injury associated with neutrophil suppression. As shown in Fig. 13.6, Lefer et al. (102) demonstrated that neutrophils accumulate within the myocardial region destined to become necrotic and that neutrophil accumulation occurs in advance of the development of necrosis, suggesting active neutrophil participation in cell demise.

The importance of neutrophils in post-bypass reperfusion injury has been well established in animal and human

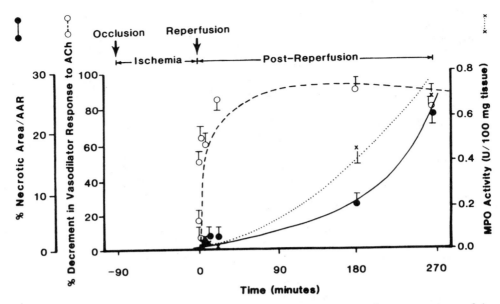

FIG. 13.6. The postischemic time course of endothelial injury measured as a percentage of decrease in vasodilator responses to agonist stimulation of nitric oxide synthase [*ACh* (acetylcholine), *dashed line*], neutrophil accumulation assessed by tissue myeloperoxidase activity (*MPO, dotted line*) and percentage of the myocardial area at risk undergoing necrosis [*necrotic area/AAR (%)*] in a model of coronary artery occlusion (ischemia) and reperfusion. (From Lefer AM, Tsai PS, Lefer DJ, et al. Role of endothelial dysfunction in the pathogenesis of reperfusion injury after myocardial ischemia. *FASEB J* 1991;5:2029–2034, with permission.)

models. The myocardium is exposed to neutrophils during the delivery of intermittent or continuous blood cardioplegia, or during reperfusion (after cross-clamp removal) following either crystalloid or blood cardioplegia. Schwartz et al. (129) showed that CPB circuitry directly "primes" neutrophils by depositing C3b on extracorporeal tubing, leading to neutrophil activation and sequestration. Further evidence for the activation of neutrophils following CPB was suggested by the finding of increased neutrophil surface expression of CD11b/CD18 and decreased surface expression of L-selectin on cells circulated in simulated CPB circuits (130,131). Studies in animal models (132,133) and humans (134–136) showed that the surface expression of CD11b/CD18 on peripheral blood neutrophils and monocytes increases following CPB (CPB). Finn et al. (135) noted in patients undergoing CPB that a rise in circulating IL-8 begins at reperfusion with rewarming of the patient after systemic hypothermia and closely correlates with the rise in neutrophil count and circulating elastase. Similarly, Schwartz et al. (129) found higher levels of soluble IL-6 and IL-8 6 hours after bypass than before bypass.

The time course for the upregulation of neutrophils and various adhesion molecules is equally important in designing treatment strategies for patients undergoing extracorporeal bypass. In a clinical study, Galiñanes et al. (137) investigated the perioperative temporal changes in the expression of various neutrophil surface adhesion molecules, concluding that downregulation of PECAM-1 is an early indicator

of neutrophil activation and may therefore represent a target for therapy aimed at reducing the inflammatory response associated with CPB.

The role of temperature in the activation of neutrophils or other inflammatory mediators following CPB in humans has not been clearly elucidated. Some investigators have reported minimal or no difference in neutrophil activation and expression of neutrophil adhesion molecules between normothermic (34° to 37°C) and hypothermic (28° to 30°C) CPB (138,139), whereas others note an attenuation in the expression of IL-8 and neutrophil elastase activity during normothermic cardiopulmonary surgery (140). In contrast, hypothermia has been shown to delay, but not prevent, the increased expression of adhesion molecules such as CD11b and CD11c (138). When measured 4 hours after bypass, the levels of IL-1ra, soluble ICAM-1 (sICAM-1), and elastase are higher after normothermic CPB than after hypothermic CPB (141,142). In conclusion, further research is required to determine the most appropriate temperature of cardioplegic administration to minimize the deleterious consequences of neutrophil-mediated damage. Interventions designed to attenuate neutrophil-related myocardial injury following CPB will be discussed later.

Complement in Cardiopulmonary Bypass and Myocardial Reperfusion Injury

The complement cascade, particularly the alternative pathway, is activated independently by myocardial ischemia–reperfusion and CPB and contributes importantly to the pathologic sequelae of CPB (133,143–145). Complement fragments such as the anaphylatoxins C3a and C5a are generated and released both systemically and locally by the ischemic–reperfused myocardium (146,147). The activation and migration of neutrophils to ischemic–reperfused myocardium requires stimulation by chemotactic factors, most notably complement fragments (C3a and C5a), eicosanoid products such as leukotriene B_4, and platelet-activating factor (148,149). Complement fragments (C5a) can be found in lymph from ischemic myocardium (150), are temporally associated with reperfusion (151), and correlate with increased neutrophil accumulation in reperfused myocardium. Furthermore, C5a directly stimulates neutrophil superoxide production and enhances adherence to coronary artery endothelium (152), whereas C3 activates monocyte adherence (153). The chemoattractant and chemotactic properties of C5a cause progressive generalized vascular leukosequestration (154) during CPB (81). The interaction between blood and extracorporeal surfaces also stimulates deposition of the complement component C3b (143,145,155), which in turn amplifies the complement alternative pathway to release C3a and C5a and subsequently form the membrane attack complex (C5b–9) (155). Accordingly, plasma levels of the anaphylatoxin C5a increase in patients undergoing CPB (155,156), which activates neutrophils to generate superoxide anions and promote adhesion to endothelial cells, stimulates degranulation of mast cells, stimulates vascular smooth-muscle contraction, and increases vascular permeability. Complement activation constitutes an early-phase response to CPB (36), which then progresses to a second, slower response phase in which *de novo* synthesis of proteins (E-selectin, ICAM, IL-8) and expression of adhesion molecules on cell surfaces occurs. The magnitude of the complement response has been linked to the duration of CPB (143) and the type of circuitry used (156). The combined stimuli of myocardial ischemia–reperfusion and CPB may synergize to exacerbate postischemic neutrophil-mediated inflammatory responses in patients undergoing CPB for myocardial revascularization. Neutrophils damage coronary vascular endothelium, myocytes, pulmonary tissue, and other organs.

Myocardial Edema

Myocardial ischemia and reperfusion are associated with unfavorable alterations in the physiologic mechanisms that regulate intracellular and interstitial fluid balance. Specifically, certain aspects of these mechanisms, including the Starling forces governing tissue fluid movement, lymphatic drainage, and cell membrane function, are altered, leading to the development of myocardial edema. The composition of cardioplegic solutions (onconicity, hemodilution) and the conditions of delivery (hypothermia, high delivery pressure) are known to exaggerate the development of edema resulting from ischemia or systemic inflammatory responses

(26,157–159). Although the pathophysiology involved in producing myocardial edema during ischemia–reperfusion injury has not been completely elucidated, Garcia-Dorado et al. (160) and others (161,162) have observed an increase in myocardial water content following coronary occlusion in animal models. Potential mechanisms of myocardial edema during ischemia–reperfusion include the following: (a) increased intracellular osmotic pressure secondary to an accumulation of metabolic end-products of anaerobic glycolysis, lipolysis, and ATP hydrolysis; (b) interference during ischemia with the maintenance of electrical potentials across cell membranes, in which an intracellular accumulation of Na^+ and Cl^- leads to a movement of water into the intracellular space (163,164); (c) increases in both microvascular permeability and osmotic pressure within the interstitial space (165).

Edema may increase microvascular resistance to a point of impeding blood flow (no-reflow phenomenon, discussed below) and increase diffusion distance to myofibrils, leading to inadequate oxygen delivery. Edema can arise with the use of cardioplegic solutions, especially in ischemic myocardium, because of (a) high delivery pressures, particularly in severely damaged myocardium; (b) hemodilution and hypoosmolarity from crystalloid primes or crystalloid cardioplegia solutions; and (c) physiologic changes in ionic pump systems (i.e., Na^+-K^+-ATPase) or Donnan equilibrium for chloride ions induced by hypothermia. Although normal myocardium tolerates relatively high infusion pressures (159,166), myocardium within (167,168) and surrounding (169) ischemic segments is vulnerable to edema induced by high delivery pressure. The extent to which reperfusion with unmodified blood following CPB induces myocardial edema depends primarily on the duration and severity of the previous ischemic episode (158,160). On reperfusion, the normo-osmotic blood quickly displaces the hyperosmotic intravascular fluid, creating an osmotic gradient between the intravascular and extravascular spaces that results in myocardial edema (170). Myocardial edema following ischemia and reperfusion is also partly caused by an influx of Na^+ ions into the cell, accompanied by interstitial water. Correspondingly, the Na^+-H^+ exchanger plays a major role in producing a net influx of Na^+ into the cell, which leads to myocardial edema (171–174). Inhibition of this Na^+-H^+ exchange system has been shown to decrease postischemic myocardial edema (175).

Microvascular Injury and the "No-Reflow" Response

One of the physiologic consequences of reperfusion injury is impaired microvascular blood flow. In 1974, Kloner et al. (176) described the "no-reflow" phenomenon as a derangement in postischemic blood flow to the myocardium at risk despite resolution of the coronary obstruction. The etiologies of the "no-reflow" or "low-reflow" phenomenon include postischemic tissue edema, interstitial hemorrhage, active vasoconstriction from loss of endothelium-derived vasodilators and release of neutrophil-derived vasoconstrictors, and capillary plugging by adherent or embolized neutrophils. Microvascular injury and postischemic defects in myocardial blood flow may be a reperfusion phenomenon because (a) the absence of a significant perfusion pressure during ischemia prevents the migration of fluid out of the extravascular space, so that edematous fluid fails to accumulate significantly (177), and (b) endothelial damage with adherence and trapping of neutrophils and loss of NO-induced regulation of vascular resistance occurs during the early moments of reperfusion (102,178,179).

Tissue edema: Ischemia places the microcirculation in a "leaky" state that allows extravasation of fluid into the extravascular spaces. With reperfusion, the Starling forces regulating transcapillary fluid movement shift in favor of the formation of interstitial edema. In addition, the combined effects of endothelial cell swelling and extravascular compression of capillaries by tissue edema may cause severe impairment of microvascular perfusion and precipitation of the no-reflow response (180).

Endothelial cell injury: Normally, the endothelium secretes vasodilators such as adenosine and NO, which help regulate microcirculatory vascular resistance. After ischemia–reperfusion injury, impaired secretion of these endothelium-derived vasodilator factors may lead to unopposed microcirculatory vasoconstriction, which perpetuates the no-reflow phenomenon (181). In addition to loss of vasodilators, the secretion of endothelin-1 by the endothelium, the most powerful vasoconstrictor yet identified, markedly increases following hypoxia and reoxygenation (182) and may contribute to collapse of the microcirculation within the no-reflow myocardial zone.

Capillary plugging: Engler and colleagues (183) showed that during reperfusion, neutrophils plugged up to 27% of the microcirculatory capillaries, thereby decreasing regional blood flow after reperfusion. This observation was not observed with leukocyte-depleted blood reperfusion.

The initial delivery pressure during reperfusion has been implicated as a potential contributor to the no-reflow phenomenon. In a canine model of 2 hours of coronary occlusion and 2 hours of reperfusion, our laboratory (167,184) has shown that abrupt restoration of coronary perfusion pressure to systemic levels is associated with a progressive diminution of early microvascular reactive hyperemia to 50% of preischemic blood flow. In contrast, gradual restoration of coronary reperfusion pressure during the first 30 minutes of reperfusion preserves postischemic reactive hyperemic flow, reduces infarct size, and improves segmental systolic and diastolic function, even after restoration of normal perfusion pressures. Therefore, although the evolution of the no-reflow or low-reflow condition is primarily a reperfusion event involved in the development of secondary ischemia (inadequate delivery of blood flow) and myocardial

infarction, it can be attenuated by controlling hydrodynamic conditions of perfusion (26,185).

MANIFESTATIONS OF REPERFUSION INJURY

The multiple etiologies of reperfusion injury following nonsurgical or surgical reperfusion can also present as numerous abnormalities in electrophysiology, contractile function, biochemistry, and morphology. The clinical manifestations of reperfusion injury, separate from those of ischemic injury, can be grouped into the categories listed below.

Reperfusion Dysrhythmias

Arrhythmias precipitated following reperfusion are expressed as premature ventricular contractions and ventricular fibrillation. Failure of spontaneous resumption of sinus rhythm, ventricular fibrillation, and persistence of dysrhythmias requiring direct-current countershock and antidysrhythmic therapy are common consequences of poor myocardial protection or injury. A number of mechanisms are involved in the genesis of reperfusion dysrhythmias. First, as with many reperfusion-related events, the incidence and severity of reperfusion dysrhythmias relate to the severity of the preceding ischemia. The relationship is characterized by a bell-shaped response curve, in which vulnerability is maximal after short intervals of normothermic ischemia induce reversible changes, then decreases as irreversible injury and electrical silence develop with more prolonged ischemia (74). Second, an accumulation of intracellular calcium during ischemia may interfere with normal calcium cycling at the level of the sarcoplasmic reticulum (calcium-dependent arrhythmias) (186). Third, oxygen-derived free radicals such as superoxide anion and hydroxyl radicals, produced as a respiratory burst by mitochondria, endothelium, or neutrophils during reperfusion, can damage membrane lipids and various transport proteins involved in ionic homeostasis, which in turn can precipitate reperfusion-related dysrhythmias (95,187–189). Current hypotheses merge the calcium-related events and the oxygen free radical events as "interacting triggers" for reperfusion dysrhythmias (190).

Postischemic Systolic and Diastolic Dysfunction

Reperfusion with unmodified blood (and minimally modified cardioplegia) following short periods of normothermic regional (124,191–193) or global (194–196) ischemia produces a severe degree of contractile dysfunction (Fig. 13.3). However, short periods of ischemia followed by unmodified reperfusion may be benign in regard to contractile function but injurious to other targets (endothelium, neutrophil accumulation) (49). Readily reversible (within hours) postischemic contractile dysfunction can occur in the absence of obvious morphologic injury and may therefore be "stunned," whereas longer periods of ischemia are associated with both morphologic injury (necrosis, creatine kinase release) and persistent contractile dysfunction. Previously, postischemic contractile dysfunction was thought to be attributable to a depletion of high-energy phosphate supply (i.e., ATP). However, numerous studies have failed to show a direct correlation between postischemic myocardial ATP levels and contractile function (abnormality or recovery) (197–199). The ATP turnover rate, roughly approximated by myocardial oxygen consumption, may be more important than the static tissue level of ATP. Postischemic regional and global oxygen consumption may be near normal (200) or augmented (46,201,202) despite significantly reduced levels of ATP. Although segmental work may account for these relatively elevated oxygen consumption values in the newly reperfused segment following reversible coronary occlusion, elevated global oxygen consumption in bypassed and vented hearts may be in part related to diversion of oxygen to support reparative processes, inefficient calcium cycling, and increased energy expenditure to reestablish ionic homeostasis. Alternatively, postischemic contractile dysfunction has been related to impairment of calcium kinetics in excitation–contraction coupling and in the sarcoplasmic reticulum (68,69,203). In addition to these pathologic origins of postischemic systolic contractile dysfunction, iatrogenic dysfunction related to CPB *per se* may occur as a result of systemic hemodilution (reduced oxygen delivery) and hyperkalemia, or as a result of systemic hypocalcemia caused by calcium-chelating agents in cardioplegia solutions (204).

Myocardial diastolic characteristics (compliance or chamber stiffness, rate of relaxation) are highly sensitive to ischemia and reperfusion (205). In the myocardial segment subjected to ischemia, there is a rightward shift in the position of the end-diastolic pressure–segment length relation, with little change in the shape or curvature of the end-diastolic pressure–segment length relation (Fig. 13.3), which is consistent with the concept of regional myocardial "creep" (123,157). Other reports show little or no change in segmental stiffness after up to 1 hour of coronary occlusion (185,193) unless the ischemia is very severe (loss of endogenous cardioprotection with autacoids adenosine or NO) (193). In contrast to ischemia, reperfusion is associated with immediate loss of myocardial compliance (193), characterized by a leftward shift and increase in slope of the exponential pressure–segment length relationship (indicating a relative degree of "contracture"). A similar pattern is observed with global ischemia. In several studies in which hearts were sensitized to ischemia–reperfusion injury by 30 minutes of normothermic ischemia preceding 1 hour of hypothermic (4°C) multidose blood cardioplegia, a rightward shift in the end-diastolic pressure–dimension relations (dilation) and increased chamber stiffness (201,206–208) were noted after blood reperfusion. Acute increases in postischemic chamber

stiffness are caused by myocardial edema and abnormal calcium handling in the myocardium. A decrease in diastolic relaxation impairs diastolic ventricular filling, which reduces stroke volume independently of any postischemia or postcardioplegia abnormalities in inotropic state or contractility.

Myocardial Necrosis

The question of whether reperfusion kills cells that at the time are reversibly damaged and theoretically salvageable before the initiation of reperfusion is at the very crux of the reperfusion injury controversy. Demonstration of cell viability and "salvage" in the multidimensional and dynamic process of myocellular necrosis is fraught with its own problems. Are markers such as released enzymes (creatine kinase, lactate dehydrogenase) accurate in assessing myocardial injury in global models and capable of providing chronologic "repeated measures" of developing injury? Does conventional electron microscopy introduce artifactual injury to the tissue and lead to the conclusion that irreversible injury has been sustained? Does a reduction in any marker of injury represent a permanent reduction in the extent of myocyte injury or simply a delay in the progression of necrosis? This latter distinction is important because some agents merely delay the time course of injury with no ultimate reduction of infarct size or salvage of myocytes, although a delay in myocyte demise does have important implications for the patient with a stormy postoperative course early after the discontinuation of bypass.

Endothelial Dysfunction

The general assumption has been that the consequences of ischemia–reperfusion injury affect primarily the cardiac myocyte. However, recent data indicate that ischemia and reperfusion affect other cell types in the heart, and that the degree of injury sustained by these other tissues partly determines the severity of postischemic myocardial injury. For example, the vascular endothelium of both arteries (102,209–211) and veins (104) sustains significant injury during ischemia and reperfusion and may be the primary site of complement activation and neutrophil activity after ischemia and reperfusion. This dysfunction may persist beyond the immediate acute phase of reperfusion (209) for days and weeks (212) following ischemia–reperfusion. Therefore, endothelial dysfunction plays a critical role in the pathogenesis of reperfusion injury in the myocardium (34,103). The vascular endothelium is not an inert "cellophane" layer separating the intravascular and interstitial compartments (213), but is rather a factory for numerous vasoactive autacoids (notably NO and adenosine) that regulate vascular tone, cell growth, and the interaction between vascular tissue and inflammatory blood cells. Ischemia–reperfusion reduces both basal and stimulated NO release by the coronary endothelium (39,127,214). Impaired release

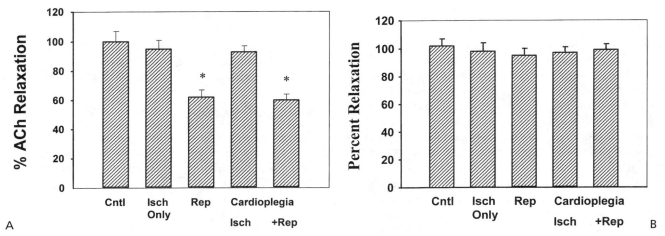

FIG. 13.7. Relaxation responses of postcardioplegia epicardial coronary arteries preconstricted with U46619 to agonist stimulators of nitric oxide synthase. **A:** Maximal relaxation responses to acetylcholine (*ACh*), an endothelium-dependent, receptor-dependent agonist. **B:** Maximal relaxation responses to the direct (endothelium-independent) vascular smooth-muscle–relaxing agent acidified $NaNO_2$. *Cntl,* normal control vessel; *Isch only,* after 45 minutes global normothermic ischemia (no reperfusion); *Rep,* ischemia followed by 1 hour of unmodified blood reperfusion; *Cardioplegia + Isch,* 45 minutes global normothermic ischemia followed by 1 hour of intermittent (every 20 minutes) 4°C hyperkalemic blood cardioplegia (four parts blood to one part crystalloid) without blood reperfusion; *Cardioplegia + Rep,* global ischemia plus 1 hour of cardioplegia as described above, followed by 1 hour of blood reperfusion. *$p < 0.05$ vs. unstarred groups. (From Nakanishi K, Zhao Z-Q, Vinten-Johansen J, et al. Coronary artery endothelial dysfunction after ischemia, blood cardioplegia, and reperfusion. *Ann Thorac Surg* 1994;58:191–199, with permission.)

of NO is expressed physiologically as an increase in the adherence of neutrophils to the surface of the endothelium and impaired vasodilator responses to endothelium-specific stimulators of NO synthase, such as acetylcholine. Decreases in *in vitro* NO, measured directly following ischemia–reperfusion, parallel the increased adherence of neutrophils to coronary artery endothelium and blunted endothelium-dependent vasodilator responses to acetylcholine and bradykinin (124,178,215,216). Figure 13.7 shows coronary artery segment function following 45 minutes of global normothermic ischemia with and without blood reperfusion. Endothelial function, assayed as maximal vasorelaxation response to the endothelium-dependent, receptor-dependent agonist acetylcholine, was not significantly reduced in hearts subjected to ischemia without subsequent reperfusion, but were significantly reduced in reperfused hearts in comparison with controls (Fig. 13.7A) (39). These data suggest that endothelial damage occurs during reperfusion rather than during short-term ischemia. More prolonged global ischemia damages the coronary endothelium (214). Similar impaired responses are observed following regional ischemia and reperfusion (124,210). At least a portion of this postcardioplegia endothelial dysfunction may be induced by CPB *per se*. Zanaboni et al. (217) reported that pulmonary endothelial function is impaired 3 to 4 days after exposure to CPB. Inflammatory mediators (218) and gaseous microemboli (219) may be involved in this endothelial injury.

Apoptosis

Apoptosis, or genetically programmed cell death, as opposed to the explosive and inflammation-initiating process of cellular necrosis (220), is known to occur in the heart during failure (221), infarction (222), and ischemia–reperfusion of the myocardium (223,224) through a change in the expression of specific gene products and production of specific cytoplasmic proteins (225). Some studies (224,226) have shown that ischemia with reperfusion, but not ischemia alone, induces apoptosis of the myocardium; hypoxia is also a stimulus for apoptosis (227). Although it is recognized that cytokines and hypoxia may stimulate myocardial apoptosis, it is not known whether apoptosis is a significant consequence of CPB or cardioplegia, or whether apoptosis contributes to endothelial dysfunction or myocardial contractile dysfunction.

STRATEGIES FOR MYOCARDIAL PROTECTION

Role of Cardioplegia in Reducing Surgical Ischemic–Reperfusion Injury

Cardioplegia offers selective perfusion to the heart and the administration of agents in higher concentrations that may not be well tolerated by other organ systems or systemically without complications (e.g., hypotension). During selective cardiac delivery, drugs at cardioactive or antiinflammatory concentrations may be rendered benign to other organs after admixture and dilution with systemic blood. This is certainly the case with the most basic component of cardioplegia, potassium, which is often administered at five times the normal blood concentration. It is important to understand that cardioplegia exerts cardioprotection during *both* ischemia and reperfusion because of the intimate link between ischemic injury (which sets the stage for later injury) and reperfusion injury. Cardioplegia exerts cardioprotection by modifying the *conditions of reperfusion* and the *composition of the reperfusate*. In its simplest formulations, cardioplegia avoids ischemic injury primarily in that it reduces oxygen demand to less than 10% of that of the working heart by (a) rapidly initiating hypothermia, (b) producing immediate asystole, (c) providing intermittent reoxygenation (multidose regimens), and (d) improving anaerobic metabolism (228). Cardioplegia also avoids reperfusion injury by targeting specifically the pathophysiologic mechanisms and mediators involved in the pathogenesis of postischemic injury. Beneficial modifications to the *conditions* of cardioplegia infusion apply to infusion pressure and volume, duration of infusion, and temperature of the solution. Modifications to the composition of cardioplegia (perfusion) and reperfusion include addition of metabolic substrates, osmotic agents, buffers, and pharmacologic agents. Finally, cardioplegia can be viewed as a vector for pharmacologic therapies to the heart with agents that target a specific aspect of either ischemic or reperfusion injury.

The inclusion of any pharmacologic agent in a cardioplegic solution should be based on scientific principles tested in the laboratory and supported by literature. There should be a defined *target(s)* toward which the agent or additive is aimed. This target can be the trigger of injury, a mechanism that perpetuates or amplifies injury, or a cellular victim of injury (myocyte, endothelium). The timing of pharmaceutical delivery is also very important (229); to administer a pharmacologic agent either before or after the occurrence of its targeted event is a missed opportunity. If the therapy is designed to exert actions on mechanisms operative during ischemia, administration of the agent at reperfusion or after declamping may be ineffective. For example, agents that activate K_{ATP} channels on myocytes may be ineffective when given during reperfusion (230,231). In addition, if an agent exerts cardioprotection during multiple time windows (before treatment, during ischemia or reperfusion), then administration at only one window truncates its effectiveness. For example, an opportunity is missed if adenosine, a potent cardioprotective autacoid, is given only before treatment and during ischemia, and not during reperfusion, timing that fails to take advantage of the potent antiinflammatory effects of adenosine (229,232). Although adenosine has been shown to exert a portion of its effects before and during ischemia, it also exerts significant cardioprotective effects during reperfusion. To target a specific mechanism, the appropriate time for action must be understood and the agent added at the appropriate time. In addition to the appropriate timing of administration, the appropriate physiologic environment, such as hypothermia versus normothermia or blood versus crystalloid, must also exist. Although hypothermia has numerous advantages, as discussed below, it also reduces membrane fluidity and potentially attenuates the ligand–receptor interactions on which the effects of many drugs depend. Therefore, the effectiveness of certain cardioprotective drugs can be attenuated when hypothermic strategies are used. Finally, adequate delivery is extremely important because the cardioplegic formulation cannot exert the effect for which it is designed if it is not adequately delivered to the target area (e.g., because of maldistribution of cardioplegia solution or shunting).

Role of the Surgeon in Myocardial Protection

As a subdiscipline of cardiac surgery, myocardial protection involves the skillful application of techniques designed to protect the heart from injury. These techniques are based on the use of solutions containing various additives at varying temperatures, with the promise of newer, more effective additives in the future. However, the skill and judgment of the surgeon in the application of available tools constitute a critical component of myocardial protection. The most sophisticated cardioplegic solution is rendered useless if it does not reach the affected myocardium. However, diligence in the application of myocardial protective techniques should not take precedence over the goals and purpose of the operation. The purpose of cardiac surgery is not to practice myocardial protection, but an appropriate protective strategy is necessary for the successful completion of any procedure.

Because the heart has enormous functional reserve, normal ventricles may tolerate injury associated with a loss of function. However, when ventricular performance is marginally matched to the physiologic needs of an individual patient, small decrements in myocardial function translate into morbidity and mortality. Four fundamental factors in myocardial protection interact with variables such as temperature, composition of the solution, state of the heart, CPB conditions, and patient-specific conditions. These factors include (a) rapid arrest, (b) prolonged electromechanical quiescence, (c) minimalization of ischemia, and (d) control of reperfusion. Each of these four factors is complex. When they are considered together with the chemical and physical options for myocardial protection, the number of variables is great, and it becomes impossible to provide a formula-driven recipe for myocardial protection. Rather, successful protection requires a combination of good myocardial physiologic preparation by the surgeon, a clear understanding of the principles of ischemia and reperfusion, and "intuition," individualized for each surgeon, that influences "surgical thinking and judgment." Individual practitioners determine which "trade-offs" they are most comfortable accepting and modify myocardial protective technique accordingly.

For example, one surgeon may enjoy the comfort associated with strongly hypothermic conditions—the diminished need to readminister cardioplegic solution in multidose fashion, the inherent protection from injury when cardioplegic solutions fail to reach their target, and the long intervals that allow attention to be focused only on the operation. Surgeons with that preference understand that myocardial protection based heavily on hypothermia may result in greater postoperative diastolic dysfunction, some stunning, longer CPB times, and other physiologic derangements that must be balanced against the security of the technique. Surgeons employing more normothermic techniques are sensitized to the need for more frequent intervals within the operation during which cardioplegia must be administered and for more monitoring of the heart to detect potential "cardioplegic escape," and to the risk for injury in myocardial regions to which cardioplegic solution is inadequately delivered. On the other hand, these surgeons appreciate the benefits of rapid restoration of cardiac performance, decreased reperfusion time, and diminished reliance on perioperative inotropic drugs and circulatory assist devices. Neither strategy is "correct," and that employed by one surgeon may not work for another.

The principle of "rapid arrest" is important. When the heart is warm and beating, high-energy phosphates are rapidly depleted. In fact, during several moments of beating at normothermia, an inadequately decompressed heart may be depleted of an amount of high-energy compounds equivalent to the amount lost during 20 minutes of perfect cardioplegic arrest. For surgeons who utilize left ventricular (or atrial) venting, cardioplegic arrest is rapidly achieved because no blood is ejected from the heart into the cross-clamped aorta, and the myocardium receives only cardioplegic solution that has been delivered into the aortic root. When surgeons do not vent the heart to prevent ejection, more thought must be given to the method of establishing initial cardioplegic arrest. Such methods include enhancing venous drainage before application of the cross-clamp, utilizing the lungs as a reservoir by synchronizing aortic cross-clamping and pulmonary deflation, and having cardioplegic solution in the aorta with appropriate concentrations of arresting agents at the moment that the cross-clamp is applied. Other surgeons may use a brief period of ventricular fibrillation associated with systemic cooling to accomplish the same effect.

Once arrest of the heart has been achieved, the extent to which expenditure of energy is minimized and "relative ischemia" is diminished is determined greatly by the extent to which unwanted cardiac contractions are avoided. The flexible delivery of potassium and supplementation with magnesium are important ways to maintain electromechanical quiescence. This is particularly true at moderate hypo-

thermia or when "tepid" cardioplegia is used. Even in hearts demonstrating no obvious mechanical activity, unrecognized electrical activity may be present that allows the slow phase of action potentials to facilitate calcium leakage into cardiomyocytes. This can set the stage for subsequent reperfusion injury by augmenting myocardial energy demands through the intracellular actions of calcium.

Inability to maintain electromechanical quiescence may signal that cardioplegic solutions are not reaching some regions of the myocardium in adequate concentration. This can be the consequence of coronary artery disease, inadequate pressure in the aortic root, or steal phenomena that divert blood away from the intended target myocardium. The supplementation of antegrade cardioplegic delivery techniques with retrograde techniques has greatly facilitated the maintenance of myocardial quiescence. Preoperative analysis of anatomy and knowledge of potential impediments to antegrade cardioplegic delivery guide the use of retrograde cardioplegia. In patients undergoing repeated coronary bypass procedures, the manipulation and transection of grafts and the risk for embolization of debris down patent grafts favor the use of retrograde cardioplegia.

It is important to recognize that retrograde delivery of cardioplegic solution may be inadequate for the inferior surface of the left and right ventricles. This can occur if the retrograde cannula is advanced too far into the great cardiac vein or if the orifice of the inferior cardiac vein is proximal to the inflating balloon on the retrograde cannula; either situation would allow the retrograde infusion of cardioplegia solution to bypass the cardiac veins that drain the septal and posterior regions of the heart. Coronary sinus catheter balloon migration, inadequate balloon inflation, and erroneous pressure readings from the tip of the catheter can also contribute to deficient delivery of retrograde cardioplegia, thereby increasing the likelihood of cardiac electrical activity rather than the desired electrical silence.

One successful cardioplegic strategy is to focus heavily on minimizing the degree of ischemia to which the heart is subjected. This strategy requires more nearly continuous delivery of cardioplegic solutions and therefore involves modification of the temperature of cardioplegic solutions. For example, warmer cardioplegic solutions are best administered more frequently and more nearly continuously, whereas cold cardioplegic solutions can be delivered more intermittently and may not provide incremental benefit if delivered continuously. Surgeons must coordinate their technique with this knowledge. If ischemia can be eliminated, reperfusion injury is by definition minimized and myocardial protection is enhanced. As described elsewhere in the chapter, myocardial ischemia and hypoxia are not synonymous. Hypoxia is better tolerated than ischemia, which suggests the importance of metabolite washout to myocardial protection. Because normothermia increases the propensity for ischemia, the greater the tendency toward normothermic protection, the greater must be the assurance that cardioplegic delivery is uniform, frequent, and abundant.

The final phase of myocardial protection is reperfusion. As described elsewhere in this chapter, the extent to which pharmacologic additives can modify the events of reperfusion is increasing rapidly. It is critically important to remember that cardioplegic solutions have evolved from near-freezing crystalloid solutions to blood-containing normothermic solutions. As more blood has been substituted for crystalloid solutions, the value of many of the additives previously deemed critical has been questioned. For example, when cardioplegia solution was based primarily on extracellular saline concentrations, the absence of hemoglobin, plasma proteins, and smaller, osmotically active components mandated the addition of buffers, free radical scavengers, and osmotic agents, and it forced the evolution of strategies to deal with solutions having high amounts of dissolved oxygen but low oxygen contents. In addition, cold solutions containing hemoglobin were adversely affected by the hypothermia-induced leftward shift in the oxyhemoglobin dissociation curve, which made release of oxygen to the tissues far less probable. In contemporary strategies, oxygen delivery is greatly enhanced by working at less cold temperatures, and surgeons may be developing strategies to utilize blood with concentrations that match those of the blood in the CPB circuit (i.e., a hemoglobin concentration of 6 to 8 g/dL).

Balanced against these newer approaches is the underlying need to complete operations in an expeditious and uncluttered fashion. To restate, the goal of the operation is not to deliver cardioplegia, but to treat the patient. Every surgeon should have an internal gauge that balances the principles of cardioplegia against an efficient performance of the procedure. The advantages of every strategic application of cardioplegic technique should be matched by the known disadvantages of that technique, and a balance should be achieved in which cardioplegia is used as an adjunct to enhance the safety of every cardiac operation while being modified in accord with the individual patient's specific physiologic needs.

Elements of Myocardial Protection: Well-established Strategies

Asystole

Ischemia rapidly depletes the myocardial high-energy phosphate pool, which initiates a complex cascade of ionic, biochemical, and morphologic sequences potentially leading to irreversible tissue injury. This rapid rate of high-energy phosphate depletion is facilitated by continued electromechanical activity after aortic cross-clamping, so that a more rapid depletion of ATP reserves occurs before anoxic arrest ensues. Biochemical changes initiated by anoxic arrest increase the severity of ischemia and consequent reperfusion

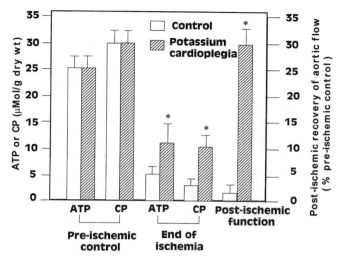

FIG. 13.8. Conservation of myocardial adenosine triphosphate (*ATP*) and creatine phosphate (*CP*) by rapid induction of diastolic arrest with chemical cardioplegia in the isolated rat heart model. One group of rat hearts (n = 6) was perfused with a cardioplegic solution containing 16 mmol of potassium per liter (*hatched bars*) to induce arrest, and a second group was perfused with a normokalemic physiologic solution (*open bars*). Both groups were then subjected to 30 minutes of normothermic ischemia. At the end of ischemia, ATP and CP levels were higher in the chemical cardioplegia group than in the anoxia-arrested group, and postischemic function was superior. (From Hearse DJ, Stewart DA, Braimbridge MV. Cellular protection during myocardial ischemia. The development and characterization of a procedure for the induction of reversible ischemic arrest. *Circulation* 1976;54:193–202, with permission.)

injury within a short period of time. The intentional induction of diastolic arrest by chemical cardioplegia solutions avoids depletion of the high-energy phosphate pool and conserves myocardial energy reserves (Fig. 13.8), which can be utilized in the interim between infusions (multidose strategies) or throughout (single-dose strategies) cardioplegic arrest to maintain ionic and metabolic homeostasis. The mechanism of conserving energy stores with immediate asystole is illustrated in Fig. 13.9. Asystole and decompression of the heart by venting heart on CPB diminishes oxygen demands (as a surrogate measure of ATP utilization) by approximately 80% to 90%; of this reduction, 30% to 40% derives from ventricular decompression *per se*, representing the energetic costs of external cardiac work; the remaining 50% arrest and comes from cessation of myofibrillar contraction against internal components (i.e., elastic compression) and the energy costs of calcium recycling and regaining ionic balance. Studies have confirmed that rapid asystole achieved by chemical cardioplegia prevents the depletion of high-energy phosphate stores otherwise caused by persistent electromechanical activity, reduces the total duration and severity of protected ischemia, and so allows greater postischemic functional recovery in comparison with applied anoxic arrest (7,233).

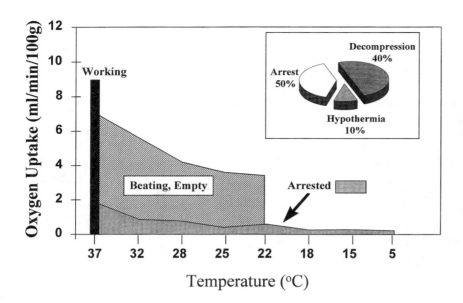

FIG. 13.9. Oxygen requirements of the continuously perfused heart at 37°C in the beating working state (*dark bar*) and at various degrees of hypothermia in the decompressed beating (beating empty; *hatched area*) and in the arrested state (*stippled area*) on cardiopulmonary bypass. Oxygen requirements of the working heart at 37°C are shown for comparison. Inset shows the percentage reduction in oxygen requirements contributed by ventricular decompression, total chemical asystole, and hypothermia to 10°C relative to those of the working heart. As discussed in the text, only minor reductions in myocardial oxygen demand are effected by hypothermia more profound than 22°C. (From Vinten-Johansen, Hammon JW Jr. Myocardial protection during cardiac surgery. In: Gravlee GP, Davis RF, Utley JR, eds. *Cardiopulmonary bypass: principles and practice.* Baltimore: Williams & Wilkins, 1993:155–206, with permission.)

Historically, rapid asystole has been achieved by a number of methods, including induction of hyperkalemia or hypocalcemia, administration of calcium channel blockers (234), and infusion of local anesthetic agents. Newer primary arresting strategies include the use of hyperpolarizing agents, such as potassium channel openers (235–237) and adenosine (238,239). Induction of hyperkalemia is the most common method employed to induce rapid arrest. Potassium depolarizes the myocyte membrane, rendering the myocardium unexcitable during the time that potassium remains within the tissue. Washout of hyperkalemic cardioplegic solutions by noncoronary collateral flow permits resumption of both electrical and mechanical activity, which may escape detection and can be counteracted by intermittent (every 20 to 30 minutes) replenishment of cardioplegic solutions. Such a multidose approach to infusion of cardioplegia solutions maintains or reestablishes electromechanical silence and pays additional dividends of restoring hypothermia, temporarily providing the ischemic myocardium with oxygen and nutrients, and washing out metabolites of anaerobiosis. Potassium concentrations in cardioplegic solutions ranging from 12 to 30 mEq/L are typically used to achieve cardiac standstill within 1 to 2 minutes under hypothermic conditions, with higher concentrations (or longer induction times) required for normothermic induction strategies. Higher potassium concentrations are used to arrest the heart with normothermic induction techniques (240,241) or to maintain arrest during a warm reperfusate cardioplegia (i.e., "hot shot") delivered just before aortic declamping, then with intermittent infusions of 4°C cardioplegia. The optimal potassium concentration is difficult to assess because prearrest function, inotropic state, and maldistribution of cardioplegia impede immediate or homogeneous arrest. However, hypothermia and hyperpolarizing agents (238) given in tandem with potassium reduce the concentration of potassium required to achieve arrest. Potassium concentrations above 40 to 50 mEq/L have been avoided because of the potential for tissue and vascular endothelial damage to coronary arteries (242) and vascular grafts, although this point remains unsettled.

Again, off-pump cardiac surgery poses a challenge to the restraint of cardiac motion and ultimately to the precision of suture placement at the anastomosis. Although various restraining devices are available and limit cardiac motion to a great extent (243), these devices also limit access to lateral and posterior target vessels. Various pharmacologic agents have been used to achieve bradycardia, including adenosine, β-blockade (esmolol) (244), the pacemaker current (diastolic potential) inhibitor S 16257-2, and hyperpolarizing ATP-sensitive potassium (K_{ATP}) channel openers. However, these agents largely fail to provide profound and consistent bradycardia, let alone complete asystole. However, asystole in off-pump cases is counterintuitive, as it is associated with cardiovascular collapse. Therefore, readily reversible asystole may be desirable in off-pump situations. Matheny et al. (245) reported that bradycardia can be achieved by vagus nerve stimulation. This technique offers the advantage of readily reversible application of electrical stimulation and resulting bradycardia, but bradycardia is inconsistent. Bufkin et al. (50) recently reported complete, transient (10 to 60 seconds), immediately reversible asystole achieved by vagal stimulation in combination with pharmacologically suppressed "escape beats." With this technique, hypotension associated with transient asystole was readily reversed, with no hemodynamic or cardiodynamic consequences in normal or jeopardized myocardium.

TABLE 13.2. POSITIVE AND NEGATIVE PHYSIOLOGIC CONSEQUENCES OF HYPOTHERMIA

Positive	Negative
Decreases metabolic rate	Decreases rate of repair
Decreases oxygen requirements	Increases intracellular swelling, Na^+ accumulation
Temporarily decreases cell–cell interactions	Decreases *rate* of contraction; increases energy demands *per beat*
Decreases rate of degradative reactions	Induces ventricular fibrillation, arrhythmias
Increases tolerance to ischemia	Impairs oxygen dissociation
Reduces $[K^+]$ necessary for arrest	Impairs coronary autoregulation
Prolongs electrical silence, cardioplegia	Potential for phrenic nerve damage
Decreases cell deformability	Promotes rouleau formation(?)
Inhibits intracellular Ca^{2+} accumulation	Decreases membrane fluidity; decreases receptor transduction , transmembrane transport
Decreases rate of NF-κB (nuclear factor) translocation	Inhibits sarcoplasmic reticulum Ca^{2+} uptake

Hypothermia

Since its initial introduction in the 1950s by Bigelow et al. (246), hypothermia has remained a cornerstone of myocardial protection. The effects of hypothermia on the myocardium are complex and must be considered in regard to their positive and negative aspects, summarized in Table 13.2. The major cardioprotective mechanisms of hypothermia center around the reduction in metabolic rate and hence oxygen demands of the myocardium. In conjunction with cardiac arrest, hypothermia reduces myocardial oxygen consumption by 97% if profound (4°C) cooling is achieved. The relationship between myocardial oxygen consumption and temperature is relatively exponential, as shown in Fig. 13.9. Generally, the relationship conforms to Van't Hoff's law or the Q_{10} effect, whereby myocardial oxygen consumption in the arrested heart decreases by 50% for every 10°C reduction in temperature. The greatest reduction in myocardial oxygen consumption in the quiescent heart occurs between 37°C and 25°C (Fig. 13.9), with a relatively small decrease in energy requirements achieved thereafter. The reduction in basal metabolic requirements of the cold asystolic heart during chemical cardioplegia increases the tolerance to ischemia for a given period of time and expands the window of "safe ischemic time" between infusions of cardioplegia solution. Therefore, 45 minutes of 4°C global ischemia is well tolerated, whereas 15 minutes of normothermic ischemia precipitates failure on reperfusion. By reducing the basal metabolic rate in proportion to the temperature achieved, myocardial hypothermia decreases the oxygen deficit during elective ischemia and thereby retards the progression of ischemia and consequent postischemic injury. The degree of protection conferred by hypothermia is related to the myocardial temperatures achieved (24,247). Figure 13.10 shows the curvilinear relationship between postischemic functional recovery of aortic flow and myocardial temperature after 60 minutes of global ischemia (24). The greatest functional recovery occurred at temperatures

below 28°C, with little additional protection achieved with lower temperatures. Rosenfeldt (247) showed a similar preservation of high-energy phosphate stores at 28°C or lower. The inflection point occurring between 24° and 28°C in the myocardial temperature versus functional recovery relation in Fig. 13.10 may be related to the greater reduction in oxygen demands that is achieved between 37° and 28°C.

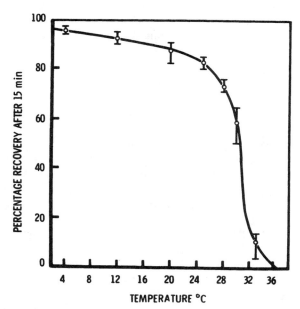

FIG. 13.10. Recovery of aortic flow after 60 minutes of global ischemia induced by hyperkalemic cardioplegia at the temperature indicated on the abscissa. The model used was the isolated perfused working rat heart ejecting against a hydrostatic pressure of 100 cm H_2O. Notice that the greatest recovery of postischemic function occurred at temperatures below 24° to 28°C. Relatively little additional protection is gained from more profound levels (<24°C). (From Hearse DJ, Stewart DA, Braimbridge MV. Cellular protection during myocardial ischemia. The development and characterization of a procedure for the induction of reversible ischemic arrest. *Circulation* 1976;54:193–202, with permission.)

Because the difference in oxygen demands between 22° and 4°C are relatively minor, small differences in regional or global myocardial temperature may be well tolerated, provided that other principles of myocardial protection (i.e., reduction of oxygen demands, hypocalcemia) are observed and impediments to the delivery of cardioplegia are overcome in a timely manner. Many reports suggest that hypothermia below 22°C does not significantly reduce the oxygen demands of the arrested heart (20) or fails to improve the degree of myocardial protection after moderate periods of arrest (24). The benefits of more profound levels of hypothermia may not be apparent unless prolonged ischemia is imposed (i.e., 4 to 6 hours), as shown in Fig. 13.3. Therefore, the surgeon does not need to be preoccupied with achieving the lowest levels of hypothermia possible, but must ensure a reasonable degree of myocardial cooling and a timely induction of local hypothermia in regions of the heart where distribution of cardioplegic solution has been compromised (i.e., infusion through grafts). Many surgeons use moderate hypothermia (approximately 24° to 28°C) for intermittent cardioplegia because significant reductions in energy demands are achieved without invoking the deleterious effects of hypothermia, listed in Table 13.2.

The benefits of simultaneous diastolic arrest and hypothermia are likely derived from complementary mechanisms that together reduce the severity of ensuing surgical ischemia. The benefits of hypothermia relate not only to reduced metabolic demands but also to other biologic reactions involved in signaling the ischemia–reperfusion injury process. Johnson et al. (248) and Haddix et al. (249) have shown that hypothermia attenuates the surface expression of adhesion molecules on the vascular endothelium and delays the translocation of the nuclear transcription factor NF-κB from the cytosol to the nucleus, thereby delaying the generation of proinflammatory mediators and synthesis of adhesion molecules. However, in this regard, hypothermia provides only a transient benefit that may offer no permanent reduction in cell activation after rewarming. The benefits of diastolic arrest and hypothermia are additive (250–253), with each component contributing to the overall protection of the heart. Hypothermia alone, without cardiac asystole, is less effective in protecting the heart because the residual contractile activity preceding anoxic arrest creates an oxygen/energy debt and places oxygen supply and demand in a vulnerable imbalance (20,254). In addition, although asystole reduces oxygen demands by 90% or more, the continued energy demands accruing over time between infusions of cardioplegia can be reduced by hypothermia.

In addition to having physiologic effects that can be used to protect the arrested myocardium, hypothermia is associated with several disadvantages, which are listed in Table 13.2. Concern has been expressed over the issue of cold injury to the heart (edema, morphologic alterations). The edema observed following infusion of hypothermic cardioplegic solutions (159,255) is of complex etiology and may

be related, in part, to the osmolality of the solution used or to sodium accumulation resulting from temporary inhibition of the Na⁺-K⁺-ATPase pump. This edema may be transient and readily reversible after reperfusion (255). In the intervals between infusions of cardioplegic solution, topical saline slush or ice chips may be applied to prevent myocardial rewarming by convection. However, application of extremely cold saline chips without saline slush (temperature 0°C) can produce epicardial freeze injury, mitochondrial damage, and severe postischemic dysfunction in the experimental setting (247).

In addition to hypothermia-induced edema in the myocardium, injury to extracardiac structures (i.e., phrenic nerve) has been a matter of concern (256–258). In a retrospective study of 505 patients who underwent coronary artery bypass in which systemic hypothermia and intermittent cold blood cardioplegia was used with or without topical cooling with iced slush, Nikas et al. (259) reported that topical hypothermia did not offer any additional cardioprotective benefit over systemic hypothermia and cold blood cardioplegia alone. In addition, patients receiving topical hypothermia had a significantly increased incidence of diaphragmatic paralysis and associated pulmonary complications. Another deleterious effect of hypothermia is potentiation of citrate toxicity, which leads to depressed myocardial contractility and thrombocytopenia (260–262).

Some of the negative aspects of hypothermia listed in Table 13.2 are essentially neutralized when cardioplegic arrest is used. For example, the paradoxical increase in inotropic state (254) and oxygen demands per beat, and the possible induction of fibrillation by hypothermia (263), are avoided when cardiac arrest is achieved before or simultaneously with the induction of hypothermia. Also, normothermic cardioplegia can be used to overcome some of the disadvantages of hypothermia (240,264). In a small series of patients who underwent coronary artery bypass, those randomized to tepid or warm antegrade or retrograde cardioplegia showed reduced anaerobic release of lactic acid during cardioplegic arrest and greater left and right ventricular cardiac function in comparison with patients who received cold cardioplegic solution (265). Furthermore, Boldt et al. (266) have shown that intricate pathways associated with the thrombomodulin–protein C–protein S system are altered such that the coagulation perturbations are greater in hypothermic patients undergoing CPB than in normothermic patients. The optimum temperature for cardioplegia in patients undergoing CPB and the overall consequences of the respective treatment modalities continue to be intensively investigated. Although a number of the physiologic effects of hypothermia appear to contradict the concepts of myocardial protection, the net myocardial protective effects are clear: the pathogenic tide of ischemia is stemmed and the unwelcome consequences of surgical ischemia–reperfusion injury are thereby limited.

Avoidance of Edema

Myocardial edema following coronary artery bypass and global ischemia can be reduced by a number of strategies that involve modifying the *conditions* of delivery and *composition* of cardioplegia solutions as they affect the movement of intracellular and interstitial fluid.

Conditions: Controlled delivery pressure—limiting the pressure at which antegrade cardioplegic solutions are infused to between 50 and 100 mm Hg—may reduce the development of edema and postischemic vascular defects (228,267,268). Constraining cardioplegia pressure within these limits may be more important in ischemically injured hearts than in normal (no antecedent ischemia) myocardium (166,168,169,269) because the vasculature of ischemic myocardium (regional or global ischemia) is sensitive to perfusion pressure (270). Vinten-Johansen and colleagues (167,184,270) showed that slowly increasing coronary pressure and blood flow (i.e., "gradual or gentle reperfusion") during the first 30 minutes of reperfusion limits infarct size and improves functional recovery of reperfused myocardium (184).

Composition (hyperosmolarity): Osmotic agents such as mannitol (159,271) and glucose have been used to prevent the development of edema. The latter component also serves as a metabolic substrate and a potential oxygen radical scavenger. Potassium cardioplegia contributes significantly to hyperosmolarity in hyperkalemic cardioplegia solutions. Although some concern has been voiced over extremely hyperosmolar solutions (>400 mOsm) because of the threat of myocardial dehydration and subsequent "rebound edema" after reperfusion with normal blood, Okamoto et al. (272) showed the greatest protection in a regionally ischemic revascularized segment with a cardioplegia solution having an osmolarity greater than 400 mOsm. Allen and colleagues (273) have demonstrated in a canine CPB model that enhancement of myocardial contractility with dobutamine following separation from bypass is associated with increased myocardial lymphatic function and leads to a significant resolution of myocardial edema.

The edema associated with postcardioplegia complications, particularly in vulnerable myocardium, can be addressed by reducing the amount of water (i.e., hemodilution) in cardioplegia solutions by using mixtures with ratios of blood to crystalloid of 1:1, 2:1, or 4:1 (274). The catalogue of cardioplegia additives, modalities of delivery, and combinations thereof may seem unnecessarily complex and daunting and threaten to interfere with the performance of the operation. Against this backdrop of increasing complexity and reduced postischemic hemodilution has risen a parallel interest in simplifying cardioplegia to its basic form while embracing the central concepts of blood as a vehicle, with its inherent oxygen-carrying capacity, physiologic buffers, and endogenous antioxidants and detoxification pathways. Menasché and colleagues have coined the term "mini-

cardioplegia" to describe a technique of administering a small quantity of a prepared arresting solution via a pump-driven syringe to otherwise unmodified blood circulating through the CPB circuit (275,276). The volume and rate of the concentrated potassium-based arresting solution is serially decreased to the lowest level possible to maintain quiescence. The key to this type of myocardial protection is the nearly continuous delivery of the blood solution to the myocardium at a tepid temperature. The continuous administration obviates the need for added buffers such as tromethamine (THAM) and citrate–phosphate dextrose because aerobic metabolism is maintained throughout the duration of arrest, resulting in sufficiently high production of energy to drive the ionic pumps responsible for Na^+, Cl^- and Ca^{2+} homeostasis and avoid intracellular acidosis. The reduction in crystalloid "dilutants" obviates progressive hemodilution. The potential benefit of minicardioplegia solutions are numerous and include (a) increased oxygen supply and increased presence of endogenous antioxidants and detoxification factors lost with hemodilution; (b) improved control of blood volume to reduce edema resulting from hypo-osmolality, bleeding complications, and cardioplegia overdose (274); (c) increased convenience and practicality; and (d) better cost effectiveness. Reports indicate good clinical satisfaction with this technique (277). This philosophy of "all-blood cardioplegia," however, does not inherently embrace the application of additives addressing mediators of ischemia–reperfusion injury that may be of clear clinical benefit. In addition, this "minicardioplegia" philosophy brings into question the need for other strategies of myocardial protection developed during the past two decades, including buffering of intracellular acidosis, calcium management, and use of hyperosmolar conditions. These issues bear repeated examination, as they relate to newer strategies of myocardial protection.

Buffering of Acidosis

During both normothermic and hypothermic ischemia, aerobic metabolism is short-lived, and the myocardium relies on the relatively low yield of ATP (2 mol/mol of glucose used) from anaerobiosis. However, tissue acidosis resulting from continued metabolism and lactate production during ischemia strongly inhibits enzymatically catalyzed metabolic reactions, further diminishing the yield of ATP. Buffering of cardioplegic solutions to counteract myocardial hydrogen ion accumulation therefore is a logical strategy for limiting the consequences of ischemia. Episodic reinfusion of cardioplegic solution further rectifies tissue acidosis by washing out metabolic by-products to reestablish acid–base homeostasis. Buffering of acidosis can be accomplished by using the cardioplegic solutions as vehicles, either exploiting the endogenous capabilities of the solution (i.e., buffering capacity of blood) or adding exogenous buffers such as histidine, bicarbonate, or THAM.

The buffering approach selected to manage the acid–base status of cardioplegic solutions should be based on the biophysical changes imposed by hypothermia and pharmacologic efforts to adjust acid–base balance, which can affect buffering capacity. In aqueous solutions, the neutral pH of water is temperature-dependent, increasing by 0.017 pH units per degree Celsius of decrease in temperature. In blood, pH is alkaline relative to the neutrality point of water, but a parallel adjustment upward in arterial pH occurs with hypothermia in that the change in pH per degree centigrade is approximately 0.0147. This thermal shift is called the *Rosenthal correction factor.* Therefore, a sample of blood cardioplegia with a pH of 7.4 as measured by electrodes warmed to 37°C would actually have a pH of 7.72 if corrected to a temperature of 10°C.

The physiologic consequences and benefits of temperature-corrected acid–base balance of fluids *in vivo* are (a) conservation of enzyme kinetics and metabolism; (b) stabilization of Donnan equilibrium of chloride, which prevents abnormal cell volume regulation and edema; and (c) conservation of ionized metabolic intermediates, which would otherwise promote metabolism during hypothermia. Blood used as a vehicle for hypothermic cardioplegic solutions may have a natural advantage over asanguineous solutions in that temperature-related pH adjustments are made in blood by both endogenous buffer systems to maintain an alkaline pH relative to the neutrality point of water and to intracellular pH.

Alkalotic cardioplegic solutions maintain better metabolism (278,279) and buffer intracellular as well as extracellular acidosis (280–283). Neethling et al. (284) report that aggressive buffering of cardioplegia solution buffers acidotic changes in interstitial pH and favorably affects postcardioplegia contractile recovery. However, a number of reports (285–287) contradict this conclusion by suggesting that acidotic solutions decrease energy demands during ischemia and attenuate intracellular Ca^{2+} accumulation during ischemia and reperfusion. Clinically, adjustments in the acid–base balance of systemic blood and cardioplegic solutions can be made either by changing P_{CO_2} levels in the arterial blood or by adding exogenous buffering agents. P_{CO_2} can be reduced by increasing the oxygenator gas flow rate (analogous to increasing minute ventilation off CPB) to achieve even greater alkalinity than that induced by hypothermia alone.

Various buffering agents have been used, either as a primary method of pH adjustment or to supplement and amplify the intrinsic buffering capabilities of the cardioplegic solution. The "ideal" buffer has a dissociation constant (pK) within 1 pH unit of the neutrality point of the solution (sanguineous or asanguineous) used at a given temperature, should be independent of changes in P_{CO_2}, and should be able to buffer the intracellular and interstitial (extracellular) compartments. Bicarbonate, THAM, histidine, and phosphate buffers are used in various cardioplegic solution formulations. Bicarbonate is a weak extracellular buffer with a pK that is both outside the desirable range of physiologic pH at lower temperatures and unable to adjust appropriately to temperature. Poor results have been obtained with bicarbonate-buffered solutions (288,289). Histidine (pK of 6.04) and the active component imidazole (pK of 6.7), the dominant buffer systems in blood, provide good buffering capacity, with an appropriate pK range and appropriate adjustment of pK to hypothermia. Experimental studies show good preservation of high-energy phosphate stores and postischemic ventricular function with these buffers (283). The imidazole–histidine buffering system may be one of the mechanisms underlying the effective buffering capacity of blood in blood cardioplegia (280,281). THAM is an excellent buffer because its pK (8.08) is nearly identical to the physiologically adjusted pH at 4° to 10°C, and it buffers both the intracellular and extracellular compartments. There are strong advocates for both THAM and histidine as "optimal" buffering agents in cardioplegia solutions.

Calcium Management

The importance of calcium in ischemia–reperfusion injury has been explained in an earlier section. Despite uniform agreement on the importance of limiting intracellular calcium during reperfusion, the optimal technique to achieve this continues to be debated (26,290–292). In addition, arriving at a uniform "solution" for calcium management may be virtually impossible because of wide variations in the composition of cardioplegia solutions used in clinical practice. However, an abundance of data is available regarding strategies of calcium management and better myocardial protection.

Ideal concentrations of calcium in cardioplegia solutions must be tailored to the type of solution used (i.e., crystalloid or blood). It should be kept in mind that the concentration-response curve for the appropriate calcium concentration is bell-shaped, with both extreme hypercalcemia and hypocalcemia (<50 μmol/L) resulting in suboptimal myocardial protection (26,290). Extreme hypocalcemia may set the stage for the calcium paradox once normal calcium levels are achieved at reperfusion. The calcium paradox is a sudden influx of calcium that occurs on normalization of calcium following a period of profound hypocalcemia. Ischemia sensitizes the myocardium to normocalcemic and hypercalcemic levels in cardioplegia solutions that are well tolerated by normal myocardium. The picture is further complicated by the dynamic interaction of calcium with other cardioplegia constituents, such as sodium (293), potassium (123,294), magnesium (294), and its behavior under conditions of hypothermia (295). In addition, the systemic release of catecholamines in response to CPB (296) alters the influx of calcium through adrenergic receptor mechanisms and, hence, increases the vulnerability of the myocardium to ischemia–reperfusion injury.

Calcium chelation: The reduction of extracellular calcium by direct chelation, which restricts transmembrane calcium influx regardless of route of entry, is a common component of myocardial protective strategies, especially when blood cardioplegia is used. Sodium citrate, often obtained in combination with phosphate and dextrose for storage of blood (CPD), is the most popular agent to chelate calcium. This agent, however, is relatively nonspecific for calcium and may chelate other divalent cations also, including magnesium. In addition, citrate is a direct inhibitor of glycolysis (297), on which the ischemic myocardium depends when tissue oxygen stores are depleted by attenuation of aerobic metabolism during ischemia. The benefits of citrate, however, seem to outweigh its negative effects, and it is a key component in many cardioprotective strategies. Other, more specific chelators of calcium are under investigation for future use in cardioplegic solutions.

Newer strategies to attenuate calcium influx during reperfusion focus on the inhibition of calcium transport into the cell through calcium channels rather than the relatively nonselective transport described earlier. Adenosine has emerged as a cardioprotective autacoid that protects in part by its ability to limit calcium influx (239). The exact mechanisms for this protection are currently poorly understood; however, opening of the K_{ATP} channel is a potential mechanism (239). Direct opening of the K_{ATP} channel with agents specifically designed for this purpose (potassium channel openers such as chromokalim and aprikalim) also attenuate calcium influx during reperfusion, but their use has met with resistance as a result of their prodysrhythmic effects. With a growing interest in the use of molecular mechanisms as a means of myocardial protection, genetic manipulation of the active calcium channels has been investigated as a way to reduce calcium influx (62). Manipulation of the ubiquitous regulatory enzyme system protein kinase C plays an important role in calcium management (62). Investigators have attempted to harness this mechanism through ischemic preconditioning, which activates protein kinase C isoforms and confers cardioprotection partially by attenuating calcium influx. Further understanding of cellular capability to regulate calcium will undoubtedly lead to improved strategies for calcium management and improved postischemic myocardial function.

Elements of Myocardial Protection: Emerging Strategies

Oxygen Radical Therapy

Therapy targeting oxygen radical-induced myocardial injury must take into consideration several factors, including (a) the time during the operative course when oxygen radicals are generated, (b) the source of the oxygen radicals (endothelial cell, neutrophil, myocyte), and (c) the species of radical toward which the intervention is directed. In general, the choice of pharmacologic intervention should consider the cascade of oxygen radical generation shown in Table 13.1. Table 13.3 summarizes the various biologic species of oxygen radicals, their sources, and their scavengers or inhibitors. The therapeutic agents targeting specific oxygen radical species are also represented in this scheme. (Although H_2O_2 is technically not an oxygen radical, it is an important transitional molecule in the oxygen radical cascade and is involved in ischemia–reperfusion injury.)

Because the infusion of cardioplegia is a form of reperfusion during which key sources for oxygen radical production (oxygen and neutrophils in blood cardioplegia) are delivered to the myocardium, scavengers and enzymes that inhibit or dismutate oxygen radicals are most effective if administered either as a pretreatment or as an additive to the cardioplegic solution. In the latter instance, the induction phase of cardioplegia delivery may be considered a pretreatment modality. An adjunct to the cardioplegic solution would allow intermittent delivery of the antioxidant agent during the period of protected arrest, with continued action in the immediate postoperative period, depending on the half-life of the agent chosen.

TABLE 13.3. SOURCES AND SCAVENGERS OR INHIBITORS OF VARIOUS SPECIES OF OXYGEN FREE RADICALS

Species	Sources	Scavenger/Inhibitor
$^-O_2^{\cdot}$	Neutrophils Endothelium Mitochondria	*SOD, allopurinol, nonsteroidal antiinflammatory agents (ibuprofen, BW755C, BAY K6575, indomethacin), α-tocopherol, ascorbate, MPG, *NO
$H_2O_2^{\cdot}$	Neutrophils Mitochondria	*catalase, *glutathione peroxidase *reduced glutathione
$^{\cdot}OH$	Mitochondria Haber-Weiss reaction	MPG, DMTU, DMSO deferroxamine, mannitol, ascorbate * methionine
Lipid peroxides	Cell membranes	α-tocopherol, *glutathione peroxidase

* Endogenous.
DMTU, dimethylthiourea; DMSO, demethylsulfoxide; SOD, superoxide dismutase; MPG, mercaptopropanyl glycine; NO, nitric oxide.

An appropriate strategy for attenuating oxygen radical-induced injury after bypass surgery should consider both the species of radical targeted and its primary source of generation. The cardioplegic vehicle must also be scrutinized for its potential to produce or exaggerate oxygen radical production. For example, crystalloid cardioplegia carries less oxygen as a substrate for oxygen radical production than its blood cardioplegia counterpart. Blood, on the other hand, contains abundant oxygen, neutrophils, lipids, and iron moieties, which may generate radicals. Reducing the participation of neutrophils by depleting blood cardioplegia solutions of neutrophils or preventing their adherence to endothelium and oxidant production (298) with agents such as adenosine has proved beneficial and further highlights the role of neutrophil-mediated damage during surgical ischemia and reperfusion (299–301). However, blood also carries important endogenous "scavengers" (i.e., super-oxide dismutase, catalase, and glutathione in erythrocytes) that may be important in counteracting radical-induced damage (302,303). Further experimental and clinical studies are necessary to determine the benefits of radical scavenger therapy, and to evaluate target-specific therapy directed toward multiple radical species and their sources.

Experiments using various animal models under a number of conditions relevant to the surgical setting have evaluated a host of oxygen radical scavengers and inhibitors as cardioplegic solution adjuvants (201,202,304–312). SOD used alone has not been shown to be beneficial, but catalase either alone (313,314) or in combination with SOD (312) has demonstrated protection beyond that provided by cardioplegic solutions alone (315–319). These observations generally reflect the consensus of extensive nonsurgical studies about short-term myocardial ischemia (93,187,320). The failure of SOD to reduce oxygen radical-related injury may be related to the proximal position of its target molecule, superoxide anion, and the fact that other radical species (i.e., H_2O_2, $^\bullet OH$) generated during ischemia–reperfusion would not be targeted by SOD. On the other hand, SOD plus catalase or catalase alone interrupts the accumulation of two radical species ($O_2^\bullet$, H_2O_2), allowing only the $^\bullet OH$ originating from sources other than the $O_2^\bullet$–H_2O_2 cascade (i.e., Haber-Weiss reaction) to persist. In addition, the relatively large peptide structure of SOD may impair its interaction with superoxide anions at the neutrophil-endothelial cell interface. SOD does not attenuate intracellular sources of superoxide anion, which may allow intracellular production of oxygen radicals by xanthine oxidase and mitochondria to go unchecked. The xanthine oxidase inhibitors allopurinol and oxypurinol improve postischemic function in experimental (202,311) and clinical (321–323) studies. The benefit to using allopurinol and oxypurinol may be derived from the accessibility of the molecules to their respective targets. *N*-(2-mercaptopropionyl) glycine (MPG) is a purported scavenger of hydroxyl radicals and superoxide anions that enters the intracellular compartment. However, when

used as an adjuvant to cardioplegia in two models of cardioplegia-based myocardial protection, MPG conferred no additional benefit to postischemic function (201,324,325).

Several clinical studies support the appearance of oxygen free radicals during CPB and cardioplegic arrest (144,326,327). Although experimental evidence strongly supports the beneficial effects of antioxidant therapy in cardioplegia, the clinical benefits of this strategy are not yet clear. Bical et al. (328) showed no attenuation of oxygen radical metabolites in patients undergoing cardioplegic arrest when crystalloid cardioplegia enhanced with allopurinol was used. Other clinical studies have failed to document improvement in postcardioplegia cardiac performance with SOD (329). This failure to reduce oxygen radicals may have been related to significant compositional differences in both the crystalloid solutions and the reperfusates, or to the inclusion of allopurinol only *after* cardioplegia (as a controlled phase of reperfusion) had been delivered, so that the generation of oxygen radicals during cardioplegia was not prevented. The latter interpretation is consistent with the study of Jolly et al. (330), who demonstrated that delivery of scavengers after the burst of oxygen radicals had occurred in early reperfusion was not myoprotective. On the other hand, Castelli et al. (331) demonstrated that allopurinol given intravenously for 1 hour after bypass improved cardiac output while decreasing plasma xanthine oxidase, implying that the protective effect was mediated through decreases in available free radicals. Allopurinol pretreatment has shown potential cardioprotective effects (323). In clinical studies in which oxygen radical scavengers (mannitol) or inhibitors (allopurinol) were delivered as additives to the cardioplegic solution, postischemic myocardial injury was reduced (332,333). The dichotomous results between studies are likely a consequence of the wide range of myocardial protective techniques employed coupled with the variability in endpoints evaluated, which makes comparisons between results difficult and leaves the question of optimal antioxidant therapies still unanswered.

Glutathione (readily available in tissue, red blood cells, and plasma) as an adjunct to both cardioplegia and transplant preservation solutions has recently received attention for its antioxidant properties (334–336). In addition to its potent antioxidant properties through glutathione peroxidase, glutathione may be involved in neutralizing peroxynitrite, a potentially injurious by-product of NO (337–339). Animal studies have demonstrated a direct correlation between endogenous glutathione production and cardioprotection by using genetic knockout and overproduction models of glutathione synthesis (336,340,341). Human studies evaluating the efficacy of glutathione in CPB patients are sparse, but numerous investigators have shown improved myocardial preservation in transplanted hearts when perfusate solutions containing glutathione were used (342,343).

Amino Acid Enhancement

Cardioplegic formulations that adequately protect the myocardium of normal hearts have often been found to provide inadequate protection for severely damaged hearts with antecedent ischemia, reperfusion injury, cardiac failure, or cardiogenic shock. Failure to protect these hearts adequately may be related to the inability to maintain sufficient levels of high-energy phosphates in the already energy-depleted myocardium, or failure to sustain adequate levels of glycolysis or other metabolic processes during the periods of hypothermic ischemia. Limitation of energy production by anaerobiosis during hypothermic ischemia may be in part related to depletion of key Krebs cycle intermediates and their precursors, glutamate and aspartate, and to the failure of the malate–aspartate shuttle mechanism to remove protons and prevent intracellular acidosis. Shorter periods of ischemia may not attenuate Krebs cycle activity *per se* (344). Both glutamate and aspartate are lost during ischemia and are actively incorporated into the myocardium when exogenously supplied (345,346). Glutamate enters into the Krebs cycle by conversion to α-ketoglutarate, whereas aspartate enters the Krebs cycle via transamination to oxaloacetic acid. Both precursors are subsequently metabolized within the Krebs cycle to succinate, each ultimately producing 1 mol of ATP by substrate-level phosphorylation independent of glycolysis (345). Therefore, high-energy phosphates can be derived from amino acid metabolism even when the level of glycolysis is reduced during ischemia. In addition, glutamate and aspartate may inhibit the mitochondrial accumulation of protons by sustaining the malate–aspartate shuttle, thereby preventing uncoupling of oxidative phosphorylation and the generation of oxygen free radicals.

Addition of glutamate and aspartate to the cardioplegic solution increases myocardial oxygen uptake during induction of cardioplegia and improves postischemic myocardial performance and oxygen utilization (347) after discontinuation of CPB. The improvement observed was greater in energy-depleted hearts (347) than in uninjured hearts (45). The study by Rosenkranz et al. (347) suggests that glutamate and aspartate used together act synergistically by providing greater protection than either amino acid alone. In addition, greater benefits may be obtained by combining amino acid supplementation with normothermic induction of cardioplegia, as both strategies augment oxygen uptake during induction of cardioplegia. Because amino acid supplementation acts mainly by replenishing lost Krebs cycle intermediates and facilitating both anaerobic and aerobic metabolism, the addition of glutamate, aspartate, or both may be indicated in other situations in which the myocardium may be extremely depressed or subjected to prolonged ischemia or hypoxia, such as hypoxia–reoxygenation injury (348), reperfusion of hypoxic or ischemic immature hearts (349,350), cardiac transplantation (351), and storage of donor hearts (352). This conclusion is not supported by Reed et al. (353), who showed no incorporation of either glutamate or aspartate into the Krebs cycle. However, amino acid supplementation has been shown to increase high-energy phosphate stores in human myocardium (354). In addition, it has been shown that glutamate administered intravenously to patients after coronary bypass operations is taken up and has a beneficial effect on oxidative metabolism, with some indication of better postcardioplegic cardiac performance (346). In agreement with the beneficial effects of intravenous amino acid supplementation, Engelman et al. (355) reported that intravenous infusion of a solution containing glutamate (3 mmol/L) and aspartate (13 mmol/L) reduced infarct size by nearly 50% and improved regional wall motion following 60 minutes of coronary artery occlusion and 6 hours of reperfusion.

Adenosine

Since the report by Olafsson et al. in 1987 (356), there has been an explosion of research focused on the mechanisms by which adenosine protects the heart from both reversible and irreversible injury after myocardial ischemia and reperfusion. Adenosine has a broad spectrum of physiologic effects that exert cardioprotection (357–359). A distinct advantage of the physiologic and pharmacologic profile of adenosine is that it exerts effects during multiple time windows that are important to the pathogenesis of ischemia–reperfusion injury (i.e., before treatment and during ischemia and reperfusion), and it acts via multiple transduction mechanisms on multiple targets (myocytes, neutrophils, endothelium). Hence, adenosine has a built-in redundancy that may at several points block the multiple mechanisms of ischemia–reperfusion injury.

Adenosine produces a majority of its physiologic effects by interacting with specific purinergic receptors. There are at least four types of adenosine receptors: A_1, A_{2a}, A_{2b}, and A_3. Stimulation of A_1 receptors, located mainly on neutrophils and myocytes, decreases adenylate cyclase activity via inhibitory G protein (G_i) or stimulates the phospholipase C–diacyl glycerol (DAG)—inositol phosphate (IP_3) pathway to cause a release of calcium from intracellular stores and a translocation of protein kinase C from the cytosol to the cell membrane. The primary effector linked to the A_1 receptor subtype may be the K_{ATP} channel, the stimulation of which induces hyperpolarization and inhibition of transmembrane calcium conductance. Physiologic effects of the adenosine A_1 receptor include negative chronotropy and dromotropy, antiadrenergic effects, increased rate of glycolysis, and stimulation of neutrophil adherence. Activation of adenosine A_2 receptors, located mainly on neutrophils, endothelial cells, vascular smooth-muscle cells, and platelets, stimulates adenylate cyclase through the stimulatory G protein (G_s), which results in vasodilation, renin release, and inhibition of neutrophil events (superoxide generation, adherence to endothelium, and endothelial dysfunction)

(360–362). The adenosine A_3 receptor has been localized in heart tissue and myocytes, yet firm data have not localized this receptor subtype to the endothelium or neutrophils. The A_3 receptor is similar to the A_1 receptor in that it inhibits adenylate cyclase, stimulates protein kinase C translocation, and may activate K_{ATP} channels. Its cardioprotective profile differs substantially from that of the A_1 receptor, however, as discussed below. In animal models of nonsurgical ischemia–reperfusion, specific activation of the adenosine A_3 receptor has been found to be cardioprotective without the untoward vasodilator effects of nonspecific adenosine agents (363). Similarly, Thourani and colleagues (364) have examined the cardiodynamic effects of a selective adenosine A_3 agonist, Cl-IB-MECA, when administered as pretreatment or as an additive to crystalloid cardioplegia in cell-free, perfused, isolated rat hearts. They found that Cl-IB-MECA administered as a pretreatment, independently of inclusion in cardioplegia, attenuated postischemic systolic and diastolic dysfunction and creatine kinase release. Adenosine A_3 supplementation of cardioplegia did not further enhance A_3 receptor-mediated cardioprotection. Further studies delineating the role and mechanism of adenosine A_3 receptor-mediated cardioprotection are warranted.

In the surgical setting, cardioprotective strategies can be applied as a pretreatment, during ischemia, and during the early phase of reperfusion. The benefit of adenosine treatment partly depends on effectively targeting the mechanism of injury operative at the time of administration (229). The pretreatment infusion of adenosine (loosely referred to as "chemical preconditioning") may protect the heart by attenuating detrimental intraoperative ischemic events. Brief pretreatment with adenosine has been shown to reduce infarct size in isolated perfused heart models (365) and *in vivo* animal models (366), and to improve postischemic contractile function (367) and preserve metabolic or energy status of the ischemic–reperfused myocardium (367). The cardioprotective effects of adenosine when administered during ischemia may be mediated primarily by activation of A_1 receptors (368) and opening of K_{ATP} channels, with the consequent reduction of cytosolic calcium overload (379). Pretreatment administration of adenosine has been reported by Lee et al. (370) in patients with poor left ventricular performance and multivessel coronary artery disease. They reported an improvement in the postsurgical cardiac index immediately after separation from CPB, which persisted for 40 hours postoperatively, in patients who received adenosine (250 to 350 μg/kg per minute for 10 minutes just before CPB, reduced as needed to sustain systolic blood pressure >70 mm Hg) in comparison with those who did not receive adenosine. Furthermore, creatine kinase levels 24 hours postoperatively were significantly lower in adenosine-treated patients. This study (370) shows that a pretreatment window is available for the effective administration of adenosine, without significant untoward complications such as hypotension or bradycardia.

One of the most obvious applications of adenosine is as an adjunct to cardioplegia solutions. In 1976, Hearse et al. (24) reported that adenosine, used either alone during ischemia or as an adjunct to cardioplegia, improved postischemic function. Since then, a plethora of studies have been performed to investigate the role of adenosine as an adjunct to crystalloid hypothermic cardioplegic solutions (371–376). Most of these studies showed that adenosine in a wide range of concentrations (100 μmol/L to 10 mmol/L) was associated with improved postischemic contractile function in comparison with unsupplemented crystalloid counterparts (371–376). The beneficial effects of adenosine-enhanced crystalloid cardioplegia have been attributed to a number of mechanisms independent of neutrophil inhibition, including improvement in the rate of anaerobic glycolysis and energy status, and reduction in calcium accumulation resulting from cell hyperpolarization. Although some studies report that adenosine restores tissue ATP content lost during ischemia (375,377), others show no correlation between tissue ATP content after reperfusion and functional recovery (198,378–381). The efficacy of adenosine in improving postischemic physiologic variables by restoring high-energy phosphate in tissues during cardioplegic arrest is not presently clear.

Adenosine as an adjunct to blood cardioplegia has been investigated by our laboratory (194,382). Hudspeth et al. (194) investigated adenosine as an adjunct to a standard hypothermic, hyperkalemic blood cardioplegic solution in

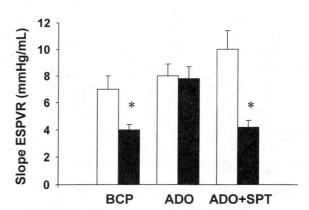

FIG. 13.11. Postcardioplegia left ventricular (*LV*) function with adenosine–blood cardioplegia. Postcardioplegia LV global function measured by slope of the end-systolic pressure–volume (impedance catheter) relations (*ESPVR*) at baseline (*clear bar*) and after 60 minutes of reperfusion (*solid bar*) following blood cardioplegia (*BCP*) alone showed significant functional deterioration. BCP supplemented with 400 μM adenosine (*ADO*) in hypothermic, hyperkalemic blood cardioplegia restored postischemic function to 95% of baseline. This cardioprotection was inhibited by the adenosine receptor antagonist 8-p-sulfophenyl theophylline (*SPT*), indicating a receptor-mediated mechanism. *p <0.05 vs. baseline value of ESPVR. (From Hudspeth DA, Nakanishi K, Vinten-Johansen J, et al. Adenosine in blood cardioplegia prevents postischemic dysfunction in ischemically injured hearts. *Ann Thorac Surg* 1994;58:1637–1644, with permission.)

ischemically injured hearts subjected to 30 minutes of normothermic global ischemia. Blood cardioplegia supplemented with adenosine (400 μmol/L) reversed the postischemic systolic dysfunction observed with unsupplemented blood cardioplegia (Fig. 13.11). The protection was inhibited with 8-*p*-sulfophenyl theophylline (8-*p*-SPT), confirming a receptor-mediated mechanism. The potent antineutrophil effects of adenosine suggest that significant cardioprotection would be exerted during reperfusion, and not necessarily during the period of cardioplegia itself. Hence, administration of the purine in hypothermic cardioplegia may not be the most optimal modality. Indeed, this has been suggested by studies by Ledingham et al. (378) and Thelin et al. (380), in which transient adenosine infusion only at the start of surgical reperfusion was associated with improved functional recovery. Recently, Thourani and colleagues (382) tested the hypothesis that adenosine given at the time of reperfusion (aortic declamping) would provide equivalent or better cardioprotection than adenosine administered as an adjunct to hypothermic, hyperkalemic blood cardioplegia. In a surgical reperfusion model of regional ischemia (75 minutes of left anterior coronary artery occlusion followed by 60 minutes of cardioplegic arrest and 2 hours of reperfusion), these investigators showed that adenosine administered either as an adjunct to blood cardioplegia (100 μmol/L) alone or as a reperfusion treatment during the terminal infusion of blood cardioplegia and during first 30 minutes after aortic declamping (140 μg/kg per minute) reduced infarct size in comparison with unsupplemented blood cardioplegia, improved postischemic contractile function, and decreased both myocardial edema and neutrophil accumulation (myeloperoxidase activity) in the area at risk (Tables 13.4 and 13.5). Furthermore, the hearts treated with adenosine only during reperfusion demonstrated preservation of postischemic coronary artery endothelial function (neutrophil adherence), which was not demonstrated by hearts subjected to either unsupplemented blood cardioplegia or adenosine-enhanced blood cardioplegia. This observation is consistent with the potent antineutrophil effects of adenosine. Human trials evaluating the role of adenosine-mediated cardioprotection when administered during reperfusion are currently under way.

Adenosine-supplemented cardioplegia has been studied in a limited number of human clinical trials. In 1996, Fremes et al. (383) reported an open-label, nonrandomized, phase I adenosine dose-ranging study in patients undergoing elective coronary artery bypass. A range of adenosine concentrations (15 to 50 μmol/L) to supplement antegrade warm blood potassium cardioplegia was tested in the initial 1,000-mL cardioplegia dose and the final 500-mL dose. It was concluded that adenosine can safely be administered during CPB and that adenosine at a concentration of 15 to 50 μmol/L is the optimal dose. In a follow-up study by the same group, Cohen and colleagues (384) performed

TABLE 13.4. BASAL ENDOTHELIAL FUNCTION, INFARCT SIZE, NEUTROPHIL ACCUMULATION, AND TISSUE WATER CONTENT AFTER ADENOSINE IN SURGICAL REPERFUSION WITH BLOOD CARDIOPLEGIA

Basal endothelial function: neutrophil adherence (PMNs/mm^2)	
Left circumflex artery (nonischemic-reperfused artery)	
SBCP	34.5 $\pm$ 3.3
ADO-BCP	29.9 $\pm$ 2.3
ADO-R	30.7 $\pm$ 1.4
Left anterior descending artery (ischemic-reperfused artery)	
SBCP	118.1 $\pm$ 3.2
ADO-BCP	113.8 $\pm$ 4.7
ADO-R	55.5 $\pm$ 2.0[+]
Infarct size (AN/AAR, %)	
SBCP	41.6 $\pm$ 4.3
ADO-BCP	29.2 $\pm$ 1.7*
ADO-R	20.7 $\pm$ 1.5*
Myeloperoxidase activity (U/min/g tissue, necrotic zone)	
SBCP	117.4 $\pm$ 5.5
ADO-BCP	20.7 $\pm$ 5.3*
ADO-R	9.6 $\pm$ 4.2*
Percentage water content (transmural ischemic zone)	
SBCP	86.4 $\pm$ 0.7
ADO-BCP	82.1 $\pm$ 0.2[@]
ADO-R	80.0 $\pm$ 0.4[+]

SBCP, standard (unsupplemented blood) cardioplegia; ADO-BCP, blood cardioplegia supplemented with adenosine; ADO-R, adenosine administered during terminal "hot shot" and intravenously after release of cross-clamp; AN/AAR, %, area of necrosis expressed as a percentage of area at risk.
[+] p <0.05 ADO-R vs. control and ADO-BCP groups; * p <0.05 vs. SBCP; [@]p <0.05 ADO-I group vs. control groups.

TABLE 13.5. REGIONAL CARDIODYNAMIC DATA WITH ADENOSINE-ENHANCED BLOOD CARDIOPLEGIA OR ADENOSINE ADMINISTERED AT THE ONSET OF REPERFUSION

	Baseline	Ischemia	W30min	W60min	W90min
%SS					
SBCP	14 ± 2[+]	−6 ± 1	−3 ± 1	−6 ± 1	−3 ± 1
ADO-BCP	13 ± 2*	−10 ± 2	2 ± 0.4	1 ± 1[^@]	2 ± 0.2[^]
ADO-R	17 ± 1*	−7 ± 0.4	5 ± 2[^@]	6 ± 2[^@]	5 ± 2[^@]
Chamber stiffness					
β-Coefficient					
Control	0.4 ± 0.2	1.0 ± 0.2	3.4 ± 0.6[^]	3.9 ± 0.6[^]	4.4 ± 0.5[^]
ADO-I	0.4 ± 0.1	0.9 ± 0.2	2.6 ± 1.4[^]	2.6 ± 0.5[^]	2.7 ± 0.3[^@]
ADO-R	0.3 ± 0.1	0.7 ± 0.3	1.4 ± 0.5[^]	1.7 ± 0.1[^@]	1.8 ± 0.3[^@]

SBCP, standard unsupplemented blood cardioplegia; ADO-BCP, blood cardioplegia supplemented with adenosine; ADO-R, adenosine administered during terminal "hot shot" and intravenously after release of cross-clamp; % SS, percentage systolic shortening; β-coefficient, unitless modulus of chamber stiffness; baseline, before normothermic left anterior descending (LAD) coronary artery occlusion; ischemia, at the end of 75 minutes of LAD ischemia; W30min, W60min, and W90min, reperfusion of the heart after 75 minutes of LAD ischemia and 60 minutes of cardioplegic arrest at 30, 60, and 90 minutes during working beating state.
[+] $p < 0.05$ vs. other time points in same group; * $p < 0.05$ vs. ischemia time point in the same group; ^ $p < 0.05$ vs. baseline and ischemia time points in the same group; [@] $p < 0.05$ vs. control within the same time point.

a double-blinded, randomized, placebo-controlled trial in patients undergoing primary, isolated, nonemergent coronary artery bypass surgery. Adenosine (15 μmol/L, 50 μmol/L, or 100 μmol/L) or placebo was added to antegrade warm blood cardioplegia in the initial 1,000 mL and last 500 mL of cardioplegia delivery. They found no significant differences between groups in the incidence of individual primary or secondary outcomes (including death, low-output syndrome, postoperative myocardial infarction, use of inotropes, or intraaortic balloon pump requirement). In contrast, Mentzer et al. (385,386) tested the efficacy of adenosine as an additive to cold blood cardioplegia in an open-labeled, randomized study of patients with ejection fractions greater than 30% undergoing elective coronary artery bypass grafting. The patients were randomized to standard antegrade cold blood cardioplegia without adenosine or to one of five adenosine doses: 100 μM, 500 μM, 1 mM, and 2 mM cardioplegia plus an intravenous pretreatment infusion of 140 μg/kg per minute. Patients were followed for 24 hours after discontinuation of CPB. Increasing concentrations of adenosine in cardioplegia were associated with lower requirements for postoperative dopamine and nitroglycerine and improved ejection fraction in comparison with placebo and 100-μM adenosine. In a follow-up study, Mentzer et al. (386) reported that the high-dose adenosine cardioplegia groups (2 mM and 200 mM followed by 140 μg/kg per minute) had significantly reduced postoperative thoracic drainage at 6 hours, 24 hours, and at the time of chest tube removal in comparison with the control and low-dose adenosine cardioplegia group (100 μM). This was associated with a significant reduction in platelet, fresh frozen plasma, and packed erythrocyte use in the high-dose adenosine cardioplegia group. Therefore, the results of clinical trials with adenosine as an adjunct to cardi-

oplegia are encouraging but as yet indicate no clear advantage to adenosine over unsupplemented cardioplegia. Clinical trials in which more sensitive indices of ventricular performance (pressure–area relations obtained with transesophageal echocardiography) are used may provide more precise measures of postoperative (vs. preoperative) cardiac performance.

Elements of Myocardial Protection: Experimental Strategies

Nitric Oxide

Two general approaches have been taken to harness the cardioprotective potential of NO: (a) modulation of endogenous NO by addition of NO precursors or agents that stimulate native NO production by NO synthase, and (b) administration of authentic NO or NO donors. These approaches can be carried out systemically (appropriate for pre-bypass or off-pump applications) or by supplementation of cardioplegia solutions. Table 13.6 lists the physiologic effects of NO that may contribute to cardioprotection.

Enhancing endogenous NO release: Enhancing the release of *endogenous* NO can be achieved by providing the precursor L-arginine. Although L-arginine appears in the blood in sufficient concentrations to saturate the endothelial isoform of NO synthase, supplemental L-arginine has been shown to increase NO release (directly or indirectly measured) by the coronary vascular endothelium (215,387,388). In isolated rat aortic endothelial cells, 1 mM L-arginine increased the release of NO by approximately 40% above basal level (215), whereas D-arginine at the same concentration did not increase NO release. In *in vitro* studies of neutrophil adherence and damage to coronary artery endothelium, sup-

TABLE 13.6. PHYSIOLOGIC EFFECTS OF NITRIC OXIDE THAT ARE POTENTIALLY RELEVANT TO MYOCARDIAL ISCHEMIA-REPERFUSION INJURY

Tissue	Effect
Endothelium	Improved vasoreactivity
	Decreased adhesion molecule expression
	Decreased adhesion molecule synthesis
	Increased vascular permeability
	Decreased platelet aggregation and adherence
Neutrophil	Decreased neutrophil-endothelial cell interaction
	Decreased superoxide generation
	Neutralization of PMN-generated superoxide
	Decreased neutrophil accumulation following I/R
Myocardium	Reduction in infarct size
	Improved post-bypass contractility(?)
	Decreased mast cell release of histamine
	Protection by preconditioning(?)

I/R, ischemia-reperfusion; PMN, polymorphonuclear leukocyte.

plementation with L-arginine in to 10-mM concentrations resulted in significantly attenuated neutrophil adherence to activated coronary artery endothelium and significantly attenuated neutrophil-mediated injury, although L-arginine did not directly attenuate neutrophil superoxide anion pro-

duction (387). Adherence was not inhibited by D-arginine (10 mM), and 600-μM carboxy-PT10, a direct scavenger of NO, reversed the effects of L-arginine (51,84). Accordingly, in surgical models of antecedent ischemia (regional or global) with subsequent cardioplegia and reperfusion, supplementation of blood cardioplegia with L-arginine has also been shown to provide significant benefit, consistent with its potent antineutrophil effects. Sato et al. (389) used a canine model of regional (left anterior descending) coronary artery ligation for 90 minutes, followed by cardioplegic arrest via blood cardioplegia without (unsupplemented) or with 10-mM L-arginine and a concomitant intravenous infusion (4 mg/kg per minute) started at release of the cross-clamp. Blood cardioplegia enhanced with L-arginine was associated with a 33% increase in postischemic systolic contractile function in the area at risk and a significant decrease in diastolic segment stiffness, a 30% reduction in infarct size, and near-normalization of postischemic left anterior descending artery endothelial function in comparison with unsupplemented blood cardioplegia (Fig. 13.12). These beneficial effects of L-arginine were also associated with a significant decrease in neutrophil accumulation in the reperfused area at risk (389). The effects of L-arginine were reversed by inclusion of the NO synthase inhibitor l-nitro-arginine before administration of L-arginine–enhanced blood cardioplegia in a separate group. These results have been corroborated by other studies in which cardioplegia solutions were supplemented with L-arginine (390,391). In-

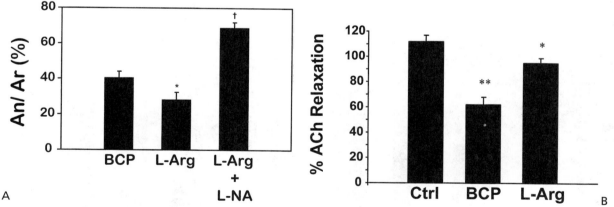

FIG. 13.12. The cardioprotective effects of blood cardioplegia (*BCP*) supplemented with L-arginine (L-*Arg*) in hearts subjected to antecedent normothermic ischemia. **A:** Infarct size, or myocardial area of necrosis expressed as a percentage of area at risk [*An/Ar (%)*], was reduced by L-arginine–supplemented BCP in comparison with unsupplemented BCP, which was reversed by the nitric oxide synthase inhibitor L-nitro-arginine (L-*NA*). $p < 0.05$ vs. L-Arg; $+p < 0.05$ vs. L-Arg and BCP. **B:** Endothelial function assessed by vasodilator responses of preconstricted postcardioplegia epicardial coronary arteries to the endothelium-dependent relaxant acetylcholine. One hundred percent indicates intact endothelial cell function. In comparison with a normal control coronary artery (*Ctrl*), unsupplemented BCP was associated with significant endothelial dysfunction, whereas L-Arg BCP prevented this dysfunction. *$p < 0.05$ vs. Ctrl; **$p < 0.05$ vs. Ctrl and L-Arg. (From Sato H, Zhao Z-Q, McGee DS, et al. Supplemental L-arginine during cardioplegic arrest and reperfusion avoids regional postischemic injury. *J Thorac Cardiovasc Surg* 1995;110:302–314, with permission.)

terestingly, 3-mM L-arginine given *after* cardioplegia was reported to be detrimental (392), a finding that may be related to (a) missing the therapeutically effective window for targets of NO therapy (neutrophil-derived superoxide anions, adherence, and neutrophil-mediated endothelial damage) or (b) the generation of deleterious decomposition products of NO (peroxynitrite).

Other studies have confirmed the cardioprotective effects of L-arginine in cardiac surgery models. Hiramatsu et al. (390,393) administered L-arginine during the early phase of reperfusion in blood-perfused isolated hearts, ostensibly to target reperfusion events, and reported better recovery of postcardioplegia systolic function in comparison with that achieved with unsupplemented perfusates. This timing of administration of L-arginine at reperfusion is consistent with its antineutrophil effect in this model. Similar beneficial effects of L-arginine administered at reperfusion were reported by Amrani et al. (394) in a cell-free perfusate system, which suggests that NO derived from supplemental L-arginine may offer protection through effects other than its antineutrophil activity (i.e., quenching of superoxide anions).

Protection by NO donors: A limitation may be encountered in utilizing the endogenous cardioprotective mechanisms evoked with L-arginine therapy in that the increased release of NO depends on the functional state of the endothelium. Consequently, an injured endothelium in which NO generation mechanisms are impaired not only may show attenuated responses to L-arginine, but also may exaggerate the phenotypic expression of postischemic injury (395). This limitation in the endogenous generation of NO can be overcome by the administration of NO donor agents. The exogenous administration of NO donors was first reported by Johnson et al. (396), who used authentic NO gas and $NaNO_2$ (397) administered only at the onset of reperfusion at subvasodilator concentrations in a feline model of regional ischemia–reperfusion. Both forms of NO therapy decreased infarct size by approximately 75% in association with decreased neutrophil accumulation in the area at risk, suggesting that NO reduces infarct size by inhibiting neutrophil-mediated damage. Subsequent studies have been performed with a variety of organic NO donor agents in nonsurgical models of coronary occlusion and reperfusion. These organic donors release NO either spontaneously or after bioconversion reactions. Nitroglycerine is the prototype NO donor agent but is a poor NO donor because of its prerequisite bioconversion by a cysteine-containing enzyme that is partially depleted in the microvasculature after ischemia–reperfusion. One such cysteine-containing compound that readily releases NO after biotransformation is SPM-5185 [*N*-(3-hydroxy-pivaloyl)-*S*-(*N'*-acetylalanoyl)-L-cysteine ethyl ester] (Schwarz Pharma AG, Monheim, Germany) (398,399). In a study by Nakanishi et al. (196) based on a canine model of CPB and cardioplegia, hearts were subjected to 30 minutes of normothermic ischemia followed by 1 hour cardioplegia (4°C multidose blood cardioplegia, blood-to-crystalloid ratio of 4:1). Hearts received either unsupplemented blood cardioplegia (BCP), or blood cardioplegia with 10-μM SPM-5185 (BCP + SPM). After 1 hour of cardioplegic arrest, the heart was reperfused for a total of 60 minutes. Left ventricular function was assessed by the slope of the end-systolic pressure–volume (imped-

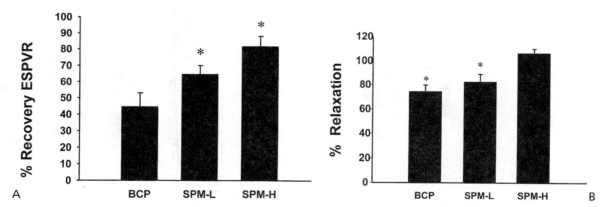

FIG. 13.13. The nitric oxide donor agent SPM-5185 in blood cardioplegia (*BCP*) at lower (*SPM-L*, 1 μM) and higher (*SPM-H*, 10 μM) concentrations administered to hearts subjected to antecedent normothermic ischemia. **A:** Left ventricular function after cardioplegia measured by slope of the end-systolic pressure–volume (impedance catheter) relations (*ESPVR*, expressed as percentage of recovery from baseline). *p <0.05 vs. unsupplemented BCP. **B:** Nitric oxide donors and postcardioplegia endothelial injury. Function measured as in Fig. 13.12. *p <0.05 vs. unsupplemented BCP. (From Nakanishi K. Zhao Z-Q, Vinten-Johansen J, et al. Blood cardioplegia enhanced with nitric oxide donor SPM-5185 counteracts postischemic endothelial and ventricular dysfunction. *J Thorac Cardiovasc Surg* 1995;109:1146–1154, with permission.)

ance catheter) relation. The postischemic end-systolic pressure–volume relation was depressed to 46.3% of preischemic values in the unsupplemented blood cardioplegia group (from 8.2 ± 1.0 to 3.8 ± 0.3 mm Hg/mL). In contrast, postischemic functional recovery was nearly complete in the SPM-enhanced blood cardioplegia group (from 7.6 ± 1.1 to 7.2 ± 1.2 mm Hg/mL) (Fig. 13.13). In postischemic coronary arteries isolated from these hearts, endothelium-dependent maximal relaxation to acetylcholine was impaired by 27% in the BCP group, but recovered to 100% or more in the BCP + SPM group (Fig. 13.13). Myeloperoxidase activity in postischemic myocardium, used as an index of neutrophil accumulation, was higher in the unsupplemented blood cardioplegia group (3.36 ± 0.58 U/100 mg of tissue) than in the SPM-enhanced blood cardioplegia group (1.27 ± 0.45 U/100 mg of tissue). Therefore, this study demonstrated that addition of a NO donor in blood cardioplegia improves postischemic ventricular performance and postcardioplegia endothelial function in ischemically injured hearts, possibly via attenuating neutrophil-mediated damage.

Potential deleterious effects of NO in cardioplegia solutions: The benefits of L-arginine or NO donor supplementation are controversial. Some experimental studies in nonsurgical models of ischemia–reperfusion report that NO has *deleterious* effects on endothelial and contractile function (337,400,401), whereas others show benefits (as described above). Deleterious effects of NO have been substantiated by other studies, which report a decrease in the time to ischemic contracture in globally ischemic hearts, a decrease in postischemic left ventricular contractile recovery, an increase in infarct size, and an increase in myocardial neutrophil accumulation (402–404).

The discrepancy in these diametrically opposed results may involve a reaction between NO and superoxide anion forming peroxynitrite. This biradical reaction proceeds at nearly diffusion-limited rates and is essentially irreversible (405,406). The dichotomy in physiologic consequences of NO (and peroxynitrite) seems to revolve around the environment in which peroxynitrite is present (i.e., a crystalloid environment or a blood environment). *In vitro* data from studies of crystalloid solutions report an increase in myocardial stunning, evidenced by decreased postischemic developed pressure in rat hearts, increased infarct size, and direct endothelial toxicity via lipid peroxidation and DNA injury (337). Other investigators have examined the effect of peroxynitrite in *in vivo* environments (i.e., blood) and have shown benefits similar to those described above with authentic NO or NO donors. Nossuli et al. (407) reported a reduction of more than 50% in infarct size in a feline model with authentic peroxynitrite in comparison with a vehicle related to higher concentrations of peroxynitrite and the presence of detoxifying agents. This dichotomy in the physiologic actions of NO through peroxynitrite has an impor-

tant impact on the surgical strategies of cardioprotection (i.e., whether crystalloid or blood cardioplegia is used as a cardioprotective agent). This important question was recently addressed by Ronson et al. (408), who determined that in a surgically relevant CPB model with 30 minutes of antecedent global ischemia, blood cardioplegia supplemented with 5-μM authentic peroxynitrite showed improved myocardial contractility in comparison with blood cardioplegia with no peroxynitrite, whereas peroxynitrite added to crystalloid cardioplegia impaired contractility relative to crystalloid cardioplegia without peroxynitrite (Fig. 13.14). This study confirms the environmental sensitivity of peroxynitrite and may have clinical implications for NO additives to crystalloid cardioplegic solutions in that appropriate adjunct detoxifying agents may be necessary to detoxify peroxynitrite if generated.

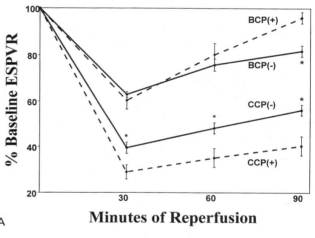

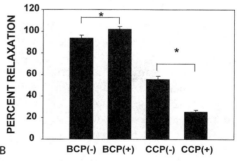

FIG. 13.14. The dichotomous effects of peroxynitrite (*ONOO⁻*) on postcardioplegia left ventricular function assessed by pressure–volume relations (**A**) and postcardioplegia coronary artery endothelial function (**B**). In panel A, left ventricular function is described as a percentage of the baseline end-systolic pressure–volume relationship (*ESPVR*) when the impedance catheter technique is used. *BCP(-)*, blood cardioplegia without ONOO⁻; *BCP(+)*, blood cardioplegia with 5 μM ONOO⁻; *CCP(-)*, crystalloid cardioplegia (Plegisol) without ONOO⁻; *CCP(+)*, crystalloid cardioplegia with 5 μM ONOO⁻. *p <0.05 vs. group with ONOO⁻. [From Ronson RS, Thourani VH, Ma X-L, et al. Peroxynitrite is beneficial in blood cardioplegia, but is deleterious in crystalloid cardioplegia *in vivo. Circulation* 1998;98:I-750(abst), with permission.]

Specific Antineutrophil Therapy in Surgical Myocardial Protection

With identification of the active role that neutrophils and endothelium play in the pathogenesis of ischemia–reperfusion injury, new myocardial protective strategies have targeted these components, either individually or as a unit (i.e., adhesion). Therapy to limit neutrophil–endothelial cell interaction could dramatically reduce myocardial dysfunction and morbidity after CPB despite the intense activation of the inflammatory cascade during coronary operations. Administering direct antibodies to cell surface adhesion molecules on both endothelium and neutrophils (to attenuate neutrophil adherence) is an area of intense investigation. Many specific monoclonal antibodies that inhibit neutrophil adherence to the endothelium are currently available, including antibodies for CD18, P-selectin, and L-selectin. However, enthusiasm for antibody therapy is mitigated by its systemic immunosuppressive effects, which may predispose to postoperative infection.

Hypothermia is the simplest method for inhibiting cell surface adhesion molecules. In addition to minimizing cellular metabolic activity, hypothermia slows the expression of endothelial adhesion molecules (248,249). Decreases in temperature to 25°C will temporarily virtually eliminate expression of E-selectin, an endothelial adherence molecule primarily responsible for firm neutrophil attachment (248). The accumulation of NF-κB, the transcription factor responsible for *de novo* adhesion molecule synthesis, in the nucleus during hypothermia results in overexpression of endothelial E-selectin and other adhesion molecules on reperfusion and rewarming, thereby increasing neutrophil adherence. These findings have been confirmed by others, but no hypothermia-induced lasting reduction of adhesion molecule expression has been observed (138,142).

The temporary effects of hypothermia highlight the time-dependent nature of adhesion molecule expression, indicating that therapy must coincide with the expression of these molecules. For example, the expression of P-selectin, an endothelial adherence molecule responsible for the initial slowing or "rolling" of neutrophils along endothelial surfaces in the early phase of reperfusion, must be addressed within the first 30 minutes of restoration of blood flow to limit neutrophil–endothelial interaction, but firmer adherence would need to be addressed with E-selectin and ICAM-1 blockade several hours later (36,409,410). This has prompted investigators to examine the transcription factors responsible for families of surface adhesion molecules. The best studied of these factors is NF-κB. Mutations in regulatory proteins for the NF-κB family of transcription factors decrease the production of both E-selectin and VCAM following endothelial activation (411,412). The clinical implications of augmentation of selectin expression are not currently known. Speculation about the potential for an increased risk for perioperative infection with systemic limi-

tation of neutrophil infiltration has slowed clinical investigation of this potentially powerful protective tool.

Targeting the neutrophil as a site for therapeutic intervention represents an alternative to attenuation of endothelial adhesion molecule expression. The transition from bubble oxygenators to the currently used membrane oxygenators was driven, in part, by the decreased complement activation and subsequent neutrophil-induced injury seen with the membrane-type devices. Like those targeting endothelial adhesion molecules, strategies to attenuate the actions of adhesion molecules on the neutrophil have been investigated with limited success. However, Flynn et al. (413) have demonstrated that an oligosaccharide that binds the sialyl Lewis^x receptor on the neutrophil is able to reduce infarct size following ischemia and reperfusion in dogs. The clinical application of this strategy remains unknown. Filtration of neutrophils with the Pall filter directly reduces neutrophil accumulation and decreases subsequent inflammatory injury (414,415). An advantage to this approach is that the filter can be interposed in the cardioplegia delivery line to filter neutrophils selectively from blood cardioplegia, rather than simply filter systemic blood (416). The clinical benefit of filtering neutrophils is still under debate, and conclusive evidence of improved patient outcome is not yet available (36).

Complement-Related Therapy

Complement is involved in the pathophysiology of myocardial postischemic injury and infarct development. As described above, both myocardial ischemia and extracorporeal circulation increase the generation of complement fragments and other components of the complement cascade, notably the terminal membrane attack complex (417). Complement products such as C3a, C5a, and C5b are activated during exposure of blood to extracorporeal surfaces, notably oxygenators, during CPB procedures. The setting of surgical revascularization of acute evolving infarction by means of CPB and cardioplegia techniques may therefore offer a strong stimulus for complement production and consequent complement-mediated injury stemming from ischemia–reperfusion and CPB (143). This complement-mediated injury may aggravate ischemia–reperfusion injury in the surgical setting and, hence, reduce the benefits of surgical revascularization. However, as Gillinov et al. (133) and others have suggested, the redundant pathways in the inflammatory cascade may require therapy that inhibits multiple arms of the inflammatory response.

A number of strategies have been adopted to attenuate complement-mediated damage in the surgical setting of CPB. Coating of extracorporeal surfaces with heparin and other agents that inhibit the inflammatory response has provided some benefit. The use of leukocyte-specific filters temporarily removes the offending neutrophils from the circulation, but this approach does not address the interaction between blood and foreign surfaces that results in complement activation, does not prevent the rapid rebound of neutrophils into the circulation after transient leukosequestration and margination, and does not prevent direct cell injury by the membrane attack complex of the complement system. Antibodies directed against cytokines, complement fragments, adhesion molecules, and the complement receptors themselves (i.e., C3 or C5a) constitute another approach to attenuating the complement-induced inflammatory component of surgical ischemia–reperfusion injury. Studies by Gillinov et al. (133) in complement (C3)-deficient dogs confirm that the absence of complement components reduces neutrophil activation (expression of CD18), neutrophil accumulation in lung tissue, and deposition of complement fragments on vascular tissue. Attenuation of complement activation with soluble human complement receptor type 1 was shown by Gillinov et al. (418) to reduce complement hemolytic activity and functional activities of C3 and C5 in a porcine model of hypothermic (28°C) CPB. Soluble complement receptor type 1 reduced post-CPB pulmonary vascular resistance but, interestingly, did not attenuate other manifestations of pulmonary injury. Finn et al. (417) also reported a reduction in complement (C3a) generation with soluble (human) complement receptor type 1, but did not find it to inhibit the generation of the terminal membrane attack complex or neutrophil activation. Tofukuji et al. (419) investigated the vasoprotective effects of a porcine anti-C5a monoclonal antibody in a surgical model of cardioplegia; this antibody would effectively deactivate C5a in the circulation, rather than inhibit the activation of complement or its interaction with receptors. In a porcine model of CPB and 60 minutes of cold K^+ crystalloid cardioplegia, pigs received intravenous anti-C5a monoclonal antibody before CPB and chemical cardioplegia. The anti-C5a monoclonal antibody (a) inhibited homotypic aggregation and chemotaxis by neutrophils, (b) attenuated endothelium-dependent microvascular dysfunction observed in unsupplemented cardioplegia, and (c) reduced neutrophil infiltration into postcardioplegia myocardium. However, the antibody did not improve postcardioplegia contractile function or reduce intramyocardial edema.

In another recent study, Riley et al. (152) investigated the cardioprotective effects of a novel C5a receptor antagonist, CGS 32359, which blocks the membrane receptor for C5a rather than binding to C5a itself. In *in vitro* studies, this antagonist in dose-dependent fashion inhibited superoxide production by human C5a-activated porcine neutrophils (18 ± 3.7 vs. 1.6 ± 0.5* nmol/5 min/5 × 10^6 neutrophils), and reduced neutrophil adherence to coronary artery endothelium (194 ± 9 vs. 43 ± 6* neutrophils/mm²). In a porcine model of simulated surgical revascularization on

CPB, the left anterior descending coronary artery was occluded for a total of 50 minutes (152). The C5a antagonist was administered intravenously (bolus of 60 mg/kg followed by 60 mg/kg hourly) before revascularization with blood cardioplegia. The intravenous administration ensured admixture of the agent in blood cardioplegia (harvested from the reservoir). After 1 hour of global cardiac arrest with multidose hypothermic (4°C) blood cardioplegia followed by 2.5 hours of reperfusion, infarct size (reported as area of necrosis as a percentage of the area at risk) was significantly reduced by the C5a antagonist (18 ± 6%*) in comparison with saline solution and unsupplemented blood cardioplegia (52 ± 3%). Systolic shortening, measured by sonomicrometry, in the area at risk was significantly greater with the C5a antagonist (expressed as a percentage of baseline, 7.3 ± 7.5*) than with saline solution (-27.8 ± 9.5) and unsupplemented blood cardioplegia. Furthermore, a significant reduction in myeloperoxidase activity of accumulated neutrophils was noted in the ischemic zone of hearts receiving C5a receptor antagonist in comparison with those receiving unsupplemented cardioplegia. Therefore, a recombinant human C5a receptor antagonist was found to be effective in inhibiting surgical ischemia–reperfusion injury after coronary occlusion and surgical reperfusion.

At this point, it is not clear how anticomplement therapy will address complement-mediated injury. The lack of consistent improvement in postcardioplegia contractile recovery in the studies by Tokufuji et al. (419) and others may be related to redundancy in the pathways of the inflammatory response and its actions on mechanisms of reversible injury (contractile function, endothelial dysfunction?) and irreversible injury (infarction, endothelial dysfunction?). A broader antiinflammatory approach may be necessary to address this point. In addition, antigen–antibody reactions of the host with peptide-related antibodies may pose a difficult problem, although humanized recombinant peptides may offer a solution (152).

Hyperpolarizing Agents

The primary goal of cardioplegic agents is to provide a quiet, nonbeating heart, which allows the cardiac surgeon to perform coronary artery bypass grafting or repair complex cardiac anomalies. Furthermore, cardioplegic agents must protect the heart during periods of global ischemia and cardiac arrest. The most commonly used arresting agents are depolarizing hyperkalemic cardioplegic and hyperpolarizing agents. In depolarizing cardioplegic solutions, potassium in high concentrations (10 to 20 mmol/L) is used as the major cardiac arresting agent; membrane depolarization results from an increase in extracellular potassium. The advantages of potassium arrest are (a) rapid arrest and (b) rapid reversibility on washout. The disadvantages include (a) potential endothelial damage with higher concentrations; (b) temperature sensitivity, requiring high concentrations for normo-

---

* Indicates p < 0.05.

thermic induction and "hot shot" or continuous cardioplegia applications; (c) the potential for systemic hyperkalemia ("overdose"), particularly with continuous cardioplegia; and (d) sustained metabolic activity. In membrane depolarization, cellular metabolic processes continue and transmembrane ionic gradients are deranged, including those of the energy-requiring calcium and sodium pumps, which continue to function and deplete critical energy supplies (420–422). The complex interactions between the sodium and calcium ion shifts following hyperkalemic cardioplegic arrest eventually result in myocyte calcium overload and a host of processes, including calcium-activated dysrhythmogenic currents, abnormal regulation of intracellular second messengers, activation of cytosolic and membrane-bound enzyme systems, impaired myocardial force production, and the potential for calcium-induced reperfusion injury. In animal infarct models, continued membrane depolarization with extracellular hyperkalemia leads to sodium and chloride influx into cells to cause an increase in water content and cell swelling (161). Similar mechanisms have been shown experimentally during hyperkalemic cardioplegic arrest (163). Consequently, it is possible that depolarized arrest with potassium may be a contributory factor toward the well-known detrimental consequence of myocardial edema following cardioplegic arrest.

It has been shown experimentally that many of the problems associated with depolarizing hyperkalemic arrest can be avoided by hyperpolarizing cardioplegia. For example, cardioplegia containing K_{ATP} channel openers provides an alternative method of achieving cardioplegic arrest (423–427). K_{ATP} channels, first described in 1983 by Noma (428), are located on vascular smooth muscle (429), cardiac myocytes (428), pancreatic β-cells (430), and neurons (431). Opening these channels induces myocyte relaxation by allowing potassium efflux from the cell, which causes membrane hyperpolarization and decreases the probability that voltage-gated calcium channels will remain open. Activation of K_{ATP} channels mediates several physiologic responses, including the vascular response to hypoxia (429), the basal level of coronary vascular tone (432), the reactive hyperemia after brief coronary occlusions (433,434), and coronary autoregulation (435,436). In addition, the opening of K_{ATP} channels mediates in part the cardioprotection effects of ischemic preconditioning (437,438) and adenosine (439,440). A variety of potassium channel openers, including diazoxide, nicorandil, minoxidil, pinacidil, cromakalim, lemakalim, and aprikalim, have been investigated in a myriad of animal models. Potassium channel openers facilitate the efflux of potassium from the myocyte, thereby arresting the myocyte at a more negative membrane potential (hyperpolarized state) that more closely resembles the normal resting potential of the cell. Proponents of hyperpolarizing cardioplegic arrest note that arrest of myocytes by potassium channel openers near their resting membrane potential may provide metabolic and ionic advantages over traditional depolarized arrest. In the hyperpolarized myocyte state, transmembrane ionic gradients are balanced, ion

channel flux is minimal, and ATP-driven pumps are largely inactive (420–422,441). A blood-perfused, parabiotic, Langendorff rabbit heart model and an *in vivo* swine model have been used to study functional recovery following hyperpolarizing cardioplegic arrest in comparison with depolarized arrest (236,423,425,426,442–445). In a recent study by Jayawant et al. (237), pinacidil cardioplegia administered continuously was superior to unsupplemented St. Thomas' Hospital cardioplegia given as either an intermittent or continuous infusion. Furthermore, in an intact CPB animal model, Jayawant et al. (442) reported that pinacidil cardioplegia resulted in the preservation of postcardioplegia contractile function following 2 hours of hypothermic global ischemia in comparison with the hyperkalemic St. Thomas' Hospital cardioplegic solution. Because they did not appreciate a correlation between contractile recovery and either high-energy nucleotide levels or a difference in myocardial edema between the depolarized and hyperpolarized groups, they hypothesized that the superior myocardial protection could be attributed to the more optimal ionic milieu in the hyperpolarized than in the depolarized hearts. Thus far, no human clinical trials evaluating myocardial protection afforded by potassium channel openers have been reported. Furthermore, the actual mechanisms by which potassium channel openers provide myocardial protection have not been clearly elucidated. Lawton et al. (443) have shown that hyperpolarized cardioplegia with pinacidil increases postcardioplegic myocardial oxygen consumption (postischemic aerobic metabolism) in comparison with hyperkalemic cardioplegia. Therefore, they hypothesize that the improved recovery seen with potassium channel opener-induced hyperpolarized arrest may be attributable to an ionic benefit provided by these drugs, largely related to the prevention of calcium overload during ischemia.

There are potential limitations to hyperpolarizing cardioplegic agents. Although potassium channel openers have been shown to have antidysrhythmic effects under conditions in which triggered dysrhythmias are produced (446), they have also been shown to be prodysrhythmic under conditions in which reentrant dysrhythmias may be generated (i.e., regional ischemia and reperfusion) (447). However, toxicity data for high concentrations of the various potassium channel openers are not yet available (448). In recent studies by Jayawant et al. (237,444) based on a blood-perfused, parabiotic, isolated rabbit model, nicorandil used as an adjunct to blood cardioplegia significantly improved postcardioplegia functional recovery and decreased myocardial edema without dysrhythmogenicity in comparison with conventional hyperkalemic cardioplegia.

Sodium–Hydrogen Exchange Inhibitors

Since Sardet and colleagues (449) isolated the first known Na^+-H^+ exchanger cDNA clone (now known as NHE-1), four isoforms (NHE-1 through NHE-4) (450) from a number of species have been described in humans, sheep, rabbits, rats, hamsters, and pigs (449,451–454). In general, the

NHE proteins are well conserved within a given isoform and among different species, and even among different isoforms of the same species. Acidosis induces negative inotropy in a variety of cardiac preparations (455–457). Because acidosis can develop quickly during myocardial ischemia, and because pH management strategies in cardioplegia solutions have been shown to be important in myocardial protection, the internal regulation of myocardial pH is especially important to the function of the postischemic heart. The Na^+-H^+ exchange system is one mechanism associated with the intrinsic regulation of acidosis in the heart. The Na^+-H^+ exchanger regulates intracellular pH by removing one intracellular H^+ in exchange for one extracellular Na^+ when intracellular pH decreases. However, the rising intracellular Na^+ concentration activates Ca^{2+} influx via the Na^+-Ca^{2+} exchangers (458,459), thereby inducing intracellular Ca^{2+} accumulation. As discussed previously, excessive intracellular Ca^{2+} accumulation leads to a host of deleterious effects on the myocardium, including uncoupling of myocardial function and metabolism, local cellular hypercontraction, triggering of dysrhythmias, and development or exaggeration of necrosis.

Under normal or even mildly acidotic physiologic conditions, the cellular regulatory balance between Na^+-H^+ exchange and intracellular Na^+ extrusion prevents Ca^{2+}-mediated myocyte injury. However, with significant intracellular acidosis (i.e., during myocardial ischemia and reperfusion), the normal regulatory mechanisms are overwhelmed, and Ca^{2+} influx and myocardial damage can result. The accumulation of lactate during ischemic anaerobic glycolysis decreases both extracellular and intracellular pH, and stimulation of the Na^+-H^+ exchanger is minimal (460–462). During reperfusion, extracellular lactate washes out first, returning the extracellular pH to physiologic values and reactivating the Na^+-H^+ exchanger, which leads to a detrimental increase in intracellular calcium and eventual cell death.

The reduction of Ca^{2+} overload within the myocardium by Na^+-H^+ exchange inhibitors is a new strategy in myocardial protection. A number of studies using first-generation Na^+-H^+ exchange (NHE) inhibitors [amiloride and its derivatives ethylisopropyl amiloride (EIPA), dimethyl amiloride (DMA), methylisobutyl amiloride (MIBA), hexamethylene amiloride (HMA), and the more specific NHE-1 inhibitor HOE-694] have demonstrated cardioprotective effects (463–466). Postischemic ventricular fibrillation has been linked to Ca^{2+} overload, and this complication has been prevented by amiloride derivatives and HOE-694 (464,467). Furthermore, studies have demonstrated a substantial reduction of postischemic contracture (468), an improvement in cardiac performance (466,469), and amelioration of myocardial stunning (470) with NHE inhibition. Myocardial protection was observed when the NHE inhibitors were given during ischemia (464,466,467,471), reperfusion (466,472,473), or both ischemia and reperfusion (466).

Although no human or large animal *in vivo* studies have evaluated NHE inhibitors as adjuncts to cardioplegia solutions, a number of isolated rat heart cardioplegic studies have been reported. The aforementioned studies have clearly shown that inhibition of the Na^+-H^+ exchanger improves postischemic ventricular function after normothermic ischemia. However, whether this beneficial effect can be used in the clinical setting to protect surgically ischemic–reperfused myocardium has only recently been investigated. In view of the nonsurgical experimental data, the cardioprotection afforded by Na^+-H^+ exchange inhibitors suggests that this potential therapy may be well suited for the episodes of ischemia and reperfusion associated with single or multidose cardioplegia. In an isolated cardioplegia rat heart model, Yamauchi et al. (173) have confirmed that activation of Na^+-H^+ exchange occurs not only during normothermia but also during hypothermic conditions (17°C). Furthermore, activation of the Na^+-H^+ exchange system leads to deterioration of ventricular function. Inhibition of the Na^+-H^+ exchanger with FR168888 before ischemia, during cardioplegic arrest, or during reperfusion significantly inhibited cell swelling and improved postischemic functional recovery after both normothermic and prolonged hypothermic cardioplegic arrest. In isolated working rat hearts, Shipolini et al. (474) reported that the NHE exchange inhibitor HOE-642 as an adjunct to cardioplegia provides significant benefits at normothermia, moderate hypothermia, and severe hypothermia. In a study by Choy et al. (475) of isolated rat hearts subjected to cardioplegic arrest and reperfusion, the addition of HOE-694 to the cardioplegic solution attenuated the increase of intracellular sodium during myocardial ischemia and early reperfusion, and this was associated with an improved recovery of contractile function.

The cardioprotection afforded by NHE exchange inhibitors also applies to the cardiac transplant model. Myers et al. (476) have shown a marked protective effect of Na^+-H^+ exchange inhibitor HOE-694 in rabbit hearts subjected to 12 hours of hypothermic ischemia. Moreover, they found significant protection when NHE inhibitors were administered only at reperfusion, but not when given only during cardioplegia.

Preconditioning and Preconditioning Mimetics

Perhaps the most revolutionary recent discovery in myocardial protection was reported in 1986 by Murry et al. (477), who showed that the myocardium exhibits endogenous cardioprotection against prolonged ischemia when given a brief, antecedent, "preconditioning" ischemic period. For the first time, it was convincingly shown that the heart is not a "bystander" to exogenous manipulation of the cellular milieu during ischemia and reperfusion, but rather that myocytes use endogenous pathways that can be exploited to protect against ischemia–reperfusion injury. Since this seminal observation, ischemia has been used as the primary trigger to initiate the protective mechanisms, which has become known as "ischemic preconditioning." This technique has provided more potent cardioprotection than pharmacotherapy. Recent studies have focused on identifying pharmacologic agents such as adenosine, NO, and potassium channel openers to harness the preconditioning potential of the myocytes without the need for inducing ischemia and incurring its potential deleterious effects (370,439,478,479).

The specific pathways involved in endogenous myocardial protection by preconditioning are numerous and redundant. Adenosine, and specifically activation of the A_1 adenosine receptor, has been shown to mimic many of the effects of preconditioning by (a) decreasing the rate of ATP depletion during prolonged ischemia, (b) releasing adenosine into the interstitial compartment, and (c) upregulating the protein kinase C enzyme system (366,480–482). Activation of the protein kinase C pathway opens the K_{ATP} channels to provide cardioprotection (479). Protein kinase C may be an important common mediator for a number of pathways that have been regarded as important to preconditioning. Although new triggers for preconditioning are being identified on a regular basis, the direct clinical application of preconditioning triggered by ischemia or hypoxia remains unclear.

Many investigators have documented reduced infarct size (366,484,485), improved endothelial function (486), and decreased neutrophil accumulation (49) in postischemic myocardium following preconditioning. However, the ability of preconditioning to restore postischemic contractility is controversial. Furthermore, the role of preconditioning as an adjunct to other protective strategies, such as cardioplegia and hypothermia, is also unclear. Except in a few studies, ischemic preconditioning does not seem to afford any additional improvement in postischemic contractile function over conventional myocardial protection techniques (489–491). Pharmacologic pretreatment before the interval of chemical cardioplegia with agents such as adenosine has afforded slightly greater protection. However, side effects such as hypotension and bradycardia have limited their clinical application (366). Perhaps the ultimate goal is to identify a chemical surrogate of preconditioning, one that can trigger the *in vivo* mechanisms that operate on end-effectors, so that long-term or "permanent" preconditioning can be imposed.

As the use of off-pump coronary surgery, without the conveniences of extracorporeal circulation and extracorporeally based myocardial protection (i.e., cardioplegia), increases, preconditioning may find a niche in protecting the myocardium from ischemic injury encountered during creation of the anastomosis. Bufkin et al. (49) have shown that 5 minutes of left anterior descending artery occlusion imposed before more prolonged occlusion in an off-pump model reduces myocardial neutrophil accumulation and improves vascular reactivity, but does not improve recovery of regional contractile function after 3 hours of reperfusion. However, the exact impact of preconditioning, either physical (ischemia) or chemical (pharmacologic) in off-pump applications, has yet to be defined.

SUMMARY

Recent advances in myocardial protection have expanded to target the molecular and cellular mechanisms of injury that occur during ischemia, cardioplegic arrest, and reperfusion. The mechanisms leading to postischemic and postcardioplegia injury (vascular dysfunction, apoptosis, necrosis, contractile and diastolic dysfunction) are essentially moving targets undergoing definition and characterization by basic science research. Their application to myocardial protection strategies, therefore, must keep pace with the basic science advances. In addition, the conventional concepts of myocardial protection are undergoing radical evolution, fueled by the desire to (a) preserve simple yet broad-spectrum approaches, (b) reduce hemodilution, and (c) curtail the use of CPB and extracorporeal equipment, which may promote the inflammatory response. Hence, off-pump cardiac surgery will challenge the fundamental concepts of myocardial protection that relies on various delivery devices and prompt redesigned strategies embracing systemic approaches or local delivery systems. Molecular approaches that intervene in the inflammatory responses may be combined with genetic approaches to alter the responses of the heart to myocardial injury. Gene therapy can be used to increase the release of endogenous cardioprotective substances such as heat shock proteins, NO, and adenosine, or reduce the insults that lead to injury. In addition, gene therapy may permit injured or dead myocytes to be replaced by healthy myocytes or by stem cells that can transform into functional myocytes. New strategies using gene therapy ("gene cuisine cardioplegia"), target-specific antibodies and autacoids, ion channel inhibitors, and cell replacements offer exciting and potentially revolutionary future prospects for myocardial protection.

KEY POINTS

- *Intraoperative myocardial injury* can occur before, during, or after cardiopulmonary bypass.
  - *Injury before cardiopulmonary bypass* is commonly "unprotected" (i.e., lacking cardiopulmonary bypass or cardioplegia).
  - *Injury during cardiopulmonary bypass* can be multifactorial, related to the composition or delivery of cardioplegic protective solutions or to the reperfusion period after cardioplegic arrest.
  - *Injury after cardiopulmonary bypass* commonly results from postischemic reperfusion.
- The degree of permanent myocardial injury after ischemia is a function of the severity and duration of ischemia, which can be modified by numerous factors.

- *Reperfusion injury* is defined as additional myocardial injury incurred after restoration of blood flow to ischemic myocardium. Important contributors to this injury include calcium influx into cells, oxygen radicals, neutrophil activation and extravasation, complement, and edema.
- Impaired microvascular blood flow ("no-reflow" response) can result from these injury mechanisms. Endothelial dysfunction and injury contribute to this phenomenon.
- Reperfusion injury can cause atrial and ventricular dysrhythmias, reversible systolic and diastolic left ventricular dysfunction (stunning), myocardial necrosis, endothelial dysfunction, and apoptosis.
- A variety of *strategies for myocardial protection* have been identified, which can be divided into established, emerging, and experimental strategies:
  - Established Strategies:
    - *Chemically induced cardiac arrest* in diastole, most often induced by controlled hyperkalemia localized to the heart.
    - *Hypothermia* to decrease myocardial oxygen consumption. The benefits of this approach appear to be optimal at myocardial temperatures between 24° and 28°C.
    - *Avoidance or reduction of myocardial edema* by limiting the pressure of cardioplegia infusions and by providing moderately hyperosmolar cardioplegia solutions that contain blood.
    - *Buffering the acidosis* that results from ischemia by including tromethamine (THAM), histidine–imidazole, or both in the cardioplegia solution.
    - Close management of *myocardial calcium balance* to avoid extremes of intracellular hypercalcemia or hypocalcemia, especially during reperfusion.
  - Emerging Strategies:
    - Therapies to avoid oxygen radical injury, such as superoxide dismutase and xanthine oxidase inhibitors.
    - Amino acid enhancement with glutamate and aspartate to sustain anaerobic glycolysis during ischemia.
    - Addition of adenosine to cardioplegia or "reperfusion" solutions.
  - Experimental Strategies:
    - These include stimulation of nitric oxide production, antineutrophil therapy, complement pathway inhibition, hyperpolarizing agents, sodium–hydrogen exchange inhibitors, ischemic preconditioning, and strategies aimed at protecting the beating heart during surgical revascularization procedures performed without cardiopulmonary bypass.

REFERENCES

1. Brock RC, Ross DN. Hypothermia. III: Clinical application of hypothermic techniques. *Guy's Hosp Rev* 1955;104:99.
2. Katz AM, Tada M. The "stone heart": a challenge to the biochemist. *American Journal Cardiology* 1972;29:578–580.
3. Katz AM, Tada M. The "stone heart" and other challenges to the biochemist. *Am J Cardiol* 1977;39:1073–1077.
4. Cooley DA, Ruel GJ, Wukasch DC. Ischemic contracture of the heart: "stone heart." *Am J Cardiol* 1972;29:575–577.
5. Melrose DG, Dreyer B, Bentall HH. Elective cardiac arrest. *Lancet* 1955;2:21–22.
6. Baker JBE, Bentall HH, Dreyer B, et al. Arrest of isolated heart with potassium citrate. *Lancet* 1957;September 21:555–559.
7. Follette DM, Mulder DG, Maloney JV Jr, et al. Advantages of blood cardioplegia over continuous coronary perfusion and intermittent ischemia. *J Thorac Cardiovasc Surg* 1978;76:604–617.
8. Sergeant CK, Geoghegan T, Lam CR. Further studies in induced cardiac arrest using the agent acetylcholine. *Surg Forum* 1957;254–257.
9. Lam CR, Gahagan T, Sergeant C, et al. Acetylcholine-induced asystole. In: Allen JG, ed. *Extracorporeal circulation.* Springfield, IL: Charles C. Thomas Publisher, 1958:451–458.
10. Sealy WC, Young WG Jr, Brown I, et al. Potassium, magnesium and neostigmine for controlled cardioplegia. *Arch Surg* 1958;77:33–38.
11. Helmsworth JA, Kaplan S, Clark LC Jr, et al. Myocardial injury associated with asystole induced with potassium citrate. *Ann Surg* 1959;149:200–206.
12. Bretschneider HJ, Hübner G, Knoll D, et al. Myocardial resistance and tolerance to ischemia: physiological and biochemical basis. *J Cardiovasc Surg* 1975;16:241–260.
13. Kirsch U, Rodewald G, Kalmár P. Induced ischemic arrest. Clinical experience with cardioplegia in open-heart surgery. *J Thorac Cardiovasc Surg* 1972;63:121–130.
14. Shumway NE, Lower RR. Topical cardiac hypothermia for extended periods of anoxic arrest. *Surg Forum* 1959;10:563–566.
15. Steare SE, Yellon DM. The potential for endogenous myocardial antioxidants to protect the myocardium against ischaemia-reperfusion injury: refreshing the parts exogenous antioxidants cannot reach? [Review]. *J Mol Cell Cardiol* 1995;27:65–74.
16. Drew CE, Anderson IM. Profound hypothermia in cardiac surgery: report of 3 cases. *Lancet* 1959;1:748–750.
17. Taber RE, Morales AR, Fine G. Myocardial necrosis and the postoperative low-cardiac-output syndrome. *Ann Thorac Surg* 1967;4:12–28.
18. Buckberg GD. Collective review: left ventricular subendocardial necrosis. *Ann Thorac Surg* 1977;24:379–393.
19. Goldstein SM, Nelson RL, McConnell DH, et al. Effects of conventional hypothermic ischemic arrest and pharmacological arrest on myocardial supply/demand balance during aortic cross-clamping. *Ann Thorac Surg* 1977;23:520–528.
20. Buckberg GD, Brazier JR, Nelson RL, et al. Studies of the effects of hypothermia on regional myocardial blood flow and metabolism during cardiopulmonary bypass. I. The adequately perfused beating, fibrillating, and arrested heart. *J Thorac Cardiovasc Surg* 1977;73:87–94.
21. Gay WA Jr, Ebert PA. Functional, metabolic, and morphologic effects of potassium-induced cardioplegia. *Surgery* 1973;74:284–290.
22. Tyers GFO, Todd GJ, Niebauer IM, et al. The mechanism of myocardial damage following potassium citrate (Melrose) cardioplegia. *Surgery* 1975;78:45–53.
23. Tyers GFO, Manley CJ, Williams EH, et al. Preliminary clinical

experience with isotonic hypothermic potassium-induced arrest. *J Thorac Cardiovasc Surg* 1977;74:674–681.

24. Hearse DJ, Stewart DA, Braimbridge MV. Cellular protection during myocardial ischemia. The development and characterization of a procedure for the induction of reversible ischemic arrest. *Circulation* 1976;54:193–202.

25. Follette D, Fey K, Becker H, et al. Superiority of blood cardioplegia over asanguinous cardioplegia: experimental and clinical study. *Chirurgisches Forum fur Experimentelle und Klinische Forschung* 1908:279–283.

26. Follette DM, Fey K, Buckberg GD, et al. Reducing postischemic damage by temporary modification of reperfusate calcium, potassium, pH, and osmolarity. *J Thorac Cardiovasc Surg* 1981; 82:221–238.

27. Jacocks MA, Weiss M, Guyton RA, et al. Regional myocardial protection during aortic cross-clamp ischemia in dogs: calcium-containing crystalloid solutions. *Ann Thorac Surg* 1981;31: 454–463.

28. Gerola LR, Oliveira SA, Moreira LF, et al. Blood cardioplegia with warm reperfusion versus intermittent aortic cross-clamping in myocardial revascularization. Randomized controlled trial. *J Thorac Cardiovasc Surg* 1993;106:491–496.

29. Wandschneider W, Winter S, Thalmann M, et al. Crystalloid versus blood cardioplegia in coronary by-pass surgery. A prospective, randomized, controlled study in 100 consecutive adults. *J Cardiovasc Surg* 1994;35:85–89.

30. Rinne T, Pehkonen E, Kaukinen S, et al. Comparison of cardioprotection with crystalloid and blood cardioplegia in CABG patients [see Comments]. *J Cardiothorac Vasc Anesth* 1993;7: 679–683.

31. Lapenna D, Mezzetti A, de Gioia S, et al. Blood cardioplegia reduces oxidant burden in the ischemic and reperfused human myocardium. *Ann Thorac Surg* 1994;57:1522–1525.

32. Calafiore AM, Teodori G, Di Giammarco G, et al. Intermittent antegrade cardioplegia: warm blood vs. cold crystalloid. A clinical study. *J Cardiovasc Surg* 1994;35:179–184.

33. Vinten-Johansen J, Hammon JW Jr. Myocardial protection during cardiac surgery. In: Utley J, Gravlee GP, eds. *Cardiopulmonary bypass: principles and practice*. Baltimore: Williams & Wilkins, 1993:155–206.

34. Boyle EM, Pohlman TH, Cornejo CJ, et al. Endothelial cell injury in cardovascular surgery: ischemia–reperfusion. *Ann Thorac Surg* 1996;62:1868–1875.

35. Sellke FW, Boyle EM, Verrier ED. Endothelial cell injury in cardiovascular surgery: the pathophysiology of vasomotor dysfunction. *Ann Thorac Surg* 1996;62:1222–1228.

36. Boyle EM, Pohlman TH, Johnson MC, et al. Endothelial cell injury in cardiovascular surgery: the systemic inflammatory response. *Ann Thorac Surg* 1997;63:277–284.

37. Hashimoto K, Pearson PJ, Schaff HV, et al. Endothelial cell dysfunction after ischemic arrest and reperfusion: a possible mechanism of myocardial injury during reflow. *J Thorac Cardiovasc Surg* 1991;102:688–694.

38. Pearson PJ, Lin PJ, Schaff HV. Global myocardial ischemia and reperfusion impair endothelium-dependent relaxations to aggregating platelets in the canine coronary artery. A possible cause of vasospasm after cardiopulmonary bypass. *J Thorac Cardiovasc Surg* 1992;103:1147–1154.

39. Nakanishi K, Zhao Z-Q, Vinten-Johansen J, et al. Coronary artery endothelial dysfunction after ischemia, blood cardioplegia, and reperfusion. *Ann Thorac Surg* 1994;58:191–199.

40. Dreyer WJ, Michael LH, West MW, et al. Neutrophil accumulation in ischemic canine myocardium: insights into time course, distribution, and mechanism of localization during early reperfusion. *Circulation* 1991;84:400–411.

41. Dreyer WJ, Smith CW, Entman ML. Invited letter concerning

neutrophil activation during cardiopulmonary bypass. *J Thorac Cardiovasc Surg* 1991;102:318–320.

42. Zhao Z-Q, Nakamura M, Wang N-P, et al. Infarct extension and dynamic coronary endothelial dysfunction in the late reperfusion phase. *Circulation* 1998;98:I-796(abst).

43. Gayheart PA, Vinten-Johansen J, Johnston WE, et al. Oxygen requirements of the dyskinetic myocardial segment. *Am J Physiol* 1989;257:H1184–H1191.

44. Allen BS, Rosenkranz ER, Buckberg GD, et al. Studies of controlled reperfusion after ischemia. VII. High oxygen requirements of dyskinetic cardiac muscle. *J Thorac Cardiovasc Surg* 1986;92:543–552.

45. Robertson JM, Vinten-Johansen J, Buckberg GD, et al. Safety of prolonged aortic clamping with blood cardioplegia. I. Glutamate enrichment in normal hearts. *J Thorac Cardiovasc Surg* 1984;88:395–401.

46. Rosenkranz ER, Okamoto F, Buckberg GD, et al. Safety of prolonged aortic clamping with blood cardioplegia. II. Glutamate enrichment in energy-depleted hearts. *J Thorac Cardiovasc Surg* 1984;88:402–409.

47. Reimer KA, Lowe JE, Rasmussen MM, et al. The wavefront phenomenon of ischemic cell death. 1. Myocardial infarct size vs. duration of coronary occlusion in dogs. *Circulation* 1977; 56:786–794.

48. Reimer KA, Jennings RB. The "wavefront phenomenon" of myocardial ischemic cell death. II. Transmural progression of necrosis within the framework of ischemic bed size (myocardial at risk) and collateral flow. *Lab Invest* 1979;40:633–644.

49. Bufkin BL, Shearer ST, Vinten-Johansen J, et al. Preconditioning during simulated MIDCABG attenuates blood flow defects and neutrophil accumulation. *Ann Thorac Surg* 1998;66: 726–732.

50. Bufkin BL, Puskas JD, Vinten-Johansen J, et al. Controlled intermittent asystole: pharmacologic potentiation of vagal-induced asystole. *Ann Thorac Surg* 1998;66:1185–1190.

51. Thourani VH, Nakamura M, Duarte IG, et al. Ischemic preconditioning attenuates postischemic coronary artery endothelial dysfunction in a model of minimally invasive direct coronary artery bypass (MIDCAB). Circulation 1997;96(8):I-680.

52. Wang N-P, Bufkin BL, Wilcox JN, et al. Ischemic preconditioning inhibits apoptosis in the area at risk of stunned myocardium. *Circulation* 1997;96:I-737.

53. Sagawa K, Suga H, Shoukas AA, et al. End-systolic pressure/volume ratio: a new index of ventricular contractility. *Am J Cardiol* 1977;40:748–753.

54. Vinten-Johansen J, Duncan HW, Finkenberg JG, et al. Prediction of myocardial O_2 requirements by indirect indices. *Am J Physiol* 1982;243:H862–H868

55. Robicsek F, Schaper J. Reperfusion Injury: fact or myth? *J Card Surg* 1997;12:133–137.

56. Kloner RA. Does reperfusion injury exist in humans? [Review]. *J Am Coll Cardiol* 1993;21:537–545.

57. Opie LH. Reperfusion injury—fad, fashion, or fact? *Cardiovasc Drugs Ther* 1991;5[Suppl 2]:223–224.

58. Przyklenk K. Lethal myocardial "reperfusion injury": the opinions of good men. *J Thromb Thrombol* 1997;4:5–6.

59. Hudson KF. A phenomenon of paradox: myocardial reperfusion injury [Review]. *Heart Lung* 1994;23:384–393; quiz: 394–396.

60. Mehta JL, Jayaram K. Reperfusion injury in humans: existence, clinical relevance, mechanistic insights, and potential therapy. *J Thromb Thrombol* 1997;4:75–77.

61. Kusuoka H, Porterfield JK, Weisman HF, et al. Pathophysiology and pathogenesis of stunned myocardium. Depressed Ca^{2+} activation of contraction as a consequence of reperfusion-induced cellular calcium overload in ferret hearts. *J Clin Invest* 1987;79:950–961.

62. Meldrum DR, Cleveland JC, Sheridan BC, et al. Cardiac surgical implications of calcium dyshomeostasis in the heart. *Ann Thorac Surg* 1996;61:1273–1280.

63. Shen AC, Jennings RB. Kinetics of calcium accumulation in acute myocardial ischemic injury. *Am J Pathol* 1972;67:441–452.

64. Walsh LG, Tormey JM. Subcellular electrolyte shifts during *in vitro* myocardial ischemia and reperfusion. *Am J Physiol* 1988;255:H917–H928.

65. Langer GA. Sodium-calcium exchange in the heart. *Ann Rev Physiol* 1982;44:435–449.

66. McCord JM. Oxygen-derived free radicals in postischemic tissue injury. *N Engl J Med* 1985;312:159–163.

67. Simpson PJ, Lucchesi BR. Free radicals and myocardial ischemia and reperfusion injury. *J Lab Clin Med* 1987;110:13–30.

68. Krause SM, Hess ML. Characterization of cardiac sarcoplasmic reticulum dysfunction during short-term normothermic global ischemia. *Circ Res* 1985;55:176–184.

69. Hess ML, Okabe E, Ash P, et al. Free radical mediation of the effects of acidosis on calcium transport by cardiac sarcoplasmic reticulum in whole heart homogenates. *Cardiovasc Res* 1984;18:149–157.

70. Gunther GR, Herring MB. Inhibition of neutrophil superoxide production by adenosine released from vascular endothelial cells. *Ann Vasc Surg* 1991;5:325–330.

71. Zhao Z-Q, McGee DS, Nakanishi K, et al. Receptor-mediated cardioprotective effects of endogenous adenosine are exerted primarily during reperfusion after coronary occlusion in the rabbit. *Circulation* 1993;88:709–719.

72. Gryglewski RJ, Palmer RMJ, Moncada S. Superoxide anion is involved in the breakdown of endothelium-derived relaxing factor. *Nature* 1986;320:454–460.

73. Ganz W, Watanabe I, Kanamasa K, et al. Does reperfusion extend necrosis? A study in a single territory of myocardial ischemia: half reperfused and half not reperfused. *Circulation* 1990;82:1020–1033.

74. Manning AS, Hearse DJ. Reperfusion-induced arrhythmias: mechanisms and prevention [Review]. *J Mol Cell Cardiol* 1984;16:497–518.

75. Hammond B, Hess ML. The oxygen free radical system: potential mediator of myocardial injury. *J Am Coll Cardiol* 1985;6:215–220.

76. Roy RS, McCord JM. Superoxide and ischemia conversion of xanthine dehydrogenase to xanthine oxidase. In: Greenwald R, Cohen G, eds. *Oxyradicals and their scavenger systems.* New York: Elsevier Science, 1983:145–153 (*Cellular and molecular aspects,* vol 2).

77. Downey JM, Hearse DJ, Yellon DM. The role of xanthine oxidase during myocardial ischemia in several species including man. *J Mol Cell Cardiol* 1988;20[SuppII]:55–63.

78. Jarasch ED, Bruder G, Heid HW. Significance of xanthine oxidase in capillary endothelial cells. *Acta Physiol Scand* 1986;548:39–46.

79. Mohazzab KM, Wolin MS. Sites of superoxide anion production detected by lucigenin in calf pulmonary artery smooth muscle. *Am J Physiol* 1994;267:L815–L822.

80. Mohazzab KM, Kaminski PM, Wolin MS. NADH oxidoreductase is a major source of superoxide anion in bovine coronary artery endothelium. *Am J Physiol* 1994;266:H2568–H2572.

81. Chenowith DE, Cooper SW, Hugli TE, et al. Complement activation during cardiopulmonary bypass: evidence for generation of C3a and C5a anaphylatoxins. *N Engl J Med* 1981;304:497–503.

82. Videm V, Fosse E, Mollnes TE, et al. Complement activation with bubble and membrane oxygenators in aortocoronary bypass grafting. *Ann Thorac Surg* 1990;50:387–391.

83. Faymonville ME, Pincemail J, Duchateau J, et al. Myeloperoxidase and elastase as markers of leukocyte activation during cardiopulmonary bypass in humans. *J Thorac Cardiovasc Surg* 1991;102:309–317.

84. Lucchesi BR, Mullane KM. Leukocytes and ischemia-induced myocardial injury. *Ann Rev Pharmacol Toxicol* 1986;26:201–224.

85. Jacob HS, Vercellotti GM. Granulocyte-mediated endothelial injury: oxidant damage amplified by lactoferrin and platelet activating factor. In: Halliwell B, ed. *Oxygen radicals and tissue injury.* Rockville, MD: FASEB Publications, 1998:57–62.

86. Guarnieri C, Flamigni F, Caldarera CM. Role of oxygen in the cellular damage induced by re-oxygenation of hypoxic heart. *J Mol Cell Cardiol* 1980;12:797–808.

87. Freeman BA, Crapo JD. Biology of disease: free radicals and tissue injury. *Lab Invest* 1982;47:412–426.

88. Rao PS, Cohen MV, Mueller HS. Production of free radicals and lipid peroxides in early experimental myocardial ischemia. *J Mol Cell Cardiol* 1983;15:713–716.

89. Zweier JL, Flaherty JT, Weisfeldt ML. Direct measurement of free radicals generated following reperfusion of ischemic myocardium. *Proc Natl Acad Sci U S A* 1987;84:1404–1407.

90. Bolli R, Jeroudi MO, Patel BS, et al. Marked reduction of free radical generation and contractile dysfunction by antioxidant therapy begun at the time of reperfusion: evidence that myocardial "stunning" is a manifestation of reperfusion injury. *Circ Res* 1989;65:607–622.

91. Bolli R, Patel BS, Jeroudi MO, et al. Demonstration of free radical generation in "stunned" myocardium of intact dogs with the use of the spin trap α-phenyl N-tert-butyl nitrone. *J Clin Invest* 1988;82:476–485.

92. Bolli R. Oxygen-derived free radicals and myocardial reperfusion injury. An overview. *Cardiovasc Drugs Ther* 1991;5:249–268.

93. Bolli R. Oxygen-derived free radicals and postischemic myocardial dysfunction ("stunned myocardium") reviews. *J Am Coll Cardiol* 1988;12:239–249.

94. Bolli R. Superoxide dismutase 10 years later: a drug in search of a use [Editorial; Comment]. *J Am Coll Cardiol* 1991;18:231–233.

95. Jeroudi MO, Hartley CJ, Bolli R. Myocardial reperfusion injury: role of oxygen radicals and potential therapy with antioxidants [Review]. *Am J Cardiol* 1994;73:2B–7B.

96. Black SC, Driscoll EM, Lucchesi BR. Inhibition of platelet-activating factor fails to limit ischemia and reperfusion-induced myocardial damage. *J Cardiovasc Pharmacol* 1992;20:997–1005.

97. Kilgore KS, Friedrichs GS, Johnson CR, et al. Protective effects of the SOD-mimetic SC-52608 against ischemia/reperfusion damage in the rabbit isolated heart. *J Mol Cell Cardiol* 1994;26:995–1006.

98. Lucchesi BR, Werns SW, Fantone JC. The role of neutrophils and free radicals in ischemic myocardial injury. *J Mol Cell Cardiol* 1989;21:1241–1251.

99. Werns SW, Shea MJ, Lucchesi BR. Free radicals and myocardial injury: pharmacologic implications. *Circulation* 1986;74:1–5.

100. Ihnken K, Morita K, Buckberg GD, et al. Controlling oxygen content during cardiopulmonary bypass to limit reperfusion/reoxygenation injury. *Transplant Proc* 1995;27:2809–2811.

101. Ihnken K, Morita K, Buckberg GD, et al. Studies of hypoxemic/reoxygenation injury with aortic clamping: XI. Cardiac advantages of normoxemic versus hyperoxemic management during cardiopulmonary bypass. *J Thorac Cardiovasc Surg* 1995;110:1255–1264.

102. Lefer AM, Tsao PS, Lefer DJ, et al. Role of endothelial dysfunc-

tion in the pathogenesis of reperfusion injury after myocardial ischemia. *FASEB J* 1991;5:2029–2034.

103. Lefer AM, Ma X-L, Weyrich A, et al. Endothelial dysfunction and neutrophil adherence as critical events in the development of reperfusion injury. *Agents Actions Suppl* 1993;41:127–135.

104. Lefer DJ, Nakanishi K, Vinten-Johansen J, et al. Cardiac venous endothelial dysfunction after myocardial ischemia and reperfusion in dogs. *Am J Physiol* 1992;263:H850–H856.

105. Lefer AM. Role of selectins in myocardial ischemia-reperfusion injury. *Ann Thorac Surg* 1995;60:773–777.

106. Lefer AM, Weyrich AS, Buerke M. Role of selectins, a new family of adhesion molecules, in ischaemia-reperfusion injury. *Cardiovasc Res* 1994;28:289–294.

107. Ley K, Tedder TF. Leukocyte interactions with vascular endothelium. New insights into selectin-mediated attachment and rolling. *J Immunol* 1995;155:525–528.

108. McEver RP. Selectins: novel receptors that mediate leukocyte adhesion during inflammation. *Thromb Haemost* 1991;65:223–228.

109. Verrier E. The microvascular cell and ischemia-reperfusion injury. *J Cardiovasc Pharmacol* 1996;27[Suppl 1]:S26–S30.

110. Gaboury JP, Anderson DC, Kubes P. Molecular mechanisms involved in superoxide-induced leukocyte-endothelial cell interactions *in vivo*. *Am J Physiol* 1994;266:H637–H642.

111. Toothill VJ, Van Mourik JA, Niewenhuis HK, et al. Characterization of the enhanced adhesion of neutrophil leukocytes to thrombin-stimulated endothelial cells. *J Immunol* 1990;145:283–291.

112. Kilbridge PM, Mayer JE Jr, Newburger JW, et al. Induction of intercellular adhesion molecule-1 and E-selectin mRNA in heart and skeletal muscle of pediatric patients undergoing cardiopulmonary bypass. *J Thorac Cardiovasc Surg* 1994;107:1183–1192.

113. Verrier ED, Shen I. Potential role of neutrophil anti-adhesion therapy in myocardial stunning, myocardial infarction, and organ dysfunction after cardiopulmonary bypass. *J Card Surg* 1993;8:309–312.

114. Abe Y, Kawakami M, Kuroki M, et al. Transient rise in serum interleukin-8 concentration during acute myocardial infarction. *Br Heart J* 1993;70:132–134.

115. Finn A, Naik S, Klein N, et al. Interleukin-8 release and neutrophil degranulation after pediatric cardiopulmonary bypass. *J Thorac Cardiovasc Surg* 1993;105:234–241.

116. Karakurum M, Shreeniwas R, Chen J, et al. Hypoxic induction of interleukin-8 gene expression in human endothelial cells. *J Clin Invest* 1994;93:1564–1570.

117. Kubes P, Jutila M, Payne D. Therapeutic potential of inhibiting leukocyte rolling in ischemia/reperfusion. *J Clin Invest* 1995;95:2510–2519.

118. Moore KL, Patel KD, Bruehl RE, et al. P-selectin glycoprotein ligand-1 mediates rolling of human neutrophils on P-selectin. *J Cell Biol* 1995;128:661–671.

119. Kukielka GL, Hawkins HK, Michael L, et al. Regulation of intercellular adhesion molecule-1 (ICAM-1) in ischemic and reperfused canine myocardium. *J Clin Invest* 1993;92:1504–1516.

120. Youker KA, Hawkins HK, Kukielka GL, et al. Molecular evidence for induction of intracellular adhesion molecule-1 in the viable border zone associated with ischemia-reperfusion injury of the dog heart. *Circulation* 1994;89:2736–2746.

121. Huber AR, Kunkel SL, Todd RF3, et al. Regulation of transendothelial neutrophil migration by endogenous interleukin-8 [published errata appear in *Science* 1991 Nov 1;254(5032):631 and 1991 Dec 6;254(5037):1435]. *Science* 1991;254:99–102.

122. Sommers HM, Jennings RB. Experimental acute myocardial infarction: histological and histochemical studies of early myo-

cardial infarcts induced by temporary or permanent occlusion of a coronary artery. *Lab Invest* 1964;13:1491–1503.

123. Nakanishi K, Lefer DJ, Johnston WE, et al. Transient hypocalcemia during the initial phase of reperfusion extends myocardial necrosis after 2 hours of coronary occlusion. *Coron Artery Dis* 1991;2:1009–1021.

124. Nakanishi K, Vinten-Johansen J, Lefer DJ, et al. Intracoronary l-arginine during reperfusion improves endothelial function and reduces infarct size. *Am J Physiol* 1992;263:H1650–H1658.

125. Lefer DJ, Nakanishi K, Johnston WE, et al. Anti-neutrophil and myocardial protecting actions of SPM-5185, a novel NO (NO) donor, following acute myocardial ischemia and reperfusion in dogs. *Biol Nitric Oxide* 1992;188–190.

126. Romson JL, Hook BG, Rigot VH, et al. The effect of ibuprofen on accumulation of indium-111-labeled platelets and leukocytes in experimental myocardial infarction. *Circulation* 1982;66:1002–1011.

127. Tsao PS, Aoki N, Lefer DJ, et al. Time course of endothelial dysfunction and myocardial injury during myocardial ischemia and reperfusion in the cat. *Circulation* 1990;82:1402–1412.

128. Flynn PJ, Becker WK, Vercellotti GM, et al. Ibuprofen inhibits granulocyte responses to inflammatory mediators. A proposed mechanism for reduction of experimental myocardial infarct size. *Inflammation* 1984;8:33–44.

129. Schwartz JD, Shamamian P, Schwartz DS, et al. Cardiopulmonary bypass primes polymorphonuclear leukocytes. *J Surg Res* 1998;75:177–182.

130. Kappelmayer J, Bernabei A, Gikakis N, et al. Upregulation of Mac-1 surface expression on neutrophils during simulated extracorporeal circulation. *J Lab Clin Med* 1993;121:118–126.

131. Finn A, Rebuck N, Moat N. Neutrophil activation during cardiopulmonary bypass. *J Thorac Cardiovasc Surg* 1992;104:1746–1748.

132. Dreyer WJ, Michael LH, Millman EE, et al. Neutrophil activation and adhesion molecule expression in a canine model of open heart surgery with cardiopulmonary bypass. *Cardiovasc Res* 1995;29:775–781.

133. Gillinov AM, Redmond JM, Winkelstein JA, et al. Complement and neutrophil activation during cardiopulmonary bypass: a study in the complement-deficient dog. *Ann Thorac Surg* 1994;57:345–352.

134. Rinder CS, Bonan JL, Rinder HM, et al. Cardiopulmonary bypass induces leukocyte-platelet adhesion. *Blood* 1992;79:1201–1205.

135. Finn A, Moat N, Rebuck N, et al. Changes in neutrophil CD11b/CD18 and L-selectin expression and release of interleukin 8 and elastase in paediatric cardiopulmonary bypass. *Agents Actions* 1993;38[Spec No]:C44–C46.

136. Gillinov AM, Bator JM, Zehr KJ, et al. Neutrophil adhesion molecule expression during cardiopulmonary bypass with bubble and membrane oxygenators. *Ann Thorac Surg* 1993;56:847–853.

137. Galiñanes M, Watson C, Trivedi U, et al. Differential patterns of neutrophil adhesion molecules during cardiopulmonary bypass in humans. *Circulation* 1996;94[9 Suppl]:II364–II369.

138. Le Deist F, Menasché P, Kucharski C, et al. Hypothermia during cardiopulmonary bypass delays but does not prevent neutrophil-endothelial cell adhesion: a clinical study. *Circulation* 1995;92[Suppl 2]:354–358.

139. Boldt J, Osmer C, Linke LC, et al. Hypothermic versus normothermic cardiopulmonary bypass: influence on circulating adhesion molecules. *J Cardiothorac Vasc Anesth* 1996;10:342–347.

140. Ohata T, Sawa Y, Kadoba K, et al. Normothermia has beneficial effects in cardiopulmonary bypass attenuating inflammatory reactions. *ASAIO J* 1995;41:M288–M291.

141. Menasche P, Peynet J, Lariviere J, et al. Does normothermia

during cardiopulmonary bypass increase neutrophil-endothelium interactions? *Circulation* 1994;90(5 Pt 2):II275–II279.

142. Menasché P, Peynet J, Haeffner-Cavaillon N, et al. Influence of temperature on neutrophil trafficking during clinical cardiopulmonary bypass. *Circulation* 1995;92:II-334–II-340.

143. Kirklin JK, Westaby S, Blackstone EH, et al. Complement and the damaging effects of cardiopulmonary bypass. *J Thorac Cardiovasc Surg* 1983;86:845–857.

144. Cavarocchi NC, England MD, Schaff HV, et al. Oxygen free radical generation during cardiopulmonary bypass: correlation with complement activation. *Circulation* 1986;74:III-130–III-133.

145. Chenoweth DE. Complement activation during cardiopulmonary bypass. In: Utley JR, Betleski R, eds. *Pathophysiology and techniques of cardiopulmonary bypass.* Baltimore: Williams & Wilkins, 1983:49–60.

146. McManus LM, Kolb WP, Crawford MH, et al. Complement localization in ischemic baboon myocardium. *Lab Invest* 1983; 48:436–447.

147. Rossen RD, Swain JL, Michael LH, et al. Selective accumulation of the first component of complement and leukocytes in ischemic canine heart muscle. *Circ Res* 1985;57:119–130.

148. Homeister JW, Satoh P, Lucchesi BR. Effects of complement activation in the isolated heart. Role of the terminal complement components. *Circ Res* 1992;71:303–319.

149. Kubes P. Polymorphonuclear leukocyte-endothelium interactions: a role for pro-inflammatory and anti-inflammatory molecules [Review]. *Can J Physiol Pharmacol* 1993;71:88–97.

150. Dreyer WJ, Michael LH, Nguyen T, et al. Kinetics of C5a release in cardiac lymph of dogs experiencing coronary artery ischemia-reperfusion injury. *Circ Res* 1992;71:1518–1524.

151. Ivey CL, Williams FM, Collins PD, et al. Neutrophil chemoattractants generated in two phases during reperfusion of ischemic myocardium in the rabbit. Evidence for a role for C5a and interleukin-8. *J Clin Invest* 1995;95:2720–2728.

152. Riley RD, Sato H, Zhao Z-Q, et al. Recombinant human complement C5a receptor antagonist reduces infarct size following surgical revascularization. *Circulation* 1997;96(8):I-679.

153. McNally AK, Anderson JM. Complement C3 participation in monocyte adhesion to different surfaces. *Proc Natl Acad Sci U S A* 1994;91:10119–10123.

154. Engler RL, Roth DM, del Balzo U, et al. Intracoronary C5a induces myocardial ischemia by mechanisms independent of the neutrophil: leukocyte filters desensitize the myocardium to C5a. *FASEB J* 1991;5:2983–2991.

155. Steinberg JB, Kapelanski DP, Olson JD, et al. Cytokine and complement levels in patients undergoing cardiopulmonary bypass. *J Thorac Cardiovasc Surg* 1993;106:1008–1016.

156. Ovrum E, Mollnes TE, Fosse E, et al. Complement and granulocyte activation in two different types of heparinized extracorporeal circuits. *J Thorac Cardiovasc Surg* 1995;110:1623–1632.

157. Vinten-Johansen J, Johnston WE, Mills SA, et al. Reperfusion injury after temporary coronary occlusion. *J Thorac Cardiovasc Surg* 1988;95:960–968.

158. Jennings RB, Reimer KA, Steenbergen C. Myocardial ischemia revisited: the osmolar load, membrane damage and reperfusion. *J Mol Cell Cardiol* 1986;18:769–780.

159. Foglia RP, Steed DL, Follette DM, et al. Iatrogenic myocardial edema with potassium cardioplegia. *J Thorac Cardiovasc Surg* 1979;78:217–222.

160. Garcia-Dorado D, Theroux P, Munoz R, et al. Favorable effects of hyperosmotic reperfusion on myocardial edema and infarct size. *Am J Physiol* 1992;262(1 Pt 2):H17–H22.

161. Tranum-Jensen J, Janse MJ, Fiolet WT, et al. Tissue osmolality, cell swelling, and reperfusion in acute regional myocardial ischemia in the isolated porcine heart. *Circ Res* 1981;49:364–381.

162. Karolle BL, Carlson RE, Aisen AM, et al. Transmural distribution of myocardial edema by NMR relaxometry following myocardial ischemia and reperfusion. *Am Heart J* 1991;122: 655–664.

163. Drewnowska K, Clemo HF, Baumgarten CM. Prevention of myocardial intracellular edema induced by St. Thomas' Hospital cardioplegic solution. *J Mol Cell Cardiol* 1991;23: 1215–1221.

164. Weng ZC, Nicolosi AC, Detwiler PW, et al. Effects of crystalloid, blood, and University of Wisconsin perfusates on weight, water content, and left ventricular compliance in an edema-prone, isolated porcine heart model. *J Thorac Cardiovasc Surg* 1992;103:504–513.

165. Dauber IM, VanBenthuysen KM, McMurtry IF, et al. Functional coronary microvascular injury evident as increased permeability due to brief ischemia and reperfusion. *Circ Res* 1990;66: 986–998.

166. Johnson RE, Dorsey LMA, Moye SJ, et al. Cardioplegic infusion. The safe limits of pressure and temperature. *J Thorac Cardiovasc Surg* 1982;83:813–823.

167. Vinten-Johansen J, Johnston WE, Lefer DJ, et al. Controlled reperfusion attenuates no-reflow and reduces infarct size. *Circulation* 1990;82[Suppl III]:286(abst).

168. Okamoto F, Allen BS, Buckberg GD, et al. Studies of controlled reperfusion after ischemia. XIV. Reperfusion conditions: importance of ensuring gentle versus sudden reperfusion during relief of coronary occlusion. *J Thorac Cardiovasc Surg* 1986;92: 613–620.

169. Gunnes S, Ytrehus K, Sorlie D, et al. Improved energy preservation following gentle reperfusion after hypothermic, ischemic cardioplegia in infarcted rat hearts. *Eur J Cardiothorac Surg* 1987;1:139–143.

170. Garcia-Dorado D, Oliveras J. Myocardial oedema: a preventable cause of reperfusion injury? [Review]. *Cardiovasc Res* 1993;27: 1555–1563.

171. Inserte J, Garcia-Dorado D, Ruiz-Meana M, et al. The Na$^+$-H$^+$ exchange occuring during hypoxia in the genesis of reoxygenation-induced myocardial oedema. *J Mol Cell Cardiol* 1997; 29:1167–1175.

172. Grinstein S, Woodside M, Sardet C, et al. Activation of the Na$^+$/H$^+$ antiporter during cell volume regulation. Evidence for a phosphorylation-independent mechanism. *J Biol Chem* 1992; 267:23823–23828.

173. Yamauchi T, Ichikawa H, Sawa Y, et al. The contribution of Na$^+$/H$^+$ exchange to ischemia-reperfusion injury after hypothermic cardioplegic arrest. *Ann Thorac Surg* 1997;63:1107–1112.

174. Fliegel L, Frohlich O. The Na$^+$/H$^+$ exchanger: an update on structure, regulation and cardiac physiology. *Biochem J* 1993; 296:273–285.

175. Tritto FP, Inserte J, Garcia-Dorado D, et al. Sodium/hydrogen exchanger inhibition reduces myocardial reperfusion edema after normothermic cardioplegia. *J Thorac Cardiovasc Surg* 1998;115:709–715.

176. Kloner RA, Ganote CE, Jennings RB. The "no-reflow" phenomenon after temporary coronary occlusion in the dog. *J Clin Invest* 1974;54:1496–1508.

177. Becker LC, Ambrosio G. Myocardial consequences of reperfusion. *Prog Cardiovasc Dis* 1987;30:23–44.

178. Tsao PS, Lefer AM. Time course and mechanism of endothelial dysfunction in isolated ischemic- and hypoxic-perfused rat hearts. *Am J Physiol* 1990;259:H1660–H1666.

179. Ma X-L, Tsao PS, Viehman GE, et al. Neutrophil-mediated vasoconstriction and endothelial dysfunction in low-flow perfusion-reperfused cat coronary artery. *Circ Res* 1991;69:95–106.

180. Becker LC, Ambrosio G, Manissi J, et al. The no-reflow phenomenon: a misnomer? In: Sideman S, ed. *Analysis and simula-*

tion of the cardiac system—ischemia. Boca Raton: CRC Press, 1989:289–309.

181. Sellke FW, Friedman M, Dai HB, et al. Mechanisms causing coronary microvascular dysfunction following crystalloid cardioplegia and reperfusion. *Cardiovasc Res* 1993;27:1925–1932.

182. Gertler JP, Ocasio VH. Endothelin production by hypoxic human endothelium. *J Vasc Surg* 1993;18:178–182.

183. Engler RL, Dahlgren MD, Peterson MA, et al. Accumulation of polymorphonuclear leukocytes during 3-h experimental myocardial ischemia. *Am J Physiol* 1986;251:H93–H100.

184. Vinten-Johansen J, Lefer DJ, Nakanishi K, et al. Controlled coronary hydrodynamics at the time of reperfusion reduces postischemic injury. *Coron Artery Dis* 1992;3:1081–1093.

185. Sato H, Jordan JE, Zhao Z-Q, et al. Gradual reperfusion reduces infarct size and endothelial injury but augments neutrophil accumulation. *Ann Thorac Surg* 1997;64:1099–1107.

186. Opie LH, Coetzee WA. Role of calcium ions in reperfusion arrhythmias: relevance to pharmacologic intervention. *Cardiovasc Drugs Ther* 1988;2:623–636.

187. Bolli R. Oxygen-derived free radicals and myocardial reperfusion injury: an overview [Review]. *Cardiovasc Drugs Ther* 1991; 5[Suppl 2]:249–268.

188. Cerbai E, Ambrosio G, Porciatti F, et al. Cellular electrophysiological basis for oxygen radical-induced arrhythmias. A patch-clamp study in guinea pig ventricular myocytes. *Circulation* 1991;84:1773–1782.

189. Tosaki A, Droy-Lefaix MT, Pali T, et al. Effects of SOD, catalase, and a novel antiarrhythmic drug, EGB 761, on reperfusion-induced arrhythmias in isolated rat hearts. *Free Radic Biol Med* 1993;14:361–370.

190. Hearse D J, Tosaki A. Free radicals and calcium: simultaneous interacting triggers as determinants of vulnerability to reperfusion-induced arrhythmias in the rat heart. *J Mol Cell Cardiol* 1988;20:213–223.

191. Jordan JE, Zhao Z-Q, Sato H, et al. Adenosine A$_2$ receptor activation attenuates reperfusion injury by inhibiting neutrophil accumulation, superoxide generation and coronary endothelial adherence. *J Pharmacol Exp Ther* 1997;280:301–309.

192. Lefer DJ, Nakanishi K, Vinten-Johansen J. Endothelial and myocardial cell protection by a cysteine-containing nitric oxide donor after myocardial ischemia and reperfusion. *J Cardiovasc Pharmacol* 1993;22:S34–S43.

193. Sato H, Zhao Z-Q, McGee DS, et al. Supplemental L-arginine during cardioplegic arrest and reperfusion avoids regional postischemic injury. *J Thorac Cardiovasc Surg* 1995;110:302–314.

194. Hudspeth DA, Nakanishi K, Vinten-Johansen J, et al. Adenosine in blood cardioplegia prevents postischemic dysfunction in ischemically injured hearts. *Ann Thorac Surg* 1994;58:1637–1644.

195. Mizuno A, Baretti R, Buckberg GD, et al. Endothelial stunning and myocyte recovery after reperfusion of jeopardized muscle: a role of L-arginine blood cardioplegia. *J Thorac Cardiovasc Surg* 1997;113:379–389.

196. Nakanishi K, Zhao Z-Q, Vinten-Johansen J, et al. Blood cardioplegia enhanced with nitric oxide donor SPM-5185 counteracts postischemic endothelial and ventricular dysfunction. *J Thorac Cardiovasc Surg* 1995;109:1146–1154.

197. Vinten-Johansen J, Edgerton TA, Howe HR, et al. Immediate functional recovery and avoidance of reperfusion injury with surgical revascularization of short-term coronary occlusion. *Circulation* 1985;72:431–439.

198. Rosenkranz ER, Okamoto F, Buckberg GD, et al. Studies of controlled reperfusion after ischemia. II. Biochemical studies: failure of tissue adenosine triphosphate levels to predict recovery of contractile function after controlled reperfusion. *J Thorac Cardiovasc Surg* 1986;92:488–501.

199. Taegtmeyer H, Roberts AF, Raine AE. Energy metabolism in reperfused heart muscle: metabolic correlates to return of function. *J Am Coll Cardiol* 1985;6:864–870.

200. Vinten-Johansen J, Gayheart PA, Johnston WE, et al. Regional function, blood flow, and oxygen utilization relations in repetitively occluded reperfused canine myocardium. *Am J Physiol* 1991;261:H538–H547.

201. Vinten-Johansen J, Chiantella V, Johnston WE, et al. Adjuvant *N*-(2-mercaptopropionyl)-glycine in blood cardioplegia does not improve myocardial protection in ischemically damaged hearts. *J Thorac Cardiovasc Surg* 1990;100:65–76.

202. Vinten-Johansen J, Chiantella V, Faust KB, et al. Myocardial protection with blood cardioplegia in ischemically injured hearts: reduction of reoxygenation injury with allopurinol. *Ann Thorac Surg* 1988;45:319–326.

203. Pridjian AK, Levitsky S, Krukenkamp I, et al. Intracellular sodium and calcium in the postischemic myocardium. *Ann Thorac Surg* 1987;43:416–419.

204. Yokoyama H, Julian JS, Vinten-Johansen J, et al. Postischemic [Ca^{2+}] repletion improves cardiac performance without altering oxygen demands. *Ann Thorac Surg* 1990;49:894–902.

205. Gaasch WH, Apstein CS, Levine HJ. Diastolic properties of the left ventricle. In: Levine HJ, Gaasch WH, ed. *The ventricle: basic and clinical aspects.* Boston: Martinus Nijboff Publishing, 1985:143–170.

206. Vinten-Johansen J, Julian JS, Yokoyama H, et al. Efficacy of myocardial protection with hypothermic blood cardioplegia depends on oxygen. *Ann Thorac Surg* 1991;52:939–948.

207. Lazar HL, Haasler GB, Collins RH, et al. Mechanisms of altered ventricular compliance following ischemia using two-dimensional echocardiography. *Curr Surg* 1982;39:253–255.

208. Starnes VA, Hammon JW Jr. The influence of acute global ischemia on left ventricular compliance in the adult and immature dog. *J Surg Res* 1981;30:281–286.

209. Pearson PJ, Schaff HV, Vanhoutte PM. Acute impairment of endothelium-dependent relaxations to aggregating platelets following reperfusion injury in canine coronary arteries. *Circ Res* 1990;67:385–393.

210. Ma X-L, Weyrich AS, Lefer DJ, et al. Diminished basal nitric oxide release after myocardial ischemia and reperfusion promotes neutrophil adherence to coronary endothelium. *Circ Res* 1993;72:403–412.

211. Nakanishi K, Zhao Z-Q, Vinten-Johansen J, et al. The effects of blood cardioplegia on the coronary vascular endothelium. *FASEB J* 1993;7:703(abst).

212. Pearson PJ, Schaff HV, Vanhoutte PM. Long-term impairment of endothelium-dependent relaxations to aggregating platelets after reperfusion injury in canine coronary arteries. *Circulation* 1995;81:1921–1927.

213. Kaiser L, Sparks HV Jr. Endothelial cells: not just a cellophane wrapper. *Arch Intern Med* 1987;147:569–573.

214. Dignan RJ, Dyke CM, Abd-Elfattah AS, et al. Coronary artery endothelial cell and smooth muscle dysfunction after global myocardial ischemia. *Ann Thorac Surg* 1992;53:311–317.

215. Guo J-P, Murohara T, Buerke M, Scalial R, et al. Direct measurement of nitric oxide release from vascular endothelial cells. *J Appl Physiol* 1996;81:774–779.

216. Engelman DT, Watanabe M, Engleman RM, et al. Constitutive nitric oxide release is impaired after ischemia and reperfusion. *J Thorac Cardiovasc Surg* 1995;110:1047–1053.

217. Zanaboni P, Murray PA, Simon BA, et al. Selective endothelial dysfunction in conscious dogs after cardiopulmonary bypass. *J Appl Physiol* 1997;82(6):1776–1784.

218. Dauber IM, Parsons PE, Welsh CH, et al. Peripheral bypass-induced pulmonary and coronary vascular injury. Association

with increased levels of tumor necrosis factor. *Circulation* 1993; 88:726–735.

219. Feerick AE, Johnston WE, Steinsland O, et al. Cardiopulmonary bypass impairs vascular endothelial relaxation: effects of gaseous microemboli in dogs. *Am J Physiol* 1994;267: H1174–H1182.

220. Hale AJ, Smith CA, Sutherland LC, et al. Apoptosis: molecular regulation of cell death. *Eur J Biochem* 1996;236:1–26.

221. Narula J, Haider N, Virmani R, et al. Apoptosis in myocytes in end-stage heart failure. *N Engl J Med* 1996;335:1182–1189.

222. Saraste A, Pulkki K, Kallajoki M, et al. Apoptosis in human acute myocardial infarction. *Circulation* 1997;95:320–323.

223. Fliss H, Gattinger D. Apoptosis in ischemic and reperfused rat myocardium. *Circ Res* 1996;79:949–956.

224. Gottlieb RA, Burleson KO, Kloner RA, et al. Reperfusion injury induces apoptosis in rabbit cardiomyocytes. *J Clin Invest* 1994; 94:1621–1628.

225. Vaux DL, Strasser A. The molecular biology of apoptosis. *Proc Natl Acad Sci U S A* 1996;93:2239–2244.

226. Maulik N, Engleman RM, Deaton D, et al. Reperfusion of ischemic myocardium induces apoptosis and DNA laddering with enhanced expression of protooncogene c-*myc* mRNA. *Circulation* 1996;94:2417(abst).

227. Tanaka M, Ito H, Adachi S, et al. Hypoxia induces apoptosis with enhanced expression of Fas antigen messenger RNA in cultured neonatal rat cardiomyocytes. *Circ Res* 1994;75: 426–433.

228. Buckberg GD. Myocardial protection: an overview. *Semin Thorac Cardiovasc Surg* 1993;5:98–106.

229. Vinten-Johansen J, Hammon JW Jr. Cardioprotection by adenosine: is it a question of effective dose, timing, or the target compartment? [Letters to the Editor]. *J Thorac Cardiovasc Surg* 1996;112:202–204.

230. Cole WC, McPherson CD, Sontag D. ATP-regulated K^+ channels protect the myocardium against ischemia/reperfusion damage. *Circ Res* 1991;69:571–581.

231. Yao Z, Cavero I, Gross GJ. Activation of cardiac K_{ATP} channels: an endogenous protective mechanism during repetitive ischemia. *Am J Physiol* 1993;264:H495–H504.

232. Vinten-Johansen J, Zhao Z-Q. Myocardial protection from reperfusion injury with adenosine. In: Mentzer RM Jr, Kitakaze M, Downey J, et al., eds. *Adenosine: cardioprotection and clinical application.* Boston: Kluwer Academic Publishers, 1997:49–70.

233. Nelson R, Fey K, Follette DM. The critical importance of intermittent infusion of cardioplegic solution during aortic cross-clamping. *Surg Forum* 1976;26:241–243.

234. Lowe JE, Kleinman LH, Reimer KA, et al. Effects of cardioplegia produced by calcium flux inhibition. *Surg Forum* 1977; 28:279–280.

235. Cohen NM, Damiano RJJ, Wechsler AS. Is there an alternative to potassium arrest? *Ann Thorac Surg* 1995;60:858–863.

236. Lawton JS, Hsia PW, Allen CT, et al. Myocardial protection in the acutely injured heart: hyperpolarizing versus depolarizing hypothermic cardioplegia. *J Thorac Cardiovasc Surg* 1997;113: 567–575.

237. Jayawant M, Stephenson ER Jr, Damiano RJJ. Advantages of continuous hyperpolarized arrest with pinacidil over St. Thomas' Hospital solution during prolonged ischemia. *J Thorac Cardiovasc Surg* 1998;116:131–138.

238. de Jong JW, van der Meer P, van Loon H, et al. Adenosine as adjunct to potassium cardioplegia: effect on function, energy metabolism, and electrophysiology. *J Thorac Cardiovasc Surg* 1990;100:445–454.

239. Terzic A, Lopez JR, Alekseev AE, et al. Adenosine prevents K^+-induced Ca^{2+} loading: insight into cardioprotection during cardioplegia. *Ann Thorac Surg* 1998;65:586–591.

240. Rosenkranz ER, Vinten-Johansen J, Buckberg GD, et al. Benefits of normothermic induction of blood cardioplegia in energy-depleted hearts, with maintenance of arrest by multidose cold blood cardioplegic infusions. *J Thorac Cardiovasc Surg* 1982; 84:667–677.

241. Teoh KH, Christakis GT, Weisel RD, et al. Accelerated myocardial metabolic recovery with terminal warm blood cardioplegia. *J Thorac Cardiovasc Surg* 1986;91:888–895.

242. He GW, Yang CQ, Rebeyka IM, Wilson GJ. Effects of hyperkalemia on neonatal endothelium and smooth muscle. *J Heart Lung Transplant* 1995;14:92–101.

243. Borst C, Santamore WP, Smedira NG, et al. Minimally invasive coronary artery bypass grafting: on the beating heart and via limited access. *Ann Thorac Surg* 1997;63:S1–S5.

244. Bel A, Perrault LP, Faris B, et al. Inhibition of the pacemaker current: a bradycardiac therapy for off-pump coronary operations. *Ann Thorac Surg* 1998;66:148–152.

245. Matheny RG, Shaar CJ. Vagus nerve stimulation as a method to temporarily slow or arrest the heart. *Ann Thorac Surg* 1997; 63:S28–S29.

246. Bigelow WG, Callaghan JC, Hopps JA. General hypothermia for experimental intracardiac surgery. *Ann Surg* 1950;132: 531–539.

247. Rosenfeldt FL. The relationship between myocardial temperature and recovery after experimental cardioplegic arrest. *J Thorac Cardiovasc Surg* 1982;84:656–666.

248. Johnson M, Haddix T, Pohlman T, et al. Hypothermia reversibly inhibits endothelial cell expression of E-selectin and tissue factor. *J Card Surg* 1995;10:428–435.

249. Haddix TL, Pohlman TH, Noel RF, et al. Hypothermia inhibits human E-selectin transcription. *J Surg Res* 1996;64:176–183.

250. Rosenfeldt FL, Hearse DJ, Cankovic-Darracott S, et al. The additive protective effects of hypothermia and chemical cardioplegia during ischemic cardiac arrest in the dog. *J Thorac Cardiovasc Surg* 1980;79:29–38.

251. Hearse DJ, Stewart DA, Braimbridge MV. The additive protective effects of hypothermia and chemical cardioplegia during ischemic cardiac arrest in the rat. *J Thorac Cardiovasc Surg* 1980; 79:39–43.

252. Kay HR, Levine FH, Fallon JT, et al. Effect of cross-clamp time, temperature, and cardioplegic agents on myocardial function after induced arrest. *J Thorac Cardiovasc Surg* 1978;76: 590–603.

253. Kenyon NM, Litwak RS, Beck HJ, et al. Preliminary observations in isolated hypothermic cardiac asystole. *Surg Forum* 1959; 10:567–570.

254. Fukunami M, Hearse DJ. The inotropic consequences of cooling: studies in the isolated rat heart. *Heart Vessels* 1989;5:1–9.

255. Swanson DK, Myerowitz PD. Distribution of adenylates, water, potassium, and sodium within the normal and hypertrophied canine heart following 2 hours of preservation. *J Surg Res* 1982; 32:515–525.

256. Speicher CE, Ferrigan L, Wolfson SK Jr, et al. Cold injury of myocardium and pericardium in cardiac hypothermia. *Surg Gynecol Obstet* 1962;114:659–665.

257. Rousou JA, Parker T, Engelman RM, et al. Phrenic nerve paresis associated with the use of iced slush and the cooling jacket for topical hypothermia. *J Thorac Cardiovasc Surg* 1985;89: 9221–9225.

258. Kohorst WR, Schonfeld SA, Altman M. Bilateral diaphragmatic paralysis following topical cardiac hypothermia. *Chest* 1984;85: 65–68.

259. Nikas DJ, Ramadan FM, Elefteriades JA. Topical hypothermia: ineffective and deleterious as adjunct to cardioplegia for myocardial protection [see Comments]. *Ann Thorac Surg* 1998;65: 28–31.

260. Khuri SF, Michelson AD, Valeri CR. The effect of cardiopulmonary bypass on hemostasis and coagulation. In: Loscalzo J, Schafer AI, eds. *Thrombosis and hemorrhage.* Cambridge, MA: Blackwell Science, 1994:1051–1073.

261. Valeri CR, Cassidy G, Khuri S, et al. Hypothermia-induced reversible platelet dysfunction. *Ann Surg* 1987;205:175–181.

262. Nakamura M, Toombs CF, Duarte IG, et al. Recombinant human megakaryocyte growth and development factor attenuates postbypass thrombocytopenia. *Ann Thorac Surg* 1998;66:1216–1223.

263. Becker H, Vinten-Johansen J, Buckberg GD, et al. Myocardial damage caused by keeping pH 7.40 during systemic deep hypothermia. *J Thorac Cardiovasc Surg* 1981;82:810–820.

264. Lichtenstein SV, Ashe KA, El Dalati H, et al. Warm heart surgery. *J Thorac Cardiovasc Surg* 1991;101:269–274.

265. Hayashida N, Ikonomidis JS, Weisel RD, et al. The optimal cardioplegic temperature. *Ann Thorac Surg* 1994;58:961–971.

266. Boldt J, Knothe C, Welters I, et al. Normothermic versus hypothermic cardiopulmonary bypass: do changes in coagulation differ? *Ann Thorac Surg* 1996;62:130–135.

267. Buckberg GD. Myocardial protection during adult cardiac operations. In: Anonymous. *Surgery for acquired heart disease.* 1993:1417–1441.

268. Buckberg GD. Strategies and logic of cardioplegic delivery to prevent, avoid, and reverse ischemic and reperfusion damage. *J Thorac Cardiovasc Surg* 1987;93:127–139.

269. Lindal S, Gunnes S, Lund I, et al. Myocardial and microvascular injury following coronary surgery and its attenuation by mode of reperfusion. *Eur J Cardiothorac Surg* 1995;9:83–89.

270. Sato H, Zhao Z-Q, Jordan JE, et al: Gradual restoration of reperfusion reduces coronary artery endothelial injury and myocardial infarction. *FASEB J* 1995;9:A421(abst).

271. Lucas SK, Gardner TJ, Flaherty JT, et al. Beneficial effects of mannitol administration during reperfusion after ischemic arrest. *Circulation* 1980;62:I-34–I-41.

272. Okamoto F, Allen BS, Buckberg GD, et al. Studies of controlled reperfusion after ischemia. XI. Reperfusate composition: interaction of marked hyperglycemia and marked hyperosmolarity in allowing immediate contractile recovery after 4 hours of regional ischemia. *J Thorac Cardiovasc Surg* 1986;92:583–593.

273. Allen SJ, Geissler HJ, Davis KL, et al. Augmenting cardiac contractility hastens myocardial edema resolution after cardiopulmonary bypass and cardioplegic arrest. *Anesth Analg* 1997;85:987–992.

274. Ihnken K, Morita K, Buckberg GD. New approaches to blood cardioplegic delivery to reduce hemodilution and cardioplegic overdose. *J Card Surg* 1994;9:26–36.

275. Menasché P. Blood cardioplegia: do we still need to dilute? *Ann Thorac Surg* 1996;62:957–960.

276. Menasché P, Touchot B, Pradier F, et al. Simplified method for delivering normothermic blood cardioplegia. *Ann Thorac Surg* 1993;55:177–178.

277. Machiraju VR, Lima CAB, Culig MH. The value of minicardioplegia in the clinical setting. *Ann Thorac Surg* 1997;64:887.

278. Buckberg GD, Becker H, Vinten-Johansen J, et al. Myocardial function resulting from varying acid–base management during and following deep surface and perfusion hypothermia and circulatory arrest. In: Rahn H, Prakash O, eds. *Acid–base regulation and body temperature.* Boston: Martinus Nijhoff, 1985:135–159.

279. McConnell DH, White F, Nelson RL, et al. Importance of alkalosis in maintenance of "ideal" blood pH during hypothermia. *Surg Forum* 1975;26:263–265.

280. Warner KG, Josa M, Marston W, et al. Reduction in myocardial acidosis using blood cardioplegia. *J Surg Res* 1987;42:247–256.

281. Warner KG, Josa M, Butler MD, et al. Regional changes in myocardial acid production during ischemic arrest: a comparison of sanguineous and asanguineous cardioplegia. *Ann Thorac Surg* 1988;45:75–81.

282. Geffin GA, Reynolds TR, Titus JS, et al. Relation of myocardial protection to cardioplegic solution pH: modulation by calcium and magnesium. *Ann Thorac Surg* 1991;52:955–964.

283. del Nido PJ, Wilson GJ, Mickle DAG, et al. The role of cardioplegic solution buffering in myocardial protection. A biochemical and histopathological assessment. *J Thorac Cardiovasc Surg* 1985;89:689–699.

284. Neethling WM, van den Heever JJ, Cooper S, et al. Interstitial pH during myocardial preservation: assessment of five methods of myocardial preservation. *Ann Thorac Surg* 1993;55:420–426.

285. Bernard M, Menasché P, Canioni P, et al. Influence of the pH of cardioplegic solutions on intracellular pH, high-energy phosphates, and postarrest performance. Protective effects of acidotic, glutamate-containing cardioplegic perfusates. *J Thorac Cardiovasc Surg* 1985;90:235–242.

286. Kitakaze M, Weisfeldt ML, Marban E. Acidosis during early reperfusion prevents myocardial stunning in perfused ferret hearts. *J Clin Invest* 1988;82:920–927.

287. Tian GH, Mainwood GW, Biro GP, et al. The effect of high buffer cardioplegia and secondary cardioplegia on cardiac preservation and postischemic functional recovery: a 31P NMR and functional study in Langendorff perfused pig hearts. *Can J Physiol Pharmacol* 1991;69:1760–1768.

288. Nugent WC, Levine FH, Liapis CD, et al. Effect of the pH of cardioplegic solution on postarrest myocardial preservation. *Circulation* 1982;66:I-68–I-72.

289. Tait GA, Booker PD, Wilson GJ, et al. Effect of multidose cardioplegia and cardioplegic solution buffering on myocardial tissue acidosis. *J Thorac Cardiovasc Surg* 1982;83:824–829.

290. Yamamoto F, Braimbridge MV, Hearse DJ. Calcium and cardioplegia: the optimal calcium content for St. Thomas' Hospital cardioplegic solution. *J Thorac Cardiovasc Surg* 1984;87:908–912.

291. Jynge P, Hearse DJ, Braimbridge MV, et al. Myocardial protection during ischemic cardiac arrest. A possible hazard with calcium-free cardioplegic infusates. *J Thorac Cardiovasc Surg* 1977;73:848–855.

292. Allen BS, Okamoto F, Buckberg GD. Studies of controlled reperfusion after ischemia. IX. Reperfusate composition: benefits of marked hypocalcemia and diltiazem on regional recovery. *J Thorac Cardiovasc Surg* 1986;92:564–572.

293. Tani M, Neely JR. Role of intracellular Na^+ in Ca^{2+} overload and depressed recovery of ventricular function of reperfused ischemic rat hearts: possible involvement of H^+/Na^+ exchange and Na^+/Ca^{2+} exchange. *Circ Res* 1989;65:1045–1056.

294. Kuroda H, Ishiguro S, Mori T. Optimal calcium concentration in the initial reperfusate for post-ischemic myocardial performance (calcium concentration during reperfusion). *J Mol Cell Cardiol* 1986;18:625–633.

295. Lahorra JA, Torchiana DF, Tolis G Jr, et al. Rapid cooling contracture with cold cardioplegia. *Ann Thorac Surg* 1997;63:1353–1360.

296. Baller D, Wolpers HG, Schrader R, et al. Paradoxical effects of catecholamines and calcium on myocardial function in moderate hypothermia. *Thorac Cardiovasc Surg* 1983;31:131–138.

297. Randle PJ, Denton RN, England PJ. Citrate as a metabolic regulator in muscle and adipose tissue. In: Goodman TW, ed. *Metabolic roles of citrate.* London: Academic Press, 1968:87–103.

298. Maggirwar SB, Dhanraj DN, Somani SM, et al. Adenosine acts as an endogenous activator of the cellular antioxidant defense system. *Biochem Biophys Res Comm* 1994;201:508–515.

299. Kofsky ER, Julia PL, Buckberg GD, et al. Studies of controlled

reperfusion after ischemia. XXII. Reperfusate composition: effects of leukocyte depletion of blood and blood cardioplegic reperfusates after acute coronary occlusion. *J Thorac Cardiovasc Surg* 1991;101:350–359.

300. O'Neill PG, Charlat ML, Michael LH, et al. Influence of neutrophil depletion on myocardial function and flow after reversible ischemia. *Am J Physiol* 1989;256:H341–H351

301. Romson JL, Hook BG, Kunkel SL, et al. Reduction of the extent of ischemic myocardial injury by neutrophil depletion in the dog. *Circulation* 1983;67:1016–1023.

302. Julia PL, Buckberg GD, Acar C, et al. Studies of controlled reperfusion after ischemia. XXI. Reperfusate composition: superiority of blood cardioplegia over crystalloid cardioplegia in limiting reperfusion damage—importance of endogenous oxygen free radical scavengers in red blood cells. *J Thorac Cardiovasc Surg* 1991;101:303–313.

303. Bing OHL, LaRaia PJ, Gaasch WH, et al. Independent protection provided by red blood cells during cardioplegia. *Circulation* 1982;66[Suppl I]:I-81–I-84.

304. Shlafer M, Kane PF, Wiggins VY, et al. Possible role for cytotoxic oxygen metabolites in the pathogenesis of cardiac ischemic injury. *Circulation* 1982;66[Suppl 1]:85–92.

305. Stewart JR, Blackwell WH, Crute SL, et al. Prevention of myocardial ischemia/reperfusion injury with oxygen free-radical scavengers. *Surg Forum* 1982;33:317–320.

306. Myers CL, Weiss SJ, Kirsh MM, et al. Effects of supplementing hypothermic crystalloid cardioplegic solution with catalase, superoxide dismutase, allopurinal, or deferoxamine on functional recovery of globally ischemic and reperfused isolated hearts. *J Thorac Cardiovasc Surg* 1986;91:281–289.

307. Menasché P, Grousset C, Gauduel Y, et al. A comparative study of free radical scavengers in cardioplegic solutions. Improved protection with peroxidase. *J Thorac Cardiovasc Surg* 1986;92:264–271.

308. Gardner TJ, Stewart JR, Casale AS, et al. Reduction of myocardial ischemic injury with oxygen-derived free radical scavengers. *Surgery* 1983;94:423–427.

309. Stewart JR, Blackwell WH, Crute SL, et al. Inhibition of surgically induced ischemia/reperfusion injury by oxygen free radical scavengers. *J Thorac Cardiovasc Surg* 1983;86:262–272.

310. Stewart JR, Crute SL, Loughlin V, et al. Prevention of free radical-induced myocardial reperfusion injury with allopurinol. *J Thorac Cardiovasc Surg* 1985;90:68–72.

311. Chambers DJ, Braimbridge MV, Hearse DJ. Free radicals and cardioplegia: allopurinol and oxypurinol reduce myocardial injury following ischemic arrest. *Ann Thorac Surg* 1987;44:291–297.

312. Chambers DJ, Braimbridge MV, Hearse DJ. Free radicals and cardioplegia: free radical scavengers improve postischemic function of rat myocardium. *Eur J Cardiothorac Surg* 1987;1:37–45.

313. Galiñanes M, Qiu Y, Ezrin A, et al. PEG-SOD and myocardial protection. Studies in the blood- and crystalloid-perfused rabbit and rat hearts. *Circulation* 1992;86:672–682.

314. Pisarenko OI, Studneva IM, Lakomkin VL, et al. Human recombinant extracellular-superoxide dismutase type C improves cardioplegic protection against ischemia/reperfusion injury in isolated rat heart. *J Cardiovasc Pharmacol* 1994;24:655–663.

315. Gharagozloo F, Melendez FJ, Hein RA, et al. The effect of oxygen free radical scavengers on the recovery of regional myocardial function after acute coronary occlusion and surgical reperfusion. *J Thorac Cardiovasc Surg* 1988;95:631–636.

316. Das DK, Engelman RM, Rousou JA, et al. Pathophysiology of superoxide radical as potential mediator of reperfusion injury in pig heart. *Basic Res Cardiol* 1986;81:155–166.

317. Shlafer M, Kane PF, Kirsh MM. Superoxide dismutase plus catalase enhances the efficacy of hypothermic cardioplegia to protect the globally ischemic, reperfused heart. *J Thorac Cardiovasc Surg* 1982;83:830–839.

318. Ytrehus K, Gunnes S, Myklebust R, et al. Protection by superoxide dismutase and catalase in the isolated rat heart reperfused after prolonged cardioplegia: a combined study of metabolic, functional, and morphometric ultrastructural variables. *Cardiovasc Res* 1987;21:492–499.

319. Greenfield DT, Greenfield LJ, Hess ML. Enhancement of crystalloid cardioplegic protection against global normothermic ischemia by superoxide dismutase plus catalase but not diltiazem in the isolated, working rat heart. *J Thorac Cardiovasc Surg* 1988;95:799–813.

320. Uraizee A, Reimer KA, Murry CE, et al. Failure of superoxide dismutase to limit size of myocardial infarction after 40 minutes of ischemia and 4 days of reperfusion in dogs. *Circulation* 1987;75:1237–1248.

321. Coghlan JG, Flitter WD, Clutton SM, et al. Allopurinol pretreatment improves postoperative recovery and reduces lipid peroxidation in patients undergoing coronary artery bypass grafting. *J Thorac Cardiovasc Surg* 1994;107:248–256.

322. Gimpel JA, Lahpor JR, Van der Molen A-J, et al. Reduction of reperfusion injury of human myocardium by allopurinol: a clinical study. *Free Radic Biol Med* 1995;19:251–255.

323. Sisto T, Paajanen H, Metsa-Ketela T, et al. Pretreatment with antioxidants and allopurinol diminishes cardiac onset events in coronary artery bypass grafting. *Ann Thorac Surg* 1995;59:1519–1523.

324. Chambers DJ, Astras G, Takahashi A, et al. Free radicals and cardioplegia: organic anti-oxidants as additives to the St. Thomas' Hospital cardioplegic solution. *Cardiovasc Res* 1989;23:351–358.

325. Das DK, Engelman RM, Flansaas D, et al. Developmental profiles of protective mechanisms of heart against peroxidative injury. *Basic Res Cardiol* 1987;82:36–50.

326. England MD, Cavarocchi NC, O'Brien JF, et al. Influence of antioxidants (mannitol and allopurinol) on oxygen free radical generation during and after cardiopulmonary bypass. *Circulation* 1986;74:III-134–III-137.

327. Weisel JW, Mickle DAG, Finkle CD, et al. Myocardial free-radical injury after cardioplegia. *Circulation* 1989;80[Suppl III]:14–18.

328. Bical O, Gerhardt M-F, Paumier D, et al. Comparison of different types of cardioplegia and reperfusion on myocardial metabolism and free radical activity. *Circulation* 1991;84[Suppl III]:III-375–III-379.

329. Flaherty JT, Pitt B, Gruber JW, et al. Recombinant human superoxide dismutase (h-SOD) fails to improve recovery of ventricular function in patients undergoing coronary angioplasty for acute myocardial infarction. *Circulation* 1994;89:1982–1991.

330. Jolly SR, Kane WJ, Bailie MB, et al. Canine myocardial reperfusion injury: its reduction by the combined administration of superoxide dismutase and catalase. *Circ Res* 1984;54:277–285.

331. Castelli P, Condemi AM, Brambillasea C, et al. Improvement in cardiac function by allopurinol on patients undergoing cardiac surgery. *J Cardiovasc Pharmacol* 1995;25:119–125.

332. Ferreira R, Burgos M, Llesuy S, et al. Reduction of reperfusion injury with mannitol cardioplegia. *Ann Thorac Surg* 1989;78:77–84.

333. Emerit I, Fabiani JN, Ponzio O, et al. Clastogenic factor in ischemia-reperfusion injury during open-heart surgery: protective effect of allopurinol. *Ann Thorac Surg* 1995;60:736–737.

334. Seiler KS, Kehrer JP, Starnes JW. Exogenous glutathione attenuates stunning following intermittent hypoxia in isolated rat hearts. *Free Radic Res* 1996;24:115–122.

335. Konorev EA, Joseph J, Tarpey MM, et al. The mechanisms of

cardioprotection by *S*-nitrosoglutathione monoethyl ester in rat isolated heart during cardioplegic ischemic arrest. *Br J Pharmacol* 1996;119:511–518.

336. Kevelaitis E, Nyborg NC, Menasché P. Protective effect of reduced glutathione on endothelial function of coronary arteries subjected to prolonged storage. *Transplantation* 1997;64: 660–663.

337. Ma X-L, Lopez BL, Liu G-L, et al. Peroxynitrite aggravates myocardial reperfusion injury in the isolated perfused rat heart. *Cardiovasc Res* 1997;36:195–204.

338. Wu M, Pritchard KA Jr, Kaminski PM, et al. Involvement of nitric oxide and nitrosothiols in relaxation of pulmonary arteries to peroxynitrite. *Am J Physiol* 1994;266:H2108–H2113.

339. Cheung P-Y, Schulz R. Glutathione causes coronary vasodilation via a nitric oxide- and soluble guanylate cyclase-dependent mechanism. *Am J Physiol* 1997;273:H1231–H1238.

340. Yoshida T, Maulik N, Engelman RM, et al. Glutathione peroxidase knockout mice are susceptible to myocardial ischemia reperfusion injury. *Circulation* 1997;96[9 Suppl]:II-216–II-220.

341. Anonymous. Transgenic mice overexpressing glutathione peroxidase are resistant to myocardial ischemia reperfusion injury. *J Mol Cell Cardiol* 1996;28:1759–1767.

342. Menasché P, Termignon JL, Pradier F, et al. Experimental evaluation of Celsior, a new heart preservation solution. *Eur J Cardiothorac Surg* 1994;8:207–213.

343. Pietri S, Culcasi M, Albat B, et al. Direct assessment of the antioxidant effects of a new heart preservation solution, Celsior. A hemodynamic and electron spin resonance study. *Transplantation* 1994;58:739–742.

344. Weiss RG, Kalil-Filho R, Herskowitz A, et al. Tricarboxylic acid cycle activity in postischemic rat hearts. *Circulation* 1993; 87:270–282.

345. Sanborn T, Gavin W, Berkowitz S, et al. Augmented conversion of aspartate and glutamate to succinate during anoxia in rabbit heart. *Am J Physiol* 1979;237:H535–H541.

346. Svedjeholm R, Vanhanen I, Hakanson E, et al. Metabolic and hemodynamic effects of intravenous glutamate infusion early after coronary operations. *J Thorac Cardiovasc Surg* 1996;112: 1468–1477.

347. Rosenkranz ER, Okamoto F, Buckberg GD, et al. Safety of prolonged aortic clamping with blood cardioplegia. III. Aspartate enrichment of glutamate-blood cardioplegia in energy-depleted hearts after ischemic and reperfusion injury. *J Thorac Cardiovasc Surg* 1986;91:428–435.

348. Morita K, Ihnken K, Buckberg GD, et al. Studies of hypoxemic/reoxygenation injury: without aortic clamping. VIII. Counteraction of oxidant damage by exogenous glutamate and aspartate. *J Thorac Cardiovasc Surg* 1995;110:1228–1234.

349. Kofsky E, Julia P, Buckberg GD, et al. Studies of myocardial protection in the immature heart. V. Safety of prolonged aortic clamping with hypocalcemic glutamate/aspartate blood cardioplegia. *J Thorac Cardiovasc Surg* 1991;101:33–43.

350. Julia P, Young HH, Buckberg GD, et al. Studies of myocardial protection in the immature heart. IV. Improved tolerance of immature myocardium to hypoxia and ischemia by intravenous metabolic support [see Comments]. *J Thorac Cardiovasc Surg* 1991;101:23–32.

351. Keith F. Oxygen free radicals in cardiac transplantation [Review]. *J Card Surg* 1993;8:245–248.

352. Tixier D, Matheis G, Buckberg GD, et al. Donor hearts with impaired hemodynamics. Benefit of warm substrate-enriched blood cardioplegic solution for induction of cardioplegia during cardiac harvesting. *J Thorac Cardiovasc Surg* 1991;102: 207–214.

353. Reed MK, Barak C, Malloy CR, et al. Effects of glutamate and aspartate on myocardial substrate oxidation during potassium arrest. *J Thorac Cardiovasc Surg* 1996;112:1651–1660.

354. Pisarenko OI, Portnoy VF, Studneva IM, et al. Glutamate-blood cardioplegia improves ATP preservation in human myocardium. *Biomed Biochim Acta* 1987;46:499–504.

355. Engelman RM, Rousou JA, Flack JE III, et al. Reduction of infarct size by systemic amino acid supplementation during reperfusion. *J Thorac Cardiovasc Surg* 1991;101:855–859.

356. Olafsson B, Forman MB, Puett DW, et al. Reduction of reperfusion injury in the canine preparation by intracoronary adenosine: importance of the endothelium and the no-reflow phenomenon. *Circulation* 1987;76:1135–1145.

357. Cronstein BN. Adenosine, an endogenous anti-inflammatory agent. *J Appl Physiol* 1994;76:5–13.

358. Vinten-Johansen J, Zhao Z-Q. Cardioprotection from ischemic-reperfusion injury by adenosine. In: Abd-Elfattah AS, Wechsler AS, eds. *Purines and myocardial protection.* Boston: Kluwer Academic Publishers, 1995:315–344.

359. Lasley RD, Mentzer RM Jr. Protective effects of adenosine in the reversibly injured heart. *Ann Thorac Surg* 1995;60:843–846.

360. Zhao Z-Q, Sato H, Williams MW, et al. Adenosine A$_2$-receptor activation inhibits neutrophil-mediated injury to coronary endothelium. *Am J Physiol* 1996;271:H1456–H1464.

361. Cronstein BN, Rosenstein ED, Kramer SB, et al. Adenosine: a physiologic modulator of superoxide anion generation by human neutrophils. Adenosine acts via an A$_2$ receptor on human neutrophils. *J Immunol* 1985;135:1366–1371.

362. Cronstein BN, Levin RI, Belanoff J, et al. Adenosine: an endogenous inhibitor of neutrophil-mediated injury to endothelial cells. *J Clin Invest* 1986;78:760–770.

363. Thourani VH, Nakamura M, Zhao Z-Q, et al. Specific adenosine A$_3$ receptor stimulation attenuates global ischemic-reperfusion injury in a neutrophil-free model. *Circulation* 1997;96:I-743(abst).

364. Thourani VH, Ronson RS, Jordan JE, et al. Pretreatment with a specific adenosine A$_3$ receptor agonist before cardioplegia arrest improves postischemic function of jeopardized myocardium. *Surg Forum* 1998;49:207–209.

365. Woolfson RG, Patel VC, Yellon DM. Pre-conditioning with adenosine leads to concentration-dependent infarct size reduction in the isolated rabbit heart. *Cardiovasc Res* 1996;31: 148–151.

366. Toombs CF, McGee DS, Johnston WE, et al. Myocardial protective effects of adenosine. Infarct size reduction with pretreatment and continued receptor stimulation during ischemia. *Circulation* 1992;86:986–994.

367. Zhou Z, Bunger R, Lasley RD, et al. Adenosine pretreatment increases cytosolic phosphorylation potential and attenuates postischemic cardiac dysfunction in swine. *Surg Forum* 1993; 249–251.

368. Thornton JD, Liu GS, Olsson RA, et al. Intravenous pretreatment with A$_1$-selective adenosine analogues protects the heart against infarction. *Circulation* 1992;85:659–665.

369. Randhawa MPS Jr, Lasley RD, Mentzer RM Jr. Adenosine and the stunned heart. *J Card Surg* 1993;8[Suppl]:332–337.

370. Lee HT, LaFaro RJ, Reed GE. Pretreatment of human myocardium with adenosine during open heart surgery. *J Card Surg* 1995;10:665–676.

371. Boehm DH, Human PA, von Oppell U, et al. Adenosine cardioplegia: reducing reperfusion injury of the ischaemic myocardium? *Eur J Cardiothorac Surg* 1991;5:542–545.

372. Schubert T, Vetter H, Owen P, et al. Adenosine cardioplegia: adenosine versus potassium cardioplegia: effects on cardiac arrest

and postischemic recovery in the isolated rat heart. *J Thorac Cardiovasc Surg* 1989;98:1057–1065.

373. Bolling SF, Bies LE, Gallagher KP, et al. Enhanced myocardial protection with adenosine. *Ann Thorac Surg* 1989;47:809–815.

374. Wyatt DA, Ely SW, Lasley RD, et al. Purine-enriched asanguineous cardioplegia retards adenosine triphosphate degradation during ischemia and improves postischemic ventricular function. *J Thorac Cardiovasc Surg* 1989;97:771–778.

375. Bolling SF, Bies LE, Bove EL, et al. Augmenting intracellular adenosine improves myocardial recovery. *J Thorac Cardiovasc Surg* 1990;99:469–474.

376. Bolling SF, Bove EL, Gallagher KP. ATP precursor depletion and postischemic myocardial recovery. *J Surg Res* 1991;50: 629–633.

377. Bolling SF, Bies LE, Bove EL. Effect of ATP synthesis promoters on postischemic myocardial recovery. *J Surg Res* 1990;49: 205–211.

378. Ledingham S, Katayama O, Lachno D, et al. Beneficial effect of adenosine during reperfusion following prolonged cardioplegic arrest. *Cardiovasc Res* 1990;24:247–253.

379. Hohlfeld T, Hearse DJ, Yellon DM, et al. Adenosine-induced increase in myocardial ATP: are there beneficial effects for the ischaemic myocardium? *Basic Res Cardiol* 1989;84:499–509.

380. Thelin S, Hultman J, Ronquist G. Effects of adenosine infusion on the pig heart during normothermic ischemia and reperfusion. *Scand J Thorac Cardiovasc Surg* 1991;25:207–213.

381. Ambrosio G, Jacobus WE, Mitchell MC, et al. Effects of ATP precursors on ATP and free ADP content and functional recovery of postischemic hearts. *Am J Physiol* 1989;256:H560–H566.

382. Thourani VH, Ronson RS, VanWylen DG, et al. Myocardial protection with adenosine given at reperfusion is superior to adenosine-enhanced cardioplegia. *Circulation* 1998;98[Suppl]: I-1–I-1016(abst).

383. Fremes SE, Levy SL, Christakis GT, et al. Phase 1 human trial of adenosine–potassium cardioplegia. *Circulation* 1996;94:II-370–II-375.

384. Cohen G, Feder-Elituv R, Iazetta J, et al. Phase 2 studies of adenosine cardioplegia. *Circulation* 1998;98:II-225–II-233.

385. Mentzer RM Jr, Rahko PS, Molina-Viamonte V, et al. Safety, tolerance, and efficacy of adenosine as an additive to blood cardioplegia in humans during coronary artery bypass surgery. *Am J Cardiol* 1997;79:38–43.

386. Mentzer RM Jr, Rahko PS, Canver CC, et al. Adenosine reduces postbypass transfusion requirements in humans after heart surgery. *Ann Surg* 1996;234:523–530.

387. Sato H, Zhao Z-Q, Vinten-Johansen J. L-Arginine inhibits neutrophil adherence and coronary artery dysfunction. *Cardiovasc Res* 1996;31:63–72.

388. Palmer RMJ, Rees DD, Ashton DS, et al. L-Arginine is the physiological precursor for the formation of nitric oxide in endothelium-dependent relaxation. *Biochem Biophys Res Comm* 1988;153:1251–1256.

389. Sato H, Zhao Z-Q, McGee DS, et al. Supplemental L-arginine during cardioplegic arrest and reperfusion avoids regional postischemic injury. *J Thorac Cardiovasc Surg* 1995;110:302–314.

390. Hiramatsu T, Forbess JM, Miura T, et al. Effect of L-arginine cardioplegia on recovery of neonatal lamb hearts after 2 hours of cold ischemia. *Ann Thorac Surg* 1995;60:1187–1192.

391. Engelman DT, Watanabe M, Maulik N, et al. L-Arginine reduces endothelial inflammation and myocardial stunning during ischemia/reperfusion. *Ann Thorac Surg* 1995;60: 1275–1281.

392. Engelman DT, Watanabe M, Maulik N, et al. Critical timing

393. Hiramatsu T, Forbess JM, Miura T, et al. Additive effects of l-arginine infusion and leukocyte depletion on recovery after hypothermic ischemia in neonatal lamb hearts. *J Thorac Cardiovasc Surg* 1995;110:172–179.

394. Amrani M, Chester AH, Jayakumar J, et al. L-Arginine reverses low coronary reflow and enhances postischaemic recovery of cardiac mechanical function. *Cardiovasc Res* 1995;30:200–204.

395. Sato H, Zhao Z-Q, Jordan JE, et al. Basal nitric oxide expresses endogenous cardioprotection during reperfusion by inhibition of neutrophil-mediated damage after surgical revascularization. *J Thorac Cardiovasc Surg* 1997;113(2):399–409.

396. Johnson G III, Tsao PS, Lefer AM. Cardioprotective effects of authentic nitric oxide in myocardial ischemia with reperfusion. *Crit Care Med* 1991;19:244–252.

397. Johnson G III, Tsao PS, Mulloy D, et al. Cardioprotective effects of acidified sodium nitrite in myocardial ischemia with reperfusion. *J Pharmacol Exp Ther* 1990;252:35–41.

398. Lefer DJ, Nakanishi K, Vinten-Johansen J. Endothelial and myocardial cell protection by a cysteine-containing nitric oxide donor after myocardial ischemia and reperfusion. *J Cardiovasc Pharmacol* 1993;22[Suppl 7]:S34–S43.

399. Lefer DJ, Nakanishi K, Johnston WE, et al. Antineutrophil and myocardial protection actions of a novel nitric oxide donor after acute myocardial ischemia and reperfusion in dogs. *Circulation* 1993;88:2337–2350.

400. Lopez BL, Christopher TA, Ma X-L. The effects of peroxynitrite on the myocardium during ischemia–reperfusion are dependent upon the biological environment. *Endothelium* 1995;3:76(abst).

401. Lopez BL, Liu G-L, Christopher TA, et al. Peroxynitrite, the product of nitric oxide and superoxide, causes myocardial injury in the isolated perfused rat heart. *Coron Artery Dis* 1997;8: 149–153.

402. Pabla R, Curtis MJ. Effect of endogenous nitric oxide on cardiac systolic and diastolic function during ischemia and reperfusion in the rat isolated perfused heart. *J Mol Cell Cardiol* 1996;28: 2111–2121.

403. Pabla R, Buda AJ, Flynn DM, et al. Nitric oxide attenuates neutrophil-mediated myocardial contractile dysfunction after ischemia and reperfusion. *Circ Res* 1996;78:65–72.

404. Hoshida S, Yamashita N, Igarashi J, et al. Nitric oxide synthase protects the heart against ischemia-reperfusion injury in rabbits. *J Pharmacol Exp Ther* 1995;274:413–418.

405. Beckman JS, Wink DA, Crow JP. Nitric oxide and peroxynitrite. In: Feelisch M, Stamler JS, eds. *Methods in nitric oxide.* West Sussex, England: John Wiley and Sons, 1996:61–70.

406. Beckman JS, Koppenol WH. Nitric oxide, superoxide, and peroxynitrite: the good, the bad, and the ugly. *Am J Physiol* 1996; 271:C1424–C1437.

407. Nossuli TO, Hayward R, Jensen D, et al. Mechanisms of cardioprotection by peroxynitrite in myocardial ischemia and reperfusion injury. *Am J Physiol* 1998;275:H509–H519.

408. Ronson RS, Thourani VH, Ma X-L, et al. Peroxynitrite is beneficial in blood cardioplegia, but is deleterious in crystalloid cardioplegia *in vivo. Circulation* 1998;98:I-750(abst).

409. Armstrong S, Ganote CE. Adenosine receptor specificity in preconditioning of isolated rabbit cardiomyocytes: evidence of A$_3$ receptor involvement. *Cardiovasc Res* 1994;28:1049–1056.

410. Sluiter W, Pietersma A, Lamers JMJ, et al. Leukocyte adhesion molecules on the vascular endothelium: their role in the pathogenesis of cardiovascular disease and the mechanisms underlying their expression. *J Cardiovasc Pharmacol* 1993;22[Suppl 4]: S37–S44.

411. Collins T, Read MA, Neish AS, et al. Transcriptional regulation of endothelial cell adhesion molecules: NF-κB and cytokine-inducible enhancers. *FASEB J* 1995;9:899–909.

412. Weber C, Erl W, Pietsch A, et al. Aspirin inhibits nuclear factor-κB mobilization and monocyte adhesion in stimulated human endothelial cells. *Circulation* 1995;91:1914–1917.

413. Flynn DM, Buda AJ, Jeffords PR. A sialyl Lewis (x)-containing carbohydrate reduces infarct size: role of selectins in myocardial reperfusion injury. *Am J Physiol* 1996;271[5 Pt 2]: H2080–H2096.

414. Gu YJ, Obster R, Haan J, et al. Biocompatibility of leukocyte removal filters during leukocyte filtration of cardiopulmonary bypass perfusate. *Artif Organs* 1993;17:660–665.

415. Wilson IC, Gardner TJ, DiNatale JM, et al. Temporary leukocyte depletion reduces ventricular dysfunction during prolonged postischemic reperfusion. *J Thorac Cardiovasc Surg* 1993;106: 805–810.

416. Gott JP, Cooper WA, Schmidt FEJ, et al. Modifying risk for extracorporeal circulation: trial of four antiinflammatory strategies. *Ann Thorac Surg* 1998;66:747–753.

417. Finn A, Morgan BP, Rebuck N, et al. Effects of inhibition of complement activation using recombinant soluble complement receptor 1 on neutrophil CD11B/CD18 and L-selectin expression and release of interleukin-8 and elastase in simulated cardiopulmonary bypass. *J Thorac Cardiovasc Surg* 1996;111: 451–459.

418. Gillinov AM, DeValeria PA, Winkelstein JA, et al. Complement inhibition with soluble complement receptor type 1 in cardiopulmonary bypass. *Ann Thorac Surg* 1993;55:619–624.

419. Tofukuji M, Stahl GL, Agah A, et al. Anti-C5A monoclonal antibody reduces cardiopulmonary bypass and cardioplegia-induced coronary endothelial dysfunction. *J Thorac Cardiovasc Surg* 1998;116:1060–1068.

420. Kleber AG, Oetliker H. Cellular aspects of early contractile failure in ischemia. In: Fozzard HA, Haber E, Jennings RB, et al., eds. *The heart and cardiovascular system.* New York: Raven Press, 1992:1975–2020.

421. Reimer KA, Jennings RB. Myocardial ischemia, hypoxia, and infarction. In: Fozzard HA, Haber E, Jennings RB, et al., eds. *The heart and cardiovascular system.* New York: Raven Press, 1992:1875–1973.

422. Damiano RJ Jr. The electrophysiology of ischemia and cardioplegia: implications for myocardial protection. *J Card Surg* 1995;10[4 Suppl]:445–453.

423. Lawton JS, Hsia PW, Damiano JrRJ. The adenosine-triphosphate-sensitive potassium-channel opener pinacidil is effective in blood cardioplegia. *Ann Thorac Surg* 1998;66:768–773.

424. Kirvaitis RJ, Krukenkamp IB, Bukhari EA, et al. Pinacidil-induced hyperpolarized cold blood cardioplegia: a novel myoprotective strategy. *Surg Forum* 1995;46:224–226.

425. Maskal SL, Cohen NM, Hsia PW, et al. Hyperpolarized cardiac arrest with a potassium-channel opener, aprikalim. *J Thorac Cardiovasc Surg* 1995;110:1083–1095.

426. Lawton JS, Harrington GC, Allen CT, et al. Myocardial protection with pinacidil cardioplegia in the blood-perfused heart. *Ann Thorac Surg* 1996;61:1680–1688.

427. He G-W, Yang C-Q. Cardiopulmonary bypass, myocardial management, and support techniques. Superiority of hyperpolarizing to depolarizing cardioplegia in protection of coronary endothelial function. *J Thorac Cardiovasc Surg* 1997;114: 643–650.

428. Noma A. ATP-regulated K+ channels in cardiac muscle. *Nature* 1983;305:147–148.

429. Daut J, Maier-Rudolph W, von Beckerath N, et al. Hypoxic dilation of coronary arteries is mediated by ATP-sensitive potassium channels. *Science* 1990;247:1341–1343.

430. Cook DL, Hales CN. Intracellular ATP directly blocks K+ channels in pancreatic B-cells. *Nature* 1984;311:271–273.

431. Schmid-Antomarchi H, Amoroso S, Fosset M, et al. K+ channel openers activate brain sulfonylurea-sensitive K+ channels and block neurosecretion. *Proc Natl Acad Sci U S A* 1990;87: 3489–3492.

432. Samaha FF, Heineman FW, Ince C, et al. ATP-sensitive potassium channel is essential to maintain basal coronary vascular tone *in vivo. Am J Physiol* 1992;262[5 Pt 1]:C1220–C1227.

433. Aversano T, Ouyang P, Silverman H. Blockade of the ATP-sensitive potassium channel modulates reactive hyperemia in the canine coronary circulation. *Circ Res* 1991;69:618–622.

434. Kanatsuka H, Sekiguchi N, Sato K, et al. Microvascular sites and mechanisms responsible for reactive hyperemia in the coronary circulation of the beating canine heart. *Circ Res* 1992;71: 912–922.

435. Komaru T, Lamping KG, Eastham CL, et al. Role of ATP-sensitive potassium channels in coronary microvascular autoregulatory responses. *Circ Res* 1991;69:1146–1151.

436. Narishige T, Egashira K, Akatsuka Y, et al. Glibenclamide, a putative ATP-sensitive K+ channel blocker, inhibits coronary autoregulation in anesthetized dogs. *Circ Res* 1993;73:771–776.

437. Grover GJ, Sleph PG, Dzwonczyk S. Role of myocardial ATP-sensitive potassium channels in mediating preconditioning in the dog heart and their possible interaction with adenosine A1 receptors. *Circulation* 1992;86:1310–1316.

438. Gross GJ, Auchampach JA. Blockade of ATP-sensitive potassium channels prevents myocardial preconditioning in dogs. *Circ Res* 1992;70:223–233.

439. Auchampach JA, Gross GJ. Adenosine A1 receptors, K_ATP channels, and ischemic preconditioning in dogs. *Am J Physiol* 1993; 264:H1327–H1336.

440. Toombs CF, McGee DS, Johnston WE, et al. Protection from ischaemic-reperfusion injury with adenosine pretreatment is reversed by inhibition of ATP-sensitive potassium channels. *Cardiovasc Res* 1993;27:623–629.

441. Katz AM. The cardiac action potential. In: Katz AM, ed. *Physiology of the heart.* New York: Raven Press, 1992:438–472.

442. Jayawant AM, Stephenson ER Jr, Matte GS, et al. Hyperpolarized arrest with pinacidil is superior to traditional St. Thomas' solution in the intact animal. *Surg Forum* 1998;49:192–194.

443. Lawton JS, Hsia PW, McClain LC, et al. Myocardial oxygen consumption in the rabbit heart after ischemia: hyperpolarized arrest with pinacidil versus depolarized hyperkalemic arrest. *Circulation* 1997;96[9 Suppl]:II-247–II-252.

444. Jayawant AM, Lawton JS, Hsia PW, et al. Hyperpolarized cardioplegic arrest with nicorandil: advantages over other potassium channel openers. *Circulation* 1997;96[9 Suppl]:II-240–II-246.

445. Lawton JS, Sepic JD, Allen CT, et al. Myocardial protection with potassium-channel openers is as effective as St. Thomas' solution in the rabbit heart. *Ann Thorac Surg* 1996;62:31–39.

446. Antzelevitch C, Di Diego JM. Role of K+ channel activators in cardiac electrophysiology and arrhythmias [Editorial; Comment]. *Circulation* 1992;85:1627–1629.

447. Chi L, Uprichard AC, Lucchesi BR. Profibrillatory actions of pinacidil in a conscious canine model of sudden coronary death. *J Cardiovasc Pharmacol* 1990;15:452–464.

448. Cohen NM, Wise RM, Wechsler AS, et al. Elective cardiac arrest with a hyperpolarizing adenosine triphosphate-sensitive potassium channel opener. *J Thorac Cardiovasc Surg* 1993;106: 317–328.

449. Sardet C, Franchi A, Pouyssegur J. Molecular cloning, primary

structure, and expression of the human growth factor-activatable Na⁺/H⁺ antiporter. *Cell* 1989;56:271–280.

450. Scheufler E, Henrichs M, Guttmann I, et al. Effect of the Na/H exchange inhibitor ethyl-isopropyl-amiloride (EIPA) during ischaemia and reperfusion. *Br J Pharmacol* 1993;108: 118P(abst).

451. Takaichi K, Wang D, Balkovetz DF, et al. Cloning, sequencing, and expression of Na(⁺)-H⁺ antiporter cDNAs from human tissues. *Am J Physiol* 1992;262[4 Pt 1]:C1069–C1076.

452. Fliegel L, Dyck JR, Wang H, et al. Cloning and analysis of the human myocardial Na⁺/H⁺ exchanger. *Mol Cell Biochem* 1993; 125:137–143.

453. Reilly RF, Hildebrandt F, Biemesderfer D, et al. cDNA cloning and immunolocalization of a Na(⁺)-H⁺ exchanger in LLC-PK1 renal epithelial cells. *Am J Physiol* 1991;261[6 Pt 2]: F1088–F1094.

454. Collins JF, Honda T, Knobel S, et al. Molecular cloning, sequencing, tissue distribution, and functional expression of a Na⁺/H⁺ exchanger (NHE-2). *Proc Natl Acad Sci U S A* 1993; 90:3938–3942.

455. Godt RE, Nosek TM. Changes of intracellular milieu with fatigue or hypoxia depress contraction of skinned rabbit skeletal and cardiac muscle. *J Physiol* 1989;412:155–180.

456. Jeffrey FM, Malloy CR, Radda GK. Influence of intracellular acidosis on contractile function in the working rat heart. *Am J Physiol* 1987;253[6 Pt 2]:H1499–H1505.

457. Malloy CR, Matthews PM, Smith MB, et al. *In vivo* phosphorus-31 nuclear magnetic resonance study of the regional metabolic response to cardiac ischemia. *Adv Myocard* 1985;6: 461–464.

458. Miura Y, Kimura J. Sodium-calcium exchange current. Dependence on internal Ca²⁺ and Na⁺ and competitive binding of external Na⁺ and Ca²⁺. *J Gen Physiol* 1989;93:1129–1145.

459. Kimura J, Norma A, Irisawa H. Na-Ca exchange current in mammalian heart cells. *Nature* 1986;319:596–597.

460. Pike MM, Luo CS, Clark MD, et al. NMR measurements of Na⁺ and cellular energy in ischemic rat heart: role of Na⁺-H⁺ exchange. *Am J Physiol* 1993;265:H2017–H2026.

461. Wallert MA, Frohlich O. Na⁺-H⁺ exchange in isolated myocytes from adult rat heart. *Am J Physiol* 1989;26:C207–C213.

462. Vaughan-Jones RD, Wu ML. Extracellular H⁺ inactivation of Na⁺-H⁺ exchange in the sheep cardiac Purkinje fibre. *J Physiol (Lond)* 1990;428:441–466.

463. Karmazyn M, Ray M, Haist JV. Comparative effects of Na⁺/H⁺ exchange inhibitors against cardiac injury produced by ischemia/reperfusion, hypoxia/reoxygenation, and the calcium paradox. *J Cardiovasc Pharmacol* 1993;21:172–178.

464. Scholz W, Albus U, Lang HJ, et al. Hoe 694, a new Na⁺/H⁺ exchange inhibitor, and its effects in cardiac ischaemia. *Br J Pharmacol* 1993;109:562–568.

465. Harper IS, Bond JM, Chacon E, et al. Inhibition of Na⁺/H⁺ exchange preserves viability, restores mechanical function, and prevents the pH paradox in reperfusion injury to rat neonatal myocytes. *Basic Res Cardiol* 1993;88:430–442.

466. Hendrikx M, Mubagwa K, Verdonck F, et al. New Na⁺/H⁺ exchange inhibitor HOE 694 improves postischemic function and high energy phosphate resynthesis and reduces Ca²⁺ overload in isolated perfused rabbit heart. *Circulation* 1994;89: 2787–2798.

467. Scholz W, Albus U, Linz W, et al. Effects of Na⁺/H⁺ exchange inhibitors in cardiac ischemia. *J Mol Cell Cardiol* 1992;24: 731–739.

468. Garcia-Dorado D, Gonzalez MA, Barrabes JA, et al. Prevention

of ischemic rigor contracture during coronary occlusion by inhibition of Na⁺-H⁺ exchange. *Cardiovasc Res* 1997;35:80–89.

469. Moffat MP, Karmazyn M. Protective effects of the potent Na/H exchange inhibitor methylisobutyl amiloride against post-ischemic contractile dysfunction in rat and guinea-pig hearts. *J Mol Cell Cardiol* 1993;25:959–971.

470. Sack S, Mohri M, Schwarz ER, et al. Effects of a new Na⁺/H⁺ antiporter inhibitor on postischemic reperfusion in pig heart. *J Cardiovasc Pharmacol* 1994;23:72–78.

471. Maron R. Functional and metabolic protection by Na⁺/H⁺ exchange inhibition in global ischemia. *J Mol Cell Cardiol* 1989; 21:1226(abst).

472. Mochizuki S, Seki S, Ejima M-A, et al. Na⁺/H⁺ exchanger and reperfusion-induced ventricular arrhythmias in isolated perfused heart: possible role of amiloride. *Mol Cell Biochem* 1993;119: 151–157.

473. Faes FC, Sawa Y, Ichikawa H, et al. Inhibition of Na⁺/H⁺ exchanger attenuates neutrophil-mediated reperfusion injury. *Ann Thorac Surg* 1995;60:377–381.

474. Shipolini AR, Galinanes M, Edmondson SJ, et al. Na⁺/H⁺ exchanger inhibitor HOE-642 improves cardioplegic myocardial preservation under both normothermic and hypothermic conditions. *Circulation* 1997;96:II-266–II-273.

475. Choy IO, Schepkin VD, Budinger TF, et al. Effects of specific sodium/hydrogen exchange inhibitor during cardioplegic arrest. *Ann Thorac Surg* 1997;64:94–99.

476. Myers ML, Karmazyn M. Improved cardiac function after prolonged hypothermic ischemia with the Na⁺/H⁺ exchange inhibitor HOE 694. *Ann Thorac Surg* 1996;61:1400–1406.

477. Murry CE, Jennings RB, Reimer KA. Preconditioning with ischemia: a delay of lethal cell injury in ischemic myocardium. *Circulation* 1986;74:1124–1136.

478. Bilinska M, Maczewski M, Beresewicz A. Donors of nitric oxide mimic effects of ischaemic preconditioning on reperfusion induced arrhythmias in isolated rat heart. *Mol Cell Biochem* 1996; 160/161:265–271.

479. Menasché P, Kevelaitis E, Mouas C, et al. Cardiopulmonary bypass, myocardial management, and support techniques. Preconditioning with potassium channel openers—a new concept for enhancing cardioplegic protection? *J Thorac Cardiovasc Surg* 1995;110:1606–1614.

480. Liu GS, Thornton J, Van Winkle DM, et al. Protection against infarction afforded by preconditioning is mediated by A₁ adenosine receptors in rabbit hearts. *Circulation* 1991;84:350–356.

481. Dana A, Baxter GF, Walker JM, et al. Prolonging the delayed phase of myocardial protection: repetitive adenosine A₁ receptor activation maintains rabbit myocardium in a preconditioned state. *J Am Coll Cardiol* 1998;31:1142–1149.

482. Tsuchida A, Thompson R, Olsson RA, et al. The anti-infarct effect of an adenosine A₁-selective agonist is diminished after prolonged infusion as is the cardioprotective effect of ischaemic preconditioning in rabbit heart. *J Mol Cell Cardiol* 1994;26: 303–311.

483. Cohen MV, Walsh RS, Goto M, et al. Hypoxia preconditions rabbit myocardium via adenosine and catecholamine release. *J Mol Cell Cardiol* 1995;27:1527–1534.

484. Liu Y, Downey JM. Ischemic preconditioning protects against infarction in rat heart. *Am J Physiol* 1992;263:H1107–H1112.

485. Schott RJ, Rohmann S, Braun ER, et al. Ischemic preconditioning reduces infarct size in swine myocardium. *Circ Res* 1990; 66:1133–1142.

486. DeFily DV, Chilian WM. Preconditioning protects coronary arteriolar endothelium from ischemia-reperfusion injury. *Am J Physiol* 1993;265:H700–H706.

487. Valen G, Takeshima S, Vaage J. Preconditioning improves cardiac function after global ischemia, but not after cold cardioplegia. *Ann Thorac Surg* 1996;62:1397–1403.

488. Kaukoranta PK, Lepojärvi MPK, Ylitalo KV, et al. Normothermic retrograde blood cardioplegia with or without preceding ischemic preconditioning. *Ann Thorac Surg* 1997;63: 1268–1274.

489. Juggi JS, Al-Awadi F, Joseph S, et al. Ischemic preconditioning is not additive to preservation with hypothermia or crystalloid cardioplegia in the globally ischemic rat heart. *Mol Cell Biochem* 1997;176:303–313.

490. Cleveland JC, Meldrum DR, Rowland RT, et al. Preconditioning and hypothermic cardioplegia protect human heart equally against ischemia. *Ann Thorac Surg* 1997;63:147–152.

491. Perrault LP, Menasche P, Bel A, et al. Cardiopulmonary bypass, myocardial management, and support techniques. *J Thorac Cardiovasc Surg* 1996;112:1378–1386.

492. Hearse DJ. The protection of the ischemic myocardium: surgical success vs. clinical failure? *Prog Cardiovasc Dis* 1988;30: 381–402.

CHANGES IN THE PHARMACOKINETICS AND PHARMACODYNAMICS OF DRUGS ADMINISTERED DURING CARDIOPULMONARY BYPASS

RICHARD I. HALL

Cardiac surgery using cardiopulmonary bypass (CPB) may profoundly affect how drugs are distributed and cleared by the body and how drugs interact with the body to produce their effects (1–4). Factors such as components of the CPB circuit (5–13), the use of hypothermia (14–23), pulsatile versus nonpulsatile flow (7,24,25), alterations in receptor density and function (26–29), and generation of the systemic inflammatory response syndrome (SIRS) (30–33) may alter drug disposition and the nature of drug actions during the conduct of cardiac surgery. This chapter reviews some basic concepts of pharmacokinetics and pharmacodynamics and then describes the role CPB may play in altering the pharmacokinetics and pharmacodynamics of drugs administered during cardiac surgery. A description of studies of pharmacokinetic and pharmacodynamic changes for individual classes of drugs is given. By understanding the effects of CPB on drug actions and elimination, it may be possible to explain apparent anomalies (e.g., continued intravenous anesthetic effect in the presence of hemodilution during CPB) (11,34–37) and to prevent adverse consequences (e.g., awareness under anesthesia due to insufficient drug administration) (38,39).

BASIC PRINCIPLES AND DEFINITION OF TERMS

To understand how CPB may alter drug effects, it is necessary to have an understanding of the basic principles of pharmacokinetics and pharmacodynamics.

R. I. Hall: Department of Anesthesiology, Pharmacology and Surgery, Dalhousie University, Queen Elizabeth II Health Sciences Centre, Halifax, Nova Scotia B3H 3A7, Canada.

Pharmacokinetics

Pharmacokinetics may be defined as the mathematical description of the processes by which a drug is handled once introduced into the body (i.e., what the body does to the drug). Because most drugs given during the conduct of cardiac surgery are given intravenously, this discussion focuses on a description of pharmacokinetic terms after intravenous administration.

After injection of a single intravenous dose of a drug (e.g., induction of the anesthetic state at the beginning of cardiac surgery), a number of processes are immediately initiated that reduce drug levels. Drug is delivered to and taken up by tissues within the body—a process known as *distribution*. Distribution occurs first to tissues that are highly perfused, such as the brain, heart, lungs, liver, and kidneys, where uptake by the tissue occurs. Tissue uptake is variable depending on protein binding and the lipid solubility of the drug. Thereafter, further uptake of drug occurs into tissues that are less well perfused, such as muscle and fat. Simultaneously, drug is delivered to organs, such as the liver, kidneys, and lungs, where *elimination* by biotransformation and excretion can occur. For most drugs used during cardiac surgery, this elimination occurs at a constant fraction of drug remaining in the body per unit of time, so-called first-order kinetics.

To provide a means of quantitating what happens to a drug once introduced into the body, various mathematical models have been developed. Figure 14.1 depicts a two-compartment model (40). After drug injection, distribution occurs within a central compartment (blood) and to peripheral compartments (tissues). Transfer of drug between the central and peripheral compartments can be described by appropriate rate constants (Fig. 14.1). Elimination occurs from the central compartment and can be described by the elimination rate constant. By measuring plasma concentrations over time from injection of the drug, it is possible to

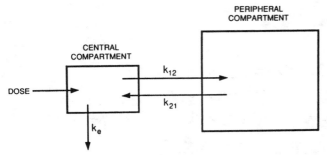

FIG. 14.1. Two-compartment pharmacokinetic model illustrating the distribution of a drug within a central compartment (blood) and peripheral compartment (tissues) and its ultimate biotransformation and elimination from the body. K_{12} and K_{21} are first-order rate constants for transfer of drug between the peripheral and central compartments, whereas K_e is the elimination rate constant. (From Hall RI, Thomas BL, Hug CC Jr. Pharmacokinetics and pharmacodynamics during cardiac surgery and cardiopulmonary bypass. In: Mora CT, ed. *Cardiopulmonary bypass. Principles and techniques of extracorporeal circulation.* New York: Springer-Verlag, 1995:56, with permission.)

describe the concentration versus time profile for the drug (Fig. 14.2) (40). Distribution and elimination phases can be determined, and a mathematical description of the change in concentration versus time can be developed. More sophisticated models can be developed [e.g., a model that characterizes distribution to *highly perfused* tissues and *less highly perfused tissues*, and the elimination phase (a three-compartment model)] and strategies exist to determine which mathematical model best describes the observed concentration versus time profile for any drug given (41). Derivation of the rate constants then allows the development of computer programs designed to produce continuous infusions of drugs at rates that produce a continuous stable targeted plasma concentration (42–44).

Characterization of concentration versus time profiles for intravenously administered drugs also allows the derivation of other pharmacokinetic parameters such as the volume of distribution, clearance, and elimination half-time.

Volume of Distribution

Volume of distribution (V_d) may be defined as that volume of fluid into which a drug would be administered to produce the observed concentration of drug in plasma. It does not correspond directly to any particular tissue compartment but rather is useful in predicting drug levels based on pharmacokinetic parameters. V_d is used to characterize the total volume of distribution, whereas V_c describes the volume of the central compartment, or the initial volume of distribution (also termed V_i). V_{ss} describes the volume of distribution when steady state plasma concentrations of drug are achieved.

Clearance

Clearance (*Cl*) refers to the removal of drug from the body, usually by way of the central compartment, and is expressed as volume of blood cleared of drug per unit of time.

Elimination Half-Time

Elimination half-time ($t_{1/2}\beta$) is the time required for the concentration of drug in plasma to decline by one half. It can be determined by examining the elimination portion of the concentration versus time curve or by substituting the relevant parameters in the equation

$$t_{1/2}\beta = \frac{0.693 \cdot V_d}{Cl}$$

Similarly, distribution half-times ($t_{1/2}p$, $t_{1/2}\alpha$) can also be determined by examining the distribution phase of the concentration versus time curve.

Drugs with short elimination half-times are characterized

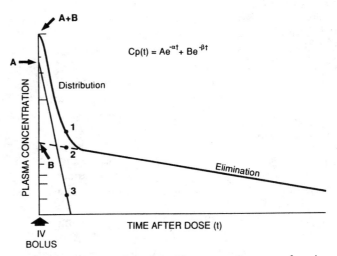

FIG. 14.2. Plasma [log] concentration versus time curve for a hypothetical drug after a single intravenous dose. The curve (*A + B*) is the sum of the contributions from the rapid distribution (*A*) phase and the slow elimination (*B*) phase to the logarithmic decline in concentration after a bolus dose. The concentration at any time is given by the equation $C_p(t) = A_e{}^{-dt} + B_e + B_t$, where $C_p(t)$ is the drug concentration in plasma at time *t*. A, constant determined from the *Y*-axis intercept (time = 0) of the distribution portion of the log concentration versus time curve, derived by subtracting the contribution of the (constant, first order) elimination phase of the curve; α, slope of the log concentration versus time curve of the distribution phase, derived by subtracting the contribution due to elimination; B, constant determined from the *Y*-axis intercept (time = 0) of the elimination phase of the log concentration versus time curve; β, slope of the log concentration versus time curve of the elimination phase. (From Hall RI, Thomas BL, Hug CC Jr. Pharmacokinetics and pharmacodynamics during cardiac surgery and cardiopulmonary bypass. In: Mora CT, ed. *Cardiopulmonary bypass. Principles and techniques of extracorporeal circulation.* New York: Springer-Verlag, 1995:56, with permission.)

by small volumes of distribution and/or rapid clearance. Drugs with a long elimination half-time tend to be highly lipid soluble (most anesthetic agents) with a large volume of distribution and/or slow rate of elimination.

The degree to which drug effect is terminated depends on the rapidity of drug redistribution to the central compartment once the injection stops and the capacity of elimination processes to clear the drug. Although important after injection of a single dose, this concept is also of importance when drugs are given by continuous infusion or in repeated doses. If drug administration is greater than the body's ability to clear it, drug accumulation will occur, leading to prolonged drug effect. At times, drug administration may completely saturate clearance mechanisms (e.g., excess alcohol ingestion), leading to a situation where clearance is no longer a function of drug level in the plasma (so-called zero-order kinetics). More commonly, as drug administration continues, there is accumulation of drug in tissues over time, which increases with the duration of drug infusion. At the time of termination of the infusion, offset of drug effect then represents redistribution of drug from tissues (greater with longer infusions) and the rate of elimination. Reliance on the elimination half-time to predict offset of drug effect will not adequately characterize the termination of drug effect under these circumstances. This has led to the introduction of the term *context-sensitive half-time* as a better description of the phenomenon of increased duration of drug effect with increased drug infusion time (Fig. 14.3) (45).

Computer-driven infusions of drugs apply the pharmacokinetic parameters previously derived from concentration versus time profiles to set their infusion rates. The accuracy of these infusions to provide the desired plasma concentrations therefore depends on the accuracy of the initial parameter estimates. Errors in these parameters can occur for a variety of reasons, including number of drug measurement points (too few), duration of the drug measurements (too short), sensitivity of the drug assay used (too low), and nature of the population studied (e.g., young healthy males versus elderly females in congestive heart failure). Other pitfalls in blood drug measurement include difficulties in measurement of the actual drug concentrations. Drug in the blood exists in several forms: free (active), bound to plasma proteins (e.g., albumin) and therefore subject to changes in plasma protein levels, and sequestered in red blood cells. CPB has the potential to alter all these factors, which makes description of pharmacokinetic parameters during CPB problematic.

Where infusions are administered at constant rates (so-called zero-order infusions), drug accumulation over time is likely. To prevent drug accumulation, it is suggested that adjustment of infusion rates according to patient response is the preferred method. This is likely to maintain the concentration in the lower therapeutic range and permit the optimum reduction in concentration once the infusion is terminated.

For drugs not administered directly into the vascular system, other variables will determine the blood concentration

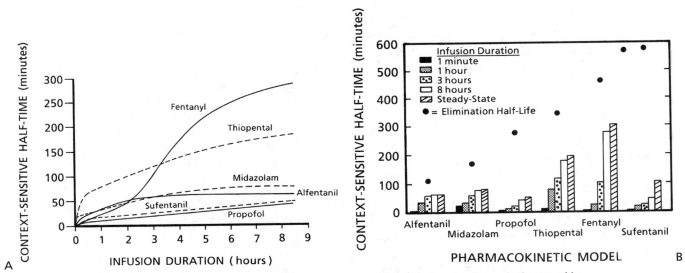

FIG. 14.3. **A:** Context-sensitive half-times as a function of infusion duration for each pharmacokinetic model simulated. *Solid and dashed lines* are used to permit overlapping lines to be distinguished. **B:** Context-sensitive half-times (*bars*) redrawn from **A** for each pharmacokinetic model after terminating a 1-minute, 1-hour, 3-hour, 8-hour, or infinitely long (i.e., to steady state) computer-designed infusion designed to instantaneously achieve and maintain a target concentration shown relative to the elimination half-life (*dots*) computed for each model. (From Hughes MA, Glass PSA, Jacobs JR. Context-sensitive half-time in multicompartment pharmacokinetic models for intravenous anesthetic drugs. *Anesthesiology* 1992;76:336, with permission.)

achieved, including the dose administered, blood flow to the site of administration, the proximity and permeability of the capillaries to the drug, the degree of tissue binding at the administration site, the local pH of the tissues, and the acid-base status of the drug.

Termination of drug effect is highly dependent on clearance mechanisms. For most drugs this involves some degree of liver metabolism and/or renal excretion. Lipophilic drugs are metabolized in the liver in two stages. Phase I reactions convert lipophilic drugs to more water-soluble compounds. This occurs through oxidation, reduction, or hydrolytic reactions. Oxidation-reduction reactions occur in the endoplasmic reticulum by mixed function oxidases (cytochrome P450) that exist in a number of isoforms with specificity for particular metabolic effects (46). These enzymes are under regulatory control by gene transcription, and their activity can be modified by drugs and disease processes (47–52). Phase II reactions couple the drug (or its metabolites) to an endogenous substrate such as sulphate, acetate, or glucuronide to form a highly polar water-soluble compound more easily excreted (53). A number of factors have been identified that may alter hepatic metabolism, including the presence of drugs that cause induction [e.g., rifampin (51)] or inhibition of cytochrome P450 enzymes [e.g., erythromycin (54), propofol (49), fluconazole (52)], and genetic predisposition [e.g., heterogeneity in the ability for some people to metabolize certain drugs (55)].

The ability of the liver to metabolize a drug in the absence of limitations imposed by hepatic blood flow or drug–protein binding is termed *intrinsic hepatic clearance*. The *hepatic extraction ratio* is the fraction of drug contained in hepatic arterial blood that is removed as it passes through the liver. For drugs with a high extraction ratio, a large percentage of the drug is removed per unit of time as it traverses the liver bed. These two concepts are related by the equation

$$Cl_{\text{hepatic}} = Q \cdot \frac{Cl_i}{(Q + Cl_i)} = \frac{Q \cdot (C_a - C_v)}{C_a} = Q \cdot E$$

where $Cl_{hepatic}$ is the hepatic clearance rate of a drug, Q is the liver blood flow, Cl_i is the intrinsic hepatic clearance, C_a is the arterial drug concentration, C_v is the venous drug concentration, and E is the hepatic extraction ratio.

Drugs with a low extraction ratio [e.g., diazepam (56)] depend on intrahepatic metabolism for their elimination and are much more affected by changes in protein binding and the liver's ability to metabolize drugs (e.g., induction or inhibition of cytochrome P450) than changes in liver blood flow. In contrast, metabolism of drugs with a moderate [e.g., alfentanil (57)] or a high extraction ratio [e.g., fentanyl (58) or papaverine (59)] may be critically affected by changes in liver blood flow.

For drugs cleared by the kidneys, excretion depends on renal blood flow, glomerular filtration rate, tubular secretion, and reabsorption. When excreted by filtration [e.g.,

mannitol (60)], the rate will depend on the plasma concentration and renal blood flow. Drugs excreted by tubular processes [tubular secretion and reabsorption, e.g., cefazolin (61)] are subject to possible saturation of active transport processes.

Pharmacodynamics

Pharmacodynamics describes how a drug interacts with the body to produce its effects. Most drugs produce these effects by interaction with a specific *receptor* (i.e., that macromolecular component of the organism with which the chemical interacts (Fig. 14.4) (62). Activation of the receptor leads to changes intracellularly, often through activation of secondary messengers, which leads to changes in cell function (e.g., muscle contraction). The most numerous type of receptor is protein, although other types exist (e.g., nucleic acids). Among protein receptors, those that serve as endogenous regulatory ligands are particularly important because drugs that interact with these receptors will produce physiologic effects similar to that which occurs in nature when an endogenous ligand stimulates the receptor (63–66). Such agents are referred to as *agonists*. Drugs that bind to the receptor but do not mimic but rather interfere with the binding of the endogenous ligand and possess no intrinsic regulatory activity of their own are termed *antagonists*.

Whether a drug acts as an agonist or antagonist depends on its structure, and this is exploited in drug design. The degree to which a compound is capable of mimicking the effect of the endogenous ligand is also a function of the number and affinity of the receptor(s) for the drug and the concentration of drug.

Receptors

Physiologic receptors serve two functions: they bind to the appropriate ligand and then the activated receptor propagates the regulatory signal to the target cell. This has led to the functional localization of two regions within the receptor—a *ligand-binding domain* and an *effector domain*.

Receptor regulatory actions may be produced by action directly on its cellular target(s), *effector proteins*, or may be conveyed to other cellular targets by intermediary cellular molecules termed *transducers* (Fig. 14.4) (62). The combination of the receptor, its target proteins, and the intermediary molecules is termed the *signal transduction pathway*. Effector proteins may not be the final cellular component affected by receptor stimulation. In some cases, the effector protein may cause synthesis or release of another signaling molecule known as a *second messenger* (Fig. 14.5) (62).

A number of families of receptors have been characterized. Receptors for peptide hormones that regulate growth, differentiation, and development take the form of membrane-bound protein kinases, which act by phosphorylating target proteins. Receptors for neurotransmitters are fre-

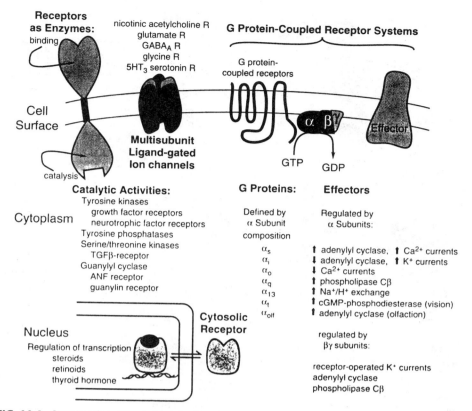

FIG. 14.4. Structural motifs of physiologic receptors and their relationships to signaling pathways. Schematic diagram of the diversity of mechanisms for control of cell function by receptors for endogenous agents acting via the cell surface or in the nucleus. (From Ross EM. Pharmacodynamics. Mechanisms of drug action and the relationship between drug concentration and effect. In: Hardman JG, Limbird LE, eds. *Goodman and Gilman's the pharmacological basis of therapeutics*, 9th ed. Montreal: McGraw-Hill, 1996:32, with permission.)

quently in the form of an agonist-regulated ion-selective channel in the plasma membrane termed *ligand-gated ion channel* (67). Stimulation of the receptor leads to alteration in the cell's membrane potential or ionic composition. Receptors in this group include nicotinic cholinergic receptors (site of skeletal muscle relaxant activity), and the GABA$_A$ receptor (benzodiazepines, propofol, barbiturates).

Many receptors take the form of *G protein-coupled receptors* (68). These receptors facilitate binding of GTP to specific G proteins causing their activation and consequent regulation of specific effectors, including enzymes such as adenyl cyclase; phospholipases A$_2$, C$_1$, and D; channels specific for Na$^+$, K$^+$, and Ca^{2+} conductance; and certain transport proteins. The G protein receptor has been well characterized and consists of seven α-helical segments spanning the plasma membrane (Fig. 14.6) (68). Ligand binding occurs at the cytoplasmic membrane and causes changes in G protein-coupled receptor polypeptides on the inner surface of the plasma membrane. These are heterotrimeric molecules designated as α, β, and δ. When receptor activation occurs, GTP binds to these subunits, resulting in disassocia-

tion of the α subunit from the $\beta\delta$ unit, and interaction with the membrane-bound effector occurs (Fig. 14.7) (68). The $\beta\delta$ subunit may also interact with and influence effector activity. Termination of signal transmission results from hydrolysis of GTP to GDP by a GTPase intrinsic to the α subunit with subsequent reassociation of α and $\beta\delta$ subunits. Several receptors in a cell may activate a single G protein and a single receptor may activate more than one G protein (Table 14.1) (68).

Soluble DNA binding proteins that regulate transcription of specific genes serve as the receptor for steroid hormones, thyroid hormone, vitamin D, and the retinoids. They are part of a larger family of transcription factors regulated by phosphorylation, association with other protein factors, or by binding to metabolites or cellular regulatory ligands. The receptor is composed of three domains: a hormone binding region near the carboxyl terminus; a central region that interacts with the nuclear DNA to activate or inhibit gene transcription, for glucocorticosteroids the so-called glucocorticoid-responsive element; and an amino-terminal region whose function is not well defined (69).

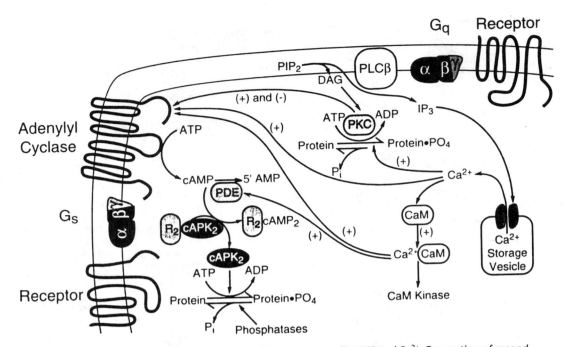

FIG. 14.5. Interactions between the second messengers cyclic AMP and Ca^{2+}. Generation of second messengers cyclic AMP (cAMP) and Ca^{2+} permits distribution of cell-surface regulatory input within the cell interior, amplification of the initial signal, and opportunities for synergistic or antagonistic regulation of other signaling pathways. *PIP$_2$*, phosphatidyl inositol-4,5 biophosphate; *DAG*, diacylglycerol; *IP$_3$*, 1,4,5-inositol triphosphate; *CaM*, calmodulin; *R$_2$*, regulatory subunits of cyclic AMP-dependent protein kinase, which bind cyclic AMP; *cAPK$_2$*, catalytic subunits of cyclic AMP-dependent protein kinase; *PKC*, protein kinase C, activated by DAG and Ca^{2+}. (From Ross EM. Pharmacodynamics. Mechanisms of drug action and the relationship between drug concentration and effect. In: Hardman JG, Limbird LE, eds. *Goodman and Gilman's the pharmacological basis of therapeutics*, 9th ed. Montreal: McGraw-Hill, 1996:34, with permission.)

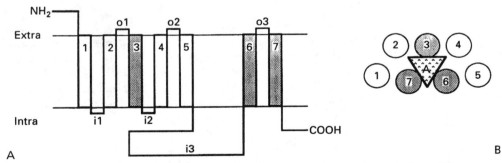

FIG. 14.6. Muscarinic receptor structure. **A:** The muscarinic receptor is a member of the seven transmembrane (*TMI-7*) spanning G protein-coupled receptors. The receptor has three intracellular (*i1–i3*) and three extracellular (*o1–o3*) loops. *i3*, site of G protein (α subunit) coupling. **B:** Helical wheel transformation of the receptor shows transmembrane domains 3, 6, and 7 forming the agonist (*A*) binding pocket. (From Lambert DG. Signal transduction: G proteins and second messengers. *Br J Anaesth* 1993;71:87, with permission.)

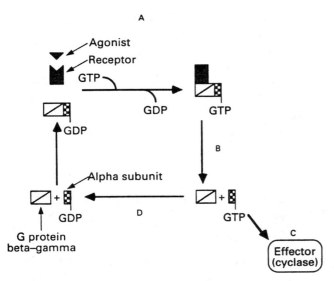

FIG. 14.7. Schematic representation of the G protein cycle. From top left, clockwise: agonist binding to its receptor promotes GDP from GTP exchange (*A*), G protein dissociation (*B*) allows the α-GTP subunit to activate the effector enzyme (*C*), an intrinsic GTPase converts GTP back to GDP (*D*), and the cycle is complete. (From Lambert DG. Signal transduction: G proteins and second messengers. *Br J Anaesth* 1993;71:88, with permission.)

Receptors are subject to regulatory and homeostatic controls. As an example, continuous stimulation of a receptor by an agonist may result in a reduced effect due to a process known as *desensitization*, where the number of cell surface receptors is reduced over time due to phosphorylation of the receptor, destruction of the receptor, or relocalization of the receptor within the cell (66).

TABLE 14.1. EXAMPLES OF G PROTEIN-COUPLED RECEPTORS AND THE INTRACELLULAR SECOND MESSENGERS THEY GENERATE

Receptor	Second Messenger
Adrenoceptors	
Alpha$_{1A/1B/1C}$	IP3 +
Alpha$_{2A/2B/2C}$	cAMP −
Beta$_{1/2/3}$	cAMP +
Bradykinin (B$_{1-3}$)	IP3 +
Calcitonin gene-related peptide	cAMP +
Dopamine (D$_{1-5}$)	IP3 +/cAMP −
Glutamate (metabotrophic)	IP3 +
Histamine	cAMP +/IP3 +
5-HT ($_{1A-1D/2/3/4}$)	cAMP −/cAMP +/IP3 +
Muscarinic (M1−5)	IP3 +/cAMP −
Opioid ($\mu/\delta/\kappa$)	cAMP −
Vasopressin (V$_{1A,1B/2}$)	IP3 +/cAMP +

cAMP +, Receptor stimulates generation of cAMP; cAMP −, receptor inhibits generation of cAMP; IP3$^+$, receptor stimulates generation of inositol (1,4,5) triphosphate (IP3).
Source: Lambert DG. Signal transduction: G protein and second messengers. *Br J Anaeth* 1993;71:86–95, with permission.

Receptor synthesis is subject to feedback regulation. In the presence of an antagonist, the number of cell surface receptors may increase. Traditionally, receptors have been classified by their physiologic effects and relative potencies. Examples include muscarinic versus nicotinic receptors in the cholinergic system and α and β receptors in the adrenergic system. Subtypes of receptors exist (e.g., α_1, α_2) and are targets for drug-selective effects. Molecular cloning techniques have allowed tissue-specific receptor subtypes to be identified and localized (63,66).

Second Messenger Systems

These systems are relatively few in number. However, their synthesis and release reflects the activity of many pathways, and each may influence the other directly by altering the other messenger's metabolism or indirectly by sharing intracellular targets (Fig. 14.5) (62).

Cyclic AMP is synthesized by adenyl cyclase in response to receptor activation. Stimulation is mediated by G_s and inhibition by G_i proteins. There are currently at least 10 tissue-specific adenyl cyclase isozymes. These isozymes may be inhibited by the G protein $\beta\delta$ subunits, stimulated by the G$\beta\delta$ subunit in the presence of stimulation by the α subunit of G_s, or may be stimulated by Ca^{2+} or Ca^{2+}–calmodulin complexes. The isozyme activity may be enhanced or attenuated by phosphorylation (Fig. 14.8) (68).

Termination of cyclic AMP activity is by hydrolysis, a process catalyzed by several phosphodiesterases. Cyclic AMP may also be extruded from the cell via a regulated active transport mechanism. Among other activities, cyclic AMP functions to activate cyclic AMP-dependent protein kinases that serve to regulate a number of intracellular proteins by catalyzing their phosphorylation.

Intracellular Ca^{2+} serves as another second messenger (70), and its intracellular concentration is controlled by regulation of several different Ca^{2+}-specific channels in the plasma membrane and by its release from intracellular storage sites (68,70). Ca^{2+}-dependent ion channels are opened by electrical depolarization, by phosphorylation by a cyclic AMP-dependent protein kinase, by G_s, by K$^+$, or by Ca^{2+} itself (70). Opening of the channel may be inhibited by other G proteins (e.g., G_i).

Release of Ca^{2+} from intracellular stores is mediated by the second messenger inositol 1,4,5-triphosphate, which is formed by hydrolysis of the membrane lipid phosphatidylinositol 4,5-bisphosphate catalyzed by phospholipase C (PLC) (Fig. 14.9) (68). Three families of PLCs exist, each with its own distinct signaling pathway: PLC-β by G proteins, PLC-γ by phosphorylation on tyrosine residues activated through the cell surface receptor-activated tyrosine kinase pathway, and PLC-δ by an unknown pathway.

Ca^{2+} regulates intracellular activity by interaction with several proteins, including protein kinase C and calmodulin.

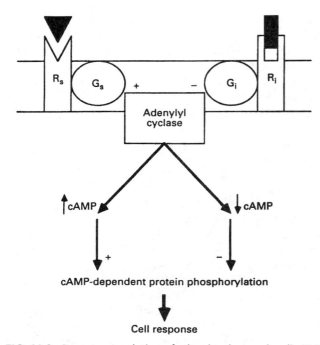

FIG. 14.8. Receptor regulation of adenyl cyclase and cyclic AMP formation. Membrane bound adenyl cyclase is activated to increase cyclic AMP via stimulatory receptors (R_s) acting through G_s (e.g., β-adrenergic receptor) or inhibited via inhibitory receptors (R_i) through G_i (e.g., opioids). Altered concentrations of cyclic AMP alter protein phosphorylation and cellular responses. (From Lambert DG. Signal transduction: G proteins and second messengers. *Br J Anaesth* 1993;71:88, with permission.)

Activation of protein kinase C by Ca^{2+} is potentiated by diacylglycerol, another second messenger released by the PLC-catalyzed reaction that liberates inositol 1,4,5-triphosphate (Fig. 14.9) (68).

The complexity of the second messenger system is obvious, and the interactions among its members are being unravelled. The internal milieu is tightly controlled by these interactions and subject to perturbation by drugs at any of the steps outlined above.

CHANGES DUE TO CARDIOPULMONARY BYPASS

Pharmacokinetics

In theory, CPB may affect the pharmacokinetics of drugs in a variety of ways, including changes due to hemodilution, hypothermia, altered organ perfusion, acid-base status, drug sequestration into lungs and the CPB circuit, and altered metabolism and clearance due to activation of SIRS.

Hemodilution

The CPB apparatus is primed with fluid, usually some combination of crystalloid $\pm$ colloid. At the time of initiation of CPB, the addition of this fluid to the circulation has several immediate effects:

1. An immediate reduction in levels of circulating proteins such as albumin and α_1-acid glycoprotein. This has implications for protein binding of drugs due to alteration

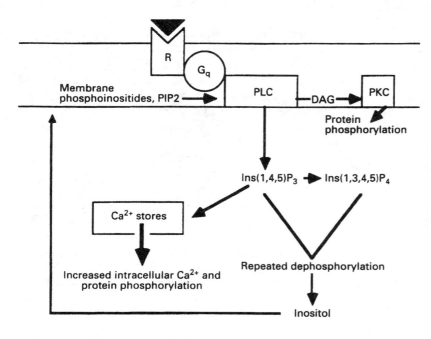

FIG. 14.9. Receptor regulation of phospholipase C activity and inositol 1,4,5-triphosphate [*Ins(1,4,5)P_3*] generation. Membrane bound phospholipase C is activated by G_q linked receptors (e.g., muscarinic M1, M3, M5) to increase phosphatidyl inositol-4,5 biophosphate hydrolysis and yield two biologically active second messengers: water-soluble Ins(1,4,5)P_3 and lipid-soluble diacylglycerol (*DAG*). The latter activates protein kinase C (*PKC*) and the former releases Ca^{2+} from an intracellular store. Ins(1,4,5)P_3 produced by receptor stimulation is either phosphorylated to Ins(1,3,4,5)P_4 (which may have some biologic activity) or dephosphorylated to inositol. Increased Ca^{2+} and PKC activity cause increased protein phosphorylation and alter cellular responsiveness. (From Lambert DG. Signal transduction: G proteins and second messengers. *Br J Anaesth* 1993;71:90, with permission.)

in the ratio of bound-to-free drug in the circulation (35–37,71–76).

2. An immediate reduction in red blood cell concentration, which has implications for compounds that are sequestered to a significant degree in red blood cells (11,77,78).

3. An immediate reduction in the amount of free drug in the circulation at the initiation of CPB. This will reduce the amount of drug available for interaction with the receptor with the potential for adverse events (e.g., lightening of the level of anesthesia) (35–37,79).

A number of studies have been carried out to examine these issues and to determine their relative importance to clinical practice (35–37,71–75). Typical findings of these studies are a reduction in total drug concentration in plasma with little change in free drug concentration over time while on CPB [Fig. 14.10 (36)] other than a transient (less than 5-min) reduction at initiation of CPB due to hemodilution. It would appear that the greatest risk for unwanted lightening of anesthesia is within this timeframe, and it might be prudent to supplement the anesthetic at this time (Fig. 14.11) (11). The explanation for why free drug levels are sustained during CPB is a pharmacokinetic one. The volume of distribution for most anesthetic agents is large relative to the volume of the CPB prime and serves as a huge reservoir for drug after intravenous administration. When plasma concentrations fall due to hemodilution, drug moves down its concentration gradient from tissue stores to plasma to rapidly reestablish the equilibrium.

Hypothermia

CPB is frequently conducted under hypothermic conditions. Hypothermia may alter drug pharmacokinetics in several ways. Hypothermia depresses metabolism by inhibiting enzyme function and reduces tissue perfusion by increasing blood viscosity and activation of autonomic and endocrine reflexes to produce vasoconstriction. As a consequence, pharmacokinetics may be altered through the following mechanisms:

1. Decreased absorption of drugs administered other than by the intravenous route (80);

2. Reduction in drug distribution from central to peripheral compartments (i.e., reduced volume of distribution, V_d) (18,19);

3. Altered central nervous system (CNS) drug penetration (80);

4. Reduction in rate of reuptake of drug from peripheral tissues to the central compartment and subsequent reductions in hepatic clearance leading to prolonged elimination half-time (18,81–84);

5. Reduced biotransformation rate with decreased clearance and increased elimination half-time (Fig. 14.12) (18,23,84–88);

6. Altered renal drug excretion as a result of decreased renal perfusion, decreased glomerular filtration rate, and decreased tubular secretion (82).

Hypothermic CPB would be expected to significantly alter the clearance of drugs with a low extraction ratio such as diazepam (56). When normothermia is reestablished, reperfusion of tissues might lead to washout of drug sequestered during the hypothermic CPB period. This may be a reason for the observation of secondary increases in opioid plasma levels during the rewarming phase (89–91).

For drugs with a low V_d, the vasoconstriction produced by hypothermia may further decrease the V_d. This may be one explanation for the increase in plasma levels of neuromuscular relaxants observed during hypothermic CPB (92–94).

Perfusion

CPB may be conducted with or without pulsatile perfusion. Nonpulsatile perfusion is associated with altered tissue perfusion (25). However, no difference in thiopental levels was detected when pulsatile versus nonpulsatile flow was studied (7). In contrast, cefamandole tissue levels were higher and elimination half-time prolonged in patients having pulsatile perfusion versus nonpulsatile perfusion (24). The degree to which pulsatile perfusion alters drug pharmacokinetics is thus variable and requires further study.

Perfusion to tissues may also be altered as a consequence of activation of the stress response during CPB (32). As a consequence of the activation of the systemic inflammatory response, a variety of autonomic, endocrine, and local cytokine reflexes are initiated that may affect not only tissue distribution of drugs but probably clearance mechanisms as well (32).

Acid-Base Status

CPB may be conducted using pH stat or alpha stat blood gas management. The change in pH with either management scheme may affect organ blood flow [e.g., increased cerebral blood flow with pH stat (95) and thus drug distribution (95,96)]. pH management may affect the degree of ionization and protein binding of certain drugs, leading to either increased or decreased free (active) drug concentrations (Fig. 14.13) (96–98).

Sequestration

During CPB, the lungs are out of circuit. Drugs, which are taken up by the lungs [e.g., opioids (90,99–102)] are therefore sequestered during CPB, and the lungs may serve as a reservoir for drug release when systemic reperfusion is established (Fig. 14.14) (90). This effect is, however, quite transient (90,101,102).

The red blood cell may serve as a reservoir for drugs,

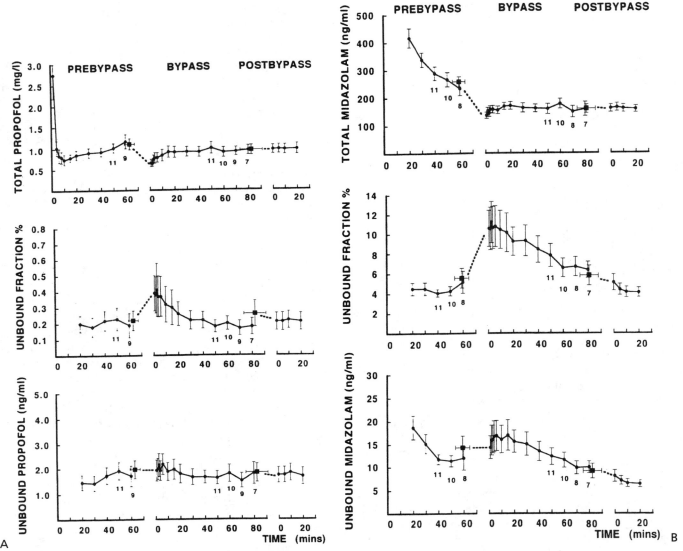

FIG. 14.10. **A:** Total plasma concentration, unbound fraction, and unbound plasma concentration for propofol as a function of time for pre-bypass, bypass, and post-bypass periods. Each data point represents $n = 12$ (mean $\pm$ SEM). Numbers adjacent to data points indicate n, where n is less than 12. The square data point to the left of $t = 0$ of the bypass time period in each graph represents the mean of the final pre-bypass samples (mean $\pm$ SEM) plotted at the time (mean $\pm$ SEM) at which they occurred. The square data point to the left of the $t = 0$ of the post-bypass time period in each graph represents the mean of the final bypass samples (mean $\pm$ SEM) plotted at the time (mean $\pm$ SEM) at which they occurred. Total plasma concentrations fall at initiation of CPB with little change in free drug concentrations leading to an increase in free fraction. **B:** Total plasma concentration, unbound fraction, and unbound plasma concentration for midazolam as a function of time for pre-bypass, bypass, and post-bypass periods. Each data point represents $n = 12$ (mean $\pm$ SEM). Numbers adjacent to data points indicate n, where n is less than 12. The square data point to the left of the $E = 0$ of the bypass time period in each graph represents the mean of the final pre-bypass samples (mean $\pm$ SEM) plotted at the time (mean $\pm$ SEM) at which they occurred. The square data point to the left of $t = 0$ of the post-bypass time period in each graph represents the mean of the final bypass samples (mean $\pm$ SEM) plotted at the time (mean $\pm$ SEM) at which they occurred. Total plasma concentrations fall at initiation of CPB with little change in free drug concentrations leading to an increase in free fraction. (From Dawson PJ, Bjorksten AR, Blake DW, et al. The effects of cardiopulmonary bypass on total and unbound plasma concentrations of propofol and midazolam. *J Cardiothorac Vasc Anesth* 1997;11:559, with permission.)

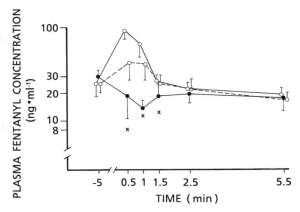

FIG. 14.11. Plasma fentanyl concentrations (mean ± SD) in patients connected to cardiopulmonary bypass (CPB) circuits with primes containing no fentanyl (●—●) or containing a calculated fentanyl concentration of 140 (○- - -○) or 280 (○—○) ng/ml. *X*, lowest drug concentration measured at each stage during the first 1.5 min of CPB in patients not receiving fentanyl in their prime. N.B.: Regardless of whether the prime is or is not supplemented, no difference exists in fentanyl concentrations within 2.5 minutes. (From Hynynen M. Binding of fentanyl and alfentanil to the extracorporeal circuit. *Acta Anaesth Scand* 1987;31:708, with permission.)

and the anemia associated with CPB may alter drug levels (11). The degree to which this is important clinically is uncertain.

Drugs may be taken up by various components of the CPB circuit itself. In vitro, various oxygenators bind lipophilic agents such as volatile anesthetic agents, propofol, opioids, barbiturates, and nitroglycerin (5–13,96, 103–105). This phenomenon has, however, never been demonstrated to be important in vivo, likely because any drug removed by the circuit is replaced from the much larger

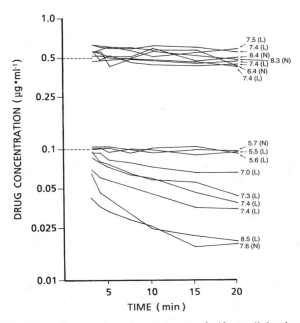

FIG. 14.13. Changes in concentrations of alfentanil (**top**) and fentanyl (**bottom**) in extracorporeal circuit prime with time (shown on the same logarithmic scale—vertical axis). *Dotted lines* represent predicted concentrations. Numbers on the right side are pH values of each priming solution: (*L*) = low temperature (24.4 to 25.70°C); (*N*) = normothermic (34.1 to 37.0°C). N.B.: The differences in binding to the cardiopulmonary bypass apparatus occurring as a result of dissimilarities in the ionization of the two drugs with changes in pH. (From Skacel M, Knott C, Reynolds F, et al. Extracorporeal circuit sequestration of fentanyl and alfentanil. *Br J Anaesth* 1986;58:948, with permission.)

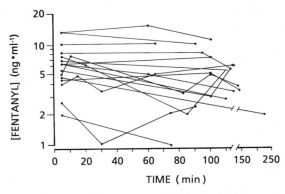

FIG. 14.12. Fentanyl plasma concentrations in 18 children during profound hypothermia (18 to 25°C). Time zero is the initiation of cardiopulmonary bypass. Total plasma fentanyl levels remain essentially unchanged. (From Koren G, Barker C, Goresky G, et al. The influence of hypothermia on the disposition of fentanyl—human and animal studies. *Eur J Clin Pharmacol* 1987;32:374, with permission.)

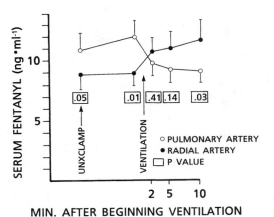

FIG. 14.14. Mean fentanyl levels in seven cardiac surgery patients as ventilation and perfusion to the lung are resumed near the end of cardiopulmonary bypass. Systemic fentanyl concentrations rise with ventilation, whereas levels in the pulmonary artery fall, suggesting washout of fentanyl sequestered in the lungs during CPB. *Unxclamp*, removal of aortic cross-clamp. (Bently JB, Canahan TJ III, Cork RC. Fentanyl sequestration in lungs during cardiopulmonary bypass. *Clin Pharmacol Ther* 1983;34:705, with permission.)

tissue reservoir (7,11,13,103). In general, sequestration likely plays a minor role in altering drug levels during CPB.

Pharmacodynamics

Changes in drug effect occurring as a result of CPB are only beginning to be explored. The ability of a drug to produce its effect is contingent on the ability of free (unbound) drug to reach its receptor and activate the receptor to transduce the signal. A number of factors may affect the ability of the drug to reach and interact with its receptor during cardiac surgery and CPB.

Protein Binding

In the blood, drugs exist as free (unbound) drug in equilibrium with bound (i.e., bound to plasma proteins) drug. It is the free drug concentration that interacts with the receptor to produce drug effect. Drugs are bound primarily to the plasma proteins albumin (acid drugs) and α_1-acid glycoprotein (basic drugs, e.g., fentanyl, lidocaine), an acute phase reactant. The concentration of α_1-acid glycoprotein is elevated during stress (32,97,98,106) and has been demonstrated to reduce lidocaine (107) and quinidine (75) free drug concentration after CPB with return of dysrhythmias despite adequate measured total drug levels.

Changes in protein binding are of clinical significance only for drugs that are highly protein bound. The degree of drug–protein binding depends on the total drug concentration, the available protein concentration, the affinity of the protein for the drug, and the presence of other substances that may compete with the drug or alter the drug-binding site (108). Measurement of total drug concentrations in plasma (free and bound) during CPB may thus fail to elucidate the true picture of changes in drug effect unless measurement of unbound concentration is also reported (Fig. 14.10) (36).

The degree of protein binding may be altered by pathologic states in existence before CPB [e.g., acute myocardial infarction (109)] or as a result of changes occurring during CPB [e.g., the development of SIRS (32)]. Renal failure and liver disease reduce plasma albumin levels (important for binding of acidic drugs) (110). The affinity of albumin for drugs such as phenytoin and thiopental may be reduced in the presence of chronic disease states (98,110). In contrast, α_1-acid glycoprotein levels are increased in chronic diseases or after acute myocardial infarction and are increased as part of SIRS developing during CPB (32,75,107,109,111). To prevent clot formation during CPB, heparin is administered. Heparin administration causes release of free fatty acids that may displace drugs from protein binding sites and increase free drug levels with resultant enhanced pharmacologic effect (76,112,113).

Tissue Binding

After drug administration, free drug penetrates into tissues where it may be bound to tissue proteins. Certain tissues (e.g., heart and lung) may have an affinity for certain drugs (42,90,99–102,114). This has two consequences of pharmacodynamic relevance. Tissue binding may limit access of drug to its receptor if located outside the bound tissue, thus potentially limiting the magnitude of effect (102), and the tissue may serve as a reservoir, thus extending drug effect, particularly if out of circuit during CPB (Fig. 14.14) (90). Changes in plasma free drug concentrations occurring as a result of protein binding (e.g., hemodilution during CPB) are buffered by redistribution of drug from tissue stores to plasma (11,13,36,37).

Age

Most adult cardiac surgical patients are elderly. Independent of pathologic processes, aging is associated with a variety of physiologic processes that may influence drug effect. The function of organs such as the heart and blood flow to the kidneys and liver are reduced (115). This has implications for the ability of the elderly to clear drugs (116). Elderly humans have increased amounts of adipose tissue, which may serve as binding sites for lipid-soluble drugs. Albumin levels may be reduced with higher free drug concentrations when standard doses are administered (116).

CNS sensitivity to drugs in the elderly has been investigated. CNS sensitivity to barbiturates may be unaltered in the elderly (117), but reductions in dose are required due to a slower return of drug from the effect site to the central compartment (a pharmacokinetic difference) (118,119). In contrast, a true difference in CNS sensitivity to opioids [fentanyl, alfentanil, and remifentanil (120–122)] and to volatile agents (123) has been described in the elderly.

For the elderly undergoing CPB, a reduction in dose to limit high levels of free drug concentrations and the potential for prolonged or toxic drug effects would seem prudent.

At the other end of the age spectrum, infants and children may have altered drug effects due to differences in distribution of body fat, immaturity of clearance mechanisms, and disease-related changes in drug handling (124–133). The degree to which they may have differences in drug sensitivity has received little scientific scrutiny.

Central Nervous System Penetration

For anesthetic agents, the site of drug effect is presumed to be the CNS. Differences in CNS pharmacodynamic effects between drugs have been measured using the time difference between peak plasma levels of drugs and their effect on the CNS reflected by changes in the electroencephalogram (134). A hysteresis has been observed between the peak plasma concentration of fentanyl versus alfentanil and the shift in the spectral edge frequency of the electroencephalogram (135). A similar time lag has been observed as drug concentrations fall and differences between drugs have been detected. Most likely this represents disposition of the more lipophilic fentanyl to highly lipophilic brain tissue preventing fentanyl concentrations from rising at the opioid receptor level and prolonging time to peak effect (i.e., a pharmacokinetic difference). This hypothesis is substantiated by the finding that the hysteresis for sufentanil (another lipophilic opioid) more closely approximates that of fentanyl than the more hydrophilic alfentanil (136). A similar rationale has been used to describe differences in onset of action between midazolam and diazepam (134,137). Use of these time differences and concentrations can be measured and modeled and has led to the development of computer programs designed to target drug concentrations at the effect site (receptor level) (138). Such programs have been used in studies of drug administration to target concentrations during cardiac surgery (128).

Temperature

Hypothermia may have a number of pharmacodynamic effects. Anesthetic requirements are reduced by hypothermia (14,139). Changes in receptor affinity [(e.g., decreased opioid receptor affinity (140) and nicotinic acetycholine receptor sensitivity (141)] occur under hypothermic conditions. Changes in the action of neuromuscular receptor blocking agents (usually enhanced with hypothermia) have been observed during CPB and may reflect both a pharmacodynamic and a pharmacokinetic effect (15,16,20–22, 94,142–144).

Use of hypothermia may attenuate release of the excitatory neurotransmitters glutamate and glycine (145), thus exerting a cerebroprotective effect. The implications of such an effect on drug action are unknown but potentially important (146) because presumably a reduction in brain injury would lead to preservation of anesthetic effect.

Acid-Base Changes

Altered tissue blood flow produces tissue acidosis during CPB (147,148). This may affect the response to catecholamines (149). The degree of ionization and protein binding (hence free drug levels) of weak acids and bases may also be affected by the blood gas management strategy used during CPB (Fig. 14.13) (96). Changes in pH may also affect electrolyte balance. Calcium, magnesium, and potassium levels decline during CPB (150–152), and associated muscle weakness, dysrhythmias, and enhanced digitalis toxicity may ensue.

Anesthetic Agents

Volatile anesthetic agents are commonly used during CPB, usually in combination with intravenous anesthetic agents

to avoid adverse hemodynamic aberrations (153–155). Volatile agents may disrupt ion channels and intracellular transduction mechanisms (156–159). The anesthetic requirements for volatile agents are reduced after CPB in dogs (160) by an as yet unidentified mechanism (146,161), although the nature of the priming solution (acetate) may prove to be important in this regard by acting as a supplemental anesthetic agent (161).

Receptor Density

The number of receptors available for interaction with a ligand will determine subsequent magnitude of drug effect. Patients presenting for cardiac surgery frequently have an element of congestive heart failure. A reduction in the number of cardiac β-receptors under these circumstances has been observed, and defects in receptor transduction, and impairment of synthesis and reuptake of norepinephrine occur (162,163). Administration of β-adrenergic agonists in this condition has been associated with further reductions in β-receptor numbers with diminished pharmacologic effect (164,165).

Removal of β-adrenergic blockade in patients treated for angina pectoris may lead to β-adrenergic receptor upregulation and increased adrenergic responsiveness (166,167). Increases in myocardial oxygen demand due to increased heart rate and contractility may lead to worsened symptomatology, and deaths are reported (168). It is generally recommended, with only rare exception, that chronic medications, including β-adrenoceptor receptor blocking agents, are continued until surgery commences (166).

Changes in receptor density and function may occur very quickly and have been observed to occur during cardiac surgery (26–29). Further work is required to elucidate the mechanisms and clinical implications of these acute changes in receptor density and function.

SYSTEMIC INFLAMMATORY RESPONSE SYNDROME

CPB and cardiac surgery initiate a systemic inflammatory response as a consequence of blood contact with a foreign surface and complement activation, development of ischemia and reperfusion injury, and the presence of endotoxin (Fig. 14.15) (32,33,169). The magnitude of the response is influenced by the use of pharmacologic agents and mechanical therapies designed to ameliorate the response, including (32) composition of the priming solution (170,171), presence of pulsatile perfusion (172,173), use of mechanical filtration (174–179), type of oxygenator (172,174,180–189), type of extracorporeal circuit (190–198), and temperature during CPB (199–203) or by the avoidance of the use of CPB altogether (204). As part of the response, cytokines are released, including tumor ne-

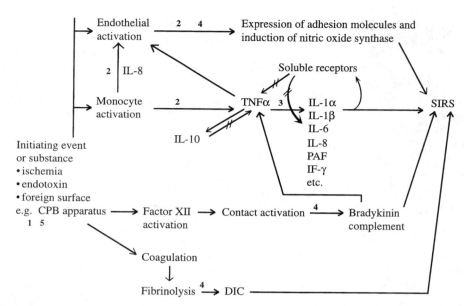

FIG. 14.15. Pathways leading to activation of the systemic inflammatory response syndrome (*SIRS*) and sites of therapeutic intervention. Therapeutic interventions: *1*, mechanical factors; *2*, glucocorticoids; *3*, pentoxyphylline; *4*, protease inhibitors; *5*, gut therapy. *TNF-α*, tumor necrosis factor-alpha; *IL*, interleukin; *CPB*, cardiopulmonary bypass; *DIC*, disseminated intravascular coagulation. (From Hall RI, Stafford Smith M, Rocker G. The systemic inflammatory response to cardiopulmonary bypass: pathophysiological, therapeutic, and pharmacological considerations. *Anesth Analg* 1997;85:767, with permission.)

crosis factor-alpha (TNF-α), interleukin (IL)-1, IL-6, IL-2, IL-8, IL-10, and nitric oxide (32). Each cytokine subserves a number of functions, but those of relevance to this discussion include the production of acute phase proteins by TNF-α (205), IL-1 (206), and IL-6 (207), which may reduce free drug levels, and myocardial depression by IL-6 (208–210) and nitric oxide (209), which may alter distribution of drugs. Activation of neutrophils with generation of oxygen-derived free radicals may injure tissue, particularly endothelium, leading to a capillary leak syndrome, which may affect volume of distribution for drugs and penetration to receptors (184,211–216). Reductions in liver blood flow may reduce clearance of drugs with a high hepatic extraction ratio (e.g., fentanyl) (23,147,217–219). Cytokines may inhibit reticuloendothelial function (220) and thus impair drug metabolism. TNF-α, IL-1β, and IL-6 are endogenous pyrogens (206,221) that may produce an anesthetic-sparing effect (222). It can be seen that the impact of the systemic inflammatory response during CPB could have a significant impact on drug pharmacokinetics and pharmacodynamics. Strategies designed to ameliorate the systemic inflammatory response require further investigation (32,33).

SPECIFIC DRUGS

The actual influence of the factors outlined above on the pharmacokinetics and pharmacodynamics of drugs admin-

istered during hypothermia and CPB have been investigated for a number of agents. An overview of the results of some of these investigations is provided below and in Table 14.2. However, caution should be exercised in the interpretation and comparison of the reported results because they may be influenced by a variety of factors, such as the coadministration of other agents (e.g., vasoconstrictors and vasodilators that might alter the volume of distribution and clearance), differences in anesthetic technique (changes in cardiac output and tissue distribution), type of oxygenator (differential drug uptake), use and magnitude of hypothermia (changes in distribution and pharmacodynamics), hemodilution (changes in protein binding), and nature of the priming solution (blood colloid or crystalloid and implications for drug binding).

Opioids

Studies of opioid administration during cardiac surgery (Table 14.1) show, in general, a rapid decline in concentrations of drug administered before CPB, a further reduction in concentrations at the initiation of CPB with rapid readjustment of free drug levels while on CPB, a relatively stable plasma level during hypothermic CPB, an increase in initial concentration after termination of CPB likely due to washout of drug sequestered in the lungs, and a reduction in elimination of drug in the post-CPB period likely as a result of an increased volume of distribution and reduced clear-

TABLE 14.2. STUDIES OF PHARMACOKINETIC AND PHARMACODYNAMIC CHANGES OF DRUGS ADMINISTERED DURING CARDIOPULMONARY BYPASS

Study	Drug (n)	Bypass Temperature	Oxygenator	Relevant Findings
			Opioids	
Lunn et al. 1979 (234)	Fentanyl 50 μg·kg^{-1} (9) induction + 25 μg·kg^{-1} post intubation @ 300 μg·min^{-1} (18)	32°C	Bentley Bubble	Patients unresponsive to verbal stimuli at [FEN] = 34 ng·mL^{-1}. Concentrations declined 40% on CPB. N$_2$O addition produced ↓CO, ↑HR, ↑SVR, ↑PVR. Only four measurements during CPB starting at 15 min.
Bovill and Sebel 1980 (235)	Fentanyl 60 μg·kg^{-1} (5)	25°C	Polystan Rygg-Kyvsgaard 5000 Bubble	[FEN] fell by 53% at onset of CPB. No consistent pattern of [FEN] vs. time while on CPB. No change in [FEN] for 2 hr post-CPB, then exponential decline. $t_{1/2}\beta\uparrow$ (423 min) post-CPB vs. values reported in healthy humans (170–356 min).
Koska et al. 1981 (219)	Group 1: Fentanyl 0.5 mg·70 kg^{-1} with CPB (6) Group 2: Fentanyl 0.5 mg·70 kg^{-1} without CPB (6)	NA	NA	$t_{1/2}\beta$ prolonged post-CPB relative to control (5.2 vs. 3.3 hr). Liver blood flow decreased by 30% during CPB.
Sprigge et al. 1982 (236)	Group 1: Fentanyl 30 μg·kg^{-1} + 0.3 μg·kg^{-1}·min^{-1} (10) Group 2: Fentanyl 40 μg·kg^{-1} + 0.4 μg·kg^{-1}·min^{-1} (10) Group 3: Fentanyl 50 μg·kg^{-1} + 0.5 μg·kg^{-1}·min^{-1} (10) until rewarming on CPB or maximum 100 μg·kg^{-1} total dose	Hypothermia	NA	Plasma levels of fentanyl decreased 30% at start of CPB but returned to pre-CPB level by 30 min. No difference in number of responses to noxious stimuli between groups (Group 1; 9; Group 2; 7; Group 3; 5). Patients with the highest dose had fewer hemodynamic changes. One patient in lowest dose group had memory of intraoperative events. Dose-dependent increase in plasma fentanyl levels.
Bentley et al. 1983 (90)	Group 1: Fentanyl 100 μg (5) Group 2: Fentanyl 100 μg (7)	30°C	NA	[FEN] ↓ 47% during CPB. [FEN] ↑ 22% with resumption of ventilation during CPB due to washout of fentanyl from lungs.
DeLange and DeBruijn 1983 (237)	Alfentanil 3 mg·min^{-1} until loss of consciousness, then 2 mg at intubation, then 50 mg·hr^{-1}, stopped during cooling on CPB, 12.5 mg·hr^{-1} during rewarming and post-CPB (14). Adjusted based on hemodynamic response with 2.5 mg bolus	26°C	Travenol Membrane (SM 1430)	Most hemodynamic responses occurred pre-CPB (average alfentanil dose 60 mg). MAP not controlled on CPB in 3 patients at maximum rate. [ALF] decreased by 53% on CPB. Reduced requirements for alfentanil post-CPB.
Wynands et al. 1983 (238)	Group 1: Fentanyl 75 μg·kg^{-1} (10) Group 2: Fentanyl 75 μg·kg^{-1} + 0.75 μg·kg^{-1}·min^{-1} (10) until rewarming	26°C	NA	No between group differences in number of hypertensive episodes requiring treatment pre-CPB. Increased requirements for vasopressors in high dose group and vasodilators in low dose group. [FEN] higher in high dose group. All patients in low dose group hypertensive during CPB. No increase in time to tracheal extubation (17 vs. 19 hr).
Koren et al. 1984 (10)	Group 1: Fentanyl 50 μg·kg^{-1} + 0.15 μg·kg^{-1}·min^{-1} (4) Group 2: Fentanyl 50 μg·kg^{-1} + 0.3 μg·kg^{-1}·min^{-1} (6) Group 3: Fentanyl 30 μg·kg^{-1} + 0.3 μg·kg^{-1}·min^{-1} (9) until onset CPB + [FEN] 20 ng·mL^{-1} in prime. Children with CHD. In vitro studies with CPB apparatus	<20°C	Sci-Med 0800-2A Membrane	[FEN] decreased by 74% at start of CPB. [FEN] = 20 ng·mL^{-1} in prime did not prevent decrease in [FEN] (76%) at time of CPB. In vitro binding studies showed oxygenator to be principle binding site.
Koren et al. 1984 (239)	Group 1: Fentanyl 50 μg·kg^{-1} + 0.15 μg·kg^{-1}·min^{-1} (4) Group 2: Fentanyl 50 μg·kg^{-1} + 0.3 μg·kg^{-1}·min^{-1} (6) Group 3: Fentanyl 30 μg·kg^{-1} + 0.3 μg·kg^{-1}·min^{-1} (9) until onset of CPB Children with CHD. In vitro studies of Fentanyl binding to CPB circuit	16–28°C	NA	[FEN] decreased by 71% with onset of CPB. Stable thereafter without additional drug. Significant binding of FEN to CPB apparatus in vitro. [FEN] higher in children with CHD at same dose rate than in adults. V_D (1,385 ml·kg^{-1}) significantly smaller with no difference in Cl (13 ml·kg^{-1}·min^{-1}) or $t_{1/2}\beta$ (141 min) vs. adult cardiac patients.

(continued)

TABLE 14.2. *Continued.*

Study	Drug (n)	Bypass Temperature	Oxygenator	Relevant Findings
Alvis et al. 1985 (240)	Group 1: Control: Fentanyl 150–250 μg bolus postinduction + 150–250 μg for response to surgical stimulation (10) Group 2: Group S: Fentanyl by CACI to 7.5 ng·mL^{-1} set point (10) Group 3: Group V: Fentanyl by CACI and varied according to stimulation (10) Sampling up to 60 min or pre-CPB if <60 min	NA	NA	Predicted *vs.* actual [FEN] closely correlated in CACI groups. More fentanyl given in Group 2. Equivalent numbers of patients demonstrated hemodynamic responses but overall better hemodynamic control in Group V. No difference in time to extubation among groups (Group 1; 14 hr; Group 2; 15 hr; Group 3; 14 hr).
Fischler et al. 1985 (241)	Phenoperidine 5 mg bolus + 5 mg·hr^{-1} until post-CPB (5)	25°C	Bentley BOS-10S	Initial decrease in concentration at initiation of CPB with return to pre-CPB concentrations within 10 min. Further increase in concentration during CPB.
Koren et al. 1986 (242)	Group 1: Fentanyl 50 μg·kg^{-1} + 0.15 μg·kg^{-1}·min^{-1} (4) Group 2: Fentanyl 50 μg·kg^{-1} + 0.3 μg·kg^{-1}·min^{-1} (6) Group 3: Fentanyl 30 μg·kg^{-1} + 0.3 μg·kg^{-1}·min^{-1} (9) until CPB onset. Children with CHD	NA	NA	V_D correlated with age in 8 Tetralogy of Fallot patients (i.e., with disease severity). Cl decreased with age.
Skacel et al. 1986 (96)	*In vitro* to circuit Alfentanil 1 mg (8) Fentanyl 200 μg (9)	Low = 25°C Normal = 37°C	Shiley S-100A Bubble	As pH of priming solution increased, [FEN] decreased over time. No effect of pH on [ALF]. No effect of temperature on concentration (i.e., no change) over time for either drug.
Davis et al. 1987 (125)	Sufentanil 15 μg·kg^{-1} Group 1: <10 mo not cooled to 32°C (7) Group 2: >10 mo not cooled to 32°C (6) Group 3: <10 mo cooled to 32°C (7) and additional sufentanil as required until 120 min or start of CPB	NA	NA	Children <10 mo $t_{1/2}\beta\downarrow$ Cl$\downarrow$ *vs.* adult reports. $V_D\downarrow$ in infants *vs.* children >10 mo and adults. $V_D\uparrow$ and $t_{1/2}\beta\uparrow$ in surface cooled children. No difference in catecholamine levels between groups.
Flezzani et al. 1987 (43)	Sufentanil to target concentration of 5 ng·mL^{-1} started by CACI 10 min pre-CPB (10)	25°C	NA	Plasma levels of sufentanil fell from 3.8 to 2.5 ng·mL^{-1} (34%) with initiation of CPB and rose to 4.7 ng·mL^{-1} during course of CPB. Plasma albumin levels decreased (24%) on CPB. Drug accumulation evident and likely due to effects of hypothermia. CACI able to achieve and maintain stable [SUF] during CPB.
Greeley et al. 1987 (126)	Sufentanil 10–15 μg·kg^{-1} pre-CPB Group 1: <30 days (9) Group 2: <24 mo (7) Group 3: <12 yr (7) Group 4: >12 yr (5) Pediatric population with CHD	NA	NA	$t_{1/2}\beta\downarrow$ Cl$\downarrow$ and $V_{Dss}\uparrow$ in neonates; Cl$\uparrow$ in infants and children relative to adolescents. Kinetics age related.
Hynynen 1987 (11)	Group 1: Fentanyl 48 μg·kg^{-1} + 0.3 μg·kg^{-1}·min^{-1} (6) Group 2: Alfentanil 48 μg·kg^{-1} + 6 μg·kg^{-1}·min^{-1} (6) Group 3: Fentanyl 48 μg·kg^{-1} + 0.3 μg·kg^{-1}·min^{-1} + 140 ng·mL^{-1} in CPB pump prime (4) Group 4: Fentanyl 48 μg·kg^{-1} + 0.3 μg·kg^{-1}·min^{-1} + 240 ng·mL^{-1} in CPB pump prime (6) Group 5: Alfentanil 48 μg·kg^{-1} + 6 μg·kg^{-1}·min^{-1} + 700 ng·mL^{-1} in CPB pump prime (5)	34°C	Shiley S-100A Bubble (21) or Bentley BOS-10 CM50 Membrane (4)	*In vitro*, perfusion for 60 min resulted in significant (73%) reduction in fentanyl level with or without blood and independent of membrane or bubble oxygenator. For alfentanil 80% of predicted concentration present in nonhemic prime and >100% present in blood prime at the end of 60 min. No effect of oxygenator type. *In vivo*, opioid concentrations decreased at onset of CPB but new steady state concentration achieved within 1.5 min. Addition of fentanyl or alfentanil to prime prevented initial decline in concentration but no difference in opioid concentration with *vs* without opioids in prime at 2.5 min.
Koren et al. 1987 (18)	Fentanyl 30 or 50 μg·kg^{-1} bolus + infusion at 0.15 or 0.30 μg·kg^{-1}·min^{-1} until onset of CPB (18) + pig study	<20°C	NA	During profound hypothermia plasma levels of fentanyl unchanged. Pig study demonstrated hypothermia caused $V_D\downarrow$ and Cl$\uparrow$ and $t_{1/2}\beta\uparrow$.

(continued)

TABLE 14.2. *Continued.*

Study	Drug (*n*)	Bypass Temperature	Oxygenator	Relevant Findings
Thomson et al. 1987 (39)	Group 1: Fentanyl 100 μg·kg^{-1} (16) Group 2: Sufentanil 15 μg·kg^{-1} (17)	Hypothermia	Bubble	No important clinical differences in hemodynamic parameters between groups. No correlation between [FEN] or [SUF] and hemodynamic responses to stimulation. Recall of intraoperative events in two patients.
Caspi et al. 1988 (91)	Fentanyl 100–135 μg·kg^{-1} (29)	24°C	NA	Development of rigidity/respiratory acidosis/hemodynamic instability 2–6 hr postop. [FEN] = 5–8 ng·mL^{-1}. Likely secondary to redistribution of fentanyl from tissue stores.
den Hollander et al. 1988 (127)	Alfentanil 20 μg·kg^{-1} + infusion of 1 μg·kg^{-1}·min^{-1} Bolus 5 μg·kg^{-1} for hemodynamic aberrations Group 1: Infants < 1 yr (6) Group 2: Children (5)	24°C	Polystan VT 1500 or 2000 Bubble	Early extubation possible. Cl↑ and V_{Dss}↑ in infants. No difference in $t_{1/2}\beta$.
Kumar et al. 1988 (37)	Alfentanil 10 μg·kg^{-1}·min^{-1} bolus + 1 μg·kg^{-1}·min^{-1} infusion (5)	28°C	COBE Optiflo II Membrane	At initiation of CPB, total alfentanil levels decreased, free alfentanil concentration increased, as did unbound fraction.
Okutani et al. 1988 (89)	Group 1: Sufentanil 30 μg·kg^{-1} (10) Group 2: Sufentanil 10 μg·kg^{-1} + 0.05 μg·kg^{-1}·min^{-1} (10) Group 3: Sufentanil 20 μg·kg^{-1} + 0.1 μg·kg^{-1}·min^{-1} (10) Group 4: Sufentanil 40 μg·kg^{-1} + 0.2 μg·kg^{-1}·min^{-1} (10)	25°C	Bentley BOS-10 Bubble	[SUF] decreased on initiation of CPB (30–55%) and increased with rewarming with further increase immediately post-CPB. No correlation between [SUF] and change (increase) in catecholamine levels. [SUF] stable on CPB.
Rosen et al. 1988 (12)	Fentanyl 125 ng·mL^{-1} (1) Fentanyl 367 ng·mL^{-1} (1) *in vitro* study	23°C 23°C	Sci-Med 2A-800 Membrane	Membrane of oxygenator identified as site of fentanyl uptake. Saturation of binding sites possible.
Stone et al. 1988 (104)	Sufentanil 30 μg·kg^{-1} (20) at induction	28°C	Membrane	Hemoconcentration with a Bentley CPB-7000 Blood Processor (3) or William Harvey H-4200 Hemoconcentrator (5) did not result in significant reduction in [SUF]. Use of cell-saver (Haemonetics) (19) removed only 0.1% sufentanil. [SUF] fell during CPB (49%).
Taeger et al. 1988 (100)	Group 1: Fentanyl base 0.3 mg (5) Group 2: Alfentanil base 8 mg (6)	NA	NA	Significant first pass uptake (43–87%) of fentanyl by the lung with washout over time. For alfentanil 36–80% sequestration demonstrated. Both drugs characterized by an initial rapid washout phase then a slower phase which could serve as a drug depot.
Newland et al. 1989 (243)	Fentanyl 5–10 μg·kg^{-1} + 5–10 μg·kg^{-1} increments to 100 μg·kg^{-1} pre-CPB Group 1: Infants <1 yr Group 2: Children <5 yr	24°C	SciMed Membrane	[FEN] fell by 57% at initiation of CPB and remained stable thereafter on CPB.
Robbins et al. 1990 (244)	Group 1: Alfentanil 250 μg·kg^{-1}·hr^{-1} × 1 hr + 2.5 μg·kg^{-1}·min^{-1} (8) Group 2: Alfentanil 300 μg·kg^{-1}·hr^{-1} × 1 hr + 3.0 μg·kg^{-1}·min^{-1} (10) Group 3: Alfentanil 350 μg·kg^{-1}·hr^{-1} × 1 hr + 3.5 μg·kg^{-1}·min^{-1} (10)	NA	NA	No difference in incidence of response to noxious stimuli between groups. No difference between groups in [ALF]. [ALF] stable during CPB. No correlation between [ALF] and noxious response. $t_{1/2}\beta$ post-CPB = 5.9 hr. Time to awakening 3.2 hr and to extubation 8.8 hr.
Kern et al. 1991 (245)	Sufentanil by CACI to 0.5–3.0 ng·mL^{-1} target concentration Midazolam by CACI to 25–100 ng·mL^{-1} target concentration (17) Children with CHD	NA	COBE Membrane	CACI overestimated [SUF] on CPB.
Mantz et al. 1991 (246)	Alfentanil 10 mg bolus + infusion of 60 mg·hr^{-1} to sternotomy, then 30 mg·hr^{-1} to end of surgery. Bolus 5 mg at incision, sternotomy, initiation of rewarming, sternal wires, transfer to ICU. Bolus 2.5 mg PRN for hemodynamic aberrations. (10)	29°C	NA	Despite high dose technique, inability to obtund all hemodynamic responses. [ALF] fell 30% at onset CPB. Possible development of acute tolerance demonstrated as awakening occurred at [ALF] = 810 ng·mL^{-1}, $t_{1/2}\beta$ = 379 min, V_D = 0.96 mL·kg^{-1}, Cl = 165 mL·min^{-1}.
den Hollander et al. 1992 (247)	Alfentanil 200 μg·kg^{-1} pre-CPB 80 μg·kg^{-1} post-CPB Group 1: Infants <1 yr (6) Group 2: Children <9 yr (6)	24°C	COBE VPCML Membrane	V_D↑ post-CPB in both age groups. No age-related differences in pharmacokinetics.

(continued)

TABLE 14.2. *Continued.*

Study	Drug (n)	Bypass Temperature	Oxygenator	Relevant Findings
Bailey et al. 1993 (42)	Sufentanil to specified target concentration by CACI (9) pre-CPB	NA	NA	Concentration *vs.* effect relationship established. For obtundation of response to intubation, incision, sternotomy Cp_{50} = 7 $ng \cdot mL^{-1}$. For mediastinal dissection Cp_{50} = 12.7 $ng \cdot mL^{-1}$.
Boer et al. 1994 (99)	Group 1: Sufentanil 1 $\mu g \cdot kg^{-1}$ (6) Group 2: Alfentanil 30 $\mu g \cdot kg^{-1}$ (8)	NA	NA	First pass uptake of sufentanil and alfentanil by the lung is not affected by the type of mechanical ventilation: apnea *vs.* IPPV *vs.* IPPV + PEEP.
Cross and Nikas 1994 (248)	Group 1: Fentanyl 50 $\mu g \cdot kg^{-1}$ at induction + 25 $\mu g \cdot kg^{-1}$ before sternotomy (α-stat) (8) Group 2: Fentanyl 50 $\mu g \cdot kg^{-1}$ at induction + 25 $\mu g \cdot kg^{-1}$ before sternotomy (pH-stat) (8) Group 3: Sufentanil 7 $\mu g \cdot kg^{-1}$ at induction + 3 $\mu g \cdot kg^{-1}$ before sternotomy (α-stat) (8) Group 4: Sufentanil 7 $\mu g \cdot kg^{-1}$ at induction + 3 $\mu g \cdot kg^{-1}$ before sternotomy (pH-stat) (8)	25°C	Maxima Membrane	Blood gas management strategy had no effect on fentanyl levels but reduced levels were found for sufentanil using pH-stat management. Not explained by changes in protein binding.
Hodges et al. 1994 (249)	Fentanyl 18–78 $\mu g \cdot kg^{-1}$ (10) Children with CHD	NA	If CPB flow rate <1,500 $mL \cdot min^{-1}$ Shiley-Dideco 701 > 1,500 $mL \cdot min^{-1}$ Maxima Hollow Fiber	Using a Gambro FH 66 polyamide filter post-CPB for ultrafiltration, no removal of fentanyl demonstrated.
Hug et al. 1994 (34)	Alfentanil 125 $\mu g \cdot kg^{-1}$ pre- and post-CPB (8)	23°C	Travenol Membrane	$V_D\downarrow$, $t_{1/2}\beta\uparrow$ post-CPB. Reduced protein binding. Minimal change (13%) in free [ALF] at CPB initiation despite 55% reduction in total [ALF] levels.
Boer et al. 1995 (102)	Sufentanil to specified target concentration by CACI (10) pre-CPB	NA	NA	First pass retention (8%) of sufentanil by the lung demonstrated. Process may be saturable.
Fiset et al. 1995 (128)	Alfentanil to target plasma concentrations CACI (14) Children with CHD	NA	NA	$Cl\downarrow$ $V_{Dss}\uparrow$ $t_{1/2}\beta\uparrow$ *vs.* previously reported parameters. New model created to account for CPB effect.
Petros et al. 1995 (250)	Alfentanil 50 $\mu g \cdot kg^{-1} \cdot min^{-1} \times 10$ min Group 1: Post-CPB Normothermic (12) Group 2: Post-CPB Hypothermic (12) Group 3: At induction Thoracotomy (12)	Hypothermic 26°C Normothermic 35°C	Bubble Oxygenator	$V_D\uparrow$ post-CPB *vs.* thoracotomy but not different for hypothermic group *vs.* normothermic group.
Borenstein et al. 1997 (251)	Group 1: Sufentanil 30 $\mu g \cdot kg^{-1} \cdot min^{-1}$ for 0.5 min (12) Group 2: Sufentanil 5 $\mu g \cdot kg^{-1} \cdot min^{-1}$ for 3 min (11) Group 3: Sufentanil 2 $\mu g \cdot kg^{-1} \cdot min^{-1}$ for 7 min (9) pre-CPB	NA	NA	No between group differences in V_D, Cl, $t_{1/2}\beta$ (40–47 min). Rate of adverse hemodynamics ↑ with ↑ time of infusion rates.
Duthie et al. 1997 (252)	Remifentanil Group 1: 1 $\mu g \cdot kg^{-1} \cdot min^{-1}$ (2) Group 2: 1.5 $\mu g \cdot kg^{-1} \cdot min^{-1}$ (4) Group 3: 2.0 $\mu g \cdot kg^{-1} \cdot min^{-1}$ (4)	28°C	Membrane	Remifentanil does not undergo significant pulmonary extraction during CPB. Cl = 2.18 $L \cdot min^{-1}$. [REMI] dose dependent over range of infusions tested.
Russell et al. 1997 (88)	Remifentanil 2–5 $\mu g \cdot kg^{-1}$ as a bolus 1. Pre-CPB 2. On CPB and hypothermic 3. On CPB and normothermic (16)	28°C	NA	Cl ↓ during hypothermic CPB by 20%.
Volatile anesthetic agents				
Loomis et al. 1986 (253)	Isoflurane to maintain MAP 50–80 mm Hg on CPB (10)	25°C	COBE Membrane	α-stat blood gas management. Concentration dependent decrease in EEG activity with ↑[ISO] until burst suppression at 46.5 $\mu g \cdot mL^{-1}$. Rapid offset of action with $t_{1/2}$ of 19 min. Hypothermia alone decreased EEG amplitude but did not produce burst suppression. Mean vaporizer setting 2.2%.
Moore et al. 1986 (254)	Halothane Group 1: Acyanotic (10) Group 2: Cyanotic (10) Children with CHD	Hypothermia	Sci-Med Membrane	Reductive metabolism significantly greater in the cyanotic group.

(continued)

TABLE 14.2. *Continued.*

Study	Drug (n)	Bypass Temperature	Oxygenator	Relevant Findings
Henderson et al. 1988 (255)	Isoflurane (14) 1% inspired	28°C	Bentley Bio Bubble (7) Terumo Capiox Membrane (7)	α-stat blood gas management. Washin of isoflurane had a rapid phase followed by a slow phase with a continued slow rise in concentration in plasma up to 48 min. Washout was characterised by a rapid phase followed by a slower elimination with a $t_{1/2}\beta$ of 9.4 min (Bubble) to 14.9 min (Membrane). Concentration fell by >50% within 2 min.
Nussmeier et al. 1988 (77)	Group 1: Isoflurane (6) Group 2: Isoflurane + Enflurane + Halothane 0.3 MAC each (5) *in vitro* study	24°C	Bentley BOS-10 Bubble	Isoflurane washin >50% equilibration by 4 min and >90% by 16 min. Washout was >75% by 4 min and >90% by 16 min. Washin was faster at higher gas flow rates as was washout. Neither washin or washout rate was affected by pump flow rates. Initial washin rates higher for isoflurane and enflurane *vs.* halothane. Isoflurane had highest washout rate.
Price et al. 1988 (256)	Isoflurane (10)	25°C	Bentley BOS-10 Bubble	Rapid washout from circuit (0.85% to <0.05% in 9 min). Time constant of approximately 2 min reflects washout from vessel rich groups.
Nussmeier et al. 1989 (78)	Isoflurane 1% to oxygenator during CPB (9)	23°C	Bentley BOS-10 Bubble	Washin 41% at 16 min, 51% at 32 min and 57% at 48 min. Washout 36% of peak at 8 min, 24% at 16 min, and 13% at 32 min. Venous concentration declined more slowly than arterial. Washin slower during hypothermic CPB due to greater tissue capacity. Washout during rewarming similar to normothermic patients.
Stern et al. 1989 (9)	Isoflurane 2% (3) *in vitro* study	NA	Sci-Med Membrane #1-35002A	α-stat blood gas management. Sci-Med oxygenator absorbs significant amounts of isoflurane. Blood equilibration affected by gas flow rates but not by blood flow rate. Time constant for Isoflurane elimination = 7 min.
Tarr and Snowden 1991 (257)	Enflurane 0.6% V/V (10)	24°C	COBE Membrane	Solubility and [ENF]↓ (25%) with onset of CPB. [ENF]↑ during hypothermic CPB. No tissue redistribution to blood phase during rewarming demonstrated.
Hickey et al. 1996 (8)	Isoflurane 1.15% Group 1: SM-35 oxygenator (4) Group 2: CML oxygenator (4) Group 3: SAFEII oxygenator (4) *in vitro* study	28°C and 37°C	SM-35 (Avecor) or CML (COBE) or SAFEII (Polystan) Membrane	α-stat blood gas management. Uptake of isoflurane was slower by the SM-35 oxygenator at both temperatures. Elimination was also slower with the SM-35 oxygenator. Elimination was faster at 37° *vs.* 28° for CML and SM-35 oxygenators but not for the SAFE II.
		Intravenous anesthetic agents		
Aaltonen et al. 1982 (258)	Group 1: Lorazepam 4 mg 1 hr pre-CPB (5) Group 2: Lorazepam 0.03 mg·kg^{-1} (14) for nasal surgery	30°C	NA	Lorazepam concentration fell at start of CPB then recovered. Lorazepam concentrations increased post-CPB. $t_{1/2}\beta$↑ from 12 (control population) to 15 hr (CPB population).
Oduro et al. 1983 (259)	Etomidate 0.15 mg·kg^{-1} + 20 μg·kg^{-1}·min^{-1} (6)	28°C	NA	Etomidate concentrations decreased (33%) at start of CPB and recovered over time during cooling with reduction again during rewarming phase. Elevated again post-CPB due to transfusion of oxygenator contents.
Boscoe et al. 1984 (260)	Group 1: Lorazepam night before surgery (12) Group 2: Lorazepam night before surgery and at induction (12) Group 3: Lorazepam night before surgery and 10 min pre-CPB (12) <60 kg = 2 mg; 60–80 kg = 3 mg; >80 kg = 4 mg	NA	Bentley BOS 10	Lorazepam levels decreased 27% at start of CPB in all groups. Only patients given lorazepam just before bypass had therapeutic concentrations (>30 μg·L^{-1}) during CPB.
Harper et al. 1985 (261)	Group 1: Midazolam 0.3 mg·kg^{-1} post-CPB (7) Group 2: Minor surgery Midazolam 0.3 mg·kg^{-1} at induction (25) Group 3: Major surgery Midazolam 0.3 mg·kg^{-1} at induction (38)	NA	NA	$t_{1/2}\beta$ prolonged relative to minor surgery subjects. Clearance increased with younger patients.
Kanto et al. 1985 (262)	Group 1: Midazolam 0.075 mg·kg^{-1} (6) Group 2: Midazolam 0.15 mg·kg^{-1} (6) at induction	NA	NA	[MID]↓ at CPB initiation. After CPB, [MID]↑ in the high dose group. $t_{1/2}\beta$↑ (281 min) relative to previous reports in normals.
Lowry et al. 1985 (263)	Group 1: Diazepam 5 mg q2hr Group 2: Midazolam 5 mg q2hr for 12 hr post-CPB	NA	NA	[MID] stable while [DIAZ] continued to rise. After discontinuation, [MID] fell rapidly while [DIAZ] still remained high.

(continued)

TABLE 14.2. *Continued*.

Study	Drug (n)	Bypass Temperature	Oxygenator	Relevant Findings
Morgan et al. 1986 (35)	Thiopental by CACI at induction + infusion to maintain target concentration 15 μg·mL^{-1} (7)	<28°C	Bentley BOS 10 or COBE Optiflo II	Total [THIO]↓ at initiation of CPB by 50% but unbound [THIO]↓ by only 30% and recovered more rapidly than total levels during CPB. Unbound fraction higher during CPB and correlated with albumin levels.
Bjorksten et al. 1988 (74)	Group 1: Methohexital 1 mg·kg^{-1} + infusion to target 5 mg·L^{-1} (10) Group 2: Thiopental 2.5 mg·kg^{-1} + infusion to target 10 mg·L^{-1} (10)	28°C	Bentley BOS 10 Bubble	[METHO]: Onset of CPB produced fall in total concentration of ~40% with gradual increase thereafter. Unbound fraction increased from 27–43% pre *vs.* on CPB with little change in absolute free concentration level. [THIO]: Onset of CPB produced fall in total concentration of ~50% with gradual increase thereafter. Unbound fraction increased from 16 to 30% pre *vs.* CPB with little change in absolute free concentration level.
Mathews et al. 1988 (129)	Midazolam 0.3 mg·kg^{-1} Group 1: Closed operation without CPB (6) Group 2: CPB (6) Group 3: CPB + Arrest (5) Group 4: Midazolam 0.05 as bolus + 0.05 mg·kg^{-1}·h^{-1} post-CPB (10) Children with CHD	NA	NA	$t_{1/2}\beta$↓ with CPB. Cl↓ with CPB. NSD in volume of distribution. Postop $t_{1/2}\beta$ 3.1 hr. Children have Cl↑ and $t_{1/2}\beta$↓ relative to reports in adults.
Hynynen et al. 1989 (7)	Thiopentone 6 mg·kg^{-1} Before CPB Group 1: Pulsatile (6) Group 2: Nonpulsatile (7) During CPB Group 3: Pulsatile (9) Group 4: Nonpulsatile (8) perfusion + *in vitro* study	29°C	Shiley S-100A Bubble	No differences in pharmacokinetics in pulsatile *vs.* nonpulsatile perfusion groups. [THIO]↓ 44% at initiation of CPB. No pulmonary sequestration detected *in vivo* but 50% bound to circuit *in vitro*. $t_{1/2}\beta$ prolonged during CPB.
Maitre et al. 1989 (264)	Midazolam 15 mg·hr^{-1} for 4 hr postop (12)	NA	NA	Protein binding 97%. $t_{1/2}\beta$ 10.6 hr. V_{Dss} 103 L. Cl 0.25 L·min^{-1}. $t_{1/2}\beta$↑ Clearance ↓ relative to reports in normal patients.
Russell et al. 1989 (79)	Propofol 10 mg·kg^{-1}·hr^{-1} for 20 min then 3 mg·kg^{-1}·hr^{-1} (10)	25°C	NA	Onset of CPB associated with a 50–78% drop in [PROP] with subsequent rapid recovery to 98% of pre-CPB levels by 20 min. Free fraction increased by 1.5–3-fold with onset of CPB.
Boer et al. 1990 (265)	Group 1: Propofol 0.2 mL·kg^{-1} (14) Group 2: Intralipid (14) Group 3: Propofol 2 mg·kg^{-1} (10) during CPB	26°C	Membrane	Propofol decreased vascular resistance and [PROP] declined slowly during CPB.
Massey et al. 1990 (266)	Propofol 4 mg·kg^{-1}·hr^{-1} (10)	28°C	Shiley M2000	[PROP] maintained at >1 μg·mL^{-1} throughout surgery. V_D 626 L Cl 2.2 L·min^{-1} $t_{1/2}\beta$ 356 min.
Kern et al. 1991 (245)	Sufentanil to target concentration 0.5–3.0 ng·mL^{-1} by CACI + Midazolam to target concentration 25–100 ng·mL^{-1} by CACI (17) Children with CHD	NA	COBE Membrane	CACI overestimated actual [MID] on CPB.
LeHot et al. 1993 (267)	Methohexital 2 mg·kg^{-1} Group 1: Hypothermic CPB (11) Group 2: Normothermic CPB (11) 10 min post-CPB Group 3: Vascular (8) post-skin incision	28°C Group 1 37°C Group 2 37°C Group 3	CML Membrane	No difference between CPB groups for [METH] and derived pharmacokinetic parameters. As compared with vascular patients, [METH] were lower, Cl and V_D were greater, but $t_{1/2}\beta$ not different.
Hynynen et al. 1994 (13)	*In vivo*: Propofol 10 mg·kg^{-1}·hr^{-1} for 20 min then 3 mg·kg^{-1}·hr^{-1} (14) *In vitro*: Propofol to achieve [PROP] of 2 μg·mL^{-1} (3)	28°C	D703 Compactflo Membrane	*In vivo*, some degree of sequestration in circuit likely as at initiation of CPB fall in concentration (45%) > degree expected by hemodilution (29%). *In vitro*, Propofol taken up by the circuit (75% uptake at 120 min of perfusion).
Lee et al. 1995 (268)	Propofol 4 mg·kg^{-1}·hr^{-1} during CPB (11)	28°C	Capiox Terumo Membrane	$t_{1/2}\beta$ = 370 min Cl 1.3 L..min^{-1} V_{Dss} 322 L
Ng et al. 1995 (269)	Group 1: Propofol 4 mg·kg^{-1}·hr^{-1} (11) Group 2: Morphine/diazepam (10) during CPB	28°C	Capiox Terumo Membrane	[PROP] 1 μg·mL^{-1} by 15 min. Concentrations of cortisol, epinephrine, norepinephrine lower in propofol group.

(continued)

TABLE 14.2. *Continued.*

Study	Drug (n)	Bypass Temperature	Oxygenator	Relevant Findings
Bailey et al. 1996 (270)	Group 1: Propofol by CACI to maintain [PROP] 3–10 μg·mL^{-1} (11) Group 2: Propofol by CACI to maintain [PROP] at 2, 4, or 6 μg·mL^{-1} (30) pre-CPB	23°C	NA	α-stat blood gas management strategy. Low values for volume of central compartment and central clearance as compared to previous studies. Model derived provided better fit of predicted vs. actual [PROP] in the pre-CPB group. Better predictive capability achieved by allowing V_1 and Cl_1 to increase with onset of CPB.
Hammaren et al. 1996 (76)	Propofol 10 mg·kg^{-1}·hr^{-1} for 20 min then 3 mg·kg^{-1}·hr^{-1} (15)	30°C	Membrane	Heparin ↑ [PROP] free fraction from 1.5–2.3%. [PROP] free fraction ↑ again during CPB from 2.3–3.5%.
McLean et al. 1996 (271)	Ketamine 2 mg·kg^{-1} + infusion of 50 μg·kg^{-1}·min^{-1} (6)	30°C	Bard HF5400 Membrane	[KET] decreased 33% with onset of CPB then increased during CPB. $t_{1/2}\beta$ = 2.1 hr.
Dawson et al. 1997 (36)	Group 1: Propofol 1 mg·kg^{-1} + 3 mg·kg^{-1}·hr^{-1} (12) Group 2: Midazolam 0.2 mg·kg^{-1} + 0.07 mg·kg^{-1}·hr^{-1} (12)	30°C	NA	Free [PROP] did not change with onset of and throughout CPB. [MID] did not change at CPB initiation but decreased during CPB.
Doi et al. 1997 (44)	Propofol by CACI + Alfentanil by CACI (12)	28°C	Membrane	Concentration of [PROP] and [ALF] stable during CPB.
		Neuromuscular receptor blocking agents		
d'Hollander et al. 1983 (15)	Pancuronium 0.07 mg·kg^{-1} at induction and thereafter to maintain 10% of control twitch height (10)	24°C	Optiflo II Bubble	Increased requirement for pancuronium to maintain blockade during cooling at initiation of CPB due to hemodilution, reduced during hypothermic period, increased during rewarming, and at pre-CPB requirements in the post-CPB period. [PANC]↓ during cooling and increased during rewarming and post-CPB periods. Temperature has a significant impact on Pancuronium effect.
Futter et al. 1983 (225)	Pancuronium 0.06–0.09 mg·kg^{-1} + infusion to maintain first twitch in train-of-four < 10% of control (8)	26°C	NA	Pancuronium requirements reduced 84% during hypothermic period. During rewarming Pancuronium requirements increased. Requirements in the post-CPB period less than in pre-CPB period.
Shanks et al. 1983 (92)	Group 1: Gallamine 480 mg (11) Group 2: Gallamine 240 mg + 240 mg pre-CPB (11)	28°C	Bentley BOS 10	$t_{1/2}\beta$↑. V_{ss}↓ and Cl↓ relative to previous reports. Relaxant not bound by CPB apparatus. Plasma levels elevated during CPB.
Walker et al. 1983 (93)	Alcuronium 0.27 mg·kg^{-1} at induction + 1 μg/kg^{-1}·min^{-1} (10)	25°C	Bentley BOS 10 or COBE-Optiflo II	[ALC]↑ above pre-CPB levels during CPB. Cl↓ and $t_{1/2}\beta$↑ relative to previous reports.
Flynn et al. 1984 (85)	Atracurium 0.6 mg·kg^{-1} at induction + infusion to maintain twitch height < 10% of control (12)	25°C	NA	Train-of-four response disappeared during hypothermia. Reduced requirements (55%) for Atracurium infusion during and after CPB.
Buzello et al. 1985 (142)	Group 1: Pancuronium 0.075 mg·kg^{-1} + 0.015 mg·kg^{-1} (10) Group 2: Vecuronium 0.075 mg·kg^{-1} + 0.015 mg·kg^{-1} maintenance dose (10) to maintain EMG response < 25% of control	26°C	NA	Recovery from neuromuscular blockade prolonged during hypothermia with no difference between agents. Some recovery with rewarming but duration of neuromuscular blockade still prolonged relative to pre-bypass and impairment of recovery persisted into post-bypass period.
Denny and Kreeshaw 1986 (272)	Group 1: Atracurium 0.5 mg·kg^{-1} + 0.4 mg·kg^{-1}·hr^{-1} (14) Group 2: Vecuronium 0.1 mg·kg^{-1} + 0.08 mg·kg^{-1}·hr^{-1} (11)	30°C	NA	Decreased requirements (Vecuronium 71% reduction and Atracurium 35%) for drug to maintain block during hypothermia.
Avram et al. 1987 (94)	Metocurine 0.3 mg·kg^{-1} + infusion at 0.04 mg·kg^{-1}·hr^{-1} Group 1: CPB (10) Group 2: Hip replacement (9)	30°C	NA	Plasma levels fell with initiation of CPB and then recovered. Disposition otherwise unaffected by CPB. Blockade intensity reduced by hypothermia.
Buzello et al. 1987 (224)	Group 1: Alcuronium 0.15 mg·kg^{-1} + 0.03 mg·kg^{-1}·hr^{-1} (10) Group 2: d-tubocurarine 0.3 mg·kg^{-1} + 0.06 mg·kg^{-1}·hr^{-1} (10) Group 3: Pancuronium 0.05 mg·kg^{-1} + 0.01 mg·kg^{-1}·hr^{-1} (10) Group 4: Vecuronium 0.05 mg·kg^{-1} + 0.05 mg·kg^{-1}·hr^{-1} (10)	26°C	NA	Effects of d-tubocurarine/alcuronium/pancuronium attenuated during hypothermic CPB. Effect of vecuronium enhanced during hypothermic CPB.
Wierda et al. 1990 (273)	Group 1: Pancuronium 200 μg·kg^{-1} (6) Group 2: Pancuronium 200 μg·kg^{-1} + Dopamine 2 μg·kg^{-1}·min^{-1} (6)	28°C	Shiley M-2000 Membrane	No change in Pancuronium pharmacokinetics with addition of Dopamine. Tubular reabsorption of Pancuronium decreased during hypothermia.

(continued)

TABLE 14.2. *Continued.*

Study	Drug (n)	Bypass Temperature	Oxygenator	Relevant Findings
Wierda et al. 1990 (274)	Group 1: Pipecuronium 200 μg·kg^{-1} (10) Group 2: Pancuronium 200 μg·kg^{-1} (10) at induction	29°C	NA	More tachycardia with pancuronium. Pharmacokinetics of pipecuronium unchanged by hypothermic CPB.
Diefenbach et al. 1992 (21)	Atracurium 460 μg·kg^{-1} + maintenance bolus 138 μg·kg^{-1} to maintain 95% twitch depression (15)	28°C	Membrane	Increased time to onset of blockade (57%) and increased duration (2×) of effect during hypothermic CPB.
Diefenbach et al. 1995 (87)	Mivacurium 150 μg·kg^{-1} + maintenance doses of 75 μg·kg^{-1} to maintain twitch depression (9)	34°C	Membrane	Cholinesterase activity reduced by 42% during CPB. Onset time 26% longer but duration of effect not increased during post-normothermic CPB.
Smeulers et al. 1995 (143)	Rocuronium 0.6 mg·kg^{-1} (10)	25°C	CML II Excel Membrane	[ROC] at time of 5% recovery of twitch function higher during normothermia than during both hypothermic CPB and rewarming. Duration of blockade significantly prolonged during hypothermia (four times). $t_{1/2}\beta$ = 97 min.
McDonagh et al. 1996 (144)	Group 1: Doxacurium 0.05 mg·kg^{-1} (10) Group 2: Doxacurium 0.075 mg·kg^{-1} (10) 10% of intubating dose when twitch recovery 25% of control	32°C	Membrane	Duration of effect ↑ with higher dose and ↑ in both groups (60–100%) relative to previous reports in other patient populations.
Kansanaho et al. 1997 (275)	Group 1: Atracurium 0.4 mg·kg^{-1} + CACI infusion (10) Group 2: Vecuronium 0.08 mg·kg^{-1} + CACI infusion (10)	28°C	Membrane	CACI performance poor during hypothermic CPB. Infusion rates reduced by 70% (Atracurium) and 90% (Vecuronium).
		Inotropic agents		
Lawless et al. 1988 (130)	Amrinone 0.75–1.1 mg·kg^{-1} + 5–10 μg·kg^{-1}·min^{-1} Children with CHD (10)	NA	NA	$t_{1/2}\beta$ = 7.8 hr Cl 2.93 mL·kg^{-1}·min^{-1} V_D 1.7 L·kg^{-1} Age-dependent kinetics. Higher doses required to achieve therapeutic concentrations in infants.
Lawless et al. 1989 (131)	Amrinone 0–2.3 mg·kg^{-1} bolus + 5–10 μg·kg^{-1}·min^{-1} Children with CHD (18)	NA	NA	Age-dependent pharmacokinetics demonstrated. Infants have higher dosing requirements than adults. Suggested dose of 3–4.5 mg·kg^{-1} bolus + 10 μg·kg^{-1}·min^{-1} for infants (<1 yr). For neonates (<4 wk), 3–4.5 mg·kg^{-1} bolus + 5 μg·kg^{-1}·min^{-1}.
Bailey et al. 1991 (276)	Group 1: Amrinone 0.75 mg·kg^{-1} (5) Group 2: Amrinone 1.5 mg·kg^{-1} (5) Group 3: Amrinone 2.0 mg·kg^{-1} (5) Group 4: Amrinone 2.5 mg·kg^{-1} (5) Group 5: Amrinone 0.75 mg·kg^{-1} + 10 μg·kg^{-1}·min^{-1} (5) Group 6: Amrinone 2.0 mg·kg^{-1} + 5 μg·kg^{-1}·min^{-1} (5) Group 7: Amrinone 2.0 mg·kg^{-1} + 10 μg·kg^{-1}·min^{-1} (5) during CPB	23°C	COBE CML Membrane	A bolus dose of 2 mg·kg^{-1} + infusion of 10 μg·kg^{-1}·min^{-1} required to achieve consistent therapeutic levels (>2 μg·mL^{-1}) during CPB.
Hayashi et al. 1993 (277)	Dopamine (48)	28°C	Membrane	α-stat blood gas management. Uptake of dopamine by the lung pre- and post-CPB demonstrated.
Lynn et al. 1993 (132)	Amrinone 4.5 mg·kg^{-1} bolus + 10 μg·kg^{-1}·min^{-1} infusion post-CPB (14) Children with CHD	NA	NA	Cl 3.4 mL·kg^{-1}·min^{-1} V_D 1.65 L·kg^{-1} $t_{1/2}\beta$ = 5.75 hr. No correlation between $t_{1/2}\beta$ and age. [AMR] 3–5 μg·mL^{-1}.
Bailey et al. 1994 (278)	Group 1: Milrinone 25 μg·kg^{-1} (5) Group 2: Milrinone 50 μg·kg^{-1} (5) Group 3: Milrinone 75 μg·kg^{-1} (5) Group 4: Milrinone 50 μg·kg^{-1} + 0.5 μg·kg^{-1}·min^{-1} (5) at rewarming Group 5: Milrinone 50 μg·kg^{-1} (5) just after CPB	23°C	COBE CML Membrane	Dose-related increases in [MIL] with rapid decline in single dose groups. [MIL] sustained by continuous infusion. No difference if given post-CPB. CPB does not substantially alter milrinone pharmacokinetics. Calculation of context-sensitive half-time showed milrinone to be more rapidly removed than Amrinone if duration of infusion < 400 min. Maintenance of therapeutic levels (>100 ng·mL^{-1}) achieved by bolus + infusion regime.
Das et al. 1994 (279)	Milrinone 50 μg·kg^{-1} + 0.5 μg·kg^{-1}·min^{-1} post-CPB (6)	28°C	NA	Cl↓ (120 mL·min^{-1}) V_D (0.31 L·kg^{-1})↑ $t_{1/2}\beta$ (1.69 hr)↑ vs. normals but similar to reports in patients with CHF. [MIL] > 100 ng·mL^{-1}.

(continued)

TABLE 14.2. *Continued.*

Study	Drug (n)	Bypass Temperature	Oxygenator	Relevant Findings
Butterworth et al. 1995 (280)	Group 1: Milrinone 25 μg·kg^{-1} (10) Group 2: Milrinone 50 μg·kg^{-1} (10) Group 3: Milrinone 75 μg·kg^{-1} (9) post-CPB	NA	NA	Milrinone increased CO. Phenylephrine required to maintain BP in most patients. Unable to define a concentration vs. effect relationship. Pharmacokinetics not affected by dose. Loading dose of 50 μg·kg^{-1} recommended.
DeHert et al. 1995 (281)	Group 1: Milrinone 20 μg·kg^{-1} (10) Group 2: Milrinone 40 μg·kg^{-1} (10) + 0.5 μg·kg^{-1}·min^{-1} during CPB	26°C	NA	More norepinephrine required to maintain BP in high dose group. [MIL] above predicted at all dose and time intervals. Cl = 1.4 L.hr^{-1} for low dose vs. 4.0 L.hr^{-1} for high dose. $t_{1/2}\beta$ 58 hr vs. 13 hr, respectively. Both clearance and elimination values changed over time likely due to alterations in renal function with CPB.
Williams et al. 1995 (133)	Amrinone to produce target [AMR] = 0.5 to 7 μg·mL^{-1} (27) before CPB termination Children with CHD + in vitro binding study	26°C	Terumo Capiox 320 or 308 Hollow Fiber	In vitro binding study showed 20% binding to CPB circuit. Mean [AMR] 180% of predicted. At Amrinone dose of 4.9 mg·kg^{-1}, mean [AMR] 5 μg·mL^{-1}. Measured to predicted ratio of [AMR]: neonates 1.37; infants 1.73; children 2.03.
Kikura et al. 1997 (282)	Group 1: Milrinone 50 μg·kg^{-1} (8) Group 2: Milrinone 50 μg·kg^{-1} + 0.5 μg·kg^{-1}·min^{-1} (9) Group 3: Control (10) post-CPB	23°C	COBE CML Membrane	Cp$_{50}$ for half maximum increase in velocity of shortening of circumference = 139 ng·mL^{-1}. All doses of milrinone effective.
		β-Adrenergic receptor blocking agents		
McAllister et al. 1979 (19)	Propranolol 40–320 mg·day^{-1} discontinued 12 hr preop (12) + dog studies	27°C	NA	[PROP]↑ during hypothermic CPB after initial fall at onset of CPB. Dog studies suggested reduction in clearance due to effect of hypothermia on in vivo metabolic activity.
Wood et al. 1979 (283)	Propranolol 80–240 mg·day^{-1} discontinued over 48 hr. Last dose at least 9 hr preop (7)	NA	NA	Heparin administration doubled the free fraction (7–14%) of Propranolol. Protamine administration decreased the free fraction from 13 to 9%. No change in free fraction during CPB. Free fatty acid levels increased with heparin administration.
Plachetka et al. 1981 (112)	Group 1: Propranolol 0.1 mg·kg^{-1} at induction (7) Group 2: Placebo (7) **NB:** all patients taking Propranolol chronically	31°C	NA	[PROP]↓ 60% with onset of CPB and ↑ 57% at CPB termination. $t_{1/2}\beta$ increased from 2–5.5 hr.
Sill et al. 1984 (228)	Group 1: Chronic therapy of Propranolol 40–240 mg·day^{-1} discontinued preop (14) Group 2: Chronic therapy + Propranolol bolus 2–7 mg + infusion 0.4–0.9 μg·kg^{-1}·min^{-1} (12)	NA	NA	[PROP]↓ 55% during onset CPB. Adverse hemodynamic responses correlated with reduced [PROP].
deBruijn et al. 1987 (284)	Esmolol given as a timed infusion of 100–500 μg·kg^{-1}·min^{-1} (19) pre-CPB study **NB:** all study subjects receiving chronic β-receptor blocking agents	NA	NA	$t_{1/2}\beta$ 9.9 min V_D (1.9 L.kg^{-1})↓ Cl (128 mL.kg^{-1}·min^{-1})↓ relative to healthy patients.
Mantz et al. 1990 (285)	Acebutalol 6 mg·kg^{-1} (7) **NB:** all study subjects receiving Acebutalol chronically	29°C	Bentley BOS10 Bubble	[AC]↓ 26% with onset of CPB, stable during CPB and for 1 hr post-CPB.
Jacobs et al. 1993 (86)	Esmolol 0.5 mg·kg^{-1} 30 min pre-CPB + 100 μg·kg^{-1}·min^{-1} (10)	26°C	COBE CML Membrane	[ESM]↑ on CPB during hypothermia. No uptake by oxygenator.
		Antibiotics		
Goldman et al. 1977 (286)	Group 1: Cephalothin 1 g i.m. preop, 2 g i.v. at induction, 2 g q6hr × 7 doses (72) Group 2: Cephalothin 1 g i.m. preop, 2 g i.v. at induction, 2 g q6hr × 23 doses (85)	NA	NA	6-day regime no more effective than 2-day regime. Prolonged procedures associated with inadequate levels.
Archer et al. 1978 (287)	Group 1: Cephalothin 20 mg·kg^{-1} i.m. at induction (15) Group 2: Cefamandole 20 mg·kg^{-1} i.m. at induction (15)	32°C	NA	[CEFAM] > [CEPHAL] but adequate serum levels during CPB < 200 min. [CEFAM] 3–5 × > [CEPHAL] in atrial and valve tissue.
Eigel et al. 1978 (288)	Group 1: Cephalothin 2 g i.v. (12) Group 2: Cefazolin 2 g i.v. (8) Group 3: Cefamandole 2 g i.v. (8) at induction	28°C	Harvey Bubble	[CEFAZ] higher and declined slower during CPB than other two agents. Adequate tissue levels achieved with all agents.

(continued)

TABLE 14.2. *Continued.*

Study	Drug (n)	Bypass Temperature	Oxygenator	Relevant Findings
Kini et al. 1978 (289)	Group 1: Cefazolin 0.5 g *i.m.* (49) Group 2: Cephalothin 1.0 g *i.m.* (50) midnight and 1 hr preop, then *i.v.* in ICU and q6hr × 5 days	NA	NA	Both effective for infection prophylaxis. [CEFAZ] stable during CPB and less variable than [CEPHAL].
Polk et al. 1978 (290)	Cefamandole 20 mg·kg⁻¹ (16)	32°C	Harvey H-1000	Cefamandole $t_{1/2}\beta$ increased during CPB. [CEFAM] concentrations adequate. Redose after 4 hr CPB time.
Miller et al. 1979 (291)	Cephalothin 2 g preop, induction and postop (5)	26°C	Bentley Q200 A	No difference in preop *vs.* 1 day postop pharmacokinetics. [CEPHAL]↓ at initiation of CPB, then plateaued. $t_{1/2}\beta$ > 50% longer than preop and postop. Cl↓.
Quintiliani et al. 1979 (292)	Group 1: Cephalothin 2 g *i.v.* 20–120 min before removal of atrial appendage (12) Group 2: Cephapirin 2 g *i.v.* 20–120 min before removal of atrial appendage (15)	NA	NA	[CEPHAP] > [CEPHAL] in atrial tissue and pericardial fluid but concentrations of both agents acceptable. Protein binding of cephapirin ↓ relative to cephalothin. Tissue concentrations decline faster than serum levels.
Akl et al. 1980 (293)	Group 1: Cefazolin 1 g (10 adults) Group 2: Cefazolin 20 mg·kg⁻¹ (10 children with CHD) *i.m.* 1 hr preop + *i.v.* q6hr × 5 days	28°C	Harvey Bubble	[CEFAZ]↓ 42–50% with start of CPB in both groups. Levels stable thereafter and adequate for antimicrobial effect.
Miller et al. 1980 (294)	Cefazolin 1 or 2 g *i.v.* preop, induction, postop (8)	26°C	Bentley Q200A	[CEFAZ]↓ with CPB then stable. Cl↓ and $t_{1/2}\beta$↑ *vs.* preop and postop. Renal clearance ↓ intraop *vs.* preop and postop but no further ↓ with CPB.
Nightingale et al. 1980 (295)	Group 1: Cefazolin 2 g *i.v.* 30–118 min before removal of right atrial appendage Group 2: Cephradine 2 g 30–118 min before removal of right atrial appendage	NA	NA	[CEFAZ] > [CEPHRA] in serum and tissue. Both provided adequate levels. Free [CEPHRA] > free [CEFAZ] in serum and pericardial fluid.
Olson et al. 1980 (296)	Cefamandole 2 g *i.v.* 20–120 min before removal of atrial appendage (23)	NA	NA	[CEFAM] adequate in atrial and pericardial fluid up to 225 min.
Mullany et al. 1982 (297)	Group 1: Ceforanide 30 mg·kg⁻¹ 32–214 min before removal of right atrial appendage (13) Group 2: Cefamandole 30 mg·kg⁻¹ 32–214 min before removal of right atrial appendage (13)	NA	NA	[CEFOR] > [CEFAM] but both adequate in atria, pericardial fluid, plasma, aorta, muscle, and sternum for duration < 200 min. Cl↓ during CPB.
Bryan et al. 1983 (298)	Group 1: Cefamandole 2 g *i.v.* 60 min before incision (16) Group 2: Cefazolin 2 g *i.v.* 60 min before incision (16)	NA	NA	[CEFAZ] > [CEFAM] but [CEFAZ] inadequate in 3/16 bone samples. Better relative tissue penetration of cefamandole.
Bergeron et al. 1985 (299)	Group 1: Cefamandole 1 g *i.v.* at induction and q4hr for 24 hr (37) Group 2: Cloxacillin 1 g *i.v.* at induction and q4hr for 24 hr (34) Group 3: Fusidic acid 580 mg *i.v.* over 2 hr then q8hr (29)	NA	NA	[CEFAM] and [FUS] adequate in cardiac tissue but [CLOX] insufficient in some patients. Cl↓ for cefamandole and cloxacillin.
Pieper et al. 1985 (300)	Cloxacillin 2 g + Benzylpenicillin 6 g at induction and 4 hr (10)	25°C	NA	Antibiotic concentrations > minimal inhibitory concentration for *Staphylococcus aureus* and *Staphylococcus epidermidis*.
Daschner et al. 1987 (301)	Vancomycin 15 mg·kg⁻¹ *i.v.* before surgery (33)	25°C	NA	Adequate valve/muscle/subcutaneous tissue and blood levels achieved.
Frank et al. 1987 (302)	Ceftazidime 2 g *i.v.* preop (24)	25°C	NA	Adequate levels achieved in serum/valve/muscle and fat.
Kaiser et al. 1987 (303)	Group 1: Cefazolin 2 g *i.v.* at induction, q4hr intraop, q6hr postop × 72 hr (255) Group 2: Cefazolin 2 g *i.v.* at induction + Gentamicin 1.5 mg·kg⁻¹ *i.v.* at induction, q4hr intraop + q6hr postop × 72 hr (253) Group 3: Cefamandole 2 g *i.v.* at induction, q2hr intraop, q4hr postop × 72 hr (259) Group 4: Cefamandole 2 g *i.v.* at induction, q2hr intraop, q4hr postop × 72 hr + Gentamicin 1.5 mg·kg⁻¹ *i.v.* at induction (263)	NA	NA	Cefamandole provided better protection than cefazolin. Gentamicin of no benefit. To ensure adequate levels during CPB, Cefamandole dosing interval should be every 2 hr.

(continued)

TABLE 14.2. *Continued.*

Study	Drug (n)	Bypass Temperature	Oxygenator	Relevant Findings
Oksenhendler et al. 1987 (304)	Ceftriaxone 2 g *i.v.* (15) at induction	NA	NA	Free fraction ↓ 61% at start of CPB. V_D↑ and $t_{1/2}\beta$↑ relative to normal values. Effective antibiotic concentration maintained throughout surgery.
Klamerus et al. 1988 (305)	Vancomycin 1 gm + Netilmicin 3 mg·kg^{-1} *i.v.* (10)	27°C	Shiley S-100A HED	Renal Cl decreased during CPB. At onset of CPB [VANCO] ↓ 17% [NETIL] ↓ 29%. [NETIL] rebounded over time during CPB. [VANCO] ↑ with removal of aortic cross-clamp.
van der Starre et al. 1988 (306)	Group 1: Cefamandole 30 mg·kg^{-1} at induction (11) Group 2: Cefamandole 30 mg·kg^{-1} at induction + 15 mg·kg^{-1} just before CPB (11)	28°C	NA	[CEFAM] ↑ with supplemental dose before CPB. Unacceptable levels in 6/11 patients in Group 1.
Weiner et al. 1988 (24)	Cefamandole 20 mg·kg^{-1} *i.v.* midnight day before surgery, 0600 hr, and just before CPB Group 1: Pulsatile perfusion (6) Group 2: Non pulsatile perfusion (6)	NA	NA	[CEFAM] adequate during CPB in both groups but higher in pulsatile perfusion group. $t_{1/2}\beta$↓ in nonpulsatile group.
Wilson et al. 1988 (307)	Group 1: Teicoplanin 400 mg *i.v.* (23) at induction + 200 mg *i.v.* 24 hr postop Group 2: Flucloxacillin 500 mg *i.v.* at induction and q6hr × 5 days + Tobramycin 1.5 mg·kg^{-1} *i.v.* (9) Group 3: Teicoplanin 400 mg *i.v.* at induction, end CPB, 24 hr (10) + PK study + tissue penetration study	NA	NA	Teicoplanin dose used in Group 1 produced inadequate [TEI] levels at 24 hr. No dose effective to achieve adequate [TEI] in fat tissue. [TEI] $t_{1/2}\beta$↑ after CPB. Inadequate [FLU] in some patients.
Jungbluth et al. 1989 (113)	Ceftriaxone 14 mg·kg^{-1} *i.v.* (7) at induction	28°C	Membrane	Free fraction increased post-heparin administration and further increased during CPB. Cl↑, V_D↑, $t_{1/2}\beta$↑ relative to previously reported normal values.
LeHot et al. 1989 (308)	Oxacillin 50 mg·kg^{-1} + Group 1: Tobramycin 1 mg·kg^{-1} (30) Group 2: Tobramycin 2 mg·kg^{-1} (15)	25°C	Bentley BOS10 Bubble	No uptake of either agent by oxygenator. [OX] adequate. [TOB] adequate in high dose only group.
Lippert et al. 1989 (309)	Gentamicin 80 mg *i.v.* + Cefuroxime 1.5 g *i.v.* at skin incision and repeated at 3 hr then before midnight, then q8hr (8)	28°C	NA	$t_{1/2}\beta$ not different during CPB *vs.* post-CPB. Adequate levels achieved.
Mini et al. 1989 (310)	Teicoplanin 600 mg *i.v.* (18) 1.5 hr pre-skin incision	25°C	NA	No change in pharmacokinetics with CPB. Adequate concentrations maintained.
Sue et al. 1989 (311)	Cefazolin 1 g *i.v.* at induction + 1 g in Prime (8)	NA	NA	$t_{1/2}\beta$ increased post-CPB. No correlation between amount of chest tube drainage and serum levels of antibiotic.
Wilson et al. 1989 (312)	Teicoplanin 12 mg·kg^{-1} *i.v.* at induction and 200 mg *i.v.* at 24 hr (10)	NA	NA	Effective concentrations achieved in plasma/fat/skin. [TEI] maintained on CPB at 40–50% of pre-CPB levels.
LeHot et al. 1990 (313)	Cefazolin 25 mg·kg^{-1} *i.v.* at induction and q8hr × 48 hr + Netilmicin 2 mg·kg^{-1} *i.v.* at induction and 1 mg·kg^{-1} q8hr × 48 hr (10)	28°C	Bentley BOS10 Bubble	Cefazolin kinetics not different during *vs.* post-CPB. Netilmicin $t_{1/2}\beta$↑ V_D↑ Cl↓ during CPB. [CEFAZ] ↓ 28% and [NET] ↓ 30% at start of CPB. Therapeutic levels achieved intraop.
Mertes et al. 1990 (314)	Group 1: Ciprofloxacin 400 mg *i.v.* at 12, 6, 3, or 1 hr preop, or arrival in OR, or induction, or incision (18) Group 2: Ciprofloxacin 750 mg *p.o.* q12hr × 48 hr + 400 mg *i.v.* as for Group 1 (18)	28°C	Shiley S100A Membrane	[CIPRO] ↑ with multiple dose regimen. Good penetration to myocardium and valve tissue but poor penetration to fat.
Kullberg et al. 1991 (315)	Cloxacillin 1 g *i.v.* at induction + 1 g in Prime (10)	26°C	Sarns Hollow Fibre Membrane	Adequate levels achieved during but not post-CPB.
Lonsky et al. 1992 (316)	Group 1: Oxacillin 2 g *i.v.* (15) Group 2: Cefazolin 1 g *i.v.* (15) during induction and at end of CPB	28°C	Polystan Venotherm Bubble	[OX] subtherapeutic at 180 min and [CEFAZ] at 150 min. Duration of CPB extended beyond the effective duration of antibiotic coverage.
Pryka et al. 1993 (317)	Ciprofloxacin 300 mg *i.v.* at 1. 24 hr preop 2. during surgery 3. 48–72 hr postop (5)	23°C	Sarns S-100 HED Membrane	Cl↓, V_D↓ during surgery.

(continued)

TABLE 14.2. *Continued.*

Study	Drug (n)	Bypass Temperature	Oxygenator	Relevant Findings
Menges et al. 1997 (318)	Group 1: Cefamandole 2 g i.v. before incision (24) Group 2: Cefamandole 2 g at induction + 2 g 10 min before aortic cannulation (22) Group 3: Cefamandole 4 g before incision (23)	NA	NA	Supplementation of dose before CPB maintained therapeutic concentrations in blood and tissue until first postop day.
		Digitalis glycosides		
Beall et al. 1963 (319)	Digoxin 1 mg i.v. (10) 6 hr preop	NA	Bubble diffusion Rotating disc	Digoxin present in oxygenator blood post-CPB. No change in myocardial digoxin levels but plasma levels decreased after CPB.
Ebert et al. 1963 (320)	Digoxin 1 mg i.m. day before surgery (8) Children with CHD	NA	NA	Right atrial concentration reduced post-CPB by 15%. Digoxin found in CPB blood post-CPB.
Hernandez et al. 1963 (321)	Digoxin 0.033 mg·kg^{-1} over 24 hr beginning 48 hr preop then 20% maintenance dose in next 24 hr preop (9) Children with CHD	NA	NA	[DIG] in atrial tissue unchanged post-CPB. Digoxin not present in CPB solution postop, i.e., no washout of digoxin evident.
Coltart et al. 1971 (114)	Digoxin 0.25–0.75 mg chronically. D/C 24 hr preop. (11)	28°C	Rygg or Baxter or Kay-Cross	[DIG] lower after CPB. Clearance decreased during CPB. Only small amounts lost to the oxygenator prime.
Morrison et al. 1973 (322)	Digoxin (20) Digitoxin (4) chronic administration	28°C	Bentley Temptrol	Plasma levels post-bypass exceeded pre-CPB levels over a 3–21 hr period. Digoxin toxic arrhythmias coincided with peak concentrations and correlated to high levels before, during, and after CPB.
Krasula et al. 1974 (323)	Group 1: Recent: Digoxin 0.046 mg·kg^{-1} over 18 hr 2–5 days preop then 25% of dose for 1–2 days (18) Group 2: Maintenance: Digoxin 0.013 mg·kg^{-1} D/C 24 hr preop (18) Children with CHD	NA	NA	[DIG] fell on CPB and increased post-CPB. No difference between groups. Atrial appendage concentrations did not change in either group over time but Group 1 levels higher than Group 2 levels. Digoxin clearance reduced post-CPB.
Carruthers et al. 1975 (324)	Group 1: Digoxin 0.25 mg D/C 24 hr preop (8) Group 2: Digoxin 0.25 mg D/C 48 hr preop (8) Group 3: Digoxin 0.5 mg D/C 24 hr preop (8) Group 4: Digoxin 0.5 mg D/C 48 hr preop (8)	NA	Rygg-Kyvsgaard Bubble	[DIG] less if drug stopped 48 vs. 24 hr preop and less in digoxin 0.5 48 hr vs. 0.25 24 hr group. Levels declined at start of CPB and recovered during CPB. Digoxin concentrated in the heart with papillary muscle concentration > atrial muscle. No correlation to plasma level. Atrial levels stable during CPB.
Storstein et al. 1979 (325)	Digitoxin 0.1 mg daily maintenance (14)	NA	NA	[DIGIT] decreased 50% on CPB. Renal clearance reduced. Unbound fraction increased after heparin administration and at start of CPB.
Koren et al. 1984 (10)	Digoxin to achieve 25 ng·mL^{-1} in CPB prime in vitro study	NA	Sci-Med 0800-2A Membrane	No binding of digoxin to CPB apparatus.
		Antiarrhythmic agents		
Morrell and Harrison 1983 (71)	Group 1: Lidocaine 1.5 mg·kg^{-1} (10) Group 2: Lidocaine 2.5 mg·kg^{-1} (9) Group 3: Lidocaine 3.5 mg·kg^{-1} (5) during hypothermic CPB	28°C	Polystan Venotherm VT 5000 Bubble	60% of patients receiving lowest dose had subtherapeutic [LID] within 2 min. 90% of patients receiving 2.5 mg.min^{-1} had subtherapeutic [LID] at 30 min. At highest dose, [LID] > 1.5 μg·mL^{-1} for 20 min. $t_{1/2}\beta$, V_D were doubled relative to previously reported values. Cl was the same.
Holley et al. 1984 (107)	Lidocaine 100 mg Group 1: Preop, 15 min postop, 1 day post-CPB (5) Group 2: Preop and days 3 and 7 postop (5) + 3 patients from Group 1 at 3 days	27°C	Harvey H-1500	No change in PK parameters post-CPB in Group 1. In Group 2, 3 days postop Cl↓ to 58%, V_{Dss}↓ to 60%. Recovered by day 7. No change in $t_{1/2}\beta$. Lidocaine free fraction fell from 30 to 16% at day 3 and remained low at day 7. α_1 acid glycoprotein levels increased 200% at day 3.
Garfunkel et al. 1987 (75)	Quinidine 200 mg bolus + 30 μg·kg^{-1}·min^{-1} postop (1)	NA	NA	Increased α_1 acid glycoprotein levels led to decreased free quinidine levels in spite of adequate/toxic total levels.
Schiavello et al. 1988 (84)	Lidocaine 2 mg·kg^{-1} at induction of anesthesia and again during CPB (10)	25°C	Harvey H-1500 Bubble	During CPB, Cl↑ and V_{Dss}↑.

(continued)

TABLE 14.2. *Continued.*

Study	Drug (n)	Bypass Temperature	Oxygenator	Relevant Findings
Landow et al. 1990 (72)	Lidocaine 1.5 mg·kg^{-1} bolus 10 s before release of the aortic cross-clamp then 2 mg·min^{-1} for 6 hr (28)	27°C	Maxima 5K 1380 or BOS CM 50 or M-2000 or Terumo 5.4	Free [LID] within therapeutic window, although total [LID] below therapeutic range from 30–120 min.
Landow and Wilson 1991 (73)	Lidocaine 1.5 mg·kg^{-1} bolus 10 s before release of aortic cross-clamp, 5 mg.min^{-1} for 1 hr then 2 mg.min^{-1} for 23 hr (10)	27°C	Maxima SK 1380 or BOS CM 50 or M-2000 or Terumo 5.4	Infusion regimen resulted in more patients with total [LID] consistently in therapeutic range. Free [LID] at therapeutic range.
		Vasodilator agents		
Dasta et al. 1983 (5)	Group 1: Nitroglycerin 100 μg·mL^{-1} to prime solution (1) Group 2: Nitroglycerin 100 μg·mL^{-1} at 90 mL.hr^{-1} added to oxygenator prime (1) *in vitro* study	32°C	Cobe Optiflo II Bubble	Significant uptake of nitroglycerin by CPB circuit, mostly by the oxygenator (65%) first pass uptake.
Kramer and Romagnoli 1984 (59)	Papaverine 1 mg·kg^{-1} Group 1: Vascular surgery (6) Group 2: Cardiac surgery (5)	NA	NA	$t_{1/2}\beta$ doubled in cardiac surgical group.
Moore et al. 1985 (17)	Nitroprusside 0.45 mg·kg^{-1}·hr^{-1} into oxygenator (6)	25°C	Bentley BOS-10 Bubble	Nonenzymatic conversion to cyanide unaffected by hypothermic CPB but enzymatic conversion of cyanide to thiocyanate delayed. Recovered with rewarming.
Dasta et al. 1986 (326)	Nitroglycerin 200 μg·mL^{-1} (7)	27°C	Bentley BOS-10S Bubble	Cl↑ 20% during CPB.
Katz et al. 1990 (327)	Nifedipine 10–20 mg chronically (10) + *in vitro* study	23°C	Shiley M2000 Membrane	[NIF] fell during CPB. Subtherapeutic in some patients pre- and at end of CPB. Not bound to oxygenator.
Booth et al. 1991 (6)	Nitroglycerin 5 mg·mL^{-1} *in vitro* study	25°C or 37°C	Bentley Spiraflow BOS-10S Bubble (4) or Maxima Hollow Fibre Membrane (4) or COBE CML Membrane (3)	Nitroglycerin uptake by oxygenator substantial: BOS-10S 67%; Cobe 47%; Maxima 21%. No effect of temperature.
Finegan et al. 1992 (328)	Diltiazem 60 or 90 mg day before surgery and day of surgery (10)	NA	NA	Dose dependent pharmacokinetics. [DIL]↓ 50% at start of CPB. Free fraction ↑ on CPB. Metabolite levels unchanged during CPB.
Booth et al. 1994 (329)	Group 1: Nitroglycerin 0.5 μg·kg^{-1}·min^{-1} pre- and post-CPB + 5 μg·kg^{-1}·min^{-1} during CPB (12) Group 2: Nitroglycerin 0.5 μg·kg^{-1}·min^{-1} Normothermic CPB (8) Group 3: Nitroglycerin 0.5 μg·kg^{-1}·min^{-1} pre- and post-CPB + 1 μg·kg^{-1}·min^{-1} during CPB Hypothermic (8)	NA	COBE CML Membrane	During hypothermic CPB [TNG]↑ Cl↓ Gender differences measured. TNG metabolism is impaired by hypothermia.
		Glucocorticoid agents		
Thompson et al. 1982 (330)	Group 1: Methylprednisolone 30 mg·kg^{-1} (10) Group 2: Saline (10) at induction and just before CPB	NA	NA	Methylprednisolone plasma levels maintained by second dose.
Kong et al. 1990 (331)	Group 1: Methylprednisolone Hemisuccinate 1.7–2.4 g in cardioplegic solution (6) Group 2: Control 50 mg (60)	28°C	Membrane(5) Bubble(1)	Converted to methylprednisolone rapidly. Methylprednisolone pharmacokinetics: Cl 181 mL·hr^{-1}·kg^{-1}; V_D 1.3 L.kg^{-1}; $t_{1/2}\beta$ 7.9 hr. As compared with normals, Cl↓ 50%, V_D unchanged, and $t_{1/2}\beta$ doubled.
		Miscellaneous		
Larach et al. 1987 (332)	Dantrolene 2.6 mg·kg^{-1} Child with CHD (1) + *in vitro* binding study	32°C	Bentley BOS-2S Bubble	[DAN] fell 54% on initiation of CPB to subtherapeutic levels. No binding to CPB circuit demonstrated.
Comunale et al. 1991 (333)	Dantrolene 2.5 mg·kg^{-1} (1)	28°C	COBE Membrane	[DAN] fell 17% on initiation of CPB. Therapeutic levels maintained.

(continued)

TABLE 14.2. *Continued.*

Study	Drug (n)	Bypass Temperature	Oxygenator	Relevant Findings
Hynynen et al. 1992 (334)	Atrial natriuretic factor 50 μg during CPB (5)	29°C	Shiley S100A Bubble	$t_{1/2}\beta$ = 14 min Cl = 3.8 $L.min^{-1}$ Urine output ↑ Relative to normal subjects $t_{1/2}\beta$↑ and Cl↓
Bennett-Guerrero et al. 1996 (335)	Aprotinin 2 × 10⁶ units at incision + 0.5 × 10⁶ units·hr⁻¹ for 4 hr on initiation of CPB + 2 × 10⁶ units added to CPB Prime (14)	28°C	Membrane	Therapeutic concentration achieved and maintained.
Bennett-Guerrero et al. 1997 (336)	Epsilon aminocaproic acid 150 mg·kg⁻¹ on incision + 30 mg·kg⁻¹ for 4 hr on initiation of CPB (27)	28°	Membrane	Therapeutic concentration achieved and maintained.

NB, unless otherwise indicated; all concentration are total drug concentrations; NA, Not available in methods of cited reference; [ ], plasma concentration of drug; CPB, cardiopulmonary bypass; CO, cardiac output; HR, heart rate; SVR, systemic vascular resistance; PVR, pulmonary vascular resistance; MAP, mean arterial pressure; $t_{1/2}\beta$, terminal elimination half-time; Cl, drug clearance; V_D, volume of distribution; V_{Dss}, volume of distribution at steady state plasma concentrations of drug; Cp_{50}, plasma concentration at which response to given stimulus abolished in 50% of patients; CHD, congenital heart disease; CACI, computer assisted continous infusion; ICU, intensive care unit; IPPV, intermittent positive pressure ventilation; PAP, pulmonary artery pressure; EEG, electroencephalogram; BP, blood pressure; OR, operating room; PK, pharmacokinetic.

ance. Changes in pH, for example due to blood gas management, are more likely to affect fentanyl and sufentanil concentrations. There is little (no) dose-response relationship for suppression of responses to noxious stimuli, and concomitant adjuvant agents are required to control hemodynamics. It is possible to develop pharmacokinetic models for use during cardiac surgery so as to permit use of computer-driven infusions. Significant binding of opioids to CPB apparatus (oxygenator) occurs but is of limited clinical importance other than during initiation of CPB due to rapid redistribution of drug from peripheral storage sites. To prevent a reduction in opioid levels at the time of initiation of CPB (which appears to be a period of risk for development of patient awareness during the surgical procedure), it is recommended that anesthetic levels are supplemented at this time point.

Volatile Anesthetic Agents

In general, washin and washout of volatile anesthetic agents are rapid, slower at hypothermic temperatures, and may be affected by the type of oxygenator used. This is of possible clinical relevance only at the initiation and termination of CPB when the possibility of awareness under anesthesia or the myocardial depressant effects of volatile agents may become an issue. For initiation of CPB, overpressurization with high inspired anesthetic concentrations and with high gas flows may increase the anesthetic level more rapidly. At termination of CPB, sufficient time should be allowed for volatile agent levels to diminish to reduce the myocardial depressant effects yet still maintain adequate levels of anesthesia to prevent awareness. It may be necessary to supplement anesthetic levels with the use of adjuvant anesthetic agents at this time.

Intravenous Anesthetic Agents

Studies of changes in pharmacokinetic parameters of intravenous anesthetic agents mirror those observed for the opioids, that is, reductions in total drug concentrations at initiation of CPB with rapid readjustment of free drug levels to approach those present before initiation of CPB and reductions in drug clearance and increased volume of distribution, leading to an increased elimination half-time (and drug effect) after termination of CPB. As for the opioids, supplementation of the anesthetic may be appropriate just before initiation of CPB to prevent the development of inadequate plasma drug concentrations when CPB is initiated and the impact of hemodilution is maximal. This time period is short (less than 5 min for most agents examined), and the agent chosen to supplement anesthetic levels should be chosen with the overall objective of the anesthetic (e.g., early tracheal extubation, etc.) in mind.

Neuromuscular Receptor Blocking Agents

Review of the studies in Table 14.2 shows the effects of neuromuscular blocking agents to be enhanced by hypothermia. This appears to be due to a synergistic effect of hypothermia itself [a pharmacodynamic effect (16,20,22, 223)] and a pharmacokinetic effect (reduced clearance and contraction of the volume of distribution).

It is perhaps in this class of pharmacologic agents where the most contradictory evidence exists for changes in pharmacokinetics and pharmacodynamics during hypothermic CPB. Examination of Table 14.2 reveals studies where requirements for muscle relaxant are increased (15,224) or reduced (225) for the same agent (pancuronium). Most likely this represents the confounding pharmacodynamic effects of hypothermia on the function of the neuromuscular junction, likely to be variable depending on magnitude and duration of hypothermia (16,20,22). For agents such as atracurium and mivacurium, changes in the level of the metabolizing enzyme cholinesterase may also play an important role (87). The importance of monitoring neuromuscular function by use of a twitch monitor is evident given the changes in function and kinetics demonstrated for this class of drugs.

Inotropic Agents

Because of the thrombocytopenia occasionally observed with the use of amrinone (226), milrinone has become the preferred phosphodiesterase III antagonist most commonly used during cardiac surgery (227). Studies (Table 14.2) suggest that although CPB affects milrinone pharmacokinetics, doses should be based on pharmacodynamic considerations. An appropriate infusion regime would be a loading dose of 50 μg·kg^{-1} with a maintenance infusion of 0.5 μg·kg^{-1}/min. One should anticipate the requirement for a vasoconstrictor such as norepinephrine to sustain the systemic blood pressure.

β-Adrenergic Receptor Blocking Agents

The importance of maintaining chronic β-adrenergic receptor blocking agent therapy is illustrated by the study of Sill et al. (228). Adverse hemodynamic responses may be associated with acute beta-blockade withdrawal. As a rule, plasma concentrations of beta-receptor blocking drugs decrease substantially with onset of CPB, likely due to hemodilution. The exception to this rule is esmolol. Plasma esterase activity decreases with hypothermia so that breakdown of esmolol decreases and increased plasma concentrations from "usual" doses may result.

Antibiotics

Infection is a devastating complication after cardiac surgery because it increases morbidity, mortality, and hospital costs. The primary causative bacteria are *Staphylococcus aureus* and *Staphylococcus epidermidis*. Although the choice of prophylactic antibiotic used often reflects the local pattern of antibiotic resistance and surgical preference, it is important to ensure that whatever drug is used as a prophylactic antibiotic achieves and sustains therapeutic serum and tissue levels against these organisms during surgery and CPB. Examination of Table 14.2 reveals that this is not always the case. Failure to achieve therapeutic plasma/serum and tissue levels may be due to inadequate dose or inappropriate timing of an otherwise adequate dose. Agents used for antibacterial prophylaxis during cardiac surgery have been examined in a recent meta-analysis (229). This review determined that prophylaxis was of benefit but could find no difference in efficacy when a short versus long period of prophylaxis (i.e., days) was used or when first- versus second-generation ceph-

alosporins were used. There may be some advantage to the use of cefamandole because it appeared to have better tissue penetration. For most second-generation cephalosporins (e.g., cefazolin, cefamandole), it is recommended that the dose given at initiation of anesthesia is supplemented before or on initiation of CPB.

Digitalis Glycosides

Results of studies listed in Table 14.2 suggest that provided digoxin is continued until the day of surgery, adequate tissue levels are sustained during CPB.

Antidysrhythmic Agents

Lidocaine is frequently administered during cardiac surgery, usually just before release of the aortic cross-clamp, to prevent ventricular ectopy. Review of data in Table 14.2 suggests that the bolus dose of lidocaine administered should be increased (from 1.5 to 2.5 mg·kg^{-1}) to ensure therapeutic levels are achieved. If an infusion is subsequently initiated, the free drug concentration may decline over time despite adequate total drug levels due to enhanced protein binding by the acute phase reactant protein α_1-acid glycoprotein. This effect appears to be maximal at 3 days in uncomplicated cases. If ectopy occurs during this time period, an increase in infusion rate is warranted.

Vasodilator Agents

For most volatile agents identified in Table 14.2, whereas significant uptake by the oxygenator can be demonstrated in vitro, this appears to be of little clinical significance in vivo.

Glucocorticoid Agents

Glucocorticoid administration may have a role to play in ameliorating the stress response associated with CPB (32,230–233). Pharmacokinetic studies suggest that methylprednisolone hemisuccinate is rapidly converted to the active agent methylprednisolone even during CPB (Table 14.2). It may be necessary to supplement the dose before CPB, although this requires further study.

SUMMARY AND CONCLUSIONS

This chapter reviews some basic pharmacologic concepts of pharmacokinetics and pharmacodynamics. The potential role of hypothermia and CPB in altering drug disposition and action has been examined and relevant studies presented. Understanding of these concepts and potential for alteration by CPB allows the appropriate adjustment in drug regimes to prevent unwanted complications, including inadequate levels of anesthesia, infectious complications, and arrhythmias. Further work to elucidate the role of ameliorating the SIRS occurring during surgery and CPB and its effects on drug pharmacokinetics and pharmacodynamics is required.

KEY POINTS

- Pharmacokinetics is the description, usually in mathematical terms, of the processes involved in handling a drug once it is introduced into the body.
  - Volume of distribution
  - Clearance
  - Elimination half-time
  - Hepatic extraction ratio
- Pharmacodynamics is the description of how a drug reacts with the body to produce its effects.
  - Receptors
  - Second messengers
  - CPB-induced changes
- Pharmacokinetic changes are induced by
  - hemodilution
  - hypothermia
  - perfusion
  - acid-base status
  - sequestration
- Pharmacodynamic properties are changed by
  - binding (to tissue, proteins, apparatus)
  - age
  - tissue penetration
  - temperature
  - receptor density
  - acid-base status
  - anesthetic agents.
- Specific drugs with CPB influenced properties
  - Opioids: concentrations decrease with onset of CPB but free drug concentrations rapidly return toward baseline during CPB.
  - Neuromuscular blocking drugs: effects markedly influenced by hypothermia.
  - Antibiotics: variable tissue penetration.
  - Lidocaine: higher loading dose is indicated (2.5 mg/kg).

REFERENCES

1. Holley FO, Ponganis KV, Stanski DR. Effect of cardiopulmonary bypass on the pharmacokinetics of drugs. *Clin Pharmacokinet* 1982;7:234–251.
2. Buylaert WA, Herregods LL, Mortier EP, et al. Cardiopulmonary bypass and the pharmacokinetics of drugs: an update. *Clin Pharmacokinet* 1989;17:10–26.
3. Hall R. The pharmacokinetic behaviour of opioids administered during cardiac surgery. *Can J Anaesth* 1991;38:747–756.
4. Gedney JA, Ghosh S. Pharmacokinetics of analgesics, sedatives and anaesthetic agents during cardiopulmonary bypass. *Br J Anaesth* 1995;75:344–351.
5. Dasta JF, Jacobi J, Wu LS, et al. Loss of nitroglycerin to cardiopulmonary bypass apparatus. *Crit Care Med* 1983;11:50–52.
6. Booth BP, Henderson M, Milne B, et al. Sequestration of glyceryl trinitrate (nitroglycerin) by cardiopulmonary bypass oxygenators. *Anesth Analg* 1991;72:493–497.
7. Hynynen M, Olkkola KT, Näveri E, et al. Thiopentone pharmacokinetics during cardiopulmonary bypass with a nonpulsatile or pulsatile flow. *Acta Anaesthesiol Scand* 1989;33:554–560.
8. Hickey S, Gaylor JDS, Kenny GNC. In vitro uptake and elimination of isoflurane by different membrane oxygenators. *J Cardiothorac Vasc Anesth* 1996;10:352–355.
9. Stern RC, Weiss CI, Steinbach JH, et al. Isoflurane uptake and elimination are delayed by absorption of anesthetic by the Scimed membrane oxygenator. *Anesth Analg* 1989;69:657–662.
10. Koren G, Crean P, Klein J, et al. Sequestration of fentanyl by the cardiopulmonary bypass (CPBP). *Eur J Clin Pharmacol* 1984;27:51–56.
11. Hynynen M. Binding of fentanyl and alfentanil to the extracorporeal circuit. *Acta Anaesthesiol Scand* 1987;31:706–710.
12. Rosen D, Rosen K, Davidson B, et al. Fentanyl uptake by the Scimed membrane oxygenator. *J Cardiothorac Anesth* 1988;2:619–626.
13. Hynynen M, Hammarén E, Rosenberg PH. Propofol sequestration within the extracorporeal circuit. *Can J Anaesth* 1994;41:583–588.
14. Antognini JF. Hypothermia eliminates isoflurane requirements at 20 C. *Anesthesiology* 1993;78:1152–1156.
15. d'Hollander AA, Duvaldestin P, Henzel D, et al. Variations in pancuronium requirement, plasma concentration, and urinary excretion induced by cardiopulmonary bypass with hypothermia. *Anesthesiology* 1983;58:505–509.
16. Buzello W, Pollmaecher T, Schluermann D, et al. The influence of hypothermic cardiopulmonary bypass on neuromuscular transmission in the absence of muscle relaxants. *Anesthesiology* 1986;64:279–281.
17. Moore RA, Geller EA, Gallagher JD, et al. Effect of hypothermic cardiopulmonary bypass on nitroprusside metabolism. *Clin Pharmacol Ther* 1985;37:680–683.
18. Koren G, Barker C, Goresky G, et al. The influence of hypothermia on the disposition of fentanyl—human and animal studies. *Eur J Clin Pharmacol* 1987;32:373–376.
19. McAllister RG Jr, Bourne DW, Tan TG, et al. Effects of hypothermia on propranolol kinetics. *Clin Pharmacol Ther* 1979;25:1–7.
20. Heier T, Caldwell JE, Sessler DI, et al. The relationship between adductor pollicis twitch tension and core, skin, and muscle temperature during nitrous oxide-isoflurane anesthesia in humans. *Anesthesiology* 1989;71:381–384.
21. Diefenbach C, Abel M, Buzello W. Greater neuromuscular blocking potency of atracurium during hypothermic than during normothermic cardiopulmonary bypass. *Anesth Analg* 1992;75:675–678.
22. Mills GH, Khan ZP, Moxham J, et al. Effects of temperature on phrenic nerve and diaphragmatic function during cardiac surgery. *Br J Anaesth* 1997;79:726–732.
23. Mathie RT, Ohri SK, Batten JJ, et al. Hepatic blood flow during cardiopulmonary bypass operations: the effect of temperature and pulsatility. *J Thorac Cardiovasc Surg* 1997;114:292–293.
24. Weiner B, Melby MJ, Faraci PA, et al. Cefamandol pharmacokinetics during standard and pulsatile cardiopulmonary bypass. *J Clin Pharmacol* 1988;28:655–659.
25. Hornick P, Taylor K. Pulsatile and nonpulsatile perfusion: the continuing controversy. *J Cardiothorac Vasc Anesth* 1997;11:310–315.

26. Schranz D, Droege A, Broede A, et al. Uncoupling of human cardiac β-adrenoceptors during cardiopulmonary bypass with cardioplegic cardiac arrest. *Circulation* 1993;87:422–426.

27. Mantz J, Marty J, Pansard Y, et al. β-Adrenergic receptor changes during coronary artery bypass grafting. *J Thorac Cardiovasc Surg* 1990;99:75–81.

28. Smiley RM, Pantuck CB, Chadburn A, et al. Down-regulation and desensitization of the β-adrenergic receptor system of human lymphocytes after cardiac surgery. *Anesth Analg* 1993;77:653–661.

29. Schwinn DA, McIntyre RW, Hawkins ED, et al. α₁-Adrenergic responsiveness during coronary artery bypass surgery: effect of preoperative ejection fraction. *Anesthesiology* 1988;69:206–217.

30. Waxman K. Shock: ischemia, reperfusion, and inflammation. *New Horiz* 1996;4:153–160.

31. Wan S, LeClerc J-L, Vincent J-L. Inflammatory response to cardiopulmonary bypass: mechanisms involved and possible therapeutic strategies. *Chest* 1997;112:676–692.

32. Hall RI, Stafford Smith M, Rocker G. The systemic inflammatory response to cardiopulmonary bypass: pathophysiological, therapeutic, and pharmacological considerations. Anesth Analg 1997;85:766–782.

33. Hill GE. Cardiopulmonary bypass-induced inflammation: is it important? *J Cardiothorac Vasc Anesth* 1998;12[Suppl 1]:21–25.

34. Hug CC Jr, Burm AGL, deLange S. Alfentanil pharmacokinetics in cardiac surgical patients. *Anesth Analg* 1994;78:231–239.

35. Morgan DJ, Crankshaw DP, Prideaux PR, et al. Thiopentone levels during cardiopulmonary bypass. Changes in plasma protein binding during continuous infusion. *Anaesthesia* 1986;41:4–10.

36. Dawson PJ, Bjorksten AR, Blake DW, et al. The effects of cardiopulmonary bypass on total and unbound plasma concentrations of propofol and midazolam. *J Cardiothorac Vasc Anesth* 1997;11:556–561.

37. Kumar K, Crankshaw DP, Morgan DJ, et al. The effect of cardiopulmonary bypass on plasma protein binding of alfentanil. *Eur J Clin Pharmacol* 1988;35:47–52.

38. Hilgenberg JC. Intraoperative awareness during high-dose fentanyl-oxygen anesthesia. *Anesthesiology* 1981;54:341–343.

39. Thomson IR, Hudson RJ, Rosenbloom M, et al. A randomized double-blind comparison of fentanyl and sufentanil anaesthesia for coronary artery surgery. *Can J Anaesth* 1987;34:227–232.

40. Hall RI, Thomas BL, Hug CC Jr. Pharmacokinetics and pharmacodynamics during cardiac surgery and cardiopulmonary bypass. In: Mora CT, ed. *Cardiopulmonary bypass: principles and techniques of extracorporeal circulation.* New York: Springer-Verlag, 1995:55–87.

41. Boxenbaum HG, Riegelman S, Elashoff RM. Statistical estimates in pharmacokinetics. *J Pharmacokinet Biopharm* 1974;2:123–148.

42. Bailey JM, Schwieger IM, Hug CC Jr. Evaluation of sufentanil anesthesia obtained by a computer-controlled infusion for cardiac surgery. *Anesth Analg* 1993;76:247–252.

43. Flezzani P, Alvis MJ, Jacobs JR, et al. Sufentanil disposition during cardiopulmonary bypass. *Can J Anaesth* 1987;34:566–569.

44. Doi M, Gajraj RJ, Mantzaridis H, et al. Effects of cardiopulmonary bypass and hypothermia on electroencephalographic variables. *Anaesthesia* 1997;52:1048–1055.

45. Hughes MA, Glass PSA, Jacobs JR. Context-sensitive half-time in multicompartment pharmacokinetic models for intravenous anesthetic drugs. *Anesthesiology* 1992;76:334–341.

46. Wrighton SA, Stevens JC. The human hepatic cytochromes P450 involved in drug metabolism. *Crit Rev Toxicol* 1992;22:1–21.

47. Park GR, Pichard L, Tinel M, et al. What changes metabolism in critically ill patients? Two preliminary studies in isolated human hepatocytes. *Anaesthesia* 1994;49:188–191.

48. Park GR, Miller E, Navapurkar V. What changes drug metabolism in critically ill patients? II. Serum inhibits the metabolism of midazolam in human microsomes. *Anaesthesia* 1996;51:11–15.

49. Chen TL, Ueng TH, Chen SH, et al. Human cytochrome P450 mono-oxygenase system is suppressed by propofol. *Br J Anaesth* 1995;74:558–562.

50. Chen TL, Wang MJ, Huang CH, et al. Difference between in vivo and in vitro effects of propofol on defluorination and metabolic activities of hamster hepatic cytochrome P450-dependent mono-oxygenases. *Br J Anaesth* 1995;75:462–466.

51. Kharasch ED, Russell M, Mautz D, et al. The role of cytochrome P450 3A4 in alfentanil clearance. Implications for interindividual variability in disposition and perioperative drug interactions. *Anesthesiology* 1997;87:36–50.

52. Palkama VJ, Isohanni MH, Neuvonen P, et al. The effect of intravenous and oral fluconazole on the pharmacokinetics and pharmacodynamics of intravenous alfentanil. *Anesth Analg* 1998;87:190–194.

53. LeGuellec C, Lacarelle B, Villard P-H, et al. Glucuronidation of propofol in microsomal fractions from various tissues and species including humans: effect of different drugs. *Anesth Analg* 1995;81:855–861.

54. Bartkowski RR, Goldberg ME, Larijani GHE, et al. Inhibition of alfentanil metabolism by erythromycin. *Clin Pharmacol Ther* 1989;46:99–102.

55. Guengerich FP, Distlerath LM, Reilly PEB, et al. Human-liver cytochromes P-450 involved in polymorphisms of drug oxidation. *Xenobiotica* 1986;16:367–378.

56. Benet LZ, Øie S, Schwartz JB. Design and optimization of dosage regimens: pharmacokinetic data (Appendix II). In: Hardman JG, Limberd LE, eds. *Goodman and Gilman's the pharmacological basis of therapeutics*, 9th ed. Montreal: McGraw-Hill, 1996:1707–1792.

57. Chauvin M, Bonnet F, Montembault C, et al. The influence of hepatic plasma flow on alfentanil plasma concentration plateaus achieved with an infusion model in humans: measurement of alfentanil hepatic extraction coefficient. *Anesth Analg* 1986;65:999–1003.

58. Scholz J, Steinfath M, Schulz M. Clinical pharmacokinetics of alfentanil, fentanyl and sufentanil. An update. *Clin Pharmacokinet* 1996;31:275–292.

59. Kramer WG, Romagnoli A. Papaverine disposition in cardiac surgery patients and the effect of cardiopulmonary bypass. *Eur J Clin Pharmacol* 1984;27:127–130.

60. Jackson EK. Diuretics. In: Hardman JG, Limberd LE, eds. *Goodman and Gilman's the pharmacological basis of therapeutics*, 9th ed. Montreal: McGraw-Hill, 1996:685–713.

61. Mandell GL, Petri WA Jr. Antimicrobial agents (continued): penicillins, cephalosporins, and other β-lactam antibiotics. In: Hardman JG, Limberd LE, eds. *Goodman and Gilman's the pharmacological basis of therapeutics*, 9th ed. Montreal: McGraw-Hill, 1996:1073–1101.

62. Ross EM. Pharmacodynamics: mechanisms of drug action and the relationship between drug concentration and effect. In: Hardman JG, Limberd LE, eds. *Goodman and Gilman's the pharmacological basis of therapeutics*, 9th ed. Montreal: McGraw-Hill, 1996:29–42.

63. Goodchild CS. GABA receptors and benzodiazepines. *Br J Anaesth* 1993;71:127–133.

64. Pleuvry BJ. Opioid receptors and their relevance to anaesthesia. *Br J Anaesth* 1993;71:119–126.

65. Hayashi Y, Maze M. Alpha₂ adrenoceptor agonists and anaesthesia. *Br J Anaesth* 1993;71:108–118.

66. Schwinn DA. Adrenoceptors as models for G protein-coupled receptors: structure, function and regulation. *Br J Anaesth* 1993; 71:77–85.

67. Daniels S, Smith EB. Effects of general anaesthetics on ligand-gated ion channels. *Br J Anaesth* 1993;71:59–64.

68. Lambert DG. Signal transduction: G proteins and second messengers. *Br J Anaesth* 1993;71:86–95.

69. Barnes PJ, Pedersen S, Busse WW. Efficacy and safety of inhaled corticosteroids: new developments. *Am J Respir Crit Care Med* 1998;157:S1–S53.

70. Kress HG, Tas PWL. Effects of volatile anaesthetics on second messenger Ca^{2+} in neurones and non-muscular cells. *Br J Anaesth* 1993;71:47–58.

71. Morrell DF, Harrison GG. Lignocaine kinetics during cardiopulmonary bypass: optimum dosage and the effects of haemodilution. *Br J Anaesth* 1983;55:1173–1177.

72. Landow L, Wilson J, Heard SO, et al. Free and total lidocaine levels in cardiac surgical patients. *J Cardiothorac Anesth* 1990; 4:340–347.

73. Landow L, Wilson J. An improved lidocaine infusion protocol for cardiac surgical patients. *J Cardiothorac Vasc Anesth* 1991; 5:209–213.

74. Bjorksten AR, Crankshaw DP, Morgan DJ, et al. The effects of cardiopulmonary bypass on plasma concentrations and protein binding of methohexital and thiopental. *J Cardiothorac Anesth* 1988;2:281–289.

75. Garfinkel D, Mamelok RD, Blaschke TF. Altered therapeutic range for quinidine after myocardial infarction and cardiac surgery. *Ann Intern Med* 1987;107:48–50.

76. Hammaren E, Yli-Hankala A, Rosenberg PH, et al. Cardiopulmonary bypass-induced changes in plasma concentrations of propofol and in auditory evoked potentials. *Br J Anaesth* 1996; 77:360–364.

77. Nussmeier NA, Moskowitz GJ, Weiskopf RB, et al. In vitro anesthetic washin and washout via bubble oxygenators: influence of anesthetic solubility and rates of carrier gas inflow and pump blood flow. *Anesth Analg* 1988;67:982–987.

78. Nussmeier NA, Lambert ML, Moskowitz GJ, et al. Washin and washout of isoflurane administered via bubble oxygenators during hypothermic cardiopulmonary bypass. *Anesthesiology* 1989;71:519–525.

79. Russell GN, Wright EL, Fox MA, et al. Propofol-fentanyl anaesthesia for coronary artery surgery and cardiopulmonary bypass. *Anaesthesia* 1989;44:205–208.

80. Ballard BE. Pharmacokinetics and temperature. *J Pharm Sci* 1974;63:1345–1358.

81. Ham J, Miller RD, Benet LZ, et al. Pharmacokinetics and pharmacodynamics of d-tubocurarine during hypothermia in the cat. *Anesthesiology* 1978;49:324–329.

82. Koren G, Barker C, Bohn D, et al. Influence of hypothermia on the pharmacokinetics of gentamicin and theophylline in piglets. *Crit Care Med* 1985;13:844–847.

83. Miller RD, Agoston S, van der Pol F, et al. Hypothermia and the pharmacokinetics and pharmacodynamics of pancuronium in the cat. *J Pharmacol Exp Ther* 1978;207:532–538.

84. Schiavello R, Mezza A, Feo L, et al. Compartmental analysis of lidocaine kinetics during extracorporeal circulation. *J Cardiothorac Anesth* 1988;2:290–296.

85. Flynn PJ, Hughes R, Walton B. Use of atracurium in cardiac surgery involving cardiopulmonary bypass with induced hypothermia. *Br J Anaesth* 1984;56:967–971.

86. Jacobs JR, Croughwell ND, Goodman DK, et al. Effect of hypothermia and sampling site on blood esmolol concentrations. *J Clin Pharmacol* 1993;33:360–365.

87. Diefenbach C, Abel M, Rump AFE, et al. Changes in plasma cholinesterase activity and mivacurium neuromuscular block in response to normothermic cardiopulmonary bypass. *Anesth Analg* 1995;80:1088–1091.

88. Russell D, Royston D, Rees PH, et al. Effect of temperature and cardiopulmonary bypass on the pharmacokinetics of remifentanil. *Br J Anaesth* 1997;79:456–459.

89. Okutani R, Philbin DM, Rosow CE, et al. Effect of hypothermic hemodilutional cardiopulmonary bypass on plasma sufentanil and catecholamine concentrations in humans. *Anesth Analg* 1988;67:667–670.

90. Bentley JB, Conahan TJ III, Cork RC. Fentanyl sequestration in lungs during cardiopulmonary bypass. *Clin Pharmacol Ther* 1983;34:703–706.

91. Caspi J, Klausner JM, Safadi T, et al. Delayed respiratory depression following fentanyl anesthesia for cardiac surgery. *Crit Care Med* 1988;16:238–240.

92. Shanks CA, Ramzan IM, Walker JS, et al. Gallamine disposition in open-heart surgery involving cardiopulmonary bypass. *Clin Pharmacol Ther* 1983;33:792–799.

93. Walker JS, Brown KF, Shanks CA. Alcuronium kinetics in patients undergoing cardiopulmonary bypass surgery. *Br J Clin Pharmacol* 1983;15:237–244.

94. Avram MJ, Shanks CA, Henthorn TK, et al. Metocurine kinetics in patients undergoing operations requiring cardiopulmonary bypass. *Clin Pharmacol Ther* 1987;42:576–581.

95. Schell RM, Kern FH, Greeley WJ, et al. Cerebral blood flow and metabolism during cardiopulmonary bypass. *Anesth Analg* 1993;76:849–865.

96. Skacel M, Knott C, Reynolds F, et al. Extracorporeal circuit sequestration of fentanyl and alfentanil. *Br J Anaesth* 1986;58: 947–949.

97. Marathe PH, Shen DD, Artru AA, et al. Effect of serum protein binding on the entry of lidocaine into brain and cerebrospinal fluid in dogs. *Anesthesiology* 1991;75:804–812.

98. Wood M. Plasma drug binding: implications for anesthesiologists. *Anesth Analg* 1986;65:786–804.

99. Boer F, Bovill JG, Burm AGL, et al. Effect of ventilation on first-pass pulmonary retention of alfentanil and sufentanil in patients undergoing coronary artery surgery. *Br J Anaesth* 1994; 73:458–463.

100. Taeger K, Weninger E, Schmelzer F, et al. Pulmonary kinetics of fentanyl and alfentanil in surgical patients. *Br J Anaesth* 1988; 61:425–434.

101. Roerig DL, Kotrly KJ, Vucins EJ, et al. First pass uptake of fentanyl, meperidine, and morphine in the human lung. *Anesthesiology* 1987;67:466–472.

102. Boer F, Engbers FHM, Bovill JG, et al. First-pass pulmonary retention of sufentanil at three different background concentrations of the opioid. *Br J Anaesth* 1995;74:50–55.

103. Rosen DA, Rosen KR. Elimination of drugs and toxins during cardiopulmonary bypass. *J Cardiothorac Vasc Anesth* 1997;11: 337–340.

104. Stone JG, Damask MC, Khambatta HJ. Is sufentanil removed by blood conservation devices? *J Cardiothorac Anesth* 1988;2: 615–618.

105. Hanowell LH, Eisele JH Jr, Erskine EV. Autotransfusor removal of fentanyl from blood. *Anesth Analg* 1989;69:239–241.

106. Booker PD, Taylor C, Saba G. Perioperative changes in α_1-acid glycoprotein concentrations in infants undergoing major surgery. *Br J Anaesth* 1996;76:365–368.

107. Holley FO, Ponganis KV, Stanski DR. Effects of cardiac surgery with cardiopulmonary bypass on lidocaine disposition. *Clin Pharmacol Ther* 1984;35:617–626.

108. Rowland M. Plasma protein binding and therapeutic drug monitoring. *Ther Drug Monitor* 1980;2:29–37.

109. Routledge PA, Stargel WW, Wagner GS, et al. Increased alpha-

1-acid glycoprotein and lidocaine disposition in myocardial infarction. *Ann Intern Med* 1980;93:701–704.

110. Piafsky KM. Disease-induced changes in plasma binding of basic drugs. *Clin Pharmacokinet* 1980;5:246–262.

111. Piafsky KM, Borgå O, Odar-Cederlöf I, et al. Increased plasma protein binding of propranolol and chlorpromazine mediated by disease-induced elevations of plasma $\alpha 1$ acid glycoprotein. *N Engl J Med* 1978;299:1435–1439.

112. Plachetka JR, Salomon NW, Copeland JG. Plasma propranolol before, during, and after cardiopulmonary bypass. *Clin Pharmacol Ther* 1981;30:745–751.

113. Jungbluth GL, Pasko MT, Beam TR, et al. Ceftriaxone disposition in open-heart surgery patients. *Antimicrob Agents Chemother* 1989;33:850–856.

114. Coltart DJ, Chamberlain DA, Howard MR, et al. Effect of cardiopulmonary bypass on plasma digoxin concentrations. *Br Heart J* 1971;33:334–338.

115. Bender AD. The effect of increasing age on the distribution of peripheral blood flow in man. *J Am Geriatr Soc* 1965;13:192–198.

116. Crooks J, O'Malley K, Stevenson IH. Pharmacokinetics in the elderly. *Clin Pharmacokinet* 1976;1:280–296.

117. Homer TD, Stanski DR. The effect of increasing age on thiopental disposition and anesthetic requirement. *Anesthesiology* 1985;62:714–724.

118. Stanski DR, Maitre PO. Population pharmacokinetics and pharmacodynamics of thiopental: the effect of age revisited. *Anesthesiology* 1990;72:412–422.

119. Avram MJ, Krejcie TC, Henthorn TK. The relationship of age to the pharmacokinetics of early drug distribution: the concurrent disposition of thiopental and indocyanine green. *Anesthesiology* 1990;72:403–411.

120. Minto CF, Schnider TW, Egan TD, et al. Influence of age and gender on the pharmacokinetics and pharmacodynamics of remifentanil. I. Model development. *Anesthesiology* 1997;86:10–23.

121. Minto CF, Schnider TW, Shafer SL. Pharmacokinetics and pharmacodynamics of remifentanil. II. Model application. *Anesthesiology* 1997;86:24–33.

122. Scott JC, Stanski DR. Decreased fentanyl and alfentanil dose requirements with age. A simultaneous pharmacokinetic and pharmacodynamic evaluation. *J Pharmacol Exp Ther* 1987;240:159–166.

123. Mapleson WW. Effect of age on MAC in humans: a meta-analysis. *Br J Anaesth* 1996;76:179–185.

124. Prandota J. Clinical pharmacokinetics of changes in drug elimination in children. *Dev Pharmacol Ther* 1985;8:311–328.

125. Davis PJ, Cook DR, Stiller RL, et al. Pharmacodynamics and pharmacokinetics of high-dose sufentanil in infants and children undergoing cardiac surgery. *Anesth Analg* 1987;66:203–208.

126. Greeley WJ, de Bruijn NP, Davis DP. Sufentanil pharmacokinetics in pediatric cardiovascular patients. *Anesth Analg* 1987;66:1067–1072.

127. den Hollander JM, Hennis PJ, Burm AGL, et al. Alfentanil in infants and children with congenital heart defects. *J Cardiothorac Anesth* 1988;2:12–17.

128. Fiset P, Mathers L, Engstrom R, et al. Pharmacokinetics of computer-controlled alfentanil administration in children undergoing cardiac surgery. *Anesthesiology* 1995;83:944–955.

129. Mathews HML, Carson IW, Lyons SM, et al. A pharmacokinetic study of midazolam in paediatric patients undergoing cardiac surgery. *Br J Anaesth* 1988;61:302–307.

130. Lawless S, Burckart G, Diven W, et al. Amrinone pharmacokinetics in neonates and infants. *J Clin Pharmacol* 1988;28:283–284.

131. Lawless S, Burckart G, Diven W, et al. Amrinone in neonates and infants after cardiac surgery. *Crit Care Med* 1989;17:751–754.

132. Lynn AM, Sorensen GK, Williams GD, et al. Hemodynamic effects of amrinone and colloid administration in children following cardiac surgery. *J Cardiothorac Vasc Anesth* 1993;7:560–565.

133. Williams GD, Sorensen GK, Oakes R, et al. Amrinone loading during cardiopulmonary bypass in neonates, infants, and children. *J Cardiothorac Vasc Anesth* 1995;9:278–282.

134. Böhrer M, Maitre PO, Hung O, et al. Electroencephalographic effects of benzodiazepines. I. Choosing an electroencephalographic parameter to measure the effect of midazolam on the central nervous system. *Clin Pharmacol Ther* 1990;48:544–554.

135. Scott JC, Ponganis KV, Stanski DR. EEG quantitation of narcotic effect: the comparative pharmacodynamics of fentanyl and alfentanil. *Anesthesiology* 1985;62:234–241.

136. Scott JC, Cooke JE, Stanski DR. Electroencephalographic quantitation of opioid effect: comparative pharmacodynamics of fentanyl and sufentanil. *Anesthesiology* 1991;74:34–42.

137. Bührer M, Maitre PO, Crevoisier C, et al. Electroencephalographic effects of benzodiazepines. II. Pharmacodynamic modeling of the electroencephalographic effects of midazolam and diazepam. *Clin Pharmacol Ther* 1990;48:555–567.

138. Shafer SL, Varvel JR. Pharmacokinetics, pharmacodynamics, and rational opioid selection. *Anesthesiology* 1991;74:53–63.

139. Vitez TS, White PF, Eger EI II. Effects of hypothermia on halothane MAC and isoflurane MAC in the rat. *Anesthesiology* 1974;41:80–81.

140. Puig MM, Warner W, Tang CK, et al. Effects of temperature on the interaction of morphine with opioid receptors. *Br J Anaesth* 1987;59:1459–1464.

141. Holmes PEB, Jenden DJ, Taylor DB. The analysis of the mode of action of curare on neuromuscular transmission: the effect of temperature changes. *J Pharmacol* 1951;103:382–402.

142. Buzello W, Schluermann D, Schindler M, et al. Hypothermic cardiopulmonary bypass and neuromuscular blockade by pancuronium and vecuronium. *Anesthesiology* 1985;62:201–204.

143. Smeulers NJ, Wierda JMKH, van den Broek L, et al. Effects of hypothermic cardiopulmonary bypass on the pharmacodynamics and pharmacokinetics of rocuronium. *J Cardiothorac Vasc Anesth* 1995;9:700–705.

144. McDonagh P, Dupuis J-Y, Curran M, et al. Pharmacodynamics of doxacurium during cardiac surgery with hypothermic cardiopulmonary bypass. *Can J Anaesth* 1996;43:134–140.

145. Illievich UM, Zornow MH, Choi KT, et al. Effects of hypothermia or anesthetics on hippocampal glutamate and glycine concentrations after repeated transient global cerebral ischemia. *Anesthesiology* 1994;80:177–186.

146. Doak GJ, Li G, Hall RI, et al. Does hypothermia or hyperventilation affect enflurane MAC reduction following partial cardiopulmonary bypass in dogs? *Can J Anaesth* 1993;40:176–182.

147. Andersen LW, Landow L, Baek L, et al. Association between gastric intramucosal pH and splanchnic endotoxin, antibody to endotoxin, and tumor necrosis factor-α concentrations in patients undergoing cardiopulmonary bypass. *Crit Care Med* 1993;21:210–217.

148. Fiddian-Green RG, Baker S. Predictive value of the stomach wall pH for complications after cardiac operations: comparison with other monitoring. *Crit Care Med* 1987;15:153–156.

149. Hindman BJ. Sodium bicarbonate in the treatment of subtypes of acute lactic acidosis: physiologic considerations. *Anesthesiology* 1990;72:1064–1076.

150. Scheinman MM, Sullivan RW, Hyatt KH. Magnesium metabolism in patients undergoing cardiopulmonary bypass. *Circulation* 1969;39[Suppl I]:I-235–I-241.

151. Lockey E, Longmore DB, Ross DN, et al. Potassium and open-heart surgery. *Lancet* 1966;1:671–675.

152. Romero EG, Castillo-Olivares JL, O'Connor F, et al. The importance of calcium and magnesium ions in serum and cerebrospinal fluid during cardiopulmonary bypass. *J Thorac Cardiovasc Surg* 1973;66:668–672.

153. Moffitt EA, Imrie DD, Scovil JE, et al. Myocardial metabolism and haemodynamic responses with enflurane anesthesia for coronary artery surgery. *Can Anaesth Soc J* 1984;31:604–610.

154. Hall RI, Murphy JT, Moffitt EA, et al. A comparison of the myocardial metabolic and haemodynamic changes produced by propofol-sufentanil and enflurane-sufentanil anaesthesia for patients having coronary artery bypass graft surgery. *Can J Anaesth* 1991;38:996–1004.

155. Hall RI, Murphy JT, Landymore R, et al. Myocardial metabolic and hemodynamic changes during propofol anesthesia for cardiac surgery in patients with reduced ventricular function. *Anesth Analg* 1993;77:680–689.

156. Eskinder H, Rusch NJ, Supan FD, et al. The effects of volatile anesthetics on L- and T-type calcium channel currents in canine cardiac purkinje cells. *Anesthesiology* 1991;74:919–926.

157. Kress HG, Müller J, Eisert A, et al. Effects of volatile anesthetics on cytoplasmic Ca^{2+} signalling and transmitter release in a neural cell line. *Anesthesiology* 1991;74:309–319.

158. Terrar DA. Structure and function of calcium channels and the actions of anaesthetics. *Br J Anaesth* 1993;71:39–46.

159. Franks NP, Lieb WR. Selective actions of volatile general anaesthetics at molecular and cellular levels. *Br J Anaesth* 1993;71:65–76.

160. Hall RI, Sullivan JA. Does cardiopulmonary bypass alter enflurane requirements for anesthesia? *Anesthesiology* 1990;73:249–255.

161. Neumeister MW, Li G, Williams G, et al. Factors influencing MAC reduction after cardiopulmonary bypass in dogs. *Can J Anaesth* 1997;44:1120–1126.

162. Fowler MB, Laser JA, Hopkins GL, et al. Assessment of the β-adrenergic receptor pathway in the intact failing human heart: progressive receptor down-regulation and subsensitivity to agonist response. *Circulation* 1986;74:1290–1302.

163. Packer M. Neurohumoral interactions and adaptations in congestive heart failure. *Circulation* 1988;77:721–730.

164. Colucci WS, Alexander RW, Williams GH, et al. Decreased lymphocyte beta-adrenergic-receptor density in patients with heart failure and tolerance to the beta-adrenergic agonist pirbuterol. *N Engl J Med* 1981;305:185–190.

165. Francis GS, Cohn JN. The autonomic nervous system in congestive heart failure. *Annu Rev Med* 1986;37:235–247.

166. Stafford Smith M, Muir H, Hall R. Perioperative management of drug therapy. *Drugs* 1996;51:238–259.

167. Hart GR, Anderson RJ. Withdrawal syndromes and the cessation of antihypertensive therapy. *Arch Intern Med* 1981;141:1125–1127.

168. Alderman EL, Coltart DJ, Wettach GE, et al. Coronary artery syndromes after sudden propranolol withdrawal. *Ann Intern Med* 1974;81:625–627.

169. Royston D. The inflammatory response and extracorporeal circulation. *J Cardiothorac Vasc Anesth* 1997;11:341–354.

170. Bonser RS, Dave JR, Davies ET, et al. Reduction of complement activation by prime manipulation. *Ann Thorac Surg* 1990;49:279–283.

171. Jansen PGM, Te Velthuis H, Wildevuur WR, et al. Cardiopulmonary bypass with modified gelatin and heparin-coated circuits. *Br J Anaesth* 1996;76:13–19.

172. Dapper F, Neppl H, Wozniak G, et al. Influence of 4 different membrane oxygenators on inflammation-like processes during extracorporeal circulation with pulsatile and non-pulsatile flow. *Eur J Cardiothorac Surg* 1992;6:18–24.

173. Driessen JJ, Dhaese H, Fransen G, et al. Pulsatile compared with nonpulsatile perfusion using a centrifugal pump for cardiopulmonary bypass during coronary bypass grafting. Effects on systemic haemodynamics, oxygenation, and inflammatory response parameters. *Perfusion* 1995;10:31–2.

174. Dutton RC, Edmunds LH, Hutchinson JC, et al. Platelet aggregate emboli produced in patients during cardiopulmonary bypass with membrane and bubble oxygenators. *J Thorac Cardiovasc Surg* 1974;67:258–265.

175. Millar AB, Armstrong L, van der Linden J, et al. Cytokine production and hemofiltration in children undergoing cardiopulmonary bypass. *Ann Thorac Surg* 1993;56:1499–1502.

176. Journois D, Pouard P, Greeley WJ, et al. Hemofiltration during cardiopulmonary bypass in pediatric cardiac surgery: effects on hemostasis, cytokines, and complement components. *Anesthesiology* 1994;81:1181–1189.

177. Journois D, Pouard P, Rolland B, et al. Ultrafiltration allows to reduce cytokine plasma concentrations during pediatric cardiopulmonary bypass. *Contrib Nephrol* 1995;116:86–88.

178. Johnson D, Thomson D, Mycyk T, et al. Depletion of neutrophils by filter during aortocoronary bypass surgery transiently improves postoperative cardiorespiratory status. *Chest* 1995;107:1253–1259.

179. Wang M-J, Chiu I-S, Hsu C-M, et al. Efficacy of ultrafiltration in removing inflammatory mediators during pediatric cardiac operations. *Ann Thorac Surg* 1996;61:651–656.

180. Videm V, Fosse E, Mollnes TE, et al. Complement activation with bubble and membrane oxygenators in aortocoronary bypass grafting. *Ann Thorac Surg* 1990;50:387–391.

181. Butler J, Chong GL, Baigrie RJ, et al. Cytokine responses to cardiopulmonary bypass with membrane and bubble oxygenation. *Ann Thorac Surg* 1992;53:833–838.

182. Gillinov AM, Bator JM, Zehr KJ, et al. Neutrophil adhesion molecule expression during cardiopulmonary bypass with bubble and membrane oxygenators. *Ann Thorac Surg* 1993;56:847–853.

183. Ferries LeRH, Marx JJJ, Ray JFIII. The effect of methylprednisolone on complement activation during cardiopulmonary bypass. *J Extracorp Technol* 1984;16:83–88.

184. Cavarocchi NC, Pluth JR, Schaff HV, et al. Complement activation during cardiopulmonary bypass: comparison of bubble and membrane oxygenators. *J Thorac Cardiovasc Surg* 1986;91:252–258.

185. Clark RE, Beauchamp RA, Magrath RA, et al. Comparison of bubble and membrane oxygenators in short and long perfusions. *J Thorac Cardiovasc Surg* 1979;78:655–666.

186. van Oeveren W, Kazatchkine MD, Descamps-Latscha B, et al. Deleterious effects of cardiopulmonary bypass: a prospective study of bubble versus membrane oxygenation. *J Thorac Cardiovasc Surg* 1985;89:888–899.

187. Nilsson L, Nilsson U, Venge P, et al. Inflammatory system activation during cardiopulmonary bypass as an indicator of biocompatibility: a randomized comparison of bubble and membrane oxygenators. *Scand J Thorac Cardiovasc Surg* 1990;24:53–58.

188. Nilsson L, Tydén H, Johansson O, et al. Bubble and membrane oxygenators-Comparison of postoperative organ dysfunction with special reference to inflammatory activity. *Scand J Thorac Cardiovasc Surg* 1990;24:59–64.

189. Videm V, Fosse E, Mollnes TE, et al. Time for new concepts about measurement of complement activation by cardiopulmonary bypass? *Ann Thorac Surg* 1992;54:725–731.

190. Videm V, Svennevig JL, Fosse E, et al. Reduced complement activation with heparin-coated oxygenator and tubings in coro-

nary bypass operations. *J Thorac Cardiovasc Surg* 1992;103: 806–813.

191. Gu YJ, van Oeveren W, Akkerman C, et al. Heparin-coated circuits reduce the inflammatory response to cardiopulmonary bypass. *Ann Thorac Surg* 1993;55:917–922.

192. Fosse E, Moen O, Johnson E, et al. Reduced complement and granulocyte activation with heparin-coated cardiopulmonary bypass. *Ann Thorac Surg* 1994;58:472–477.

193. Hatori N, Yoshizu H, Haga Y, et al. Biocompatibility of heparin-coated membrane oxygenator during cardiopulmonary bypass. *Artif Organs* 1991;18:904–910.

194. Pekna M, Hagman L, Halden E, et al. Complement activation during cardiopulmonary bypass: effects of immobilized heparin. *Ann Thorac Surg* 1994;58:421–424.

195. Pekna M, Borowiec J, Fagerhol MK, et al. Biocompatibility of heparin-coated circuits used in cardiopulmonary bypass. *Scand J Thorac Cardiovasc Surg* 1994;28:5–11.

196. Sellevold OFM, Berg TM, Rein KA, et al. Heparin-coated circuit during cardiopulmonary bypass. *Acta Anaesth Scand* 1994; 38:373–379.

197. Weerwind PW, Maessen JG, van Tits LJH, et al. Influence of Duraflo II heparin-treated extracorporeal circuits on the systemic inflammatory response in patients having coronary bypass. *J Thorac Cardiovasc Surg* 1995;110:1633–1641.

198. Moen O, Høgåsen K, Fosse E, et al. Attenuation of changes in leukocyte surface markers and complement activation with heparin-coated cardiopulmonary bypass. *Ann Thorac Surg* 1997; 63:105–111.

199. Menasché P, Peynet J, Larivière J, et al. Does normothermia during cardiopulmonary bypass increase neutrophil-endothelium interactions? *Circulation* 1994;90[Part II]:II-275–II-279.

200. Menasché P, Haydar S, Peynet J, et al. A potential mechanism of vasodilation after warm heart surgery: the temperature-dependent release of cytokines. *J Thorac Cardiovasc Surg* 1994; 107:293–299.

201. Ohata T, Sawa Y, Kadoba K, et al. Normothermia has beneficial effects in cardiopulmonary bypass attenuating inflammatory reactions. *ASAIO J* 1995;41:M288–M291.

202. Tönz M, Mihaljevic T, von Segesser LK, et al. Normothermia versus hypothermia during cardiopulmonary bypass: a randomized, controlled trial. *Ann Thorac Surg* 1995;59:137–143.

203. Boldt J, Osmer C, Linke LC, et al. Hypothermic versus normothermic cardiopulmonary bypass: influence on circulating adhesion molecules. *J Cardiothorac Vasc Anesth* 1996;10:342–347.

204. Fann JI, Stevens JH, Pompili MF, et al. Minimally invasive coronary artery bypass grafting. *Curr Opin Cardiol* 1997;12: 482–487.

205. Blick M, Sherwin SA, Rosenblum M, et al. Phase I study of recombinant tumor necrosis factor in cancer patients. *Cancer Res* 1987;47:2986–2989.

206. Smith JW II, Urba WJ, Curti B, et al. The toxic and hematologic effects of interleukin-1 alpha administered in a phase I trial to patients with advanced malignancies. *J Clin Oncol* 1992; 10:1141–1152.

207. Pullicino EA, Carli F, Poole S, et al. The relationship between the circulating concentrations of interleukin 6 (IL-6), tumor necrosis factor (TNF) and the acute phase response to elective surgery and accidental injury. *Lymphokine Res* 1990;9:231–238.

208. Hennein HA, Ebba H, Rodriguez JL, et al. Relationship of the proinflammatory cytokines to myocardial ischemia and dysfunction after uncomplicated coronary revascularisation. *J Thorac Cardiovasc Surg* 1994;108:626–635.

209. Finkel MS, Oddis CV, Jacob TD, et al. Negative inotropic effects of cytokines on the heart mediated by nitric oxide. *Science* 1992;257:387–389.

210. Finkel MS, Hoffman RA, Shen L, et al. Interleukin-6 (IL-6) as a mediator of stunned myocardium. *Am J Cardiol* 1993;71: 1231–1232.

211. Tönz M, Mihaljevic T, von Segesser LK, et al. Acute lung injury during cardiopulmonary bypass: are the neutrophils responsible? *Chest* 1995;108:1551–1556.

212. Sinclair DG, Haslam PL, Quinlan GJ, et al. The effect of cardiopulmonary bypass on intestinal and pulmonary endothelial permeability. *Chest* 1995;108:718–724.

213. Kharazmi A, Andersen LW, Baek L, et al. Endotoxemia and enhanced generation of oxygen radicals by neutrophils from patients undergoing cardiopulmonary bypass. *J Thorac Cardiovasc Surg* 1989;98:381–385.

214. Cavarocchi NC, England MD, Schaff HV, et al. Oxygen free radical generation during cardiopulmonary bypass: correlation with complement activation. *Circulation* 1986;74[Suppl III]: III-130–III-133.

215. Elliott MJ, Finn AHR. Interaction between neutrophils and endothelium. *Ann Thorac Surg* 1993;56:1503–1508.

216. Davies SW, Underwood SM, Wickens DG, et al. Systemic pattern of free radical generation during coronary bypass surgery. *Br Heart J* 1990;64:236–240.

217. Landow L, Phillips DA, Heard SO, et al. Gastric tonometry and venous oximetry in cardiac surgery patients. *Crit Care Med* 1991;19:1226–1233.

218. Hampton WW, Townsend MC, Schirmer WJ, et al. Effective hepatic blood flow during cardiopulmonary bypass. *Arch Surg* 1989;124:458–459.

219. Koska AJ III, Romagnoli A, Kramer WG. Effect of cardiopulmonary bypass on fentanyl distribution and elimination. *Clin Pharmacol Ther* 1981;29:100–105.

220. Stadler J, Bentz BG, Harbrecht BG, et al. Tumor necrosis factor alpha inhibits hepatocyte mitochondrial respiration. *Ann Surg* 1992;216:539–546.

221. Coceani F, Lees J, Mancilla J, et al. Interleukin-6 and tumor necrosis factor in cerebrospinal fluid: changes during pyrogen fever. *Brain Res* 1993;612:165–171.

222. Pollmacher T, Schreiber W, Gudewill S, et al. Influence of endotoxin on nocturnal sleep in humans. *Am J Physiol* 1993; 264:R1077–R1083.

223. Shearer ES, Russell GN. The effect of cardiopulmonary bypass on cholinesterase activity. *Anaesthesia* 1993;48:293–296.

224. Buzello W, Schluermann D, Pollmaecher T, et al. Unequal effects of cardiopulmonary bypass-induced hypothermia on neuromuscular blockade from constant infusion of alcuronium, d-tubocurarine, pancuronium, and vecuronium. *Anesthesiology* 1987;66:842–846.

225. Futter ME, Whalley DG, Wynands JE, et al. Pancuronium requirements during hypothermic cardiopulmonary bypass in man. *Anaesth Intens Care* 1983;11:216–219.

226. Ross MP, Allen-Webb EM, Pappas JB, et al. Amrinone-associated thrombocytopenia: pharmacokinetic analysis. *Clin Pharmacol Ther* 1993;53:661–667.

227. Kikura M, Lee MK, Safon RA, et al. The effects of milrinone on platelets in patients undergoing cardiac surgery. *Anesth Analg* 1995;81:44–48.

228. Sill JC, Nugent M, Moyer TP, et al. Influence of propranolol plasma levels on hemodynamics during coronary artery bypass surgery. *Anesthesiology* 1984;60:455–463.

229. Kreter B, Woods M. Antibiotic prophylaxis for cardiothoracic operations. Metaanalysis of thirty years of clinical trials. *J Thorac Cardiovasc Surg* 1992;104:590–599.

230. Hill GE, Alonso A, Spurzem JR, et al. Aprotinin and methylprednisolone equally blunt cardiopulmonary bypass-induced inflammation in humans. *J Thorac Cardiovasc Surg* 1995;110: 1658–1662.

231. Hill GE, Alonso A, Thiele GM, et al. Glucocorticoids blunt

neutrophil CD11b surface glycoprotein upregulation during cardiopulmonary bypass in humans. *Anesth Analg* 1994;79: 23–27.

232. Hill GE, Snider S, Galbraith TA, et al. Glucocorticoid reduction of bronchial epithelial inflammation during cardiopulmonary bypass. *Am J Respir Crit Care Med* 1995;152:1791–1795.

233. Chaney MA, Nikolov MP, Blakeman B, et al. Pulmonary effects of methylprednisolone in patients undergoing coronary artery bypass grafting and early tracheal extubation. *Anesth Analg* 1998;87:27–33.

234. Lunn JK, Stanley TH, Eisele J, et al. High dose fentanyl anesthesia for coronary artery surgery: plasma fentanyl concentrations and influence of nitrous oxide on cardiovascular responses. *Anesth Analg* 1979;58:390–395.

235. Bovill JG, Sebel PS. Pharmacokinetics of high-dose fentanyl. A study in patients undergoing cardiac surgery. *Br J Anaesth* 1980; 52:795–801.

236. Sprigge JS, Wynands JE, Whalley DG, et al. Fentanyl infusion anesthesia for aortocoronary bypass surgery: Plasma levels and hemodynamic response. *Anesth Analg* 1982;61:972–978.

237. de Lange S, de Bruijn NP. Alfentanil-oxygen anaesthesia: plasma concentrations and clinical effects during variable-rate continuous infusion for coronary artery surgery. *Br J Anaesth* 1983;55: 183S–189S.

238. Wynands JE, Townsend GE, Wong P, et al. Blood pressure response and plasma fentanyl concentrations during high- and very high-dose fentanyl anesthesia for coronary artery surgery. *Anesth Analg* 1983;62:661–665.

239. Koren G, Goresky G, Crean P, et al. Pediatric fentanyl dosing based on pharmacokinetics during cardiac surgery. *Anesth Analg* 1984;63:577–582.

240. Alvis JM, Reves JG, Govier AV, et al. Computer-assisted continuous infusions of fentanyl during cardiac anesthesia: comparison with a manual method. *Anesthesiology* 1985;63:41–49.

241. Fischler M, Levron JC, Trang H, et al. Pharmacokinetics of phenoperidine in patients undergoing cardiopulmonary bypass. *Br J Anaesth* 1985;57:877–882.

242. Koren G, Goresky G, Crean P, et al. Unexpected alterations in fentanyl pharmacokinetics in children undergoing cardiac surgery: age related or disease related? *Dev Pharmacol Ther* 1986; 9:183–191.

243. Newland MC, Leuschen P, Sarafian LB, et al. Fentanyl intermittent bolus technique for anesthesia in infants and children undergoing cardiac surgery. *J Cardiothorac Vasc Anesth* 1989;3: 407–410.

244. Robbins GR, Wynands JE, Whalley DG, et al. Pharmacokinetics of alfentanil and clinical responses during cardiac surgery. *Can J Anaesth* 1990;37:52–57.

245. Kern FH, Ungerleider RM, Jacobs JR, et al. Computerized continuous infusion of intravenous anesthetic drugs during pediatric cardiac surgery. *Anesth Analg* 1991;72:487–492.

246. Mantz J, Abi-Jaoudé F, Ceddaha A, et al. High-dose alfentanil for myocardial revascularization: a hemodynamic and pharmacokinetic study. *J Cardiothorac Vasc Anesth* 1991;5:107–110.

247. den Hollander JM, Hennis PJ, Burm AGL, et al. Pharmacokinetics of alfentanil before and after cardiopulmonary bypass in patients undergoing cardiac surgery: part I. *J Cardiothorac Vasc Anesth* 1992;6:308–312.

248. Cross DA, Nikas D. The effects of carbon dioxide management on plasma levels of fentanyl and sufentanil during hypothermic cardiopulmonary bypass. *J Cardiothorac Vasc Anesth* 1994;8: 649–652.

249. Hodges UM, Berg S, Naik SK, et al. Filtration of fentanyl is not the cause of the elevation of arterial blood pressure with post-bypass ultrafiltration in children. *J Cardiothorac Vasc Anesth* 1994;8:653–657.

250. Petros A, Dunne N, Mehta R, et al. The pharmacokinetics of alfentanil after normothermic and hypothermic cardiopulmonary bypass. *Anesth Analg* 1995;81:458–464.

251. Borenstein M, Shupak R, Barnette R, et al. Cardiovascular effects of different infusion rates of sufentanil in patients undergoing coronary surgery. *Eur J Clin Pharmacol* 1997;51:359–366.

252. Duthie DJR, Stevens JJWM, Doyle AR, et al. Remifentanil and pulmonary extraction during and after cardiac anesthesia. *Anesth Analg* 1997;84:740–744.

253. Loomis CW, Brunet D, Milne B, et al. Arterial isoflurane concentration and EEG burst suppression during cardiopulmonary bypass. *Clin Pharmacol Ther* 1986;40:304–313.

254. Moore RA, McNicholas KW, Gallagher JD, et al. Halothane metabolism in acyanotic and cyanotic patients undergoing open heart surgery. *Anesth Analg* 1986;65:1257–1262.

255. Henderson JM, Nathan HJ, Lalande M, et al. Washin and washout of isoflurane during cardiopulmonary bypass. *Can J Anaesth* 1988;35:587–590.

256. Price SL, Brown DL, Carpenter RL, et al. Isoflurane elimination via bubble oxygenator during extracorporeal circulation. *J Cardiothorac Anesth* 1988;2:41–44.

257. Tarr TJ, Snowdon SL. Blood/gas solubility coefficient and blood concentration of enflurane during normothermic and hypothermic cardiopulmonary bypass. *J Cardiothorac Vasc Anesth* 1991; 5:111–115.

258. Aaltonen L, Kanto J, Arola M, et al. Effect of age and cardiopulmonary bypass on the pharmacokinetics of lorazepam. *Acta Pharmacol Toxicol* 1982;51:126–131.

259. Oduro A, Tomlinson AA, Voice A, et al. The use of etomidate infusions during anaesthesia for cardiopulmonary bypass. *Anaesth* 1983;38[Suppl]:66–69.

260. Boscoe MJ, Dawling S, Thompson MA, et al. Lorazepam in open-heart surgery—plasma concentrations before, during and after bypass following different dose regimens. *Anaesth Intens Care* 1984;12:9–13.

261. Harper KW, Collier PS, Dundee JW, et al. Age and nature of operation influence the pharmacokinetics of midazolam. *Br J Anaesth* 1985;57:866–871.

262. Kanto J, Himberg JJ, Heikkilä H, et al. Midazolam kinetics before, during and after cardiopulmonary bypass surgery. *Int J Clin Pharm Res* 1985;5:123–126.

263. Lowry KG, Dundee JW, McClean E, et al. Pharmacokinetics of diazepam and midazolam when used for sedation following cardiopulmonary bypass. *Br J Anaesth* 1985;57:883–885.

264. Maitre PO, Funk B, Crevoisier C, et al. Pharmacokinetics of midazolam in patients recovering from cardiac surgery. *Eur J Clin Pharmacol* 1989;37:161–166.

265. Boer F, Ros P, Bovill JG, et al. Effect of propofol on peripheral vascular resistance during cardiopulmonary bypass. *Br J Anaesth* 1990;65:184–189.

266. Massey NJA, Sherry KM, Oldroyd S, et al. Pharmacokinetics of an infusion of propofol during cardiac surgery. *Br J Anaesth* 1990;65:475–479.

267. Lehot J-J, Boulieu R, Foussadier A, et al. Comparison of the pharmacokinetics of methohexital during cardiac surgery with cardiopulmonary bypass and vascular surgery. *J Cardiothorac Vasc Anesth* 1993;7:30–34.

268. Lee H-S, Khoo Y-M, Chua B-C, et al. Pharmacokinetics of propofol infusion in Asian patients undergoing coronary artery bypass grafting. *Ther Drug Monitor* 1995;17:336–341.

269. Ng A, Tan SSW, Lee HS, et al. Effect of propofol infusion on the endocrine response to cardiac surgery. *Anaesth Intens Care* 1995;23:543–547.

270. Bailey JM, Mora CT, Shafer SL, et al. Pharmacokinetics of propofol in adult patients undergoing coronary revascularization. *Anesthesiology* 1996;84:1288–1297.

271. McLean RF, Baker AJ, Walker SE, et al. Ketamine concentrations during cardiopulmonary bypass. *Can J Anaesth* 1996;43: 580–584.

272. Denny NM, Kneeshaw JD. Vecuronium and atracurium infusions during hypothermic cardiopulmonary bypass. *Anaesthesia* 1986;41:919–922.

273. Wierda JMKH, van der Starre PJA, Scaf AHJ, et al. Pharmacokinetics of pancuronium in patients undergoing coronary artery surgery with and without low dose dopamine. *Clin Pharmacokinet* 1990;19:491–498.

274. Wierda JMKH, Karliczek GF, Vandenbrom RHG, et al. Pharmacokinetics and cardiovascular dynamics of pipecuronium bromide during coronary artery surgery. *Can J Anaesth* 1990; 37:183–191.

275. Kansanaho M, Hynynen M, Olkkola KT. Model-driven closed-loop feedback infusion of atracurium and vecuronium during hypothermic cardiopulmonary bypass. *J Cardiothorac Vasc Anesth* 1997;11:58–61.

276. Bailey JM, Levy JH, Rogers HG, et al. Pharmacokinetics of amrinone during cardiac surgery. *Anesthesiology* 1991;75: 961–968.

277. Hayashi Y, Sumikawa K, Yamatodani A, et al. Quantitative analysis of pulmonary clearance of exogenous dopamine after cardiopulmonary bypass in humans. *Anesth Analg* 1993;76: 107–112.

278. Bailey JM, Levy JH, Kikura M, et al. Pharmacokinetics of intravenous milrinone in patients undergoing cardiac surgery. *Anesthesiology* 1994;81:616–622.

279. Das PA, Skoyles JR, Sherry KM, et al. Disposition of milrinone in patients after cardiac surgery. *Br J Anaesth* 1994;72:426–429.

280. Butterworth JF, Hines RL, Royster RL, et al. A pharmacokinetic and pharmacodynamic evaluation of milrinone in adults undergoing cardiac surgery. *Anesth Analg* 1995;81:783–792.

281. De Hert S, Moens MM, Jorens PG, et al. Comparison of two different loading doses of milrinone for weaning from cardiopulmonary bypass. *J Cardiothorac Vasc Anesth* 1995;9:264–271.

282. Kikura M, Levy JH, Michelsen LG, et al. The effect of milrinone on hemodynamics and left ventricular function after emergence from cardiopulmonary bypass. *Anesth Analg* 1997;85:16–22.

283. Wood M, Shand DG, Wood AJJ. Propranolol binding in plasma during cardiopulmonary bypass. *Anesthesiology* 1979;51: 512–516.

284. de Bruijn NP, Reves JG, Croughwell N, et al. Pharmacokinetics of esmolol in anesthetized patients receiving chronic beta blocker therapy. *Anesthesiology* 1987;66:323–326.

285. Mantz J, Blanchot G, Marty J, et al. Acebutolol and diacetolol plasma levels in patients undergoing myocardial revascularization with hypothermic cardiopulmonary bypass. *J Cardiothorac Anesth* 1990;4:577–581.

286. Goldman DA, Hopkins CC, Karchmer AW, et al. Cephalothin prophylaxis in cardiac valve surgery. A prospective, double-blind comparison of two-day and six-day regimens. *J Thorac Cardiovasc Surg* 1977;73:470–479.

287. Archer GL, Polk RE, Duma RJ, et al. Comparison of cephalothin and cefamandole prophylaxis during insertion of prosthetic heart valves. *Antimicrob Agents Chemother* 1978;13:924–929.

288. Eigel P, Tschirkov A, Satter P, et al. Assays of cephalosporin antibiotics administered prophylactically in open heart surgery. Determination of serum and tissue levels before, during and after cardiopulmonary bypass. *Infection* 1978;6:23–28.

289. Kini PM, Fernandez J, Causay RS, et al. Double-blind comparison of cefazolin and cephalothin in open-heart surgery. *J Thorac Cardiovasc Surg* 1978;76:506–509.

290. Polk RE, Archer GL, Lower R. Cefamandole kinetics during cardiopulmonary bypass. *Clin Pharmacol Ther* 1978;23: 473–480.

291. Miller KW, Chan KKH, McCoy HG, et al. Cephalothin kinetics: before, during, and after cardiopulmonary bypass surgery. *Clin Pharmacol Ther* 1979;26:54–62.

292. Quintiliani R, Klimek J, Nightingale CH. Penetration of cephapirin and cephalothin into the right atrial appendage and pericardial fluid of patients undergoing open-heart surgery. *J Infect Dis* 1979;139:348–352.

293. Akl BF, Richardson G. Serum cefazolin levels during cardiopulmonary bypass. *Ann Thorac Surg* 1980;29:109–112.

294. Miller KW, McCoy HG, Chan KKH, et al. Effect of cardiopulmonary bypass on cefazolin disposition. *Clin Pharmacol Ther* 1980;27:550–556.

295. Nightingale CH, Klimek JJ, Quintiliani R. Effect of protein binding on the penetration of nonmetabolized cephalosporins into atrial appendage and pericardial fluids in open-heart surgical patients. *Antimicrob Agents Chemother* 1980;17:595–598.

296. Olson NH, Nightingale CH, Quintiliani R. Penetration characteristics of cefamandole into the right atrial appendage and pericardial fluid in patients undergoing open-heart surgery. *Ann Thorac Surg* 1980;29:104–108.

297. Mullany LD, French MA, Nightingale CH, et al. Penetration of ceforanide and cefamandole into the right atrial appendage, pericardial fluid, sternum, and intercostal muscle of patients undergoing open heart surgery. *Antimicrob Agents Chemother* 1982;21:416–420.

298. Bryan CS, Smith CW Jr, Sutton JP, et al. Comparison of cefamandole and cefazolin during cardiopulmonary bypass. *J Thorac Cardiovasc Surg* 1983;86:222–225.

299. Bergeron MG, Desaulniers D, Lessard C, et al. Concentrations of fusidic acid, cloxacillin, and cefamandole in sera and atrial appendages of patients undergoing cardiac surgery. *Antimicrob Agents Chemother* 1985;27:928–932.

300. Pieper R, Henze A, Josefsson K, et al. Penetration of penicillins into cardiac valves and auricles of patients undergoing open-heart surgery. *Scand J Thorac Cardiovasc Surg* 1985;19:49–53.

301. Daschner FD, Frank U, Kümmel A, et al. Pharmacokinetics of vancomycin in serum and tissue of patients undergoing open-heart surgery. *J Antimicrob Chem* 1987;19:359–362.

302. Frank U, Kappstein I, Schmidt-Eisenlohr E, et al. Penetration of ceftazidime into heart valves and subcutaneous and muscle tissue of patients undergoing open-heart surgery. *Antimicrob Agents Chemother* 1987;31:813–814.

303. Kaiser AB, Petracek MR, Lea JW IV, et al. Efficacy of cefazolin, cefamandole, and gentamicin as prophylactic agents in cardiac surgery. *Ann Surg* 1987;206:791–797.

304. Oksenhendler G, Leroy A, Schleifer D, et al. Ceftriaxone pharmacokinetics during cardiopulmonary bypass. *Chemioterapia* 1987;6[Suppl 2]:271–272.

305. Klamerus KJ, Rodvold KA, Silverman NA, et al. Effect of cardiopulmonary bypass on vancomycin and netilmicin disposition. *Antimicrob Agents Chemother* 1988;32:631–635.

306. van der Starre PJA, Trienekens PH, Harinck-de Weerd JE, et al. Comparative study between two prophylactic antibiotic regimens of cefamandole during coronary artery bypass surgery. *Ann Thorac Surg* 1988;45:24–27.

307. Wilson APR, Taylor B, Treasure T, et al. Antibiotic prophylaxis in cardiac surgery: serum and tissue levels of teicoplanin, flucloxacillin and tobramycin. *J Antimicrob Chem* 1988;21:201–212.

308. Lehot JJ, Reverdy ME, Etienne J, et al. Oxacillin and tobramycin serum levels during cardiopulmonary bypass. *J Cardiothorac Anesth* 1989;3:163–167.

309. Lippert S, Josephsen SD, Jendresen M, et al. Elimination of cefuroxime and gentamicin during and after open heart surgery. *J Antimicrob Chem* 1989;24:775–780.

310. Mini E, Mazzei T, Reali EF, et al. Pharmacokinetics of tei-

coplanin during cardiopulmonary bypass surgery. *Int J Clin Pharm Res* 1989;10:287–292.

311. Sue D, Salazar TA, Turley K, et al. Effect of surgical blood loss and volume replacement on antibiotic pharmacokinetics. *Ann Thorac Surg* 1989;47:857–859.

312. Wilson APR, Shankar S, Felmingham D, et al. Serum and tissue levels of teicoplanin during cardiac surgery: the effect of a high dose regimen. *J Antimicrob Chem* 1989;23:613–617.

313. Lehot J-J, Reverdy M-E, Etienne J, et al. Cefazolin and netilmicin serum levels during and after cardiac surgery with cardiopulmonary bypass. *J Cardiothorac Anesth* 1990;4:204–209.

314. Mertes PM, Voiriot P, Dopff C, et al. Penetration of ciprofloxacin into heart valves, myocardium, mediastinal fat, and sternal bone marrow in humans. *Antimicrob Agents Chemother* 1990; 34:398–401.

315. Kullberg BJ, Mattie H, Huysmans HA, et al. Evaluation of cloxacillin concentrations in plasma and muscle tissue during cardiopulmonary bypass. *Scand J Infect Dis* 1991;23:233–238.

316. Lonsky V, Mandák J, Lonská V, et al. Serum oxacillin and cephazolin levels during cardiopulmonary bypass. *Perfusion* 1992;7:115–118.

317. Pryka RD, Rodvold KA, Ting W, et al. Effects of cardiopulmonary bypass surgery on intravenous ciprofloxacin disposition. *Antimicrob Agents Chemother* 1993;37:2106–2111.

318. Menges T, Sablotzki A, Welters I, et al. Concentration of cefamandole in plasma and tissues of patients undergoing cardiac surgery: the influence of different cefamandole dosage. *J Cardiothorac Vasc Anesth* 1997;11:565–570.

319. Beall AC Jr, Johnson PC, Driscoll T, et al. Effect of total cardiopulmonary bypass on myocardial and blood digoxin concentration in man. *Am J Cardiol* 1963;11:194–200.

320. Ebert PA, Morrow AG, Austen WG. Clinical studies of the effect of extracorporeal circulation on myocardial digoxin concentration. *Am J Cardiol* 1963;11:201–204.

321. Hernandez A Jr, Kouchoukos N, Burton RM, et al. The effect of extracorporeal circulation upon the tissue concentration of digoxin-h^3. *Pediatrics* 1963;31:952–957.

322. Morrison J, Killip T. Serum digitalis and arrythmia in patients undergoing cardiopulmonary bypass. *Circulation* 1973;47: 341–352.

323. Krasula RW, Hastreiter AR, Levitsky S, et al. Serum, atrial, and urinary digoxin levels during cardiopulmonary bypass in children. *Circulation* 1974;49:1047–1052.

324. Carruthers SG, Cleland J, Kelly JG, et al. Plasma and tissue digoxin concentrations in patients undergoing cardiopulmonary bypass. *Br Heart J* 1975;37:313–320.

325. Storstein L, Nitter-Hauge S, Fjeld N. Effect of cardiopulmonary bypass with heparin administration on digitoxin pharmacokinetics, serum electrolytes, free fatty acids, and renal function. *J Cardiovasc Pharmacol* 1979;1:191–204.

326. Dasta JF, Weber RJ, Wu LS, et al. Influence of cardiopulmonary bypass on nitroglycerin clearance. *J Clin Pharmacol* 1986;26: 165–168.

327. Katz RI, Kanchuger MS, Patton KF, et al. Effect of cardiopulmonary bypass on plasma levels of nifedipine. *Anesth Analg* 1990;71:411–414.

328. Finegan BA, Hussain MD, Tam YK. Pharmacokinetics of diltiazem in patients undergoing coronary artery bypass grafting. *Ther Drug Monitor* 1992;14:485–492.

329. Booth BP, Brien JF, Marks GS, et al. The effects of hypothermic and normothermic cardiopulmonary bypass on glyceryl trinitrate activity. *Anesth Analg* 1994;78:848–856.

330. Thompson MA, Broadbent MP, English J. Plasma levels of methylprednisolone following administration during cardiac surgery. *Anaesthesia* 1982;37:405–407.

331. Kong A-N, Jungbluth GL, Pasko MT, et al. Pharmacokinetics of methylprednisolone sodium succinate and methylprednisolone in patients undergoing cardiopulmonary bypass. *Pharmacotherapy* 1990;1:29–34.

332. Larach DR, High KM, Larach MG, et al. Cardiopulmonary bypass interference with dantrolene prophylaxis of malignant hyperthermia. *J Cardiothorac Anesth* 1987;1:448–453.

333. Communale ME, DiNardo JA, Schwartz MJ. Pharmacokinetics of dantrolene in an adult patient undergoing cardiopulmonary bypass. *J Cardiothorac Vasc Anesth* 1991;5:153–155.

334. Hynynen M, Olkkola KT, Palojoki R, et al. Pharmacokinetics and effects of atrial natriuretic factor during hypothermic cardiopulmonary bypass. *Eur J Clin Pharmacol* 1992;43:647–650.

335. Bennett-Guerrero E, Sorohan JG, Howell ST, et al. Maintenance of therapeutic plasma aprotinin levels during prolonged cardiopulmonary bypass using a large-dose regimen. *Anesth Analg* 1996;83:1189–1192.

336. Bennett-Guerrero E, Sorohan JG, Canada AT, et al. ε-Aminocaproic acid plasma levels during cardiopulmonary bypass. *Anesth Analg* 1997;85:248–251.

15

IMMUNE AND INFLAMMATORY RESPONSES AFTER CARDIOPULMONARY BYPASS

PHILIP HORNICK
KENNETH M. TAYLOR

Immune responses offer protection to the organism from a variety of pathologic insults. The immune system comprises two fundamental features that act to effect such protection by generating both innate and acquired responses to the insult. *Innate* immunity depends on a variety of immunologic effector mechanisms that are neither specific for a particular infectious agent nor improved by repeated encounters with the same agent. In contrast to the innate system with its phagocytic and natural killer cells and soluble factors such as complement, lysozyme, and acute phase proteins, the adaptive immune system concerns T- and B-cell function and soluble factors such as antibody. *Adaptive* (or acquired) immunity is specific for the inducing agent and is marked by an enhanced response upon repeated encounters with that agent. The key features of the adaptive immune response are therefore memory and specificity. In practice, there is considerable overlap between these two types of immunity, because the adaptive immune system can direct elements of the innate system, such as phagocytes or complement factors.

Cardiopulmonary bypass (CPB) impinges on these two elements of the immune response. CPB generates an unphysiologic innate immune response manifested as a whole body systemic inflammatory response. At the same time, CPB also induces the cellular and humoral constituents of the adaptive immune system to undergo quantitative and qualitative changes, leading to a temporary immunodeficiency.

Because CPB induces a nonphysiologic (detrimental) inflammatory response, additional specific immunologic deficit has the potential to further increase the adverse effects of CPB by reducing susceptibility to infection.

P. H. Hornick and K. M. Taylor: Department of Cardiac Surgery, National Heart and Lung Institute, Imperial College School of Medicine at Hammersmith Hospital, London, W12 ONN United Kingdom.

SYSTEMIC INFLAMMATORY RESPONSE TO CARDIOPULMONARY BYPASS

Definition

At the outset, it is important to define what is meant by the systemic inflammatory response in the context of CPB. A variety of terms are used to describe this pathologic condition: "sepsislike" syndrome; hyperdynamic circulation; postperfusion syndrome; disseminated intravascular postpump syndrome; and pathologic similarities to the "systemic inflammatory response syndrome" (SIRS); adult respiratory distress syndrome; and multiple system organ failure.

It is generally accepted that CPB produces a "whole body" inflammatory response. In its most severe form, a spectrum of injury may be observed that includes one or more of the following clinical manifestations: pulmonary, renal, gut, central nervous system, and myocardial dysfunction; coagulopathy; vasoconstriction; capillary permeability; vasodilatation; accumulation of increased interstitial fluid; hemolysis; pyrexia; and increased susceptibility to infections and leukocytosis (1–6). Certainly this "post-bypass" syndrome would come within the rather loose and unsatisfactory catch-all term of SIRS (7). However, the breadth of the diagnostic criteria that permit inclusion and the absence of CPB in the terminology leads to the suggestion of yet another acronym to indicate the systemic inflammatory response after bypass, SIRAB. The potential diagnostic criteria for SIRAB would at least combine the noninfectious clinical picture(s) mentioned above with certain hemodynamic and hematologic parameters together with specific biochemical markers of inflammation. An obvious pitfall here is distinguishing end-organ damage due to inflammatory phenomena per se (microemboli, hyperdynamic circulation, etc.) versus that due to suboptimal perfusion during CPB of an organ system that already has a compromised vascular supply and little endogenous reserve.

Until we define specific criteria for the inflammatory response after CPB, it will remain difficult to accurately define its incidence and prevalence and to properly apportion its pathologic effects in terms of patient morbidity and mortality. Moreover, any strategies aimed at either therapy or prevention can only be properly assessed in the light of any established criteria.

Spectrum of Response

Most patients who undergo operations requiring CPB experience few clinically identifiable adverse sequelae and convalesce normally (8,9). One could almost be forgiven for viewing CPB as near perfect. That significant clinical morbidity is relatively unusual probably is due to the patient's innate ability to compensate for the damaging effects of CPB than to extracorporeal circulatory perfection or to any specific therapy aimed at abrogating the inflammatory response.

There appears to be an inevitability about the occurrence of the inflammatory response, and once again confusion abounds as to what exactly is meant until the diagnostic criteria are properly defined. It is clear that if the definition for SIRS is used, most if not all post-bypass patients would be included. Indeed, Cremer et al. (10) estimated its occurrence in approximately 10% of all their open heart operations. However, we previously emphasized that the inflammatory response demonstrates a spectrum of severity (11). The severity of this response is not predictable nor are its clinical sequelae. The length of CPB is frequently but not necessarily (10) regarded as a risk factor. The adverse sequelae of SIRAB do in fact account for substantial morbidity in pediatric surgery, the aged or infirm, and in patients undergoing long complex surgical procedures (3,12,13).

Initiation of Systemic Inflammatory Response After Bypass

Normal blood flow is altered by nonpulsatile perfusion. This is most commonly used in most cardiac surgical units worldwide. The relative benefits of pulsatile and nonpulsatile perfusion systems are an issue beset by controversy (14). The initial unsuccessful attempts at the inception of cardiac surgery to develop pulsatile systems that would reproduce normal physiologic pulsatile blood flow led to the adoption of nonpulsatile CPB. These systems were compatible with patient survival (15), and as confidence increased, nonpulsatile perfusion has become routinely established. As William Harvey might have predicted, it appears that there are distinct benefits to pulsatile flow that may prove advantageous to particular high-risk patient subgroups (14).

The damaging effects of CPB are most reasonably attributed to altered arterial blood flow patterns and to the exposure of blood to abnormal surfaces and substances during the period of bypass. The pathophysiologic responses that are responsible for SIRAB may continue long after the discontinuation of CPB.

SIRAB is initiated by a number of injurious processes that impinge on both cellular and noncellular (humoral) elements of blood. These processes generate microemboli, disrupt hemostasis, and lead to a generalized whole body inflammatory response. Most importantly, they set in motion a sequence of cytokine-mediated events that activate vascular endothelium, allowing further neutrophil-mediated inflammatory injury. It is important to appreciate that none of these events occur in isolation but that they are simultaneous and frequently stimulate or catalyze other reactions in the pathologic cycle of SIRAB. The scenario may be further compounded by cardiogenic shock and also endotoxemia.

Damaging Process

Shear stress forces are generated by blood pumps, cardiotomy suction devices (including intracardiac venting), and cavitation around the tip of the arterial cannula. The greatest hematologic damage and activation of formed and unformed blood components and vascular endothelium during CPB, however, derives from the repeated passage of the patients blood volume through the extracorporeal circuit. Contact activation is a series of host-defense mechanisms designed to isolate and destroy the foreign surface and gaseous interface that the various blood components recognize. Synthetic materials that comprise the membrane in membrane oxygenators and abnormal blood–gas interfaces in bubble oxygenators are far removed from the normal, physiologic, endothelial cell contact.

Cellular Components of Blood

Red Blood Cell

Erythrocytes are mainly damaged during CPB by sheer stresses (16). Red cell deformability is reduced by CPB, possibly due to mechanical damage to red cells. This has the effect of inducing changes to ionic pumps at the cell surface, leading to abnormal accumulations of intracellular cations (17). Another damaging factor is produced by the membrane and is attacked by the membrane attack complex (MAC) generated from the activation of complement (1). Red cell lifespan is reduced, and this may be one reason for the anemia frequently seen in the postoperative period (18). Red cell injury is deleterious through a number of mechanisms. Free hemoglobin in plasma may be damaging to tissue function by increasing plasma oncotic pressure and viscosity. Cytotoxic oxygen free radicals are also released after autooxidation of hemoglobin. ADP released from red cell lysis may alter platelet function (19). In addition, arrhythmias may also develop as a result of potassium released from the red blood cell. Lipid red cell membrane ghosts may occlude the microcirculation and lead to organ dysfunction. Decreased red cell deformability can also lead to reduced tissue flow by alteration of the rheologic properties of the blood. This leads to reductions in tissue metabolism and oxygenation.

Neutrophil and Vascular Endothelium

Leukocytes are particularly sensitive to shear stresses that cause destruction or functional impairments such as decreased aggregation, decreased chemotactic migration, and impaired phagocytosis (20).

The neutrophil is a central cell type in the mediation of the inflammatory response, and its recruitment, activation, and cytotoxic capability are an essential aspect of the body's ability to ward off infection. Neutrophil activation through interaction with activated vascular endothelium may be responsible for much of the clinical sequelae of SIRAB. The inextricable physiologic association between the endothelium and neutrophils is important. CPB initiates a humoral cascade that results in activation of vascular endothelium. This process results in the expression of adhesion molecules that promote adhesion of leukocytes to the vascular endothelium. Once adherent to the endothelium, neutrophils release cytotoxic proteases and oxygen-derived free radicals that produce some of the end-organ damage after CPB. Neutrophil-mediated injury can occur from both activation of complement and endothelial adhesion. Neutrophil-derived proteases have been demonstrated in the circulation after CPB. These proteases break down extracellular structure and matrix, which contributes to the capillary leakage that results in extracellular volume overload and imbalance of electrolytes postoperatively (21).

Under resting conditions, the vascular endothelium offers a relatively inert surface that regulates the passage of intravascular substrates to the extravascular space and ensures the unhindered flow of cellular and serum components through the capillary network. Inflammatory signals, which include complement activation products, hypoxia, cytokines, oxygen-derived free radicals, and lipopolysaccharide (endotoxin), result in changes in gene expression, leading to activation of the endothelium with ensuing cytokine release and protein expression. These cytokines and proteins promote inflammatory reactions and thrombosis (22,23). Under normal physiologic circumstances, endothelial activation is crucial in neutrophil recruitment and promoting coagulation to limit the spread of local infection. CPB, however, induces this response at a systemic level with the release of cytokines; endothelial activation over large areas; and the recruitment, margination, and degranulation of neutrophils on a larger scale. Attenuation of this systemic response by feedback mechanisms appears to function less well when compared with the local level. The result of endothelial activation is widespread leukocyte adhesion molecule and tissue factor expression, resulting in end-organ damage, microemboli, and consumption of clotting factors, which contributes to the coagulopathy that frequently complicates cardiac operations (24–27).

The recruitment of leukocytes from the circulation to an inflammatory site is a three-stage process (Fig. 15.1, A and B) involving members of several adhesion receptor families (28,29). The first stage is the activation of the vascular

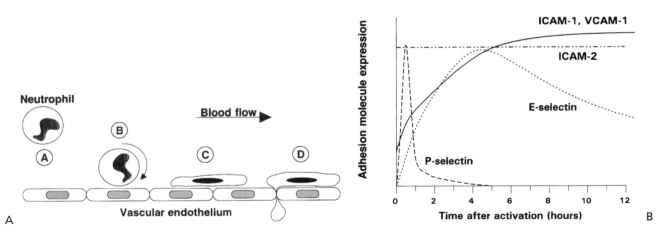

FIG. 15.1. A: Adherence of circulating neutrophils (*A*) is triggered by activation of the endothelial cells, which causes the neutrophils to roll along the endothelium (*B*), a process mediated by selectin interaction with carbohydrate ligands. Activation of the neutrophils (e.g., by interleukin-8, C5a, or PAF) results in activation of integrin molecules (e.g., by LFA-1) on the neutrophil surface. This results in firm adhesion of the neutrophils to activated endothelium (*C*) through receptors belonging to the Ig family (e.g., ICAMs). Activated adherent neutrophils extravasate through the endothelium into the tissue interstitial space (*D*). **B:** Activation of the endothelium is associated with expression of a range of adhesion molecules, including selectins (P and E) and the Ig superfamily (ICAM-1, -2, -3, and VCAM-2). Each molecule has its own kinetics of expression. The rapid response of P-selectin is achieved through release of preformed molecules. Ig superfamily molecules are synthesized with endothelial activation. Many are either not expressed at all or only at low levels before endothelial activation.

endothelium that leads to the rapid expression of members of the selectin family (30). First is P-selectin, which is stored, preformed, in Weibel-Palade bodies within the endothelial cell and is released by exocytosis within minutes of activation by agents such as histamine, thrombin, H_2O_2, and C5a. This is followed by the expression of the related E-selectin. Both molecules interact with Sialyl Lewis^X carbohydrate groups expressed by leukocytes and lymphocytes, causing the free flow of the cells to be slowed down, initiating a rolling of the cells along the endothelial surface. In addition to E- and P-selectin interactions, L-selectin expressed on the cells can interact with charged fucosylated carbohydrate groups on the endothelium.

The second stage of the recruitment process is activation of the leukocytes. This typically occurs through interaction of the cells with C5a, members of the chemokine family of cytokines [such as interleukin (IL)-8 and MIP-1b], which bind to the proteoglycan groups expressed on the surface of the endothelium (31–33), or with molecules such as platelet-activating factor produced by activated endothelial cells. All these molecules interact with a family of receptors on the leukocytes, the seven-transmembrane domain rhodopsin-like G protein-coupled receptors (34). These molecules also act as chemoattractant agents, in some cases by creating a gradient of the agent immobilized to the surface of the vascular endothelium. Interaction of receptors with the chemokines leads to activation of the integrin family of proteins expressed on the cells (e.g., LFA-1 and Mac-1), causing them to interact with their ligand (ICAM-1, -2, and -3).

Activation of neutrophils during CPB is shown by loss of L-selectin and upregulation of CD11b/CD18 (Mac-1). Increased production of reactive oxygen intermediates (35) and neutrophil-derived elastase, and similar molecules, have also been reported (35–38). Studies in complement-deficient dogs suggest that at least some of the neutrophil activation seen in CPB is due to complement activation (24). In addition to the presence of activated complement products during CPB, increased expression of neutrophil activating cytokines, such as IL-8, is also observed (39).

This process of neutrophil activation, firm adhesion, and sequestration can lead to obstruction of capillaries and local ischemia (40). In addition, the release by activated cells of cytotoxic products can cause direct cellular damage. These cytotoxins include both preformed agents that are present in the granules of neutrophils and newly synthesized molecules. There are two forms of neutrophil granules. The primary, or azurphil, granules have a predominantly intracellular role. These granules contain various proteases and myeloperoxidase that convert hydrogen peroxide to hypochlorous acid. Neutrophil secondary granules are released from the neutrophil and function primarily extracellularly. The secondary granules contain a number of cell surface molecules, such as the receptor for breakdown products of C3b and for chemoattractants. They also contain soluble

mediators of inflammation, including activators of the C5 complement component and macrophage chemotactic agents.

In addition to causing obstruction in small vessels and the release of preformed molecules, neutrophils (and mononuclear phagocytes) synthesize novel substances including leukotrienes (38) and reactive oxygen intermediates (35). This synthesis can be readily detected by a dramatic increase in the oxygen consumption of the cells. These species are largely responsible for the so-called ischemia-reperfusion injury. Ischemic injury results when the blood supply to a tissue is impaired or suboptimal, which may occur with CPB. The paradox is that a more severe tissue injury occurs when blood flow is restored on reperfusion. The onset of ischemia is accompanied by the depletion of cellular adenosine triphosphate as a result of its degradation by hypoxanthine. Normally, hypoxanthine is oxidized by the enzyme xanthine dehydrogenase to xanthine using NAD in a reaction converting NAD to NADH. During ischemia however, xanthine dehydrogenase, which is usually present in large quantities, is converted to xanthine oxidase.

Also, anaerobic metabolism results in the production of lactic acid and altered cellular homeostasis with the loss of ion gradients across cell membranes. Reperfusion injury is initiated by a series of biochemical events that result in the generation of reactive oxygen metabolites. Reduction of oxygen leads to the production of the superoxide anion (Fig. 15.2, reaction 1), which is able to penetrate through cell membranes where it is converted into other more toxic oxygen species. Thus, the dismutase reaction (catalyzed by superoxide dismutase) leads to the conversion of the superoxide anion into hydrogen peroxide (Fig. 15.2, reaction 2). This can lead to the production of hypochlorous acid (the major bactericidal component of domestic bleach) by action of myeloperoxidase (Fig. 15.2, reaction 3) or, via interaction with iron salts, in the Haber-Weiss reaction to generate the highly toxic hydroxyl radical (Fig. 15.2, reaction 4). The toxicity of the hydroxyl radical results from its ability to take electrons from a wide range of molecules, leading to the formation of a new radical that can continue the reaction (Fig. 15.2, reaction 5).

$$O_2 + e^- \rightarrow O_2^- \cdot \tag{1}$$

$$HO_2^\cdot + O_2^- \cdot + H^+ \rightarrow O_2 + H_2O_2 \tag{2}$$

$$H_2O_2 + Cl^- \xrightarrow{\text{MPO}} H_2O + HOCl \tag{3}$$

$$Fe^{2+} + H_2O_2 \rightarrow Fe^{3+} + OH^- + \cdot OH \tag{4}$$

$$\cdot OH + R \rightarrow OH^- + R^\cdot \tag{5}$$

FIG. 15.2. The five principle reactions leading to the production of the superoxide anion (*1*), hydrogen peroxide (*2*), hypochlorous acid (catalyzed by myeloperoxidase, *MPO*) (*3*), the hydroxyl radical (*4*), and oxidation of other cellular molecules (*R*), leading to new free radical species (*5*).

This family of reactive oxygen intermediates exert their toxic effect through being highly reactive agents that oxidize or chlorinate a wide range of molecules, including proteins and membrane lipids. This leads to disruption of cellular function and, eventually, cell death. In addition, low nontoxic concentrations of some reactive oxygen intermediates participate in cellular activation pathways, such as the NF-κB system (41), thereby potentially activating a wide range of cell types.

Platelet

CPB is associated with a transient deficit in platelet function and number. These effects are manifest as a derangement in postoperative hemostasis. The normal platelet is able to adhere to a damaged endothelial cell or the subendothelial layer. Adherence is achieved by a bridge of a molecule of the multimeric form of the von Willebrand factor from the endothelium to the platelet at the glycoprotein (GpIb) receptor site. The platelet then undergoes a conformational change with exposure of different glycoproteins that include the complex GpIIb/IIIa, which can bind to fibrinogen. Fibrinogen is an important cofactor in platelet adhesion and is essential for platelet to platelet binding that occurs during irreversible aggregation. The aggregate is stabilized by the protein complex thrombospondin. Thromboxane A_2 is also released, which produces vasoconstriction and platelet aggregation. Platelet response to a foreign surface is different in that platelet reactivity is related to fibrinogen. Mechanisms responsible are direct activation of the platelet, ADP release from granules of activated and damaged platelets, and stimulation of the platelet receptor to thrombin. Binding sites are subsequently exposed and platelets subsequently attach to the fibrinogen on the surface of the bypass circuit. Much evidence shows abnormalities of platelet numbers and function associated with CPB, including a rapid consumption of platelets during bypass (42), a decreased reactivity to known agonists (43), an increase in the concentration of the α-granule compounds in plasma (43), and an increase in the stable metabolite of thromboxane A_2 (thromboxane $_B$) released from aggregating platelets (44). The observation that the bleeding time is prolonged after a period of extracorporeal circulation has been directly related to the time on bypass; however, the time course of these observations and the precise mechanism is less clear (45). It has been observed that platelets of patients deficient in the GpIIb/IIIa complex did not bind to a foreign surface and that the proteins adherent to the extracorporeal system were primarily made up of fragments of the GpIIb receptor (46). This suggests that the GpIIb/IIIa complex is the adhesive glycoprotein most affected by extracorporeal circulation and therefore most likely to be associated with platelet aggregation and activation. Other authors have suggested that any platelet stimulation associated with the initial phase of bypass is of little consequence and that only a small proportion of the platelets proceed beyond the initial contact phase. The argument is based on a number of observations. Zilla et al. (47) found that platelet release reaction products, such as α-granule constituents and thromboxane, increase progressively during the course of bypass, suggesting that platelets are undergoing a lytic process throughout the period of perfusion (47). Whatever the case, all studies do agree that platelet functions are abnormal during the period of extracorporeal circulation.

Humoral Components of Blood

Kirklin (3) initially hypothesized that the deleterious effects of CPB were secondary to the exposure of blood to nonendothelial surfaces in the bypass circuit, initiating a "whole body inflammatory response." He noted that this response was characterized by activation of coagulation, the kallikrein system, fibrinolysis, and complement (3,13,48). We now recognize the importance of cytokines (49) and the combined effects of this humoral cascading in the activation of endothelial cells and neutrophil adhesion.

Inflammatory Cascades

The principal event is the activation of factor XII (Hageman factor) to factor XIIa, which stimulates a number of inflammatory systems (Fig. 15.3). After surface contact, factor XII undergoes a conformational change and becomes attached to a high-molecular-weight kininogen. This complex attaches itself to the foreign surface and, after limited proteolysis, releases kallikrein and also bradykinin. In addition, limited proteolysis of factor XII releases factor XIIa. This active proteolytic factor can initiate the intrinsic coagulation cascade by direct effects on factor XI, which binds to the foreign surface and can also induce activation of factor VII, thereby further augmenting the intrinsic cascade of coagulation. Factor XIIa is also involved in a positive feedback system involving kallikrein. Factor XIIa releases kallikrein from prekallikrein, and the former is in turn able to act on factor XII to produce factor XIIa (50). Kallikrein can further activate neutrophils and in so doing can produce further activation of inflammatory cascades by producing oxygen free radicals and proteolytic enzymes. Furthermore, kallikrein and bradykinin can stimulate the fibrinolytic system. Kallikrein stimulates plasmin production by its action on pro-urokinase and bradykinin by releasing tissue-type plasminogen activator from the endothelium.

Complement System

One of the most important immunologic mechanisms involved in the inflammatory process is the complement system. This consists of more than 30 proteins that serve both as an effector arm of the immune response and as a primitive recognition system capable of self-/non–self-discrimination

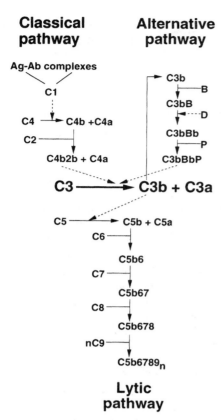

FIG. 15.3. Contact activation cascade systems that result in the production of the systemic inflammatory response after bypass (*SIRAB*).

(51). Its functions include mediating inflammation, opsonization of antigenic particles, and causing membrane damage to pathogens. The complement components interact with each other so that the products of one reaction form the enzyme for the next. Thus, a small initial stimulus can trigger a cascade of activity with consequent biologic activation. The importance of the complement system is seen in the fact that 5% to 10% of serum proteins are complement components.

There are three major pathways to the complement system consisting of a series of preformed, inactive, proteins that, upon activation, activate the next protein in the pathway. This results in massive amplification of the initial activating event and to a cascade of different members being activated, such that the primary trigger leads to the production of a large number of different effector functions. Such an amplification system needs tight control, and so it is no surprise that nearly half the proteins in the complement system are regulatory molecules.

There are two activation pathways in the system, the classic and the alternative pathway. Both pathways culminate in the production of C3 convertase molecules, which cleave the central component of the complement system,

C3, into the active C3a and C3b fragments. The classic pathway, which is probably the least important to the present discussion, is initiated by the binding of antibodies to target antigens on an appropriate surface. The clustered Fc regions of the antibodies are recognized by the first component of the classic pathway, C1, thus initiating the cascade of activation leading to the production of the classic pathway C3 convertase, C4b2b (Fig. 15.4). The alternative pathway, which is the most primitive part of the system, operates by a feedback loop in which the C3b component interacts with factor B (and subsequent activation of factor B by factor D) to generate the alternative pathway C3 convertase, C3bBb (Fig. 15.4). Thus, C3 acts as both a substrate and a component of the alternative pathway. The original C3b that initiates the alternative pathway can be generated either as a product of the classic pathway (in which case the alternative pathway acts as an amplification loop for complement activation) or through the spontaneous activation of C3 that occurs at a low level on a continuous basis. This "tickover" of C3 activation means that the complement system is continually being triggered, and to prevent the consequent activation of the whole cascade, it is necessary for cells to express regulatory proteins that inactivate the alternative pathway C3 convertase. This system provides the complement cascade with its primitive self-/non–self-recognition system in which surfaces (e.g., those of viruses and bacteria) that lack the necessary regulatory components are "recognized" by the alternative pathway, leading to the activation of the complement cascade and generation of inflammatory effector mechanisms, as discussed below.

The final pathway of the complement system is the lytic or terminal pathway. This pathway is initiated by C3b, produced by either the classic or alternative pathway C3 convertase. C3b activates C5 to generate C5a, a soluble molecule, and C5b, which is bound to the cell surface. This leads to the subsequent binding to the surface of C6, C7, and C8 and the polymerization of C9 to form a pore through the membrane that can result in target cell lysis (MAC). The MAC thus forms a transmembrane channel that allows the influx of ions and water into the cell, which is unable to maintain osmotic and chemical equilibrium (52).

There are a number of effects of activation of the complement system. First, a number of proteins, most notably the anaphylatoxins C3a, C4a, and C5a, are produced. These molecules act through receptors on mast cells and basophils, leading to their degranulation and release of a wide range of inflammatory mediators (including histamine). They also act directly on smooth muscle and endothelium, leading to muscle contraction and an increase in vascular permeability. In addition, C5a acts as a chemotactic and activating agent for neutrophils and other myeloid cells, leading both to their recruitment and release of lysosomal enzymes, reactive oxygen species, and other inflammatory mediators (53).

In addition to the production of soluble molecules, a number of components bind to surfaces after activation,

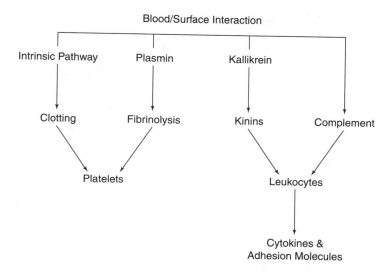

Blood/Surface Interaction

Intrinsic Pathway   Plasmin   Kallikrein

Clotting   Fibrinolysis   Kinins   Complement

Platelets   Leukocytes

Cytokines &
Adhesion Molecules

FIG. 15.4. Three pathways of the complement system. Conversion or interaction of serum components is indicated by solid lines; enzymatic reactions are shown as broken lines. The classic pathway leads to the conversion of C3 to C3b, which triggers the lytic pathway. The alternate pathway can be initiated as an amplification loop for the classic pathway by means of C3b or by C3b, resulting from the spontaneous hydrolysis of C3, in combination with factors B and D, to produce C3bBb, which is stabilized by properdin (*P*) to yield C3bBbP, which is capable of hydrolyzing C3 to produce more C3b.

including the MAC, whose role has already been mentioned. In addition, there are receptors for C4b and, more importantly, C3b and its breakdown products. These are involved in the opsonization of complement coated particles and the clearance of immune complexes.

During CPB, activation of the complement system is observed, as shown both by consumption of complement components (54) and the appearance in the circulation of C3a and C5a and the MAC. This activation of the cascade is probably due to a number of causes, including the bioincompatible nature of the surfaces encountered in the CPB apparatus and the release of endotoxin into the systemic circulation (55,56). Furthermore, physical effects of CPB may be responsible, for example, interaction with bubbles of oxygen have been shown to cause the breakdown of C3 (57).

Further Contributions to Systemic Inflammatory Response After Bypass

In addition to the inflammatory interactions that result from the bypass circuit, cardiogenic shock and endotoxemia may further compound the response (58). Cardiogenic shock can further contribute to SIRAB, and prolonged nonpulsatile perfusion or periods of circulatory arrest can lead to diffuse end-organ ischemia as well (59). The end-organ hypoxic insult likely causes endothelial cells, circulating monocytes, and tissue-fixed macrophages to release cytokines and oxygen-derived free radicals that drive this response. Once the patient is resuscitated from shock and after hypoxic end organs are reperfused, a form of systemic ischemic-reperfusion injury results (58).

Another form of inflammatory activation that results from extracorporeal circulation and episodes of systemic ischemia-reperfusion is endotoxemia. Endotoxin is frequently detected in high concentration in the systemic circulation after CPB (60). Endotoxin is a potent stimulant of both complement and of endothelial cell activation, resulting in the surface upregulation of adhesion molecules and tissue factor (23). Endotoxin is a potent agonist of macrophage tumor necrosis factor release, which may explain why the level of this cytokine is elevated in some patients after CPB. Although the precise mechanism of endotoxemia after CPB is unclear, this may derive from a translocation of bacteria from the gut, resulting from the systemic stress of CPB and splanchnic ischemia (see below) coupled with impaired Kupfer cell function (56). The result is a transient endotoxemia that contributes to the overall state of systemic inflammation after CPB.

Endotoxin is also relevant in considering the "hyperdynamic circulation" and the associated profound fall in systemic vascular resistance, which is sometimes seen after CPB (10). This condition is very similar to the early phases of sepsis or endotoxemia (11). Until recently it was thought that endotoxin exerted its myocardial depressant effects by reducing the response to adrenergic stimulation by desensitization of the B-1 receptor. Recent data indicate that G proteins (guanine nucleotide binding proteins) may in fact be the mediators of endotoxin-induced defects in inotropic regulation (61).

Organ Dysfunction and Cardiopulmonary Bypass

Lung and Pulmonary Circulation

The pulmonary circulation takes the whole of the cardiac output as the patient is weaned from CPB. This results in a high load of activated cells passing through this region. In addition, evidence suggests that activated neutrophils will preferentially lodge in the pulmonary circulation (62,63) and that free radicals derived from activated neutrophils are responsible for lung injury. Royston et al. (64) showed evidence for increased oxygen-derived free radical activity. This study demonstrated an increase in the peroxides of the polyunsaturated lipids of the cell membrane as a result of their reaction with free radicals. The rise in peroxidized products also showed a very close temporal relationship with the sequestration of neutrophils in the lung. However, other authors have provided evidence that there is in fact a reduction in the neutrophil-derived free radical output during bypass and that release of the aortic clamp and reperfusion of the lungs is associated with release of the superoxide anion by neutrophils (65).

Intravenous infusions of complement activated plasma result in an increase in pulmonary vascular resistance, a fall in arterial oxygen tension, and sequestration of neutrophils within the pulmonary vascular bed (66,67). Further experimental studies have shown that intravascular complement activation can result in pulmonary endothelial injury, leading to an increase in vascular permeability and interstitial pulmonary edema (66). The central role of neutrophils in complement-induced lung injury can be demonstrated by depletion experiments (68). It has been demonstrated that complement-induced neutrophil-dependent lung injury could be attenuated with scavengers of oxygen radicals.

Renal Function and Cardiopulmonary Bypass

Renal function is influenced by hemodilution, hypothermia, and endocrine effects during nonpulsatile perfusion. Changes in the rennin–angiotensin–aldosterone system promote an increase in renal vascular resistance and a tendency to sodium and water retention. The vasoconstrictive effects of hypothermia reduce renal cortical blood flow, glomerular filtration rate, tubular function, and free water and osmolar clearance. Hemodilution protects against renal damage during CPB by increasing outer cortical renal plasma flow and increasing sodium, potassium, osmolar, and free water clearance (5). In general, urine output will be diminished during hypothermia and improved at normothermia and after the resumption of pulsatile perfusion. Renal dysfunction may also result from microemboli (including lipid membrane ghosts) that lodge within the microcirculation and also from hemoglobinuria.

Brain and Cardiopulmonary Bypass

A range of neurologic and neuropsychological abnormalities are seen after coronary artery bypass graft. The incidence of these complications has been recorded by Shaw et al. (69–73). As a result of autoregulation of the cerebral circulation, cerebral perfusion is assumed to be adequate when the mean arterial pressure is above 50 to 60 mm Hg. This is assuming that there is no flow limiting carotid stenosis or that the patient is not chronically hypertensive. In these

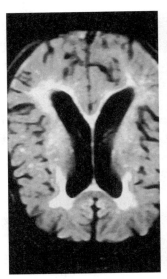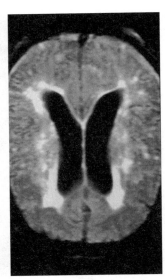

Preoperative   Postoperative

FIG. 15.5. Periventricular and deep white matter lesions consistent with ischemic disease were seen in all patients on the preoperative scans. All patients showed brain swelling with reduction in size or even obliteration of cerebral sulci fissures and cisterns on the early postoperative scans.

situations, the minimally acceptable cerebral perfusion pressure is higher than normal, because the cerebral blood flow autoregulation curve shifts to the right and cerebral blood flow (CBF) therefore becomes pressure dependent at a higher than normal perfusion pressure. Postoperative cerebral dysfunction in the absence of the aforementioned conditions is commonly attributed to macro- and microembolization during surgery. Studies using intraoperative transcranial Doppler and fluorescein retinal angiography have documented a high incidence of cerebral and retinal microemboli of blood cell aggregates during CPB (74–76). Magnetic resonance imaging identifies brain swelling after coronary artery bypass graft (Fig. 15.5) (77). In this pilot series of six patients, no major neurologic deficits were seen. The mechanism of the swelling is uncertain. Hypotheses include stasis of interstitial fluid caused by an absence in arterial pulsations but not of flow during aortic cross clamping (78) and increased cerebral blood flow due to postbypass hyperemia (79). Brain swelling may provide further insight into the cause of neuropsychological deficits seen after coronary artery bypass surgery.

Gut and Cardiopulmonary Bypass

Gut mucosal ischemia is common during CPB but rarely produces clinical evidence of gastrointestinal disease in the absence of postoperative low cardiac output syndrome (80). Factors that contribute include splanchnic vasoconstriction induced by elevated angiotensin II levels during nonpulsatile perfusion, splanchnic shunting during rewarming from systemic hypothermia, microemboli comprising platelet or leukocyte aggregates with the release of vasoactive substances, and preexisting atherosclerotic disease in the splanchnic bed (81).

Therapeutic Avenues

Effective amelioration of SIRAB has yet to become a reality. Certain proactive strategies may be instituted when there is difficulty in maintaining an adequate perfusion pressure before the discontinuation of bypass, which may indicate a profoundly low systemic vascular resistance. The only current therapy in this situation is vasoconstrictor and inotropic drugs, recognizing that such treatment does not address the pathologic basis of the hypotension.

The recognition that the deleterious effects of SIRAB are of lesser magnitude and shorter duration in the presence of robust postoperative cardiac performance suggests that at least an optimal cardiac output increases the clearance of inflammatory proteins and mediators. Accordingly, improved methods of myocardial preservation and organ perfusion offer the possibility of ameliorating, at least to some extent, the deleterious effects of humoral activation.

To prevent or ameliorate SIRAB, the optimal strategy would be to develop a CPB system that does not produce contact activation of blood components rather than to systemically administer anti-inflammatory therapeutic agents because of their potential to render the patient more susceptible to postoperative infection.

In terms of technical advances in relation to the CPB circuit, pulsatile perfusion may have beneficial effects compared with nonpulsatile flow (14). There is increasing clinical and experimental evidence for the benefit of membrane oxygenators over bubble oxygenators (48,82). The membrane oxygenator system provides superior oxygenation compared with a bubble oxygenator and produces less trauma to blood elements during prolonged use. In addition, membrane oxygenators are associated with a reduction in microembolism when compared with bubble oxygenators (83). By reducing complement activation (84), the membrane oxygenator may reduce the incidence of pulmonary dysfunction after CPB (85). It seems unlikely that modifications of bypass equipment alone will provide a unique solution to the problem of contact activation in the absence of any other manipulations.

In contrast to the aforementioned, Videm et al. (86) showed that the MAC (terminal effector unit, C5-C9) is increased in the plasma to a similar degree no matter what type of oxygenator was used. Other interventions include the coating of membranes and CPB apparatus with heparin. This coating appears to provide a more biocompatible surface and to decrease complement activation (87–89). Another strategy makes use of hemofiltration. This allows the removal of neutrophils from the circulation. In so doing,

their biologic availability to promote inflammatory injury is decreased (90). The problem appears to revolve around a return of leukocytes to the circulation when the filter is discontinued. Use of heparin-bonded circuits and hemofiltration is still far from routine in clinical practice.

In terms of pharmacologic manipulation of SIRAB, many strategies have been proposed to inhibit complement activation, but such is the complexity of the complement pathways that an agent has yet to be found that can inhibit effectively all aspects of the system. Many agents have a limited inhibitory action *in vitro* but are often restricted to one or other of the complement pathways. Corticosteroids inhibit the formation of C3 and C5 convertases *in vitro*, but there have been conflicting reports as to their efficacy at inhibiting complement activation during CPB (91). A number of protease inhibitors, for example FUT-175, have been proposed as effective inhibitors of the complement pathways (92). It is nonspecific in that it also inhibits factor XIIa, kallikrein, and thrombin. It is, however, a much more potent inhibitor of the classic pathway than the alternative pathway and is therefore of limited interest in regard to the prevention of the complement activation that accompanies CPB. Pharmacologic agents, such as corticosteroids, may be useful in preventing activation, though the results are conflicting. At the present time, their function as routine prophylaxis has not found clinical use because there is no evidence of effective *in vivo* complement inhibition, cellular host defense mechanisms are impaired, and elevated endotoxin levels have been reported in treated patients (93).

Aprotinin (Trasylol) is a serine protease inhibitor isolated from bovine lung. It inhibits several proteinases, including trypsin, plasmin, and kallikrein. In view of its antiplasmin effect, it is also considered to be an antifibrinolytic agent. The precise mechanism of action of aprotinin is still unclear. The broad range of antiprotease activity might indicate several potentially interlinked mechanisms (94–97). Aprotinin has been used in the past in a variety of clinical situations, including acute pancreatitis, adult respiratory distress syndrome, septic shock, and hemorrhagic shock. In 1963, Tice et al. (98) reported its use in cardiac surgical patients. Despite subsequent use by others indicating that it might be effective in reducing bleeding after cardiac surgery (99), aprotinin's potential role in cardiac surgery was largely ignored for many years. The Hammersmith group found that high-dose aprotinin therapy, which they used in an attempt to block complement and kallikrein-induced lung damage, showed remarkable efficacy in reducing blood loss and blood transfusion requirements in cardiac surgical patients (100–102). The experience with aprotinin has recently been extended and confirmed in a larger study in the United Kingdom (103). Aprotinin has been suggested to have a dose-responsive inhibitory effect on complement activation *in vivo* (104). However, a detailed study by Blauhut et al. (105) demonstrated no inhibitory effect on complement cascades during CPB. Aprotinin has, however, been shown to reduce plasma concentrations of neutrophil elastase after aortic cross-clamp removal (94). The fact that aprotinin acts as a nonspecific antiprotease and blocks the action of kallikrein and the fibrinolytic pathway does nonetheless offer considerable potential for the role of this drug as an inhibitor of SIRAB and as a hemostatic agent.

The prevention of neutrophil activation would be of use in preventing many problems associated with CPB. A number of pharmacologic agents, such as glucocorticoids and other inflammatory agents, have been used that reduce neutrophil activation (25,106,107). These reports suggest that some specific antineutrophil therapy may be possible to prevent tissue injury in the future.

Lowering the temperature of the patient has also been shown to reduce adherence of neutrophils to the endothelium (108); however, although hypothermia is beneficial when the patient is cold, the benefits are rapidly lost when the patient rewarms (109,110).

Techniques designed to impair neutrophil-endothelial cell interaction have the potential to make a substantial difference if not actually attenuate SIRAB. There is much interest currently in the use of monoclonal antibodies as therapeutic agents to block specific adhesion molecules expressed by activated endothelium. Such an approach, or similar strategies using soluble ligands of the adhesion molecules, has been shown to block neutrophil recruitment in a number of experimental systems, including CPB (25,59). A further therapeutic avenue is the use of monoclonal antibodies directed against cytokine receptors. Such antibodies directed against tumor necrosis factor and IL-1 receptors in animal models of sepsis appear to prevent endotoxin-induced shock (111,112). Such interventions may result in inhibition of T- and B-cell proliferation and lymphokine generation. This will likely result in a diminution of host defense mechanisms and hence make the patient more vulnerable to severe infection. Similarly, adhesion molecule blockade has been shown to increase the body's susceptibility to infection, an effect that severely limits this approach as a therapeutic strategy (113). At this time a multiplicity of monoclonal antibodies exists with the capability to block adhesion molecules. Boyle et al. (58) emphasized the importance of addressing the time courses of expression of specific endothelial adherence molecules so that interventions can be directed to each specific adhesion molecule at the time when it can be expected to be maximally expressed. Other approaches that appear attractive include the inhibition of adhesion molecule expression. Efforts to characterize the molecular events that result in endothelial activation genes could conceivably result in utilization of gene-based therapies to modulate or attenuate SIRAB.

The ability to produce novel molecules using recombinant DNA technology has also shown some promise for the future. In an animal model, a soluble version of the complement receptor 1 (sCR1, normally a cell surface inhibitor of complement activation) has been shown to de-crease complement activation during CPB (114). It is likely that an increasing number of similar molecules will be produced and tested in both preclinical and clinical settings over the next few years. Furthermore, it is possible to envisage incorporation of such molecules onto the surfaces of membranes and tubes to prevent local activation.

IMMUNE RESPONSE AFTER CARDIOPULMONARY BYPASS

The cellular and humoral constituents of the adaptive immune system undergo changes in both function and number after CPB. The concern is that postoperative morbidity and mortality related to infection is partially due to a loss of T and B cells and immunoglobulin consumption resulting from CPB. This section examines the effect of CPB on adaptive immunity and, specifically, T-cell function.

Immunodeficiency and Cardiopulmonary Bypass

Numerous studies have demonstrated that a depression of the acquired immune response occurs after surgical procedures (115–124). The degree of immunosuppression is directly related to the magnitude and duration of the surgical procedure and to the volume of transfused blood (123). Therefore, one would expect that cardiac operations would be highly immunosuppressive. The clinical prevalence of infections after cardiac surgery indicates that prolonged operating time and duration of CPB are significantly correlated to the incidence of infections (125,126). The risk factors for the development of infections identified in general surgical patients are applicable to cardiac surgery (127,128). However, it has been shown that anesthesia in open heart surgery has only minor immunologic effects (129,130).

The result of CPB is a depression of immunologic reactivity, which makes patients susceptible to perioperative infections with the development of septic shock as a possible, and frequently fatal, result (131). In one cardiac institution, 55% of perioperative mortality was due to multisystem organ failure associated with sepsis (132). Whether sepsis was the primary factor initiating the multisystem organ failure or was the result of endotoxin and bacterial translocation produced by a primary circulatory abnormality could not be determined. With the advent of interventional catheterization laboratory techniques and better medical management of patients with coronary artery disease, older and sicker patients are being referred for operation. These patients comprise a group that is at higher risk for the development of infections in the postoperative period. Of additional concern is that any depression of the acquired immune response may be detrimental because it could increase the susceptibility of cardiac surgical patients (many of whom have prosthetic material in the vascular system) to endocarditis.

Under normal conditions, relatively low levels of immunoglobulins and complement are sufficient for adequate opsonization of bacteria (133). However, if the load of infectious microorganisms increases, as may occur in patients undergoing open heart surgical procedures (134), then an imbalance may develop in the homeostasis of the host defense. The quantitative and qualitative exhaustion of humoral and cell-mediated immune mechanisms may have an adverse effect on clinical outcome when an additional injury occurs to a patient with a downregulated immune system in the early postoperative period. It is therefore not surprising that opportunistic pathogens are frequently found in cardiac surgical patients experiencing one or more perioperative complications, for example renal failure or low cardiac output. This patient group is likely to develop sepsis-related multisystem organ failure that can account for a high proportion of perioperative fatalities (135). At the present time, the lack of correlation between laboratory data and clinical findings in surgical patients with or without CPB has been noted by several groups of investigators (124,130,136,137). It may be possible to relate clinical outcome and laboratory results if more discriminative tests are applied and by using large patient numbers.

Humoral Immunity

In patients undergoing CPB, serum levels of immunoglobulins and complement are markedly reduced (3,4,48, 136,138–140). As a consequence, the contribution of these proteins to host defense is quantitatively affected, resulting, for example, in reduced opsonization of bacteria *in vitro* (139). Bubble oxygenators produce a greater deleterious effect in this regard than membrane oxygenators (141,142). Leukocyte counts fall with the onset of CPB. The sequestration of leukocytes in tissue is increased after their activation by anaphylatoxins C3a and C5a. After CPB, the chemotactic ability of granulocytes is impaired (141–144), which may also contribute to a higher susceptibility to bacterial infections. Other studies show that not only the phagocytic function but also the metabolic function of leukocytes is impaired after CPB (145).

It is unclear what happens to B-cell numbers after CPB. Some investigators report no change (6) and others a decrease (146). Roth et al. (137) reported that relative levels (percentage) of B cells increase after CPB with no significant increase in absolute numbers. The secretion of IgG, IgM, and IgA by B cells in response to pokeweed mitogen is diminished after CPB (137). The bactericidal activity of serum is depressed after CPB. Complement is consumed, and all components of humoral immunity are decreased as a consequence of the hemodilution caused by bypass (147). The denaturation, flocculation, and clearing of these microparticles by the reticuloendothelial system is responsible for

the continued fall in concentration of the immune proteins during bypass (148). Exposure of immune proteins to contact with gaseous and foreign surfaces results in denaturation. Surface depolarizing forces result in the disruption of the sulphydryl and hydrogen bonds that stabilize the secondary and tertiary structure of the protein molecules. The resulting unfolding of globular protein molecules may expose otherwise masked chemical groups and create a randomly coiled molecule. The macromolecules thus formed then tend to flocculate. These changes in plasma proteins may also lead to coalescence of serum lipids and an increase in plasma viscosity because of protein denaturation (6,149).

Natural Killer Cells

Natural killer cells are a heterogeneous subpopulation of lymphoid cells that are not T or B lymphocytes. Natural killer cells have been shown to produce cytotoxic responses in virus-infected cells and transformed target cells (e.g., tumor cells). Decreases in both number and function of natural killer cells have been shown after CPB (139,150, 151).

Reticuloendothelial System

The reticuloendothelial system is made up of tissue macrophages in the spleen, lymph nodes, lung, and liver. These cells are initially derived from bloodborne monocytes. The normal function of the reticuloendothelial system includes clearing of bacteria, endotoxin, platelets, denatured proteins, chylomicrons, plasma hemoglobin, thrombin, fibrin, fibrin degradation products, thromboplastin, and plasminogen activator from the circulating blood. The function of the reticuloendothelial system has been shown to be depressed after CPB. The microparticles generated by CPB are a major factor in the depression of this system (152).

T Cells

T cells are lymphocytes that develop in the thymus. This organ is seeded by lymphocytic stem cells from the bone marrow during embryonic development. These cells then develop their T-cell antigen receptors and differentiate into the two major peripheral T-cell subsets, one of which expresses the CD4+ marker (helper cells) and the other CD8+ (cytotoxic cells). T helper cells play a central role in the initiation and regulation of the acquired immune response. T helper cells recognize antigen presented on the surface of antigen presenting cells in association with class II molecules encoded by the major histocompatibility complex (MHC). T-cell activation requires other specific costimulatory signals generated by the antigen presenting cell. Cytotoxic T cells recognize antigen presented on the surface of antigen presenting cells in association with class I molecules encoded by the MHC. T helper cells provide "help" in the form of lymphokine secretion. Such lymphokines help B cells to divide, differentiate, and produce antibody. The lymphokines also are required for the development of leukocyte lines from hematopoietic stem cells and development of cytotoxic T cells. They also cause activation of macrophages, allowing them to destroy the pathogens they have taken up. Cytotoxic T cells are capable of destroying virus-infected target cells or allogeneic (transplanted) cells.

Quality and Quantity

Phenotypic changes induced by CPB have been investigated using standard commercially available leukocyte labeling monoclonal antibodies together with flow cytometric analysis. There is a decrease in CD3+, CD4+, and CD8+ cells with a reversal of the normal CD4+/CD8+ ratio. Such changes are maximal on postoperative day 1 and remain low for approximately 1 week (151,153–155). T lymphocytes are significantly reduced in numbers [relative and absolute (137)].

The capacity to counteract microbial infection by the innate immune system is reduced in patients after cardiac operation due to a waste of complement factors (3,48,140) and a decrease in the cellular elements of the innate immune response, for example neutrophils and natural killer cells (137,150,156). Hisatomi et al. (157) showed in patients having cardiac operations that lymphocyte response to the mitogen phytohemagglutinin (PHA) was low on the first and seventh days after operation and that IL-2 production was greater than 90% depressed on the first postoperative day. There was no significant change in a control group of patients who underwent cholecystectomy. Furthermore, improvement in IL-2 production occurred immediately in patients without blood transfusion from random donors and reached normal levels by postoperative day 3. However, IL-2 production remained depressed on day 3 in all patients with transfusion from random donors and remained significantly diminished on day 7 in patients in NYHA classes III and IV.

Markewitz et al. (135) showed a similar depression of the response to PHA and a specific antigen cocktail (purified protein derivative, tetanus toxoid, streptolysin, mumps, and vaccinia antigen). Using *in vitro* cytolytic assays, Nguyen et al. (151) showed a decrease in cytotoxic T cell activity that was maximal on postoperative day 1 with a return to baseline values on postoperative day 3.

Morphologic Correlation

Scanning electron microscopy of T cells after CPB shows profound alterations to the plasma membrane of the T cells. There is a decreased number of microvilli and a decrease in the folded aspect of the lymphocyte surface. Furthermore, after CPB, the membrane does not accommodate monoclonal microbeads.

Mechanisms

The mechanism responsible for the decrease in T lymphocytes in circulating blood after CPB is not defined. A high level of cortisol probably plays an important role in postoperative immunosuppression, yet it is unlikely to be the only factor in this complex phenomenon (158). Elevation of serum corticosteroids may cause a decrease in circulating T-cell levels by causing a redistribution to lymphoid tissues, although this is usually mild and transient (153,159). Lymphocyte transformation by PHA is retarded by corticosteroids. Although serum cortisol levels are elevated after operation, the lack of correlation between changes in serum cortisol and changes in lymphocyte number and function suggests that serum cortisol is not an etiologic factor in postoperative immunosuppression (137). Blood dilution as a consequence of CPB, fluid shifts between extravascular and intravascular compartments, and mechanical destruction and consumption are likely causes of quantitative and qualitative change (160). Ide et al. (155) suggested T-cell redistribution between bone marrow, lymphoid tissue, and peripheral blood may occur.

Perspectives

T cells are quantitatively reduced and qualitatively affected by CPB. The literature does not, however, address two fundamental issues. First, one of the main factors that determines the magnitude of an immune response is the number of antigen or allo-specific lymphocytes available to respond at the time of antigenic or allogeneic challenge. The experiments described thus far give no more than an overall impression of the diminution in quality of the immune response and have inherently poor quantitation. The qualitative defect has, therefore, not been quantified at the cellular level. Such quantification is essential if one is to compare the immunomodulatory effect of certain agents or to make appropriate judgments regarding the effects of CPB on the T-cell response. Furthermore, it is not possible to make any judgments as to the effect of CPB on the T-cell response to nominal as opposed to allo-antigen, the latter being of importance in the context of cardiac transplantation. The second issue is the assessment of whether CPB affects the ability of antigen presenting cells (macrophages, B cells, and dendritic cells) to present antigen to T cells. This would also affect the quality of the T-cell response. Because all other aspects of the immune response appear to be affected by CPB, it would not be surprising to find out that such a defect was produced by CPB. This could also be quantified and the impact of putative immunomodulatory agents properly assessed.

The most sensitive and quantitative technique for measuring reactive T cells at a population level is to determine their frequencies by limiting dilution. Limiting dilution analysis defines a previously unknown frequency in a population of cells and is the only way to quantitate the immune response in humans at the cellular level. It is used both as a research tool and clinically in the context of bone marrow transplantation to predict the risk of developing graft-versus-host disease. Methods are established for assaying the frequencies of reactive cytotoxic T lymphocytes and IL-2 secreting T helper cells (161,162). These assays, however, are able to estimate the frequency of T helper cells or cytotoxic T cells to a specific nominal or allo-antigen. This technique alone could provide powerful information as to the impact of CPB on the ability of patient T cells to respond to antigen and also antigen presenting cells to present antigen, or both. In a less quantitative manner, antigen presenting function of patient cells could be assessed by performing bulk culture experiments. In these, a T-cell clone, restricted for the patient's class II MHC and specific for a peptide (e.g., hemagglutinin), is used. The patients antigen presenting cells present peptide to this clone, and proliferation of the T-cell clone is measured by tritiated thymidine incorporation into replicating DNA. The assumption is that if the antigen presenting cells are affected by CPB, the clone will proliferate to a different extent compared with pre-bypass proliferation. In this manner, more accurate quantitative comparisons may be made.

SUMMARY

It is clear that the inflammatory and immunologic sequelae of CPB are not responsible for a large morbidity or mortality per se. However, they assume more importance in longer more complex surgery performed on patients who are at the extremes of age and who have significant comorbid conditions. Furthermore, the contribution that the inflammatory and immunologic sequelae to CPB make to postoperative infection remains unknown. At this time, CPB is far from perfect. Despite some technologic improvement in CPB equipment, no single anti-inflammatory or immunologic therapy has yet found routine use in clinical practice. Until more is known about the specific time course of SIRAB and which molecules assume central importance, pharmacologic therapy (including the future promise offered by monoclonal antibodies and gene-based strategies) should be treated with caution due to the risk of compounding postoperative immunodeficiency and thus increasing postoperative sepsis.

KEY POINTS

- Systemic Inflammatory Response After Bypass (SIRAB)
- CPB induces a whole body inflammatory response involving cellular and noncellular elements of blood.

- Red cell damage is due to shear stress and produces cell lysis, release of hemoglobin, and production of membrane "ghosts."
- Both neutrophils and vascular endothelial cells are activated by CPB.
  - Neutrophils adhere to endothelium and degranulate, releasing cytotoxic substances and causing small vessel obstruction.
- Platelets activate, degranulate, and adhere to CPB components.
- Humoral inflammatory cascade begins with activation of Hageman factor (factor XII).
  - Factor XII activates the intrinsic coagulation cascade, kallikrein, bradykinin, and plasmin (through kallikrein).
  - Complement is activated, leading to formation of the MAC.
  - Endotoxin circulates in high concentrations after CPB.
- SIRAB is associated with significant pulmonary, renal, and central nervous system pathology.
- Heparin coating of CPB circuitry and use of protease inhibitors (e.g., aprotinin) may ameliorate SIRAB.
- Cellular and humoral immune function is depressed after CPB.
- Numbers and function of T and B lymphocytes, killer T cells, RES cells decrease after CPB.
  - Altered T-cell plasma membrane after CPB.
  - Decreased lymphocyte response to PHA and decreased IL-2 production by lymphocytes after CPB.

REFERENCES

1. Westaby S. Complement and the damaging effects of cardiopulmonary bypass. *Thorax* 1983;38:321–325.
2. Kirklin JW, Donald DE, Harshbarger HG, et al. Studies in extracorporeal circulation 1. Applicability of Gibbon-type pump-oxygenator to human intracardiac surgery: 40 cases. *Ann Surg* 1956;144:2–8.
3. Kirklin JK, Westaby S, Blackstone EH, et al. Complement and the damaging effect of cardiac surgery. *J Thorac Cardiovasc Surg* 1983;86:845–852.
4. Van Velzen-Blad H, Dijkstra YJ, Heijnen CJ, et al. Cardiopulmonary bypass and host defense functions in human beings, lymphocyte function. *Ann Thorac Surg* 1985;39:212–217.
5. Utley JR. Renal effects of cardiopulmonary bypass. In: Utley JR, ed. *Pathophysiology and techniques of cardiopulmonary bypass.* Vol. 1. Baltimore: Williams & Wilkins, 1982:40–54.
6. Utley JR. Pathophysiology of cardiopulmonary bypass: a current review. *Aust J Cardiac Thorac Surg* 1992;1:46–52.
7. American College of Chest Physicians/Society of Critical Care Medicine. Consensus Conference: definition for sepsis and organ failure and guidelines for the use of innovative therapies in sepsis. *Crit Care Med* 1992;20:864–868.
8. Kirklin J, McGriffin D. Early complications following cardiac surgery. *Cardiovasc Clin* 1987;17:321–343.

9. Miedzinsky L, Karen G. Serious infectious complications of open heart surgery. *Can J Surg* 1987;30:103–107.

10. Cremer J, Martin M, Redl H, et al. Systemic inflammatory response after cardiac operations. *Ann Thorac Surg* 1996;61: 1714–1720.

11. Taylor K. SIRS—the systemic inflammatory response syndrome after cardiac operations. *Ann Thorac Surg* 1996;61: 1607–1608.

12. Elliot M. Perfusion for pediatric open heart surgery. *Semin Thorac Cardiovasc Surg* 1990;2:332–340.

13. Kirklin J. Prospects for understanding and eliminating the deleterious effects of cardiopulmonary bypass [editorial comment]. *Ann Thorac Surg* 1991;51:529–531.

14. Hornick P, Taylor K. Pulsatile and non-pulsatile perfusion: the continuing controversy. *J Cardiothorac Vasc Anesth* 1997;11: 310–315.

15. Taylor K. The present status of pulsatile perfusion. *Curr Med Lit Cardiovasc Med* 1984;3:66–69.

16. Hirayama T, Yamaguchi H, Allers M, et al. Evaluation of red cell damage during cardiopulmonary bypass. *Scand J Cardiovasc Surg* 1985;19:263–265.

17. Hoffman J. Cation transport and structure of the red cell plasma membrane. *Circulation* 1962;26:1201–1213.

18. Kreel I, Zaroff L, Canter J, et al. A syndrome following total body perfusion. *Surg Gynecol Obstet* 1960;111:317–321.

19. Scmid-Schonbein H, Born G, Richardson P, et al. ADP release from red cells subjected to high shear stress. In: Scmid-Schonbein H, Teitel P, eds. *Basic aspects of blood trauma.* The Hague, The Netherlands: Nijhoff, 1979:99.

20. Martin R. Alterations in leukocyte structure and function due to mechanical trauma. In: Hwang N, Gross D, Patel D, eds. *Quantitative cardiovascular studies: clinical and research applications of engineering principles.* Baltimore: University Park Press, 1979:419.

21. Faymonville M, Pincemail J, Duchateau J, et al. Myeloperoxidase and elastase as markers of leukocyte activation during cardiopulmonary bypass in humans. *J Thorac Cardiovasc Surg* 1991;102:309–312.

22. Albelda S, Smith C, Ward P. Adhesion molecules and inflammatory injury. *FASEB J* 1994;8:504–512.

23. Crossman D, Tuddenham E. Procoagulant functions of the endothelium. In: Warren J, ed. *The endothelium: an introduction to current research.* New York: Wiley-Liss, 1990:119–128.

24. Gillinov AM, Redmond JM, Winkelstein JA, et al. Complement and neutrophil activation during cardiopulmonary bypass: a study in the complement-deficient dog. *Ann Thorac Surg* 1994; 57:345–352.

25. Gillinov AM, Redmond JM, Zehr KJ, et al. Inhibition of neutrophil adhesion during cardiopulmonary bypass. *Ann Thorac Surg* 1994;57:126–133.

26. Kilbridge P, Mayer J, Newburger J, et al. Induction of intercellular adhesion molecule-1 and E-selectin mRNA in heart and skeletal muscle of pediatric patients undergoing cardiopulmonary bypass. *J Thorac Cardiovasc Surg* 1994;107:1183–1192.

27. Wilson I, Gillinov A, Curtis W, et al. Inhibition of neutrophil adherence improves postischemic ventricular performance in the neonatal heart. *Circulation* 1993;88[Suppl 2]:372–379.

28. Bevilacqua MP. Endothelial-leukocyte adhesion molecules. *Annu Rev Immunol* 1993;11:767–804.

29. Bevilacqua MP, Nelson RM, Mannori G, et al. Endothelial-leukocyte adhesion molecules in human disease. *Annu Rev Med* 1994;45:361–378.

30. McEver RP. Selectins. *Curr Opin Immunol* 1994;6:75–84.

31. Rot A. Endothelial binding of NAP-1/IL-8: role in neutrophil emigration. *Immunol Today* 1992;13:291–294.

32. Tanaka Y, Adams DH, Shaw S. Proteoglycans on endothelial cells present adhesion-inducing cytokines to leukocytes. *Immunol Today* 1993;14:111–115.

33. Tenaka Y, Adams DH, Hubscer S, et al. T-cell adhesion induced by proteoglycan-immobilized cytokine MIP-1 beta. *Nature* 1993;361:79–82.

34. Murphy PM. The molecular biology of leukocyte chemo-attractant receptors. *Annu Rev Immunol* 1994;12:593–633.

35. Haga Y, Hatori N, Yoshizu H, et al. Granulocyte superoxide anion and elastase release during cardiopulmonary bypass. *Artif Organs* 1993;17:837–842.

36. Colman RW. Platelet and neutrophil activation in cardiopulmonary bypass. *Ann Thorac Surg* 1990;49:32–34.

37. Faymonville ME, Pincemail J, Duchateau J, et al. Myeloperoxidase and elastase as markers of leukocyte activation during cardiopulmonary bypass. *J Thorac Cardiovasc Surg* 1991;102: 309–317.

38. Gadaleta D, Fahey AL, Verma M, et al. Neutrophil leukotriene generation after cardiopulmonary bypass. *J Thorac Cardiovasc Surg* 1994;108:642–647.

39. Frering B, Philip I, Dehoux M, et al. Circulating cytokines in patients undergoing normothermic cardiopulmonary bypass. *J Thorac Cardiovasc Surg* 1994;108:642–647.

40. Anderson LW, Baek L, Degn H, et al. Presence of circulating endotoxins during cardiac operations. *J Thorac Cardiovasc Surg* 1987;93:115–119.

41. Baeuerle PA, Henkel T. Function and activation of NF-kappa B in the immune system. *Annu Rev Immunol* 1994;12:141–179.

42. Hennessy VL, Hicks RE, Niewiarowski S, et al. Function of human platelets during extracorporeal circulation. *Am J Physiol* 1977;232:622–628.

43. Salzman EW. Blood platelets and extracorporeal circulation. *Transfusion* 1963;3:274–277.

44. Watkins DM, Peterson MB, Kong DL, et al. Thromboxane and prostacycline changes during cardiopulmonary bypass with and without pulsatile flow. *J Thorac Cardiovasc Surg* 1982;84: 250–256.

45. Harker LA, Malpass TW, Branson HE, et al. Mechanism of abnormal bleeding in patients undergoing cardiopulmonary bypass, acquired transient platelet defect associated with alpha granule release. *Blood* 1980;56:824–834.

46. Musial J, Niewiarowski S, Hershock D, et al. Loss of fibrinogen receptors from the platelet surface during simulated extracorporeal circulation. *J Lab Clin Med* 1985;105:514–526.

47. Zilla P, Fasol R, Groscurth P, et al. Blood platelets in cardiopulmonary bypass operations. *J Thorac Cardiovasc Surg* 1989;97: 379–388.

48. Chenoweth DE, Cooper SW, Hugli TE, et al. Complement activation during cardiopulmonary bypass: evidence for generation of C3a and C5a anaphylatoxins. *N Engl J Med* 1981;304: 497–503.

49. Pober J, Cotran R. Cytokines and endothelial cell biology. *Physiol Rev* 1990;70:427–451.

50. Kluft C, Dooijewaard G, Emeis J. Role of the contact system in fibrinolysis. *Semin Thromb Hemost* 1987;13:50–68.

51. Paul WE. *Fundamental immunology.* New York: Raven Press, 1993.

52. Muller-Eberhard H. The membrane attack complex. *Semin Immunopathol* 1984;73:93–141.

53. Gerard C, Gerard NP. C5a anaphylatoxin and its seven transmembrane-segment receptor. *Annu Rev Immunol* 1994;12: 775–808.

54. Parker DJ, Cantrell JW, Karp RB, et al. Changes in serum complement and immunoglobulins following cardiopulmonary bypass. *Surgery* 1972;71:824–827.

55. Jansen NJ, van-Oeveren W, Gu YJ, et al. Endotoxin release

and tumor necrosis factor formation during cardiopulmonary bypass. *Ann Thorac Surg* 1992;54:744–747.

56. Taggart DP, Sundaram S, McCartney C, et al. Endotoxemia, complement, and white blood cell activation in cardiac surgery: a randomized trial of laxatives and pulsatile perfusion. *Ann Thorac Surg* 1994;57:376–382.

57. Pekna M, Nilsson L, Nilsson-Ekdahl K, et al. Evidence for iC3 generation during cardiopulmonary bypass as the result of blood-gas interaction. *Clin Exp Immunol* 1993;91:404–409.

58. Boyle E, Pohlman T, Johnson M, et al. The systemic inflammatory response. *Ann Thorac Surg* 1997;64:531–537.

59. Verrier ED, Shen I. Potential role of neutrophil anti-adhesion therapy in myocardial stunning, myocardial infarction, and organ dysfunction after cardiopulmonary bypass. *J Card Surg* 1993;8:309–312.

60. Nilsson L, Kulander L, Nystrom S, et al. Endotoxins in cardiopulmonary bypass. *J Thorac Cardiovasc Surg* 1990;100: 777–780.

61. Campbell K, Forse R. Endotoxic rat atria show G-protein based deficits in inotropic regulation. *Surgery* 1993;114:471–479.

62. Ratcliff NB, Young WG, Hackett DB, et al. Pulmonary injury secondary to extracorporeal circulation. *J Thorac Cardiovasc Surg* 1973;65:425–431.

63. Haslett C, Worthen GS, Giclas PC, et al. The pulmonary vascular sequestration of neutrophils in endotoxemia is initiated by an effect of endotoxin on the neutrophil in the rabbit. *Am Rev Respir Dis* 1987;136:11–19.

64. Royston D, Fleming JS, Desai JB, et al. Increased peroxide generation associated with open heart surgery: evidence for free radical generation. *J Thorac Cardiovasc Surg* 1986;91:759–766.

65. Kharazmi A, Andersen LW, Baek L. Endotoxemia and enhanced generation of oxygen radicals by neutrophils from patients undergoing cardiopulmonary bypass. *J Thorac Cardiovasc Surg* 1989;98:381–385.

66. Fountain SW, Martin BA, Musclow CE, et al. Pulmonary leukostasis and its relationship to pulmonary dysfunction in sheep and rabbits. *Circ Res* 1980;46:175–180.

67. McDonald JW, Ali M, Morgan E, et al. Thromboxane synthesis by sources other than platelets in association with complement-induced pulmonary leukostasis and pulmonary hypertension in sheep. *Circ Res* 1983;52:1–6.

68. Till GO, Johnson KJ, Kunkel R. Intravascular activation of complement and acute lung injury. Dependency on neutrophils and toxic oxygen metabolites. *J Clin Invest* 1982;69: 1126–1135.

69. Shaw PJ, Bates D, Cartlidge NEF, et al. Early neurological complications of coronary bypass surgery. *Br Med J* 1985;291: 1384–1387.

70. Shaw PJ, Bates D, Cartlidge NEF, et al. Early intellectual dysfunction following coronary bypass surgery. *Q J Med* 1986;225: 59–68.

71. Shaw PJ, Bates D, Cartlidge NEF, et al. Natural history of neurological complications of coronary bypass surgery: a sixth month follow-up study. *Br Med J* 1986;293:165–167.

72. Shaw PJ, Bates D, Cartlidge NEF, et al. Neuro-ophthalmological complications of coronary artery bypass graft surgery. *Acta Neurol Scand* 1987;99:1–7.

73. Shaw PJ, Shaw DA. Psychiatry morbidity following cardiac surgery: a review. In: Davidson K, Kerr A, eds. *Contemporary themes in psychiatry.* London: Gaskell, 1989.

74. Blauth C, Koner EM, Arnold J, et al. Retinal microembolism during cardiopulmonary bypass demonstrated by fluorescein angiography. *Lancet* 1986;2:837–839.

75. Blauth CI, Arnold JV, Shulenberg WE, et al. Cerebral microembolism during cardiopulmonary bypass. Retinal microvascular studies in vivo with fluorescein angiography. *J Thorac Cardiovasc Surg* 1988;95:668–676.

76. Smith PLC, Newman S, Treasure T, et al. Cerebral consequences of cardiopulmonary bypass. *Lancet* 1986;1:823–824.

77. Harris DNF, Bailey SM, Smith PLC, et al. Brain swelling in the first hour after coronary artery bypass surgery. *Lancet* 1993; 342:586–587.

78. Wolbers JG. Brain swelling and coronary artery bypass surgery. *Lancet* 1993;343:62.

79. Cook DJ, Bryce RD, Oliver WC, et al. Brain swelling after coronary artery surgery. *Lancet* 1993;342:1370.

80. Ohri S, Desai J, Gaer J, et al. Intraabdominal complications following cardiopulmonary bypass. *Ann Thorac Surg* 1991;52: 826–831.

81. Fiddian-Green RG. Gut mucosal ischemia during cardiac surgery. *Semin Thorac Cardiovasc Surg* 1990;2:389–399.

82. Nilsson L, Tyd'en H, Johansson O, et al. Bubble and membrane oxygenators-comparison of postoperative organ dysfunction with special reference to inflammatory activity. *Scand J Thorac Cardiovasc Surg* 1990;24:59–64.

83. Blauth C, Smith P, JV A, et al. Influence of oxygenator type on the prevalence and extent of microembolic retinal ischemia during cardiopulmonary bypass. Assessment by digital image analysis. *J Thorac Cardiovasc Surg* 1990;99:61–69.

84. Cavarocchi N, Pluth J, Schaff H, et al. Complement activation during cardiopulmonary bypass. *J Thorac Cardiovasc Surg* 1986; 91:252–258.

85. Gu YJ, Wang YS, Chiang BY, et al. Membrane oxygenator prevents lung reperfusion injury in canine cardiopulmonary bypass. *Ann Thorac Surg* 1991;51:573–578.

86. Videm V, Fosse E, Mollnes TE, et al. Different oxygenators for cardiopulmonary bypass lead to varying degrees of complement activation. *J Thorac Cardiovasc Surg* 1989;97:764–770.

87. Gu YJ, van-Oeveren W, Akkerman C, et al. Heparin-coated circuits reduce the inflammatory response to cardiopulmonary bypass. *Ann Thorac Surg* 1993;55:917–922.

88. Jones D, Hill R, Hollingsed M, et al. Use of heparin-coated circuits reduce the inflammatory response to cardiopulmonary bypass. *Ann Thorac Surg* 1993;56:566–568.

89. Fosse E, Moen O, Johnson E, et al. Reduced complement and granulocyte activation with heparin-coated cardiopulmonary bypass. *Ann Thorac Surg* 1994;58:472–477.

90. Gu Y, Obster R, Haan J, et al. Biocompatibility of leukocyte removal filters during leukocyte filtration of cardiopulmonary bypass perfusate. *Artif Organs* 1993;17:660–665.

91. Moore FDJ, Warner KG, Assousa S, et al. The effects of complement activation during cardiopulmonary bypass. Attenuation by hypothermia, heparin, and hemodilution. *Ann Surg* 1988; 208:95–103.

92. Miyamoto Y, Hirose H, Matsuda H, et al. Analysis of complement activation profile during cardiopulmonary bypass and its inhibition by FUT-175. *Trans Am Soc* 1989;31:508–511.

93. Anderson LW, Baek L, Thomsen BS, et al. Effect of methylprednisolone on endotoxemia and complement activation during cardiac surgery. *J Cardiothorac Anesth* 1989;3:544–549.

94. Van Oeveren W, Jansen NJG, Bidstrup BP, et al. Effects of aprotinin on hemostatic mechanisms in cardiopulmonary bypass. *Ann Thorac Surg* 1987;44:610–615.

95. Van Oeveren W, Eijsman L, Roozendaal KJ, et al. Platelet preservation by aprotinin during cardiopulmonary bypass. *Lancet* 1988;1:644–648.

96. Hunt BJ, Cottam S, Segal H, et al. Inhibition of tPA-mediated fibrinolysis during orthotopic liver transplantation. *Lancet* 1990;336:381.

97. Tice DA, Worth M, Clauss RH. The inhibition by Trasylol of

fibrinolytic activity associated with cardiovascular operations. *Surg Gynecol Obstet* 1964;119:71–74.

98. Tice DA, Reed GE, Clauss RH, et al. Hemorrhage due to fibrinolysis occurring with open heart operations. *J Thorac Cardiovasc Surg* 1963;46:673–676.

99. Mammen EF. Natural protease inhibitors in extracorporeal circulation. *Ann NY Acad Sci* 1968;146:754–762.

100. Bidstrup BP, Royston D, Sapsford RN, et al. Reduction in blood loss and blood use after cardiopulmonary bypass with high dose aprotinin (Trasylol). *J Thorac Cardiovasc Surg* 1989; 97:364–372.

101. Royston D, Bidstrup BP, Taylor KM, et al. Effect of aprotinin on the need for blood transfusions after repeat open heart surgery. *Lancet* 1987;2:1289–1291.

102. Bidstrup BP, Royston D, Taylor KM, et al. Effect of aprotinin on need for blood transfusion in patients with septic endocarditis having open heart surgery. *Lancet* 1988;1:366–367.

103. Bidstrup BP, Harrison J, Royston D, et al. Aprotinin therapy in cardiac operations: a report on use in 41 cardiac centres in the United Kingdom. *Ann Thorac Surg* 1993;55:971–976.

104. Dietrich W, Spannagl M, Jochum M. Influence of high dose aprotinin treatment on blood loss and coagulation pattern in patients undergoing myocardial revascularization. *Anesthesiology* 1990;73:1119–1126.

105. Blauhut B, Gross C, Necek S, et al. Effects of high dose aprotinin on blood loss, platelet function, fibrinolysis, complement, and renal function after cardiopulmonary bypass. *J Thorac Cardiovasc Surg* 1991;101:958–967.

106. Hill GE, Alonso A, Thiele GM, et al. Glucocorticoids blunt neutrophil CD11b surface glycoprotein upregulation during cardiopulmonary bypass in humans. *Anesth Analg* 1994;79: 23–27.

107. Mathew JP, Rinder CS, Tracey JB, et al. Acadesine inhibits neutrophil CD11b up-regulation in vitro and during in vivo cardiopulmonary bypass. *J Thorac Cardiovasc Surg* 1995;109: 448–456.

108. Menasche P, Peynet J, Lariviere J, et al. Does normothermia during cardiopulmonary bypass increase neutrophil-endothelium interactions? *Circulation* 1994;90:275–279.

109. Johnson M, Haddix T, Pohlman T, et al. Hypothermia reversibly inhibits endothelial expression of E-selectin and tissue factor. *J Card Surg* 1995;10:428–435.

110. Le Deist, Menasche P, Kucharski C, et al. Hypothermia during cardiopulmonary bypass delays but does not prevent neutrophil-endothelial cell adhesion: a clinical study. *Circulation* 1995; 92[Suppl 2]:354–358.

111. Tracey KJ, Fong Y, Hesse DG, et al. Anti-cachectin/TNF monoclonal antibodies prevent septic shock during lethal bacteremia. *Nature* 1987;330:662–664.

112. Ohlsson K, Bjork P, Bergenfeldt M, et al. Interleukin-1 receptor antagonist reduces mortality from endotoxic shock. *Nature* 1990;348:550–552.

113. Sharar S, Winn R, Murry C, et al. A CD18 monoclonal antibody increases the incidence and severity of subcutaneous abscess formation after high-dose *Staphylococcus aureus* injection in rabbits. *Surgery* 1991;110:213–219.

114. Gillinov AM, DeValeria PA, Winkelstein JA, et al. Complement inhibition with soluble complement receptor type 1 in cardiopulmonary bypass. *Ann Thorac Surg* 1993;55:619–624.

115. Cochran A, Spilg W, RM M, et al. Post-operative depression of tumor-directed cell-mediated immunity in patients with malignant disease. *Br Med J* 1972;4:67–70.

116. Cullen B, Van Belle G. Lymphocyte transformation and changes in leukocyte count: effects of anesthesia and operation. *Anesthesiology* 1975;43:563–567.

117. Han T. Postoperative immunosuppression in patients with breast cancer. *Lancet* 1974;1:742–746.

118. Hofmann J, Helm L, Boulanger W, et al. The effect of surgery on cellular immunity. *Wis Med J* 1973;72:249–255.

119. Jubert A, Lee E, Hersh E, et al. Effects of surgery, anesthesia and intraoperative blood loss on immunocompetence. *J Surg Res* 1973;15:399–402.

120. Lee Y-TN. Effect of anesthesia and surgery on immunity. *J Surg Oncol* 1977;9:425–429.

121. Park S, Brady J, Wallace H, et al. Immuno-suppressive effect of surgery. *Lancet* 1971;1:53–57.

122. Riddle P, Berenbaum M. Postoperative depression of lymphocyte response to phytohemagglutinin. *Lancet* 1967;2:746–749.

123. Roth J, Golub S, Grimm E, et al. Effect of surgery on in vitro lymphocyte function. *Surg Forum* 1974;25:102–106.

124. Slade M, Simmons R, Yunis E, et al. Immunodepression after major surgery in normal patients. *Surgery* 1975;78:363–367.

125. Ulicny K, Hiratzka L. The risk factors of median sternotomy infection: a current review. *J Card Surg* 1991;6:338–351.

126. Loop F, Lytle B, Cosgrove D, et al. Sternal wound complications after isolated coronary artery bypass grafting. Early and late mortality, morbidity and cost of care. *Ann Thorac Surg* 1990; 49:179–187.

127. Bucknall T. Factors affecting healing. In: Bucknall T, Ellis H, eds. *Wound healing for surgeons*. London: Balliere Tindall, 1987: 42ff.

128. Serry C, Bleck P, Javid H, et al. Sternal wound complications: management and results. *J Thorac Cardiovasc Surg* 1980;80: 861–867.

129. Eskola J, Salo M, Viljanem K, et al. Impaired B lymphocyte function during open heart surgery. *Br J Anaesth* 1984;56: 333–337.

130. Salo M, Seppi E, Lassila O, et al. Effect of anesthesia and open-heart surgery on lymphocyte responses to phytohemagglutinin and concavalin A. *Acta Anaesth Scand* 1978;22:471–475.

131. Goris J, Boeckhorst T, Nuytinck J, et al. Multiple organ failure generalized autodestructive inflammation. *Arch Surg* 1985;120: 1109–1115.

132. Markewitz A, Faist E, Lang S, et al. Successful restoration of cell mediated immune response after cardiopulmonary bypass by immunomodulation. *J Thorac Cardiovasc Surg* 1993;105: 15–24.

133. Alexander J. The role of host defense functions in surgical infections. *Surg Clin North Am* 1980;60:107–111.

134. Dankert J. The use of a mobile cross-flow unit in open-heart surgery: a bacteriological evaluation. *Antonie Van Leeuwenhoek* 1978;44:247–253.

135. Markewitz A, Faist E, Niesel S, et al. Changes in lymphocyte subsets and mitogen responsiveness following open heart surgery and possible therapeutic approaches. *Thorac Cardiovasc Surg* 1992;40:14–18.

136. Gierhake F, Johannsen P, Stocker R, et al. Immuno-suppressive Wirkungen bei Operationen und Moglichkeiten ihrer Begrenzung. *Immun Infekt* 1975;3:116–119.

137. Roth J, Golub S, Cuckingnan R, et al. Cell-mediated immunity is depressed following cardiopulmonary bypass. *Ann Thorac Surg* 1981;31:350–356.

138. Parker FB, Marvast MA, Bove EL. Neurologic complications following coronary artery bypass: the role of atherosclerotic emboli. *Thorac Cardiovasc Surg* 1985;33:207–209.

139. Van Velzen-Blad H, Dijkstra Y, Schurink G, et al. Cardiopulmonary bypass and host defense functions in human beings: serum levels and the role of immunoglobulins and complement in phagocytosis. *Ann Thorac Surg* 1985;39:207–213.

140. Hammerschmidt D, Strcek D, Bowers T, et al. Complement

activation and neutropoenia occurring during cardiopulmonary bypass. *J Thorac Cardiovasc Surg* 1981;81:370–377.

141. Mayer J, McCullough J, Weiblen B, et al. Effects of cardiopulmonary bypass on neutrophil chemotaxis. *Surg Forum* 1976; 27:285–289.

142. Boonstra P, Vermeulen F, Leusink J, et al. Hematological advantage of a membrane oxygenator over a bubble oxygenator in long perfusion. *Ann Thorac Surg* 1986;41:297–300.

143. Bubenink O, Meakins J. Neutrophil chemotaxis in surgical patients: effect of cardiopulmonary bypass. *Surg Forum* 1976;27: 267–269.

144. Burrows F, Steele R, Marmer D, et al. Influence of operations with cardiopulmonary bypass on polymorphonuclear leukocyte function in infants. *J Thorac Cardiovasc Surg* 1987;93:253–260.

145. van Oeveren W, Dankert J, Wildevuur C. Bubble oxygenation and cardiotomy suction impair the host defense during cardiopulmonary bypass, a study in dogs. *Ann Thorac Surg* 1987;44: 523–528.

146. De Palma L, YU M, McIntosh C, et al. Changes in lymphocyte subpopulations as a result of cardiopulmonary bypass. *J Thorac Cardiovasc Surg* 1991;101:240–244.

147. Kress HG, Gehrsitz P, Elert O. Predictive value of skin test in neutrophil migration and C-reactive protein for post-operative infections in cardiopulmonary bypass patients. *Acta Anaesth Scand* 1987;31:397–404.

148. Larmi TKI, Karkola P. Plasma protein electrophoresis during a three hour cardiopulmonary bypass in dogs. *Scand J Thorac Cardiovasc Surg* 1974;8:152–157.

149. Lee WHJ, Krumhaar D, Fonkalsrud EW, et al. Denaturation of plasma proteins as a cause of morbidity and death after intracardiac operations. *Surgery* 1961;50:29–33.

150. Ryhaenen P, Huttunen K, Llonen J. Natural killer cell activity after open heart surgery. *Acta Anaesth Scand* 1984;28:490–492.

151. Nguyen D, Mulder D, Shennib H. Effect of cardiopulmonary bypass on circulating lymphocyte function. *Ann Thorac Surg* 1992;53:611–616.

152. Subramanian V, Lowman J, Gans H. Effect of extracorporeal circulation on recticuloendothelial function. Impairment and its relationship to blood trauma. *Arch Surg* 1968;97:330–334.

153. Brody H, Pickering N, Fink G, et al. Altered lymphocyte subsets during cardiopulmonary bypass. *Am J Clin Pathol* 1987;87: 626–628.

154. Pollock R, Ames R, Rubio P, et al. Protracted severe immune deregulation induced by cardiopulmonary bypass: a predisposing etiologic factor in blood transfusion-related AIDS? *J Clin Lab Immunol* 1987;22:1–5.

155. Ide H, Kackiuchi T, Furata N, et al. The effect of cardiopulmonary bypass on T cells and their subpopulations. *Ann Thorac Surg* 1987;44:277–282.

156. Ryhaenen P, Herna E, Hollmen A, et al. Changes in peripheral blood leukocyte counts, lymphocyte subpopulations and in vitro transformation after heart valve replacement. *J Thorac Cardiovasc Surg* 1979;77:259–266.

157. Hisatomi K, Isomura T, Kawara T, et al. Changes in lymphocyte subsets, mitogen responsiveness, and interleukin 2 production after cardiac operations. *J Thorac Cardiovasc Surg* 1989; 98:580–591.

158. Keller S, Weiss J, Scheifer S, et al. Stress-induced suppression of immunity in adrenalectomized rats. *Science* 1983;221: 1301–1303.

159. Yu D, Clements P, Paulus H, et al. Human lymphocyte subpopulations: effect of corticosteroids. *J Clin Invest* 1974;53: 565–568.

160. Tajima K, Yamamoto F, Kawazoe K, et al. Cardiopulmonary bypass and cellular immunity: changes in lymphocyte subsets and natural killer cell activity. *Ann Thorac Surg* 1992;55: 625–630.

161. Hornick P, Brookes P, Mason P, et al. Optimising a limiting dilution culture system for quantifying the frequency of IL-2 producing alloreactive helper T lymphocytes. *Transplantation* 1997;64:472–479.

162. Sharrock C, Kaminski E, Man S. Limiting dilution analysis of human T cells: a useful clinical tool. *Immunol Today* 1990;11: 281.

EMBOLIC EVENTS

BRUCE D. BUTLER
MARK KURUSZ

The word embolus is derived from the two Greek words *en* (in) and *ballein* (to throw); the combination *embolos* originally was used to describe a wedge-shaped object or stopper. The modern standard medical definition of embolism is "a sudden blocking of an artery by a clot or foreign material which has been brought to its site of lodgment by the blood current" (1).

Embolic events associated with cardiopulmonary bypass (CPB) have been a concern from the earliest clinical applications to the present time. Gross air embolism was one of the first identified risks of open heart surgery, but in the 1960s emboli composed of blood-derived material became increasingly recognized as etiologic factors in adverse postoperative sequelae. Improved techniques for anticoagulation management in the 1970s and a growing acceptance of blood filtration in the 1980s probably contributed to a decrease in morbidity and mortality during CPB procedures. Although current technologies, such as microporous membrane oxygenation, improved arterial line filters, and blood surface coatings, have decreased the incidence of microemboli even further, subtle embolic events still occur whenever CPB is used.

The production of emboli during CPB, whether gross or microscopic, has been causally linked to numerous perioperative and postoperative complications, patient characteristics such as age, technical features relating to the type of oxygenator, pump, reservoir, or CPB circuit, and the surgical procedure (2). Emboli fall into three general categories: biologic, foreign material, and gaseous. By definition, each type has the propensity to distribute into and ultimately obstruct microvessels (3 to 500 μm in diameter) of any number of tissues. Because of their small size, vast

quantities (namely, hundreds of thousands to hundreds of millions) are required to cause detectable organ injury (3,4).

Each of the three categories of emboli has been addressed to some degree by device design changes, adaptation of specific surgical or therapeutic procedures, or enhanced removal and preventive efforts by surgeons and perfusionists. These efforts have likely contributed to an appreciable decline in morbidity associated with CPB. In spite of this, emboli continue to be a topic of concern with all medical uses of extracorporeal circulation and open heart surgery. Of particular concern is the susceptibility of the brain to embolic damage. This condition is the subject of numerous reports demonstrating varying degrees of neurologic dysfunction after CPB (5–8).

The purpose of this chapter is to review the various types of emboli associated with CPB, their detection and pathophysiology, preventive measures and treatment, and future trends.

TYPES OF EMBOLI
Bloodborne

Bloodborne microemboli associated with CPB consist primarily of autologous cellular products or aggregates of various cell types (9,10). Cellular products include microthrombi containing fibrin/fibrinogen, lipid material, protein (denatured or not), bone or muscle fragments, and so forth. Platelet, neutrophil, and red cell aggregates also are commonly observed during and after bypass. Bloodborne emboli can derive from homologous transfused blood that accumulate proportionally with storage time (11,12). Fibrin formation occurs when inadequately anticoagulated blood contacts a foreign surface, thereby activating factor XII to factor XIIa and thus initiating the coagulation cascade. Heparin blocks coagulation within the cascade at multiple points, mainly by potentiating antithrombin III (13). An initial rapid adsorption of protein material, predominantly fibrinogen, occurs on foreign surfaces (14,15). Fibrin deposits likely form in areas of stagnant blood flow or where turbulence or cavitation phenomena exist and on roughened

B. D. Butler: Department of Anesthesiology, Hermann Center for Environmental, Aerospace and Industrial Medicine, University of Texas-Houston Medical School, Houston, Texas 77030.

M. Kurusz: Department of Surgery, Division of Cardiothoracic Surgery, University of Texas Medical Branch at Galveston, Galveston, Texas 77555-0528.

surfaces (14,16). Specific sites include intraluminal projections (17), oxygenator connectors (18), within bubble oxygenators (19), or within arterial line filters (20).

Anticoagulation therapy with heparin is usually assessed by measurement of the activated coagulation time, which, if greater than 300 to 400 seconds, is considered adequate for prevention of fibrin formation within circuits (21,22). Activated coagulation time measurement is necessary because the rate of heparin metabolism may vary with different patients (23); thus, dosage or plasma levels may not accurately predict the degree of anticoagulation (24).

Macroembolic and microembolic particles of fat are generated during CPB and are found in capillaries of the kidneys, lungs, heart, brain, liver, spleen (25), and in pericardial blood (26). These emboli are released as a result of trauma to the fat cells in the epicardium and surgical wound (27,28) and can occur without CPB after median sternotomy or thoracotomy (27). Fat emboli may be observed directly using microscopy or possibly inferred from increases in serum levels of total lipids, free fatty acids, triglycerides, or lipases. It has been estimated that two thirds of the fat emboli developed within a CPB circuit enter via cardiotomy suction (28). Fat emboli are commonly observed with bubble oxygenators (26,28,29) and to a lesser degree with membrane-type oxygenators (28), although this claim is not without challenge (30).

Fat emboli are typically formed with denaturation of plasma lipoproteins and lipids. The fat molecules that come out of solution consist of chylomicron aggregates (29) or free fat-containing triglycerides and cholesterol (28). Fat emboli may vary from 4 to 200 μm in diameter (26). A number of fatty acids and other lipid molecules have been linked with postperfusion lung parenchymal damage or alterations in surface properties (31,32). Generation of immiscible fat, however, is reduced by hemodilution (27).

As plasma proteins come into contact with foreign surfaces within the extracorporeal circuit, denaturation can occur (29). This process results in alterations in immunologic and complement proteins (33,34). Blood contact with foreign surfaces also activates platelets, which leads to aggregate formation and subsequent thrombocytopenia as platelets are consumed in this process (35–38). Membrane oxygenators reportedly produce fewer aggregates than bubble oxygenators (35). Platelet aggregates also are commonly observed in stored whole blood, packed red cells, and stored platelet concentrates (12). Although many aggregates are likely to disperse within the circulation (38), their embolic potential has been manifested in various organs, including the brain.

Significant decreases (30% to 50%) from preoperative platelet counts are usually observed early in the procedure as the platelets adhere to the surfaces within the circuit (39) or to the gas–blood interface of gaseous microemboli (40). Functional changes and decreased platelet counts have been associated with postoperative bleeding, whereas the circulat-

ing aggregates may provide a causative link with postoperative neurologic dysfunction (41). Preservation of platelet numbers has been reported with prostacyclin use and a reduction in aggregate formation (42,43). Reducing platelet sensitivity to aggregation with heparin (44) may be assisted with prostacyclin therapy, thus reducing the microembolic risk associated with bypass (45,46).

Platelet aggregation is associated with release of biogenic amines such as serotonin and other bioactive mediators such as thromboxane, which not only produce vasoconstriction but also may further promote adhesiveness and aggregate formation. Release of histamine from platelets and mast cells may promote changes in microvascular membrane permeability to plasma proteins, promoting interstitial edema formation (47).

Neutrophil aggregation during CPB may lead to complement activation (34). Hicks et al. (38) and Ratliff et al. (48) found aggregated leukocytes in the lungs of dogs undergoing bypass, and their presence was difficult to prevent clinically, although damage to other organs was not reported. Complement-mediated neutrophil aggregation appears to depend on the nature of the foreign material that the neutrophils contact (49). After aggregation, lysosomal enzyme release increases microvascular endothelial permeability to protein, especially in the lungs, contributing to the postperfusion lung syndrome (50). Upregulation of adhesion molecules and the subsequent adherence and activation of neutrophils with CPB is reviewed by Hall et al. (51).

Patients who possess cold-reacting antibodies, usually of the IgM class, may be at risk for red cell aggregate microembolization with cold cardioplegia or other hypothermic techniques used during open heart surgery (52–54).

Foreign Material

Foreign material emboli may consist of cotton fibers, plastic or metal particles from connectors or housings of disposable devices, filter material, tubing, talc, or surgical thread. Pulmonary embolism from bone wax used as a hemostatic agent with sternotomy incisions in experimental studies has been suggested as a potential contributor to pulmonary complications after open heart surgery (55). Obviously, some of the material described above may be present on artificial surfaces that come into contact with blood during CPB or result from inadvertent inclusion within the circulating blood (56). Braun et al. (57) reported elevated serum aluminum levels postoperatively in patients who had undergone CPB. Such aluminum contamination was associated with use of specific manufacturers' aluminum heat exchangers. When a stainless steel heat exchanger was used, there was no elevation in plasma aluminum levels. More recently, Challa et al . (58) elevated levels of aluminum and silicone in the brains of patients who died after CPB.

Microemboli that are usually relatively large in diameter (greater than 300 μm) may be released into the circuit from tubing (e.g., by spallation). These emboli are more common with silicone-based rubber tubing than with tubing of polyvinyl chloride or polyurethane base (59–62). Another known foreign material is microfibrillar collagen used for surgical hemostasis. Used topically, this material has been shown to pass through autotransfusion devices and oxygenators, and although effectively removed by filtration, the ability of platelets to aggregate seems to persist. This effect has resulted in the recommendation that blood from treated patients should not be returned to the extracorporeal circuit (63).

Microparticles (10 μm and greater) of silicone antifoam A (Dow Corning Corp., Midland, MI) have been observed after bypass in the adrenal gland and pancreas (64). Antifoam is composed of a liquid polymer (dimethylpolysiloxane) and particulate silica. The polymer material is the defoaming agent, whereas the silica provides for blood dispersion.

In the early 1960s, a number of studies demonstrated antifoam emboli in experimental animals and patients undergoing bypass. The amount of defoamer material and methods of incorporation were less understood during that period. Orenstein et al. (64) reported particle-droplet complexes incorporating antifoam in patients up to 8 months after open heart surgery. The ultimate fate of antifoam in the body is not clear. Some reports have described particles in the phagocytic cells of the spleen or lymph nodes, whereas others have reported continuous recirculation for prolonged periods (65). Tissue reaction to silicone or antifoam has not been reported to any significant degree. Wells et al. (66), however, reported that the antifoam polymethylsiloxane magnified the hemolytic phenomena attributed to oxygenators primarily by decreasing the resistance of red cells to mechanical stress. In earlier experimental studies on dogs, antifoam emboli were found in the brain, kidneys, and occasionally in the spleen and liver (67–69).

Gupta et al. (70) reported a significant yet transient rise in pulmonary artery pressure with antifoam injections in dogs, demonstrating the capacity of these microparticles to obstruct pulmonary microvascular blood flow. Washoff of antifoam material from the oxygenator and cardiotomy reservoir has been shown to decrease the surface tension of the pre-CPB prime solution, which has important implications for gaseous microembolus stability or removal by arterial line filters (71). Further reductions in post-CPB plasma surface tension were not observed, and the values did not correlate with the duration of bypass or plasma-free hemoglobin (72). Design changes and a better understanding of the amounts and methods of applications of antifoam material and the use of membrane oxygenators have enabled significant reductions in the occurrence of embolic risk from these particles. Table 16.1 summarizes the reported types of nongaseous emboli associated with CPB.

TABLE 16.1. NONGASEOUS MICROEMBOLI REPORTED DURING CARDIOPULMONARY BYPASS

Microthrombi (e.g., fibrin)	Cotton fibers
Platelet aggregates	Plastic particles
Neutrophil aggregates	Filter material
Red cell aggregates	Tubing fragments
Denatured protein	Metal
Fat or lipids	Talc
Cold-reacting antibodies	Thread
Bone fragments	Bone wax
Muscle fragments	Microfibrillar collagen
Calcium particles	Silicone antifoam

Gaseous

Gaseous microemboli originate from a number of sources during bypass; however, oxygen microbubbles generated by bubble oxygenators have historically been the most commonly reported source. Gaseous microemboli produced in these devices are usually 400 μm or less in diameter and consist primarily of oxygen, although other gases, including carbon dioxide, nitrogen, or nitrous oxide, may exchange with the bubbles once they are formed and perfused into the patient (73–80). Gaseous microemboli size may be quite variable, with most in the 10- to 100-μm range. Bubbles with diameters greater than 35 to 40 μm are reportedly associated with CPB morbidity, unlike those of smaller diameters (3,81). Table 16.2 compares bubble diameters with volume and surface area. By the mid-1980s, bubble oxygenators had been designed to minimize gaseous microemboli production while maintaining oxygen transfer characteristics at lower gas-to-blood flow ratios (82–85). These design changes, along with chemical defoaming agents and arterial line filtration, significantly reduced the numbers and sizes of gaseous microemboli produced by bubble oxygenators. Gaseous microemboli with diameters below 40 μm are still reported, however, even with arterial line filtration (86,87).

Production of gaseous microemboli depends in part on the methods of operation of the bubble oxygenator. Maintaining a low gas-to-blood flow ratio will reduce the number of microbubbles released into the arterial line (88,89). Current oxygenators operate efficiently at ratios approximating 1:1. This represents a significant advance over earlier models requiring ratios 10-fold greater (4). The enhanced efficiency is largely because of the production of smaller oxygen bubbles. The smaller size increases the total area of the contact surface of the oxygen bubble and the blood (82). These smaller microbubbles are more difficult to remove, however, and often require arterial line filtration. Arterial and venous blood reservoir levels have been shown to be inversely related to gaseous microemboli production (74,90–93). With increased fluid levels, the time available for gas dissipation and defoamer action increases. Persistent gaseous microem-

TABLE 16.2. RELATIONSHIP OF DIAMETER, VOLUME, AND SURFACE AREA

Diameter of Each Bubble	Volume of Each Bubble	No. of Bubbles	Total Volume (Volume of Each Bubble × No. of Bubbles)	Surface Area of Each Bubble	Total Surface Area (Surface Area × No. of Bubbles)
1 cm = 10 mm	0.5 mL	1	0.5 mL	3.14 cm²	3.14 cm²
0.1 cm = 1 mm	0.5 μL	1,000	0.5 mL	3.14 mm²	31.4 cm²
0.01 cm = 100 μm	5×10^{-4} μL	1,000,000	0.5 mL	31,400 μm²	314 cm²
0.001 cm = 10 μm	5×10^{-7} μL	1,000,000,000	0.5 mL	314 μm²	3,140 cm²

Source: Tovar EA, Del Campo C, Borsari A, et al. Postoperative management of cerebral air embolism: gas physiology for surgeons. *Ann Thorac Surg* 1995;60:1138–1142, with permission.

boli often adhere to the artificial surfaces in quiescent areas of the oxygenator and reservoir, and any unnecessary jarring or abrupt shock releases these bubbles into the arterial line (75).

The production of gaseous microemboli by membrane-type blood oxygenators is significantly reduced or, by some accounts, nonexistent (74,84,94). Physical damage to the membrane material may allow release of gas bubbles into the blood, or areas with elevated transmembrane pressure ratios may cause bubble formation on the blood side. Graves et al. (95) described a counter-diffusion phenomenon whereby bubbles would be formed at the membrane surface.

Regardless of oxygenator type, the solubility characteristics of gases are such that the colder the solution, the greater the number of molecules dissolved within the liquid phase. The solubility of oxygen, for example, is 2.6 volume percent in water at 30°C and 4.9 volume percent at 0°C. While warming from hypothermia, gaseous microemboli will form in the blood if the warming gradient exceeds a certain critical threshold (96). This relationship is most evident when the subsequent rewarming gradient is in excess of 10 to 17°C (3,94,97,98), which can cause gaseous microemboli to be released in the heat exchanger. Another condition could also occur whereby gaseous microemboli are released into the blood during the cooling phase when the saturated cold arterial blood exiting the heat exchanger is warmed upon mixture with the patient's warm blood (99). The opposite situation also has been described, whereby the warm arterial blood coming from the heat exchanger is circulated into a hypothermic patient and the increased solubility of the gases in the cold blood prevents the evolution of bubbles (100). Any existent bubbles likewise would be expected to dissolve under these conditions.

Based on these principles, Edmunds and Williams (3) concluded that the greatest chance of gaseous microemboli production as a result of temperature changes most likely occurs during the cooling phase, where bubbles are released directly into the patient's circulation. Almond et al. (101) reported ischemic cerebral injury in dogs with cooling gradients of 13 to 15°C. However, their studies did not involve the search for or detection of circulating bubbles. Circumstantial evidence lending support to these phenomena has

been reported clinically with rapid induction of hypothermia in patients undergoing CPB (102–104). Geissler et al. (105) studied cooling gradients and gaseous microemboli formation in dogs undergoing CPB using membrane oxygenators. With transesophageal echocardiography and Doppler ultrasound sensors located on the CPB circuit and carotid arteries, they reported that rapid cooling did not result in gaseous microemboli formation when the cooled perfusate entered the subject, even when temperature gradients between the water bath and core (esophageal) temperatures exceeded 20°C. It was observed, however, that the actual determinative gradient site for the formation of gaseous microemboli was in the aortic arch where the blood and perfusate first mix. Gaseous microemboli were detected in small quantities when the temperature gradient was preestablished and exceeded 10°C. The incidence of gaseous microemboli was directly correlated with the extent of the temperature gradient, and in no cases were bubbles detected in the carotid arteries. Although currently available bubble oxygenators incorporate the heat exchanger directly into the oxygenating column, thereby enabling the defoamer action to minimize gaseous microemboli production, standard operating procedures should continue to require that heating or cooling gradients not exceed 10°C (4,98).

Gaseous and particulate emboli are commonly reported with cardiotomy suction (36,106). Inherent to all suctioning procedures is the mixing of air with the blood, forming relatively large bubbles, often in a foamlike matrix. These bubbles are not only larger than the gaseous microemboli produced by the oxygenator but consist of air (mostly nitrogen) and hence are more stable and often associated with other blood products or aggregate material (107). The increased stability is due not only to the larger volume of gas in the bubbles that must be reabsorbed, but also to the differences in solubility of nitrogen in blood as compared with oxygen or carbon dioxide. Because of their greater stability, these bubbles present a significant risk to the patient if filtration techniques are inadequate. Previously, it has been demonstrated that bubbles can pass through a cardiotomy reservoir (108,109); however, newer design changes incorporating improved defoamer material, unique flow patterns, and integral filters have significantly reduced the incidence of this phenomenon.

The process of suctioning also results in significant blood trauma, which causes cellular aggregation and gas foam formation. Efforts to reduce the amount of air aspirated with operative field blood and care in monitoring suction pump speed will reduce blood cell trauma and decrease the likelihood of embolization.

Gaseous emboli also can be produced by processes known as gaseous or vaporous cavitation (110,111). Cavitation involves hydrodynamic phenomena that consist of bubble nucleation, growth in volume, and then ultimate collapse (112). The bubbles or cavities contain gas or vapor. True vaporous cavitation is an extremely transient phenomenon. Gaseous cavitation, similar to effervescence, is more common in gas-nucleated fluids, including blood, that are subjected to tensile, ultrasonic, or supersaturating pressures (113). In these conditions, bubble growth is achieved by mass transfer of gas molecules by diffusive mechanisms and occurs with lesser pressure reductions. Vaporous cavitation occurs when a vacuous space is created in blood, for example, within the negative pressure regions that develop behind the roller pump heads, and the sudden pressure reduction creates a drop to below liquid vapor pressure (114,115). Early model centrifugal pumps reportedly produce fewer gaseous microemboli than roller pump heads (116).

Similar cavitating phenomena can occur at arterial injection sites or at stenotic regions in the circuit where vortices are created with turbulent flow and negative pressures spontaneously develop (117–119). In their review of cavitation phenomena during CPB, Kuntz and Maurer (120) evaluated a number of factors involved with gaseous microemboli production at the arterial cannula site. Such factors include Reynolds' number, kinetic energy, hydrostatic and line pressure, temperature, PO_2 levels, cannula size, and fluid flow rate. The authors concluded that excess blood gas tensions should be avoided and that larger bore arterial cannulas were less likely to be associated with gaseous microemboli production at cavitating velocities. In addition to the formation of gaseous microemboli, cavitating phenomena are extremely traumatic to red cells and can cause platelet activation, granule release, and cell lysis (112). Vapor bubbles are also reported with transmyocardial laser revascularization, as detected with transesophageal echo and transcranial Doppler (121,122). Although both studies detected cerebral vascular emboli, neither reported adverse gross neurologic deficits or decreases in mean cerebral blood flow velocity or jugular bulb oxygen saturation.

Air emboli can be introduced into the patient's arterial blood when the cardiac chambers are opened to the atmosphere for valvular, atrial septal, or ventricular septal repair. Pearson (79) characterized "surgical air" as that entering the arterial circulation from cannulation of the heart and aorta, after removal of the aortic clamp, air entrainment at the site of venous cannulation, after restoration of cardiac function, and during left atrial catherization. Air may be introduced with insertion of the aortic, caval, or right atrial cannulas. In the presence of an atrial septal defect or with placement of a left atrial or left ventricular vent cannula, air may be introduced directly into the systemic circulation (123).

With open heart procedures, air often is entrained on the luminal surfaces of the heart or trapped within the muscular trabeculae. Cardiac ejection should be avoided until complete blood filling occurs. Residual air has been reported for 30 to 45 minutes using transesophageal echocardiography even with careful deairing attempts (124,125), and upon resumption of cardiac contractions cerebral vascular gas was detected with transcranial Doppler (124). Prevention of systemic air embolism can be accomplished by insertion of a vent into the left ventricle (126) or needle aspiration of the pulmonary veins and cardiac chambers (127). Another technique reported to reduce air embolism at the operative site is flooding the surgical field with carbon dioxide (128–130). Recent reports on cardiac valve operations have demonstrated with transesophageal echocardiography that carbon dioxide field flooding caused residual gas, remaining after careful deairing maneuvers, to disappear within 1 minute in 86% of cases and within 1 to 24 minutes in the remaining cases (125). Other maneuvers include closure of the left atrium under blood, lung expansion to clear pulmonary venous blood, and placement of the patient in the Trendelenburg position or allowing the right lung to collapse (131), thus preventing air from entering pulmonary veins on the right side. Details of ventricular venting have been described by Utley and Stephens (132) and are discussed more fully in Chapter 6. Both advantages and disadvantages of venting and explicit procedures have been described by these authors for operative ways to prevent or remove surgical air.

As previously mentioned, gaseous microemboli produced by bubble oxygenators usually consist of oxygen, and because of the solubility/diffusibility of this gas, their longevity and pathophysiology are limited to some degree. Experimentally, animals embolized intravascularly with gases of high solubility, such as carbon dioxide or oxygen, tolerate the insult better than those embolized with air or nitrogen bubbles (133–135). Bubbles will pass into the systemic vasculature, causing blood flow obstruction, until the volume decreases by mass diffusion across the gas–blood interface and further movement within the microcirculation ensues. In the case of oxygen bubbles, the diffused gas will combine with unsaturated hemoglobin while carbon dioxide may be absorbed within the plasma. Yang et al. (136,137) studied stationary and moving bubbles in whole blood and plasma and found that dissolution rates were proportional to the fluid flow rate. The outward diffusion of the gas was largely assisted by the convective effects of the flowing blood and subsequent thinning of the boundary layer (138). A small

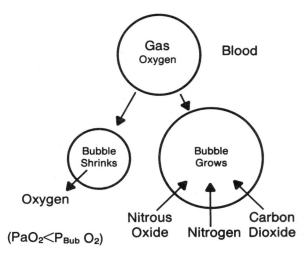

FIG. 16.1. Bubble in blood showing the effects of gas diffusion on size. Oxygen diffuses out and nitrogen, carbon dioxide, and nitrous oxide diffuse in, according to partial pressure gradients. (From Butler BD. Biophysical aspects of gas bubbles in blood. *Med Instrum* 1985;19:59–62, with permission.)

microbubble has an increased degree of curvature that accelerates the dissolution rates as surface tension increases and pressure within the bubble rises (Fig. 16.1).

Because gaseous microemboli are likely to occur with bypass, it has been shown that ventilation with highly soluble gases more soluble than nitrogen, such as nitrous oxide, may cause existing bubbles to grow. Some therefore recommend that nitrous oxide should be discontinued at least 10 minutes before establishing CPB (139–141). Wells et al. (142) confirmed the benefit of this practice by measuring cerebrospinal fluid markers of ischemia in 20 patients, 10 of whom received 50% to 60% nitrous oxide until CPB was begun. Lactate levels were significantly elevated in these 10 patients. Several extensive reviews cover the behavior of gas bubbles in fluids (143–149).

Free microbubbles in blood provide a foreign surface that initiates microthrombus formation (150), activates platelets and leukocytes, and alters erythrocyte count (150–152). These gas–liquid interfaces also cause the adsorption and denaturation of plasma proteins (150,151,153) subsequent to formation of a lipoprotein layer (154). This lipoprotein coat has been described as a layer 40 to 100 Å thick, within which physical forces exist that cause disruption of the secondary and tertiary protein configurations. Release of bound lipids is likely to occur as well (155). This includes phospholipids, which may have a polar attraction to the gas–liquid interface. Activation of the Hageman factor and acceleration of coagulation also are reported with intravascular bubbles (153).

Adherence of platelets to bubble interfaces has been observed microscopically, which apparently forms a thin outer layer that contains fibrinogen (40,150,156). Figure 16.2 is a photomicrograph of cellular adhesion to a gas bubble. As the first protein layered onto a bubble surface, fibrinogen has nonpolar hydrophilic groups that are exposed as possible binding sites for other bloodborne products, including fatty acids (153) and large lipid particles that may further promote platelet adhesion and spreading (157). Ultrastructural changes of microbubble-activated platelets resemble those following activation with thrombin, adenosine diphosphate, or collagen (158). Accumulation of platelets within the interstices between bubbles may also play a role in foam stabilization where excess bubbling occurs.

Microbubble-activated platelet density is greater when bubbles are 40 μm or more in diameter, suggesting a dependency on size rather than on total bubble count (157). This may be partly because of the lesser degree of curvature with larger bubbles, which could facilitate platelet adhesion and spreading (158), thereby initiating aggregate formation (153). Table 16.3 summarizes the reported causes of gaseous microemboli during CPB. Direct action of gaseous emboli on the vascular endothelium reportedly includes functional changes, denudation and herniation of the cells, and leukocyte and platelet aggregation and activation (40,149, 159–162). Release of inflammatory mediators from activated cells, including leukotrienes, thromboxanes, and prostaglandins, is also reported with gas embolism and causally linked to changes in microvascular permeability (163–166). Because the endothelial cells are also responsible for release of other vasoactive mediators such as nitric oxide, the degree of injury caused by the gas emboli can affect vessel diameter and flow (161,167–169). Table 16.4 lists mediators that are released during bubble–blood interactions. Contrasting evidence indicating no adverse effect of gaseous microemboli on cerebral blood flow or metabolism or arterial vasospasm was partially explained by differences in size and total amount of emboli involved (161,170). Table 16.5 summarizes both direct and indirect bubble–blood interactions.

DETECTION

Detection of microemboli associated with bypass has been described using histologic techniques (18,79), direct visual or optical methods (171–173), radiography (127), computed tomography (174), particle sizing using resistance or laser devices (12,175), screen filtration pressure (176), screen sampling (35), bulk compressibility (177), fluorescein angiography (178,179), and ultrasound (180). Each of the above techniques has afforded some degree of precision in its ability to size or count microemboli; however, more often than not, one parameter is gained at the expense of another. Optical detection devices, including particle-size analyzers and screen sampling, usually require a small sample volume obtained through a sidestream suitably narrow for light and optical through-transmission. Such techniques may be reliable for sizing, but not counting, the microem-

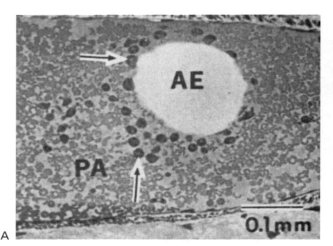

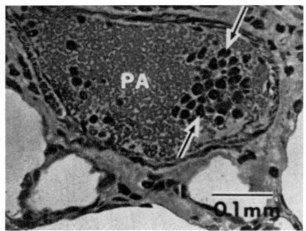

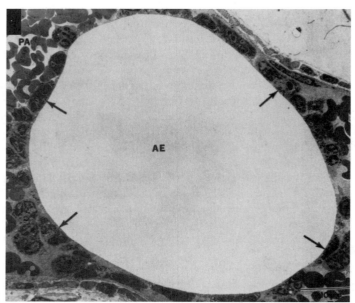

FIG. 16.2. Air embolism in sheep blood. **A:** Single air embolism (*AE*) 4 hours after pulmonary artery (*PA*) embolization. Note dark cells (neutrophils) aggregated around the AE. **B:** Clumps of neutrophils believed to be remnants of the air bubble–blood interface after the air bubble was resorbed. **C:** Transmission electron micrograph of an AE nearly completely surrounded by neutrophils at the AE–blood interface. (From Albertine KH, Weiner-Kronish JP, Koike K, et al. Quantitation of damage by air emboli to lung microvessels in anesthetized sheep. *J Appl Physiol* 1984;57: 1360–1368, with permission.)

TABLE 16.3. KNOWN CAUSES OF GASEOUS MICROEMBOLI

Bubble oxygenation
High gas-to-blood flow ratio (bubble oxygenator)
Low CPB reservoir level
Excessive cooling and heating gradients (i.e., >10°C)
Drug injections into circuit
Mechanical jarring of circuit
Inadequate debubbling (especially of arterial filter)
Gaseous or vaporous cavitation
Damaged membrane material
Counter-diffusion phenomena
Overoccluded roller pump
Excessive cardiotomy/vent suction
Pulsatile flow through microporous membrane oxygenator

CPB, cardiopulmonary bypass.

TABLE 16.4. MEDIATOR RELEASE FROM GASEOUS EMBOLIZATION

ADP
Catecholamines
Histamine
Hydrogen peroxide
Hydroxy radicals
Leukotrienes
Prostaglandins
Serotonin
Superoxide anions
Thromboxanes

ADP, adenosine diphosphate.

TABLE 16.5. BLOOD: BUBBLE INTERACTIONS (DIRECT AND INDIRECT)

Adsorption/denaturation of plasma proteins
Adsorption of phospholipids
Adsorption of fibrinogen
Activation of Hageman factor
Complement activation
Clumping of red cells
Leukocyte activation/adherence
Lipid peroxidation
Microthrombi production
Platelet activation/adherence
Thrombin activation
Phospholipase activation
Endothelial cell damage

---

boli (181). Sequential sampling of aliquots of blood can be used with settling or rising chambers (in the case of gaseous microemboli) to determine bulk volume or total gas phase using dilatometry but are less reliable for size determination (182,183). This same analogy applies to screen filtration techniques. Bulk compressibility takes advantage of the compressible nature of gas bubbles dispersed within a fluid to determine total volume but not size or count of total numbers. More recently described techniques for detecting microembolism during or resulting from CPB surgery are magnetic resonance imaging (184) and the potential for combined use of single-photon emission computed tomography with transcranial Doppler to evaluate subclinical effects (185).

Of all emboli detection techniques, ultrasonic devices are the most commonly used today. These devices include transcranial, transesophageal, and Doppler flow devices (pulsed and continuous wave) and echo machines using both M- and B-modes. The enthusiasm for using ultrasound to detect microemboli is based in part on the ability to discriminate the circulating particles from the background blood flow using usually noninvasive techniques. Ultrasound devices work by emitting a sound signal from a piezoelectric crystal that is reflected from the moving blood cells. The frequency of the reflected signals differs from that of the transmitted signal in proportion to the blood velocity. With Doppler devices, these frequency shifts typically occur within the audible range (0 to 10 kHz). The audio signal contains both amplitude and frequency information, and the degree of reflection of the sound waves is a function of the difference in acoustic properties of the reflecting particles.

Microemboli, whether solid or gaseous, are more effective in scattering sound because of the difference in density between the particle and the surrounding blood or tissue. Gas bubbles are much more efficient at scattering ultrasound than more rigid particles, such as red cell aggregates or microthrombi, especially at the smaller diameters (150).

This difference is due to the acoustic properties of nongaseous emboli being similar to those of blood. Additionally, gas bubbles have the propensity to resonate as the ultrasonic wave causes pressure oscillations and hence vibration of the gas inside the bubble. At the resonance frequency of a bubble of a particular size, the scattering of sound is maximal (186). The reflection of sound waves also is influenced by the frequency of the ultrasonic wave as it passes through the tissue and fluid and by the diameter of the microembolus itself (108). Gaseous microemboli as small as 1 μm have been detected with ultrasound (186) in tissues, whereas other authors have detected circulating microbubbles of 20 to 50 μm (186–188).

Ultrasonic Doppler devices used for detection of microemboli used pulsed or continuous-wave transmission. With pulsed systems, short energy bursts (about 2 μs) are emitted at rates on the order of 1,000 pulses per second. Particles along the beam path are then set in motion, reflecting the sound waves, whereas the regions in front of or behind it are not affected. This technique enables the operator to focus the beam to a specified depth. Using pulsed Doppler systems for microemboli detection highly depends on the particle diameter (189,190), angulation of the ultrasonic transducer (75,108,191), and incident pulse length (189,190). Blood flow rate also has an important influence on pulsed Doppler systems in that the pulse echoes usually represent the product of the pulse frequency and the time that the bubble resides within the sampling field (190). Some devices take this feature into consideration by making the pulse-repetition frequency proportional to the blood flow (192). With continuous-wave ultrasound, the emitted beam is continuous, and the particles are sonified along the entire length of beam penetration. Continuous-wave Doppler devices are currently used in a number of clinical diagnostic devices and are commonly used for microemboli detection.

Echo imaging systems have gained widespread support in recent years in detecting circulating microemboli. Transthoracic, transesophageal, and transcranial ultrasound devices enable localization of microemboli within each of the respective acoustic fields. The B-mode enables the operator to view the emboli within the heart chambers, although some degree of quantitation may be obtained by M-mode, because the x-axis represents the time scale and relative counts are possible (193). Transesophageal echocardiography has been shown to be particularly effective in detecting gaseous microemboli during and after CPB and is useful in determining the adequacy of deairing maneuvers (194–198). The closeness of the esophagus to the myocardium and aorta enable transesophagal echo to obtain an acoustic window without interference from the chest wall, ribs, and lungs and does not interfere with the surgical field (199,200). It also represents one of the most sensitive modalities for gas embolus detection of volumes as small as 0.0001 mL/kg within the left ventricle (196) or of individual bubbles ranging in size from 25 to 225 μm (mean, 70 ± 49) in diameter (201).

Transcranial Doppler has been used for detection of perioperative cerebral microemboli, for evaluation of arterial line filtration (202), for valve replacement monitoring (124), and for its original application during carotid endarterectomy (203,204). These devices not only enable the detection and visualization of bubbles or particulate matter in the cranial arteries but also determine blood flow characteristics (124,202–205).

Yao et al. (206) compared the efficacy of simultaneous embolic monitoring using transcranial Doppler of the middle cerebral artery and transesophageal echocardiography of the aortic arch in 20 patients undergoing CPB. Emboli signals were obtained from all patients, with the mean total signal counts of the aorta being 77% greater than the cerebral emboli. Overall, 83% of the emboli signals were detected during the aortic cross-clamp and partial occlusion clamp placement. Both techniques were recommended as effective emboli monitors. Because fewer emboli circulate into the cerebral vessels, Droste et al. (207) suggested that monitoring times last at least 1 hour when using transcranial Doppler to allow greater specificity.

Clark et al. (208) combined data on stroke with coma and inappropriate behavior to validate these effects against total microembolic counts measured with transcranial Doppler in patients undergoing CPB. The Doppler device was used to evaluate the various surgical maneuvers and their role in emboli generation. Seventy percent of the patients that demonstrated cerebral dysfunction had embolic counts greater than 60. Those patients with the highest incidence of surgical air had the highest incidence of cerebral dysfunction, whereas those with the higher counts of CPB-generated emboli had greater decrements in cognitive function compared with those with fewer. Overall, the CPB-generated emboli were relatively well tolerated.

Quantitation of microemboli is difficult with any ultrasonic device because of certain limitations inherent to their proper operation (192,209,210). These limitations involve characteristics such as the frequency requirements, transducer angulation, and electrical circuitry used for signal analysis and sampling area (85,88,181,192,209). Calibration of the devices, although often overlooked, is very important. Use of solid artificial microparticles of plastic or glass is common for calibration; however, their acoustic properties are usually different than those of bloodborne or gaseous microemboli (75,148,211), and clumping or settling may further complicate any sort of accurate calibration. For accurate gaseous microemboli quantification, calibrated microbubbles are more reliable because of their similarities in acoustic properties (150,175,190,209,211–213).

Despite these calibration procedures, certain limitations exist with any attempt to quantitate the size or number of microemboli present in vessels or the bypass circuit (180,208,213,214). Figure 16.3 depicts potential causes for signal differences from bubbles detected by Doppler ultrasound. Current trends are to develop techniques to both discriminate between gaseous and solid microemboli and to quantitate them in terms of size and/or numbers. Using multifrequency devices or sophisticated signal analysis of spectral patterns, some investigators have undertaken efforts to accomplish these goals (215–219). Other efforts have been made to determine the nature and size of the emboli using the intensity of the reflected signals (220–221); however, features relevant to the composition of the embolus may be more difficult to characterize (222). Dual frequency,

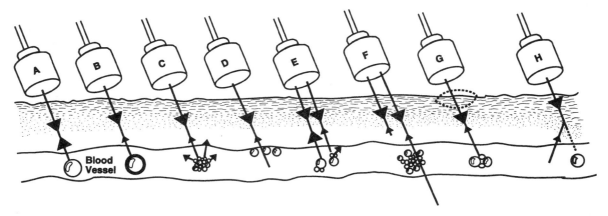

FIG. 16.3. Potential causes for signal differences from bubbles detected by Doppler ultrasound: **(A)** encapsulated bubble; **(B)** ideal condition with signal reflected back from discrete bubble; **(C)** multiple bubbles with scattered signals; **(D)** different location of bubbles within sample beam; **(E)** bubbles of different sizes blocking sound waves of others; **(F)** probe operated at different frequencies; **(G)** artifact due to gross movement of skin/surface probe interface; and **(H)** refraction of beam due to density differences at tissue interfaces. (Modified from Butler BD. Biophysical aspects of gas bubbles in blood. *Med Instrum* 1985;19:59–62, with permission.)

multifrequency, second harmonic, pattern recognition, and artificial neural network using ultrasound devices have also recently been tested for further refinement of the embolus characteristics (223–229).

PATHOPHYSIOLOGY

It is generally accepted that postoperative diffuse cerebral dysfunction after the use of CPB is largely attributable to microembolism and/or compromise of cerebral blood flow (223). Individual differences in patient tolerance to bypass make it difficult to universally define safe thresholds for flow, pressure, and pulsatility (170,230,231). The brain has been the focus of most studies evaluating negative surgical outcome after CPB, principally because of the variety of sensitive tests capable of implicating cerebral damage (232,233). Histologic studies have also shown embolic material in the kidneys, heart, liver, lungs, and spleen after CPB (25,26). Histology of the brains of patients who died after open heart surgery has demonstrated fibrin, fat, muscle fragments, calcium, and platelet aggregate microemboli in the vasculature (30). In these studies, fat emboli were detected in 80% of the cases and their presence was independent of perfusion variables, whereas nonfat emboli were related to the length of perfusion time. Thus, the period of greatest risk of cerebral injury is likely to be at the beginning of CPB when the patient is susceptible to both hypotension and microemboli initially released from the perfusion circuit (234,235).

Postoperative cerebral dysfunction after bypass, as demonstrated with psychomotor tests, may persist from a few hours to days or weeks (236–239). Some misinterpretation of the etiology of the injury may occur because similar changes in cerebral function are reported not only after microembolization but also with anxiety, sleep deprivation, drugs, cerebral edema, or hypoxemia (7,210,240,241).

Additional reasons for the wide range of reported incidences of neurologic dysfunction after CPB include the variability commonly observed when comparing prospective and retrospective studies, the time lapse between pre- and postsurgical evaluation, and the thoroughness of the tests conducted (6,242). In their retrospective evaluation of postoperative neurologic dysfunction, Bojar et al. (243) and Coffey et al. (244) reported incidence rates of 1% to 5%. This is in contrast to reported incidence rates in prospective studies as high as 30% to 61% (245–247). Incidence of stroke has been reported in approximately 5% of coronary artery bypass procedures in two prospective studies. Shaw (6), Newman (7), Smith (248), and Campbell and Raskin (249) have published excellent reviews on the subject of neurologic and neuropsychologic morbidity and its prevention during cardiac surgery. Johnston et al. (170) reported increases in gaseous microemboli during hypothermia with

a bubble oxygenator in dogs; however, global cerebral blood flow and regional brain perfusion were not affected.

Adverse neurologic outcome after bypass also has been correlated with arterial line microemboli (250). Earlier, Lee et al. (241) found postoperative deficits in 23% of their patients after open heart surgery, 14% of whom had psychiatric findings. Carlson et al. (236) found a greater percentage of patients with decreased Bender-Gestalt visual motor test scores when a bubble oxygenator was used instead of a membrane-type or without use of an arterial line filter. These results correlated with ultrasonic detection of circulating microemboli. Levels of the brain-specific enzymes of creatine phosphokinase were significantly elevated in patients undergoing open heart surgery (251–253), and this effect was preventable in dogs with use of an arterial filter (254). Other cerebrospinal fluid and serum enzymatic protein markers of brain injury have been reported in 6% to 50% of cardiac surgery patients (253,255,256). Moody et al. (258) detected focal small cerebral capillary and arteriolar dilations in dogs and patients after bypass that they attributed to microemboli, the identity of which was suggested as either silicone antifoam (258) or air (259). In earlier studies, cardiotomy suction was implicated as an important source of lipid emboli (36) that can lead to formation of small capillary and arterial dilatations (260) found in brain and other organs (257,261). They suggested that these focal dilations could be the equivalent of an anatomic correlate to neurologic deficits.

In the case of gas emboli, the topic of pathophysiology has been studied for more than three centuries (262). A number of reports and reviews have described the outcome of arterial air embolism with cardiac surgery involving gaseous microemboli and gross air (3,4,79,209,210,214, 263–265). Cerebral gas embolism can cause transient changes in the electroencephalogram that may persist from seconds to hours, in addition to the neurologic dysfunction described for nongaseous microemboli. Coronary air is associated with impaired left and right ventricular function and with numerous electrocardiographic changes, including ventricular dysrhythmias, atrioventricular dissociation, QRS complex widening, and ST segment and T wave changes (264,266). Clearance of coronary air while on CPB can be accomplished with the use of certain drugs, surface-active chemicals (267,268), aortic clamping with ventricular or aortic compression, or retrograde cerebral perfusion (269,270). Figure 16.4 illustrates the major mechanisms of CPB air embolism as reported in 1986 (271). More recent surveys (272,273) have indicated that iatrogenic air embolism continues to occur during CPB, but the incidence of patient injury is greatly reduced from the earlier survey data (271).

Arteriolar obstruction by gaseous emboli may be associated with vascular spasm followed by hyperemia (266) and perivascular hemorrhage (274). Immediately after occlusion, vasodilation occurs in the arteries and venules, fol-

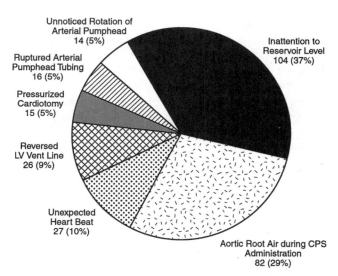

FIG. 16.4. Major mechanisms of gas embolism. Survey respondents who observed 284 incidents of air embolism during clinical cardiopulmonary bypass reported these etiologies. *CPS*, cardioplegic solution; *LV*, left ventricular. (From Kurusz M, Wheeldon DR. Risk containment during cardiopulmonary bypass. *Semin Thorac Cardiovasc Surg* 1990;2:400–409, with permission.)

lowed by congestion and stasis. These responses represent a direct action or injury to the vascular endothelium (265). Cerebral pathology may include many features of infarction or ischemia such as hemorrhage, edema, astrocyte and neuronal swelling, vacuolation, and necrosis (40,275–280).

Visual abnormalities manifested as occult visual field defects after cardiac surgery may be explained by ocular embolization with subsequent microvessel obstruction of the retina (179,281).

PREVENTION

It is unlikely today that even with the most current bypass devices, all embolic events can be totally eliminated. However, an awareness of those factors responsible for their production and interaction with the blood (282), as previously described, may allow perfusion teams to minimize the numbers generated and consequences during clinical bypass. Undoubtedly, filtration has been the single most important technique used to reduce all types of emboli, whereas the current near-universal acceptance of membrane oxygenators has led to dramatic decreases in gaseous microemboli production.

The technique of blood filtration began with the development of modern blood banking and blood transfusion practices in the 1930s (283,284). An early blood collection/transfusion apparatus incorporating a 250-μm reusable stainless steel filter was reported by Cooksey (285) and was later modified and used successfully on more than 11,000 transfusions.

Early laboratory experience with extracorporeal circulation confirmed the superior filtration characteristics of the pulmonary bed, and blood was often precirculated through the animal's lungs before beginning perfusion. Bjork (286) and Miller et al. (287) used filters with pores 300 × 300 μm in the arterial line during early clinical applications. The original Lillehei-DeWall bubble oxygenator incorporated four standard infusion set screen filters on the outflow side of the arterial settling reservoir (288). The early CPB experience of Kolff et al. (289) and Gross et al. (290) also relied on arterial filters for particulate trapping and air removal.

The seminal work of Swank et al. (291,292) in the mid-1960s led to the use in 1970 by Hill et al. (293) and others of the Swank depth filter for filtration of cardiotomy blood first (292) and later arterial blood (294). The hospital mortality for patients decreased significantly in those on whom filters were used. Also, in the early 1970s, Patterson and Twichell (295) described a 40-μm pleated polyester mesh filter that functioned with low pressure drop at clinical flow rates.

Solis et al. (36) evaluated the effectiveness of both types of filters using a microparticle counter and concluded that microaggregates in the cardiotomy-suctioned blood comprised a tremendously greater volume than those found in arterial or venous blood. Figure 16.5 compares the volume of particulates detected in venous, arterial, and cardiotomy return blood during CPB. Further, such microaggregates found in the cardiotomy-return blood were more resistant

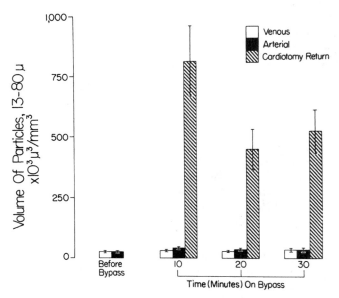

FIG. 16.5. Largest volume of particulates detected in cardiotomy blood and a small gradient between venous and arterial blood that disappears by 30 minutes on cardiopulmonary bypass. (From Solis RT, Noon GP, Beall AC, et al. Particulate microembolism during cardiac operation. *Ann Thorac Surg* 1974;17:332–344, with permission.)

to deaggregation and thus posed the greatest risk to the patient. Page et al. (296) confirmed the benefit of depth filtration of cardiotomy-suctioned blood during clinical perfusion to reduce embolus transmission to patients.

The extent of filter use by cardiac surgical teams nationwide was reported in 1983 (297). Ninety-four percent reported the practice of filtering bank blood added to the CPB circuit. Ninety-seven percent filtered cardiotomy-suctioned blood, and 78% filtered blood in the arterial line during both adult and pediatric perfusion. Because of the potential for filter occlusion with inadequate anticoagulation, several questions on this survey were posed regarding its management. Blood coagulation status was measured by greater than 95% of the respondents, who most often performed the activated coagulation time at least every 30 minutes during CPB. Forty percent also reported filtration of the cardioplegic solution after earlier reports of particulate emboli contained in these solutions (298–301). The importance of rinsing and filtering the circuit with crystalloid solution before establishing bypass was emphasized by Reed et al. (56) in 1974 and was performed by most perfusionists in 1982 (297). Subsequent surveys (273,302) have shown the near universal use of arterial line filtration during CPB.

The benefit of arterial line filtration, in conjunction with either bubble or membrane oxygenation, has been confirmed in several reports using Doppler or transesophageal echocardiographic detection of decreased quantities of microemboli (303–306) or improved patient scores on neuropsychologic tests after CPB (307). Figure 16.6 is a scanning electron photomicrograph of a heparin-coated screen arterial filter after clinical bypass.

Pharmacologic interventions to minimize emboli during bypass consist primarily of ensuring adequate heparin anticoagulation (22,24,308,309). Close monitoring of the activated coagulation time during CPB, as previously described, is now nearly universally practiced. Although controversial, administration of isoflurane has been shown by some to afford better tolerance for cerebral ischemia and would therefore appear potentially useful in minimizing the effects of cerebral emboli (310–312). Barbiturates also have been used by some (313) to improve the cerebral outcome after open heart surgery, but their use as prophylaxis against emboli appears less clearly defined. Royston (314) reviewed pharmacologic interventions aimed at reducing platelet and neutrophil emboli during CPB.

Acid-base management using alpha-stat was popularized in the early 1980s (315–317), and more recent survey results (318) indicate its use in most CPB cases. Alpha-stat management more closely maintains cerebral autoregulation in contrast to pH-stat management, during which enhanced cerebral blood flow occurs. Decreased transmission of microemboli per unit volume of blood flow, therefore, favors the alpha-stat approach to minimize the embolic "load" in perfused tissue beds (319). In a recent study on swine, Plochl and Cook (281) introduced the physiologic interven-

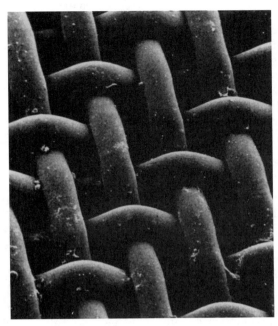

FIG. 16.6. Scanning electron micrograph (original magnification, ×300) of mesh of 40-μm heparin-coated screen arterial line filter after approximately 90 minutes of cardiopulmonary bypass. Note relatively clean surfaces with sparse depositions of amorphous debris and absence of occluded filter pores or platelet/neutrophil adhesion. (From Borowiec JW, Bylock A, Van der Linden J, Thelin S. Heparin coating reduces blood cell adhesion to arterial filters during coronary bypass: a clinical study. *Ann Thorac Surg* 1993;55:1540–1545, with permission.)

tion of $PaCO_2$ manipulation to control cerebral blood flow during periods of high embolic risk.

Prevention of gross air embolism from either the bypass circuit or operative field has been the subject of numerous reports (270,320,321). A variety of safety devices with proven efficacy is available for the circuit and includes arterial line filters, bubble traps, air bubble detectors, low-level alarms, and one-way valves for the vent or arterial filter purge line. The arterial line filter and air bubble detector have been reported to be highly effective in prevention of air embolism originating in the extracorporeal arterial line (271). Equally important in prevention of air embolism are clear lines of communication and use of protocols during CPB (322). Prebypass checklists have gained wide acceptance by teams and are effective in uncovering unsafe conditions before initiating bypass (323) (see Chapter 27 for a more detailed discussion).

Another less appreciated source of emboli during cardiac surgery relates to the status of the patient's ascending aorta, which usually must be cannulated, cross-clamped, and manipulated during the procedure. Atheromatous plaques that are present may be dislodged during these maneuvers (324,325). The recent multicenter study investigating adverse cerebral outcomes after coronary bypass surgery (8) found the presence of proximal aortic atherosclerosis to be a strong predictor of stroke. Alternative cannulation (326–328) or venting sites have been proposed, as well as the so-called no-touch technique (329). Intraoperative epiaortic echocardiography is becoming increasingly popular to define the extent of disease in the aorta. (See Chapter 28 for further discussion of management of the atherosclerotic aorta.)

TREATMENT

There is no specific treatment for microemboli per se; instead, prevention, as discussed previously, has received the most attention and appears to be the most rational approach in decreasing the risk. However, when gross air embolism occurs, definite treatment protocols have been proposed (330,331) and used with remarkable success (332–335). The importance of having a plan for this rare event has been emphasized and can often make the difference between severe injury or death and an uneventful recovery (322,330,336). Hyperbaric oxygenation is considered the most effective treatment of gross air embolism (337–344), although access to such a treatment facility may be limited (271). Detection of cerebral air embolism by computed tomography often indicates that a large volume of gas remains. Dexter and Hindman (345) modeled the absorption rates of cerebral gas emboli and determined that volumes in excess of 1.0×10^{-3} will remain for periods from 1.6 to 4.9 hours depending on the breathing gases, oxygen or air. Larger volumes remain proportionally longer, indicating that postsurgical hyperbaric oxygenation treatment may remain effective even hours or days after the initial insult (346).

A treatment modality for gas embolism studied in animals but not yet tested in humans is hemodilution with perfluorocarbon emulsions, which aids in the absorption of the vascular bubbles (347). Another treatment modality is systemic heparinization, especially with air embolism to reduce thrombi and other blood–bubble interactions, although it may be deleterious if cerebral infarction has already occurred (348). If the air embolization occurs during open chest procedures, direct aspiration of the cardiac chambers or great vessels is possible, as well as venting, direct cardiac massage to mobilize the emboli, induction of hypothermia for cerebral protection, or retrograde coronary sinus or cerebral perfusion (270,331,349–355). If air is suspected as the embolizing gas, 100% oxygen ventilation should be implemented to achieve favorable bubble resolution conditions and to limit cerebral ischemia and use of nitrous oxide should be discontinued to avoid bubble growth (356,357). Use of the Trendelenburg position or other patient repositioning techniques have been previously advocated to aid in the removal or prevention of arterial bubbles entering the brain. These techniques, however, have been shown ex-

perimentally using *in vivo* and *in vitro* techniques to offer little or no protection (358,359). Recently, Dexter et al. (360) verified this finding using maximum gas bubble absorption rates to indicate no benefit in absorption of air bubbles. Reviews of this topic describe various effective treatment modalities (223,274,330).

The use of transesophageal echocardiography and transcranial Doppler has been reported to aid in the identification of intraventricular or intravascular bubbles, primarily during valvular procedures or when the heart chambers have been opened (361). Rigorous deairing techniques may be assessed in this manner to decrease the persistence of entrapped surgical air emboli (195,350,362–365).

CONCLUSIONS AND FUTURE TRENDS

The subject of cerebral reactions to open heart surgery continues to receive much attention (366–369), and further improvements in CPB techniques (370) and patients' neurologic outcomes appear likely to emerge in the coming years. Although controversy sometimes continues regarding what are the optimal specific devices, a consensus now clearly favors incorporating membrane oxygenation and filtration of blood and all fluids during bypass. The chemical modification of blood-contacting surfaces used in extracorporeal devices may further decrease blood-derived microemboli from blood–foreign surface interaction. The current predominance of membrane oxygenation over that of bubble oxygenation has undoubtedly reduced gaseous microembolic phenomena in patients during bypass. Finally, ongoing research and continuing education will increase our understanding of the problems of embolic events and CPB and should further reduce levels of patient morbidity and mortality.

KEY POINTS

- The three categories of emboli are biologic, foreign material, and gaseous.
- Bloodborne emboli consist of cellular and noncellular products or aggregates.
- Most fat emboli are derived from cardiotomy-suctioned blood.
- Platelet aggregates are present in bank blood and are generated by CPB foreign surface contact.
- Platelet and neutrophil activation releases biogenic amines and other bioactive mediators that promote adhesion, further aggregation, and changes in microvascular endothelial permeability.
- Foreign material emboli are derived from the CPB circuit and from materials and debris in the operative field.
- Antifoam emboli were more prevalent with bubble oxygenators but are still present in smaller quantities in most circuits using membrane oxygenators.

- Generation of gaseous microemboli is greatly reduced when using membrane oxygenators.
- Gaseous microemboli production is minimized by adherence to cooling and warming gradients that do not exceed 10°C.
- Gaseous microemboli may be produced by rapid injection of drugs or blood into the CPB circuit.
- Cardiotomy-suctioned blood contains the greatest volume of both gaseous and particulate emboli.
- Cavitation refers to transient hydrodynamic phenomena that consists of bubble nucleation, growth, and collapse and is produced by extreme (positive and negative) pressure changes within blood.
- Surgical air refers to gas bubbles that enter the bloodstream when native vessels or chambers are opened during cannulation for CPB or application of vascular clamps.
- Depending on gas composition and bubble volume, bubbles will persist in the blood for long periods or resolve quickly, with air (composed mostly of nitrogen) resolving slowest and carbon dioxide resolving most quickly.
- Free microbubbles in blood are a foreign surface that promote cellular and protein activation at the bubble–blood interface.
- Bubble contact with vascular walls alters endothelial cells that further promotes release of vasoactive mediators and platelet and neutrophil adhesion.
- Ultrasonic detection (including transcranial, transesophageal, and Doppler) of microemboli is the most frequently used clinical modality.
- Ultrasonic detection devices are limited in their ability to quantitate sizes or emboli count.
- The most common manifestation of emboli after CPB is cerebral injury or dysfunction.
- The pathophysiology of arterial and venous gas embolism has been well studied in the laboratory.
- Filtration of bank, cardiotomy, and arterial blood is the most important technique to reduce emboli during CPB.
- Maintenance of adequate anticoagulation can decrease CPB-generated microemboli.
- Hyperbaric oxygenation is considered the most effective treatment for gross air embolism.
- Transesophageal echocardiography is an effective tool to assess thoroughness of cardiac deairing techniques.

REFERENCES

1. *Dorland's illustrated medical dictionary*, 27th ed. Philadelphia: W.B. Saunders, 1988:542.
2. Stump DA, Tegeler CH, Newman SP, et al. Older patients have more emboli during coronary artery bypass graft surgery [abstract]. *Anesthesiology* 1992;77:A52.
3. Edmunds LH Jr, Williams W. Microemboli and the use of filters during cardiopulmonary bypass. In: Utley JR, ed. *Pathophysiology and techniques of cardiopulmonary bypass.* Vol. 2. Baltimore: Williams & Wilkins, 1983:101–114.
4. Kurusz M. Gaseous microemboli: sources, causes, and clinical considerations. *Med Instrum* 1985;19:73–76.
5. Wong DHW. Perioperative stroke. Part II. Cardiac surgery and cardiogenic embolic stroke. *Can J Anaesth* 1991;38:471–488.
6. Shaw PJ. The incidence and nature of neurological morbidity following cardiac surgery: a review. *Perfusion* 1989;4:83–91.
7. Newman S. The incidence and nature of neuropsychological morbidity following cardiac surgery. *Perfusion* 1989;4:93–100.
8. Roach GW, Kanchuger M, Mangano CM, et al. Adverse cerebral outcomes after coronary bypass surgery. *N Engl J Med* 1996;335:1857–1863.
9. Solis RT, Kennedy PS, Beall AC, et al. Cardiopulmonary bypass—microembolization and platelet aggregation. *Circulation* 1975;52:103–108.
10. Clark RE. Microemboli: an overview. *Med Instrum* 1985;19:53–54.
11. Swank RL. Alteration of blood on storage: measurement of adhesiveness of "aging" platelets and leukocytes and their removal by filtration. *N Engl J Med* 1961;265:728–733.
12. Solis RT, Gibbs MB. Filtration of the microaggregates in stored blood. *Transfusion* 1972;12:245–250.
13. Rosenberg RD. Heparin action. *Circulation* 1974;49:603–605.
14. Zapol WM, Levy RI, Kolobow T, et al. In vitro denaturation of plasma alpha lipoproteins by bubble oxygenator in the dog. *Curr Top Surg Res* 1969;1:449–467.
15. Baier RE, Dutton RC. Initial events in interaction of blood with a foreign surface. *J Biomed Mater Res* 1969;3:191–206.
16. Kurusz M, Williams DR. Blood surfaces in the extracorporeal circuit: a scanning electron microscopic study. *J Extra-Corp Technol* 1975;7:186–198.
17. Davies GC, Sobel M, Salzman EW. Elevated plasma fibrinopeptide A and thromboxane A_2 levels during cardiopulmonary bypass. *Circulation* 1980;61:808–814.
18. Allardyce DB, Yoshida SH, Ashmore PG. The importance of microembolism in the pathogenesis of organ dysfunction caused by prolonged use of the pump oxygenator. *J Thorac Cardiovasc Surg* 1966;52:706–715.
19. Ashmore PG, Cvitek V, Ambrose P. The incidence and effects of particulate aggregation and microembolism in pump oxygenator systems. *J Thorac Cardiovasc Surg* 1968;55:691–697.
20. Dutton RC, Edmunds LH Jr. Measurement of emboli in extracorporeal perfusion systems. *J Thorac Cardiovasc Surg* 1973;65:523–530.
21. Bull BS, Huse WM, Brauer FS, et al. Heparin therapy during extracorporeal circulation. II. The use of a dose-response curve to individualize heparin and protamine dosage. *J Thorac Cardiovasc Surg* 1975;69:685–689.
22. Young JA, Kisker CT, Doty DB. Adequate anticoagulation during cardiopulmonary bypass determined by activated clotting time and the appearance of fibrin monomer. *Ann Thorac Surg* 1978;26:231–240.
23. Bull BS, Korpman RA, Huse WM, et al. Heparin therapy during extracorporeal circulation. I. Problems inherent in existing heparin protocols. *J Thorac Cardiovasc Surg* 1975;69:674–684.
24. Esposito RA, Culliford AT, Colvin SB, et al. The role of the activated clotting time in heparin administration and neutralization for cardiopulmonary bypass. *J Thorac Cardiovasc Surg* 1983;85:174–185.
25. Evans EA, Wellington JS. Emboli associated with cardiopulmonary bypass. *J Thorac Cardiovasc Surg* 1964;48:323–330.
26. Wright ES, Sarkozy E, Dobell ARC, et al. Fat globulinemia in extracorporeal circulation. *Surg* 1963;53:500–504.
27. Arrants JE, Gadsden RH, Huggins MB, et al. Effects of extracor-

poreal circulation upon blood lipids. *Ann Thorac Surg* 1973; 15:230–242.

28. Clark RE, Margraf HW, Beauchamp RA. Fat and solid filtration in clinical perfusion. *Surgery* 1975;77:216–224.

29. Lee WH Jr, Krumhaar D, Fonkalsrud E, et al. Denaturation of plasma proteins as a cause of morbidity and death after intracardiac operation. *Surgery* 1961;50:29–39.

30. Hill JD, Aguilar MJ, Baranco A, et al. Neuropathological manifestations of cardiac surgery. *Ann Thorac Surg* 1969;7:409–419.

31. Jefferson NC, Necheles H. Oleic acid toxicity and fat embolism. *Proc Soc Exp Biol Med* 1948;68:248–250.

32. Tieney DF, Johnson RP. Surface tension of lung extracts [abstract]. *Federation Proc* 1963;22:339.

33. Clark RE, Beauchamp RA, Magrath RA, et al. Comparison of bubble and membrane oxygenators in short and long perfusions. *J Thorac Cardiovasc Surg* 1979;78:655–666.

34. Chenoweth DE, Cooper SW, Hugli TE, et al. Complement activation during cardiopulmonary bypass. *N Engl J Med* 1981; 304:497–503.

35. Dutton RC, Edmunds LH Jr, Hutchinson JC, et al. Platelet aggregate emboli produced in patients during cardiopulmonary bypass with membrane and bubble oxygenators and blood filters. *J Thorac Cardiovasc Surg* 1974;67:258–265.

36. Solis RT, Noon GP, Beall AC, et al. Particulate microembolism during cardiac operation. *Ann Thorac Surg* 1974;17:332–344.

37. McKenna R, Bachmann F, Whittaker B, et al. The hemostatic mechanism after open-heart surgery. II. Frequency of abnormal platelet functions during and after extracorporeal circulation. *J Thorac Cardiovasc Surg* 1975;70:298–308.

38. Hicks RE, Dutton RC, Reis CA, et al. Production and fate of platelet aggregate emboli during veno-venous perfusion. *Surg Forum* 1973;24:250–252.

39. Ward CA, Ruegsegger B, Stanga D, et al. Reduction in platelet adhesion to biomaterials by removal of gas nuclei. *Trans Am Soc Artif Intern Organs* 1974;20A:77–84.

40. Warren BA, Philp RB, Inwood MJ. The ultrastructural morphology of air embolism: platelet adhesion to the interface and endothelial damage. *Br J Exp Pathol* 1973;54:163–172.

41. Preston FE, Martin JF, Stewart RM, et al. Thrombocytosis, circulating platelet aggregates and neurological dysfunction. *Br Med J* 1979;2:156–158.

42. Longmore DB, Gueierrara D, Bennett G, et al. Prostacyclin: a solution to some problems of extracorporeal circulation. *Lancet* 1979;1:1002–1005.

43. Aren CA, Fedderson K, Radegran K. Effects of prostacyclin infusion on platelet activation and post-operative blood loss in coronary bypass. *Ann Thorac Surg* 1983;36:49–54.

44. Ellison N, Edmunds LH Jr, Colman RW. Platelet aggregation following heparin and protamine administration. *Anesthesiology* 1978;48:65–68.

45. Faichney A, Davidson KG, Wheatley DJ, et al. Prostacyclin in cardiopulmonary bypass operations. *J Thorac Cardiovasc Surg* 1982;84:601–608.

46. Royston D. Aprotinin in open-heart surgery: background and results in patients having aortocoronary bypass grafts. *Perfusion* 1990;5[Suppl]:63–72.

47. Hovig T. The role of platelets in thrombosis. *Thromb Diathes Haemorrhag* 1970;42[Suppl]:137–153.

48. Ratliff NB, Young WG Jr, Hackel BB, et al. Pulmonary injury secondary to extracorporeal circulation ultrastructural study. *J Thorac Cardiovasc Surg* 1973;65:425–432.

49. Kurusz M, Schneider B, Conti VR, et al. Scanning electron microscopy of arterial line filters following clinical cardiopulmonary bypass. *Proceedings of the First World Congress on Extracorporeal Technology.* Brighton, UK. London: Franklin Scientific Products, 1981:17–23.

50. Hammerschmidt DE, Stroncek DF, Bowers TK, et al. Complement activation and neutropenia occurring during cardiopulmonary bypass. *J Thorac Cardiovasc Surg* 1981;81:370–377.

51. Hall RI, Smith MS, Rocker G. The systemic inflammatory response to cardiopulmonary bypass: pathophysiological, therapeutic, and pharmacological considerations. *Anesth Analg* 1997; 85:766–782.

52. Pruzanski W, Shumak KH. Biologic activity of cold-reacting autoantibodies [first of two parts]. *N Engl J Med* 1977;297: 538–542.

53. Pruzanski W, Shumak KH. Biologic activity of cold-reacting autoantibodies [second of two parts]. *N Engl J Med* 1977;297: 583–589.

54. Moore RA, Geller EA, Matthews ES, et al. The effects of hypothermic cardiopulmonary bypass on patients with low-titer, nonspecific cold agglutinins. *Ann Thorac Surg* 1984;37: 233–238.

55. Robicsek F, Masters TN, Littman L, et al. The embolization of bone wax from sternotomy incisions. *Ann Thorac Surg* 1981; 31:357–359.

56. Reed CC, Romagnoli A, Taylor DE, et al. Particulate matter in bubble oxygenators. *J Thorac Cardiovasc Surg* 1974;68: 971–974.

57. Braun PR, L'Hommedieu BD, Klinedinst WJ. Aluminum contamination by heat exchangers during cardiopulmonary bypass. *Proc Am Acad Cardiovasc Perfus* 1988;9:69–72.

58. Challa VR, Lovell MA, Moody DM, et al. Laser microprobe mass spectrometric study of aluminum and silicon in brain emboli related to cardiac surgery. *J Neuropathol Exp Neurol* 1998; 57:140–147.

59. Hubbard LC, Kletschka HD, Olsen DA, et al. Spallation using roller pumps and its clinical implications. *AmSECT Proc* 1975; 3:27–32.

60. Kurusz M, Christman EW, Williams EH, et al. Roller pump induced tubing wear: another argument in favor of arterial line filtration. *J Extra-Corp Technol* 1980;12:115–119.

61. Israel AL, Walton RM, Crane TN, et al. Comparison study of polyvinyl chloride versus silicone rubber tubing. *Proc Am Acad Cardiovasc Perfus* 1983;4:47–52.

62. Uretsky G, Landsburg G, Cohn DD, et al. Analysis of microembolic particles originating in extracorporeal circuits. *Perfusion* 1987;2:9–17.

63. Robicsek F, Duncan GD, Born GVR, et al. Inherent dangers of simultaneous application of microfibrillar collagen hemostat and blood-saving devices. *J Thorac Cardiovasc Surg* 1986;92: 766–770.

64. Orenstein JM, Sato N, Aaron B, et al. Microemboli observed in deaths following cardiopulmonary bypass surgery: silicone antifoam agents and polyvinyl chloride tubing as sources of emboli. *Hum Pathol* 1982;13:1082–1090.

65. Smith WT. Cerebral lesions due to emboli of silicone antifoam in dogs subjected to cardiopulmonary bypass. *J Pathol Bacteriol* 1960;90:9–18.

66. Wells R, Bygdeman MS, Shahriari AA, et al. Influence of a defoaming agent upon hematological complications of pump oxygenators. *Circulation* 1968;37:638–647.

67. Penry JK, Cordell AR, Johnston FR, et al. Cerebral embolism by Antifoam A in a bubble oxygenator system experimental and clinical study. *Surgery* 1960;47:84–94.

68. Cassie AB, Riddel AG, Yates PO. Hazard of antifoam emboli from a bubble oxygenator. *Thorax* 1960;15:22–29.

69. Thomassen RW, Howbert JP, Winn DF Jr, et al. The occurrence and characterization of emboli associated with the use of a silicone antifoaming agent. *J Thorac Cardiovasc Surg* 1961; 41:611–622.

70. Gupta S, Dandapat R, Maitra TK. Effects of silicone antifoam

on the pulmonary vasculature. *J Thorac Cardiovasc Surg* 1972; 63:714–719.

71. Kurusz M, Conti VR, Speer D, et al. Surface tension changes of perfusates: implications for gaseous microemboli during cardiopulmonary bypass. *J Extra-Corp Technol* 1985;17:138–142.

72. Butler BD, Kurusz M, Conti VR. Postbypass plasma surface tension and its role in bubble filtration. *Perfusion* 1986;1: 187–191.

73. Jordan P Jr, Tolstedt GE, Beretta FF. Micro-bubble formation in artificial oxygenation. *Surgery* 1957;43:266–269.

74. Kessler J, Patterson RH Jr. The production of microemboli by various blood oxygenators. *Ann Thorac Surg* 1970;9:221–228.

75. Patterson RH Jr, Kessler J. Microemboli during cardiopulmonary bypass detected by ultrasound. *Surg Gynecol Obstet* 1969; 129:505–510.

76. Krebber HJ, Hill JD, Osborn JJ, et al. Microemboli during extracorporeal circulation. *Thorac Cardiovasc Surg* 1980;28: 249–252.

77. Krebber HJ, Hanrath P, Janzen R, et al. Gas emboli during open-heart surgery. *Thorac Cardiovasc Surg* 1982;30:401–404.

78. Pearson DT, Holden MP, Poslad SJ. Gaseous microemboli production of bubble and membrane oxygenators. In: Lautier A, Gille JP, eds. *Extracorporeal gas exchange. Design and techniques.* London: W.B. Saunders, 1986:198–234.

79. Pearson DT. Microemboli: gaseous and particulate. In: Taylor KM, ed. *Cardiopulmonary bypass. Principles and management.* London: Chapman and Hall, 1986:313–353.

80. Hill AG, Groom RC, Tewksbury L, et al. Sources of gaseous microemboli during cardiopulmonary bypass. *Proc Am Acad Cardiovasc Perfus* 1988;9:122–130.

81. Brennan RW, Patterson RH, Kessler J. Cerebral blood flow and metabolism during cardiopulmonary bypass. *Neurology* 1971; 21:665–672.

82. Hammond GL, Bowley WW. Bubble mechanics and oxygen transfer. *J Thorac Cardiovasc Surg* 1976;71:422–428.

83. Reed CC, Miller D, Stafford TB, et al. Microemboli emission of extracorporeal oxygenators. *Les Cahiers du CECEC* 1984;22: 35–40.

84. Pearson DT, McArdle B, Poslad SJ, et al. A clinical evaluation of the performance characteristics of one membrane and five bubble oxygenators: gas transfer and gaseous microemboli production. *Perfusion* 1986;1:15–26.

85. Pearson DT, Clayton R, Murray A, et al. Blood gas control in bubble and membrane oxygenators. *Proc Am Acad Cardiovasc Perfus* 1987;8:190–199.

86. Chan R, Tidwell R. Study of gaseous microemboli removal capabilities of five different arterial filters in vitro. *Proc Am Acad Cardiovasc Perfus* 1983;4:53–55.

87. Massimino RM, Dyer RK, Martin J Jr, et al. Microemboli in the arterial line and the carotid artery during perfusion with a bubble oxygenator. *ASAIO J* 1984;7:155–159.

88. Pearson DT, Holden MP, Poslad SJ, et al. A clinical evaluation of the gas transfer characteristics and gaseous microemboli production of two bubble oxygenators. *Life Support Syst* 1984;2: 252–266.

89. Pearson DT. Blood gas control during cardiopulmonary bypass. *Perfusion* 1988;3:113–133.

90. Selman MW, McAlpine WA, Ratan RS. The effectiveness of various heart-lung machines in the elimination of microbubbles from the circulation. *J Thorac Cardiovasc Surg* 1967;53: 613–617.

91. Clark RE, Dietz DR, Miller JG. Continuous detection of microemboli during cardiopulmonary bypass in animals and man. *Circulation* 1976;54:74–78.

92. Mitchell SJ, Willcox T, McDougal C, et al. Emboli generation by the Medtronic Maxima hard-shell adult venous reservoir in

cardiopulmonary bypass circuits-a preliminary study. *Perfusion* 1996;11:145–155.

93. Mitchell SJ, Willcox T, Gorman DF. Bubble generation and venous air filtration by hard-shell venous reservoirs: a comparative study. *Perfusion* 1997;12:325–333.

94. Katoh S, Yoshida F. Physical factors affecting microembolus formation in extracorporeal circulation. *Ann Biomed Eng* 1976; 4:60–67.

95. Graves DJ, Quinn JA, Smock RA. Supersaturation and bubble formation in membrane oxygenators [Abstract]. *Proceedings of the 27th Annual Meeting of the Alliance for Engineering in Medicine and Biology,* 1974:197.

96. Severinghaus JW. Temperature gradients during hypothermia. *Ann NY Acad Sci* 1959;80:515–521.

97. Donald DE, Fellows JL. Physical factors relating to gas emboli in blood. *J Thorac Cardiovasc Surg* 1961;42:110–118.

98. Pollard HS, Fleischaker RJ, Timmes JJ, et al. Blood-brain barrier studies in extracorporeal cooling and warming. *J Thorac Cardiovasc Surg* 1961;42:772–778.

99. Gibbon JH Jr. Maintenance of cardiorespiratory function by extracorporeal circulation. *Circulation* 1959;19:646–656.

100. Gollan F. Physiology of deep hypothermia by total body perfusion. *Ann NY Acad Sci* 1959;80:301–334.

101. Almond CH, Jones JC, Snyder HM, et al. Cooling gradients and brain damage with deep hypothermia. *J Thorac Cardiovasc Surg* 1964;48:890–905.

102. Ehrenhaft JL, Claman MA. Cerebral complications of open-heart surgery: further observations. *J Thorac Cardiovasc Surg* 1961;42:514–526.

103. Ehrenhaft JL, Claman MA. Cerebral complications of open-heart surgery. *J Thorac Cardiovasc Surg* 1961;41:503–508.

104. Bjork VO, Hultquist G. Contraindications to profound hypothermia in open-heart surgery. *J Thorac Cardiovasc Surg* 1962; 44:1–13.

105. Geissler HJ, Allen SJ, Mehlhorn U, et al. Cooling gradients and formation of gaseous microemboli with cardiopulmonary bypass: an echocardiographic study. *Ann Thorac Surg* 1997;64: 100–104.

106. Miller DR, Allbritton FF. "Coronary suction" as a source of air embolism: an experimental study using the Kay-Cross oxygenator. *Ann Surg* 1960;151:75–84.

107. Wright G, Sanderson JM. Cellular aggregation and trauma in cardiotomy suction systems. *Thorax* 1979;34:621–628.

108. Loop FD, Szabo J, Rowlinson RD, et al. Events related to microembolism during open-heart surgery: effectiveness of in-line filtration recorded by ultrasound. *Ann Thorac Surg* 1976;21: 412–420.

109. Gallagher EG, Pearson DT. Ultrasonic identification of sources of microemboli during open-heart surgery. *Thorax* 1973;28: 295–305.

110. Chahine GL. Cavitation dynamics at microvascale level. *J Heart Valve Dis* 1994;3[Suppl 1]:S102–S116.

111. Kuhl T, Ruths M, Chen YL, et al. Direct visualization of cavitation and damage in ultra thin liquid films. *J Heart Valve Dis* 1994;3[Suppl 1]:S117–S127.

112. Freed D, Walker WE, Dube CM, et al. Effects of vaporous cavitation near prosthetic surfaces. *Trans Am Soc Artif Intern Organs* 1981;27:105–109.

113. Yount DE. On the evolution, generation, and regeneration of gas cavitation nuclei. *J Acoust Soc Am* 1982;71:1473–1481.

114. Bass RM, Longmore DB. Cerebral damage during open-heart surgery. *Nature* 1969;222:30–33.

115. Hannemann RE, Barile RG. Bubble formation in the roller infusion pump. *Am J Dis Child* 1973;125:706–708.

116. Mandl JP. Comparison of emboli production between a con-

strained force vortex pump and a roller pump. *AmSECT Proc* 1977;5:27–31.

117. Ross J Jr. Factors influencing the formation of bubbles in blood. *Trans Am Soc Artif Intern Organs* 1959;5:140–147.

118. Baird RJ, Miyagishima RT. The danger of air embolism through pressure-perfusion cannula. *J Thorac Cardiovasc Surg* 1963;46:212–219.

119. Kort A, Kronzon I. Microbubble formation: in vitro and in vivo observation. *J Clin Ultrasound* 1982;10:117–120.

120. Kuntz RA, Maurer WG. An examination of cavitation as it relates to the extracorporeal arterial infusion model. *J Extra-Corp Technol* 1982;14:345–354.

121. Knobelsdorff GV, Brauer P, Tonner PH, et al. Transmyocardial laser revascularization induces cerebral microembolization. *Anesthesiology* 1997;87:58–62.

122. Lee J, Murkin JM, McKenzie FN, et al. Cerebral emboli during transmyocardial revascularization as viewed by transcranial Doppler. *Outcomes 97, The Key West Meeting.* [abstract]. 1997.

123. Feerick AE, Church JA, Zwischenberger J, et al. Systemic gaseous microemboli during left atrial catheterization: a common occurrence? *J Cardiothorac Vasc Anesth* 1995;9:395–398.

124. Van der Linden J, Casimir-Ahn H. When do cerebral emboli appear during open-heart operations? A transcranial Doppler study. *Ann Thorac Surg* 1991;51:237–241.

125. Webb WR, Harrison LH, Helmake FR, et al. Carbon dioxide field flooding minimizes residual intracardiac air after open heart operation. *Ann Thorac Surg* 1997;64:1489–1491.

126. Miller BJ, Gibbon JH Jr, Greco VR, et al. The use of a vent for the left ventricle as a means of avoiding air embolism to the systemic circulation during open cardiotomy with the maintenance of the cardiorespiratory function of animals by a pump oxygenator. *Surg Forum* 1953;4:29–33.

127. Taber RE, Maraan BM, Tomatis L. Prevention of air embolism during open heart surgery; a study of the role of trapped air in the left ventricle. *Surgery* 1970;68:685–691.

128. Burbank A, Ferguson TB, Burford TH. Carbon dioxide flooding of the chest in open-heart surgery. *J Thorac Cardiovasc Surg* 1965;50:691–698.

129. Ng WS, Rosen M. Carbon dioxide in the prevention of air embolism during open-heart surgery. *Thorax* 1968;23:19–26.

130. Nichols HT, Morse DP, Hirose T. Coronary and other air embolization occurring during open heart surgery prevention by use of gaseous carbon dioxide. *Surgery* 1958;43:236–244.

131. Kalkunte JR. Air embolism prevention [letter]. *Ann Thorac Surg* 1988;45:586–587.

132. Utley JR, Stephens DB. Venting during cardiopulmonary bypass. In: Utley JR, ed. *Pathophysiology and techniques of cardiopulmonary bypass.* Vol. 2. Baltimore: Williams & Wilkins, 1983:115–127.

133. Weathersby PK, Homer LD. Solubility of inert gases in biological fluids and tissues: a review. *Undersea Biomed Res* 1980;7:227–296.

134. Spencer MP, Oyama Y. Pulmonary capacity for dissipation of venous gas emboli. *Aerospace Med* 1971;42:822–827.

135. Harkins HN, Harmon PH. Embolism by air and oxygen comparative studies. *Proc Soc Exp Biol* 1934;32:178–181.

136. Yang WJ, Echigo R, Wotton DR, et al. Experimental studies of the dissolution of gas bubbles in whole blood and plasma. I. Stationary bubbles. *J Biomech* 1971;4:275–281.

137. Yang WJ, Echigo R, Wotton DR, et al. Experimental studies of the dissolution of gas bubbles in whole blood and plasma. II. Moving bubbles or liquids. *J Biomech* 1971;4:283–288.

138. Hlastala MP, Van Liew HD. Absorption of in vivo inert gas bubbles. *Respir Physiol* 1975;24:147–158.

139. Munson ES, Merrick HC. Effect of nitrous oxide on venous air embolism. *Anesthesiology* 1966;27:783–787.

140. Bethune DW. Organ damage after heart surgery. *Lancet* 1976;2:1410–1411.

141. Tisovec L, Hamilton WK. Newer considerations in air embolism during operation. *JAMA* 1967;201:376–377.

142. Wells DG, Podolakin W, Mohr M, et al. Nitrous oxide and cerebrospinal fluid markers of ischaemia following cardiopulmonary bypass. *Anaesth Intens Care* 1987;15:431–435.

143. Epstein PS, Plesset MS. On the stability of gas bubbles in liquid-gas solutions. *J Chem Physics* 1950;18:1505–1509.

144. Liebermann L. Air bubbles in water. *J Appl Physics* 1957;28:205–211.

145. Turner WR. Microbubble persistence in fresh water. *J Acoust Soc Am* 1961;33:1223–1233.

146. Tanasawa I, Wotton DR, Yang W, et al. Experimental study of air bubbles in a simulated cardiopulmonary bypass system with flow constriction. *J Biomech* 1970;3:417–424.

147. Hlastala MP, Fahri LE. Absorption of gas bubbles in flowing blood. *J Appl Physiol* 1973;35:311–316.

148. Ward CA, Tikuisis P, Venter RD. Stability of bubbles in a closed volume of liquid-gas solution. *J Appl Physiol* 1975;24:147–158.

149. Feinstein SB, Shah PM, Bing RJ, et al. Microbubble dynamics visualized in the inert capillary circulation. *J Am Coll Cardiol* 1984;4:595–600.

150. Philp RB, Inwood MJ, Warren BA. Interactions between gas bubbles and components of the blood: implications in decompression sickness. *Aerospace Med* 1972;43:946–953.

151. Philp RB. A review of blood changes associated with compression-decompression: relationship to decompression sickness. *Undersea Biomed Res* 1974;1:117–150.

152. Philp RB, Bennett PB, Andersen JC, et al. Effects of aspirin and dipyridamole on platelet function, hematology, and blood chemistry of saturation divers. *Undersea Biomed Res* 1979;6:127–140.

153. Vroman L, Adams AL, Klings M. Interactions among human blood proteins at interfaces. *Federation Proc* 1971;30:1494–1502.

154. Harvey EN, Barnes DK, McElroy WD, et al. Bubble formation in animals. I. Physical factors. *J Cell Comp Physiol* 1944;24:1–22.

155. Butler BD, Hills BA. Role of lung surfactant in cerebral decompression sickness. *Aviat Space Environ Med* 1973;54:11–15.

156. Philp RB, Schacham P, Gowdey CW. Involvement of platelets and microthrombi in experimental decompression sickness: similarities with disseminated intravascular coagulation. *Aerospace Med* 1971;42:494–502.

157. Thorsen T, Brubakk A, Ovstedal T, et al. A method for production of N_2 microbubbles in platelet-rich plasma in an aggregometer-like apparatus, and effect on the platelet density in vitro. *Undersea Biomed Res* 1986;13:271–288.

158. Thorsen T, Dalen H, Bjerkvig R, et al. Transmission and scanning electron microscopy of microbubble-activated human platelets in vitro. *Undersea Biomed Res* 1987;14:45–58.

159. Furchgott RF. The discovery of endothelium-dependent relaxation. *Circulation* 1993;87:V3–V8.

160. Perrson LL, Johansson BB, Hansson HA. Ultrastructural studies on blood-brain barrier dysfunction after cerebral air embolism in the rat. *Acta Neuropathol* 1978;44:53–56.

161. Feerick AE, Johnston WE, Steinsland O, et al. Cardiopulmonary bypass impairs vascular endothelial relaxation: effects of gaseous microemboli in dogs. *Am J Physiol* 1994;267:H1174–H1182.

162. Albertine KH, Weiner-Kronish JP, Koike K, et al. Quantification of damage by air emboli to lung microvessels in anesthetized sheep. *J Appl Physiol* 1984;57:1360–1368.

163. Bonsignore MR, Rice TR, Dodek PM, et al. Thromboxane and

prostacyclin in acute lung injury caused by venous air emboli in anesthetized sheep. *Microcirc Endothel Lymph* 1986;3:187–212.

164. Fukushima M, Kobayashi T. Effects of thromboxane synthase inhibition on air emboli lung injury in sheep. *J Appl Physiol* 1986;60:1828–1833.

165. Butler BD, Little T. Effects of venous air embolism and decompression on thromboxane and leukotriene levels in dogs. *Undersea Hyp Med* 1994;215:21–22.

166. Butler BD, Powell M, Little T. Dose response levels of 11-dehydrothromboxane B_2 (TXB_2) and leukotriene E_4 (LTE4) with venous air embolism. [abstract] *Undersea Hyp Med* 1995; 22[Suppl 40].

167. Busse RA, Müisch A, Fleming I, et al. Mechanisms of nitric of oxide release from the vascular endothelium. *Circulation* 1993; 87:V18–V25.

168. Stewart DJ, Baffour R. Functional state of the endothelium in coronary circulation. *Cardiovasc Res* 1990;24:7–12.

169. Helps SC, Parsons DW, Reilly PL, et al. The effect of gas emboli on rabbit cerebral blood flow. *Stroke* 1990;21:94–99.

170. Johnston WE, Stump DA, DeWitt DS, et al. Significance of gaseous microemboli in the cerebral circulation during cardiopulmonary bypass in dogs. *Circulation* 1993;88[part 2]: 319–329.

171. Tepper R, Gelman S, Lowenfelds AB, et al. A method for the detection of microbubbles resulting from passage of blood through heart-lung machines. *Surg Forum* 1958;9:171–174.

172. Selman MW, McAlpine WA, Ratan RS. The effectiveness of various heart-lung machines in the elimination of microbubbles from the circulation. *J Thorac Cardiovasc Surg* 1967;53: 613–617.

173. Padula RT, Eisenstat TE, Bronstein MU, et al. Intracardiac air following cardiotomy. *J Thorac Cardiovasc Surg* 1971;62: 736–742.

174. Muraoka R, Yokata M, Aoshima M, et al. Subclinical changes in brain morphology following cardiac operations as reflected by computed tomographic scans of the brain. *J Thorac Cardiovasc Surg* 1981;81:346–349.

175. Grulke DC, Marsh NR, Hills BA. Measurement of microbubbles using the Coulter counter. *Br J Exp Pathol* 1973;54: 684–691.

176. Swank RL. The screen filtration pressure method in research: significance and interpretation. *Series Haematol* 1968;1: 146–167.

177. Sakauye LM, Servas FM, O'Connor KK, et al. An in vitro method to quantitate gaseous microemboli production of bubble oxygenators. *J Extra-Corp Technol* 1982;14:445–452.

178. Blauth C, Arnold J, Kohner EM, et al. Preliminary communication. Retinal microembolism during cardiopulmonary bypass demonstrated by fluorescein angiography. *Lancet* 1986;2: 837–839.

179. Blauth CI, Arnold JV, Schulenberg WE, et al. Cerebral microembolism during cardiopulmonary bypass. Retinal microvascualr studies in vivo with fluorescein angiography. *J Thorac Cardiovasc Surg* 1988;95:668–676.

180. Austen WA, Howry DH. Ultrasound as a method to detect bubbles or particulate matter in the arterial line during cardiopulmonary bypass. *J Surg Res* 1965;5:283–284.

181. Richardson PD. Qualitative and quantitative methods for investigating gas emboli in blood. *Med Instrum* 1985;19:55–58.

182. Sellman M, Ivert T, Stensved P, et al. Doppler ultrasound estimation of microbubbles in the arterial line during extracorporeal circulation. *Perfusion* 1990;5:23–32.

183. De Somer F, Dierickx P, DuJardin D, et al. Can an oxygenator design potentially contribute to air embolism in cardiopulmonary bypass: a novel method for the determination of the air

184. Moody DM, Brown WR, Challa VR, et al. Brain microemboli associated with cardiopulmonary bypass: a histologic and magnetic resonance imaging study. *Ann Thorac Surg* 1995;59: 1304–1307.

185. Marochnik S, Alexandrov AV, Anthone D, et al. Feasibility of SPECT for studies of brain perfusion during cardiopulmonary bypass. *J Neuroimaging* 1996;6:243–245.

186. Hartveit F, Lystad H, Minken A. The pathology of venous air embolism. *Br J Exp Pathol* 1968;49:81–86.

187. Rubbisow GJ, Mackay RS. Decompression study and control using ultrasonics. *Aerospace Med* 1974;45:476–478.

188. Butler BD, Hills BA. The lung as a filter for microbubbles. *J Appl Physiol* 1979;47:537–543.

189. Hickling R. Analysis of echoes from a solid elastic sphere in water. *J Acoust Soc Am* 1962;34:1582–1592.

190. Furness A, Wright G. Microbubble detection during cardiopulmonary bypass for open-heart surgery. *Life Support Syst* 1985; 3:103–109.

191. Hatteland K, Pedersen T, Semb BKH. Comparison of bubble release from various types of oxygenators. *Scand J Thorac Cardiovasc Surg* 1985;19:125–130.

192. Wright G, Furness A, Haigh S. Integral pulse frequency modulated ultrasound for the detection and quantification of gas microbubbles in flowing blood. *Perfusion* 1987;2:131–138.

193. Ikeda T, Suzuki S, Shinizu K, et al. M-mode detection of microbubbles following saturation diving; a case report and proposal for a new grading system. *Aviat Space Environ Med* 1989;60: 160–169.

194. Duff HJ, Buda AJ, Kramer R, et al. Detection of entrapped intracardiac air with intraoperative echocardiography. *Am J Cardiol* 1980;46:255–260.

195. Oka Y, Inoue T, Hong Y, et al. Retained intracardiac air; transesophageal echocardiography for definition of incidence and monitoring removal by improved techniques. *J Thorac Cardiovasc Surg* 1986;91:329–338.

196. Furuya, Suzuki T, Okamura F, et al. Detection of air embolism by transesophageal echocardiography. *Anesthesiology* 1983;58: 124–129.

197. Zhou JL, Chen XF, Zhang QP. Detection and removal of intracardiac residual air during open heart surgery with CPB under the guidance of echocardiography. *Acta Acad Med Wuhan* 1984; 4:56–60.

198. Padayachee TS, Parsons S, Theobold R, et al. The detection of microemboli in the middle cerebral artery during cardiopulmonary bypass: a transcranial Doppler ultrasound investigation using membrane and bubble oxygenators. *Ann Thorac Surg* 1987;44:298–302.

199. Cicek S, Demirkilic U, Tatar H. Intraoperative echocardiography: techniques and current applications. *J Card Surg* 1993;8: 678–692.

200. Schluter M, Langenstein BA, Poister J, et al. Transesophageal cross-sectional echocardiography with a phased array transducer system: technique and initial clinical results. *Br Heart J* 1982; 48:67–72.

201. Morris WP, Tonnesen AS, Butler BD. Transesophageal echocardiographic study of venous air embolism following pneumomediastinum in dogs. *Intensive Care Med* 1995;21:790–796.

202. Pugsley W. The use of Doppler ultrasound in the assessment of microemboli during cardiac surgery. *Perfusion* 1989;4: 115–122.

203. Padayachee TS, Gosling RG, Bishop CC, et al. Monitoring middle cerebral artery blood velocity during carotid endarterectomy. *Br J Surg* 1986;73:98–100.

204. Spencer MP. Transcranial Doppler monitoring and causes of stroke from carotid endarterectomy. *Stroke* 1997;28:685–691.

205. Spencer MP, Thomas GI, Nicholls SC, et al. Detection of middle cerebral artery emboli during carotid endarterectomy using transcranial Doppler ultrasonography. *Stroke* 1990;21: 415–423.

206. Yao FS, Barbut D, Hager DN, et al. Comparison of transcranial Doppler and transesophageal echocardiography to monitor emboli during coronary artery bypass surgery. [abstract] *Anesth Analg* 1996;82:SCA61.

207. Droste DW, Decker W, Siemens HJ, et al. Variability in occurrence of embolic signals in long term transcranial Doppler recordings. *Neurol Res* 1996;18:25–30.

208. Clark RE, Brillman J, Davis DA, et al. Microemboli during coronary artery bypass grafting: genesis and effect on outcome. *J Thorac Cardiovasc Surg* 1995;109:249–258.

209. Butler BD. Gaseous micro emboli: concepts and considerations. *J Extra-Corp Technol* 1983;15:148–155.

210. Butler BD, Kurusz M. Gaseous microemboli: a review. *Perfusion* 1990;5:81–99.

211. Abts LR, Beyer RT, Galletti PM, et al. Computerized discrimination of microemboli in extracorporeal circuits. *Am J Surg* 1978;135:535–538.

212. Butler BD. Production of microbubbles for use as echo contrast agents. *J Clin Ultrasound* 1986;14:408–412.

213. Horton JW, Wells CH. Resonance ultrasonic measurements of microscopic gas bubbles. *Aviat Space Environ Med* 1976;47: 777–781.

214. Butler BD. Biophysical aspects of gas bubbles in blood. *Med Instrum* 1985;19:59–62.

215. Wright G, Furness A. Gaseous microembolism—validity of bubble counting systems. *Perfusion* 1986;1:217–219.

216. Moehring MA. Discrimination of air bubbles and red cell aggregate emboli using the embolus-to-blood (EBR) power ratio measurement [abstract]. *Proceedings of the Ninth International Cerebral Hemodynamics Symposium, Charleston, SC,* 1995:113.

217. Hanzawa K, Ohzeki H, Hayashi J, et al. Distinguish between solid micro-embolic signal and micro-gaseous signal by HITS spectra during cardiac surgery [abstract]. *Outcomes 97, The Key West Meeting.* 1997.

218. Ries F, Tiemann K, Pohl C, et al. High resolution emboli detection and differentiation by characteristic postembolic spectral patterns. *Stroke* 1998;29:668–672.

219. Lui P-W, Chan BCB, Chan FHY, et al. Wavelet analysis of embolic heart sound detected by precordial Doppler ultrasound during continuous venous air embolism in dogs. *Anesth Analg* 1998;86:325–331.

220. Russell D, Madden KP, Clark WM, et al. Detection of arterial emboli using Doppler ultrasound in rabbits. *Stroke* 1991;22: 253–281.

221. Markus H. Transcranial Doppler detection of circulating cerebral emboli: a review. *Stroke* 1993;24:1246–1250.

222. Markus HS, Broen MM. Differentiation between different pathological cerebral embolic materials using transcranial Doppler in an in vitro model. *Stroke* 1993;24:1–5.

223. Kurusz M, Butler BD, Katz J, et al. Air embolism during cardiopulmonary bypass. *Perfusion* 1995;10:361–391.

224. Newhouse VL, Shankar PM. Bubble size measurement using the nonlinear mixing of two frequencies. *J Acoust Soc Am* 1984; 75:1473–1477.

225. Spencer MP, Granado L. Ultrasonic frequency and Doppler sensitivity to arterial microemboli [abstract]. *Stroke* 1993;24: 5120.

226. Christman CL, Catron PW, Flynn ET, et al. In vivo microbubble detection in decompression sickness using a second harmonic resonant bubble detector. *Undersea Biomed Res* 1986;13: 1–18.

227. Brucher R, Russell D. Automatic embolus detection with artifact suppression [abstract]. *J Neuroimaging* 1993;3:77.

228. Magari PJ, Kline-Schoder RJ, Stoedefalke BH, et al. A noninvasive, in-vivo bubble sizing instrument. *Proceedings of the IEEE Ultrasonics Symposium,* Ontario, Canada, 1997: 1205–1210.

229. Strong K, Westenkow DR, Fine PG, et al. A preliminary laboratory investigation of air embolus detection and grading using an artificial neural network. *Int J Clin Monit Comp* 1997;14: 103–107.

230. Taylor KM. Brain damage during open heart surgery [editorial]. *Thorax* 1982;37:873–876.

231. Taylor KM. Assessment of cerebral damage during cardiopulmonary bypass with particular reference to perfusion and microembolic damage. *Proc Am Acad Cardiovasc Perfus* 1983;4: 110–113.

232. Stump DA, Kon NA, Rogers AT, et al. Emboli and neuropsychological outcome following cardiopulmonary bypass. *Echocardiography* 1996;13:555–558.

233. Stump DA, Rogers AT, Hammon JW, et al. Cerebral emboli and cognitive outcome after cardiac surgery. *J Cardiothorac Vasc Anesth* 1996;10:113–119.

234. Branthwaite MA. Detection of neurological damage during open heart surgery. *Thorax* 1973;28:464–472.

235. Branthwaite MA. Prevention of neurological damage during open heart surgery. *Thorax* 1975;30:258–261.

236. Carlson RG, Lande AJ, Landis B, et al. The Lande-Edwards membrane oxygenator during heart surgery: oxygen transfer, microemboli counts and Bender-Gestalt visual motor test scores. *J Thorac Cardiovasc Surg* 1973;66:894–905.

237. Savageau JA, Stanton BA, Jenkins CD, et al. Neuropsychological dysfunction following elective cardiac operation. I. Early assessment. *J Thorac Cardiovasc Surg* 1982;84:585–594.

238. Savageau JA, Stanton BA, Jenkins CD, et al. Neuropsychological dysfunction following elective cardiac operation. II. A six-month reassessment. *J Thorac Cardiovasc Surg* 1982;84: 595–600.

239. Landis B, Baxter J, Patterson RH Jr, et al. Bender-Gestalt evaluation of brain dysfunction following open-heart surgery. *J Personality Assess* 1974;38:556–562.

240. Aberg T, Kilgren M. Cerebral protection during open heart surgery. *Thorax* 1977;32:525–533.

241. Lee WH Jr, Miller W, Rowe J, et al. Effects of extracorporeal circulation on personality and cerebration. *Ann Thorac Surg* 1969;7:562–570.

242. Sotaniemi KA. Cerebral outcome after extracorporeal circulation: comparison between prospective and retrospective evaluations. *Arch Neurol* 1983;40:75–77.

243. Bojar RM, Najafi H, Delaria GA, et al. Neurological complications of coronary revascularization. *Ann Thorac Surg* 1983;36: 427–432.

244. Coffey CE, Massey W, Roberts KB, et al. Natural history of cerebral complications of coronary bypass graft surgery. *Neurology* 1983;33:1416–1421.

245. Breuer AC, Furlan AJ, Hanson MR, et al. Neurologic complications of open-heart surgery. *Cleve Clin Q* 1981;48:205–206.

246. Breuer AC, Furlan AJ, Hanson MR, et al. Neurologic complications of coronary artery bypass graft surgery: a prospective analysis of 421 patients. *Stroke* 1983;14:682–687.

247. Shaw PJ, Bates D, Cartlidge NEF, et al. Early neurological complications of coronary artery bypass surgery. *Br Med J* 1985; 291:1384–1386.

248. Smith PL. Brain injury and protection. *Semin Thorac Cardiovasc Surg* 1990;2:381–388.

249. Campbell DE, Raskin SA. Cerebral dysfunction after cardiopulmonary bypass: aetiology, manifestations and interventions. *Perfusion* 1990;5:251–260.

250. Pugsley W, Klinger L, Paschalis C, et al. The impact of microemboli during cardiopulmonary bypass on neuropsychological functioning. *Stroke* 1994;25:1393–1399.

251. Aberg T, Ronquist G, Tyden H, et al. Release of adenylate kinase into cerebrospinal fluid during open-heart surgery and its relation to postoperative intellectual function. *Lancet* 1982; 1:1139–1142.

252. Lundar T, Stokke O. Total creatine kinase activity in cerebrospinal fluid as an indicator of brain damage during open-heart surgery. *Scand J Thorac Cardiovasc Surg* 1983;17:157–161.

253. Aberg T, Ronquist G, Tyden H, et al. Adverse effects on the brain in cardiac operations as assessed by biochemical, psychometric, and radiologic methods. *J Thorac Cardiovasc Surg* 1984; 87:99–105.

254. Taylor KM, Devlin BJ, Mittra SM, et al. Assessment of cerebral damage during open-heart surgery: a new experimental model. *Scand J Thorac Cardiovasc Surg* 1980;14:197–203.

255. Steinberg GK, De LaPaz R, Mitchell RS, et al. MR and cerebrospinal fluid enzymes as sensitive indicators of subclinical cerebral injury after open-heart valve replacement surgery. *Am J Neuroradiol* 1996;17:205–212.

256. Johansson P. Markers of cerebral ischemia after cardiac surgery. *J Cardiothorac Vasc Anesth* 1996;10:120–126.

257. Moody DM, Bell MA, Challa VR, et al. Brain microemboli during cardiac surgery or aortography. *Ann Neurol* 1990;28:477–486.

258. Williams IM, Stephens JF, Richardson EP, et al. Brain and retinal microemboli during cardiac surgery [letter]. *Ann Neurol* 1991;29:736–737.

259. Moody DM, Bell MA, Challa VR. Reply. [letter] *Ann Neurol* 1992;30:737.

260. Brooker RF, Brown WR, Moody DM, et al. Cardiotomy suction: a major source of brain lipid emboli during cardiopulmonary bypass. *Ann Thorac Surg* 1998;65:1651–1655.

261. Challa VR, Moody DM, Troost BT. Brain emboli phenomena associated with cardiopulmonary bypass. *J Neurol Sci* 1993;117:224–231.

262. Boyle R. New pneumatical experiments about respiration. *Philos Trans R Soc Lond B Biol Sci* 1670;62:2011–2049.

263. Nicks R. Air embolism in cardiac surgery: incidence and prophylaxis. *Aust NZ J Surg* 1969;38:328–332.

264. Durant TM, Oppenheiner MJ, Webster MR, et al. Arterial air embolism. *Am Heart J* 1949;38:481–500.

265. Fries CC, Levowitz B, Adler S, et al. Experimental cerebral gas embolism. *Ann Surg* 1957;145:461–470.

266. Utley JR, Stephens DB. Air embolus during cardiopulmonary bypass. In: Utley JR, ed. *Pathophysiology and techniques of cardiopulmonary bypass.* Vol. 2. Baltimore: Williams & Wilkins, 1983: 78–100.

267. Malette WA, Fitzgerald JB, Eiseman B. Aeroembolus: a protective substance. *Surg Forum* 1960;11:155–156.

268. Eiseman B, Baxter BJ, Prachuabmoh K. Surface tension reducing substances in the management of coronary air embolism. *Ann Surg* 1959;149:374–380.

269. Geohegan T, Lam CR. The mechanism of death from intracardiac air and its reversibility. *Ann Surg* 1953;138:351–359.

270. Mills NL, Ochsner JL. Massive air embolism during cardiopulmonary bypass. *J Thorac Cardiovasc Surg* 1980;80:708–717.

271. Kurusz M, Conti VR, Arens JF, et al. Perfusion accident survey. *Proc Am Acad Cardiovasc Perfus* 1986;7:57–65.

272. Jenkins OF, Morris R, Simpson JM. Australasian perfusion incident survey. *Perfusion* 1997;12:279–288.

273. Mejak BL, Stammers A, Rauch E, et al. A retrospective study on perfusion accidents and safety devices. *Perfusion* 2000;15: 51–61.

274. Chase WH. Anatomical experimental observations on air embolism. *Surg Gynecol Obstet* 1934;49:569–577.

275. Orebaugh SL, Grenvik A. Air embolization. In: Ayres SM, Grenvik A, Holbrook PR, et al., eds. *Textbook of critical care,* 3rd ed. Philadelphia: W.B. Saunders, 1995:617–627.

276. Peirce EC II. Cerebral gas embolism (arterial) with special reference to iatrogenic accidents. *HBO Rev* 1980;1:161–184.

277. Hallenbeck JM, Bradley ME. Experimental model for systematic study of impaired microvascular reperfusion. *Stroke* 1977; 8:238–243.

278. Brierly JB. Neuropathological findings in patients dying after open heart surgery. *Thorax* 1963;18:291–304.

279. Rapoport S, Thompson H. Osmotic opening of the blood-brain barrier in the monkey without associated neurologic deficits. *Science* 1973;180:971–979.

280. Peirce EC II, Jacobson JH II. Cerebral edema. In: Davis JC, Hunt TK, eds. *Hyperbaric oxygen therapy.* Bethesda: Undersea Medical Society, 1977:287–301.

281. Plochl W, Cook DJ. Quantification and distribution of cerebral emboli during cardiopulmonary bypass in swine. *Anesthesiology* 1999;90:183–190.

282. Royston D. Blood cell activation. *Semin Thorac Cardiovasc Surg* 1990;2:341–357.

283. Wilson TI, Jamieson JMM. Transfusion with stored blood. *Br Med J* 1938;1:1207.

284. Fantus B. The therapy of the Cook County Hospital. *JAMA* 1938;111:317–321.

285. Cooksey WB. New apparatus for storing, filtering and administering blood. *Am J Surg* 1940;49:526–527.

286. Bjork VO. An artificial heart or cardiopulmonary machine. *Lancet* 1948;2:491–493.

287. Miller BJ, Gibbon JH Jr, Gibbon MH. An improved mechanical heart and lung apparatus. *Med Clin North Am* 1953;37: 1603–1624.

288. Lillehei CW, Warden HE, DeWall RA, et al. Cardiopulmonary bypass in surgical treatment of congenital or acquired cardiac disease. *Arch Surg* 1957;75:928–945.

289. Kolff WJ, Effler DB, Groves LK, et al. Disposable membrane oxygenator (heart-lung machine) and its use in experimental surgery. *Cleve Clin Q* 1956;23:69–97.

290. Gross RE, Sauvage LR, Pontius RG, et al. Experimental and clinical studies of a syphon-filling disc-oxygenator system for complete cardiopulmonary bypass. *Ann Surg* 1960;151: 285–302.

291. Swank RL, Hirsch H, Breuer M, et al. Effect of glass wool filtration on blood during extracorporeal circulation. *Surg Gynecol Obstet* 1963;117:547–552.

292. Swank RL, Porter GA. Disappearance of microemboli transfused into patients during extracorporeal circulation. *Transfusion* 1963;3:192–197.

293. Hill JD, Osborn JJ, Swank RL, et al. Experience using a new Dacron wool filter during extracorporeal circulation. *Arch Surg* 1970;101:649–652.

294. Osborn JJ Swank RL, Hill JD, et al. Clinical use of a Dacron wool filter during perfusion for open-heart surgery. *J Thorac Cardiovasc Surg* 1970;60:575–581.

295. Patterson RW Jr, Twichell JB. Disposable filter for microemboli in cardiopulmonary bypass and massive transfusion. *JAMA* 1971;215:76–80.

296. Page US, Bigelow JC, Carter CR, et al. Emboli (debris) produced by bubble oxygenators: removal by filtration. *Ann Thorac Surg* 1974;18:164–170.

297. Kurusz M, Schneider B, Brown JP, et al. Filtration during open-

heart surgery: devices techniques, opinions, and complications. *Proc Am Acad Cardiovasc Perfus* 1983;4:123–129.

298. MacDonald JL. Is crystalloid cardioplegia a source of particulate debris? *Proc Am Acad Cardiovasc Perfus* 1981;2:20–24.

299. Robinson LA, Braimbridge MV, Hearse DJ. The potential hazard of particulate contamination of cardioplegic solutions. *J Thorac Cardiovasc Surg* 1984;87:48–58.

300. Kurusz M, Speer D, Coughlin TR, et al. In-line filtration of crystalloid cardioplegic solution. *Proc Am Acad Cardiovasc Perfus* 1985;6:123–125.

301. Palanzo DA, O'Neill MJ, Harrison LH Jr. An effective 0.2 micron filter for the administration of crystalloid cardioplegia. *Proc Am Acad Cardiovasc Perfus* 1987;8:182–185.

302. American Society of Extra-Corporeal Technology. Perfusion practice survey, September, 1993. *Perfusion Life* 1994;11: 42–45.

303. Smith PLC. Interventions to reduce cerebral injury during cardiac surgery—introduction and the effect of oxygenator type. *Perfusion* 1989;4:139–145.

304. Meloni L, Abbruzzese PA, Cardu G, et al. Detection of microbubbles released by oxygenators during cardiopulmonary bypass by intraoperative transesophageal echocardiography. *Am J Cardiol* 1990;66:511–514.

305. Griffin S, Pugsley W, Treasure T. Microembolism during cardiopulmonary bypass: a comparison of bubble oxygenator with arterial line filter and membrane oxygenator alone. *Perfusion* 1991;6:99–103.

306. Abbruzzese PA, Meloni L, Cardu G, et al. Role of arterial filters in the prevention of systemic embolization by microbubbles released by oxygenators [letter]. *Am J Cardiol* 1991;67: 911–912.

307. Treasure T. Interventions to reduce cerebral injury during cardiac surgery—the effect of arterial line filtration. *Perfusion* 1989;4:147–162.

308. Verska JJ. Control of heparinization by activated clotting time during bypass with improved postoperative hemostasis. *Ann Thorac Surg* 1977;24:170–174.

309. Cohen JA. Activated coagulation time method for control of heparin is reliable during cardiopulmonary bypass. *Anesthesiology* 1984;60:121–124.

310. Newberg LA, Michenfelder JD. Cerebral protection by isoflurane during hypoxemia or ischemia. *Anesthesiology* 1983;59: 29–35.

311. Newman B, Gelb AW, Lam AM. The effect of isoflurane-induced hypotension on cerebral blood flow and cerebral metabolic rate for oxygen in humans. *Anesthesiology* 1986;64: 307–310.

312. Woodcock TE, Murkin JM, Farrar JK, et al. Pharmacologic EEG suppression during cardiopulmonary bypass: cerebral heodynamic and metabolic effects of thiopental or isoflurance during hypothermia and normothermia. *Anesthesiology* 1987;67: 218–224.

313. Nussmeir NA, Arlund C, Slogoff S. Neuropsychiatric complications after cardiopulmonary bypass: cerebral protection by a barbiturate. *Anesthesiology* 1986;64:165–170.

314. Royston D. Interventions to reduce cerebral injury during cardiac surgery—the effect of physical and pharmacological agents. *Perfusion* 1989;4:153–161.

315. White FN. A comparative physiological approach to hypothermia [editorial]. *J Thorac Cardiovasc Surg* 1981;82:821–831.

316. Ream AK, Reitz BA, Silverberg G. Temperature correction of pCO_2 and pH in estimating acid base status: an example of the emperor's new clothes? *Anesthesiology* 1982;56:41–44.

317. Swan H. The importance of acid-base management for cardiac and cerebral preservation during open heart operations. *Surg Gynecol Obstet* 1984;158:391–414.

318. Groom RC, Hill AG, Akl BF, et al. Pediatric perfusion survey. *Proc Am Acad Cardiovasc Perfus* 1990;11:78–84.

319. Henriksen L, Hjims E, Lindeburgh T. Brain hyperperfusion during cardiac operations. *J Thorac Cardiovasc Surg* 1983;86: 202–208.

320. Stoney WS, Alford WC Jr, Burrus GR, et al. Air embolism and other accidents using pump oxygenators. *Ann Thorac Surg* 1980; 29:36–40.

321. Kurusz M, Wheeldon DR. Risk containment during cardiopulmonary bypass. *Semin Thorac Cardiovasc Surg* 1990;2:400–409.

322. Bayindir O, Paker T, Akpinar B, et al. Case conference: a 58-year old man had a massive air embolism during cardiopulmonary bypass. *J Cardiothorac Vasc Anesth* 1991;5:627–634.

323. American Society of Extra-Corporeal Technology. Suggested pre-bypass perfusion checklist. *Perfusion Life* 1990;7:76–77.

324. Tobler HG, Edwards JE. Frequency and location of atherosclerotic plaques in the ascending aorta. *J Thorac Cardiovasc Surg* 1988;96:304–306.

325. Wareing TH, Davila-Roman VG, Barzilai B, et al. Management of the severely atherosclerotic ascending aorta during cardiac operations. *J Thorac Cardiovasc Surg* 1992;103:453–462.

326. Golding LAR. New cannulation technique for the severely calcified ascending aorta. *J Thorac Cardiovasc Surg* 1985;90: 626–627.

327. Culliford AT, Colvin SB, Rohrer K, et al. The atherosclerotic ascending aorta and transverse arch: a new technique to prevent cerebral injury during bypass: experience with 13 patients. *Ann Thorac Surg* 1986;41:27–35.

328. Groom RC, Hill AG, Kuban B, et al. Aortic cannula velocimetry. *Perfusion* 1995;10:183–188.

329. Mills NL, Everson CT. Atherosclerosis of the ascending aorta and coronary artery bypass: pathology, clinical correlates, and operative management. *J Thorac Cardiovasc Surg* 1991;102: 546–553.

330. Brenner WI. A battle plan in the event of massive air embolism during open heart surgery. *J Extra-Corp Technol* 1985;17: 133–137.

331. Mills NL, Morris JM. Air embolism associated with cardiopulmonary bypass. In: Waldhausen JA, Orringer MB, eds. *Complications in cardiothoracic surgery.* St. Louis: Mosby Year Book, 1991:60–67.

332. Toscano M, Chiavarelli R, Ruvalo G, et al. Management of massive air embolism during open heart surgery with retrograde perfusion of the cerebral vessels and hyperbaric oxygenation. *Thorac Cardiovasc Surg* 1983;31:183–184.

333. Hendriks FFA, Bogers AJJC, de la Riviere AB, et al. The effectiveness of venoarterial perfusion in treatment of arterial air embolism during cardiopulmonary bypass. *Ann Thorac Surg* 1983;36:433–436.

334. Stark J, Hough J. Air in the aorta: treatment by reversed perfusion. *Ann Thorac Surg* 1986;41:337–338.

335. Brown JW, Dierdorf SF, Moorthy S, et al. Venoarterial cerebral perfusion for treatment of massive arterial air embolism. *Anesth Analg* 1987;66:673–674.

336. Tovar EA, DelCampo C, Borsari A, et al. Postoperative management of cerebral air embolism: gas physiology for surgeons. *Ann Thorac Surg* 1995;60:1138–1142.

337. Meijne NG, Schoemaker G, Bulterijs AB. The treatment of cerebral gas embolism in a high pressure chamber: an experimental study. *J Cardiovasc Surg* 1963;4:757–763.

338. Takita H, Olszewski W, Schimert G, et al. Hyperbaric treatment of cerebral air embolism as a result of open-heart surgery: report of a case. *J Thorac Cardiovasc Surg* 1968;55:682–685.

339. Peirce EC II. Specific therapy for arterial air embolism [editorial]. *Ann Thorac Surg* 1980;29:300–303.

340. Murphy BP, Harford FJ, Cramer FS. Cerebral air embolism

resulting from invasive medical procedures: treatment with hyperbaric oxygen. *Ann Surg* 1985;201:242–245.

341. Lar LW, Lai LC, Ren LW. Massive arterial air embolism during cardiac operation: successful treatment in a hyperbaric chamber under 3ATA. *J Thorac Cardiovasc Surg* 1990;100:928–930.

342. Armon C, Deschamps C, Adkinson C, et al. Hyperbaric treatment of cerebral air embolism sustained during an open-heart surgical procedure. *Mayo Clin Proc* 1991;66:565–571.

343. Bitterman H, Melamed Y. Delayed hyperbaric treatment of cerebral air embolism. *Israel J Med Sci* 1993;29:22–26.

344. Kol S, Ammar R, Weisz G, et al. Hyperbaric oxygenation of arterial air embolism during cardiopulmonary bypass. *Ann Thorac Surg* 1993;55:401–403.

345. Dexter F, Hindman BJ. Recommendations for hyperbaric oxygen therapy of cerebral air embolism based on a mathematical model of bubble absorption. *Anesth Analg* 1997;84:1203–1207.

346. Mader JT, Hulet WH. Delayed hyperbaric treatment of cerebral air embolism: report of a case. *Arch Neurol* 1979;36:504–505.

347. Cochran RP, Kunzelman KS, Vocelka CR, et al. Perfluorocarbon emulsion in the cardiopulmonary bypass prime reduces neurologic injury. *Ann Thorac Surg* 1997;63:1326–1332.

348. Dutka AJ. A review of the pathophysiology and potential application of experimental therapies for cerebral ischemia to the treatment of cerebral arterial gas embolism. *Undersea Biomed Res* 1985;12:403–421.

349. Milsom FP, Mitchell SJ. A novel dual vent left heart de-airing technique markedly reduces carotid artery micro emboli. *Ann Thorac Surg* 1998;66:785–791.

350. Spampinato N, Stassano P, Gagliardi C, et al. Massive air embolism during cardiopulmonary bypass; successful treatment with immediate hypothermia and circulatory support. *Ann Thorac Surg* 1981;32:602–603.

351. Steward D, Williams WG, Freedom R. Hypothermia in conjunction with hyperbaric oxygenation in the treatment of massive air embolism during cardiopulmoinary bypass. *Ann Thorac Surg* 1977;24:591–593.

352. Fundaro P, Santoil C. Massive coronary gas embolism managed by retrograde coronary sinus perfusion. *Tex Heart Inst J* 1984; 11:172–174.

353. Alvaran SB, Toung JK, Graaff TE, et al. Venous air embolism-comparative merits of external cardiac massage, intracardiac aspiration, and left lateral decubitus position. *Anesth Analg* 1978; 57:166–170.

354. Sandhu AA, Spotnitz HM, Dickstein ML, et al. Cardiopulmonary bypass, myocardial management and support techniques. Retrograde cardioplegia preserves myocardial function after in-duced coronary air embolism. *J Thorac Cardiovasc Surg* 1997; 113:917–922.

355. Yerlioglu ME, Wolfe D, Mezrow CK, et al. The effect of retrograde cerebral perfusion after particulate embolization to the brain. *J Thorac Cardiovasc Surg* 1995;110:1470–1485.

356. Munson ES. Transfer of nitrous oxide into body air cavities. *Br J Anaesth* 1974;46:202–209.

357. Presson RG Jr, Kirk KR, Haselby KA, et al. Effect of ventilation with soluble and diffusible gases on the size of air emboli. *J Appl Physiol* 1991;70:1068–1074.

358. Butler BD, Laine GA, Leiman GC, et al. Effect of Trendelenburg position on the distribution of arterial air emboli in dogs. *Ann Thorac Surg* 1988;45:198–202.

359. Mehlhorn U, Burke EJ, Butler BD, et al. Body position does not affect the hemodynamic response to venous air embolism in dogs. *Anesth Analg* 1994;79:734–739.

360. Dexter F, Hindman BJ, Marshall JS. Estimate of the maximum absorption rate of microscopic arterial air emboli after entry into the arterial circulation during cardiac surgery. *Perfusion* 1996;11:445–450.

361. Diehl JT, Ramos D, Dougherty F, et al. Intraoperative, two-dimensional echocardiography-guided removal of retained intracardiac air. *Ann Thorac Surg* 1987;43:674–675.

362. Tingleff J, Joyce FS, Pettersson G. Intraoperative echocardiography study of air embolism during cardiac operations. *Ann Thorac Surg* 1995;60:673–677.

363. Orihashi K, Matsuura T, Hamanaka T, et al. Retained intracardiac air in open-heart operations examined by transesophageal echocardiography. *Ann Thorac Surg* 1993;55:1467–1471.

364. Dalmas J-P, Eker A, Girard C, et al. Intracardiac air clearing in valvular surgery guided by transesophageal echocardiography. *J Heart Valve Dis* 1996;5:553.

365. Salzano RP Jr, Khachane VB. Simple system for deairing the heart after cardiopulmonary bypass. *Ann Thorac Surg* 1996;62: 1537–1538.

366. Taylor KM. The cerebral consequences of cardiac surgery [editorial]. *Perfusion* 1989;4:83.

367. Mills SA. Cerebral injury and cardiac operations. *Ann Thorac Surg* 1993;56:S86–S91.

368. Murkin JM, ed. Proceedings, Conference on Cardiopulmonary Bypass, CNS Dysfunction after Cardiac Surgery: defining the problem. *Ann Thorac Surg* 1995;59:1288–1362.

369. Aberg T. Signs of brain cell injury during open heart operations: past and present. *Ann Thorac Surg* 1995;59:1312–1315.

370. Taylor RL, Borger MA, Weisel RD, et al. Cerebral microemboli during cardiopulmonary bypass: increased emboli during perfusionist interventions. *Ann Thorac Surg* 1999;68:89–93.

17

ENDOCRINE, METABOLIC, AND ELECTROLYTE RESPONSES

JOHN F. BUTTERWORTH
RICHARD C. PRIELIPP

Surgical procedures using cardiopulmonary bypass (CPB) produce physiologic alterations not found in other major surgical procedures. During total CPB, the heart and lungs are not perfused and can neither secrete hormones nor make their normal contributions to drug metabolism. Exposure to the pump-oxygenator and its tubing traumatizes cellular blood elements, causes plasma proteins to be adsorbed and removed from the circulation, and stimulates an immune response, as is well described in other chapters in this volume. Hemodilution (from blood-free priming solutions) and heparin anticoagulation alter blood concentrations of electrolytes, hormones, and serum proteins during CPB. Finally, moderate to profound hypothermia is generally used, reducing the rates of biochemical reactions and further perturbing hormonal responses.

Additional characteristics of extracorporeal perfusion contribute to the endocrine, metabolic, and electrolyte alterations produced. Nonpulsatile perfusion may change the distribution of flow both among and within organs. As a consequence, some hormonal alterations during CPB can be lessened or prevented by pulsatile perfusion. CPB increases "stress" hormones disproportionate to the apparent levels of physiologic disturbance, and it remains unclear which factor—hypothermia, hemodilution, decreased perfusion of endocrine glands, or denaturation of hormones by foreign surfaces—most contributes to these changes. Additionally, some hormone concentrations increase above normal levels after termination of bypass with the return of pulsatile warm perfusion to endocrine glands (1). Consistent with expectations, one study shows that deeper planes of anesthesia attenuate or eliminate the exaggerated endocrine responses to CPB and reduce mortality (2). Finally, interest in the use of spinal and epidural anesthesia for cardiac surgery has recently developed, and these techniques have long been known to inhibit the neuroendocrine response to abdominal and lower extremity surgery.

The literature regarding endocrine, metabolic, and electrolyte responses to CPB is difficult to summarize because of marked variations in patient populations, perfusion and cardioplegia techniques, perfusate temperatures, priming solutions, and anesthetic and adjuvant drugs. Early hormone assays often were not specific for intact active hormones. When possible, this chapter emphasizes the most recent studies in which current anesthesia, cardioplegia, perfusion, and hormone measurement techniques were used.

PITUITARY HORMONES

The anterior portion of the pituitary gland secretes hormones that regulate the adrenal cortex, thyroid, ovaries, and testes. Several aspects of pituitary response are considered in subsequent sections. Gonadotropin responses during CPB have not been reported.

Pituitary apoplexy, a rare but potentially devastating complication, has been reported after CPB (3–7), typically in patients with pituitary adenomas. These patients demonstrated varying combinations of ptosis, ophthalmoplegia, nonreactive and dilated pupils, decreased visual acuity, and visual field defects in addition to the characteristic hormonal deficits. Ischemia, hemorrhage, and edema of the gland appear to be the mechanisms for pituitary failure after bypass. The diagnosis can be confirmed with cranial computed tomography or magnetic resonance imaging (Fig. 17.1). Hormonal replacement and prompt hypophysectomy are indicated, and experience suggests that the latter may be safely performed early after cardiac surgery (3).

Vasopressin

Vasopressin, or antidiuretic hormone (ADH), secreted by the posterior pituitary gland, is a potent regulator of renal water excretion (8). At high concentrations, ADH may in-

J. F. Butterworth and R. C. Prielipp: Department of Anesthesiology, Wake Forest University School of Medicine, Winston-Salem, North Carolina 27157-1009.

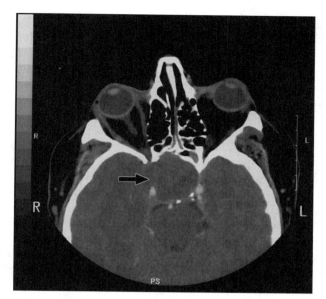

FIG. 17.1. Cranial tomographic scan of a 56-year-old man 3 days after mitral valve repair. The patient presented with unilateral pupillary mydriasis, complete ophthalmoplegia, and loss of sensation in divisions I and II or cranial nerve V upon extubation several hours after his surgery. Note the mass in the sella turcica and bony erosion of the sphenoid "wing," as indicated by the *arrows*. (From Meek EN, Butterworth J, Kon ND, et al. New onset of cranial nerve palsies immediately following mitral valve repair. *Anesthesiology* 1998;89:1580–1582, with permission.)

crease peripheral vascular resistance, decrease cardiac contractility, and decrease coronary blood flow (8,9). ADH increases renal vascular resistance, reducing renal blood flow (9), and stimulates the release of the von Willebrand factor, perhaps improving hemostasis during and after cardiac surgery (see Chapter 28). Stimuli provoking ADH release include increased plasma osmolality, decreased blood volume or blood pressure, hypoglycemia, angiotensin, stress, and pain (8). General anesthesia and surgery are associated with moderate increases in ADH (10,11). Cardiac surgery with CPB is associated with striking increases in ADH concentration, far above those seen during other major surgical procedures (11–15), and these effects may persist for hours postoperatively (12–15) (Fig. 17.2).

The exaggerated ADH response to CPB could be initiated by any number of stimuli, including the decrease in circulating blood volume upon initiating bypass. Left atrial pressure decreases markedly, especially with left ventricular venting, thereby simulating volume depletion, which is a potent stimulus for ADH release. The transient hypotension normally occurring at the onset of bypass may lead to increased ADH secretion. Pulsatile perfusion during CPB attenuates the exaggerated ADH response, particularly after bypass, but does not eliminate it (13,15,16) (Fig. 17.3). Pulsatile perfusion does not seem to significantly increase urinary output, despite reduced ADH concentrations (15).

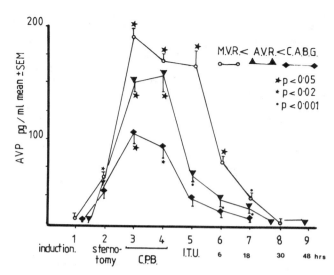

FIG. 17.2. Plasma concentration of arginine vasopressin (*AVP*) during nonpulsatile bypass for mitral valve replacement (*MVR, n* = 8), aortic valve replacement (*AVR, n* = 5), or coronary artery bypass grafting (*CABG, n* = 5). Data are presented as means ± SEM. As indicated, measurements were obtained at *1*) anesthesia induction, *2*) sternotomy, *3*) 10 minutes after initiation of cardiopulmonary bypass, *4*) 10 minutes before termination of cardiopulmonary bypass, *5*) upon arrival in the critical care unit, *6*) 6 hours after bypass, *7*) 18 hours after bypass, *8*) 30 hours after bypass, and *9*) 48 hours after bypass. All three groups of patients demonstrated significant increases in AVP concentrations during bypass. Only at sample 5 did the mitral valve patients demonstrate significantly greater AVP concentration than the CABG patients. *p* values on the figure indicate comparisons between sample 1 and subsequent samples in the same surgical group. (From Kaul TK, Swaminathan R, Chatrath RR, et al. Vasoactive pressure hormones during and after cardiopulmonary bypass. *Int J Artif Organs* 1990; 13:293–299, with permission.)

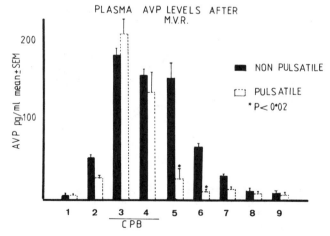

FIG. 17.3. Effect of pulsatile (*n* = 5) or nonpulsatile (*n* = 8) perfusion on arginine vasopressin (*AVP*) responses to mitral valve replacement. See legend to Figure 17.1 for measurement times. Significant differences between the two groups were observed after cardiopulmonary bypass (sample 5 and later). In this study, pulsatile bypass did not attenuate AVP responses during coronary bypass or aortic valve replacement. (From Kaul TK, Swaminathan R, Chatrath RR, et al. Vasoactive pressure hormones during and after cardiopulmonary bypass. *Int J Artif Organs* 1990;13: 293–299, with permission.)

Certain anesthetic techniques, for example, maintenance of anesthesia with large doses of synthetic opioids (fentanyl or sufentanil) or with regional anesthesia, attenuate the hormonal responses associated with noncardiac surgical procedures. Indeed, Kuitunen et al. (17) found that patients anesthetized with 50 μg/kg fentanyl demonstrated significantly reduced arginine vasopressin concentration after bypass than patients who received a lighter plane of general anesthesia using inhaled enflurane. However, even opioid anesthesia will not completely ablate the release of ADH at the onset of CPB (14,18). Unfortunately, multiple studies provide conflicting data as to whether higher peak ADH concentrations occur in patients undergoing coronary surgery or valve surgery during and after CPB (12,13,15) (Fig. 17.2). In summary, ADH concentrations increase markedly during CPB irrespective of the anesthesia or perfusion technique.

ADRENAL HORMONES

Catecholamines

The catecholamines epinephrine and norepinephrine are products of the adrenal medulla and (in the latter case) of peripheral sympathetic and central nerve terminals. Marked elevations of plasma epinephrine and norepinephrine concentrations occurring during CPB may underlie many hemodynamic sequelae of bypass, including peripheral vasoconstriction and shifts in intraorgan blood flow (16,19–22). With hypothermia, the plasma epinephrine concentrations may increase as much as 10-fold over the pre-bypass concentrations; norepinephrine concentrations typically increase to a lesser extent (4-fold) (2,16,20,22), and deepening hypothermia attenuates these (Table 17.1). In early studies, peak increases in both norepinephrine and epinephrine occurred when the heart and lungs were excluded from the circulation (21,22). However, norepinephrine and epinephrine were found to peak at different times. In a recent study, patients

undergoing cardiac surgery were randomly assigned to have CPB with mild (34°C) or moderate (28°C) hypothermia. With both bypass temperatures, peak norepinephrine concentrations were observed after release of the aortic crossclamp and rewarming, whereas peak epinephrine concentrations were observed at the target hypothermic temperature (23). Neonates, infants, and young children, much like adults, demonstrate marked increases in catecholamine concentrations during CPB (2,24,25).

"Deeper" planes of general anesthesia (whether accomplished with larger doses of synthetic opioids, addition of a propofol infusion, higher concentrations of volatile anesthetic vapors, or addition of epidural anesthesia) significantly reduce the catecholamine concentrations of patients undergoing coronary artery bypass surgery compared with patients less deeply anesthetized (26–29). Furthermore, in critically ill neonates undergoing correction of congenital heart disease, deeper planes of general anesthesia from large intravenous doses of sufentanil not only produced lower catecholamine concentrations in response to CPB (Fig. 17.4) but also reduced mortality compared with lighter planes of general anesthesia with halothane/morphine (2). Consistent with these observations regarding anesthetic depth, infusion of propofol during bypass (4 mg/kg/hr) resulted in markedly reduced concentrations of epinephrine and norepinephrine compared with a single bolus injection of diazepam 0.1 mg/kg (27). Addition of thoracic epidural anesthesia to a "high-dose opioid" general anesthetic, including either fentanyl or sufentanil, significantly reduces catecholamine concentrations during and after bypass relative to concentrations measured without thoracic epidural anesthesia (28,29) (Fig. 17.5).

The effect of pulsatile perfusion on catecholamine concentrations during CPB remains controversial (16,30). Although early studies demonstrated that catecholamine concentrations were increased during bypass whether or not pulsatile perfusion was used (16), a more recent study of elective coronary surgery patients showed significant reductions in epinephrine and norepinephrine concentrations with pulsatile perfusion (30) (Fig. 17.6).

TABLE 17.1. BLOOD PRESSURE AND PLASMA CATECHOLAMINE CONCENTRATIONS DURING EXTRACORPOREAL PERFUSION IN PATIENTS UNDERGOING AORTOCORONARY BYPASS GRAFTING

Time Sequence	Before Anesthesia	After Intubation	On Bypass	Core Tmperature (32°C)	Core Temperature (28°C)	Core Temperature (24°C)
Core Temperature; °C	37.0 ± 0	36.1 ± .5[a]	34.7 ± .4[a]	31.5 ± .5[a]	27.8 ± .4[a]	24.1 ± .2[a]
MAP, mm Hg	86 ± 3	76 ± 1	70 ± 4[a]	73 ± 3[a]	60 ± 3[a]	60 ± 2[a]
NE, pg/mL	287 ± 40	360 ± 94	416 ± 83	662 ± 172[a]	540 ± 153	312 ± 86
EPI, pg/mL	50 ± 15	29 ± 8	138 ± 47	506 ± 191[a]	267 ± 136	130 ± 62

Catecholamine concentrations were not corrected for hemodilution.
[a] $p < 0.05$ compared with preinduction values.
Core temperature, rectal temperature; EPI, plasma epinephrine concentration; MAP, mean arterial pressure; NE, plasma norepinephrine concentration.
Source: Reed HL, Chernow B, Lake CR, et al. *Chest* 1989;95:616–622, with permission.

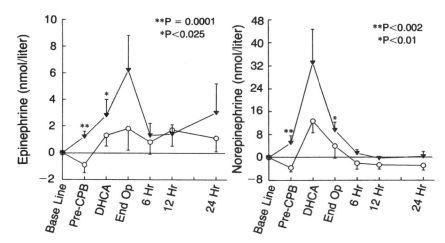

FIG. 17.4. Perioperative changes in plasma epinephrine and norepinephrine in neonates undergoing cardiac surgery with either high-dose sufentanil (○; *n* = 30) or halothane-morphine (▼; *n* = 15) anesthesia. *Pre CPB*, before bypass; *DHCA*, after deep hypothermic circulatory arrest; *End OP*, end of operation; *6 hr, 12 hr, 24 hr*, 6, 12, or 24 hours after operation. *p* values determined with Mann-Whitney U test. (From Anand KJS, Hickey PR. Halothane-morphine compared with high-dose sufentanil for anesthesia and postoperative analgesia in neonatal cardiac surgery. *N Engl J Med* 1992;326:1–9, with permission.)

Some increase in catecholamine concentrations during and after bypass may be unavoidable with current anesthetic and surgical techniques; nevertheless, higher doses of opioids, inhaled general anesthetics, and epidural local anesthesia can limit the increases.

Adrenal Cortical Hormones

Secretion of cortisol is one of the central features of the metabolic stress response (18). In the classic studies by

Hume et al. (31) of patients undergoing major surgery (without bypass perfusion), cortisol concentrations rose quickly to a maximum and then slowly returned to baseline 24 hours postoperatively. CPB modifies cortisol responses to surgery. Total plasma cortisol concentrations typically decrease immediately upon initiation of bypass, likely as a consequence of hemodilution (32–35) (Fig. 17.7). During bypass, cortisol concentrations return to values significantly above baseline values (2,32–36). After CPB, patients exhibit

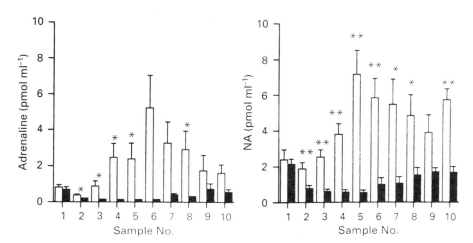

FIG. 17.5. Effects of thoracic epidural anesthesia with bupivacaine 0.5% (■, *n* = 8) versus control (□, *n* = 9) on catecholamine concentrations measured during coronary artery surgery. All 17 patients studied received general anesthesia with sufentanil 20 μg/kg. Samples were obtained *1)* before anesthesia, *2)* after anesthesia induction, *3)* after 30 min of surgery, *4)* after 30 min of cardiopulmonary bypass (CPB), *5)* after 60 min of CPB, *6)* 1 hr after CPB, *7)* 2 hr after CPB, *8)* 4 hr after CPB, *9)* 6 hr after CPB, and *10)* 24 hr after CPB. *$p < 0.05$, **$p < 0.01$ for between group differences. *Adrenaline*, epinephrine; *NA*, noradrenaline or norepinephrine. (From Moore CM, Cross MH, Desborough JP, et al. Hormonal effects of thoracic extradural analgesia for cardiac surgery. *Br J Anaesth* 1995;75:387–393, with permission.)

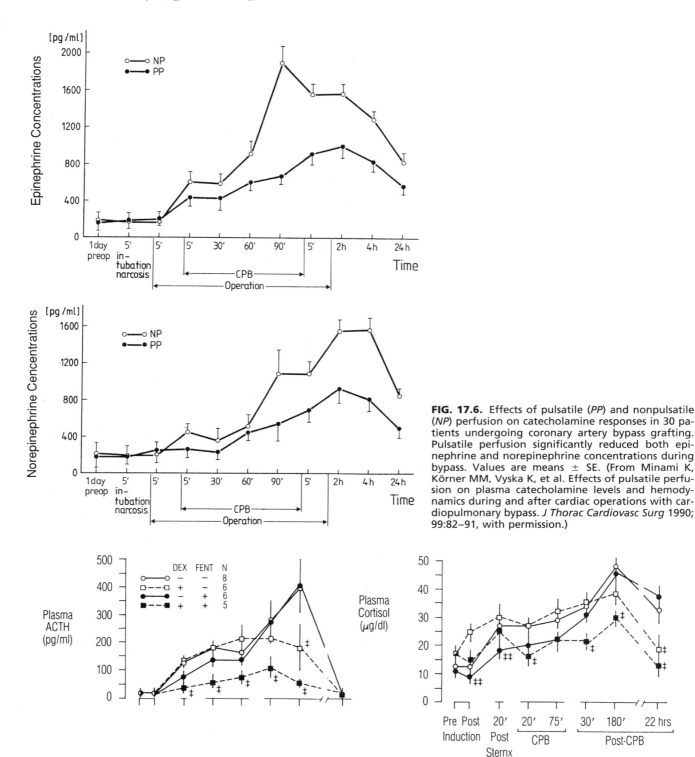

FIG. 17.6. Effects of pulsatile (*PP*) and nonpulsatile (*NP*) perfusion on catecholamine responses in 30 patients undergoing coronary artery bypass grafting. Pulsatile perfusion significantly reduced both epinephrine and norepinephrine concentrations during bypass. Values are means ± SE. (From Minami K, Körner MM, Vyska K, et al. Effects of pulsatile perfusion on plasma catecholamine levels and hemodynamics during and after cardiac operations with cardiopulmonary bypass. *J Thorac Cardiovasc Surg* 1990; 99:82–91, with permission.)

FIG. 17.7. The effects of either enflurane or fentanyl anesthesia with or without dexamethasone treatment on cortisol and adrenocorticotropic hormone responses to cardiac surgery. All groups demonstrated significant increases in both cortisol and adrenocorticotropic hormone in response to surgery. The combination of fentanyl and dexamethasone significantly attenuated the adrenocorticotropic hormone response to surgery relative to the other three groups (‡ = $p < 0.05$ compared with the no dexamethasone, no fentanyl group; ‡‡ = $p < 0.05$ compared with the dexamethasone-treated, no fentanyl group). (From Raff H, Norton AJ, Flemma RJ, et al. Inhibition of the adrenocorticotropin response to surgery in humans: interaction between dexamethasone and fentanyl. *J Clin Endocrinol Metab* 1987;65:295–298, with permission.)

markedly elevated concentrations of cortisol (both free and total) for more than 48 hours (35–37). Free cortisol remains elevated for 24 hours. Tinnikov et al. (38) studied 14 children undergoing repair of ventricular septal defects with deep hypothermia and circulatory arrest without the use of extracorporeal circulation. Maximal perioperative concentrations of cortisol and minimal perioperative concentrations of cortisol binding globulin were recorded at the first assessment after circulatory arrest. Thus, hypothermia and circulatory arrest initiate a cortisol-stress response even in the absence of bypass perfusion.

Cortisol responses during bypass appear to be perfusion temperature-dependent. Taggart et al. (39) showed that the rise in cortisol concentration during CPB can be blunted by perfusion with blood at 20°C rather than at the more usual 28°C. Cortisol concentrations during bypass were decreased by deeper planes of anesthesia in both adults and children (2,35,36) (Fig. 17.8). Stenseth et al. (28) found that compared with high-dose fentanyl anesthesia alone, high-dose fentanyl anesthesia plus thoracic epidural anesthesia resulted in a delayed increase in cortisol concentrations during coronary artery surgery and lower concentrations during bypass. Similarly, Moore et al. (29) found that thoracic epidural anesthesia combined with sufentanil 20 μg/kg was associated with markedly lower cortisol concentrations compared with sufentanil anesthesia alone.

CPB modifies adrenocorticotropic hormone responses in

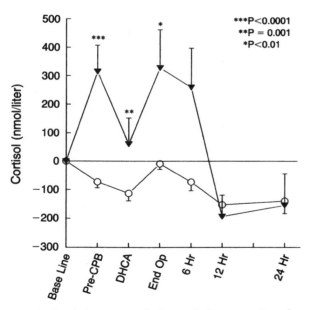

FIG. 17.8. Cortisol responses during and after correction of congenital heart lesions with either halothane-morphine (*n* = 15, ▲) or sufentanil (*n* = 30, ○) anesthesia. The narcotic-based techniques significantly attenuated the "stress" response to cardiac surgery. (From Anand KJS, Hickey PR. Halothane-morphine compared with high-dose sufentanil for anesthesia and postoperative analgesia in neonatal cardiac surgery. *N Engl J Med* 1992;326: 1–9, with permission.)

surgical patients. In the previously mentioned study by Hume et al. (31), surgical patients not undergoing bypass showed no increase in cortisol concentrations after an injection of adrenocorticotropic hormone, indicating that adrenal secretion of cortisol was already maximal. Amado and Diago (40) observed a blunted response to corticotropin-releasing hormone during bypass, similar to responses seen in patients with hypothalamic corticotropin-releasing hormone deficiency. In contrast, when patients undergoing extracorporeal perfusion received adrenocorticotropic hormone, cortisol concentrations increased (32). Taylor et al. (41) measured a progressive fall in adrenocorticotropic hormone concentrations during bypass, with a subsequent increase 1 hour after pulsatile perfusion was restored. More recently, Raff et al. (34) showed that although neither high-dose fentanyl anesthesia nor dexamethasone 40 mg alone blunted the increase in adrenocorticotropic hormone concentration in response to CPB, concurrent administration of both agents significantly reduced the adrenocorticotropic hormone concentration (Fig. 17.7).

Unlike some other hormones, cortisol and adrenocorticotropic hormone responses to CPB have generally not been influenced by pulsatile perfusion. To be sure, one study found that total plasma cortisol rose during pulsatile bypass but fell dramatically in patients undergoing nonpulsatile perfusion (33). In another study, patients with and without pulsatile perfusion showed initial increases in cortisol, adrenocorticotropic hormone, and aldosterone, followed by a gradual decline in concentrations of all three hormones during bypass and then a subsequent increase in all three hormones after bypass perfusion (42). After correction for the effect of hemodilution, there was no decrease in calculated free cortisol concentrations and a slight increase in adrenocorticotropic hormone concentrations, irrespective of whether pulsatile perfusion was used. In children undergoing bypass with either pulsatile or nonpulsatile perfusion, Pollock et al. (43) found large increases in cortisol and adrenocorticotropic hormone during CPB, followed by a slow decline toward baseline concentrations of both hormones over 24 hours with both pulsatile and nonpulsatile CPB techniques.

Although there is no evidence for true adrenocortical hypofunction during or after CPB, the inflammatory response initiated by the triad of blood contact with the foreign surfaces of the extracorporeal membrane, reperfusion injury, and endotoxemia may be attenuated by large doses of exogenous glucocorticoids (44). This inflammatory response triggers tissue injury in the heart, kidneys, hemostatic system, and especially the lung, which is the only organ exposed to the entire cardiac output. Previous investigations have studied small numbers of cardiac surgery patients randomized to variable doses of different corticosteroids (most commonly 1 mg/kg dexamethasone or 30 mg/kg methylprednisolone) initiated at varying intervals between induction of anesthesia and the start of CPB (44). Unfortunately, few if any of these studies have addressed outcome issues such as morbidity and mortality, intensive care unit or hospital length of stay, and other aspects of hospital resource utilization. Rather, process variables of the inflammatory pathways were used as surrogate endpoints. Thus, results generally demonstrate an amelioration of the inflammatory response, with decreases in cytokine formation (tumor necrosis factor and the interleukin-1, -6, and -8) but inconsistent effects on C3a and elastase concentrations. Leukotrienes such as LTB_4 are decreased in a dose-dependent fashion (44). In addition, large doses of methylprednisolone can block upregulation of neutrophil integrin adhesion receptors, whereas dexamethasone decreases endothelial production of certain adhesion molecules (45). Clinically, glucocorticoid therapy may result in an increased cardiac index and decreased systemic vascular resistance (46). Dietzman et al. (47) showed improvement in tissue perfusion and a decrease in peripheral vascular resistance when a large dose of glucocorticoid was given just before bypass (48). Routine glucocorticoid supplementation has also been advocated as part of an accelerated recovery program (49), albeit without much supporting evidence.

In summary, current data nearly uniformly demonstrate large increases in cortisol and adrenocorticotropic hormone concentrations with initiation of bypass. These rises may be attenuated by deeper planes of general anesthesia or addition of thoracic epidural anesthesia to general anesthesia. Pulsatile perfusion does not appear to reduce these exaggerated responses. Moreover, it is not clear whether elevated corticosteroid concentrations during bypass are deleterious or beneficial.

Glucose Homeostasis

Carbohydrate metabolism is regulated by insulin, glucagon, cortisol, growth hormone, and epinephrine, the concentrations of which are generally perturbed during and after CPB. After onset of CPB, blood glucose concentrations rise steadily (50–52). Despite marked hyperglycemia, insulin concentrations decline from their control values during hypothermic bypass (50–52). Normoglycemia can be maintained only with great difficulty during hypothermic nonpulsatile CPB in nondiabetic adults, even with large doses of insulin. Thus, hyperglycemia, hypoinsulinemia, and insulin resistance are produced by hypothermic nonpulsatile CPB in adults (50–52).

Counter-regulatory hormones also decline from pre-bypass concentrations during hypothermic bypass (53). With rewarming, insulin concentrations rise spontaneously to appropriate high levels; nonetheless, blood glucose remains elevated (51). Normoglycemia is better preserved in children undergoing hypothermic CPB when washed red blood cells rather than conventional packed cells (suspended in adenine-glucose-mannitol-saline) are used in the pump priming solution (53,54). Blood glucose concentrations in packed red cells range from 400 to 700 mg/dL (54).

Concentrations of glucose, insulin, and glucagon are higher during normothermic than hypothermic CPB (52,55). Nagaoka et al. (50) compared pulsatile with nonpulsatile perfusion in patients undergoing cardiac surgery with moderate hypothermia (body temperature approximately 26°C). In both groups, blood glucose concentrations increased with CPB and rose further with hypothermia, reaching values greater than 200 mg/dL (Table 17.2). Blood glucose concentrations remained elevated for at least 5 hours postoperatively, but the patients receiving pulsatile perfusion showed a more rapid return to baseline glucose concentration than did patients receiving nonpulsatile perfusion. Insulin concentration, C peptide concentration, and the insulin-to-glucagon molar ratio increased significantly compared with baseline during pulsatile but not during nonpulsatile CPB. Type I ("juvenile onset") diabetics require no greater doses of insulin to control blood glucose during CPB

TABLE 17.2. EFFECT OF NONPULSATILE (*n* = 18) OR PULSATILE (*n* = 20) CARDIOPULMONARY BYPASS ON GLUCOSE METABOLISM

Variable	Group	Preoperative	CPB	Postoperative (hr) 1	5	24	48
Blood glucose, mg/dL	P	83 ± 18	206 ± 44[a]	253 ± 51[a]	235 ± 52[a]	125 ± 46	115 ± 27
	NP	87 ± 27	254 ± 92[a]	281 ± 67[a]	271 ± 60[a]	208 ± 72[a]	149 ± 25
Immunoreactive insulin, mIU/L	P	16 ± 9	72 ± 39[a]	71 ± 34[a]	89 ± 36[a]	72 ± 42	64 ± 35
	NP	13 ± 5	24 ± 15	29 ± 20[b]	40 ± 27[b]	31 ± 23	27 ± 18
Immunoreactive glucagon, ng/L	P	98 ± 34	150 ± 81	148 ± 73	202 ± 101	225 ± 88	220 ± 91
	NP	107 ± 45	200 ± 96	197 ± 88	221 ± 79	175 ± 80	156 ± 66

Values are means ± SEM.
[a] $p < 0.05$ vs. preoperative value; [b] $p < 0.05$ vs. group P.
CPB, cardiopulmonary bypass; P, pulsatile CPB; NP, nonpulsatile CPB.
Source: Nagaoka H, Innami R, Watanabe M, et al. *Ann Thorac Surg* 1989;48:798–802, with permission.

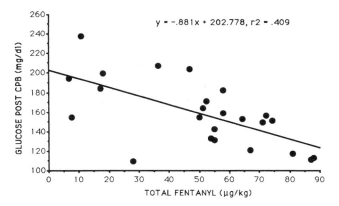

FIG. 17.9. Total fentanyl dose is inversely correlated with blood glucose concentrations in 24 children undergoing correction of congenital heart disease with hypothermic circulatory arrest (but without profound hypothermia or circulatory arrest). Blood samples were withdrawn within 30 minutes after cessation of bypass. $p = 0.0007$ for the slope of the regression line. (From Ellis DJ, Steward DJ. Fentanyl dosage is associated with reduced blood glucose in pediatric patients after hypothermic cardiopulmonary bypass. *Anesthesiology* 1990;72:812–815, with permission.)

than do nondiabetic control subjects, whereas type II ("adult onset") diabetics exhibit marked insulin resistance compared with type I diabetics and nondiabetic control patients during CPB (52). Children receiving deeper anesthesia demonstrated lower blood glucose concentrations upon termination of bypass than did children receiving lighter anesthetic techniques (2,56) (Fig. 17.9).

In patients undergoing coronary artery surgery, growth hormone was found to increase significantly during and after CPB (57,58). The increase in growth hormone could be prevented using opioid general anesthetic techniques (58). The physiologic significance of this growth hormone response is unclear, because it can be inhibited by prior administration of somatostatin without an effect on glucose or glutamine metabolism.

ATRIAL NATRIURETIC FACTOR

Atrial natriuretic factor denotes a family of biologically active peptides first isolated from cardiac atria (59). These peptides, released in response to atrial distention, increase glomerular filtration; inhibit renin release; reduce aldosterone concentrations in blood; antagonize renal vasoconstrictors such as vasopressin, norepinephrine, and angiotensin; and reduce arterial blood pressure. Atrial natriuretic factor regulates vascular volume by increasing sodium excretion and decreasing vasomotor tone (59).

Plasma atrial natriuretic factor has been measured before, during, and after CPB, with conflicting conclusions. Patients with cardiac valve lesions, especially those with arrhythmias and congestive failure, may demonstrate elevated

preoperative atrial natriuretic factor concentrations, whereas coronary artery surgery patients may have normal preoperative atrial natriuretic factor concentrations (60–64). In one study, no significant changes were noted during induction of anesthesia or during CPB; however, after separation from CPB, both arterial and venous concentrations of atrial natriuretic factor increased in these patients having coronary artery surgery (64). In contrast, most other studies found significant alterations of atrial natriuretic factor concentrations during bypass, particularly during aortic cross-clamping. Curello et al. (62) measured atrial natriuretic factor in patients undergoing either coronary artery bypass or mitral valve replacement for mitral stenosis (Fig. 17.10). Although there was no change in atrial natriuretic factor concentrations during bypass in the coronary surgery group, patients undergoing mitral valve replacement demonstrated significantly reduced concentrations during CPB. After release of the aortic clamp, atrial natriuretic factor concentrations in both groups of patients rose to values equal to those found preoperatively in the mitral valve patients (62).

Nearly identical responses were observed by Northridge et al. (65) in their study of 12 patients undergoing aortocoronary bypass grafting with hypothermic nonpulsatile perfusion. In another study, arterial concentrations of atrial natriuretic factor decreased significantly after aortic cross-clamping (66). Interestingly, this study also found evidence for atrial natriuretic factor release from the brain during bypass. Ashcroft et al. (61) found a significant reduction in atrial natriuretic factor concentrations during bypass, with return to baseline values postoperatively. Haug et al. (67) studied 33 patients undergoing coronary artery surgery and found significantly increased concentrations of atrial natriuretic factor after CPB, with a further increase measured at the end of surgery that was maintained in measurements 24 hours after the operation. Pasaoglu et al. (68) found that atrial natriuretic factor concentrations were elevated (relative to normal values) before induction of anesthesia for coronary artery surgery. Atrial natriuretic factor concentrations increased significantly (relative to baseline values) after surgical incision and remained elevated during and after surgery, with the highest mean values recorded on the fifth postoperative day; however, no measurements were made during CPB. In 16 patients undergoing aortocoronary bypass grafting or mitral valve replacement, atrial natriuretic factor concentrations decreased significantly during hypothermic extracorporeal perfusion and aortic cross-clamping (63).

Two recent studies comparing atrial natriuretic factor concentrations in systemic and pulmonary venous and arterial blood identified secretion of atrial natriuretic factor into the left atrium and its clearance by the lungs in adults and children (66,69). Atrial natriuretic factor concentrations declined significantly during aortic cross-clamping, but rebounded rapidly after release of the aortic clamp (62,65,66).

Multiple studies of both children and adults demonstrated no correlation between atrial pressure and atrial na-

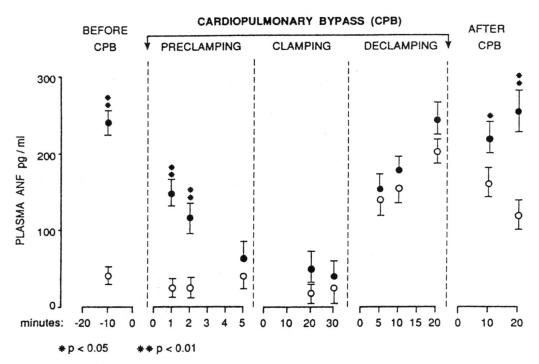

FIG. 17.10. Measurements of plasma atrial natriuretic factor (*ANF*) in six patients undergoing aortocoronary bypass (○) and eight patients undergoing mitral valve replacement (●). Data are presented as means ± SEM. Despite large differences between the groups before aortic clamping, differences were minimal during and early after the ischemic period. (From Curello S, Ceconi C, De Giuli F, et al. Time course of human atrial natriuretic factor release during cardiopulmonary bypass in mitral valve and coronary artery diseased patients. *Eur J Cardiothorac Surg* 1991;5: 205–210, with permission.)

triuretic factor concentration during and after cardiac surgery. This is particularly apparent when patients demonstrated paradoxical increased atrial natriuretic factor concentrations during rewarming, despite reduced atrial pressure at the time (60,62,63,65,66,69,70). After CPB, urine flow and sodium excretion increased concurrently with increased atrial natriuretic factor and normal vasopressin concentrations; thus, this diuresis could be the result of elevated atrial natriuretic factor concentrations (70). The relationship between atrial natriuretic factor concentration and atrial pressure remained abnormal in the first few hours after bypass but returned to normal after 24 hours (60,63). Despite no correlation between atrial pressure and atrial natriuretic factor concentrations during bypass, a 30-minute infusion of atrial natriuretic factor (1.67 μg/min) significantly increased urinary output and sodium excretion compared with placebo, indicating preserved end-organ responses to the hormone during bypass (71) (Fig. 17.11).

Amano et al. (72) infused 1 mL/kg of 10% saline to patients before and after heart or lung operations. Patients having lung surgery showed normal atrial natriuretic factor responses to saline before and after surgery; conversely, patients showed a normal increase in atrial natriuretic factor with saline infusion before undergoing cardiac surgery but

had no significant response to the same stimulus delivered after surgery (72).

In summary, the preponderance of recent evidence suggests that atrial natriuretic factor concentrations are reduced during CPB, especially during hypothermia and aortic cross-clamping. Decreases in hormone concentration are most evident in patients with preoperative elevations in atrial natriuretic factor, which is especially common with valvular heart disease. Most patients will demonstrate distinctly elevated atrial natriuretic factor concentrations (relative to those measured during aortic cross-clamping) during rewarming and after discontinuation of bypass. Finally, patients will fail to demonstrate the normal relationship between atrial natriuretic factor concentrations and atrial pressure during bypass and the early postoperative period or the normal response of atrial natriuretic factor to saline infusion after bypass.

RENIN-ANGIOTENSIN-ALDOSTERONE AXIS

The renin-angiotensin-aldosterone axis regulates arterial blood pressure, intravascular volume, and electrolyte balance (73). The renal juxtaglomerular apparatus secretes renin in response to sodium depletion, falls in blood volume, or reduced renal perfusion. Conversely, factors that

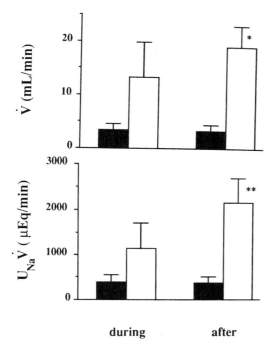

FIG. 17.11. Diuresis and natriuresis in response to atrial natriuretic factor ($n = 6$, □) or placebo ($n = 6$, ■) infused during cardiopulmonary bypass. Responses were recorded during and after drug administration. V, urine volume; $U^{Na}V$, urine sodium concentration times urine volume. (From Hynynen M, Palojoki R, Heinonen J, et al. Renal and vascular effects of atrial natriuretic factor during cardiopulmonary bypass. *Chest* 1991;100: 1203–1209, with permission.)

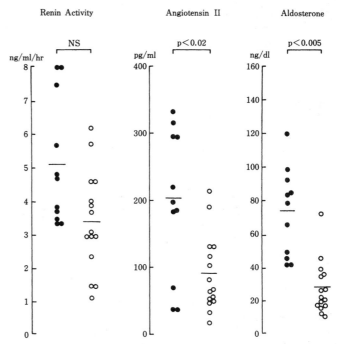

FIG. 17.12. Pulsatile perfusion (○) reduces concentrations of angiotensin II and aldosterone (versus nonpulsatile perfusion, ●) during cardiopulmonary bypass. (From Nagaoka H, Innami R, Arai H. Effects of pulsatile cardiopulmonary bypass on the renin-angiotensin-aldosterone system following open heart surgery. *Jpn J Surg* 1988;18:390–396, with permission.)

increase blood volume, renal perfusion, and sodium load inhibit the release of renin. The sympathetic nervous system stimulates renin release in response to pain, emotion, and stress. Renin catalyzes the conversion of angiotensinogen to the decapeptide angiotensin I in the blood. Angiotensin-converting enzyme, present in blood vessel walls (particularly of the pulmonary vasculature), catalyzes the conversion of angiotensin I to angiotensin II (an octapeptide). Conversion of angiotensin I to angiotensin II is nearly complete during a single pass through the lungs. Angiotensin II raises blood pressure through two mechanisms: direct vasoconstriction and stimulation of aldosterone secretion by the adrenal glands. Aldosterone stimulates the renal distal tubules to reabsorb sodium and secrete potassium and hydrogen ions into tubular fluid.

Serial measurements taken before, during, and after CPB have shown that renin activity increases during and shortly after CPB (64). Similarly, angiotensin II and aldosterone concentrations rise significantly during and shortly after bypass in patients undergoing nonpulsatile perfusion (74–77). Pulsatile perfusion during CPB eliminates the intraoperative and postoperative increases in plasma renin activity and postoperative increases in both angiotensin II and aldosterone (77,78) (Fig. 17.12). Goto et al. (79) found no significant differences between pulsatile and nonpulsatile perfu-

sion on concentrations of renin, angiotensin II, or aldosterone, with concentrations of all three hormones declining upon initiation of CPB and only aldosterone increasing during and after CPB.

Angiotensin-converting enzyme concentrations change markedly during and after cardiac surgery; however, if corrected for hemodilution, minimal response to CPB or hypothermia is observed (22). Absolute and corrected concentrations of angiotensin-converting enzyme are depressed during rewarming, after separation from bypass, and during the first 24 hours of recovery (22,80,81). By 24 hours after bypass, angiotensin-converting enzyme concentrations recover to baseline values (80,81). Secretion of angiotensin-converting enzyme into the vascular compartment by the lungs remains diminished in the period immediately after CPB (22,80,81). These studies suggest that depression of angiotensin-converting enzyme activity during CPB begins after the induction of hypothermia but before rewarming (22). Angiotensin-converting enzyme concentration may also serve as a biologic marker of thyroid hormone [free triiodothyronine (T_3)] action during and after cardiac surgery (81).

The role of the renin-angiotensin-aldosterone axis in the maintenance of blood pressure and peripheral vascular resistance during and after CPB remains unclear (82). Preoperative administration of an angiotensin-converting enzyme inhibitor did not impair blood pressure regulation during anesthesia and CPB (83). Two studies have documented that concentrations of renin, angiotensin II, and aldosterone during bypass did not correlate with intraoperative or postoperative hypertension (75,76). In another study, postoperative hypertension and the need for vasodilators were associated with high vasopressin concentrations but not with angiotensin II concentrations (82). A fourth study found that postoperative hypertension could not be related to elevated renin levels; moreover, hypertension was not treated effectively by saralasin blockade of angiotensin II (84). Similarly, preoperative administration of angiotensin-converting enzyme inhibitors failed to prevent hypertension after coronary artery bypass grafting (83). Thus, the preponderance of evidence would suggest that both intraoperative and postoperative hypertension is at best only loosely related to the abnormal concentrations of renin, angiotensin II, or aldosterone seen during and after bypass.

THYROID

A variety of acute illnesses leads to alterations of peripheral thyroid hormone metabolism. Characteristically, serum concentrations of T_3 (the active thyroid hormone species) are reduced, thyroxine (T_4) is normal or reduced, free thyroxine is reduced, and thyrotropin (thyroid-stimulating hormone) concentrations are normal, producing the so-called sick euthyroid syndrome (85). Multiple studies have documented the presence of this syndrome during and after CPB in adults and children. Recent evidence confirms the sick euthyroid syndrome also is seen in patients undergoing normothermic (35 ± 1°C) CPB (86). In theory, the concentration of T_3 would be especially important for patients having cardiac surgery because T_3 regulates the number of β-adrenergic receptors and their sensitivity to agonists (87). Jones et al. (88) demonstrated a frequent (greater than 10%) incidence of preoperative abnormalities in thyroid function in patients undergoing CPB. Nevertheless, there appeared to be no association between abnormal laboratory results and adverse outcome (88).

Before CPB, administration of heparin leads to small increases in free T_3 and free T_4, because heparin displaces hormones from binding proteins (89–92). Total T_3 concentrations drop precipitously with bypass and remain depressed 24 hours after surgery (22,87,93,94) (Fig. 17.13). T_3 values corrected for hemodilution (using albumin concentration) are not altered by the initiation of CPB or by the initiation of hypothermic perfusion (22). Similarly, the free and the dialyzable fractions of T_3 increase after the onset of bypass and hypothermia (22,89). These alterations in T_3 and T_4 during bypass are independent of thyrotropin-stimulating hormone secretion because adjustments in T_3 and T_4 concentrations normally are delayed by 2 to 4 hours after a change in thyrotropin-stimulating hormone concentration (95). Absolute thyrotropin-stimulating hormone and total T_3 concentrations return to normal after surgery, at a time that varies from study to study (94,96).

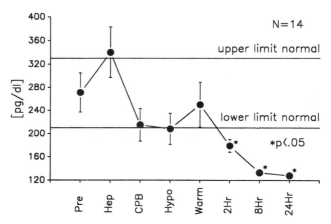

FIG. 17.13. Response of free T_3 concentration to cardiovascular surgery in 14 patients. T_3 declined during cardiopulmonary bypass (CPB) and then declined further during the first 24 hours after operation. Concentrations of free T_3 during cardiac surgery in 14 patients. Concentrations were measured preoperatively (*Pre*), after administration of heparin (*Hep*), after initiation of CPB (*CPB*), at the nadir of hypothermia (*Hypo*), after rewarming (*Warm*), and at 2 (*2 Hr*), 8 (*8 Hr*), and 24 hours (*24 Hr*) after CPB. Statistical comparisons were made between the preoperative and subsequent measurements. (From Holland FW II, Brown PS Jr, Weintraub BD, et al. Cardiopulmonary bypass and thyroid function: a "euthyroid sick syndrome." *Ann Thorac Surg* 1991;52: 46–50, with permission.)

The central regulating mechanism for thyroid hormone is the thyrotropin-releasing hormone-thyrotropin axis in the hypothalamus and pituitary gland. In adults, thyrotropin concentrations are unchanged during normothermic bypass; however, thyrotropin declines upon initiation of hypothermic bypass and then steadily rises during perfusion (89,93) (Fig. 17.14). During the first postoperative day, thyrotropin concentrations decline below baseline values (81,93,97). During and shortly after CPB, the normal increase in thyrotropin concentration in responses to exogenous administration of thyrotropin-releasing hormone is blunted (97–99) (Fig. 17.15). Because of the reduced total T_3 concentrations during bypass, an increased sensitivity to thyrotropin-releasing hormone might have been anticipated. The cause of this pituitary hypofunction remains unknown; however, rises in endogenous dopamine (100) or somatostatin (101) concentrations or nonpulsatile blood flow to the anterior pituitary gland are possible etiologies (99).

Children undergoing correction of congenital heart disease demonstrate thyroid hormonal responses similar to those of adults, demonstrating the sick euthyroid syndrome at 24 hours after surgery (102) (Fig. 17.16). Curiously, patients having deep hypothermia and circulatory arrest demonstrate better preservation of the relationship between thyrotropin and T_3 during and early after CPB than do patients undergoing cardiac repair without circulatory arrest. Deep hypothermia with circulatory arrest may better preserve the hypothalamo-pituitary axis than conventional hypothermic bypass without circulatory arrest (102). Nevertheless, any

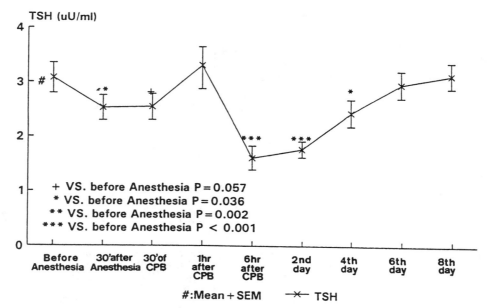

FIG. 17.14. Effect of cardiovascular surgery on thyroid-stimulating hormone (*TSH*) concentration in 44 patients. TSH reached its nadir 6 hours after bypass and remained low through the fourth postoperative day. Statistical comparisons (as indicated on the figure) all compare subsequent TSH concentrations versus those measured before anesthesia. (From Chu S-H, Huang T-S, Hsu R-B, et al. Thyroid hormone changes after cardiovascular surgery and clinical implications. *Ann Thorac Surg* 1991;52:791–796, with permission.)

benefit is only transitory: At 24 hours patients demonstrate decreased thyrotropin and T$_3$ concentrations whether or not circulatory arrest was used (102). Murzi et al. (103) measured concentrations of thyroid hormones for up to 8 days after correction of congenital heart defects and observed return of thyrotropin concentrations to baseline pre-operative values by the third postoperative day; nevertheless, T$_3$ concentrations continued to be depressed below baseline values at the seventh postoperative day. Mainwaring et al. (104) studied 10 neonates undergoing either repair of D-transposition of the great arteries or total anomalous pulmonary venous drainage. Free T$_3$ was unchanged immediately

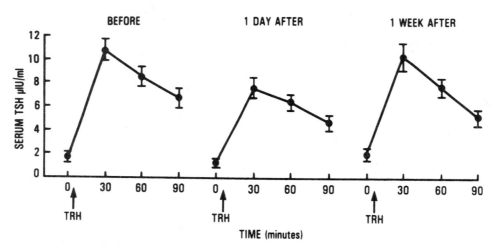

FIG. 17.15. Serum thyrotropin hormone response to thyrotropin-releasing hormone (TRH) in euthyroid subjects before, 1 day after, and 1 week after coronary bypass surgery with hypothermic nonpulsatile perfusion. TSH, thyroid stimulating hormone. (From Zaloga GP, Chernow B, Smallridge RC, et al. A longitudinal evaluation of thyroid function in critically ill surgical patients. *Ann Surg* 1985;201:456–464, with permission.)

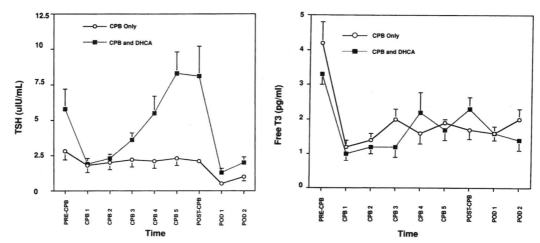

FIG. 17.16. Concentrations of free triiodothyronine (T₃) and thyrotropin (TSH) in infants and young children undergoing correction of congenital heart disease with cardiopulmonary bypass (CPB) (*n* = 12) or CPB and deep hypothermic circulatory arrest (DHCA) (*n* = 11). Blood samples were obtained *PreCPB*, after anesthesia induction before heparin; *CPB1*, immediately after onset of bypass; *CPB2*, during cooling, halfway to the target temperature; *CPB3*, at the lowest core temperature (CPB group); *CPB4*, during rewarming; *CPB5*, just before separation from CPB; *PostCPB*, after placement of sternal wires; *POD1*, on the morning after surgery; *POD2*, on the second morning after surgery. Note that both groups have inappropriately low TSH concentrations given the free T₃ concentrations on the first and second postoperative days. (From Ririe DG, Butterworth JF, Hines M, et al. Effects of cardiopulmonary bypass and deep hypothermic circulatory arrest on the thyroid axis during and after repair of congenital heart defects: preservation by deep hypothermia? *Anesth Analg* 1998;87:543–548, with permission.)

after institution of bypass but was significantly reduced 1 hour and 1 day after surgery. Five days after surgery, free T₃ was increasing but remained significantly less than baseline values. Thyrotropin was significantly reduced relative to baseline during CPB, 1 hour and 1 day after the operation. Five days postoperatively, the thyrotropin concentration was significantly increased relative to baseline, consistent with a normal relationship between thyrotropin and T₃. Saatvedt and Lindberg (105) associated depressed concentrations of T₃ after CPB in children with elevated concentrations of interleukin-6, an inflammatory cytokine that has been shown to decrease secretion of thyrotropin, T₃, and T₄ in rats (106).

In an early study, pulsatile flow during bypass maintained a normal thyrotropin response to exogenously administered thyrotropin-releasing hormone, contrasting with the abnormal responses observed during nonpulsatile perfusion (107). In a more recent study of pulsatile flow in 30 patients undergoing coronary artery surgery, Buket et al. (108) found sharp decreases in free and total T₃ and thyrotropin upon initiation of bypass whether or not pulsatile perfusion was used. Later measurements demonstrated a lesser decrease in free and total T₃ in patients undergoing pulsatile bypass compared with nonpulsatile bypass (108). Patients making an uncomplicated recovery from surgery demonstrated a sharp increase in thyrotropin, total T₃, and total T₄ on day 4 after surgery, whereas patients with complications after surgery did not demonstrate such pronounced increases in these hormone concentrations (94).

These studies of thyroid function during and after CPB may have important clinical implications. T₃ serves to regulate cardiac rate, contractility, and oxygen consumption. Cyclic AMP production in response to β-adrenergic receptor agonists is markedly reduced in hypothyroid cardiac, adipose, and hepatic tissue. Cyclic AMP regulates intracellular calcium transients and myocardial contractility (109,110). Experimental studies have shown improved myocardial contractility in animals receiving T₃ after CPB (111,112). Patients with preoperative left ventricular ejection fraction greater than 40% receiving T₃ demonstrated significantly greater cardiac outputs after CPB than control patients. Patients with preoperative left ventricular ejection fraction less than 40% receiving T₃ required much less dobutamine and furosemide than did control patients (113). On the other hand, two recent controlled clinical trials failed to show that patients receiving T₃ prophylactically were less likely to require inotropic drug support than those receiving placebo (114,115).

Caution must be exercised in considering thyroid replacement in patients with concurrent hypothyroidism and chronic ischemic heart disease, however. Levothyroxine or T₃ hormone replacement therapy may precipitate myocardial ischemia and infarction, or even adrenal insufficiency. Indeed, patients with mild to moderate hypothyroidism appear to tolerate cardiac surgery without excess morbidity or mortality, though practitioners must be cognizant of the potential for delayed emergence from anesthesia, hypotension, bleeding, and the need for exogenous corticosteroids (116).

EICOSANOIDS

The lungs are actively involved in the metabolism of vasoactive substances, including eicosanoids; thus, the separation of the lungs from the circulation during extracorporeal perfusion may significantly alter the plasma concentrations and kinetics of prostaglandins and thromboxanes (117). The endoperoxide prostaglandin H_2 can isomerize (catalyzed by isomerases) into PGE_2, $PGF_{2\alpha}$, or PGD_2, or be chemically converted (catalyzed by either prostacyclin or thromboxane synthetase, respectively), into either prostacyclin (PGI_2) or thromboxane (TXA_2). The predominant prostaglandins formed in the bronchial tree and in the pulmonary vasculature are prostaglandin E_2 and prostacyclin (PGI_2) (117,118). PGEs are dilators in most vascular beds. PGD_2 and $PGF_{2\alpha}$ are pulmonary vasoconstrictors. In addition to synthesis and release of prostaglandins, the lungs are a major site for metabolism of prostaglandins of the E and F types (117). These substances are nearly completely cleared during a single passage through the pulmonary circulation. PGI_2 can disaggregate platelets and act as a potent vasodilator (117). Conversely, thromboxane A_2 potently stimulates platelet aggregation and vasoconstricts.

Concentrations of 6-keto-prostaglandin $F_{1\alpha}$ (the stable metabolite of prostacyclin) rose significantly after aortic and atrial cannulation and remained elevated during CPB in children and adults (118–124). 6-Keto-prostaglandin $F_{1\alpha}$ concentrations rose at the beginning of bypass, continued rising upon aortic clamping, but decreased progressively after termination of bypass and reperfusion of the lungs. There were no significant differences between patients undergoing cardiac surgery with or without bypass (122).

Thromboxane B_2 (the stable metabolite of thromboxane A_2) concentrations increased and reached peak arterial levels just before termination of bypass, a markedly different pattern from that seen in patients undergoing cardiac surgery without bypass (122) (Fig. 17.17). After completion of the cardiac repair and discontinuation of CPB, concentrations

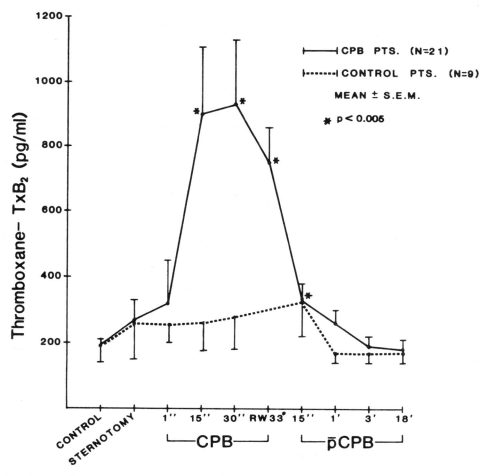

FIG. 17.17. Thromboxane metabolite (TxB_2) concentrations in children undergoing correction of congenital heart defects either with ($n = 21$) or without ($n = 9$) cardiopulmonary bypass (CPB). See the legend to Figure 17.12 for details of sampling. The CPB group demonstrated significantly elevated concentration compared with the non-bypass (control) group. (From Greeley WJ, Bushman GA, Kong DL, et al. Effects of cardiopulmonary bypass on eicosanoid metabolism during pediatric cardiovascular surgery. *J Thorac Cardiovasc Surg* 1988;95:842–849, with permission.)

of prostacyclin and thromboxane metabolites decreased progressively (118–121,123,124). Compared with adults, children have greater and more sustained increases in thromboxane metabolites (121,123). Infants undergoing extracorporeal membrane oxygenation, a form of long-term CPB, demonstrate increased prostacyclin metabolite concentrations after initiation of therapy (125). With continued use of extracorporeal membrane oxygenation, prostacyclin metabolite concentrations slowly fell. Prostacyclin metabolite concentrations rose again as the patients were weaned from extracorporeal membrane oxygenation; concentrations remained elevated for about a day thereafter (125).

Although increased concentrations of prostacyclin and thromboxane during bypass may have important effects on systemic and pulmonary vascular resistance and vasoreactivity, studies have not shown a consistent effect (118,121). Administration of the protease inhibitor aprotinin reduces the surge in thromboxane B_2 associated with bypass but has no effect on 6-keto-prostaglandin $F_{1\alpha}$ concentrations (122). These aprotinin-induced changes in prostaglandin metabolism were associated with better preserved platelet function, potentially significant in preventing postoperative hemorrhage.

A rapid increase in prostaglandin E_2 concentrations at the onset of CPB has been confirmed in several studies (118,120) (Fig. 17.18). Minimal differences between arterial and venous concentrations confirm limited prostaglan-

din E_2 metabolism in the lungs during CPB (120). Prostaglandin E_2 concentrations fall promptly after termination of bypass and reinstitution of pulmonary perfusion. Aspiration of shed pulmonary venous blood from open pleural cavities reduces mean arterial pressure during CPB and increases systemic concentrations of prostaglandin E_2 and 6-keto-prostaglandin $F_{1\alpha}$, probably as a consequence of the high concentrations of prostaglandin E_2 and 6-keto-prostaglandin $F_{1\alpha}$ measured in shed pulmonary venous blood (126).

In summary, the role of prostanoids and thromboxanes in producing desired or adverse effects during bypass remains controversial. Perhaps most significant in maintaining this controversy is the usual practice of measuring agent concentrations in systemic blood, which ignores the importance of prostanoids and thromboxanes in local regulation of blood flow within organs.

OTHER HUMORAL EFFECTS

Histamine

Elevated blood concentrations of histamine may produce vasodilation and hypotension. Numerous drugs administered to patients undergoing cardiac surgery will induce histamine release, including opioids (especially morphine and meperidine), muscle relaxants (especially tubocurarine), antibiotics, heparin, and protamine (127). Current anesthetic practice favors the use of agents that have negligible likelihood of inducing histamine release. In adults, plasma histamine concentrations rise at the time of systemic heparinization and remain elevated throughout the period of CPB (128). Comparable measurements of histamine concentration in children are problematic because, unlike adults, children often have blood products added to priming solutions used for CPB to prevent excessive hemodilution (54,129). Marath et al. (129) measured markedly elevated histamine concentrations in over 70% of blood product-containing priming solutions before their use during pediatric CPB, prompting speculation by these authors that the delivery of this massive histamine load to patients could have adverse effects. In children, particularly striking increases in histamine concentrations occur at the time the aortic cross-clamp is released, probably from reperfusion of the lungs (130). Infusion of prostacyclin during CPB diminishes the concentrations of histamine (128). van Overveld et al. (131) prevented elevated concentrations of histamine in serum during and after CPB for coronary artery surgery by administering methylprednisolone 30 mg/kg during induction of anesthesia. Histamine concentrations in patients with the cold urticaria syndrome, a relatively rare disorder, are increased nearly 10-fold during hypothermic CPB (132). In current practice, elevated histamine concentrations may be of great-

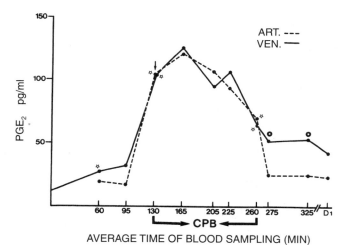

FIG. 17.18. Prostaglandin E_2 concentration in arterial and venous plasma samples before, during, and after cardiopulmonary bypass (CPB) in seven patients having coronary bypass. Stars indicate a significant change from the preceding measurement. Circled stars indicate a significant difference between arterial and venous values. (From Faymonville ME, Deby-Dupont G, Larbuisson R, et al. Prostaglandin E_2, prostacyclin, and thromboxane changes during nonpulsatile cardiopulmonary bypass in humans. *J Thorac Cardiovasc Surg* 1986;91:858–866, with permission.)

est concern when blood-containing priming solutions are used or when histamine-releasing agents must be administered.

CALCIUM

The availability of calcium ions in the sarcoplasmic reticulum determines the magnitude of the increased intracellular calcium concentrations during depolarizations, which regulates the inotropic state of the heart (133). Calcium ions are also necessary for normal electrical conduction and rhythm of the heart. Calcium in blood exists in three fractions: ionized (approximately 50%), protein bound (approximately 40%), and chelated (approximately 10%). The free ionized fraction is the physiologically active component. In critical illnesses, the distribution of calcium among these forms can be altered; thus, measurements of total calcium may be misleading (134). The blood calcium concentration is maintained within the normal range by parathormone and 1,25-dihydroxycholecalciferol (calcitriol or vitamin D) actions on bone and kidney. Parathormone secretion is stimulated by decreasing ionized calcium concentration, overt hypocalcemia, and by mild hypomagnesemia. Parathormone secretion is suppressed by rising or normal (unchanging) ionized calcium concentrations and by severe hypomagnesemia.

Changes in the total and ionized calcium fractions during and after CPB are influenced by the inclusion of exogenous calcium salts or blood products in the pump priming solution and by the frequent administration of calcium salts at discontinuation of extracorporeal perfusion. Clinical studies uniformly demonstrate a fall in ionized calcium concentration upon initiation of CPB (135–148). When blood-free priming solutions are used during bypass, both total and ionized calcium decrease as a consequence of hemodilution; ionized calcium concentrations may further decrease if albumin (which binds calcium) is added to priming solutions (147). Total calcium, total magnesium, ultrafiltrable magnesium (analogous to ionized magnesium), and total protein likewise decline upon initiation of CPB (147). During cardiac surgery, parathormone concentrations rise appropriately in response to declines in ionized calcium concentration and in response to rising ionized calcium concentrations.

As has been demonstrated in other circumstances, there is hysteresis in the relationship between parathormone and ionized calcium concentrations measured intraoperatively (147–149). Change in ionized calcium concentration and the absolute concentration regulates parathormone secretion. When ionized calcium concentration is rising in response to increased concentrations of parathormone, secretion of parathormone will *decrease* at ionized calcium concentrations below "normal" that would elicit *increased*

parathormone secretion if approached from a higher rather than a lower initial ionized calcium concentration.

Studies of parathormone concentrations using assays sensitive only to the intact hormone have found reductions at the beginning of bypass, increases to maximal concentrations during hypothermia, and a slow return toward normal values as ionized calcium concentrations approach normal values during rewarming (147). It should be noted that some early studies, using assays sensitive to both parathormone and its biologically inactive fragments, have reported falls in parathormone concentration upon initiation of bypass without appropriate increases in response to hypocalcemia thereafter (138).

Studies in adults have demonstrated that reduced magnesium concentrations do not influence the response of the calcium-parathyroid-vitamin D axis during CPB (147). Calcium and parathormone concentrations and responses were identical in patients receiving magnesium salt supplementation during bypass and in control patients in which magnesium concentrations were permitted to fall without correction. Calcitriol (vitamin D) is a fat-soluble vitamin; thus, it is not surprising that calcitriol concentrations are minimally altered by hemodilution and CPB and that this vitamin plays a minimal role in the alterations in calcium concentration seen during cardiac surgery (147).

CPB is managed differently in infants and young children than in adults. Even with the use of smaller sized extracorporeal circuits, priming solution volumes represent a much greater fraction of the pediatric patient's blood volume, and blood products are often included in the priming solutions to avoid excessive degrees of hemodilution (53,54). However, the responses of the calcium-parathyroid-calcitriol axis in 12 infants and 6 young children were similar to those of adults (148). Despite demonstrating much greater declines in ionized calcium concentration upon initiation of CPB, infants' parathyroid hormone concentrations peaked at values similar to those achieved by children and adults (147,148) (Fig. 17.19). Moreover, parathyroid gland "sensing" of increasing and decreasing ionized calcium concentrations was also similar, with infants and young children demonstrating hysteresis in a similar manner to adults (147–149). Infants and young children differed from adults in that ionized calcium concentrations did not recover as completely before termination of CPB. This was likely a consequence of the considerably shorter duration of bypass in the children compared with the adults that were studied, although impaired bone reabsorption in response to parathyroid hormone could not be ruled out. There are important clinical implications from these studies. Unlike the case for many other hormones, parathormone secretion is minimally altered by hypothermic CPB (147,148). Ionized hypocalcemia, even to severe degrees, produced no obvious adverse effects during these studies (143,147,148).

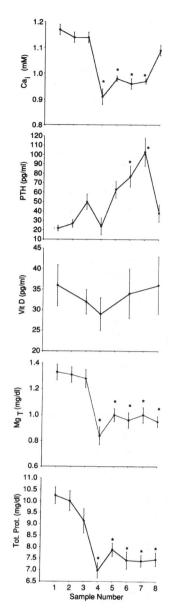

FIG. 17.19. Response of the calcium-magnesium-parathormone-calcitriol axis to coronary artery bypass grafting. *Ca$_i$*, ionized calcium; *PTH*, parathormone; *Vit D*, calcitriol; *Mg$_T$*, total magnesium; *Tot. prot*, total protein. Measurements were performed *1)* before anesthesia, *2)* after induction of anesthesia, *3)* after heparin administration, *4)* 2 minutes after initiation of bypass, *5)* 5 minutes after aortic cross-clamping, *6)* early during rewarming, *7)* shortly before separation from bypass, and *8)* during sternal closure after bypass. Data are presented as means ± SEM. Asterisks denote significant deviation from control values. (From Robertie PG, Butterworth JF IV, Royster RL, et al. Normal parathyroid hormone responses to hypocalcemia during cardiopulmonary bypass. Anesthesiology 1991;75:43–48, with permission.)

Moreover, hypercalcemia may lead to accelerated adenosine triphosphate breakdown (a calcium-dependent process) and unnecessarily increase contractility and myocardial oxygen consumption (150). Systemic hypocalcemia coupled with anoxic cardiac arrest and calcium-free cardioplegia may lead to a beneficial reduction in adenosine triphosphate breakdown (151). Rewarming and reperfusion after aortic clamp removal, essential for resynthesis of high energy phosphates, should be accompanied by minimal myocardial oxygen consumption. Exogenous calcium during this time might unnecessarily increase the myocardial inotropic state, leading to depletion of adenosine triphosphate.

The empirical use of calcium salts at the end of CPB (supposedly for inotropic support) is almost a tradition in cardiac surgery, despite limited evidence of clinical efficacy in controlled trials and the usual absence of serious hypocalcemia in adult patients. In addition, excessive use of calcium salts is a possible cause of perioperative pancreatitis (147,152–159) and may also reduce the efficacy of β-adrenergic receptor agonists (152–155,160). Ideally, calcium salts should be administered only when all of the following three conditions are met: bypass is about to be terminated, ionized calcium concentration is reduced, and increased inotropy and blood pressure are needed for resumption of full myocardial activity.

MAGNESIUM

Magnesium is the second most abundant intracellular cation (after potassium) and is a key cofactor in enzyme systems maintaining transmembrane electrolyte gradients and energy metabolism, enzymes involved in synthesis of second messengers (e.g., adenylyl cyclase), ion channels, and hormone secretion and action (e.g., insulin and parathormone) (161). Much like calcium, magnesium in the blood exists in three fractions: ionized (approximately 55%), chelated (approximately 15%), and protein bound (approximately 30%). The ultrafiltrable fraction includes only the ionized and chelated fractions and, due to the small contribution from the chelated ions, approximates the ionized fraction (162). Because there is a dynamic equilibrium between intracellular and extracellular magnesium, the magnesium concentration in blood may be normal in the presence of magnesium depletion.

Cardiac surgery patients frequently develop hypomagnesemia, which may be due to insufficient dietary intake, increased excretion (secondary to diuretics), diabetes, aminoglycoside antibiotics, cardiac glycosides, ethanol abuse, pancreatic disease, or administration of citrated blood products or albumin (161,163–165). Blood magnesium concentrations decrease during and after CPB in adults and children (147,148,163–167). During CPB, total magnesium concentrations decline in concert with the ultrafiltrable fraction as a consequence of chelation by albumin and other blood products and hemodilution (147). Urinary excretion of magnesium during bypass is not increased (164). Magnesium concentrations, unlike calcium concentrations, once reduced during CPB, return to normal only slowly in the absence of active treatment because of the lack of a specific hormonal regulatory system (147,148) (Fig. 17.19).

Hypomagnesemia in the post-bypass period commonly contributes to cardiac dysrhythmias (165,167). Infusion of magnesium salts prevents hypomagnesemia and its complications during and after CPB (147,167). During CPB, cardiac muscle is preferentially depleted of magnesium (compared with skeletal muscle). Magnesium may suppress arrhythmias by multiple mechanisms that include a direct myocardial membrane effect, a direct or indirect effect on cellular potassium and sodium concentrations, antagonism of calcium entry into cells, prevention of coronary artery vasospasm, antagonism of catecholamine action (168), or improvement of the myocardial oxygen supply/demand ratio (169). In addition, magnesium may also inhibit the calcium current during the plateau phase of the myocardial action potential. Finally, magnesium may also inhibit dysrhythmias by antagonizing accumulation of excess intracellular calcium induced by ischemia-related mediators such as lysophosphatidylcholine (170).

Supplemental magnesium decreases the incidence of dysrhythmias after cardiac surgery as noted above and during myocardial ischemia or infarction (171–173). The Leicester Intravenous Magnesium Intervention II Trial used 8 mmol of magnesium sulfate acutely, followed by 65 mmol as a continuous infusion over 24 hours in patients having an acute myocardial infarction (174). This intervention significantly reduced both mortality ($p = 0.04$) and left ventricular failure ($p = 0.009$) without producing excess hypotension. A meta-analysis of 930 patients with myocardial infarction concluded that intravenous magnesium reduced ventricular tachycardia and fibrillation by 49% and decreased overall mortality by 54% (175).

Magnesium is a critical cofactor for numerous cellular enzymes and partially regulates transmembrane calcium movement (176). Magnesium salts dilate coronary arteries (177), regulate myocardial metabolism (176), lower systemic vascular resistance, protect against catecholamine-induced myocardial necrosis (178), and modify platelet aggregation and thrombus formation. Clinically, magnesium salts are used for the treatment of both atrial and ventricular dysrhythmias (167,171–173,179), coronary artery vasospasm, myocardial ischemia (167,179), myocardial infarction (171–173), pregnancy-induced hypertension, and even therapy of bronchospasm (180).

Moderate magnesium supplementation (1 to 2 g magnesium sulfate intravenously per hour of CPB maintains serum magnesium concentrations greater than 1 mM) has minimal effects on blood pressure in normotensive patients. Renal insufficiency may predispose to magnesium toxicity exhibited as deep tendon hyporeflexia, somnolence, and even respiratory insufficiency. However, only very high concentrations of extracellular magnesium directly depress myocardial contractility. Of special note, though, magnesium potentiates neuromuscular blocking drugs, which may produce clinical weakness and respiratory insufficiency in patients with residual paralysis from previous administration of neuromuscular blocking drugs. Overall, magnesium salts are safe, effective, low-cost therapy that may be used on a routine basis for prevention or treatment of many atrial and ventricular arrhythmias. The routine occurrence of hypomagnesemia during CPB and rapid renal excretion of magnesium allows the clinician to administer moderate doses of magnesium salts empirically without the need for frequent measurement of magnesium blood concentrations.

POTASSIUM

Maintaining normal blood potassium concentrations is important in cardiac surgical patients. Patients receiving diuretics may come to operation hypokalemic; those with renal failure may be hyperkalemic. During and after CPB, potassium flux is also influenced by myocardial protectant solutions (cardioplegia), anesthetic drugs, priming solutions, renal function, carbon dioxide tension, arterial pH, hypothermia, insulin treatment of hyperglycemia, catecholamine infusion, and mineralocorticoids.

Potassium depletion may occur in as many as 40% of patients having valve surgery (181,182). Hypokalemia, the most frequent abnormality of potassium concentration observed after CPB, is common (183–186). Before the era of potassium cardioplegia, hyperkalemia was uncommon except in patients with diabetes or renal failure. Currently, brief episodes of hyperkalemia may be more common, especially immediately after the release of the aortic cross-clamp. Hyperkalemia may also be more common during normothermic than hypothermic bypass, likely due to the increased volumes of cardioplegic solutions that are required during normothermic bypass (187). Potassium loss during CPB is related to urine flow, implying that urine potassium concentration must remain nearly constant (188). Bumetanide produces less kaliuresis during CPB than furosemide for a similar diuretic response (189). Increased urinary potassium loss is characteristic of the post-bypass period (190).

Moffitt et al. (191) reported that whole blood priming may cause greater decreases in serum potassium than blood-free priming solutions. Maintenance of normocalcemia during CPB may better maintain potassium concentration than the more usual techniques that tolerate hypocalcemia

(192,193). The ionic constituents of blood-free priming solutions (other than calcium and potassium ions) have little effect on potassium concentration. Careful studies of potassium intake and output and red blood cell potassium, rates of hemolysis, and serum hemoglobin have shown that much of the fall in serum potassium concentration is not accounted for by dilution or excretion. Likewise, repeated studies have failed to identify the organ into which potassium is lost from blood (194).

In the absence of potassium cardioplegia, the fall in potassium concentration during clinical CPB appears to be proportional to the decrease in body temperature (195). Conversely, potassium concentration increases with warming (196). Blood glucose rises and insulin falls during hypothermic CPB (see previous glucose metabolism discussion). Insulin favors intracellular transport of glucose and potassium.

Increased concentrations of cortisol, aldosterone, and catecholamines during CPB may contribute to hypokalemia. Cortisol and aldosterone increase the urinary excretion of potassium. Catecholamines increase potassium uptake by skeletal muscle and decrease serum potassium (197). β-Adrenergic blockade with propranolol inhibits the uptake of potassium by skeletal muscle but does not inhibit the hepatic release of potassium by β-adrenergic stimulation and may contribute to hyperkalemia (198). Hypokalemia during CPB may be lessened if albumin is added to the priming solution, because the negatively charged albumin molecules help maintain adequate blood concentrations of positively charged potassium (199).

Potassium concentrations are usually monitored frequently during CPB, although strict normokalemia need be present only when normal cardiac electrical activity is desired (200). Increases in systemic vascular resistance have been observed with bolus intravenous potassium injections of 8 mEq or greater during CPB. With smaller bolus doses, an initial fall followed by a slight rise in systemic vascular resistance is common (201).

In summary, potassium concentrations rarely remain constant during or after CPB. Hypokalemia, formerly a frequent problem during bypass, now is uncommon due to the widespread use of multiple doses of potassium-containing cardioplegic solutions. Postoperative potassium loss and hypokalemia continues to be common after CPB.

METAL IONS: ZINC, COPPER, AND IRON

Reductions in blood iron and zinc concentrations and increases in copper concentrations occur as part of the nonspecific "acute phase reaction" to trauma, prolonged infections, burns, and major surgery (202). In adults, zinc concentrations decline at the onset of CPB and remain low for 1 to 3 days postoperatively (203–205). Zinc concentrations usually return to normal by the seventh postoperative day. Urinary excretion of zinc is unaffected by cardiac surgery. Taggart et al. (206) monitored iron and zinc concentrations before, during, and after coronary surgery in 20 patients perfused at either 20 or 28°C. Significant alteration of the metal-to-protein molar binding ratios preceded falls in the concentrations of both ions as a consequence of the acute phase reaction to surgical trauma. Patients perfused at 20°C had less alterations of iron and zinc metabolism during surgery than those perfused at 28°C. No differences were seen after surgery, when both groups demonstrated reduced serum iron and zinc concentrations. However, a reduced concentration of iron in blood may be advantageous. Administration of deferoxamine (an iron chelator) was associated with reduced production of free radicals during CPB (207).

Copper concentrations fell rapidly at the onset of bypass but usually returned to normal by the third postoperative day (203,205,206). The alterations in copper concentration appear to be caused by hemodilution (203). Zhao (204) found a more transient (relative to other authors) nadir in blood copper concentration 30 minutes after perfusion, with a return to normal concentrations 1 to 2 days postoperatively and a rise to supranormal concentrations between postoperative days 3 and 9.

Alterations in zinc and copper concentrations in blood were studied in 13 children undergoing correction of congenital heart disease (208). Concentrations of both zinc and copper were markedly reduced (compared with preoperative measurements) 6 hours after CPB. Recovery toward baseline values was not seen in the first postoperative 24 hours but was nearly complete 48 hours after bypass (208).

CONCLUSIONS

CPB produces widespread alterations in endocrine, humoral, and metabolic functions, some of which may be lessened by the use of pulsatile CPB, larger doses or higher concentrations of general anesthetic drugs, or addition of thoracic epidural anesthesia. The magnitude and direction of these changes may be influenced by the duration of bypass and the techniques used (such as the degree of hypothermia, cardiac venting, and contents of the priming solution). For the most part, the mechanisms for these neuroendocrine alterations during bypass are poorly understood. In only rare patients will endocrine alterations influence the likelihood of successful recovery from surgery. However, the importance of these changes may increase with longer durations of CPB or extracorporeal circulatory support.

KEY POINTS

- A variety of pituitary-related hormonal activities is influenced by CPB: ADH and adrenocorticotropin levels increase markedly and thyroid-stimulating hormone levels are typically normal, but T_3 and T_4 responses to TSH are reduced, consistent with "sick euthyroid syndrome."
- Adrenal responses affected by CPB include marked increases in catecholamine, aldosterone, and cortisol levels that can be attenuated to varying degrees by deeper anesthesia, thoracic epidural anesthesia, and pulsatile perfusion; and the rise in aldosterone levels is stimulated by activation of the renin-angiotensin system.
- Hyperglycemia, hypoinsulinemia, and insulin resistance occur with hypothermic nonpulsatile CPB.
- Atrial natriuretic factor concentrations decrease early in CPB but typically increase during rewarming. The secretion of atrial natriuretic factor in response to the usual physiologic stimuli is blunted during and after CPB.
- Ionized calcium concentrations decrease at the onset of CPB and then rise slowly toward normal, with physiologic parathormone responses to these changes. Routine calcium supplementation upon emergence from CPB is not recommended.
- Hypomagnesemia commonly occurs during CPB, and prophylactic treatment of this deficiency with intravenous magnesium supplementation reduces the incidence of post-CPB atrial and ventricular dysrhythmias and may reduce the incidences of coronary vasospasm and myocardial ischemia.
- Plasma potassium concentrations fluctuate during CPB under the influence of a variety of factors, especially cardioplegia composition and dosing.

REFERENCES

1. Malatinsky J, Vigas M, Jezova D, et al. The effects of open heart surgery on growth hormone, cortisol and insulin levels in man. Hormone levels during open heart surgery. *Resuscitation* 1984;11:57–68.
2. Anand KJS, Hickey PR. Halothane-morphine compared with high-dose sufentanil for anesthesia and postoperative analgesia in neonatal cardiac surgery. *N Engl J Med* 1992;326:1–9.
3. Cooper DM, Bazaral MG, Furlan AJ, et al. Pituitary apoplexy: a complication of cardiac surgery. *Ann Thorac Surg* 1986;41: 547–550.
4. Meek EN, Butterworth J, Kon ND, et al. New onset of cranial nerve palsies immediately following mitral valve repair. *Anesthesiology* 1998;89:1580–1582.
5. Slavin ML, Budabin M. Pituitary apoplexy associated with cardiac surgery. *Am J Ophthalmol* 1984;98:291–296.
6. Absalom M, Rogers KH, Moulton RJ, et al. Pituitary apoplexy after coronary artery surgery. *Anesth Analg* 1993;76:648–649.
7. Savage EB, Gugino L, Starr PA, et al. Pituitary apoplexy following cardiopulmonary bypass: considerations for a staged cardiac and neurosurgical procedure. *Eur J Cardiothorac Surg* 1994;8: 333–336.
8. Baylis PH. Vasopressin and its neurophysin. In: DeGroot LJ, ed. *Endocrinology*, 3rd ed. Vol. 1. Philadelphia: W.B. Saunders, 1995:406–420.
9. Heyndrickx GR, Boettcher DH, Vatner SF. Effects of angiotensin, vasopressin, and methoxamine on cardiac function and blood flow distribution in conscious dogs. *Am J Physiol* 1976; 231:1579–1587.
10. Cochrane JPS, Forsling ML, Gow NM, et al. Arginine vasopressin release following surgical operations. *Br J Surg* 1981;68: 209–213.
11. Knight A, Forsling M, Treasure T, et al. Changes in plasma vasopressin concentration in association with coronary artery surgery or thymectomy. *Br J Anaesth* 1986;58:1273–1277.
12. Wu W, Zbuzek VK, Bellevue C. Vasopressin release during cardiac operation. *J Thorac Cardiovasc Surg* 1980;79:83–90.
13. Philbin DM, Levine FH, Emerson CW, et al. Plasma vasopressin levels and urinary flow during cardiopulmonary bypass in patients with valvular heart disease: effect of pulsatile flow. *J Thorac Cardiovasc Surg* 1979;78:779–783.
14. Viinamaki O, Nuutinen L, Hanhela R, et al. Plasma vasopressin levels during and after cardiopulmonary bypass in man. *Med Biol* 1986;64:289–292.
15. Kaul TK, Swaminathan R, Chatrath RR, et al. Vasoactive pressure hormones during and after cardiopulmonary bypass. *Int J Artif Organs* 1990;13:293–299.
16. Landymore RW, Murphy DA, Kinley CE, et al. Does pulsatile flow influence the incidence of postoperative hypertension? *Ann Thorac Surg* 1979;28:261–268.
17. Kuitunen A, Hynynen M, Salmenpera M, et al. Anaesthesia effects plasma concentrations of vasopressin, von Willebrand factor and coagulation factor VIII in cardiac surgical patients. *Br J Anaesth* 1993;70:173–180.
18. Kehlet H. Surgical stress: the role of pain and analgesia. *Br J Anaesth* 1989;63:189–195.
19. Balasaraswathi K, Glisson SN, El-Etr AA, et al. Effect of priming volume on serum catecholamines during cardiopulmonary bypass. *Can Anaesth Soc J* 1980;27:135–139.
20. Hirvonen J, Huttunen P, Nuutinen L, et al. Catecholamines and free fatty acids in plasma of patients undergoing cardiac operations with hypothermia and bypass. *J Clin Pathol* 1978; 31:949–955.
21. Reves JG, Karp RB, Buttner EE, et al. Neuronal and adrenomedullary catecholamine release in response to cardiopulmonary bypass in man. *Circulation* 1982;66:49–55.
22. Reed HL, Chernow B, Lake CR, et al. Alterations in sympathetic nervous system activity with intraoperative hypothermia during coronary artery bypass surgery. *Chest* 1989;95:616–622.
23. Sun LS, Adams DC, Delphin E, et al. Sympathetic response during cardiopulmonary bypass: mild versus moderate hypothermia. *Crit Care Med* 1997;25:1990–1993.
24. Firmin RK, Bouloux P, Allen P, et al. Sympathoadrenal function during cardiac operations in infants with the technique of surface cooling, limited cardiopulmonary bypass, and circulatory arrest. *J Thorac Cardiovasc Surg* 1985;90:729–735.
25. Anand KJ, Hansen DD, Hickey PR. Hormonal-metabolic stress responses in neonates undergoing cardiac surgery. *Anesthesiology* 1990;73:661–670.
26. Samuelson PN, Reves JG, Kirklin JK, et al. Comparison of sufentanil and enflurane-nitrous oxide anesthesia for myocardial revascularization. *Anesth Analg* 1986;65:217–226.
27. Ng A, Tan SSW, Lee HS, et al. Effect of propofol infusion on

the endocrine response to cardiac surgery. *Anaesth Intens Care* 1995;23:543–547.

28. Stenseth R, Bjella L, Berg EM, et al. Thoracic epidural analgesia in aortocoronary bypass surgery II: effects on the endocrine metabolic response. *Acta Anaesthesiol Scand* 1994;38:834–839.

29. Moore CM, Cross MH, Desborough JP, et al. Hormonal effects of thoracic extradural analgesia for cardiac surgery. *Br J Anaesth* 1995;75:387–393.

30. Minami K, Körner MM, Vyska K, et al. Effects of pulsatile perfusion on plasma catecholamine levels and hemodynamics during and after cardiac operations with cardiopulmonary bypass. *J Thorac Cardiovasc Surg* 1990;99:82–91.

31. Hume DM, Bell CC, Bartter F. Direct measurement of adrenal secretion during operative trauma and convalescence. *Surgery* 1962;52:174–186.

32. Taylor KM, Jones JV, Walker MS, et al. The cortisol response during heart-lung bypass. *Circulation* 1976;54:20–25.

33. Taylor KM, Wright GS, Reid JM, et al. Comparative studies of pulsatile and nonpulsatile flow during cardiopulmonary bypass. II. The effects on adrenal secretion of cortisol. *J Thorac Cardiovasc Surg* 1978;75:574–578.

34. Raff H, Norton AJ, Flemma RJ, et al. Inhibition of the adrenocorticotropin response to surgery in humans: interaction between dexamethasone and fentanyl. *J Clin Endocrinol Metab* 1987;65:295–298.

35. Flezzani P, Croughwell ND, McIntyre RW, et al. Isoflurane decreases the cortisol response to cardiopulmonary bypass. *Anesth Analg* 1986;65:1117–1122.

36. Lacoumenta S, Yeo TH, Paterson JL, et al. Hormonal and metabolic responses to cardiac surgery with sufentanil-oxygen anaesthesia. *Acta Anaesthesiol Scand* 1987;31:258–263.

37. Uozumi T, Manabe H, Kawashima Y, et al. Plasma cortisol, corticosterone, and non-protein-bound cortisol in extra-corporeal circulation. *Acta Endocrinol* 1972;69:517–525.

38. Tinnikov AA, Legan MV, Pavlova IP, et al. Serum corticosteroid-binding globulin levels in children undergoing heart surgery. *Steroids* 1993;58:536–539.

39. Taggart DP, Fraser WD, Borland WW, et al. Hypothermia and the stress response to cardiopulmonary bypass. *Eur J Cardiothorac Surg* 1989;3:359–363.

40. Amado JA, Diago MC. Delayed ACTH response to human corticotropin releasing hormone during cardiopulmonary bypass under diazepam-high dose fentanyl anaesthesia. *Anaesthesia* 1994;49:300–303.

41. Taylor KM, Walker MS, Rao LG, et al. Proceedings: plasma levels of cortisol, free cortisol, and corticotrophin during cardiopulmonary by-pass. *J Endocrinol* 1975;67:29P–30P.

42. Kono K, Philbin DM, Coggins CH, et al. Adrenocortical hormone levels during cardiopulmonary bypass with and without pulsatile flow. *J Thorac Cardiovasc Surg* 1983;85:129–133.

43. Pollock EM, Pollock JC, Jamieson MP, et al. Adrenocortical hormone concentrations in children during cardiopulmonary bypass with and without pulsatile flow. *Br J Anaesth* 1988;60:536–541.

44. Hall RI, Smith MS, Rocker G. The systemic inflammatory response to cardiopulmonary bypass: pathophysiologic, therapeutic, and pharmacologic considerations. *Anesth Analg* 1997;85:66–82.

45. Miller BE, Levy JH. The inflammatory response to cardiopulmonary bypass. *J Cardiothorac Vasc Anesth* 1997;11:355–366.

46. Niazi Z, Flodin P, Joyce L, et al. Effects of glucocorticosteroids in patients undergoing coronary artery bypass surgery. *Chest* 1979;76:262–268.

47. Dietzman RH, Lunseth JB, Goott B, et al. The use of methylprednisolone during cardiopulmonary bypass. A review of 427 cases. *J Thorac Cardiovasc Surg* 1975;69:870–873.

48. Motsay GJ, Alho A, Jaeger T, et al. Effects of methylprednisolone, phenoxybenzamine, and epinephrine tolerance in canine endotoxin shock: study of isogravimetric capillary pressures in forelimb and intestine. *Surgery* 1971;70:271–279.

49. Engelman RM. Fast-track recovery in the elderly patients. *Ann Thorac Surg* 1997;63:606–607.

50. Nagaoka H, Innami R, Watanabe M, et al. Preservation of pancreatic beta cell function with pulsatile cardiopulmonary bypass. *Ann Thorac Surg* 1989;48:798–802.

51. Rogers AT, Zaloga GP, Prough DS, et al. Hyperglycemia during cardiac surgery: central vs peripheral mechanisms [abstract]. *Anesth Analg* 1990;70:S328.

52. Kuntschen FR, Galletti PM, Hahn C. Glucose-insulin interactions during cardiopulmonary bypass. Hypothermia versus normothermia. *J Thorac Cardiovasc Surg* 1986;91:451–459.

53. Ridley PD, Ratcliffe JM, Alberti KGMM, et al. The metabolic consequences of a "washed" cardiopulmonary bypass pump-priming fluid in children undergoing cardiac operations. *J Thorac Cardiovasc Surg* 1990;100:528–537.

54. Hosking MP, Beynen FM, Raimundo HS, et al. A comparison of washed red blood cells versus packed red blood cells (AS-1) for cardiopulmonary bypass prime and their effects on blood glucose concentration in children. *Anesthesiology* 1990;72:987–990.

55. Lehot JJ, Piriz H, Villard J, et al. Glucose homeostasis: comparison between hypothermic and normothermic cardiopulmonary bypass. *Chest* 1992;102:106–111.

56. Ellis DJ, Steward DJ. Fentanyl dosage is associated with reduced blood glucose in pediatric patients after hypothermic cardiopulmonary bypass. *Anesthesiology* 1990;72:812–815.

57. Powell H, Castell LM, Parry-Billings M, et al. Growth hormone suppression and glutamine flux associated with cardiac surgery. *Clin Physiol* 1994;14:569–580.

58. Desborough JP, Hall GM, Hart G, et al. Hormonal responses to cardiac surgery: effects of sufentanil, somatostatin and ganglion block. *Br J Anaesth* 1990;64:688–695.

59. Atlas SA, Maack T. Effects of atrial natriuretic factor on the kidney and the renin-angiotensin-aldosterone system. *Endocrinol Metab Clin North Am* 1987;16:107–143.

60. Dewar ML, Walsh G, Chiu RC, et al. Atrial natriuretic factor: response to cardiac operation. *J Thorac Cardiovasc Surg* 1988;96:266–270.

61. Ashcroft GP, Entwisle SJ, Campbell CJ, et al. Peripheral and intracardiac levels of atrial natriuretic factor during cardiothoracic surgery. *Thorac Cardiovasc Surg* 1991;39:183–186.

62. Curello S, Ceconi C, De Giuli F, et al. Time course of human atrial natriuretic factor release during cardiopulmonary bypass in mitral valve and coronary artery diseased patients. *Eur J Cardiothorac Surg* 1991;5:205–210.

63. Kharasch ED, Yeo KT, Kenny MA, et al. Influence of hypothermic cardiopulmonary bypass on atrial natriuretic factor levels. *Can J Anaesth* 1989;36:545–553.

64. Hedner J, Towle A, Saltzman L, et al. Changes in plasma atrial natriuretic peptide-immunoreactivity in patients undergoing coronary artery bypass graft placements. *Regul Pept* 1987;17:151–157.

65. Northridge DB, Jamieson MP, Jardine AG, et al. Pulmonary extraction and left atrial secretion of atrial natriuretic factor during cardiopulmonary bypass surgery. *Am Heart J* 1992;123:698–703.

66. Teran N, Rodriguez Iturbe B, Parra G, et al. Atrial natriuretic peptide levels in brain venous outflow during cardiopulmonary bypass in humans: evidence for extracardiac hormonal production. *J Cardiothorac Vasc Anesth* 1991;5:343–347.

67. Haug C, Bergmann KP, Hannekum A, et al. Influence of coro-

nary artery bypass graft operation on plasma atrial natriuretic peptide concentrations. *Horm Metab Res* 1993;25:399–400.

68. Pasaoglu I, Erbas B, Varoglu E, et al. Changes in the circulating endothelin and atrial natriuretic peptide levels during coronary artery bypass surgery. *Jpn Heart J* 1993;34:693–706.

69. Pfenninger J, Shaw S, Ferrari P, et al. Atrial natriuretic factor after cardiac surgery with cardiopulmonary bypass in children. *Crit Care Med* 1991;19:1497–1502.

70. Schaff HV, Mashburn JP, McCarthy PM, et al. Natriuresis during and early after cardiopulmonary bypass: relationship to atrial natriuretic factor, aldosterone, and antidiuretic hormone. *J Thorac Cardiovasc Surg* 1989;98:979–986.

71. Hynynen M, Palojoki R, Heinonen J, et al. Renal and vascular effects of atrial natriuretic factor during cardiopulmonary bypass. *Chest* 1991;100:1203–1209.

72. Amano J, Suzuki A, Sunamori M, et al. Attenuation of atrial natriuretic peptide response to sodium loading after cardiac operation. *J Thorac Cardiovasc Surg* 1995;110:75–80.

73. Miller ED Jr. The role of the renin-angiotensin-aldosterone system in circulatory control and hypertension. *Br J Anaesth* 1981;53:711–718.

74. Diedericks BJ, Roelofse JA, Shipton EA, et al. The renin-angiotensin-aldosterone system during and after cardiopulmonary bypass. *S Afr Med J* 1983;64:946–949.

75. Weinstein GS, Zabetakis PM, Clavel A, et al. The renin-angiotensin system is not responsible for hypertension following coronary artery bypass grafting. *Ann Thorac Surg* 1987;43:74–77.

76. Taylor KM, Morton IJ, Brown JJ, et al. Hypertension and the renin-angiotensin system following open-heart surgery. *J Thorac Cardiovasc Surg* 1977;74:840–845.

77. Canivet JL, Larbuisson R, Damas P, et al. Plasma renin activity and urine β_2-microglobulin during and after cardiopulmonary bypass: pulsatile vs non-pulsatile perfusion. *Eur Heart J* 1990; 11:1079–1082.

78. Nagaoka H, Innami R, Arai H. Effects of pulsatile cardiopulmonary bypass on the renin-angiotensin-aldosterone system following open heart surgery. *Jpn J Surg* 1988;18:390–396.

79. Goto M, Kudoh K, Minami S, et al. The renin-angiotensin-aldosterone system and hematologic changes during pulsatile and nonpulsatile cardiopulmonary bypass. *Artif Organs* 1993; 17:318–322.

80. Gorin AB, Liebler J. Changes in serum angiotensin-converting enzyme during cardiopulmonary bypass in humans. *Am Rev Respir Dis* 1986;134:79–84.

81. Smallridge RC, Chernow B, Snyder R, et al. Angiotensin-converting enzyme activity. A potential marker of tissue hypothyroidism in critical illness. *Arch Intern Med* 1985;145: 1829–1832.

82. Feddersen K, Aurell M, Delin K, et al. Effects of cardiopulmonary bypass and prostacyclin on plasma catecholamines, angiotensin II and arginine-vasopressin. *Acta Anaesthesiol Scand* 1985; 29:224–230.

83. Colson P, Grolleau D, Chaptal PA, et al. Effect of preoperative renin-angiotensin system blockade on hypertension following coronary surgery. *Chest* 1988;93:1156–1158.

84. Townsend GE, Wynands JE, Whalley DG, et al. Role of renin-angiotensin system in cardiopulmonary bypass hypertension. *Can Anaesth Soc J* 1984;31:160–165.

85. Hays JH. Thyroid disease. *Probl Crit Care Endocr Emerg* 1990; 4:325–341.

86. Thrush DN, Austin D, Burdash N. Cardiopulmonary bypass temperature does not affect postoperative euthyroid sick syndrome? *Chest* 1995;108:1541–1545.

87. Polikar R, Kennedy B, Maisel A, et al. Decreased adrenergic sensitivity in patients with hypothyroidism. *J Am Coll Cardiol* 1990;15:94–98.

88. Jones TH, Hunter SM, Price A, et al. Should thyroid function be assessed before cardiopulmonary bypass operations? *Ann Thorac Surg* 1994;58:434–436.

89. Bremner WF, Taylor KM, Baird S, et al. Hypothalamo-pituitary-thyroid axis function during cardiopulmonary bypass. *J Thorac Cardiovasc Surg* 1978;75:392–399.

90. Saeed uz Zafar M, Miller JM, Breneman GM, et al. Observations on the effect of heparin on free and total thyroxine. *J Clin Endocrinol Metab* 1971;32:633–640.

91. Hershman JM, Jones CM, Bailey AL. Reciprocal changes in serum thyrotropin and free thyroxine produced by heparin. *J Clin Endocrinol Metab* 1972;34:574.

92. Schwartz HL, Schadlow AR, Faierman D, et al. Heparin administration appears to decrease cellular binding of thyroxine. *J Clin Endocrinol Metab* 1973;36:598–600.

93. Holland FW II, Brown PS Jr, Weintraub BD, et al. Cardiopulmonary bypass and thyroid function: a "euthyroid sick syndrome." *Ann Thorac Surg* 1991;52:46–50.

94. Chu S-H, Huang T-S, Hsu R-B, et al. Thyroid hormone changes after cardiovascular surgery and clinical implications. *Ann Thorac Surg* 1991;52:791–796.

95. Lawton NF, Ellis SM, Sufi S. The triiodothyronine and thyroxine response to thyrotrophin-releasing hormone in the assessment of the pituitary-thyroid axis. *Clin Endocrinol* 1973;2: 57–63.

96. Reinhardt W, Mocker V, Jockenhövel F, et al. Influence of coronary artery bypass surgery on thyroid hormone parameters. *Horm Res* 1997;47:1–8.

97. Zaloga GP, Chernow B, Smallridge RC, et al. A longitudinal evaluation of thyroid function in critically ill surgical patients. *Ann Surg* 1985;201:456–464.

98. Taylor KM. Proceedings: pituitary-adrenal axis during cardiopulmonary bypass. *Br Heart J* 1976;38:321.

99. Robuschi G, Medici D, Fesani F, et al. Cardiopulmonary bypass: a low T_4 and T_3 syndrome with blunted thyrotropin (TSH) response to thyrotropin-releasing hormone (TRH). *Horm Res* 1986;23:151–158.

100. Cooper DS, Klibanski A, Ridgway EC. Dopaminergic modulation of TSH and its subunits: in vivo and in vitro studies. *Clin Endocrinol* 1983;18:265–275.

101. DeRuyter H, Burman KD, Wartofsky L, et al. Thyrotropin secretion in starved rats is enhanced by somatostatin antiserum. *Horm Metab Res* 1984;16:92–96.

102. Ririe DG, Butterworth JF, Hines M, et al. Effects of cardiopulmonary bypass and deep hypothermic circulatory arrest on the thyroid axis during and after repair of congenital heart defects: preservation by deep hypothermia? *Anesth Analg* 1998;87: 543–548.

103. Murzi B, Iervasi G, Masini S, et al. Thyroid hormones homeostasis in pediatric patients during and after cardiopulmonary bypass. *Ann Thorac Surg* 1995;59:481–485.

104. Mainwaring RD, Lamberti JJ, Billman GF, et al. Suppression of the pituitary thyroid axis after cardiopulmonary bypass in the neonate. *Ann Thorac Surg* 1994;58:1078–1082.

105. Saatvedt K, Lindberg H. Depressed thyroid function following paediatric cardiopulmonary bypass: association with interleukin-6 release? *Scand J Thorac Cardiovasc Surg* 1996;30:61–64.

106. Onoda N, Tsushima T, Isozaki O, et al. Effect of interleukin-6 on hypothalamic-pituitary-thyroid axis in rat. In: Nagataski S, Mori T, Torizuka K, eds. *80 Years of Hashimoto's disease.* Amsterdam: Elsevier Science, 1993:355.

107. Taylor KM, Wright GS, Bain WH, et al. Comparative studies of pulsatile and nonpulsatile flow during cardiopulmonary bypass. III. Response of anterior pituitary gland to thyrotropin-releasing hormone. *J Thorac Cardiovasc Surg* 1978;75:579–584.

108. Buket S, Alayunt A, Ozbaran M, et al. Effect of pulsatile flow

during cardiopulmonary bypass on thyroid hormone metabolism. *Ann Thorac Surg* 1994;58:93–96.

109. Bilezikian JP, Loeb JN. The influence of hyperthyroidism and hypothyroidism on α- and β-adrenergic receptor systems and adrenergic responsiveness. *Endocrinol Rev* 1983;4:378–388.

110. Sperelakis N, Wahler GM. Regulation of Ca^{2+} influx in myocardial cells by beta adrenergic receptors, cyclic nucleotides, and phosphorylation. *Mol Cell Biochem* 1988;82:19–28.

111. Novitzky D, Human PA, Cooper DK. Inotropic effect of triiodothyronine following myocardial ischemia and cardiopulmonary bypass: an experimental study in pigs. *Ann Thorac Surg* 1988;45:50–55.

112. Novitzky D, Human PA, Cooper DK. Effects of triiodothyronine (T_3) on myocardial high energy phosphates and lactate after ischemia and cardiopulmonary bypass. An experimental study in baboons. *J Thorac Cardiovasc Surg* 1988;96:600–607.

113. Novitzky D, Cooper DK, Barton CI, et al. Triiodothyronine as an inotropic agent after open heart surgery. *J Thorac Cardiovasc Surg* 1989;98:972–977.

114. Bennett-Guerrero E, Jimenez JL, White WD, et al. Cardiovascular effects of intravenous triiodothyronine in patients undergoing coronary artery bypass graft surgery. A randomized, double-blind, placebo-controlled trial. Duke T3 Study Group. *JAMA* 1996;275:687–692.

115. Klemperer JD, Klein I, Gomez M, et al. Thyroid hormone treatment after coronary-artery bypass surgery. *N Engl J Med* 1995;333:1522–1527.

116. Becker C. Hypothyroidism and atherosclerotic heart disease: pathogenesis, medical management, and the role of coronary artery bypass surgery. *Endocrinol Rev* 1985;77:261–265.

117. Myers A, Uotila P, Foegh ML, et al. The eicosanoids: prostaglandins, thromboxane, and leukotrienes. In: DeGroot LJ, ed. *Endocrinology*, 2nd ed. Vol. 3. Philadelphia: W.B. Saunders, 1989:2480–2490.

118. Ylikorkala O, Saarela E, Viinikka L. Increased prostacyclin and thromboxane production in man during cardiopulmonary bypass. *J Thorac Cardiovasc Surg* 1981;82:245–247.

119. Fleming WH, Sarafian LB, Leuschen MP, et al. Serum concentrations of prostacyclin and thromboxane in children before, during, and after cardiopulmonary bypass. *J Thorac Cardiovasc Surg* 1986;92:73–78.

120. Faymonville ME, Deby-Dupont G, Larbuisson R, et al. Prostaglandin E2, prostacyclin, and thromboxane changes during nonpulsatile cardiopulmonary bypass in humans. *J Thorac Cardiovasc Surg* 1986;91:858–866.

121. Greeley WJ, Bushman GA, Kong DL, et al. Effects of cardiopulmonary bypass on eicosanoid metabolism during pediatric cardiovascular surgery. *J Thorac Cardiovasc Surg* 1988;95:842–849.

122. Nagaoka H, Innami R, Murayama F, et al. Effects of aprotinin on prostaglandin metabolism and platelet function in open heart surgery. *J Cardiovasc Surg* 1991;32:31–37.

123. Watkins WD, Peterson MB, Kong DL, et al. Thromboxane and prostacyclin changes during cardiopulmonary bypass with and without pulsatile flow. *J Thorac Cardiovasc Surg* 1982;84:250–256.

124. Ritter JM, Hamilton G, Barrow SE, et al. Prostacyclin in the circulation of patients with vascular disorders undergoing surgery. *Clin Sci* 1986;71:743–747.

125. Leuschen MP, Ehrenfried JA, Willett LD, et al. Prostaglandin F1 alpha levels during and after neonatal extracorporeal membrane oxygenation. *J Thorac Cardiovasc Surg* 1991;101:148–152.

126. Lavee J, Naveh N, Dinbar I, et al. Prostacyclin and prostaglandin E2 mediate reduction of increased mean arterial pressure during cardiopulmonary bypass by aspiration of shed pulmonary venous blood. *J Thorac Cardiovasc Surg* 1990;100:546–551.

127. Levy JH. *Anaphylactic reactions in anesthesia and intensive care*, 2nd ed. Boston: Butterworth-Heinemann, 1992.

128. Man WK, Branna JJ, Fessatidis I, et al. Effect of prostacyclin on the circulatory histamine during cardiopulmonary bypass. *Agents Actions* 1986;18:182–185.

129. Marath A, Man W, Taylor KM. Histamine release in paediatric cardiopulmonary bypass—a possible role in the capillary leak syndrome. *Agents Actions* 1987;20:299–302.

130. Withington DE, Elliot M, Man WK. Histamine release during paediatric cardiopulmonary bypass. *Agents Actions* 1991;33:200–202.

131. van Overveld FJ, De Jongh RF, Jorens PG, et al. Pretreatment with methylprednisolone in coronary artery bypass grafting influences the levels of histamine and tryptase in serum but not in bronchoalveolar lavage fluid. *Clin Sci* 1994;86:49–53.

132. Johnston WE, Moss J, Philbin DM, et al. Management of cold urticaria during hypothermic cardiopulmonary bypass. *N Engl J Med* 1982;306:219–221.

133. Reiter M. Calcium mobilization and cardiac inotropic mechanisms. *Pharmacol Rev* 1988;40:189–217.

134. Zaloga GP. Calcium disorders. *Probl Crit Care Endocr Emerg* 1990;4:382–401.

135. Das JB, Eraklis AJ, Adams JG Jr, et al. Changes in serum ionic calcium during cardiopulmonary bypass with hemodilution. *J Thorac Cardiovasc Surg* 1971;62:449–453.

136. Moffitt EA, Tarhan S, Goldsmith RS, et al. Patterns of total and ionized calcium and other electrolytes in plasma during and after cardiac surgery. *J Thorac Cardiovasc Surg* 1973;65:751–757.

137. Yoshioka K, Tsuchioka H, Abe T, et al. Changes in ionized and total calcium concentrations in serum and urine during open heart surgery. *Biochem Med* 1978;20:135–143.

138. Gray R, Braunstein G, Krutzik S, et al. Calcium homeostasis during coronary bypass surgery. *Circulation* 1980;62:I57–I61.

139. Auffant RA, Downs JB, Amick R. Ionized calcium concentration and cardiovascular function after cardiopulmonary bypass. *Arch Surg* 1976;116:1072–1076.

140. Catinella FP, Cunningham JN Jr, Strauss ED, et al. Variations in total and ionized calcium during cardiac surgery. *J Cardiovasc Surg* 1983;24:593–602.

141. Abbott TR. Changes in serum calcium fractions and citrate concentrations during massive blood transfusions and cardiopulmonary bypass. *Br J Anaesth* 1983;55:753–759.

142. Hysing ES, Kofstad J, Lilleaasen P, et al. Ionized calcium in plasma during cardiopulmonary bypass. *Scand J Clin Lab Invest* 1986;184:119–123.

143. Westhorpe RN, Varghese Z, Petrie A, et al. Changes in ionized calcium and other plasma constituents associated with cardiopulmonary bypass. *Br J Anaesth* 1978;50:951–957.

144. Davies AB, Poole-Wilson PA. Whole blood calcium activity during cardiopulmonary bypass. *Intensive Care Med* 1981;7:213–216.

145. Chambers DJ, Dunham J, Braimbridge MV, et al. The effect of ionized calcium, pH, and temperature on bioactive parathyroid hormone during and after open-heart operations. *Ann Thorac Surg* 1983;36:306–313.

146. Heining MPD, Linton RAF, Band DM. Plasma ionized calcium during open-heart surgery. *Anaesthesia* 1985;40:237–241.

147. Robertie PG, Butterworth JF IV, Royster RL, et al. Normal parathyroid hormone responses to hypocalcemia during cardiopulmonary bypass. *Anesthesiology* 1991;75:43–48.

148. Robertie PG, Butterworth JF IV, Prielipp RC, et al. Parathyroid hormone responses to marked hypocalcemia in infants and

young children undergoing repair of congenital heart disease. *J Am Coll Cardiol* 1992;20:672–677.

149. Conlin PR, Fajtova VT, Mortensen RM, et al. Hysteresis in the relationship between serum ionized calcium and intact parathyroid hormone during recovery from induced hyper- and hypocalcemia in normal humans. *J Clin Endocrinol Metab* 1989; 69:593–599.

150. Butterworth JF IV, Royster RL, Prielipp RC, et al. Should calcium be administered prior to separation from cardiopulmonary bypass [reply]? *Anesthesiology* 1991;75:1121–1122.

151. Lefer DJ, Nakanishi K, Johnston WE, et al. Transient regional hypocalcemia during the initial phase of reperfusion does not reduce myocardial necrosis. *FASEB J* 1991;5:A1048.

152. Zaloga GP, Strickland RA, Butterworth JF IV, et al. Calcium attenuates epinephrine's beta-adrenergic effects in postoperative heart surgery patients. *Circulation* 1990;81:196–200.

153. Butterworth JF IV, Strickland RA, Mark LJ, et al. Calcium does not augment phenylephrine's hypertensive effects. *Crit Care Med* 1990;18:603–606.

154. Royster RL, Butterworth JF IV, Prielipp RC, et al. A randomized, blinded, placebo-controlled evaluation of calcium chloride and epinephrine for inotropic support after emergence from cardiopulmonary bypass. *Anesth Analg* 1992;74:3–13.

155. Butterworth JF IV, Zaloga GP, Prielipp RC, et al. Calcium inhibits the cardiac stimulating properties of dobutamine but not amrinone. *Chest* 1992;101:174–180.

156. Johnston WE, Robertie PG, Butterworth JF IV, et al. Is calcium or ephedrine superior to placebo for emergence from cardiopulmonary bypass? *J Cardiothorac Vasc Anesth* 1992;6:528–534.

157. Castillo CF del, Harringer W, Warshaw AL. Risk factors for pancreatic cellular injury after cardiopulmonary bypass. *N Engl J Med* 1991;325:382–387.

158. Prielipp RC, Butterworth J. Con: calcium is not routinely indicated during separation from cardiopulmonary bypass. *J Cardiothorac Vasc Anesth* 1997;11:908–912.

159. DiNardo JA. Pro: calcium is routinely indicated during separation from cardiopulmonary bypass. *J Cardiothorac Vasc Anesth* 1997;11:905–907.

160. Abernethy WB, Butterworth JF IV, Prielipp RC, et al. Calcium entry attenuates adenylyl cyclase activity. A possible mechanism for calcium-induced catecholamine resistance. *Chest* 1995;107: 1420–1425.

161. Zaloga GP, Roberts JE. Magnesium disorders. *Probl Crit Care Endocr Emerg* 1990;4:425–436.

162. Zaloga GP, Wilkens R, Tourville J, et al. A simple method for determining physiologically active calcium and magnesium concentrations in critically ill patients. *Crit Care Med* 1987;15: 813–816.

163. Turnier E, Osborn JJ, Gerbode F, et al. Magnesium and open-heart surgery. *J Thorac Cardiovasc Surg* 1972;64:694–705.

164. Scheinman MM, Sullivan RW, Hyatt KH. Magnesium metabolism in patients undergoing cardiopulmonary bypass. *Circulation* 1969;39:I235–I241.

165. Aglio LS, Stanford GG, Maddi R, et al. Hypomagnesemia is common following cardiac surgery. *J Cardiothorac Vasc Anesth* 1991;5:201–208.

166. Lum G, Marquardt C, Khuri SF. Hypomagnesemia and low alkaline phosphatase activity in patients' serum after cardiac surgery. *Clin Chem* 1989;35:664–667.

167. Harris MN, Crowther A, Jupp RA, et al. Magnesium and coronary revascularization. *Br J Anaesth* 1988;60:779–783.

168. Prielipp RC, Zaloga GP, Butterworth JF IV, et al. Magnesium inhibits the hypertensive but not the cardiotonic actions of low-dose epinephrine. *Anesthesiology* 1991;74:973–979.

169. Friedman HS, Nguyen TN, Mokraoui AM, et al. Effects of

magnesium chloride on cardiovascular hemodynamics in the neurally intact dog. *J Pharmacol Exp Ther* 1987;243:126–130.

170. Prielipp RC, Butterworth JV IV, Roberts PR, et al. Magnesium antagonizes the actions of lysophosphatidyl choline (LPC) in myocardial cells: a possible mechanism for its antiarrhythmic effects. *Anesth Analg* 1995;80:1083–1087.

171. Abraham AS, Rosenmann D, Kramer M, et al. Magnesium in the prevention of lethal arrhythmias in acute myocardial infarction. *Arch Intern Med* 1987;147:753–755.

172. Rasmussen HS, Suenson M, McNair P, et al. Magnesium infusion reduces the incidence of arrhythmias in acute myocardial infarction. A double-blind placebo-controlled study. *Clin Cardiol* 1987;10:351–356.

173. Rasmussen HS, McNair P, Norregard P, et al. Intravenous magnesium in acute myocardial infarction. *Lancet* 1986;1:234–236.

174. Woods KL, Fletcher S, Roffe C, et al. Intravenous magnesium sulphate in suspected myocardial infarction: results of the second Leicester Intravenous Magnesium Intervention Trial (LIMIT-2). *Lancet* 1992;339:1553–1558.

175. Horner SM. Efficacy of intravenous magnesium in acute myocardial infarction in reducing arrhythmias and mortality. Meta-analysis of magnesium in acute myocardial infarction. *Circulation* 1992;86:774–779.

176. Garfinkel L, Garfinkel D. Magnesium regulation of the glycolytic pathway and the enzymes involved. *Magnesium* 1985;4: 60–72.

177. Altura BM, Altura BT. Magnesium, electrolyte transport and coronary vascular tone. *Drugs* 1984;28:120–142.

178. Altura BM, Turlapaty PD. Withdraw of magnesium enhances coronary arterial spasms produced by vasoactive agents. *Br J Pharmacol* 1982;77:649–659.

179. Schwieger I, Kopel ME, Finlayson DC. Magnesium reduces incidence of postoperative dysrhythmias in patients after cardiac surgery. *Anesthesiology* 1989;71:A1163.

180. Mathew R, Altura BM. Magnesium and the lungs. *Magnesium* 1988;7:173–187.

181. Walesby RK, Goode AW, Bentall HH. Nutritional status of patients undergoing valve replacement by open heart surgery. *Lancet* 1978;1:76–77

182. Morgan DB, Mearns AJ, Burkinshaw L. The potassium status of patients prior to open-heart surgery. *J Thorac Cardiovasc Surg* 1978;76:673–677

183. Ebert PA, Jude JR, Gaertner RA. Persistent hypokalemia following open-heart surgery. *Circulation* 1965;31:I137–I143.

184. Bozer AY, Ilicin G, Apikoglu A, et al. Serum electrolyte changes during extracorporeal circulation. *Jpn Heart J* 1972;13: 195–200.

185. Regensburger D, Paschen K, Fuchs C. Changes in the electrolyte and acid-base balance in operations with cardiopulmonary bypass and haemodilution. *Thoraxchir Vask Chir* 1972;20: 473–479.

186. Marcial MB, Vedoya RC, Zerbini EJ, et al. Potassium in cardiac surgery with extracorporeal perfusion. *Am J Cardiol* 1969;23: 400–408.

187. Bert AA, Stearns GT, Feng W, et al. Normothermic cardiopulmonary bypass. *J Cardiothorac Vasc Anesth* 1997;11:91–99.

188. Patrick J, Sivpragasam S. The prediction of postoperative potassium excretion after cardiopulmonary bypass. *J Thorac Cardiovasc Surg* 1977;73:559–562.

189. Wilson GM, Dunn FG, McQueen MJ, et al. Comparison of intravenous bumetanide and frusemide during open heart surgery. *Postgrad Med J* 1975;51:72.

190. Cohn LH, Angell WW, Shumway NE. Body fluid shifts after cardiopulmonary bypass. I. Effects of congestive heart failure and hemodilution. *J Thorac Cardiovasc Surg* 1971;62:423–430.

191. Moffitt EA, White RD, Molnar GD, et al. Comparative effects

of whole blood, hemodiluted, and clear priming solutions on myocardial and body metabolism in man. *Can J Surg* 1971;14: 382–391.

192. Johnston AE, Radde IC, Steward DJ, et al. Acid-base and electrolyte changes in infants undergoing profound hypothermia for surgical correction of congenital heart defects. *Can Anaesth Soc J* 1974;21:23–45.

193. Johnston AE, Radde IC, Nisbet HI, et al. Effects of altering calcium in haemodiluted pump primes on sodium and potassium in children undergoing open-heart operations. *Can Anaesth Soc J* 1972;19:517–528.

194. Taggart P, Slater JD. Some effects of bypass surgery on myocardial and skeletal muscle electrolytes and their clinical importance. *Br Heart J* 1969;31:393.

195. Munday KA, Blane GF, Chin EF, et al. Plasma electrolyte changes in hypothermia. *Thorax* 1958;13:334–342.

196. Lim M, Linton RA, Band DM. Rise in plasma potassium during rewarming in open-heart surgery [letter]. *Lancet* 1983;1: 241–242.

197. Weber DO, Yarnoz MD. Hyperkalemia complicating cardiopulmonary bypass: analysis of risk factors. *Ann Thorac Surg* 1982;34:439–445.

198. Bethune DW, McKay R. Paradoxical changes in serum-potassium during cardiopulmonary bypass in association with noncardioselective beta blockade [letter]. *Lancet* 1978;2:380.

199. Henney RP, Riemenschneider TA, DeLand EC, et al. Prevention of hypokalemic cardiac arrhythmias associated with cardiopulmonary bypass and hemodilution. *Surg Forum* 1970;21: 145–147.

200. Manning SH, Angaran DM, Arom KV, et al. Intermittent intravenous potassium therapy in cardiopulmonary bypass patients. *Clin Pharmacol* 1982;1:234–238.

201. Schwartz AJ, Conahan TJ III, Jobes DR, et al. Peripheral vascular response to potassium administration during cardiopulmonary bypass. *J Thorac Cardiovasc Surg* 1980;79:237–240.

202. Watters JM, Wilmore DW. The metabolic responses to trauma and sepsis. In: DeGroot LJ, ed. *Endocrinology*, 2nd ed. Vol. 3. Philadelphia: W.B. Saunders, 1989:2367–2392.

203. Fuhrer G, Heller W, Hoffmeister HE, et al. Levels of trace elements during and after cardiopulmonary bypass operations. *Acta Pharmacol Toxicol* 1986;59:352–357.

204. Zhao L. Changes in blood zinc and copper and their clinical significance in patients undergoing open-heart surgery. *Chung Hua I Hsueh Tsa Chih* 1989;69:76–78.

205. Sjogren A, Luhrs C, Abdulla M. Changed distribution of zinc and copper in body fluids in patients undergoing open-heart surgery. *Acta Pharmacol Toxicol* 1986;59:348–351.

206. Taggart DP, Fraser WD, Shenkin A, et al. The effects of intraoperative hypothermia and cardiopulmonary bypass on trace metals and their protein binding ratios. *Eur J Cardiothorac Surg* 1990;4:587–594.

207. Menasche P, Pasquier C, Bellucci S, et al. Deferoxamine reduces neutrophil-mediated free radical production during cardiopulmonary bypass in man. *J Thorac Cardiovasc Surg* 1988;96: 582–589.

208. Mitchell IM, Brady L, Black J, et al. The acute phase response to cardiopulmonary bypass in children. *Perfusion* 1996;11: 103–112.

CARDIOPULMONARY BYPASS
AND THE LUNG

JONATHAN B. OSTER
ROBERT N. SLADEN
DANIEL E. BERKOWITZ

In 1977 Pennock et al. (1) wrote "pulmonary problems remain the most significant cause of morbidity following cardiopulmonary bypass today." Although this statement may no longer hold true, the impact of cardiopulmonary bypass (CPB) on lung function is still of considerable physiologic and pathologic consequence.

The lung is at risk of injury during CPB because of collapse and pleural disruption. The effects of these mechanical changes depend on the patient's underlying pulmonary reserve. The lung is also at risk to an inflammatory response mediated by contact activation of blood components during extracorporeal circulation. Its severity may vary from microscopic changes of no clinical consequence to a fulminating capillary leak syndrome and acute respiratory failure. In addition, important metabolic functions provided by the lung are bypassed by extracorporeal circulation.

This chapter addresses the pathophysiology of these processes, correlates them with clinical pulmonary syndromes during and after CPB, and outlines therapeutic approaches to the management of the lungs during CPB.

MECHANICAL ALTERATIONS IN LUNG FUNCTION

Pathophysiology of Atelectasis

Atelectasis is the most common pulmonary complication after cardiac surgery, occurring in about 70% of cases. During CPB, the lungs are not perfused and are usually allowed to collapse to functional residual capacity (FRC). When the lungs are subsequently reexpanded and ventilated toward

J. B. Oster and R. N. Sladen: Department of Anesthesiology, College of Physicians and Surgeons, Columbia University, New York Presbyterian Medical Center, New York, New York 10032.

D. S. Berkowitz: Department of Anesthesiology, The Johns Hopkins Hospital, Baltimore, Maryland 21287.

the end of CPB, a variable degree of pulmonary atelectasis remains. It ranges in severity from microatelectasis, a radiographically detectable decrease in lung volume, to complete collapse of a lobe. Intermediate degrees of atelectasis—plate, subsegmental, and segmental—are common. Atelectasis results in deterioration of FRC, lung compliance (C_L), venoarterial admixture, and alveolar arterial oxygen gradient ($AaDo_2$). However, it is difficult to distinguish the mechanical changes in lung function induced by CPB from those related to thoracotomy, pleural resection, and pleural effusion. A large number of factors predispose to postoperative pulmonary atelectasis, some of which operate during CPB, but others exist before surgery or occur after CPB.

Factors Predisposing to Atelectasis

Several preexisting conditions promote development of atelectasis and hinder its resolution in the post-CPB period (Table 18.1). Heavy smokers with chronic bronchitis develop metaplasia of ciliated columnar epithelium in the tracheal-bronchial tree. Anterograde cilial clearance of mucus and debris is impaired, surfactant production is diminished, and small airways and alveoli tend to collapse. Obesity causes a reduction in FRC and predisposes to atelectasis before and after CPB. An increase in extravascular lung water, whether due to congestive heart failure or pulmonary edema, increases the tendency for small airways to collapse.

During mechanical ventilation in the anesthetized paralyzed patient, the diaphragm is passively displaced cephalad by the abdominal contents and gas flow is preferentially distributed to the nondependent regions of the lung. This causes ventilation-perfusion mismatch and promotes hypoventilation and collapse of the dependent areas. Any monotonous ventilatory pattern without "sighs," such as that provided by a mechanical ventilator in the anesthetized patient, results in progressive microatelectasis of the dependent lung zones.

Pulmonary surfactant (dipalmitoyl lecithin) is a lipopro-

TABLE 18.1. ETIOLOGY OF PULMONARY ATELECTASIS

Preoperative factors
  Smoking, chronic bronchitis (mucus cell hyperplasia, surfactant depletion)
  Obesity (decreased FRC)
  Cardiogenic pulmonary edema
Intraoperative factors
  Passive ventilation of paralyzed diaphragm
  Monotonous ventilatory pattern
CPB factors
  Surfactant inhibition—plasma, lung distension, lung ischemia
  Increased extravascular lung water (complement activation)
  Heart rests on immobile left lower lobe
  Blind bronchial suctioning—preferential right bronchial drainage, mucosal damage
  Open pleural cavity—blood, fluid

FRC, functional residual capacity; CPB, cardiopulmonary bypass.

tein produced by alveolar granular epithelium (type II pneumocytes) that lowers surface tension in alveoli and prevents alveolar and small airway collapse. Exposure of surfactant to plasma from normal adults and children inhibits its action (2). Entrance of plasma components into air spaces through leaking lung membranes could thereby contribute to atelectasis. Mandelbaum and Giammona (3) suggested that lung distension during CPB depletes surfactant, and subsequent animal studies have confirmed that positive-pressure ventilation during CPB decreases C_L and increases intrapulmonary shunt after CPB (4).

Pharmacologic preparations containing surfactant have been used clinically in the treatment of hyaline membrane disease in premature infants. It was postulated that exogenous surfactant treatment might be valuable in the prevention or treatment of CPB-related adult respiratory distress syndrome (ARDS). A study in adult patients undergoing CPB by Macnaughton and Evans (5) and a study in pigs by Haslam et al. (6) showed exogenously administered surfactant unable to improve lung function. In fact, both studies suggested that the surfactant might be deleterious in its effects on gas transfer.

During CPB, the heart rests on the immobile left lower lobe. With blind bronchial suctioning, the suction catheter usually enters the more direct right mainstem bronchus, resulting in preferential right bronchial drainage. Traumatic mucosal "pitting" induced by the suction catheter at the carina causes secretions to dam up and promotes airway collapse (7). When the pleural cavity is opened, blood and fluid can enter and compress the adjacent lung. In patients undergoing coronary revascularization, dissection of the left internal mammary artery may require entry into the left pleural space. All these factors account for the 60% to 70% preponderance of left lower lobe atelectasis after CPB (8).

Effects on Oxygenation

$AaDO_2$ is consistently increased above normal after CPB (9–13). The $AaDO_2$ increases to a maximum about 48 hours postoperatively, does not return to normal for at least 7 days, and is detectable for weeks after surgery (14). It is generally assumed that this is due to varying degrees of lung collapse on CPB, ranging from diffuse microatelectasis to lobar atelectasis. FRC declines by about 20% after CPB (15). Although intrapulmonary shunt and venoarterial admixture are increased after CPB, there is a poor correlation between decreases in measured FRC and increases in intrapulmonary shunt (3,16).

Altered Mechanical Properties of the Lung

A number of investigators have found significant changes in pulmonary mechanics induced by CPB (12,17–21). C_L is decreased, and airway resistance (R_{AW}) and work of breathing are increased (for an explanation of the tests described, see Appendix 1). In some studies, however, alterations in pulmonary mechanics induced by CPB have been negligible (22–24).

Andersen and Ghia (12,21) assessed the effect of CPB on total R_{AW}, total compliance of the lungs and chest wall (static thoracic compliance, C_{TH}), $AaDO_2$, and the ratio of dead space to tidal volume. Although they did find some deterioration in these functions during CPB, they were of the same nature as those occurring in patients undergoing thoracic procedures without CPB. Stratification of data from patients between those whose pleura was violated versus inviolate implicated active lung retraction and pleurotomy, rather than CPB itself, as the major architects of disturbed lung mechanics during cardiac surgery. These authors also demonstrated a close relationship between poor preoperative pulmonary and cardiac function and deterioration in pulmonary function in the postoperative period.

Magnusson et al. (25) investigated general anesthesia alone versus sternotomy with CPB in a pig model. They found that atelectasis was produced to a much larger extent in the CPB group. These were, however, healthy animals, and it is not clear whether these same results can be extrapolated to patients with preexisting pulmonary pathology that might render the lung more susceptible to damage after surgical manipulations.

Sullivan et al. (22) attempted to exclude the impact of pleural violation, with its attendant pneumothorax and effusion, from the effects of CPB alone. They studied patients undergoing median sternotomy for correction of acquired valvular heart disease in whom neither pleural space was entered. Measurement of dynamic compliance, elastic and flow resistive work of breathing, and intrapulmonary shunt revealed no significant differences before and after CPB. Karlson et al. (24) were also not able to demonstrate any significant change in compliance, nonelastic resistance, or the work/volume ratio of the lung before and after CPB. However, there was a significant decline in C_L by the time patients were extubated and breathing spontaneously after surgery, compared with the preoperative level. Again, this suggests a greater contribution to pulmonary complications from the effects of anesthesia and thoracotomy than CPB itself. CPB appears to have little adverse effect on pediatric pulmonary mechanics (23). In patients with a lesion such as an endocardial cushion defect that causes pulmonary vascular engorgement, repair corrects the pulmonary hyperemia so that C_L is actually improved after CPB.

Clinical Features

During CPB, atelectasis can be directly visualized in the exposed lung, although large parts of the dependent lung fields are not in view. After the chest is closed, significant atelectasis is usually first recognized by a decrease in C_L that results in the generation of increased peak airway pressure (P_{PK}) with normal tidal volume (e.g., 35 cm H_2O at tidal volume of 10 mL/kg). This is associated with an increased $AaDO_2$ (e.g., P_aO_2 of less than 200 mm Hg on inspired oxygen fraction of 1.0), although it will be detected by pulse oximetry only when the P_aO_2 falls to less than 90 mm Hg and the arterial oxygen saturation declines below 98%. After surgery, careful auscultation of the chest reveals bronchial breathing and crackles, usually in the dependent lung fields, but clinical signs may underestimate the extent of atelectasis, and radiologic confirmation is essential.

Together the decline in FRC and C_L increases the work of breathing required to distend the alveoli. If this is severe enough, it can lead to acute hypoxemic respiratory failure and continued requirement for mechanical ventilation. Collapsed airways compromise secretion clearance and predispose to pulmonary superinfection and pneumonia.

Prevention and Treatment of Atelectasis

Prevention

Attempts have been made to prevent atelectasis from occurring during CPB by the provision of positive-pressure ventilation, sighs, or static inflation at 5 to 10 cm H_2O pressure. However, Ellis et al. (26) found that C_L deteriorated during CPB, whether the lungs were mechanically ventilated, statically inflated, or allowed to deflate. Ghia and Andersen (12) claimed that the use of static inflation plus an intermittent sigh every 10 minutes to an airway pressure of 25 to 30 cm H_2O prevented decreases in R_{AW}, C_{TH}, and increases in ratio of dead space to tidal volume and $AaDO_2$. Contrasting arguments were presented by Stanley et al. (4), who evaluated C_L and intrapulmonary shunt before and after CPB in 132 calves undergoing artificial heart implantation with halothane-O_2 anesthesia. The provision of positive-pressure ventilation during CPB caused a greater increase in shunt

and decrease in compliance after CPB, probably through depletion of surfactant. These variables were not influenced by the gas inflating the lungs (100% O_2 or 50% O_2/N_2O). Static pulmonary inflation [continuous positive airway pressure (CPAP)] offered no advantage over allowing the lungs to remain collapsed.

Berry et al. (27) contrasted three techniques of lung management during CPB. Groups were randomized to either deflated lungs, CPAP of 5 with inspired oxygen fraction 1.0, or CPAP of 5 with inspired oxygen fraction of 0.21. Although they demonstrated some reduction in $AaDO_2$ 30 minutes after CPB in the CPAP groups, all groups had similar gradients by 4 hours and the time to extubation was not affected. In a similar study, Cogliati et al. (28) showed that the group inflated with air had a preservation of pulmonary mechanics. They suggested that this might be secondary to a preservation of bronchial perfusion by the lung expansion itself. They emphasized again that CPB itself has negative effects on gas exchange regardless of the technique of lung management.

Weedn et al. (29) suggested that static inflation of the lungs with oxygen might prevent ultrastructural damage by sustaining cellular oxidative metabolism. In studies on small animals, the use of CPAP during CPB was associated with lower pulmonary lactate/pyruvate ratios and greater highenergy phosphate concentrations than the use of lung collapse (30). However, these findings have not been correlated with significant changes in gross lung function.

There is reasonable evidence that the avoidance of entry into the pleural spaces will prevent a large amount of the decrease in C_L seen after CPB (12,21,22). However, it may be impossible to avoid left pleurotomy with internal mammary artery dissection, so that this point remains moot for many patients undergoing coronary revascularization.

Treatment

It is possible that a series of sighs (i.e., slow sustained inspiratory maneuvers to a P_{PK} of 25 to 30 cm H_2O) could be given just before weaning from CPB. This may reverse atelectasis and improve C_L. Lung inflation for 15 seconds to 40 cm H_2O at the end of bypass was shown by Magnusson et al. (25) to prevent post-CPB atelectasis in a pig model. Identical Valsalva maneuvers are routinely used after open heart procedures to expel air from the left atrium and ventricle. However, there is a risk of disruption of an internal mammary graft by excessive distension of the left lung or rupture of a lung bleb or weakened area. Sighs given after separation from CPB impede venous return and add to hemodynamic instability.

Clinically, the most effective means of reversing decreased FRC and atelectasis after CPB is to provide mechanical ventilation with positive end-expiratory pressure (PEEP), which is continued into the postoperative period (16). However, the improvement in measured FRC does not directly correlate with improvement in intrapulmonary shunt or AaDo$_2$. Dobbinson and Miller (15) found that FRC increased postoperatively only when levels of PEEP of 6 cm H$_2$O or greater were used, at the expense of cardiac performance. The adverse effects of PEEP on cardiac output can easily be overcome with modest inotropic support (e.g., dopamine 5 μg/kg/min) or preload augmentation (31,32).

In our experience, we have found that the combination of large tidal volumes (12 to 15 mL/kg), moderate levels of PEEP (5 to 8 cm H$_2$O), and, importantly, adequate time (4 to 8 hours) are successful in improving oxygenation, AaDo$_2$, and C$_L$ in most cases. A clinical guide to reasonable delivered tidal volume is provided by P$_{PK}$: Ideally, it should be approximately 25 cm H$_2$O. If P$_{PK}$ is less than 20 cm H$_2$O and a system air leak has been excluded, the delivered tidal volume is probably inadequate and should be increased. If P$_{PK}$ is greater than 35 cm H$_2$O, either the delivered tidal volume is excessive or there is another cause of high airway pressure that requires investigation (e.g., endobronchial intubation, bronchospasm, or pulmonary edema). The size of the delivered tidal volume should be limited to about 12 mL/kg in patients who have undergone internal mammary grafting and where it has been noted intraoperatively that lung expansion tends to displace the graft. A large AaDo$_2$ that is unresponsive to these measures (and that does not have an obvious underlying cause) is usually due to intrinsic lung disease or pulmonary edema.

ACUTE LUNG INJURY AND CARDIOPULMONARY BYPASS

Pathophysiology of Acute Lung Injury

Soon after the advent of CPB in the 1950s, it became apparent that a substantial proportion of deaths after cardiac surgery was related to a syndrome of acute respiratory failure referred to as "pump lung" (33). Biopsy or autopsy specimens from patients revealed striking morphologic changes (34). The lungs were diffusely congested, with intraalveolar and interstitial edema and hemorrhagic atelectasis, a picture not unlike "shock lung." Electron microscopy revealed that vessel lumina were packed with neutrophils; there was diffuse swelling of the endothelial cells, including mitochondria in the endoplasmic reticulum, and cytoplasmic swelling in the membranous pneumocytes.

Microembolic Theory

Initially it was considered that this lesion was due to immobilization of particulate debris during CPB, including aggregated protein, disintegrated platelets, damaged neutrophils and fibrin, or even fat globules, a picture similar to that found with massive blood transfusion (35–40). The Dacron wool filter was introduced by Swank in 1961 (41), and Hill et al. (37) demonstrated that it could dramatically decrease the intensity of nonfat cerebral embolism. Connell et al. (39) found that Dacron wool filtration during CPB removed platelet-leukocyte aggregates and reduced the extent of the degenerative lesions in the lung: The more complete the filtration, the more normal the lungs appeared.

Despite these findings, it became apparent that striking pulmonary damage could occur even when all the perfusate is filtered, suggesting other etiologies for pump lung. Indeed, the nature of the lesion we see today may be considerably different from that described in an era when the CPB circuit was primed with whole blood (which, depending on its age, would be laden with platelet-neutrophil microaggregates), when disc or bubble oxygenators caused denaturation of plasma proteins, and when in-line arterial filters were not commonplace.

Complement Activation

Complement activation and the potential for pulmonary dysfunction appears to be a consistent response to contact activation of blood in extracorporeal circuits, such as leukophoresis and hemodialysis (42,43). Some susceptible patients have developed life-threatening bronchospasm, with urticaria, angioedema, hypotension, and cardiopulmonary collapse on first use of hemodialysis.

The complement system performs three vital functions in the body's defense against invading microorganisms: leukocyte activation, cytolysis, and opsonization. The last renders bacterial cells vulnerable to phagocytosis by the adherence of opsonins or complement components. Complement is activated through two interrelated cascades termed the classic and alternate pathways, which ultimately lead to cleavage of C3, the central component of the system (Fig. 18.1). The enzyme cascade is generated by the activation of enzyme precursors, which are fixed to biologic membranes. Each component, a highly specialized proteinase, activates the next enzyme precursor to its catalytically active state by limited proteolysis. A small peptide fragment is cleaved and a nascent membrane-binding site is exposed, so forming the next active complement enzyme of the sequence. Because each component can activate many enzyme precursors, the whole system forms an amplification cascade akin to the coagulation cascade (44).

During the activation of the complement system via either the classic or the alternate pathway, C3a and C5a anaphylotoxins are generated. C3a causes smooth muscle contraction in a wide variety of animal tissues. C5a is 10 to 20 times more active than C3a on a molar basis and has wider biologic activity. It is a major chemotactic factor for neutrophils, resulting in their margination in vessels and neutropenia. C5a activates neutrophils by triggering the bactericidal oxidative burst and causes the release of arachidonic acid metabolites such as leukotriene B4, which increases vascular permeability. C5a also provokes mast cell degranulation and smooth muscle contraction.

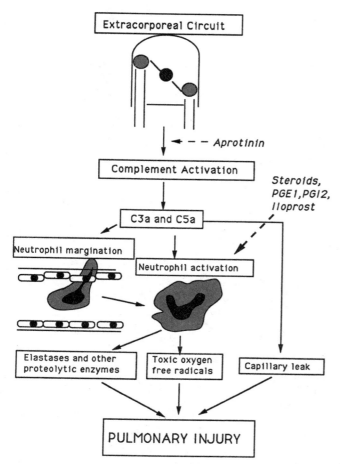

FIG. 18.1. Cascade of pathophysiologic events initiated by cardiopulmonary bypass and leading to pulmonary injury. *Dashed arrows* indicate inhibitory actions.

The striking similarities between the biologic activities of anaphylotoxins C3a and C5a, the capillary leak syndrome, and organ dysfunction associated with CPB prompted Chenoweth et al. (45) to investigate complement activation as a cause of pump lung. They demonstrated a correlation between the duration of CPB, the degree of elevation of C3a levels, and post-CPB organ dysfunction. Animal studies revealed that intravenous infusion of activated complement produces pulmonary leukocyte trapping with transient leukopenia and transpulmonary release of thromboxane A₂, leading to pulmonary vasoconstriction and hypertension. Concomitantly, there is an increase in the pulmonary microvascular permeability (46). This process can be attenuated by superoxide dismutase, which suggests that free oxygen radicals play a role in tissue injury after activated complement infusion (47).

Hammerschmidt and Jacob (48) randomized 28 patients to CPB with membrane or bubble oxygenators, with or without steroid pretreatment. A marked leukopenia occurred in all patients. Total complement showed no decline

in the first hour of CPB and only a slight decline in the group without steroid pretreatment. However, C3a and C5a could not be detected. The membrane oxygenator produced a significantly greater degree and duration of neutropenia consistent with the fact that its materials include silicone, expanded Teflon, and polypropylene, which activate complement *in vitro*. The failure to demonstrate increased circulating C3a and C5a may have been due to their rapid clearance, the detection limits of the assay, or the fact that C5a binds so avidly to human neutrophils that it may not be detectable free in the plasma.

In contrast, Howard et al. (49) demonstrated marked increases in C3a levels within 2 minutes of the onset of CPB, an increase in C5a levels toward the end of CPB, and increased C4a levels in the postoperative period. Lung biopsy specimens, which were normal before CPB, were radically altered, with an increased number of neutrophils in the pulmonary arterioles and adhering to capillary walls. The finding of a transpulmonary gradient of neutrophils suggested that they were sequestered in the pulmonary vasculature. Collett et al. (50) used sensitive assays to determine which pathway is responsible for activation of complement during CPB. They demonstrated a rapid rise in fragment Ba within 90 seconds of initiation of CPB, indicating activation of the alternate pathway. The polymers incorporated into the extracorporeal circuit are known to activate the alternate pathway *in vitro* (45,51). However, there is also activation of the common pathway because C3d increases with a concomitant decline in C3.

Inflammatory Response

During aortic cross-clamping on CPB, the neutrophil count in right and left atrial blood increases. After aortic cross-clamp release and as blood flow is restored to the pulmonary vasculature, the right atrial neutrophil count increases but the left atrial count declines: Neutrophils appear to be trapped in the pulmonary capillaries (51). Tonz et al. found a positive correlation between plasma elastase concentration (a measure of neutrophil activation) and respiratory index and intrapulmonary shunt (51A). Products of lipid peroxidation measured by the thiobarbituric acid reaction also reach a peak after aortic cross-clamp release. This implies a direct relationship between neutrophil trapping and oxygen free radical peroxidation of membrane lipids. Of course, reperfusion injury after ischemia generates oxygen free radicals and may also contribute to lipid peroxidation at this time. Braude et al. (46) confirmed that CPB in dogs is associated with neutrophil sequestration and egress from the lung of products of lipid peroxidation. They also demonstrated profound pulmonary vascular permeability by finding significantly increased lung transvascular protein flux as measured by In¹¹³ᵐ-transferrin.

Chenoweth et al. (45) demonstrated that complement is activated by the nylon mesh of the bubble oxygenator and by vigorous bubbling of oxygen through the blood. Van Oeveren et al. (52) investigated whether complement activation could be lessened by the use of hollow-fiber membrane oxygenators. Hemolysis, thrombocytopenia, β-thromboglobulin release (a marker of platelet activation), and generation of reactive oxygen species in leukocytes was significantly greater with the bubble oxygenator. However, the rate of complement activation was similar with the membrane oxygenator, casting doubt on whether its use appreciably alters pulmonary morbidity on CPB.

Jansen et al. (53) noted a significant increase in C3a and elastase (evidence of activated leukocytes) after the onset of CPB, which was exacerbated after aortic cross-clamp release. This was associated with increases in leukotriene B4 (an eicosanoid that induces capillary leak) and tissue plasminogen activator (which enhances fibrinolysis).

The role of the eicosanoids thromboxane and prostacyclin in this acute inflammatory response is yet unclear (54). There is an increased systemic level of thromboxane during CPB. Thromboxane is released from platelets activated by the extracorporeal circuit, and its profound effects on vasoconstriction and platelet aggregation could further injure the microcirculation (55). Differential measurement of thromboxane B_2 in the right and left atria has indicated that the rise in thromboxane levels during CPB reflects production in the lungs, either from ischemic pulmonary tissue or intravascular hematologic components (56). Aspirin, a cyclooxygenase inhibitor, was able to blunt this increase in thromboxane. Inhibition of thromboxane synthetase reduced lung injury related to CPB in sheep (57). Thromboxane A_2 has been implicated in the increase in pulmonary artery pressures, which follow CPB. This increase in pulmonary artery pressure was prevented in a rabbit model with cyclooxygenase inhibition and with thromboxane A_2 synthetase inhibition (58). Prostacyclin, which has the opposite actions, is released especially during pulsatile perfusion on CPB, perhaps because of increased shear stress on the endothelium (59). However, the benefits of pulsatile perfusion in prevention of acute lung injury during CPB remain unknown.

The cytokines are a group of polypeptides or glycopeptides produced primarily by macrophages and monocytes in response to tissue injury. Advances in immunochemical techniques have allowed measurement of minute concentrations of cytokines. Tumor necrosis factor-alpha and the interleukin (IL)-1beta, IL-6, and IL-8 have received a great deal of attention as potential contributors to post-CPB inflammation and pulmonary injury. Recent studies have all shown increased levels of IL-6 and IL-8. Plasma tumor necrosis factor-alpha and IL-1 do not appear to increase in response to bypass, but a local production of these cytokines cannot be excluded, as they are known to stimulate cellular production of IL-6 and IL-8 (60–65). Work is presently under way to use pharmacologic interventions and alterations in the CPB technique in efforts to blunt the increases

in interleukins. Whether decreased productions of these factors will correlate with improved lung function after CPB has also yet to be shown.

In summary, contact activation of the blood by the extracorporeal circuit triggers a series of amplification cascades mediated by proteolytic enzymes, especially serine proteases. It results in the activation of complement, especially C5a anaphylatoxin. C5a is a potent bioactive molecule that normally mediates the acute inflammatory response, which has spasmogenic and leukocyte-activating properties that cause degranulation and release of toxic oxygen free radicals (66). Complement-exposed neutrophils are stimulated to adhere to surfaces and to aggregate, resulting in margination of blood vessels and leukoembolization. These neutrophils markedly increase their production of oxygen free radicals and release proteolytic enzymes, which damage endothelial cells. Complement activation and neutrophil arachidonic acid metabolites cause increased vascular permeability with capillary leak.

Other Factors Contributing to Acute Lung Injury

Hypoxia of Lung Parenchyma

During CPB, the lungs are isolated from the pulmonary circulation. Mandelbaum and Giammona (67) demonstrated that collateral blood flow from the bronchial circulation passes through the pulmonary capillary bed and participates in cellular respiration. Attempts have been made to evaluate the nature of bronchial collateral blood flow, metabolic oxygen consumption of the lung parenchyma, and the effects of pulmonary arterial occlusion and hypoxia on the lung tissue. Loer et al. (68) determined lung oxygen consumption at 36°C to be about 11 mL/min and about 5 to 6 mL/min at 28°C. Balis et al. (69) found that perfusion of the canine pulmonary artery with oxygenated blood protects against hemorrhagic atelectasis during CPB. Although this suggests that hypoxia may contribute to acute lung injury, during CPB the pulmonary artery is not perfused with oxygenated blood either. Nahas et al. (70) perfused one lung with half the CPB venous return and ventilated both lungs. They observed a greater degree of damage in the perfused lung, which implied that acute lung injury is more likely to be due to humoral factors such as complement than direct tissue hypoxia.

Hemodilution

When the extracorporeal circuit is primed with a hypooncotic solution of colloid or crystalloid, there is an immediate decrease in the colloid oncotic pressure (COP) at the onset of CPB. Thereafter, an incomplete compensatory increase in COP occurs, due to an efflux of water from the intravascular to extravascular space and to an influx of albumin from peripheral albumin stores. The decrease in microvascular oncotic pressure caused by hemodilution increases transcapillary fluid flux. However, double dilution indicator techniques have indicated that as much as a 50% decrease in COP may be required to produce significant increases in pulmonary extravascular water. Byrick et al. (72) determined that accumulation of pulmonary extravascular water after coronary revascularization is not affected by priming the circuit with colloid or crystalloid solutions. Hemodilution on CPB with colloid or crystalloid does not appear to harm the lungs; indeed, it may be protective because it prevents impairment of surfactant.

Elevated Pulmonary Artery Pressure

In 1958 Kolff et al. (71) called attention to the danger of overfilling of the vascular bed as a possible cause of pulmonary complications after CPB: "Overfilling of the pulmonary vascular bed during operations using extracorporeal circulation is most likely to occur when the heart chambers are not open. It can be avoided by placing an adequate drainage tube in the left atrium." Elevated pulmonary artery pressure during CPB was presented as the possible cause of a case of acute pulmonary edema by Byrick et al. (72). The patient had persistent increases in pulmonary artery pressure during CPB due to inadequate venting of the left ventricle, as a result of aortic incompetence and poor left ventricular function. This was associated with a significant increase in extravascular lung water and calculated intrapulmonary shunt fraction.

Effective left ventricular venting protects the heart and lungs during CPB by reducing hydrostatic pressure in the pulmonary capillary bed. This curtails the transfer of water and electrolytes across the lung by Starling's forces in patients who are already hemodiluted and have a low COP. Increased pulmonary artery pressure is avoided if the heart is adequately vented via the pulmonary artery, right superior pulmonary vein, left atrium, left ventricle, or aortic root.

It is now apparent that inadequate venting of the left ventricle with the concomitant increase in pulmonary hydrostatic is only one of the possible etiologies for the pulmonary hypertension and the increase in pulmonary vascular reactivity that is so commonly seen after CPB. In a rabbit model of severe CPB-induced increased pulmonary vascular resistance, histologic examination showed marked intravascular neutrophil aggregation and vasoconstriction (58). Complement activation and decreased oxygen tension may be mediated by the observed increases in thromboxane release by this neutrophil-laden pulmonary vascular bed (73). Thromboxane has also been proposed as the etiology of the protamine-induced increase in pulmonary pressures (74). Plasma levels of endothelin-1, a potent vasoactive substance, is increased after CPB and has been implicated in the ensuing pulmonary hypertension (75). Probably the most talked about possible etiology for the increased pulmonary artery pressures after CPB has been the reduction of nitric oxide production secondary to pulmonary endothelial dysfunction (76–78). Inhaled nitric oxide has been shown to be an excellent selective pulmonary vasodilator and its use as

a treatment for severe pulmonary hypertension after cardiac surgery continues to gain acceptance (78–86).

Clinical Syndromes of Acute Lung Injury

Noncardiogenic Pulmonary Edema

Pathophysiology

Fulminant noncardiogenic pulmonary edema after CPB is an infrequent but life-threatening event, occurring in less than 1% of cases but associated with a mortality rate of 30% to 50% (87,88). After Llamas et al. (89) reported ARDS after CPB, Olinger et al. (90) described four patients who experienced severe ARDS and peripheral vascular collapse after an otherwise uneventful CPB. Culliford et al. (91) presented three successfully treated cases in which fulminant pulmonary edema manifested within 6 hours of uneventful CPB. Since then, multiple reports have appeared in the literature which have attempted to postulate the etiology and define the therapy for this syndrome.

Noncardiogenic pulmonary edema occurs when the permeability characteristics of the alveolar capillary membrane are dramatically altered, creating a capillary leak syndrome with net migration of water and protein into the alveolar space. In its most dramatic form, it presents as the acute onset of a massive outpouring of proteinaceous fluid from the endotracheal tube. This is associated with an increase in intraalveolar fluid, pulmonary vascular resistance, intrapulmonary shunt, and hypoxemia. C_L is markedly decreased. Diffuse bilateral infiltrates are seen on chest radiograph. Noncardiogenic pulmonary edema is distinguished from cardiac failure by the finding of normal or low left atrial or pulmonary artery wedge pressures and a high protein concentration in the edema fluid (albumin concentration is 90% or greater than that of serum albumin).

The most important etiologic factor is complement activation, which has been previously discussed. Noncardiogenic pulmonary edema probably occurs more often with the administration of blood products and fresh frozen plasma after CPB than during CPB itself (92–94). Although the exact mechanism of this process is unclear, antileukocyte antibodies have been isolated from both donors and recipients (95,96). The antibodies probably bind to the leukocyte, activate the cell, and result in the release of proteolytic enzymes with subsequent endothelial damage and capillary leak. The antigen-antibody complex may also directly activate complement and complement-mediated injury of the endothelium (48). Protamine-induced noncardiogenic pulmonary edema may be due to an immune-mediated hypersensitivity reaction (type I) to its direct activation of the complement system or by its enhancement of heparin's ability to activate complement (90,97).

Management

The treatment of noncardiogenic pulmonary edema after CPB must take into consideration that enormous amounts of fluid are lost from the intravascular space because of the profound capillary leak syndrome. Hashim et al. (92) pointed out that all three patients who died in their series of nine reactions to fresh frozen plasma after CPB succumbed to low cardiac output syndrome rather than hypoxemia. Even in patients who have diffuse pulmonary edema with a severe intrapulmonary shunt and high $AaDo_2$, aggressive restoration of intravascular volume with red cells, colloid, or crystalloid is required, guided by left ventricular filling pressure monitoring. Pulmonary management consists of positive pressure ventilation with high levels of airway pressure (98,99). This may be provided as volume-controlled ventilation with extrinsic PEEP or pressure-controlled ventilation with inverse inspiratory to expiratory ratio and intrinsic or auto-PEEP. In either event, the goals are to support the FRC, to decrease intrapulmonary shunt, and to wean a high inspired oxygen fraction. Blood transfusion and inotropic support of the cardiovascular system, with calculation of oxygen-derived variables, is necessary to maintain cardiac output and oxygen delivery. Steroid therapy is not indicated. Ultimate resolution involves healing of the injured lung, which is essentially a function of time.

Pilato et al. (100) reported a case of severe ARDS in which conventional treatment was inadequate and venovenous extracorporeal membrane oxygenation was instituted. Because of compromised cardiac function and deteriorating pulmonary function, the patient could not tolerate maximal conventional ventilator support. Extracorporeal membrane oxygenation improved oxygenation, enabling decrease in ventilator support and concomitant increase in cardiac output by minimizing the effects of mechanical ventilation on ventricular function. The increase in cardiac output decreased the intrapulmonary shunt with a further dramatic improvement in oxygenation.

Acute Bronchospasm

Severe bronchospasm during CPB is an unusual event, even though many patients with chronic obstructive pulmonary disease and asthma undergo cardiac surgery.

Case Reports

Tuman and Ivankovich (101) reported three cases of bronchospasm on CPB. None of the patients had a history of asthma. In all cases, expiratory wheezing was heard and it was impossible to deflate the lungs on resumption of ventilation at the end of CPB. The lungs became greatly distended and bulged into the surgical field. Cardiac filling pressures were normal. In two, fiberoptic bronchoscopy was performed, revealing no abnormalities. No patient developed urticaria or erythema. All patients were given bronchodilator therapy (atropine, aminophylline, steroids, epinephrine, and ketamine) plus halothane or isoflurane on CPB; all recovered.

Durant and Joucken (102) reported the remarkable case

of an asthmatic hypertensive patient who was receiving cimetidine 400 mg twice daily for a gastric ulcer. The patient was given 650 mg labetalol intravenously over 15 hours for preoperative control of hypertension and unstable angina. During the first hour of CPB, he was given 14 mg phenylephrine for hypotension (mean arterial pressure of 40 to 45 mm Hg); during rewarming, mean arterial pressure overshot to 150 mm Hg. On cessation of CPB, protracted bronchospasm occurred. Fiberoptic bronchoscopy revealed some mucous plugging and widespread edema. After aminophylline and steroids, the bronchospasm was finally relieved by an infusion of epinephrine. The authors questioned whether cimetidine had decreased labetalol clearance and whether the combination of labetalol-induced beta-blockade and phenylephrine-induced α-adrenergic stimulation caused bronchospasm.

Casella and Humphrey (103) reported severe bronchospasm in the denervated lung of a heart–lung transplant recipient. The recipient had a history of severe exercise-induced asthma and a positive family history. The donor had no history of lung disease. The recipient developed profound airway obstruction in the donor lungs after CPB, with a P_{PK} greater than 100 cm H_2O. The left lung could be inflated but not deflated. Fiberoptic bronchoscopy was negative. Treatment consisted of isoproterenol, steroids, aminophylline, halothane, atropine, and furosemide. This resulted in improvement, but the patient succumbed to a fatal postoperative pneumonia.

Kyosola et al. (104) reported two cases of bronchospasm after CPB. Neither patient had a history of asthma or chronic bronchitis. In their second case, the bulging left lung disrupted the internal mammary graft, leading to a perioperative myocardial infarction, postoperative low cardiac output syndrome, pulmonary embolism, and death.

Etiology of Bronchospasm during Cardiopulmonary Bypass

The most likely cause of fulminant bronchospasm on CPB is activation of human C5a anaphylatoxin by the extracorporeal circuit (66). A number of other potential causes exist. Acute cardiogenic pulmonary edema is frequently associated with bronchospasm ("cardiac asthma"), but there is obvious evidence of elevated left ventricular filling pressures, ventricular dysfunction, and alveolar edema. The cold urticaria syndrome is a rare disorder characterized by the release of histamine on exposure to cold, resulting in laryngospasm, bronchospasm, and hypotension. It may be prevented by pretreatment with H_1 and H_2 blockers. Bronchospasm might occur as a simple exacerbation of preexisting bronchospastic disease or may be triggered by instrumentation, secretions, or cold anesthetic gas in patients with hyperreactive airways, especially after a recent respiratory infection. β-Adrenergic blockade, even with a so-called selective (β_1) antagonist, may induce bronchospasm in susceptible individuals. Allergic reactions to antibiotics or protamine may cause acute bronchospasm in association with other manifestations of a hypersensitivity response, including hypotension, tachycardia, erythema, and urticaria. Drugs that induce histamine release, such as morphine or atracurium, are likely to exacerbate bronchospasm only when given in high doses.

Management of Bronchospasm on Cardiopulmonary Bypass

The most immediate response should be to attempt maximum hand ventilation with 100% oxygen. The anesthesia ventilator will not be able to cope with the rapid inspiratory flow and long expiratory time required to avoid further air trapping. Although bronchospasm may have been induced by CPB, it is important not to attempt to come off CPB—and it may be necessary to go back on CPB—until the severe attack has been broken. The airway should be examined from machine to patient and a suction catheter passed down the endotracheal tube to exclude mechanical obstruction. Blood must be drawn for arterial blood gas analysis because the end-tidal CO_2 will grossly underestimate P_aCO_2. A chest radiograph should be obtained to exclude pneumothorax and identify pulmonary edema. Cardiac asthma is usually accompanied by elevated left atrial and pulmonary artery pressures and pulmonary edema fluid in the endotracheal tube. Fiberoptic bronchoscopy is very helpful in excluding mechanical causes for wheezing, but it may further irritate the airways and exacerbate bronchospasm.

Specific treatment includes administration of β_2 selective agonists (albuterol, metaproterenol) directly into the endotracheal tube by metered dose inhaler. Even with the use of airway adapters, several puffs should be given because less than 15% of the bronchodilator is delivered to the small airways. If this is not effective, small intravenous boluses of epinephrine (5 to 10 μg) may be given, followed by a continuous low-dose infusion (0.01 to 0.02 μg/kg/min). Intravenous lidocaine (1.5 mg/kg) will not reverse an acute attack but should be given to decrease airway hyperreactivity before any airway manipulation.

Other pharmacologic interventions are less likely to be effective. Steroid therapy (e.g., 125 mg methylprednisolone i.v.) takes about 4 to 5 hours for onset of its effect. Ipratropium (Atrovent), an anticholinergic drying agent, is not effective in acute bronchospasm. Ketamine (25 to 150 mg) has bronchodilator activity and potentiates the effect of epinephrine on the airway. Addition of aminophylline, a nonselective phosphodiesterase inhibitor, is unlikely to enhance bronchodilation already achieved with albuterol or epinephrine and has a high risk of toxic effects such as tachydysrythmias, especially in an acidotic hypoxemic milieu. Volatile anesthetic agents are potent bronchodilators and can be used via the anesthesia machine or the pump oxygenator. However, halothane sensitizes the myocardium to catecholamines and there is a high risk of tachydysrythmias; the threshold is significantly lower with isoflurane or enflurane, which have equivalent bronchodilator properties. Combined administration of an H_1 blocker (diphenhydramine) and H_2 blocker (ranitidine) could prevent some hypersensitivity responses but is not indicated for treatment of acute bronchospasm.

Prevention and Treatment of Acute Lung Injury

Blood Filtration

Use of extracorporeal Dacron polyester blood filters decreases lung damage by reducing pulmonary microembolism by microthrombi and by filtering leukocytes and damaged platelets that promote acute inflammatory responses (36–39,105). Filters capable of extracting specific cell types are also now being experimented with. Examination of plasma before and during CPB shows an increase in neutrophil activation and neutrophil adhesion molecule expression. Continuous depletion of leukocyte and platelets with a blood separator during CPB reduced postoperative pulmonary dysfunction (54,106). Leukocyte removal in blood used to prime the bypass pump was found to be protective in patients undergoing repair of ventricular septal defects (107). Leukocyte depletion of the residual blood in the CPB pump at the completion of the bypass before reinfusion also had positive effects on postoperative lung gas exchange (108). A randomized study of 32 patients in Switzerland, however, was unable to demonstrate this beneficial effect in postoperative lung function with the use of continuous leukocyte filtration during CPB (55).

Membrane Oxygenators

Membrane oxygenators avoid potential damage to blood components and plasma proteins caused by gas bubbling. The risk of microembolization, sludging and capillary occlusion, hemolysis, thrombocytopenia, and leukocyte activation, although not overall complement activation, is significantly less than that caused by the bubble oxygenator (52). In a study of 500 patients who were randomly assigned to either membrane or bubble oxygenators for CPB, there were no demonstrable differences in duration of ventilation, intensive care unit stay, or mortality. Although the membrane group had significantly less extravascular lung water and less atelectasis evident on initial postoperative chest x-ray (CXR), the type of oxygenator used for CPB influenced neither intrapulmonary shunting nor clinical outcome (109).

Hemodilution

Hemodilution and avoidance of homologous blood prime during CPB appear to have a protective effect on lung function. One of the benefits of hemodilution may be greater preservation of surfactant. Animals in which a blood-free pump prime was used developed a significantly smaller intrapulmonary shunt than those animals in which homologous blood was used (110).

Avoidance of Pulmonary Vascular Distension

Every effort should be made to avoid left ventricular and pulmonary vascular distension, which results in pulmonary hemorrhage and acute lung injury. Pressure can be decompressed by venting either the left ventricle, left atrium, pulmonary veins, or pulmonary artery (71,72) (See Chapter 6.)

Pharmacologic Protection

Steroids

Intravenous dexamethasone and high-dose methylprednisolone are effective in inhibiting the increase in leukotriene B4 and tissue plasminogen activator after aortic cross-clamp release in patients undergoing CPB (53). However, corticosteroids do not prevent C3a activation or leukocyte elastase release. Boscoe et al. (111) found that women receiving high-dose methylprednisolone had significantly greater complement activation than men. In a study comparing 50 patients with historical control subjects, Coffin et al. (112) administered a single dose of methylprednisolone (30 mg/kg) at the start of anesthesia. Not only did this not confer any improvement on post-CPB lung function or complication rate, but patients receiving steroids did more poorly with regard to blood loss, low cardiac output syndrome, and requirement for postoperative mechanical ventilation.

Prostaglandins

Vasodilator prostaglandins such as PGE_1 may actually be more protective on CPB than corticosteroids, with greater inhibition of intravascular pulmonary leukocyte aggregation, activation, and free radical production (113). PGE_1 increases cyclic AMP formation, which stabilizes leukocyte lysosomes. PGE_1, prostacyclin, and Iloprost (a more stable prostacyclin analogue) have been infused during CPB to prevent platelet aggregation, thromboxane release, and decrease operative bleeding (114,115). However, use of these agents is somewhat limited by their hypotensive effect, and it is not clear whether their platelet-sparing actions also protect against acute lung injury on CPB. PGI_2, a known platelet inhibitor, was shown to prevent occlusive fibrin, leukocyte, and platelet-based aggregates in pulmonary arterioles in dogs without significant hypotension (116).

Aprotinin (Trasylol)

Aprotinin (Trasylol) is a naturally occurring 58-amino acid polypeptide that inhibits serine proteases such as plasmin and kallikrein (117). It has been known for a number of years that aprotinin infusion prevents the activation of ki-

ninogen and the formation of bradykinin on CPB (118). When CPB lasts longer than 60 minutes, the amounts of bradykinin released (4.6 to 18.0 ng/mL) are sufficient to increase capillary permeability and decrease peripheral vascular resistance and may thereby increase extravascular lung water and lung dysfunction. Kallikrein activates leukocytes to release free oxygen radicals. In exploring the possibility that infusion of high-dose aprotinin during CPB might prevent acute lung injury, Royston et al. (119) serendipitously found a dramatic reduction in surgical blood loss during the procedure. The primary mechanisms appear to be prevention of platelet aggregation and inhibition of fibrinolysis. The antifibrinolytic and hemostatic properties of aprotinin in the reduction of operative bleeding during cardiac and liver surgery have subsequently received a great deal of attention (120–124).

O'Brian et al. (125) found that aprotinin was able to attenuate bradykinin-induced increases in vascular permeability in rats. This effect itself was attenuated when platelets or neutrophils were depleted; they postulated that the maintenance of platelets and neutrophils after CPB might enhance the protective effects of aprotinin.

In investigating possible mechanisms for aprotinin's anti-inflammatory effects, Hill et al. (126) conducted numerous experiments in patients undergoing CPB and with cultured murine lung epithelial cells. They postulated that one mechanism of aprotinin's anti-inflammatory effects might be via moderation of the cytokine-induced form of nitric oxide synthase. *In vivo*, aprotinin was able to decrease lung nitric oxide production, whereas *in vitro* it reduced cytokine-induced nitric oxide synthase expression. In another study, Hill et al. (127) showed aprotinin able to blunt IL-8 production, which in turn reduced lung neutrophil accumulation after CPB. Aprotinin was also effective in blunting CPB-induced systemic tumor necrosis factor-alpha release and the neutrophil surface adhesive glycoprotein integrin CD11b upregulation (128).

EFFECTS OF CARDIOPULMONARY BYPASS ON LUNG METABOLIC FUNCTION

The lung plays an important function in the uptake and release of vasoactive substances. Because the lung is the only organ that receives the entire circulation, it is uniquely suited to this function. The lung is an important site for both activation and inactivation of prostaglandins. Prostacyclin (PGI_2) is primarily synthesized and released by pulmonary vascular endothelium, although it is not metabolized by the lungs. Prostaglandins of the E and F class are almost completely metabolized in a single passage through the lungs. An enzyme located in pulmonary endothelial cells converts the relatively inactive polypeptide, angiotensin I, to the potent vasoconstrictor and aldosterone stimulator, angiotensin II. The lung also inactivates circulating serotonin (5-hydroxy tryptamine) and bradykinin and participates in the uptake of norepinephrine to some degree.

Pitt et al. (129) hypothesized that systemic hypertension after CPB is caused by depressed clearance of neurohumoral substances, particularly norepinephrine, by the damaged lung after CPB. Their data suggest that the diminution in the lung's ability to remove norepinephrine from the circulation was directly related to the duration of CPB. This is supported by a recent study in which awake goats were supported for up to 336 hours on CPB. The arterial levels of prostaglandin E_2 and norepinephrine, which are both inactivated in the pulmonary circulation, increased significantly (130). Claremont and Branthwaite (131) measured the activity of angiotensin-converting enzyme and α_1-antitrypsin, a protease inhibitor thought to exert a protective effect on pulmonary tissue by inactivating proteases and elastases liberated from leukocytes and macrophages. Angiotensin-converting enzyme activity declined after CPB, possibly due to pulmonary damage. Decreased pulmonary extraction of serotonin after CPB may also play a role in postoperative pulmonary complications (132).

Evidence shows that the lungs play a role in coagulation under normal and abnormal conditions. There are a large number of mast cells containing heparin in the interstitium of the lung. The lung is able to secrete immunoglobulins in the bronchial mucus, which contribute to defense against infection. The effects of CPB on these functions have not been studied.

KEY POINTS

- The lung is a target organ for injury induced by CPB.
  - Atelectasis
  - Smoking, chronic bronchitis, chronic obstructive pulmonary disease, and obesity all predispose patients to atelectasis.
  - Atelectasis decreases oxygenation and C_L.
- Acute lung injury
  - Lung injury related to CPB and microemboli is decreased by blood filtration.
  - Complement activation correlates with lung dysfunction after CPB.
  - Inflammatory response produced by "contact activation" of blood (activation of neutrophils and endothelium, generation of complement and cytokines) contributes to lung injury after CPB.
- Noncardiogenic pulmonary edema is rare but has a high mortality rate, is most commonly associated with complement activation and protamine, and is treated by volume expansion, mechanical ventilation, and cardiac support.

- Acute bronchospasm
  - Acute bronchospasm is related to complement activation.
  - Cold urticaria can be treated with H_1 and H_2 blockade.
  - Inaccuracy of $EtCO_2$
- Prevention of lung injury is by:
  - Blood filtration
  - Membrane oxygenators
  - Hemodilution
  - Pharmacology, such as steroids (controversial), prostaglandins (i.e., leukocyte and platelet inhibition), and aprotinin (inhibits plasmin, kallikrein, bradykinin).
- Exclusion of lung circulation during CPB impairs normal metabolic functions, such as clearance of prostaglandins, serotonin, bradykinin, and norepinephrine and generation of prostaglandins and angiotensin.

APPENDIX 1

Gas Exchange

Dead space to tidal volume ratio (V_D/V_T) is calculated by the Bohr equation:

$$V_D/V_T = P_aCO_2 - P_ECO_2 \div P_aCO_2$$

where P_aCO_2 is arterial CO_2 tension and P_ECO_2 is mixed expired CO_2 tension.

Normal V_D/V_T is 0.3.

Lung Mechanics

Lung impedance describes the pressures required to effect flow and volume. These include the pressure to effect flow through the major conducting airways, which is dependent on R_{AW}, and the pressure to distend the lungs, which is dependent on C_L.

R_{AW} (cm $H_2O/L/s$) is determined by dividing the difference between peak and plateau airway pressure by air flow in L/s:

$$R_{AW} = peak - plateau\ pressure \div flow\ rate$$

Conductance (G) is the reciprocal of resistance:

$$G_{AW} = 1 \div R_{AW}$$

C_L reflects lung stiffness and expresses the volume of lung expanded per unit transpulmonary pressure applied. C_L (mL/cm H_2O) is determined by dividing the exhaled tidal volume by the difference between plateau airway pressure and end-expiratory pressure:

$$C_L = exhaled\ volume \div plateau\ pressure \\ - end\text{-}expiratory\ pressure$$

However, unless the patient is paralyzed, the pressure required to distend the chest wall is significant. Because the lung and chest wall are mechanically in series,

$$C_{TH} = C_L + C_{CW}$$

where C_{TH}, C_L, and C_{CW} are the thoracic, lung, and chest wall compliances, respectively.

Elastance (E) is the reciprocal of compliance:

$$E_L = 1 \div C_L$$

"Dynamic" compliance (C_{DYN}) is a term used, somewhat inappropriately, to describe the relationship between exhaled tidal volume and P_{PK}:

$$C_{DYN} = \text{exhaled tidal volume} \div P_{PK}$$

It cannot therefore distinguish between alterations in impedance due to airway resistance or C_L.

REFERENCES

1. Pennock J, Pierce W, Waldhausen J. The management of the lungs during cardiopulmonary bypass. *Surg Gynecol Obstet* 1977;145:917–927.
2. Phang P, Keough K. Inhibition of pulmonary surfactant by plasma from normal adults and from patients having cardiopulmonary bypass. *J Thorac Cardiovasc Surg* 1986;91:248–251.
3. Mandelbaum I, Giammona S. Extracorporeal circulation, pulmonary compliance and pulmonary surfactant. *J Thorac Cardiovasc Surg* 1964;48:881–889.
4. Stanley T, Liu W-S, Gentry S. Effects of ventilatory techniques during cardiopulmonary bypass on post-bypass and postoperative pulmonary compliance and shunt. *Anesthesiology* 1977;46:391–395.
5. Macnaughton PD, Evans TW. The effect of exogenous surfactant therapy on lung function following cardiopulmonary bypass. *Chest* 1994;105:421–425.
6. Haslam PL, Baker CS, Hughes DA, et al. Pulmonary surfactant composition early in the development of acute lung injury after cardiopulmonary bypass: prophylactic use of surfactant therapy. *Int J Exp Pathol* 1997;78:277–289.
7. Lindholm C, Ollman B, Snyder J, et al. Flexible fiberoptic bronchoscopy in critical care medicine; diagnosis, therapy and complications. *Crit Care Med* 1974;2:250–261.
8. Sladen R, Jenkins L. Intermittent mandatory ventilation and controlled mechanical ventilation without positive end-expiratory pressure following cardiopulmonary bypass. *Can Anaesth Soc J* 1978;25:166–172.
9. Osborn J, Popper R, Keith W, et al. Respiratory insufficiency following open heart surgery. *Ann Surg* 1962;156:638.
10. Hedley-Whyte J, Corning H, Lauer M, et al. Pulmonary ventilation-perfusion relations after heart valve replacement or repair in man. *J Clin Invest* 1965;44:406.
11. Geha AS, Sessler AD, Kirklin JW. Alveolar-arterial oxygen gradients after open intracardiac surgery. *J Thorac Cardiovasc Surg* 1966;51:609–615.
12. Ghia J, Andersen N. Pulmonary function and cardiopulmonary bypass. *JAMA* 1970;212:593–597.
13. Barat G, DeVillota E, Avello F, et al. A study of the oxygenation of cardiac patients submitted to extracorporeal circulation. *Br J Anaesth* 1972;44:817–825.
14. Turnbull K, Miyagishima R, Gerein A. Pulmonary complica-
tions and cardiopulmonary bypass. A clinical study in adults. *Can Anaesth Soc J* 1974;21:181.
15. Dobbinson T, Miller J. Respiratory and cardiovascular responses to PEEP in artificially ventilated patients after cardiopulmonary bypass surgery. *Anaesth Intens Care* 1981;9:307–313.
16. Downs J, Mitchell L. Pulmonary effects of ventilatory pattern following cardiopulmonary bypass. *Crit Care Med* 1976;4:295–300.
17. Garzon A, Seltzer B, Karlson K. Respiratory mechanics following open-heart surgery for acquired valvular disease. *Circulation* 1966;33:57–64.
18. Lesage A, Tsuchioka H, Young W, et al. Pathogenesis of pulmonary damage during extracorporeal circulation. *Arch Surg* 1966;93:1002–1008.
19. Shimizu T, Lewis F. An experimental study of pulmonary function following cardiopulmonary bypass. *J Thorac Cardiovasc Surg* 1966;52:565–570.
20. Garzon A, Seltzer B, Lichtenstein S, et al. Influence of open-heart surgery on respiratory work. *Dis Chest* 1967;52:392–396.
21. Andersen N, Ghia J. Pulmonary function, cardiac status, and postoperative course in relation to cardiopulmonary bypass. *J Thorac Cardiovasc Surg* 1970;59:474–483.
22. Sullivan S, Patterson R, Malm J, et al. Effect of heart-lung bypass on the mechanics of breathing in man. *J Thorac Cardiovasc Surg* 1966;51:205–212.
23. Deal C, Osborn J, Miller CJ, et al. Pulmonary compliance in congenital heart disease and its relation to cardiopulmonary bypass. *J Thorac Cardiovasc Surg* 1968;55:320–327.
24. Karlson K, Saklad M, Paliotta J, et al. Computerized on-line analysis of pulmonary mechanics in patients undergoing cardiopulmonary bypass. *Bull Soc Int Chir* 1975;2:121–124.
25. Magnusson L, Zemgulis V, Tenling A, et al. Use of a vital capacity maneuver to prevent atelectasis after cardiopulmonary bypass: an experimental study. *Anesthesiology* 1998;88:134–142.
26. Ellis EL, Brown A, Osborn JJ, et al. Effect of altered ventilation patterns on compliance during cardiopulmonary bypass. *Anesth Analg* 1969;48:947–952.
27. Berry CB, Butler PJ, Myles PS. Lung management during cardiopulmonary bypass: is continuous positive airways pressure beneficial? *Br J Anaesth* 1993;71:864–868.
28. Cogliati AA, Menichetti A, Tritapepe L, et al. Effects of three techniques of lung management on pulmonary function during cardiopulmonary bypass. *Acta Anaesth Belg* 1996;47:73–80.
29. Weedn R, Coalson J, Greenfield L. Effects of oxygenation and ventilation on pulmonary mechanics and ultrastructure during cardiopulmonary bypass. *Am J Surg* 1970;120:584–590.
30. Hewson J, Shaw M. Continuous airway pressure with oxygen minimizes the metabolic lesion of "pump lung." *Can Anaesth Soc J* 1983;30:37–47.
31. Hemmer M, Suter P. Treatment of cardiac and renal effects of PEEP with dopamine in patients with acute respiratory failure. *Anesthesiology* 1979;50:399–403.
32. Venus B, Mathru M, Smith R, et al. Renal function during application of positive end-expiratory pressure in swine: effects of hydration. *Anesthesiology* 1985;62:765–769.
33. Dodrill F. The effects of total body perfusion upon the lungs. In Allen JG, ed. *Extracorporeal circulation*. Springfield, IL: Charles C Thomas, 1958:327–335.
34. Asada S, Yamaguchi M. Fine structural changes in the lung following cardiopulmonary bypass. *Chest* 1971;59:478–483.
35. Jevevien E, Weiss D. Platelet microemboli associated with massive blood transfusion. *Am J Pathol* 1964;45:313–321.
36. Allardyce D, Yoshida S, Ashmore P. The importance of mi-

croembolism in the pathogenesis of organ dysfunction caused by prolonged use of the pump oxygenator. *J Thorac Cardiovasc Surg* 1966;52:706–715.

37. Hill J, Osborn J, Swank R. Experience using a new Dacron wool filter during extracorporeal circulation. *Arch Surg* 1970; 101:649–652.

38. Ashmore P, Swank R, Gallery R, et al. Effect of Dacron wool filtration on the microemboli phenomenon in extracorporeal circulation. *J Thorac Cardiovasc Surg* 1972;63:240–248.

39. Connell R, Page S, Bartley T, et al. The effect on pulmonary ultrastructure of Dacron wool filtration during cardiopulmonary bypass. *Ann Thorac Surg* 1973;15:217–229.

40. Hodge AJ, Dymock RB, Sutherland HD. A case of fatal fat embolism syndrome following cardiopulmonary bypass. *J Thorac Cardiovasc Surg* 1976;72:202–205.

41. Swank R. Alteration of blood on storage: measurement of adhesiveness of "aging" platelets and leukocytes and their removal by filtration. *N Engl J Med* 1961;265:728.

42. Craddock PR, Fehr J, Brigham KL, et al. Complement and leukocyte-medicated pulmonary dysfunction in hemodialysis. *N Engl J Med* 1977;296:769–774.

43. Fountain S, Martin B, Musclow E, et al. Pulmonary leukostatis and its relationship to pulmonary dysfunction in sheep and rabbits. *Circ Res* 1980;46:175–180.

44. Roitt I, Brostoff J, Male D. *Immunology.* St Louis, MO: C.V. Mosby, pp 7–14

45. Chenoweth DE, Cooper SW, Hugli TE, et al. Complement activation during cardiopulmonary bypass: evidence for generation of C3a and C5a anaphylotoxins. *N Engl J Med* 1981;304: 497–502.

46. Braude S, Nolop K, Fleming J, et al. Increased pulmonary transvascular protein flux after canine cardiopulmonary bypass. Association with lung neutrophil sequestration and tissue peroxidation. *Am Rev Respir Dis* 1986;134:867–872.

47. Perkowski, et al. *Circ Res* 53;576.

48. Hammerschmidt D, Jacob H. Adverse pulmonary reactions to transfusion. *Adv Intern Med* 1982;27:511–530.

49. Howard R, Crain C, Franzini D, et al. Effects of cardiopulmonary bypass on pulmonary leukostatis and complement activation. *Arch Surg* 1988;123:1496–1501.

50. Collett B, Alhaz A, Abdullah A, et al. Pathways of complement activation during CPB. *Br Med J* 1984;289:1251–1254.

51. Westaby S. Complement and the damaging effects of cardiopulmonary bypass. *Thorax* 1983;38:321–325.

51A. Tonz M, Mihaljevic T, von Segesser LK, et al. Acute lung injury during cardiopulmonary bypass. Are the neutrophils responsible? *Chest* 1995 Dec;108(6):1551–1556.

52. Van Oeveren W, Kazatchkine M, Descamps-Latscha B, et al. Deleterious effect of cardiopulmonary bypass. A prospective study of bubble versus membrane oxygenation. *J Thorac Cardiovasc Surg* 1985;89:888–899.

53. Jansen NJ, van OW, van VM, et al. The role of different types of corticosteroids on the inflammatory mediators in cardiopulmonary bypass. *Eur J Cardiothorac Surg* 1991;5:211–217.

54. Hachida M, Hanayama N, Okamura T, et al. The role of leukocyte depletion in reducing injury to myocardium and lung during cardiopulmonary bypass. *ASAIO J* 1995;41:M291–M294.

55. Mihaljevic T, Tonz M, von Segesser LK, et al. The influence of leukocyte filtration during cardiopulmonary bypass on postoperative lung function. A clinical study. *J Thorac Cardiovasc Surg* 1995;109:1138–1145.

56. Erez E, Erman A, Snir E, et al. Thromboxane production in human lung during cardiopulmonary bypass: beneficial effect of aspirin? *Ann Thorac Surg* 1998;65:101–106.

57. Friedman M, Wang SY, Selke FW, et al. Pulmonary injury after total or partial cardiopulmonary bypass with thromboxane synthesis inhibition. *Ann Thorac Surg* 1995;59:598–603.

58. Cave AC, Manche A, Derias NW, et al. Thromboxane A_2 mediates pulmonary hypertension after cardiopulmonary bypass in the rabbit. *J Thorac Cardiovasc Surg* 1993;106:959–967.

59. Watkins W, Peterson M, Kong D, et al. Thromboxane and prostacyclin changes during cardiopulmonary bypass with and without pulsatile flow. *J Thorac Cardiovasc Surg* 1982;84: 250–256.

60. Nathan N, Denizot Y, Cornu E, et al. Cytokine and lipid mediator blood concentrations after coronary artery surgery. *Anesth Analg* 1997;85:1240–1246.

61. Kawahito K, Kawakami M, Fujiwara T, et al. Proinflammatory cytokine levels in patients undergoing cardiopulmonary bypass. Does lung reperfusion influence the release of cytokines? *ASAIO J* 1995;41:M775–M778.

62. Steinberg JB, Kapelanski DP, Olson JD, et al. Cytokine and complement levels in patients undergoing cardiopulmonary bypass. *J Thorac Cardiovasc Surg* 1993;106:1008–1016.

63. Frering B, Philip I, Dehoux M, et al. Circulating cytokines in patients undergoing normothermic cardiopulmonary bypass. *J Thorac Cardiovasc Surg* 1994;108:636–641.

64. Kawamura T, Wakusawa R, Okada K, et al. Elevation of cytokines during open heart surgery with cardiopulmonary bypass: participation of interleukin 8 and 6 in reperfusion injury. *Can J Anaesth* 1993;40:1016–1021.

65. Ashraf S, Butler J, Tian Y, et al. Inflammatory mediators in adults undergoing cardiopulmonary bypass: comparison of centrifugal and roller pumps. *Ann Thorac Surg* 1998;65:480–484.

66. Chenoweth DE. The properties of human C5a anaphylatoxin. The significance of C5a formation during hemodialysis. *Contrib Nephrol* 1987;59:51–71.

67. Mandelbaum I, Giammona S. Bronchial circulation during cardiopulmonary bypass. *Ann Surg* 1966;164:985–989.

68. Loer SA, Scheeren TW, Tarnow J. How much oxygen does the human lung consume? *Anesthesiology* 1997;86:532–537.

69. Balis JU, Cox WD, Pifarre R, et al. The role of pulmonary hypoxia in the post- perfusion lung syndrome. *Surg Forum* 1969;20:205–207.

70. Nahas R, Melrose D, Sykes M, et al. Postperfusion lung syndrome, role of circulatory exclusion. *Lancet* 1965;2:251–253.

71. Kolff WJ, Effler DB, Groves LK, et al. Pulmonary complications of open-heart operations: their pathogenesis and avoidance. *Cleve Clin Q* 1958;25:65–83.

72. Byrick R, Finlayson D, Noble W. Pulmonary arterial pressure increases during cardiopulmonary bypass, a potential cause of pulmonary edema. *Anesthesiology* 1977;46:433–435.

73. Smith WJ, Murphy MP, Appleyard RF, et al. Prevention of complement-induced pulmonary hypertension and improvement of right ventricular function by selective thromboxane receptor antagonism. *J Thorac Cardiovasc Surg* 1994;107: 800–806.

74. Sugi K, Esato K. Effect of a thromboxane synthetase inhibitor on protamine-induced circulatory changes in sheep. *Surgery* 1993;114:586–590.

75. Kirshbom PM, Tsui SS, DiBernardo LR, et al. Blockade of endothelium-converting enzyme reduces pulmonary hypertension after cardiopulmonary bypass and circulatory arrest. *Surgery* 1995;118:440–444.

76. Seghaye MC, Duchateau J, Bruniaux J, et al. Endogenous nitric oxide production and atrial natriuretic peptide biological activity in infants undergoing cardiac operations. *Crit Care Med* 1997;25:1063–1070.

77. Morita K, Ihnken K, Buckberg GD, et al. Pulmonary vasoconstriction due to impaired nitric oxide production after cardiopulmonary bypass. *Ann Thorac Surg* 1996;61:1775–1780.

78. Kirshbom PM, Jacobs MT, Tsui SS, et al. Effects of cardiopulmonary bypass and circulatory arrest on endothelium-dependent vasodilation in the lung. *J Thorac Cardiovasc Surg* 1996; 111:1248–1256.

79. Bender KA, Alexander JA, Enos JM, et al. Effects of inhaled nitric oxide in patients with hypoxemia and pulmonary hypertension after cardiac surgery. *Am J Crit Care* 1997;6:127–131.

80. Bichel T, Spahr-Schopfer I, Berner M, et al. Successful weaning from cardiopulmonary bypass after cardiac surgery using inhaled nitric oxide. *Paediatr Anaesth* 1997;7:335–339.

81. Beghetti M, Habre W, Friedli B, et al. Continuous low dose inhaled nitric oxide for treatment of severe pulmonary hypertension after cardiac surgery in paediatric patients. *Br Heart J* 1995; 73:65–68.

82. Tonz M, von Segesser LK, Schilling J, et al. Treatment of acute pulmonary hypertension with inhaled nitric oxide. *Ann Thorac Surg* 1994;58:1031–1035.

83. Snow DJ, Gray SJ, Ghosh S, et al. Inhaled nitric oxide in patients with normal and increased pulmonary vascular resistance after cardiac surgery. *Br J Anaesth* 1994;72:185–189.

84. Schranz D, Huth R, Wippermann CF, et al. Nitric oxide and prostacyclin lower suprasystemic pulmonary hypertension after cardiopulmonary bypass. *Eur J Pediatr* 1993;152:793–796.

85. Wessel DL. Inhaled nitric oxide for the treatment of pulmonary hypertension before and cardiopulmonary bypass. *Crit Care Med* 1993;21:S344–S345.

86. Rich GF, Murphy GDJ, Roos CM, et al. Inhaled nitric oxide. Selective pulmonary vasodilation in cardiac surgical patients. *Anesthesiology* 1993;78:1028–1035.

87. Fowler A, Baird M, Eberle D, et al. Attack rates and mortality of the adult respiratory distress syndrome in patients with known predispositions. *Am Rev Respir Dis* 1983;125:77.

88. Hashim S, Kay H, Hammond G, et al. Noncardiogenic pulmonary edema after cardiopulmonary bypass: an anaphylactic reaction to fresh frozen plasma. *Am J Surg* 1984;147:560–564.

89. Llamas R, Forthman H. Respiratory distress in the adult after cardiopulmonary bypass. A successful therapeutic approach. *JAMA* 1973;225:1183–1186.

90. Olinger G, Becker R, Bonchek L. Noncardiogenic pulmonary edema and peripheral vascular collapse following cardiopulmonary bypass. Rare protamine reaction? *Ann Thorac Surg* 1980; 29:20–25.

91. Culliford A, Thomas S, Spencer F. Fulminating non-cardiogenic pulmonary edema. *J Thorac Cardiovasc Surg* 1980;80: 868–875.

92. Hashim SW, Kay HR, Hammond GL, et al. Noncardiogenic pulmonary edema after cardiopulmonary bypass. An anaphylactic reaction to fresh frozen plasma. *Am J Surg* 1984;147: 560–564.

93. Popovsky M, Moore S. Diagnostic and pathogenetic considerations in transfusion-related acute lung injury. *Transfusion* 1984; 24:433.

94. Latson T, Kickler T, Baumgarter W. Pulmonary hypertension and non-cardiogenic pulmonary edema following cardiopulmonary bypass associated with antigranulocyte antibody. *Anesthesiology* 1986;64:106–111.

95. Levy G, Shabot M, Hart M, et al. Transfusion associated non-cardiogenic pulmonary edema. *Transfusion* 1986;26:278–281.

96. Ward H. Pulmonary infiltrates associated with leukoagglutinin transfusion reactions. *Ann Intern Med* 1970;73:689–694.

97. Best N, Teisner B, Grudzinkas J, et al. Classical pathway activation during an adverse response to protamine sulphate. *Br J Anaesth* 1983;55:1149–1153.

98. Lloyd J, Newman J, Brigham K. Permeability pulmonary edema: diagnosis and management. *Arch Intern Med* 1984;144: 143–147.

99. Maggart M, Stewart S. The mechanisms and management of non-cardiogenic pulmonary edema following cardiopulmonary bypass. *Ann Thorac Surg* 1987;43:231–236.

100. Pilato M, FLeming N, Katz N, et al. Treatment of non-cardiogenic pulmonary edema following cardiopulmonary bypass with veno-venous extracorporeal membrane oxygenation. *Anesthesiology* 1988;69:609–614.

101. Tuman KJ, Ivankovich AD. Bronchospasm during cardiopulmonary bypass. Etiology and management. *Chest* 1986;90: 635–637.

102. Durant P, Joucken K. Bronchospasm and hypotension during cardiopulmonary bypass after preoperative cimetidine and labetolol therapy. *Br J Anaesth* 1984;56:917–920.

103. Casella ES, Humphrey LS. Bronchospasm after cardiopulmonary bypass in a heart-lung transplant recipient. *Anesthesiology* 1988;69:135–138.

104. Kyosola K, Takkunen O, Maamies T, et al. Bronchospasm during cardiopulmonary bypass—a potentially fatal complication of open-heart surgery. *Thorac Cardiovasc Surgeon* 1987;35: 375–377.

105. Osborn J, Swank R. Experience using a new dacron wool filter during extracorporeal circulation. *Arch Surg* 1970;101: 649–652.

106. Morioka K, Muraoka R, Chiba Y, et al. Leukocyte and platelet depletion with a blood cell separator: effects on lung injury after cardiac surgery with cardiopulmonary bypass. *J Thorac Cardiovasc Surg* 1996;111:45–54.

107. Komai H, Naito Y, Fujiwara K, et al. The protective effect of a leukocyte removal filter on the lung in open-heart surgery for ventricular septal defect. *Perfusion* 1998;13:27–34.

108. Gu YJ, de Vries AJ, Boonstra PW, et al. Leukocyte depletion results in improved lung function and reduced inflammatory response after cardiac surgery. *J Thorac Cardiovasc Surg* 1996; 112:494–500.

109. Reeve WG, Ingram SM, Smith DC. Respiratory function after cardiopulmonary bypass: a comparison of bubble and membrane oxygenators. *J Cardiothorac Vasc Anesth* 1994;8:502–508.

110. Nahas RA, Melrose DG, Sykes MK, et al. Postperfusion lung syndrome: effect of homologous blood. *Lancet* 1965;2: 254–257.

111. Boscoe MJ, Yewdall VM, Thompson MA, et al. Complement activation during cardiopulmonary bypass: quantitative study of effects of methylprednisolone and pulsatile flow. *Br Med J* 1983;287:1747–1750.

112. Coffin LH, Shinozaki T, DeMeules JE, et al. Ineffectiveness of methylprednisolone in the treatment of pulmonary dysfunction after cardiopulmonary bypass. *Am J Surg* 1975;130:555–559.

113. Bolanowski PJ, Bauer J, Machiedo G, et al. Prostaglandin influence on pulmonary intravascular leukocytic aggregation during cardiopulmonary bypass. *J Thorac Cardiovasc Surg* 1977;73: 221–224.

114. Addonizio V, Fisher C, Jenkin B, et al. Iloprost (ZK36374), a stable analogue of prostacyclin, preserves platelets during simulated extracorporeal circulation. *J Thorac Cardiovasc Surg* 1985; 89:926–933.

115. Fish K, Sarnquist F, Van Steennis C, et al. A prospective, randomized study of the effects of prostacyclin on platelets and blood loss during coronary bypass operations. *J Thorac Cardiovasc Surg* 1986;91:436–442.

116. Fessatidis IT, Brannan JJ, Taylor KM, et al. Effect of prostacyclin PGI$_2$ on cardiopulmonary bypass-induced lung injury. *Perfusion* 1994;9:23–33.

117. Royston D. High-dose aprotinin therapy: a review of the first five years' experience. *J Cardiothorac Vasc Anesth* 1992;6: 76–100.

118. Nagaoka H, Yamada T, Hatano R, et al. Clinical significance

of bradykinin liberation during cardiopulmonary bypass and its prevention by a kallikrein inhibitor. *Jpn J Surg* 1975;5:222–233.

119. Royston D, Bidstrup B, Taylor K, et al. Effect of aprotinin on the need for blood transfusion after repeat open heart surgery. *Lancet* 1987;2:1289–1291.

120. Bidstrup BP, Royston D, Sapsford RN, et al. Reduction in blood loss and blood use after cardiopulmonary bypass with high dose aprotinin (Trasylol). *J Thorac Cardiovasc Surg* 1989; 97:364–372.

121. Bo L, Belboul A, al KN, et al. High-dose aprotinin (Trasylol) in reducing bleeding and protecting lung function in potential bleeders undergoing cardiopulmonary bypass. *Chin Med J* 1991; 104:980–985.

122. Deleuze P, Loisance DY, Feliz A, et al. Reduction of per- and postoperative blood loss with aprotinin (Trasylol) during extra-corporeal circulation. *Arch Mal Coeur Vaiss* 1991;84: 1797–1802.

123. Havel M, Teufelsbauer H, Knobl P, et al. Effect of intraoperative aprotinin administration on postoperative bleeding in patients undergoing cardiopulmonary bypass operation. *J Thorac Cardiovasc Surg* 1991;101:968–972.

124. Mallett SV, Cox D, Burroughs AK, et al. The intra-operative use of trasylol (aprotinin) in liver transplantation. *Transplant Int* 1991;4:227–230.

125. O'Brian JG, Battistini B, Farmer P, et al. Aprotonin, an antifi-brinolytic drug, attenuates bradykinin-induced permeability in conscious rats via platelets and neutrophils. *Can J Physiol Pharmacol* 1997;75:741–749.

126. Hill GE, Springall DR, Robins RA. Aprotinin is associated with a decrease in nitric oxide production during cardiopulmonary bypass. *Surgery* 1997;121:449–455.

127. Hill GE, Pohorecki R, Alonso A, et al. Aprotinin reduces interleukin-8 production and lung neutrophil accumulation after cardiopulmonary bypass. *Anesth Analg* 1996;83:696–700.

128. Hill GE, Alonso A, Spurzem JR, et al. Aprotinin and methyl-prednisolone equally blunt cardiopulmonary bypass-induced inflammation in humans. *J Thorac Cardiovasc Surg* 1995;110: 1658–1662.

129. Pitt B, Gillis N, Hammond G. Depression of pulmonary metabolic function by cardiopulmonary bypass procedures increases levels of circulating norepinephrine. *J Thorac Surg* 1984;38: 508–613.

130. Eya K, Tatsumi E, Taenaka Y, et al. Importance of metabolic function of the natural lung evaluated by prolonged exclusion of pulmonary circulation. *ASAIO J* 1996;42:M805–M809.

131. Claremont D, Branthwaite M. Metabolic indices of pulmonary damage. *Anaesthesia* 1980;35:863–868.

132. Gillis LN, Greene NM, Cronau LH, et al. Pulmonary extraction of 5-hydroxytryptamine and norepinephrine before and after cardiopulmonary bypass in man. *Circ Res* 1972;30:666.

CARDIOPULMONARY BYPASS
AND THE KIDNEY

V. SIMON ABRAHAM
JULIE A. SWAIN

The kidney is the central organ in regulating body fluid composition, intravascular volume, and excretion of metabolic byproducts. Renal function has been studied extensively in patients undergoing cardiopulmonary bypass (CPB). CPB causes a number of changes in the quantity and distribution of renal blood flow, especially in patients with abnormal renal function. Many physiologic alterations (such as nonpulsatile perfusion, hypothermia, and hemodilution) occur during CPB and may alter renal function. Controversy continues regarding the relative importance of CPB versus predisposing patient factors in causing renal dysfunction after cardiac operations.

The incidence of renal complications in both infant and adult cardiac surgery is reported to be decreasing with improved patient preparation, perfusion techniques, and cardiac performance postoperatively (1–4). Once renal failure is established, however, the mortality rate continues to be over 50% despite supportive care and renal replacement therapy (5–8). In addition, renal dysfunction significantly lengthens hospitalization, length of stay in critical care units, and total medical cost of cardiac surgical procedures (6).

ANATOMY AND PHYSIOLOGY

The basic functional unit of the kidney is the nephron, and each kidney contains over one million of these structures. Anatomically, the kidney is divided into two zones: the cortex, which contains most of the glomeruli, and the medulla, which comprises the collecting system and loops of Henle. The nephron consists of two main structures: a specialized capillary network, the glomerulus, that allows filtration of fluid from plasma devoid of formed cellular components

and plasma proteins and a tubular system that collects the filtered fluid and alters its composition to convert the plasma filtrate to urine (Fig. 19.1) (9).

Blood flowing via the renal artery into the kidney passes through an efferent arteriole to the glomerulus and then exits via an efferent arteriole. Renal blood flow (RBF) accounts for approximately 20% of resting cardiac output. It can be diminished by atherosclerosis of the renal vasculature or increased vasomotor tone due to low cardiac output or in response to administered inotropic agents. The renal vascular bed responds to α-adrenergic stimuli with vasoconstriction that may decrease RBF while maintaining blood pressure. The renal vasculature also contains dopaminergic receptors and is responsive to analogues of atrial natriuretic peptide (ANP), which may specifically alter flow dynamics within the kidney.

Intraglomerular blood pressure (the difference between the pressures in the efferent and afferent arterioles) drives the filtration of fluid through the capillary endothelium and into Bowman's capsule. The endothelium of the glomerulus has a permeability that is 100 times greater than normal capillaries and is perforated by multiple fenestrations, which are approximately 80 Å in diameter. These fenestrations prevent the exodus of formed cellular elements from the blood. Glycoproteins guard these exit points electrostatically, repelling negatively charged plasma proteins from the collecting system. The fluid that enters the tubule is an ultrafiltrate similar in composition to plasma but without significant protein content.

The glomerular filtration rate (GFR) is normally 100 to 200 mL/min in the adult. The GFR is well preserved over a wide range of arterial pressures (Fig. 19.2) by autoregulation of glomerular blood pressure. Over 99% of the volume of glomerular filtrate is reabsorbed during its journey from Bowman's capsule, through the loop of Henle, to the collecting ducts at the pelvis of the renal hilum. The reabsorption of water is by passive osmotic diffusion. Certain substances of nutritional value, such as glucose and amino acids, are reabsorbed by active transport and are almost completely

V. S. Abraham: Children's Heart Center, St. Vincent Hospital, Indianapolis, IN 46260.

J. A. Swain: Department of Surgery and the Gill Heart Institute, University of Kentucky, Lexington, KY 40536-0084.

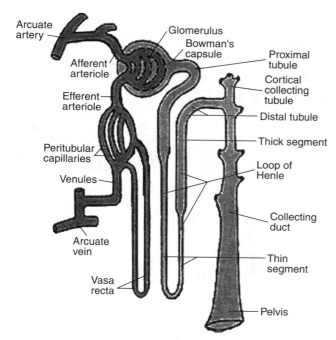

FIG. 19.1. The functional nephron showing the glomerulus through which blood is filtered and the collecting system beginning with Bowman's capsule that collects the ultrafiltrate and converts it into urine. (From Guyton AC. *Human physiology and mechanisms of disease*, 4th ed. Philadelphia: W.B. Saunders, 1987: 703, with permission.)

conserved by their removal from urine. Proteins finding their way into the glomerular filtrate are often too large to be reabsorbed via conventional transport mechanisms. Reclamation occurs by pinocytosis by tubular epithelia cells with subsequent breakdown of the protein into amino acids

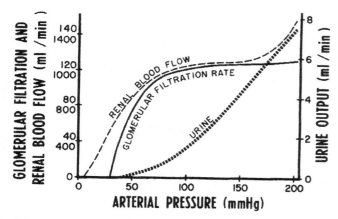

FIG. 19.2. Autoregulation maintains glomerular filtration rate and renal blood flow over a wide range of arterial blood pressures. Urine output, however, is not regulated to allow increased volume excretion as a method of circulatory control. (From Guyton AC. *Human physiology and mechanisms of disease*, 4th ed. Philadelphia: W.B. Saunders, 1987:703, with permission.)

that are returned to the bloodstream. In brief, the nephron filters the plasma and then selectively reabsorbs a significant proportion of the filtrate to produce urine.

Although GFR is autoregulated across a wide range of arterial blood pressures, urine output is not. Urine output (Fig. 19.2) rises in a nearly linear fashion with arterial blood pressure. A rise in arterial blood pressure from 100 to 200 mm Hg will cause a sevenfold increase in urinary output, whereas decreasing blood pressure to 50 mm Hg will cause urine output to nearly cease. The lack of autoregulation of urinary output results in long-term control of blood pressure. As blood pressure rises, urinary output is increased until intravascular volume is depleted and pressure falls to normal levels. The physiologic basis of the relationship between blood pressure and urine output rests both in a slight rise in GFR and more importantly in the rise in peritubular vascular pressures that decreases the reabsorption of filtrate from the tubule.

In addition to filtering the blood and preventing the loss of important substances from the body by reabsorption, the kidney can significantly alter the excretion of water by creating dilute or concentrated urine. The mechanism by which urine concentration is altered rests in the permeability of the distal collecting system and its response to antidiuretic hormone (ADH). Normally, in the absence of ADH, the distal collecting system is impermeable to water, thus preventing its reabsorption and producing dilute urine. However, in response to increasing osmolarity, ADH release increases the permeability of the distal collecting system of the nephron, allowing reabsorption of water and the production of concentrated urine. Thus, the kidney maintains blood volume within a narrow range by selective reabsorption of solute and controls osmolarity by altering water reabsorption and as a result the concentration of urine via its response to ADH. Stress, which occurs with surgical trauma and CPB, dramatically increases the circulating ADH levels (9) independent of osmolarity and may thus affect water balance perioperatively.

INCIDENCE

The incidence of acute renal failure (ARF) requiring dialysis after routine coronary revascularization is approximately 1%. Although length of CPB has been associated with the incidence of ARF, this finding is likely to be associated with more difficult procedures. As the complexity of the cardiac operation increases to include valve replacement and combined coronary and valve procedures, renal dysfunction is more common (2,7,10). These findings probably reflect increased perioperative cardiac dysfunction and the need for postoperative vasoactive drug support, thus resulting in renal hypoperfusion and ischemia.

Patient Factors

The risk of developing renal failure requiring dialysis after cardiac surgery is low. A greater proportion of patients will have transient dysfunction not necessitating dialysis. Most patients who develop new renal dysfunction after cardiac surgery have a number of comorbid conditions, including cardiac failure or diminished renal reserve, diabetes, and peripheral vascular disease (11–13). There is an association between a history of rheumatic fever and renal dysfunction after cardiac valve operations.

Chertow et al. (14) prospectively studied a large group of patients undergoing adult coronary and valve surgery to test the hypothesis that the two major factors responsible for renal dysfunction were renal ischemia due to poor cardiac output or renovascular disease and reduced renal functional reserve. In their cohort of over 42,000 patients, they found an overall incidence of renal failure requiring dialysis to be 1.1%. Using a multivariate analysis, they found several important independent risk factors. Patients undergoing surgery for valvular disease had roughly twice the risk of ARF compared with patients undergoing coronary artery bypass grafting (CABG). Findings suggesting significant reduction in cardiac performance, such as NYHA class IV heart failure, ejection fraction less than 35%, pulmonary rales, and the need for an intraaortic balloon pump, increased the risk of ARF. The incidence of ARF was correlated in an inverse fashion with creatinine clearance. The authors suggested that their finding confirmed that most risk of renal failure was due to poor cardiac output or vascular disease leading to renal ischemia or due to preexisting diminution in renal functional reserve. Interestingly, diabetes mellitus was not an independent risk factor in their analysis.

The Society of Thoracic Surgeons Cardiac Surgery Database (15) documents the incidence of renal failure requiring dialysis as 0.9% for patients undergoing first-time CABG (Fig. 19.3A). The incidence after isolated first-time aortic valve replacement is similar. Approximately 1.9% of patients undergoing mitral valve replacement required dialysis. However, patients requiring combined CABG and mitral valve replacement had an incidence of dialysis of 5.0%. Univariate analysis of the data from the Society of Thoracic Surgeons shows a strong correlation between the need for dialysis and mortality. Patients requiring dialysis had a mortality of between 44.7% and 64%, which was at least a 10-fold increase over patients in which dialysis was not needed (Fig. 19.3B). In a smaller retrospective study, Mangos et al. (7) evaluated the incidence of ARF in the Australian population. They found that ARF developed in 1.1% of patients with normal preoperative renal function but increased to an incidence of 16% in patients with impaired renal function (serum creatinine at least 0.13 mmol/L). In addition, ARF was more likely in patients over 65 years, in cases of valve surgery, and with prolonged CPB times. They

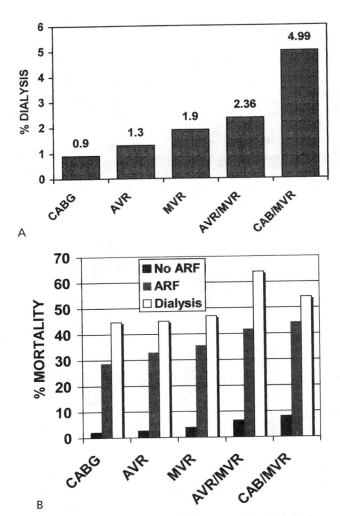

FIG. 19.3. **A:** Incidence of renal failure requiring dialysis rises as the complexity of cardiac operation increases. **B:** Mortality increases with acute renal failure and dialysis-dependent renal failure for all cardiac operations. (From *Data analysis of the STS Cardiac Surgery database.* Chicago: Society of Thoracic Surgeons, 1998, with permission.)

also recorded prolonged length of stay and increased mortality in affected patients.

Mangano et al. (6) studied the incidence of postoperative renal failure after coronary revascularization in a prospective randomized fashion. They found a 1.4% incidence of oliguric renal failure requiring dialysis. Five independent preoperative risk factors were predictive of renal dysfunction: age greater than 70, congestive heart failure, previous myocardial revascularization, diabetes mellitus, and elevated preoperative creatinine. Prolonged CPB times (more than 3 hours) and ventricular dysfunction were perioperative risk factors. Mortality among patients without renal dysfunction was 0.9% with an increase to 63% for patients requiring dialysis. Length of stay in the critical care unit and overall hospital length of stay was increased to 15 and 29 days, respectively, nearly threefold increases over patients without renal problems.

These studies and others suggest preoperative renal dysfunction is the most significant risk factor for postoperative renal failure. In addition, cardiac dysfunction and valvular heart disease increase the risks of developing renal dysfunction. Some studies have found age, diabetes, and peripheral vascular disease to be additional risk factors (6,12). Whether these are independent risk factors or merely proxies for renovascular disease and subclinical preoperative renal dysfunction is not clear.

There are fewer studies evaluating the risks of ARF after surgery in children. This patient population usually does not have underlying renal dysfunction, diabetes, or vascular disease. Picca et al. (16) performed a retrospective case-controlled study over a 10-year period on 2,262 children with a variety of diagnoses. The incidence of ARF requiring peritoneal dialysis was 2.7% and the mortality rate was 79% in patients needing peritoneal dialysis. They found that central venous hypertension, arterial hypotension, and high-dose inotropic support were independent risk factors for ARF consistent with the thesis that the underlying cause of ARF was usually low cardiac output. Preoperative serum creatinine level, cyanosis, and the use of vasodilators were not significant risk factors.

CARDIOPULMONARY BYPASS PROCEDURAL FACTORS

Numerous procedural factors have been associated with post-CPB renal dysfunction. Inherent in most CPB procedures is the use of hemodilution, hypothermia, nonpulsatile perfusion, and, in certain procedures, low flow or circulatory arrest. However, there is little conclusive evidence that modern extracorporeal perfusion per se causes renal dysfunction. Although a number of older studies have suggested that CPB may be harmful, more recent studies have failed to show a clear association between CPB and renal dysfunction (2,10,13,17).

Hemodilution

Hemodilution is thought to increase blood flow and oxygen delivery by reducing blood viscosity, and it produces its most pronounced effect in the microcirculation. The apparent viscosity of blood rises because flow depends on the deformation of blood cells passing through vessels less than 4 μm in diameter. In addition, aggregation of red cells occurs at sites of low shear stress such as postcapillary venules and is attenuated by hemodilution. Both the apparent viscosity of blood and the degree of red cell aggregation are important determinants of blood flow through the microcirculation (18). These phenomena may not be of clinical significance at normal flow rates but become increasingly im-

portant as flow rates are decreased, as they may be during CPB. The oxygen-carrying capacity of blood has a direct linear relationship to hematocrit (hemoglobin concentration), suggesting that hemodilution reduces oxygen transport. However, the viscosity of blood is lowered exponentially by hemodilution (Fig. 19.4) (19). The net result of these two opposing forces is significantly enhanced oxygen delivery to the tissues at all but the extreme of hemodilution.

In addition to enhancement of microcirculatory flow, hemodilution tends to lower afterload and increase venous return to the heart, thereby increasing cardiac output and renal blood flow. Afterload reduction is mediated by decreased shear stress on the arterial side of the circulation. Transfer of interstitial fluid into the vascular space enhances venous return. It may seem counterintuitive that hemodilution should improve the transfer of fluid from the interstitium to the vasculature. However, by reducing the aggregation of red cells in postcapillary venules, the transcapillary gradient is decreased. In this fashion, hemodilution may also decrease the fluid overload often seen in post-CPB patients.

Hemodilution is associated with a significant increase in cardiac output and peripheral vasodilatation. In experimental canine studies, cardiac output increased by 93% with

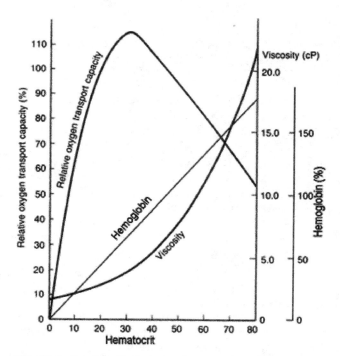

FIG. 19.4. Relationship between hematocrit and oxygen-carrying capacity of blood demonstrating a nonlinear relationship. Because of the inverse relationship between viscosity and blood flow velocity and the exponential relationship between hematocrit and viscosity, optimal oxygen-carrying capacity does not continue to rise for hematocrits above approximately 30%. (From Hint H. The pharmacology of dextran and the physiological background for the clinical use of Rheomacrodex and Macrodex. *Acta Anaesth Belg* 1968;19:119–138, with permission.)

hemodilution when hematocrit was lowered from 51% to 13% (20). Although this increase in output provides increased flow to many end-organ vascular beds, experimental studies suggest that flow to the kidney was not increased with a net decrement in oxygen delivery to the kidney (21).

The composition of the priming solution for CPB is not thought to have a significant effect on renal dysfunction. However, the degree of extracellular fluid accumulation does vary depending on whether the prime is composed purely of crystalloid, colloid, blood, or a combination of these solutions (22). Although the advantage of crystalloid versus colloid volume replacement has been debated for some time without resolution, it is clear that crystalloid prime results in greater interstitial fluid volume when compared with colloid (23,24). A number of studies have looked at prime composition and have found increased organ water content in patients with a crystalloid prime but have found no significant clinical benefit in patients with good ventricular function (25,26). Scott et al. (27) compared albumin, polygeline, and crystalloid prime in patients undergoing CABG and found significantly greater fluid requirements in patients using only crystalloid. The work by Foglia et al. (28) showed a significant increase in myocardial edema when crystalloid prime was used. The authors suggest that in patients with decreased ventricular function, the use of crystalloid prime may lead to increased edema and be detrimental.

Hypothermia

Hypothermia is used to lower end-organ metabolic requirements during CPB. It provides protection for the brain by several mechanisms, including lowering metabolic rate, increasing intracellular pH, and increasing high energy phosphate content (29). This allows decreased perfusion flows during hypothermia. With the introduction of "warm heart surgery," there has been some concern about an increased incidence of renal dysfunction. Initial studies using this method have used warm continuous cardioplegia with high potassium and volume loads, making comparisons difficult.

Several randomized studies have been performed using similar warm perfusion and cardioplegic techniques. Arom et al. (30) found that strokes and renal failure occurred more frequently in patients undergoing adult cardiac procedures at 37°C than at 34°C, but these differences did not reach statistical significance. The normothermic bypass group required significantly greater use of phenylephrine to combat peripheral vasodilatation inherent to this technique. Lehot et al. (31) evaluated the perioperative effects of hypothermic versus normothermic bypass on the kidney in 20 patients undergoing CABG/valve surgery. Patients were randomized to undergo bypass at either 27 or 37°C. There were no differences in plasma renin activity or concentrations of arginine vasopressin or ANP. Urinary output and concentration of sodium, potassium, and urea were similar in both

groups. This study was limited to the day of surgery, and no later data points were reported. Regragui et al. (32) randomized 30 patients undergoing CABG into three groups with perfusion temperatures of 28, 32, and 37°C. They found that creatinine clearance and other indices of renal clearance increased while on bypass at all temperatures and returned to normal after bypass. They concluded that perfusion temperature did not have a lasting influence on renal function. In summary, these studies suggest that hypothermia is not detrimental to renal function.

Pulsatile Perfusion

The effects of nonpulsatile perfusion have been studied extensively both in animal models and in comparison with pulsatile CPB in the clinical situation. Some studies suggest that pulsatile perfusion provides significant advantages over nonpulsatile flow, whereas an equal number of studies show no advantage in using pulsatile flow (33–38). There are, however, no studies showing pulsatile perfusion to be detrimental to renal function. Proponents of pulsatile flow argue that it is more physiologic and point to a body of experimental evidence showing improved microcirculatory flow and cerebral and renal perfusion (39). A large part of the variable results in these studies may be due to differing methodology and experimental conditions (40). Flow produced as a simple sine wave may not deliver the power, differential pressure, or rate of rise of pressure necessary to produce physiologic effects. However, clinical investigations have largely failed to show any significant advantage (34–36). Given the added complexity of providing pulsatile flow and the relative safety of current techniques, it is unlikely that pulsatile flow will become used more frequently.

Oxygenators and Filters

During the era of cardiac surgery when bubble oxygenators were used, patients were found at autopsy to have multiple emboli to the brain, heart, and kidneys. Studies into the source of these emboli found both gaseous and particulate macroemboli were responsible for these phenomena (41–44). With the increased use of membrane oxygenators and arterial line filters, the incidence of emboli and their clinical consequences have decreased greatly. Treasure et al. (45) suggested that arterial filtration should be a standard practice, and currently most centers use both of these adjuncts to reduce embolic load during CPB. The exception to this may be in pediatric cardiac surgical units. Elliot (46) reported that only one third of units use arterial filtration because of the large volumes required to prime the filter.

In summary, although there are multiple experimental and clinical studies suggesting that various procedural aspects of CPB may be detrimental to the kidney, there is no clear consensus that CPB per se causes renal failure clinically. Certainly most patients who develop renal dysfunction postoperatively suffer from preexisting renal disease or have compromised renal perfusion secondary to low cardiac output in the perioperative period. Hemodilution and hypothermia probably have salutary effects on renal perfusion, and there is little evidence that nonpulsatile perfusion is harmful to the kidney.

THERAPY

Although the treatment of established renal failure involves the use of dialysis, there are a number of therapies being evaluated to diminish the incidence of renal failure after CPB. Underlying several of these treatments is the assumption that ARF is caused in large part by renal hypoperfusion created either by low renal perfusion pressures while on CPB or in the perioperative period by renal vasoconstriction in low cardiac output states. Conger (47) reviewed therapies for prophylaxis and treatment of established acute renal failure and found no significant benefit from diuretics, including mannitol, in the prophylaxis or treatment of ARF. Other pharmacologic interventions reviewed below may have some effects either as prophylaxis or treatment of established renal failure. Dialysis is discussed in Chapter 7 and is not examined in this chapter.

Dopamine

The use of low-dose dopamine to improve renal blood flow by activating specific renal dopaminergic receptors is a common clinical intervention. Dopamine at 1 to 3 μg/kg/min may increase renal blood flow, GFR, and naturisms out of proportion to increases in cardiac output (48). The sites of action are the DA-1 and DA-2 receptors. Stimulation of the DA-1 receptors causes vasodilatation of the renal arterial vasculature. The DA-2 receptors are at the postsynaptic junction of sympathetic postganglionic neurons, and their stimulation diminishes the release of norepinephrine, thereby reducing renal vasoconstriction.

Dopamine infusion at low doses increases urine output. However, its effects are probably not due to selective enhancement of renal blood flow but rather to its renal effect as a diuretic and its cardiac effect as an inotrope, thereby improving overall cardiac output. The use of low or "renal" dose dopamine in the prevention or treatment of ARF is common and controversial. Myles et al. (49) studied the perioperative use of low-dose dopamine in patients with normal creatinine undergoing CABG and were unable to find any improvement in renal function in this group of patients. Reviews by Cotte and Saul (51) and Perdue et al. (50) concluded that in human studies there is no good evidence that dopamine administration either before or after an acute renal insult results in improved renal function or converts oliguric to nonoliguric renal failure.

Clonidine

More recently, the use of clonidine, an α-adrenergic (α_1 and α_2) agonist, has been tested in patients undergoing CABG. Clonidine inhibits ADH production (a central α_1 effect) and reabsorption of Na and H_2O (a peripheral α_2 effect) and may reduce renal hypoperfusion by blocking adrenergic vasoconstrictor stimuli to surgical stress. Kulka et al. (52) performed a prospective clinical trial using a single 4-μg/kg dose of clonidine. Although patients receiving placebo had a decrease in creatinine clearance in the early postoperative period, treated patients remained unchanged. By the third postoperative night there was no significant difference between the two groups. These patients had normal renal function and were excluded if they required intensive care unit care for more than 24 hours, so that it remains to be seen if this therapy will be of clinical benefit in the group of sicker patients who would benefit most.

Calcium Channel Blockers

Calcium channel antagonists have also been advocated for renal protection after open heart surgery. These drugs have had their greatest clinical use in patients with renal dysfunction secondary to diabetes and cyclosporin nephrotoxicity. Calcium channel blockers have been shown to be protective during infrarenal aortic surgery and CPB. Bertolossi et al. (53) prospectively evaluated 20 patients undergoing CABG to study the effect of nifedipine on renal function while controlling blood pressure under 70 mm Hg. They found in nifedipine-treated patients a significant increase in creatinine clearance and GFR comparing pre-CPB with post-CPB determinations, whereas placebo-treated patients showed no difference. However, this study excluded patients if the cardiac index was less than 2 or if they had hemorrhagic or respiratory complications. There were no clinical endpoints showing improvement. The study did not evaluate a group of patients that may benefit most from this therapy, patients with renal dysfunction or low cardiac output requiring significant inotropic support.

Diltiazem has also been shown to be a renal protectant. Experimental studies in animal models suggest that in ischemic renal failure, diltiazem increases GFR (54,55). Several clinical studies have suggested that similar increases in GFR are found in diltiazem-treated patients undergoing CPB (56,57). However, clinical endpoints showing clear improvements in morbidity and mortality in treated patients are lacking.

Atrial Natriuretic Peptide Analogues

ANP is produced in response to volume overload and activation of stretch receptors in the atria. ANP causes a marked natriuresis and is thought to help regulate blood volume. Its effect on the kidney is to increase GFR by selectively dilating afferent arterioles while constricting efferent arterioles (58). In animals with acute renal dysfunction, ANP analogues improve GFR and increases urine output (54). Several clinical studies of ANP and its analogues have provided provocative if inconclusive data. Rahman et al. (59) found that ANP given to patients with ARF showed improvement in creatinine clearance and a significant decrease in the need for dialysis. Although mortality was halved in the ANP-treated group, the difference was not statistically significant. In a large multicenter prospective trial of Anaritide, a synthetic analogue of ANP, there was improved mortality in treated patients with oliguria (58).

Even more promising are the initial reports of studies with urodilatin, a natriuretic peptide found in human urine. In comparison with circulating ANP, urodilatin exerts greater diuretic properties. Its method of action is thought to involve both improving renal blood flow and acting upon the distal collecting system. Studies in heart and liver transplantation in patients with oliguria suggest some improve-

ment in renal function (60,61). Wiebe et al. (62) performed a small randomized trial in oliguric patients after cardiac surgery. They found that administration of urodilatin caused a rapid improvement in urine output and reductions in blood urea nitrogen and creatinine (Fig. 19.5, A and B). Six of seven untreated patients required dialysis, and four of these placebo-treated patients succumbed during follow-up. They concluded that administration of urodilatin is beneficial in oliguric patients after cardiac surgery and significantly reduces mortality and the need for dialysis.

SUMMARY

Clinically important renal failure is a relatively rare occurrence after cardiac surgery, but mild renal dysfunction is common. In its most severe form, where patients require dialysis, renal failure is associated with a 10-fold increase in surgical mortality. Although CPB is a nonphysiologic state that alters renal blood flow and many neuroendocrine responses affecting the kidney, there is little clear-cut evidence that CPB per se is responsible for renal dysfunction. The bulk of the available evidence suggests that preexisting renal disease and renal hypoperfusion secondary to circulatory failure are the most important factors contributing to renal dysfunction in the postoperative period.

Therapies aimed at avoiding renal failure post-CPB all aim at maximizing cardiac output to avoid renal hypoperfusion. Most strategies intended to maximize renal blood flow in low output states probably increase RBF by increasing overall cardiac output. The use of dopamine may fit into this category. Vasodilators may preferentially relax the renal vasculature as a form of renal protection, but there is no good evidence that either calcium channel blockers or clonidine act in a specific manner. ANP analogues, however, do have specific effects on the kidney and may prove to be of great benefit in low output states. These hormones seem to have specific differential actions upon efferent and afferent arterioles in the glomerulus and may provide renal protection when overall cardiac output is diminished. Further studies are required to elucidate their mechanism and clinical efficacy before their use becomes widespread.

ACKNOWLEDGMENT

We acknowledge Dr. Wade McKweon, Department of Medicine, University of Kentucky College of Medicine, for helpful comments during preparation of this manuscript.

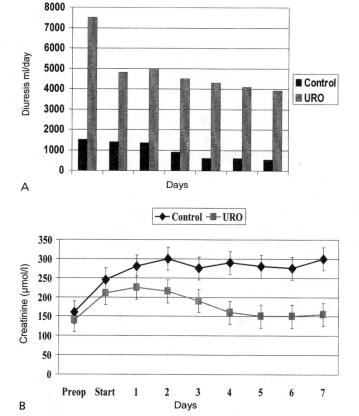

FIG. 19.5. URO (urodilation)/placebo infusion. **A:** Diuresis during the 7-day period of urodilatin infusion after cardiac surgery. **B:** Serum creatinine in patients undergoing cardiac surgery receiving urodilation (URO) and placebo. (From Wiebe K, et al. Acute renal failure following cardiac surgery is reverted by administration of urodilatin (INN: ularitide). *Eur J Med Res* 1996;1:259–265, with permission.)

KEY POINTS

- The incidence of renal failure requiring dialysis after CABG is approximately 1%, but is 2.7% in congenital heart surgery.

- Mortality rate from postoperative renal failure after CPB is more than 50%.
    - Lesser degrees of renal impairment still increase intensive care unit and total hospital length of stay significantly.
- Preoperative renal function impairment and length of CPB correlate with postoperative renal impairment.
    - Low cardiac output (and surrogates such as low ejection fraction, NYHA class IV congestive heart failure, use of intra-aortic balloon counter-pulsation, IABP) and advanced age are also predictive of postoperative renal failure.
    - Diabetes is not a consistent predictor.
- CPB procedural factors that influence renal function are as follows: hemodilution is protective, pulsatile perfusion is theoretically protective, and membrane oxygenators and arterial line filters may be protective.
- Prophylactic therapies to decrease the risk of renal failure after CPB are as follows:
    - Dopamine stimulates DA-1 receptors to increase renal blood flow and may improve GFR and tubular function.
    - Dopamine benefit is separate from inotropic effect and increased cardiac output is controversial.
    - Clonidine and calcium channel blockers may be protective.
    - ANPs and analogues appear to be protective.

REFERENCES

1. Werner H, et al. Peritoneal dialysis in children after cardiopulmonary bypass. *J Thorac Cardiovasc Surg* 1997;1:64–68.
2. Settergren G, Ohqvist G. Renal dysfunction during cardiac surgery. *Curr Opin Anesthesiol* 1994;7:59–64.
3. Asfour B, et al. Renal insufficiency in neonates after cardiac surgery. *J Cardiothorac Vasc Anesth* 1996;10:603–608.
4. Bruker A, et al. Renal insufficiency in neonates after cardiac surgery. *Clin Nephrol* 1996;46:59–63.
5. Fleming F, et al. Renal replacement therapy after repair of congenital heart disease in children. *J Thorac Cardiovasc Surg* 1995;109:322–331.
6. Mangano C, et al. Renal dysfunction after myocardial revascularization: risk factors, adverse outcomes, and hospital resource utilization. The Multicenter Study of Perioperative Ischemia Research Group. *Anesth Analg* 1998;1:3–8.
7. Mangos GJ, et al. Acute renal failure following cardiac surgery: incidence, outcomes and risk factors. *Aust NZ J Med* 1995;25:284–289.
8. McCullough P, et al. Acute renal failure after coronary intervention: incidence, risk factors, and relationship to mortality. *Am J Med* 1997;103:368–375.
9. Guyton AC. *Human physiology and mechanisms of disease*, 4th ed. Philadelphia: W.B. Saunders, 1987:703.
10. Zanardo G, et al. Acute renal failure in the patient undergoing cardiac operation. Prevalence, mortality rate, and main risk factors. *J Thorac Cardiovasc Surg* 1994;107:1489–1495.
11. Butterworth JI, et al. Factors that predict the use of positive inotropic drug support after cardiac valve surgery. *Anesth Analg* 1998;86:461–467.
12. Cohen Y, et al. Comparison of factors associated with 30-day mortality after coronary artery bypass grafting in patients with versus without diabetes mellitus. *Am J Cardiol* 1998;81:7–11.
13. Lema G, et al. Effects of extracorporeal circulation on renal function in coronary surgical patients. *Anesth Analg* 1995;81:46–451.
14. Chertow G, et al. Preoperative renal risk stratification. *Circulation* 1997;95:878–884.
15. *Data analysis of the STS Cardiac Surgery database*. Chicago: Society of Thoracic Surgeons, 1998.
16. Picca S, et al. Risks of acute renal failure after cardiopulmonary bypass surgery in children: a retrospective 10-year case-control study. *Nephrol Dialys Transplant* 1995;10:630–636.
17. Murkin JM, et al. A randomized study of the influence of perfusion technique and pH management strategy in 316 patients undergoing coronary artery bypass surgery. *J Thorac Cardiovasc Surg* 1995;110:340–348.
18. Cooper MM, Elliott M. Haemodilution. In: Jonas RA, Elliot MJ, eds. *Cardiopulmonary bypass in neonates, infants and young children*. Oxford: Butterworth-Heinemann, 1994:82–99.
19. Hint H. The pharmacology of dextran and the physiological background for the clinical use of Rheomacrodex and Macrodex. *Acta Anaesth Belg* 1968;19:119–138.
20. Bassenge E, et al. Effect of haemodilution on coronary hemodynamics in conscious dogs. A preliminary report. In: Messmer K, Schmid-Schonbein H, ed. *Haemodilution. Theoretical basis and clinical application.* New York: Karger, 1972:174–183.
21. Crystal GJ, Salem MR. Myocardial and systemic hemodynamics during isovolemic hemodilution alone and combined with nitroprusside-induced controlled hypotension. *Anesth Analg* 1991;72:227–237.
22. Beall AC, et al. Effects if temporary cardiopulmonary bypass on extracellular fluid volume and total body water in man. *Circulation* 1964;29[Suppl]:59–62.
23. Huskisson L, Elliot MJ. Prime composition. In: Jonas RA, Elliot MJ, eds. *Cardiopulmonary bypass in neonates, infants and young children.* Oxford: Butterworth-Heinemann, 1994:186–197.
24. Ross AD, Angaran DM. Colloids versus crystalloids—a continuing controversy. *Drug Intell Clin Pharm* 1984;18:202–212.
25. Hoeft A, et al. Priming of cardiopulmonary bypass with human albumin or Ringers lactate: effect on colloid osmotic pressure and extravascular lung water. *Br J Anaesth* 1991;66:73–80.
26. Ohqvist G, et al. Pulmonary oxygenation, central haemodynamics and glomerular filtration following cardiopulmonary bypass with colloid or non-colloid priming solution. *Scand J Thorac Cardiovasc Surg* 1981;15:257–262.
27. Scott DA, et al. A comparison of albumin, polygeline and crystalloid priming solutions for cardiopulmonary bypass in patients having coronary artery bypass graft surgery. *Perfusion* 1995;10:415–424.
28. Foglia PR, et al. Iatrogenic myocardial edema with crystalloid primes. Effects on left ventricular compliance, performance and perfusion. *Curr Stud Hematol Blood Transf* 1986;53:53–63.
29. Swain JA, et al. Low-flow hypothermic cardiopulmonary bypass protects the brain. *J Thorac Cardiovasc Surg* 1991;102:76–83; discussion 83–84.
30. Arom K, Emery R, Northrup W. Warm heart surgery: a prospective comparison between normothermic and tepid temperature. *J Card Surg* 1995;10:221–226.
31. Lehot JJ, et al. Hemodynamic and hormonal responses to hypothermic and normothermic cardiopulmonary bypass. *J Cardiothorac Vasc Anesth* 1992;6:132–139.
32. Regragui I, et al. Cardiopulmonary bypass perfusion temperature does not influence perioperative renal function. *Ann Thorac Surg* 1995;60:160–164.
33. Taylor KM, et al. Comparative studies of pulsatile and nonpulsatile flow during cardiopulmonary bypass. I. Pulsatile system em-

ployed and its hematologic effects. *J Thorac Cardiovasc Surg* 1978; 75:569–573.

34. Dapper F, et al. Effects of pulsatile and nonpulsatile perfusion mode during extracorporeal circulation—a comparative clinical study [see comments]. *Thorac Cardiovasc Surg* 1992;40:345–351.

35. Lindberg H, et al. Pulsatile vs. non-pulsatile flow during cardiopulmonary bypass. A comparison of early postoperative changes. *Scand J Thorac Cardiovasc Surg* 1984;18:195–201.

36. Frater RW, et al. Pulsatile cardiopulmonary bypass: failure to influence hemodynamics or hormones. *Circulation* 1980;62(2 Pt 2):I19–I25.

37. Shen J, et al. The effects of pulsatile pumping on tissue perfusion and renal function during deep hypothermic low flow perfusion. *Kyobu Geka* 1990;43:707–711.

38. Gaer JA, et al. Effect of cardiopulmonary bypass on gastrointestinal perfusion and function. *Ann Thorac Surg* 1994;57:371–375.

39. Taylor KM. Pulsatile cardiopulmonary bypass. A review. *J Cardiovasc Surg* 1981;22:561–568.

40. Hickey PR, Buckley MJ, Philbin DM. Pulsatile and nonpulsatile cardiopulmonary bypass: review of a counterproductive controversy. *Ann Thorac Surg* 1983;36:720–737.

41. Moody DM, et al. Brain microemboli during cardiac surgery or aortography. *Ann Neurol* 1990;28:477–486.

42. Pugsley W, et al. The impact of microemboli during cardiopulmonary bypass on neuropsychological functioning. *Stroke* 1994; 25:1393–1399.

43. Kurusz M. Gaseous microemboli: sources, causes, and clinical considerations. *Med Instrum* 1985;19:73–76.

44. Johnston WE, et al. Significance of gaseous microemboli in the cerebral circulation during cardiopulmonary bypass in dogs. *Circulation* 1993;88(5 Pt 2):II319–II329.

45. Treasure T, et al. Impairment of cerebral function following cardiac and other major surgery. *Eur J Cardiothorac Surg* 1989;3: 216–221.

46. Elliot MJ. Minimizing the bypass circuit: a rational step in the development of pediatric perfusion. *Perfusion* 1993;8:81–86.

47. Conger J, Interventions in clinical acute renal failure: what are the data? *Am J Kidney Dis* 1995;26:565–576.

48. Carcoana O, Hines R. Is renal dose dopamine protective or therapeutic? Yes. *Controvers Crit Care Med* 1996;12:677–685.

49. Myles PS, et al. Effect of "renal-dose" dopamine on renal function following cardiac surgery. *Anaesth Intens Care* 1993;21: 56–61.

50. Perdue PW, et al. "Renal dose" dopamine in surgical patients; dogma or science? *Ann Surg* 1998;227:470–473.

51. Cottee D, Saul WP. Is renal dose dopamine protective or therapeutic? No. *Controvers Crit Care Med* 1996;12:687–695.

52. Kulka P, Tryba M, Zenz M. Preoperative α2-adrenergic receptor agonists prevent the deterioration of renal function after cardiac surgery: results of a randomized, controlled trial. *Crit Care Med* 1996;24:947–952.

53. Bertolissi M, et al. Effects on renal function of a continuous infusion of nifedipine during cardiopulmonary bypass. *J Cardiothorac Vasc Anesth* 1996;10:238–242.

54. Schramm L, et al. Toxic acute renal failure in the rat: effects of diltiazem and urodilatin on renal function. *Nephron* 1994;68: 454–461.

55. Sandin R, et al. Effects of diltiazem on post-ischemic renal cortical microcirculation in the pig. *Acta Anaesthesiol Scand* 1991;35: 424–429.

56. Amano J, et al. Effect of calcium antagonist diltiazem on renal function in open heart surgery. *Chest* 1995;107:1260–1265.

57. Zanardo G, et al. Effects of a continuous diltiazem infusion on renal function during cardiac surgery. *J Cardiothorac Vasc Anesth* 1993;7:711–716.

58. Allgren R, et al. Anaritide in acute tubular necrosis. *N Engl J Med* 1997;336:828–834.

59. Rahman S, et al. Effects of atrial natriuretic peptide in clinical acute renal failure. *Kidney Int* 1994;45:1731–1738.

60. Brenner P, et al. Significance of prophylactic urodilatin (INN: ularitide) infusion for the prevention of acute renal failure in patients after heart transplantation. *Eur J Med Res* 1995;1: 137–143.

61. Langrehr J, et al. Prophylactic use of low-dose urodilatin for prevention of renal impairment following liver transplantation: a randomized placebo-controlled study. *Clin Transplant* 1997; 11:593–598.

62. Wiebe K, et al. Acute renal failure following cardiac surgery is reverted by administration of urodilatin (INN: ularitide). *Eur J Med Res* 1996;1:259–265.

SPLANCHNIC, HEPATIC, AND VISCERAL EFFECTS

ROBERT E. SHANGRAW

The monitoring of visceral organ perfusion and function during surgical procedures involving cardiopulmonary bypass (CPB) is less intensive than the monitoring of many other organ systems. Major limiting factors during thoracic operations include the closed abdomen, which precludes direct access to the abdominal viscera, and the cumbersome and expensive nature of available noninvasive monitoring techniques to assess the splanchnic circulation, for which there is still little evidence of altered clinical outcome in cardiovascular surgery. The purpose of this chapter is to provide a detailed review of the data available on CPB-induced functional alterations and complications in the splanchnic viscera—stomach, intestines, liver, and pancreas.

SPLANCHNIC CIRCULATION DURING CARDIOPULMONARY BYPASS

Animal Studies

The importance of adequate splanchnic circulation during CPB was underscored in the 1930s by the pathologic changes observed in "irreversible hemorrhagic shock" (1). In a large series of experiments, Wiggers and his colleagues showed that animals underwent a progressive, ultimately fatal deterioration of cardiovascular status after having initially recovered from a period of controlled hemorrhagic hypotension. At autopsy, these animals exhibited several pathologic changes in visceral organs that were dependent upon the splanchnic circulation, including capillary congestion, small hemorrhages, and early necrosis in the small intestine, stomach, liver, and pancreas (1). Therefore, early animal studies on the effects of CPB focused on the adequacy of splanchnic regional perfusion during bypass to ascertain whether a shocklike state was being created (2). CPB is often accompanied by hypotension and induced hypo-

thermia, two factors that markedly affect the regional distribution of blood flow and the amount of flow required to maintain cellular viability. The mechanism by which hypotension is produced is of critical importance to visceral organ viability: Yokoyama et al. (3) found that hepatic energy metabolism was well preserved for 3 hours during trimetaphan-induced hypotension to a mean arterial pressure of 60 mm Hg in dogs. In contrast, comparable hypotension and compromise of systemic and total hepatic blood flow produced by controlled hemorrhage was accompanied by a progressive decline in the ratio of hepatic adenosine triphosphate to inorganic phosphate (ATP/Pi), in the arterial ketone body ratio (reflecting the balance of reductive and oxidative metabolic reactions at the mitochondrial level), and in the overall hepatic energy charge (3).

Halley et al. (2) directly measured the intestinal blood flow of dogs during normothermic "high-flow" (>50 mL/kg per minute) and "low-flow" (<50 mL/kg per minute) CPB. Intestinal blood flow was increased 45% during high-flow and 27% during low-flow CPB, in association with decreased regional vascular resistance. Despite the augmented blood flow, intestinal oxygen consumption was diminished by 20% to 30% during CPB and did not correlate with changes in temperature or pH. In contrast, Desai et al. (4), using electromagnetic probes to measure hepatic blood flow in dogs, found that animals subjected to 60 minutes of CPB had a decrease in hepatic arterial flow of 46%, in portal vein flow of 44%, and in total liver flow of 45% in comparison with animals who underwent thoracotomy without CPB. The decreased portal and hepatic arterial flows were ascribed to an *increased* vascular resistance, although the variations between individuals precluded statistical significance. Mean arterial pressure fell from 110 to 56 mm Hg during CPB, but cardiac output of animals undergoing thoracotomy was not reported, precluding a comparison of total systemic flow between the two groups (4).

Lees et al. (5) used radiolabeled microspheres in 27 rhesus monkeys to compare regional blood flow in awake animals with that in animals undergoing general anesthesia alone, thoracotomy without CPB, or CPB. Total systemic flow

R. E. Shangraw: Department of Anesthesiology, Oregon Health Sciences University, Portland, Oregon 97203.

during CPB was regulated to equal that of awake animals. Mean arterial pressure decreased from 144 mm Hg in awake animals to 75 mm Hg during CPB, accompanied by a large decrease in systemic vascular resistance (5). In comparison with awake animals, animals who underwent CPB exhibited a threefold to fourfold hyperemia through the gastrointestinal tract, spleen, and mesentery. Oxygen-rich hepatic arterial flow decreased by 35%, although the calculated total hepatic perfusion—including portal vein perfusion—nearly doubled (5). Pancreatic perfusion, in contrast, was not altered by high-flow CPB (5). Rudy et al. (6) confirmed the increased gastric and intestinal blood flow during high-flow CPB but did not measure hepatic or pancreatic perfusion. The weight of experimental animal evidence, although findings are not completely unanimous, indicates that normothermic CPB with either high or low flow increases gastrointestinal blood flow but decreases hepatic arterial flow and exerts a variable effect on pancreatic perfusion.

Influence of Carbon Dioxide

The effects of arterial carbon dioxide tension (P_aCO_2) on hepatic arterial blood flow and hepatic function are controversial. Fujita et al. (7) reported that hypocapnia decreases hepatic artery flow in dogs, whereas Gelman et al. (8) found a hypocapnia-induced increase in hepatic arterial flow in monkeys. Gelman and colleagues subsequently attempted to reconcile these differences by noting that the canine experiments were performed during laparotomy while those in monkeys were not, and they suggested that the surgical stimulation of laparotomy augmented hepatic artery flow to a higher baseline before the onset of hypocapnia (9). It is also possible that the effects of the open abdomen may have contributed to a decreased venous return during the hypocapnic period.

Hypercapnia augments cardiac output in addition to portal and total hepatic circulation, probably through enhancement of sympathoadrenal activity (7). Portal venous pressure is also increased, at least partially because of increased mesenteric blood flow. Although there is no apparent decrease in hepatic arterial flow during marked hypercapnia at a P_aCO_2 of 59 mm Hg, both hepatic oxygen consumption and indocyanine green dye uptake are decreased, indicating a possible hepatocellular dysfunction during laparotomy coupled with hypercapnia (7). The studies by Fujita et al. did not control for acidosis *per se*, leaving unsettled the question of whether carbon dioxide or hydrogen ion is responsible for the observed alterations in splanchnic perfusion. However, the possibility exists that hypercapnia augments intrahepatic shunt flow, impairing nutritional microcirculation in the liver. There are no reports on the influence of P_aCO_2 on splanchnic and hepatic circulation, and their dependent cellular functions, during CPB. This

leaves unsettled the question of whether alpha-stat or pH stat acid–base management during CPB better optimizes splanchnic perfusion.

Influence of Temperature

Mori et al. (10), using a hydrogen clearance technique, examined liver and pancreatic blood flow during CPB in dogs. Flow measurements were made during cooling and warming at 5°C intervals, with an intervening total circulatory arrest at 20°C for 40 minutes. Total hepatic perfusion progressively decreased during cooling, such that flow at 20°C was only 54% of that at 35°C. Pancreatic flow concomitantly decreased by 33%. However, the pump flow rate was also decreased, from 100 mL/kg per minute at 35°C to 60 mL/kg per minute at 20°C, which makes uncertain the extent to which decreased systemic pump flow affected perfusion pressure. It is therefore impossible to discern whether the observed decrease in regional blood flow was a consequence of decreased systemic blood flow or of changes in temperature. The data do indicate, however, that neither hepatic nor pancreatic blood flow is autoregulated during hypothermic CPB. No control group, such as thoracotomy without CPB, was included, which would have enabled determination of whether there exists a baseline autoregulation of splanchnic perfusion that is lost consequent to CPB.

Effect of Pharmacologic Agents

Dopamine is used during cardiac surgery, both as a cardiac inotrope and to preserve renal function. Dopamine has an important effect on nonrenal splanchnic circulation in dogs, pigs, and humans (11–13). In anesthetized dogs without CPB, an intravenous bolus of dopamine (12.8 μg/kg) dilated the superior and inferior mesenteric arteries, left gastric artery, and superior pancreatoduodenal artery (11). In contrast, it did not dilate the canine hepatic artery, which Van Kesteren et al. (11) interpreted as indicating an absence or paucity of dopamine receptors in the hepatic artery. This interpretation is weakened, however, because dopamine also failed to dilate the renal artery in the same dogs, despite a well-documented abundance of dopamine receptors in the canine renal artery and an observed 50% increase in urine flow (11). One possible explanation for the discrepancy is that dopamine stimulates both vasodilator dopamine-1 (DA-1) and vasoconstrictor dopamine-2 (DA-2) receptors, which are both present in the renal artery. The net effect of dopamine on renovascular tone may reflect the relative numbers of the two receptor subtypes. Dopamine increases superior mesenteric arterial and portal venous flow in pigs, increasing total hepatic blood flow and total hepatic oxygen delivery despite no apparent change in hepatic arterial flow (12). The stimulatory effect of dopamine on hepatic oxygen delivery contrasts with that of norepinephrine, which decreases it, and of dobutamine, which has no effect, when each catecholamine is infused at doses producing similar effects on systemic hemodynamics (12).

Lundberg et al. (13) directly assessed the influence of dopamine on splanchnic blood flow with electromagnetic flow probes in nine patients undergoing abdominal aortic aneurysm repair without CPB. Epidural anesthesia moderately decreased splanchnic perfusion, systemic perfusion, and perfusion pressure. Dopamine (4 μg/kg per minute) reversed epidural anesthesia-induced impairment of splanchnic perfusion without altering systemic or superior mesenteric artery hemodynamics (13). Equally important, dopamine abolished the increase in lactate production by ischemic intestine. Elimination of the difference between intestinal and systemic lactate production by dopamine was interpreted to indicate that its effect is specific to preservation of splanchnic perfusion (13). These studies, although performed during an abdominal procedure rather than during CPB, underscore the inability of systemic clinical indices to detect splanchnic perfusion abnormalities. They initially provided support for optimism that the splanchnic circulation might be optimized with infusion of low-dose dopamine, which is frequently used in cardiac surgery. However, in a more recent study of pigs undergoing normothermic CPB, dopamine (5 μg/kg per minute) failed to increase splanchnic perfusion across a wide range of systemic flow rates (14). The inability of dopamine to alter splanchnic perfusion during CPB indicates that much of its effect when the cardiovascular system is intact can be attributed to an increase in cardiac output. Increasing arterial pressure with phenylephrine during CPB instead of increasing pump flow actually compromises splanchnic perfusion (15). This serves to emphasize that the use of α-adrenergic stimulation to maintain perfusion pressure during CPB can produce a paradoxical hypoperfusion of visceral organs despite an acceptable systemic arterial pressure.

Dopexamine and fenoldopam are newly introduced, specific DA-1 receptor agonists with the potential to preserve splanchnic perfusion during CPB. Both agents increase splanchnic and renal blood flow under nonoperative conditions by a mechanism that includes DA-1 stimulation and α-adrenergic stimulation (16). Berendes et al. (17) reported that dopexamine increased creatinine clearance and reduced indicators of systemic inflammation, but did not alter splanchnic oxygenation or alter gastric mucosal pH, during normothermic CPB in humans. Because of its concomitant β-adrenergic activity, dopexamine induces tachycardia, which may contraindicate its use in patients with coronary artery disease (17). In contrast, neither β-adrenergic stimulation nor tachycardia has been reported with fenoldopam. Data comparing the relative efficacy of dopamine, dopexamine, and fenoldopam in preserving splanchnic blood flow during CPB remain scarce.

Problems with Clinical Monitoring

Animal studies indicate that gross splanchnic circulation is adequately maintained during CPB, but neither the adequacy of the microcirculation nor the preservation of cellular viability and physiologic function has been assessed. Furthermore, the young adult primate may not be an ideal model for study of the circulatory effects of CPB in elderly humans with diffuse atherosclerotic disease, who constitute a growing segment of the patients undergoing CPB. One major difficulty in CPB has been the inability to monitor clinically the integrity of perfusion and physiologic function in splanchnic organs. A few attempts have been made to assess hepatic perfusion by observing the movement of dyes specifically taken up by hepatocytes, such as Bromosulphalein (sulfobromophthalein sodium) (18), or by continuously monitoring hepatic venous oxygen saturation (19), but the results of these studies have not been integrated into routine clinical management during CPB. One factor underlying the limited use of dye uptake or routine oximetry during CPB is that it is not known how well dye uptake (or oxygen consumption) reflects perfusion adequacy in the anesthetized patient (20). Hepatic vein oximetry also requires that the hepatic vein be catheterized under fluoroscopic guidance, which limits its attractiveness to the clinician. A third monitoring technique is continuous measurement of gastrointestinal pH by tonometry (21–24). Gastric tonometry has received limited acceptance, however, because it is difficult to perform and also to interpret the data generated by this technique. Recent technologic improvements have made gastric tonometry easier to carry out and more reliable, which may ultimately lead to its more widespread acceptance as a clinical monitoring tool (25). Nevertheless, gastric tonometry monitors only gastric and possibly intestinal tissues and cannot be used to assess the adequacy of pancreatic or hepatic perfusion. One reproducible finding in both human and animal studies is a decrease in gastric mucosal pH during CPB, a finding that is consistent with, but not definitive evidence of, gastric ischemia. In pigs, the decreased gastric mucosal pH during normothermic CPB appears to be secondary to decreased gastrointestinal blood flow concomitant with increased oxygen demand in mesenteric tissues (26).

Cardiopulmonary Bypass Studies in Humans

Preliminary human studies indicate that splanchnic perfusion is well maintained during normothermic CPB, given the limitation of monitoring techniques available (17,27). Berendes et al. (17) found no decrease in hepatic venous oxygen saturation during normothermic, high-flow (2.4 L/m^2 per minute) CPB in 14 patients undergoing coronary artery bypass grafting. Similarly, Haisjackl et al. (27) found that blood flow, oxygen delivery, and oxygen consumption of the splanchnic bed were unchanged in 12 patients during CPB under comparable conditions. On the other hand, both groups of investigators detected a decrease in gastric mucosal pH that persisted after separation from CPB and into the postoperative setting (17,27). Haisjackl et al. (27) also found that hepatic clearance of indocyanine green dye, but not of lactate, was diminished by CPB and remained low postoperatively. The authors ascribed the changes in indocyanine green clearance and gastric mucosal pH to systemic inflammation triggered by CPB. It should be noted that none of the patients in either study sustained an intra-abdominal complication.

LIVER FUNCTION AND CARDIOPULMONARY BYPASS

The liver performs many different functions, specifically the following: (a) produces glucose and clears lactate in the Cori cycle; (b) synthesizes plasma proteins such as albumin, coagulation factors, and plasma cholinesterase; (c) maintains immune function via Kupffer cell-mediated clearance of intravascular debris and microorganisms; and (d) metabolizes many drugs and potential toxins (such as bilirubin and ammonia) by a variety of mechanisms, including cytochrome P_{450} oxidation. The multiple distinct functions of the liver preclude global assessment of liver function with a single method. The term *liver function test* is largely a misnomer. Most of these tests reflect the leak of enzymes found in high concentration in hepatocytes into the plasma; they serve better as markers of hepatocellular injury than as measures of true hepatic function. The relationship between enzyme leak and preservation of liver function remains unclear. In contrast, plasma accumulation of bilirubin may reflect a defect in hepatic function.

Substrate Metabolism by the Liver

Waldhausen et al. (28), studying the relationship between hepatic blood flow and oxygen consumption in dogs undergoing normothermic CPB, found that hepatic oxygen consumption is preserved at pump flow rates down to 2.2 L/m^2 per minute. Below this perfusion rate, which corresponds to a hepatic blood flow of approximately 110 mL per 100 g of liver per minute, both hepatic blood flow and oxygen consumption were markedly curtailed (28). The authors did not assess consequent hepatocellular damage resulting from hypoperfusion during CPB. It is unclear whether these relationships between systemic flow, liver perfusion, and hepatic oxygen consumption are maintained under hypothermic conditions.

The liver regulates plasma glucose concentration by varying its glucose production rate. Glucagon is a pancreatic hormone that, when administered as the *glucagon challenge*

test, stimulates hepatic glucose production and consequent hyperglycemia. Kuntschen et al. (29) demonstrated that the hyperglycemic response to glucagon challenge is impaired during CPB in humans, and interpreted this observation as evidence of compromised liver function. However, they did not measure glucose *production* but instead measured only the change in plasma glucose concentration. Glucose production may already be maximally stimulated by the markedly increased plasma concentrations of cortisol and epinephrine that occur during CPB (30). Without direct assessment, it is unclear that hepatic glucose production is abnormal during CPB, but it is unlikely to be decreased during CPB for two reasons. First, there is already a marked hyperglycemia during CPB; second, the endocrine environment during CPB favors glucose production by gluconeogenesis and glycogenolysis. Glycogenolysis is stimulated by epinephrine, even without exogenous glucagon (30). There are counteracting factors that would tend to decrease hepatic glucose production. For instance, general anesthesia with pentobarbital decreases hepatic glucose production by 30% in rats (31). One can only speculate about the role of other potential underlying mechanisms, such as hypothermia and nonpulsatile or reduced hepatic blood flow.

Plasma lactic acid concentration consistently rises during and after CPB (27,32). Anderson et al. (18) demonstrated that hepatic lactate clearance is maintained during normothermic CPB in dogs despite a rising plasma concentration, indicating that CPB stimulates peripheral lactate production. However, the CPB conditions used by Anderson et al. differed from those of common clinical practice in that they maintained a high mean arterial pressure (75 to 110 mm Hg) and pump flow (50 to 60 mL/kg per minute) (18). In humans, there is evidence that splanchnic lactate clearance is actually *increased* during normothermic, high-pressure, high-flow CPB (27). This suggests that the increased plasma lactate concentration during CPB reflects accelerated lactate flux, but the tissue source of the lactate remains unknown. Hepatic lactate clearance and lactate production rates have not been reported under hypothermic, low-flow conditions. Alterations in glucose–lactate (Cori) cycling during CPB have received only scant attention to date. This could serve as a probe for examining the preservation of overall hepatic function under the unusual physiologic circumstances of CPB.

Protein Synthesis

An iatrogenic heparin-induced coagulopathy is currently a clinical standard immediately before the onset of CPB. Subsequent commencement of extracorporeal circulation of CPB dilutes, by approximately 40%, the plasma concentration of all coagulation factors except factors VIII and XI (33). Although protamine administration after discontinuance of CPB reverses the coagulopathy, decreased plasma concentration of coagulation factors persists into the early postoperative period. Accompanying the decreased procoagulant factor concentrations is a parallel decrease in concentration of anticoagulation factors antithrombin III and plasminogen (33).

The plasma concentration of fibrinogen, a protein synthesized by the liver with a moderately rapid turnover, is highly variable in the postoperative setting. In a study by Wolk et al. (33), a greater than 50% average reduction in plasma fibrinogen concentration did not achieve statistical significance because of the high variability. It is unknown whether decreased plasma fibrinogen concentration reflects increased consumption or decreased hepatic synthesis in affected patients. It would be interesting to compare plasma fibrinogen concentrations with results of standard liver function tests, such as measurement of serum glutamic–pyruvic transaminase (SGPT) or bilirubin. The test could also be performed simultaneously with an assessment of hepatic fibrinogen synthesis (34,35) to determine the extent to which liver injury and functional impairment correspond to decrease fibrinogen concentration after CPB.

Plasma fibronectin is a glycoprotein that facilitates phagocytic clearance of debris and microorganisms from the vascular compartment. Although it is synthesized by several tissues *in vitro*, the liver is the principal tissue site of plasma fibronectin synthesis *in vivo* (36). Several investigators have shown that CPB decreases the plasma fibronectin concentration (37–42), but the etiology remains uncertain. Potential responsible mechanisms are "losses" through hemodilution, bleeding, and redistribution into extravascular fluids. Fibronectin is also consumed as it binds to heparin, fibrin, and cellular debris to facilitate phagocytosis (42). A third potential mechanism depleting plasma fibronectin concentration is intravascular proteolysis by abnormally high levels of serum proteases (43). The mechanisms by which a normal plasma fibronectin concentration is restored in the hours after separation from CPB are equally complex. Extravascular fibronectin stores can be mobilized into the vascular compartment (42), and diuresis reverses the effects of hemodilution. The effects of CPB initiation and discontinuation on fibronectin *synthesis* are unknown. However, fibronectin has a very high fractional synthetic rate, approximately 30% daily, in normal humans (34,35). The high turnover rate means that changes in synthesis are rapidly reflected as changes in plasma concentration. Fibronectin synthesis is exquisitely sensitive to acute physiologic changes such as trauma (34), exercise (35), and starvation (44). Studies examining hepatic fibronectin synthesis during and after CPB remain to be performed. A functional implication of fibronectin synthesis is that fibronectin mediates Kupffer cell clearance of particulate debris and microorganisms, which are present in increased concentration as a result of CPB. The role of fibronectin in the impaired postoperative phagocytic function of Kupffer cells after CPB remains to be explored (45). Impairment of the reticuloendothelial system to handle a bacterial challenge increases the risk for systemic infection or an uncontrolled inflammatory response. Plasma cholinesterase concentration is decreased during CPB, at least partially because of hemodilution (46). Plasma cholinesterase normally recovers to preoperative values by the first or second postoperative day. It is likely that the return of the plasma cholinesterase concentration occurs through diuresis and fluid redistribution rather than increased synthesis because, unlike the synthesis rate for fibronectin, that for plasma cholinesterase is slow (46,47).

The liver is the source of several, but not all, cytokines that play a role in the inflammatory response to CPB. The systemic inflammatory response to CPB has been the subject of much recent investigation. Of particular importance to a discussion of liver function is the antiinflammatory cytokine interleukin-10, which is produced by the liver; its release is stimulated by steroid pretreatment (48).

The conclusion to be drawn from the currently available data is that although hypothermic CPB produces a mild and temporary impairment of plasma protein synthesis, it appears to be without clinical significance in the short term. Furthermore, it usually reverses completely, at least by indirect assessment, by the first postoperative day. Further work is necessary to determine the extent to which accelerated hepatic synthesis plays a role in the recovery of apparently normal levels of plasma proteins in the postoperative setting.

Hepatic Drug Metabolism

The liver metabolizes many drugs administered to patients undergoing cardiac surgery. Formation of drug metabolites can serve as an index of hepatic function during and after CPB. For instance, Autschbach et al. (49) reported that the formation of MEGX (monoethyl-glycinexylidide) from lidocaine is decreased during CPB, but they did not assess the duration of impairment after CPB was discontinued. Formation of metabolites of allopurinol, caffeine, methacetin, or aminopyrine remains to be evaluated in cardiac surgery patients (50). A more common way to evaluate hepatic drug metabolism is through the disappearance of drug from the plasma. The hepatic metabolism of fentanyl is decreased during hypothermic CPB (51–53). Koren et al. (53) reported that CPB at 20°C virtually arrests the uptake of fentanyl, a drug with a high rate of hepatic extraction, for up to 2 hours in children. There have been several attempts to distinguish the effects of hypothermia from those of altered hepatic blood flow during CPB. Koska et al. (51) correlated the increased plasma half-life of fentanyl with a comparable 30% decrease in hepatic blood flow during normothermic CPB. Alternatively, Koren et al. (53) demonstrated that hypothermia without CPB decreases fentanyl clearance by more than 70% in piglets, concomitant with a 42% decrease in hepatic blood flow. Presumably, the effect of CPB on the hepatic metabolism of sufentanil and alfentanil would approximate that on the metabolism of fentanyl. In contrast to fentanyl, theophylline is poorly extracted by the liver, and its metabolism is relatively unaffected by hypothermia (54). It is possible that (a) drugs with a high rate of hepatic extraction, such as fentanyl, are more sensitive to temperature-mediated changes in hepatic blood flow, or (b) different hepatic enzyme systems have different temperature sensitivities.

Midazolam clearance is impaired during and after CPB in both adults and children (55,56). Similarly, the hepatic metabolism of propofol is inhibited after CPB (57). The role of hypothermia in the metabolism of midazolam or propofol has not been addressed, nor has the post-CPB duration of impaired hepatic metabolism of fentanyl, midazolam, and propofol. Fentanyl is a good candidate for assessing liver function because its metabolism is sensitive to changes associated with CPB and hypothermia, but other drugs may be used to probe different enzyme systems (50).

Hepatic metabolism of nitroglycerin and lorazepam (58,59) does not appear to be reduced by cardiopulmonary bypass. Dasta et al. (58) reported that CPB causes a 20% apparent *increase* in nitroglycerin metabolism, but they could not exclude nonhepatic factors, such as adhesion of nitroglycerin to elements of the bypass circuit and metabolism by erythrocytes and endothelial cells. Failure of CPB to alter lorazepam elimination (59), in contrast to its inhibition of midazolam clearance, may relate to different metabolic pathways for the two benzodiazepines. Lorazepam is primarily conjugated intact with glucuronide (a process relatively resistant to liver disease), whereas midazolam must first be oxidized by hepatic mixed function oxidase before conjugation. Thus, identification of a particular enzyme system may be important in the evaluation of hepatic function.

Markers of Hepatocellular Injury

Hepatic blood flow is not autoregulated during CPB, although hepatic oxygen consumption is maintained at systemic flows as low as 2.2 L/m^2 per minute (10,28,60). There is no currently accepted method to assess hepatic perfusion during CPB other than careful regulation of systemic flow. The traditional "liver function tests" of plasma concentrations of bilirubin and enzymes found in high concentration in the liver actually serve better as an index of hepatocellular injury than of function. Studies of intraoperative serum bilirubin concentration during CPB have not been reported, although it is likely to decrease from pre-bypass levels because of hemodilution by the extracorporeal system.

Welbourn et al. (61) found a rise in plasma concentrations of lactic dehydrogenase, hydroxybutyrate dehydrogenase, isocitrate dehydrogenase, and glutamic–oxaloacetic transaminase (SGOT) in 22 patients during "mildly" hypothermic CPB (nadir 19° to 34°C), after correction for hemodilution. This constellation of increased plasma enzyme concentrations persisted in the postoperative setting (61). However, the source of the enzyme leak could not be ascribed to the liver; rather, it appeared to be largely a consequence of myocardial damage (61). Serum glutamic–pyruvic transaminase (SGPT) and ornithine carbamyl transferase, which are more specific markers of liver damage, are generally not elevated during or after CPB (61,62).

Dyes specifically taken up by the liver, such as Bromosulphalein or indocyanine green, have been used to assess the effects of CPB (18,49). However, it is impossible to distinguish between the effects of hepatic hypoperfusion and hepatocellular dysfunction despite "adequate" perfusion by using a dye uptake technique alone. Under normal circumstances, Bromosulphalein uptake is considered a better marker of hepatic perfusion than is indocyanine green, but this has not been verified under conditions of hypothermic CPB. Alternatively, hepatic blood flow estimated by indocyanine green clearance correlates poorly with that directly measured by flowmeter in awake healthy volunteers or subjects with liver disease (20). Dye uptake methods for assessing either liver perfusion or function must be carefully validated when they are applied to patients undergoing CPB. From a purely clinical perspective, the available evidence indicates that CPB is not detrimental to the liver in the majority of patients, but that does not obviate the need for better hepatic monitoring during cardiac surgery.

Postoperative liver dysfunction is often heralded by the appearance of jaundice ("post-pump jaundice"), which has an incidence of 10% to 20% (63–65). Post-pump jaundice is usually caused by conjugated (direct) hyperbilirubinemia (65), which indicates a defect in biliary excretion rather than hepatocellular dysfunction. This hyperbilirubinemia reaches a peak on the second postoperative day and resolves in most patients within the first week. In a prospective study of 248 patients, Collins et al. (65) found multiple valve procedures (with high right atrial pressure), a large transfusion requirement, and long duration of CPB to be risk factors for the development of post-pump jaundice. On the other hand, post-pump jaundice was not related to preoperative ethanol intake or the intraoperative occurrence of hypoxia, hypotension, or hypothermia (65). Hyperbilirubinemia can be caused by hepatocellular failure to clear a normal bilirubin challenge or by an excessive bilirubin load overwhelming a normal hepatic function. Therefore, the role of excessive bilirubin challenge secondary to massive transfusion in patients in whom post-pump jaundice develops but who are otherwise without evidence of hepatic injury or failure should be considered as a separate entity. On the other hand, a long duration of CPB is also a risk factor for specific markers of hepatocellular damage, such as elevated plasma concentration of isocitrate dehydrogenase (61).

The occurrence of post-pump jaundice in patients who have undergone uncomplicated operations raises the question of how its incidence could be reduced with better intraoperative monitoring of hepatic function. The appearance of jaundice 2 days or more following cardiac surgery is accompanied by a 25-fold increase in mortality (65,66). The postoperative progression of jaundice to fulminant hepatic failure is almost uniformly fatal (67).

Frank hepatic trauma during cardiac surgery has been reported as a result of inadvertent puncture during placement of thoracotomy tubes (68) or direct manipulation to augment venous return to the heart during placement of a right atrial line (69). Hepatic trauma can rapidly lead to unexplained hypovolemia that requires immediate abdominal exploration.

PANCREATIC FUNCTION AND CARDIOPULMONARY BYPASS
Exocrine and Endocrine Pancreas

The pancreas has two broad functions, defined as "exocrine" and "endocrine" in nature. Exocrine pancreatic function involves the synthesis and secretion of digestive enzymes and other alimentary factors. A key enzyme in this system is amylase, which is released as a proenzyme and activated in the pancreatic duct. The serum amylase concentration is normally low, but because pancreatic injury leads to intravascular leak of the enzyme, an elevated amylase concentration is an index of pancreatic injury. Pancreatic amylase must be distinguished from its salivary isoenzyme for maximal utility as a marker of pancreatic injury. Also, because the amylase concentration is affected by renal function, it has been proposed that the relationship between amylase and creatinine clearance (the amylase-to-creatinine clearance ratio, or ACCR) is a more specific indicator of pancreatic injury (70). This method has been criticized, however, because CPB-associated alterations in ACCR can be produced by alterations in renal function rather than by pancreatic injury (71). Exocrine pancreatic function *per se* is difficult to assess in the acute intraoperative and postoperative settings.

Endocrine pancreatic function largely involves α-cell secretion of glucagon and β-cell secretion of insulin. The endocrine pancreatic response to CPB is discussed in detail in Chapter 17. Briefly, both insulin and glucagon secretion are suppressed during hypothermic CPB (29,72–75). Hypothermia and altered perfusion potentially contribute to suppress pancreatic hormone secretion (29,76). Insulin secretion is specifically inhibited by high circulating concentrations of catecholamines (77), which are observed during and after CPB, but this reflects an intact physiologic control mechanism rather than impaired pancreatic function. In contrast, catecholamines normally *stimulate* glucagon secretion (78). Recovery of insulin secretion appropriate for the prevailing blood glucose concentration occurs within 1 hour after separation from CPB and remains appropriate in the postoperative setting (72,73,76,79). Plasma glucagon concentration, in contrast, reaches a maximum on the first postoperative day (80). It is unclear whether the slower glucagon secretion response relative to the insulin secretion response

represents a difference in the functional recovery of α-cells versus β-cells from the effects of CPB, hypothermia, and general anesthesia.

Markers of Pancreatic Injury

The pancreas resembles the liver by virtue of its high metabolic rate (81) and poor intrinsic autoregulation of blood flow during CPB (10,82). This combination makes the pancreas vulnerable to ischemic injury, which is especially difficult to monitor in the pancreas either by perfusion or function. A spectrum of pancreatic injury is associated with CPB. Hypothermic CPB is followed by an asymptomatic hyperamylasemia in 30% to 70% of patients (83–86). The ACCR is also elevated in 31% to 90% of patients undergoing normothermic CPB (87). The serum concentration of pancreatic isoamylase was elevated in 27% and pancreatic ribonuclease in 13% of 30 postoperative patients without clinical pancreatitis studied by Haas et al. (88). In the largest prospective series to date, Fernandez-del Castillo et al. (86) studied 300 consecutive patients undergoing CPB and found a 27% incidence of pancreatic cellular injury, defined as hyperamylasemia accompanied by a rise in pancreatic isoamylase (30%), lipase (10%), or both (60%). Ninety-nine percent of these patients with laboratory evidence of pancreatic injury were completely asymptomatic.

The incidence of clinical pancreatitis ("post-pump pancreatitis") is 0.1% to 1% by either prospective or retrospective analysis (86,88–90). Cardiac surgery patients who do not survive, as might be expected, more commonly exhibit pathologic evidence of pancreatitis. In 209 patients who died within 10 days of cardiac surgery, Feiner (91) reported a 16% incidence of pancreatitis, and Warshaw and O'Hara (92) found an 11% incidence in 101 autopsies. Pathologic findings in both series were consistent with intraoperative pancreatic ischemia (91,92).

Risk factors for post-pump pancreatitis include prolonged duration of CPB, perioperative hypotension or use of inotropic agents, low postoperative cardiac output, renal failure, and perioperative calcium administration (86,88,90). Calcium administration appears to be a risk factor independently of its possible use as a treatment for hypotension. For instance, pancreatitis has been reported secondary to hypercalcemia in a variety of medical conditions not accompanied by hypotension, including multiple myeloma (93), hyperparathyroidism (94), breast cancer (95), iatrogenic calcium overload in hyperalimentation (96), and vitamin D intoxication (97). Moreover, large replacements of calcium to replenish depleted plasma ionized calcium accompanying massive transfusion during liver transplantation results in rebound hypercalcemia as the citrate is metabolized. This rebound hypercalcemia can be associated with development of clinical pancreatitis, even in the absence of intraoperative hemodynamic instability.

A putative mechanism whereby calcium induces pancreatitis is emerging. Because calcium chloride administered to rats increased the intracellular concentration of trypsinogen activation peptide, induced pathologic changes in the pancreas, and increased serum amylase, Mithofer et al. (98) suggested that ectopic trypsin activation is involved in development of calcium-induced pancreatitis. Alternatively, it has been proposed that increased cytosolic calcium concentrations dysregulate intracellular oxygen radicals, damaging the pancreatic acinar cells (99). Regardless of the exact molecular mechanism, the data indicate that injudicious use of calcium is contraindicated in cardiac surgery patients. Hypothermia is another potential cause of pancreatitis, but the studies linking hypothermia to pancreatitis (100,101) were not controlled for the preservation of either total or splanchnic blood flow during hypothermia, which is well maintained during hypothermic CPB.

Post-pump pancreatitis has dire consequences. Severe postoperative pancreatitis has a mortality rate of 67% to 100%, and a mortality rate of 26% to 70% accompanies even mild forms (86,89,90). In a retrospective study of 5,621 patients, Lefor et al. (90) found a 44% mortality associated with clinically evident pancreatitis after CPB. Rapid intraoperative or even postoperative diagnosis of pancreatic injury occurring with cardiac surgery is hampered by inadequate monitoring techniques.

GASTROINTESTINAL COMPLICATIONS

Good parameters of perioperative gastrointestinal function and specific enzymes to indicate gastrointestinal injury in the perioperative setting are unknown, which precludes the intraoperative diagnosis of gastrointestinal ischemia and dysfunction. Even postoperative signs of gastrointestinal dysfunction are very subtle, contributing to delays in diagnosis and treatment. Thus, assessment of the effects of CPB on the gastrointestinal system has been limited to case reports of severe injury, often resulting in resection of infarcted tissue or death of the patient. Several retrospective analyses, of more than 13,000 cases, reveal a gastrointestinal complication rate of 1% to 2% for cardiac surgery with CPB (67,102–104). The gastrointestinal complication rate approximates that for pancreatitis, although either can occur independently.

The most frequent complication is bleeding, usually duodenal or gastric, which accounts for 25% to 60% of gastrointestinal complications (67,102–105). Mortality accompanying gastrointestinal hemorrhage is 33% to 53% (67,103,104). Less common complications are duodenal ulcers, diverticulitis, colonic pseudo-obstruction, mesenteric ischemia or infarction, and splenic infarction (67,106–108). The mortality associated with these complications is comparable to that observed with gastrointestinal hemorrhage. In contrast, acalculous cholecystitis, which occurs in five patients per 1,000, has a mortality rate of 86% (67).

Risk factors for gastrointestinal complications include prolonged duration of CPB, low perioperative cardiac output, postoperative requirement for vasopressor therapy, advanced age, emergent surgery, and valve surgery (with possible portal congestion) (67,104,109). Several of these risk factors have also been identified as risk factors for "post-pump jaundice" and "post-pump pancreatitis." It is therefore not unexpected that concomitant jaundice or pancreatitis in patients with "post-pump" gastrointestinal complications is frequent (67,102). It is therefore reasonable to propose that intraoperative or postoperative splanchnic ischemia underlies many of the visceral complications associated with CPB (109,110). Technical limitations in monitoring splanchnic perfusion make it difficult to prove this tempting hypothesis conclusively.

The intestinal wall normally prevents intraluminal bacteria and endotoxin from entering the vasculature. There has been considerable interest in studying whether the barrier function of the intestine is interrupted during and after CPB. Such interruption combined with the impairment of clearance by hepatic Kupffer cells (45) would imply at least a transient bacteremia or endotoxemia associated with CPB. Endotoxin, in turn, would stimulate the systemic inflammatory response, leading to multiple systems organ failure in susceptible patients. The relationship between splanchnic ischemia and multiple systems organ failure has been reviewed by Landow and Anderson (111). Rocke et al. (112) reported that the plasma endotoxin concentration was transiently increased after release of the aortic cross-clamp in nine patients undergoing CPB. All patients had an uneventful intraoperative and postoperative course, which prevented an analysis of the role of endotoxin in subsequent postoperative complications. It is still noteworthy that the magnitude of endotoxemia was directly related to the duration of CPB (112). Further, the magnitude and time course of endotoxemia in these patients closely resembled the effects of 1-hour superior mesenteric artery occlusion in cats (113). Riddington et al. (114) detected endotoxemia and labeled EDTA (ethylenediamine-tetraacetic acid) leak from the intestine during CPB in 21 of 50 patients undergoing elective cardiac surgery without any change in gastric mucosal pH. Bowel decontamination with nonabsorbable antibiotics decreased the incidence and magnitude of the endotoxemia and also limited the rise of plasma concentrations of the proinflammatory cytokines tumor necrosis factor and interleukin-6 (115). The patient's preoperative immune status with respect to endotoxin also affects outcome. Bennett-Guerrero and associates (116), in a study of 301 patients undergoing cardiac surgery with CPB, found that low preoperative serum concentration of the immunoglobulin M antibody to endotoxin core increased the serious postoperative complication rate sixfold above that for patients with high preoperative antibody concentration. The significance of endotoxin leak into the circulation is that the largest endotoxin challenge occurs in patients with the longest CPB times, which also increases the risk for direct gastrointestinal, pancreatic, and hepatic injury. These factors may converge in the development of postoperative sepsis, pulmonary or cardiac dysfunction, and multiple systems organ failure.

Seen concomitantly with the increased movement of endotoxin from the intestine to the plasma is an increased opposite flux of plasma proteins into the intestinal interstitium. CPB thus produces an abnormal bidirectional increase in material flux across the intestinal wall. Smith et al. (117) showed that intestinal permeability to plasma proteins increases to four times the control value during normothermic CPB at 2.2 L/m^2 per minute in dogs. The increased permeability is most pronounced for large molecules. Augmented protein influx into the intestinal interstitium increases tissue edema, rendering the intestine more sensitive to compromised perfusion.

The most likely mechanisms leading to hepatic, pancreatic, and gastrointestinal complications are hypoperfusion and the unexplained increased permeability of the intestine. Defining adequate splanchnic perfusion in a given patient is problematic because of the difficulty in monitoring intraoperatively and postoperatively either flow or indicators of physiologic organ function. One monitoring approach is to measure the intraluminal pH of either stomach or colon by tonometry, as acidosis of either stomach or colon is reasonably predictive of tissue ischemia (21–24). However, tonometry is relatively difficult to master from both the technical and interpretative standpoints at this time. Perhaps continued development would allow it to be simplified into a more practicable clinical tool, as has been the case with pulse oximetry. The most reliable way to optimize splanchnic perfusion during CPB remains to utilize a high rate of pump flow, which is a reasonable strategy, especially in the patient at high risk for visceral complications.

SUMMARY

Surgery with CPB produces marked alterations in the splanchnic circulation and its dependent organs. Today, most of these alterations are invisible to the physician caring for the patient because of significant limitations in the monitoring of regional blood flow and sophisticated assessment of visceral organ viability and function. Because most patients appear to do well postoperatively, there has not been a rush to improve the system of monitoring. However, the changes in perioperative splanchnic perfusion are profoundly important. These must be better understood to improve care in the future. Improved monitoring of splanchnic perfusion and cellular viability may reduce the incidence of visceral complications from the present 1% to 2% of patients. Although the relative number of patients affected at first appears to be small, the absolute number is substantial,

and the outcome of visceral complications can be devastating.

KEY POINTS

- Adverse effects of CPB specifically involving the splanchnic viscera (gut, liver, and pancreas) are relatively uncommon but remain important because they have grave consequences.
- Visceral perfusion during both normothermic and hypothermic CPB usually appears to be well preserved, but:
  - Gastric mucosal pH declines in humans during CPB.
  - Pharmacologic manipulation of perfusion pressure with vasopressor during CPB may have paradoxical effects on visceral perfusion.
  - Clinical monitoring tools are inadequate.
- Hepatic function is altered by CPB.
  - Cori cycle function is abnormal.
  - Protein synthesis is decreased.
  - Drug metabolism is altered.
  - Direct hepatocellular injury is uncommon.
- Pancreatic function is altered by CPB.
  - Both exocrine and endocrine function is altered.
  - The risk for pancreatitis relates to length of CPB, hypotension, low cardiac output, and calcium therapy.
- CPB can cause gastrointestinal complications.
  - Gastrointestinal bleeding is the most common, accounting for 25% to 60% of all complications.
  - Acalculous cholecystitis is infrequent (five patients per 1,000) but severe; the mortality is approximately 86%.
  - Risk factors are long CPB, vasopressor use, low cardiac output, advanced age, emergency procedure, and valve surgery.

REFERENCES

1. Wiggers CJ. The present status of the shock problem. *Physiol Rev* 1942;22:74–123.
2. Halley MM, Reemtsma K, Creech O Jr. Hemodynamics and metabolism of individual organs during extracorporeal circulation. *Surgery* 1959;46:1128–1134.
3. Yokoyama T, Okamoto R, Yamamoto Y, et al. Hepatic energy status in hypotension of different aetiologies in dogs. *Clin Sci* 1991;81:627–633.
4. Desai JB, Mathie RT, Taylor KM. Hepatic blood flow during cardiopulmonary bypass in the dog: a comparison between pulsatile and nonpulsatile perfusion. *Life Support Systems* 1984; 2[Suppl 1]:303–305.
5. Lees MH, Herr RH, Hill JD, et al. Distribution of systemic blood flow of the rhesus monkey during cardiopulmonary bypass. *J Thorac Cardiovasc Surg* 1971;61:570–586.

6. Rudy LW Jr, Heymann MA, Edmunds LH Jr. Distribution of systemic blood flow during cardiopulmonary bypass. *J Appl Physiol* 1973;34:194–200.

7. Fujita Y, Sakai T, Ohsumi A, et al. Effects of hypocapnia and hypercapnia on splanchnic circulation and hepatic function in the beagle. *Anesth Analg* 1989;69:152–157.

8. Gelman S, Fowler KC, Bishop SP, et al. Cardiac output distribution and regional blood flow during hypocarbia in monkeys. *J Appl Physiol* 1985;58:1225–1230.

9. Gelman S. Carbon dioxide and hepatic circulation. *Anesth Analg* 1989;69:149–151.

10. Mori A, Watanabe K, Onoe M, et al. Regional blood flow in the liver, pancreas and kidney during pulsatile and nonpulsatile perfusion under profound hypothermia. *Jpn Circ J* 1988;52:219–227.

11. Van Kesteren RG, van Alphen MMA, Charbon GA. Effects of dopamine on intestinal vessels in anesthetized dogs. *Circ Shock* 1988;25:41–51.

12. Priebe H-J, Noldge GFE, Armbruster K, et al. Differential effects of dobutamine, dopamine, and noradrenaline on splanchnic haemodynamics and oxygenation in the pig. *Acta Anaesthesiol Scand* 1995;39:1088–1096.

13. Lundberg J, Lundberg D, Norgren L, et al. Intestinal hemodynamics during laparotomy: effects of thoracic epidural anesthesia and dopamine in humans. *Anesth Analg* 1990;71:9–15.

14. Mackay JH, Feerick AE, Woodson LC, et al. Increasing organ blood flow during cardiopulmonary bypass in pigs: comparison of dopamine and perfusion pressure. *Crit Care Med* 1995;23:1090–1098.

15. O'Dwyer C, Woodson LC, Conroy BP, et al. Regional perfusion abnormalities with phenylephrine during normothermic bypass. *Ann Thorac Surg* 1997;63:728–735.

16. Mousdale S, Clyburn PA, Mackie AM, et al. Comparison of the effects of dopamine, dobutamine, and dopexamine upon renal blood flow: a study in normal healthy volunteers. *Br J Clin Pharmacol* 1988;25:555–560.

17. Berendes E, Mollhoff T, Van Aken H, et al. Effects of dopexamine on creatinine clearance, systemic inflammation, and splanchnic oxygenation in patients undergoing coronary artery bypass grafting. *Anesth Analg* 1997;84:950–957.

18. Andersen MN, Norberg B, Senning A. Studies of liver function during extracorporeal circulation with low flow rate. *Surgery* 1958;43:397–407.

19. Kainuma M, Fujiwara Y, Kimura N, et al. Monitoring hepatic venous hemoglobin oxygen saturation in patients undergoing liver surgery. *Anesthesiology* 1991;74:49–52.

20. Skak C, Keiding S. Methodological problems in the use of indocyanine green to estimate hepatic blood flow and ICG clearance in man. *Liver* 1987;7:155–162.

21. Fiddian-Green RG, Amelin PM, Herrmann JB, et al. Prediction of the development of sigmoid ischemia on the day of aortic operations. Indirect measurements of intramural pH in the colon. *Arch Surg* 1986;121:654–660.

22. Fiddian-Green RG, Baker S. Predictive value of the stomach wall pH for complications after cardiac operations: comparison with other monitoring. *Crit Care Med* 1987;15:153–156.

23. Landow L, Phillips DA, Heard SO, et al. Gastric tonometry and venous oximetry in cardiac surgery patients. *Crit Care Med* 1991;19:1226–1233.

24. Gutierrez G, Bismar H, Dantzker DR, et al. Comparison of gastric intramucosal pH with measures of oxygen transport and consumption in critically ill patients. *Crit Care Med* 1992;20:451–457.

25. Garrett SA, Pearl RG. Improved gastric tonometry for monitoring tissue perfusion: the canary sings louder. *Anesth Analg* 1996;83:1–3.

26. Tao W, Zwischenberger JB, Nguyen TT, et al. Gut mucosal ischemia during normothermic cardiopulmonary bypass results from blood flow redistribution and increased oxygen demand. *J Thorac Cardiovasc Surg* 1995;110:819–828.

27. Haisjackl M, Birnbaum J, Redlin M, et al. Splanchnic oxygen transport and lactate metabolism during normothermic cardiopulmonary bypass in humans. *Anesth Analg* 1998;86:22–27.

28. Waldhausen JA, Lombardo CR, McFarland JA, et al. Studies of hepatic blood flow and oxygen consumption during total cardiopulmonary bypass. *Surgery* 1959;46:1118–1127.

29. Kuntschen FR, Galletti PM, Hahn C. Glucose–insulin interactions during cardiopulmonary bypass. Hypothermia versus normothermia. *J Thorac Cardiovasc Surg* 1986;91:451–459.

30. Meyerholz H-H, Gardemann A, Jungermann K. Control of glycogenolysis and blood flow by arterial and portal adrenaline in perfused liver. *Biochem J* 1991;275:609–616.

31. Penicaud L, Ferre P, Kande J, et al. Effect of anesthesia on glucose production and utilization in rats. *Am J Physiol* 1987;252:E365–E369.

32. Toffaletti J, Christenson RH, Mullins S, et al. Relationship between serum lactate and ionized calcium in open-heart surgery. *Clin Chem* 1986;32:1849–1853.

33. Wolk LA, Wilson RF, Burdick M, et al. Changes in antithrombin, antiplasmin, and plasminogen during and after cardiopulmonary bypass. *Am Surg* 1985;51:309–313.

34. Thompson C, Blumenstock FA, Saba TM, et al. Plasma fibronectin synthesis in normal and injured humans as determined by stable isotope incorporation. *J Clin Invest* 1989;84:1226–1235.

35. Carraro F, Hartl WH, Stuart CA, et al. Whole body and plasma protein synthesis in exercise and recovery in human subjects. *Am J Physiol* 1990;258:E821–E831.

36. Tamkun JW, Hynes RO. Plasma fibronectin is synthesized and secreted by hepatocytes. *J Biol Chem* 1983;258:4641–4647.

37. Gandhi JG, Vander Salm T, Szymanski IO. Effect of cardiopulmonary bypass on plasma fibronectin, IgG, and C3. *Transfusion* 1983;23:476–479.

38. Snyder EL, Barash PG, Mosher DF, et al. Plasma fibronectin level and clinical status in cardiac surgery patients. *J Lab Clin Med* 1983;102:881–889.

39. Pourrat E, Sie PM, Desrez X, et al. Changes in plasma fibronectin levels after cardiac and pulmonary surgery: role of cardiopulmonary bypass. *Scand J Thorac Cardiovasc Surg* 1985;19:63–67.

40. Labrousse F, Dequirot A, Sos P, et al. Plasma fibronectin depletion after cardiac surgery in children with or without cardiopulmonary bypass. *J Clin Chem Clin Biochem* 1986;24:441–444.

41. Gotta AW, Carsons S, Abrams L, et al. Fibronectin levels during cardiopulmonary bypass. *NY State J Med* 1987;87:493–496.

42. Saba TM. Fibronectin deficiency following cardiopulmonary bypass. *NY State J Med* 1987;87:487–489.

43. Haniuda M, Morimoto M, Sugenoya A, et al. Suppressive effect of ulinastatin on plasma fibronectin depression after cardiac surgery. *Ann Thorac Surg* 1988;45:171–173.

44. Howard L, Dillon B, Saba TM, et al. Decreased plasma fibronectin during starvation in man. *J Parenter Enter Nutr* 1984;8:237–244.

45. Shimono T, Yada I, Kanamori Y, et al. Reticuloendothelial function following cardiopulmonary bypass. *J Surg Res* 1994;56:446–451.

46. Roelofse JA, van der Bijl P. Plasma cholinesterase levels during cardiopulmonary bypass. A report on 10 cases. *S Afr Med J* 1987;71:662–664.

47. Eicher O, Farah A. *Cholinesterases and anticholinesterase agents.* New York: Springer-Verlag, 1963:63.

48. Wan S, LeClerc JL, Schmartz D, et al. Hepatic release of interleukin-10 during cardiopulmonary bypass in steroid-pretreated patients. *Am Heart J* 1997;133:335–339.

49. Autschbach R, Falk V, Lange H, et al. Assessment of metabolic liver function and hepatic blood flow during cardiopulmonary bypass. *Thorac Cardiovasc Surgeon* 1996;44:76–80.

50. Barstow L, Small RE. Liver function assessment by drug metabolism. *Pharmacotherapy* 1990;10:280–288.

51. Koska AJ III, Romagnoli A, Kramer WG. Effect of cardiopulmonary bypass on fentanyl distribution and elimination. *Clin Pharmacol Ther* 1981;29:100–105.

52. Holley FO, Ponganis KV, Stanski DR. Effect of cardiopulmonary bypass on the pharmacokinetics of drugs. *Clin Pharmacokinet* 1982;7:234–251.

53. Koren G, Barker C, Goresky G, et al. The influence of hypothermia on the disposition of fentanyl—human and animal studies. *Eur J Clin Pharmacol* 1987;32:373–376.

54. Koren G, Barker C, Bohn D, et al. Influence of hypothermia on the pharmacokinetics of gentamicin and theophylline in piglets. *Crit Care Med* 1985;13:844–847.

55. Kanto J, Himberg JJ, Heikkila H, et al. Midazolam kinetics before, during and after cardiopulmonary bypass surgery. *Int J Clin Pharmacol Res* 1985;2:123–126.

56. Mathews HML, Carson IW, Lyons SM, et al. A pharmacokinetic study of midazolam in paediatric patients undergoing cardiac surgery. *Br J Anaesth* 1988;61:302–307.

57. McMurray TJ, Collier PS, Carson IW, et al. Propofol sedation after open heart surgery. A clinical and pharmacokinetic study. *Anaesthesia* 1990;45:322–326.

58. Dasta JF, Weber RJ, Wu LS, et al. Influence of cardiopulmonary bypass on nitroglycerin clearance. *J Clin Pharmacol* 1986;26:165–168.

59. Aaltonen L, Kanto J, Arola M, et al. Effect of age and cardiopulmonary bypass on the pharmacokinetics of lorazepam. *Acta Pharmacol Toxicol* 1982;51:126–131.

60. Mathie RT. Hepatic blood flow during cardiopulmonary bypass. *Crit Care Med* 1993;21:S72–S76.

61. Welbourn N, Melrose DG, Moss DW. Changes in serum enzyme levels accompanying cardiac surgery with extracorporeal circulation. *J Clin Pathol* 1966;19:220–232.

62. Norberg B, Senning A. A study of serum enzymes during and after open heart surgery with the Crafoord-Senning heart–lung machine. *Acta Chir Scand* 1959;245[Suppl]:275–284.

63. Lockey E, McIntyre N, Ross DN, et al. Early jaundice after open-heart surgery. *Thorax* 1967;22:165–169.

64. Sanderson RG, Ellison JH, Benson JA, et al. Jaundice following open heart surgery. *Ann Surg* 1967;165:217–224.

65. Collins JD, Ferner R, Murray A, et al. Incidence and prognostic importance of jaundice after cardiopulmonary bypass surgery. *Lancet* 1983;1:1119–1123.

66. Ryan TA, Rady MY, Bashour CA, et al. Predictors of outcome in cardiac surgical patients with prolonged intensive care stay. *Chest* 1997;112:1035–1042.

67. Krasna MJ, Flancbaum L, Trooskin SZ, et al. Gastrointestinal complications after cardiac surgery. *Surgery* 1988;104:773–780.

68. Robinson G, Brodman R. Going down the tube. *Ann Thorac Surg* 1981;31:400–401.

69. Eugene J, Ott RA, Stemmer EA. Hepatic trauma during cardiac surgery. *J Cardiovasc Surg* 1986;27:100–102.

70. Warshaw AL, Fuller AF. Specificity of increased renal clearance of amylase in diagnosis of acute pancreatitis. *N Engl J Med* 1975;292:325–328.

71. Smith CR, Schwartz SI. Amylase:creatinine clearance ratios, serum amylase, and lipase after operations with cardiopulmonary bypass. *Surgery* 1983;94:458–463.

72. Allison SP, Prowse K, Chamberlain MJ. Failure of insulin response to glucose load during operation and after myocardial infarction. *Lancet* 1967;1:478–481.

73. Malatinsky J, Vigas M, Jezova D, et al. The effects of open heart surgery on growth hormone, cortisol and insulin levels in man. Hormone levels during open heart surgery. *Resuscitation* 1984;11:57–68.

74. Benzing G III, Francis PD, Kaplan S, et al. Glucose and insulin changes in infants and children undergoing hypothermic open-heart surgery. *Am J Cardiol* 1983;52:133–136.

75. Kuntschen FR, Galletti PM, Hahn C, et al. Alterations of insulin and glucose metabolism during cardiopulmonary bypass under normothermia. *J Thorac Cardiovasc Surg* 1985;89:97–106.

76. Abe T. Influence of cardiac surgery using cardiopulmonary bypass on metabolic regulation. *Jpn Circ J* 1974;38:13–21.

77. Porte D Jr, Graber AL, Kuzuya T, et al. The effect of epinephrine on immunoreactive insulin levels in man. *J Clin Invest* 1966;45:228–236.

78. Gerich JE, Karam JH, Forsham PH. Stimulation of glucagon secretion by epinephrine in man. *J Clin Endocrinol Metab* 1973;37:479–481.

79. Brandt MR, Korshin J, Hansen AP, et al. Influence of morphine anaesthesia on the endocrine-metabolic response to open-heart surgery. *Acta Anaesthesiol Scand* 1978;22:400–412.

80. McKnight CK, Elliott M, Pearson DT, et al. The effect of four different crystalloid bypass pump-priming fluids upon the metabolic response to cardiac operation. *J Thorac Cardiovasc Surg* 1985;90:97–111.

81. Harper SL, Pitts VH, Granger DN, et al. Pancreatic tissue oxygenation during secretory stimulation. *Am J Physiol* 1986;250:G316–G322.

82. Kvietys PR, McLendon JM, Bulkley GB, et al. Pancreatic circulation: intrinsic regulation. *Am J Physiol* 1982;242:G596–G602.

83. Moores WY, Gago O, Morris JD, et al. Serum and urinary amylase levels following pulsatile and continuous cardiopulmonary bypass. *J Thorac Cardiovasc Surg* 1977;74:73–76.

84. Missavage AE, Weaver DW, Bouman DL, et al. Hyperamylasemia after cardiopulmonary bypass. *Am Surg* 1984;50:297–300.

85. Rattner DW, Gu Z-Y, Vlahakes GJ, et al. Hyperamylasemia after cardiac surgery. *Ann Surg* 1989;209:279–283.

86. Fernandez-del Castillo C, Harringer W, Warshaw AL, et al. Risk factors for pancreatic cellular injury after cardiopulmonary bypass. *N Engl J Med* 1991;325:382–387.

87. Murray WR, Mittra S, Mittra D, et al. The amylase-creatinine clearance ratio following cardiopulmonary bypass. *J Thorac Cardiovasc Surg* 1981;82:248–253.

88. Haas GS, Warshaw AL, Daggett WM, et al. Acute pancreatitis after cardiopulmonary bypass. *Am J Surg* 1985;149:508–515.

89. Rose DM, Ranson JHC, Cunningham JN, et al. Patterns of severe pancreatic injury following cardiopulmonary bypass. *Ann Surg* 1984;199:168–172.

90. Lefor AT, Vuocolo P, Parker FB Jr, et al. Pancreatic complications following cardiopulmonary bypass. Factors influencing mortality. *Arch Surg* 1992;127:1225–1231.

91. Feiner H. Pancreatitis after cardiac surgery. A morphologic study. *Am J Surg* 1976;131:684–688.

92. Warshaw AL, O'Hara PJ. Susceptibility of the pancreas to ischemic injury in shock. *Ann Surg* 1978;188:197–201.

93. Meltzer LE, Palmon FP Jr, Paik YK, et al. Acute pancreatitis secondary to hypercalcemia of multiple myeloma. *Ann Intern Med* 1962;57:1008–1012.

94. Mixter CG Jr, Keynes WM, Cope O. Further experience with pancreatitis as a diagnostic clue to hyperparathyroidism. *N Engl J Med* 1962;266:265–272.

95. Gafter U, Mandel EM, Har-Zahav L, et al. Acute pancreatitis secondary to hypercalcemia: occurrence in a patient with breast carcinoma. *JAMA* 1976;235:2004–2005.

96. Izsak EM, Shike M, Roulet M, et al. Pancreatitis in association with hypercalcemia in patients receiving total parenteral nutrition. *Gastroenterology* 1980;79:555–558.

97. Waele BD, Smitz J, Willems G. Recurrent pancreatitis secondary to hypercalcemia following vitamin D poisoning. *Pancreas* 1989;4:378–380.

98. Mithofer K, Fernandez-del Castillo C, Frick TW, et al. Acute hypercalcemia causes acute pancreatitis and ectopic trypsinogen activation in the rat. *Gastroenterology* 1995;109:239–246.

99. Weber H, Roesner JP, Nebe B, et al. Increased cytosolic Ca^{2+} amplifies oxygen radical-induced alterations of the ultrastructure and the energy metabolism of isolated rat pancreatic acinar cells. *Digestion* 1998;59:175–185.

100. MacLean D, Morrison J, Griffiths PD. Acute pancreatitis and diabetic ketoacidosis in accidental hypothermia and hypothermic myxoedema. *BMJ* 1973;4:757–761.

101. Savides EP, Hoffbrand BI. Hypothermia, thrombosis and acute pancreatitis. *BMJ* 1974;1:614.

102. Hanks JB, Curtis SE, Hanks BB, et al. Gastrointestinal complications after cardiopulmonary bypass. *Surgery* 1982;92:394–400.

103. Heikkinen LO, Ala-Kulju KV. Abdominal complications following cardiopulmonary bypass in open-heart surgery. *Scand J Thorac Cardiovasc Surg* 1987;21:1–7.

104. Leitman IM, Paull DE, Barie PS, et al. Intra-abdominal complications of cardiopulmonary bypass operations. *Surg Gynecol Obstet* 1987;165:251–254.

105. Decker GAG, Josselsohn E, Svensson L, et al. Acute gastroduodenal complications after cardiopulmonary bypass surgery. *S Afr J Surg* 1984;22:261–264.

106. Burton NA, Albus RA, Graeber GM, et al. Acute diverticulitis following cardiac surgery. *Chest* 1986;89:756–757.

107. Evora PRB, Moraes MMFS, Ribeiro PJF, et al. Nonocclusive intestinal ischemia and necrosis after correction of interatrial communication with cardiopulmonary bypass. *J Cardiovasc Surg* 1989;30:1002–1005.

108. Allen KB, Salam AA, Lumsden AB. Acute mesenteric ischemia after cardiopulmonary bypass. *J Vasc Surg* 1992;16:391–395.

109. Moneta GL, Misbach GA, Ivey TD. Hypoperfusion as a possible factor in the development of gastrointestinal complications after cardiac surgery. *Am J Surg* 1985;149:648–650.

110. Christenson JT, Schmuziger M, Maurice J, et al. Postoperative visceral hypotension the common cause for gastrointestinal complications after cardiac surgery. *Thorac Cardiovasc Surgeon* 1994;42:152–157.

111. Landow L, Andersen LW. Splanchnic ischaemia and its role in multiple organ failure. *Acta Anaesthesiol Scand* 1994;38:626–639.

112. Rocke DA, Gaffin SL, Wells MT, et al. Endotoxemia associated with cardiopulmonary bypass. *J Thorac Cardiovasc Surg* 1987;93:832–837.

113. Gathiram P, Gaffin SL, Wells MT, et al. Superior mesenteric artery occulsion shock in cats: modification of the endotoxemia by antilipopolysaccharide antibodies. *Circ Shock* 1986;19:231–237.

114. Riddington DW, Venkatesh B, Boivin CM, et al. Intestinal permeability, gastric intramucosal pH, and systemic endotoxemia in patients undergoing cardiopulmonary bypass. *JAMA* 1996;275:1007–1012.

115. Martinez-Pellus AE, Merino P, Bru M, et al. Endogenous endotoxemia of intestinal origin during cardiopulmonary bypass. Role of type of flow and protective effect of selective digestive decontamination. *Intensive Care Med* 1997;23:1251–1257.

116. Bennett-Guerrero E, Ayuso L, Hamilton-Davies C, et al. Relationship of preoperative antiendotoxin core antibodies and adverse outcomes following cardiac surgery. *JAMA* 1997;277:646–650.

117. Smith EEJ, Naftel DC, Blackstone EH, et al. Microvascular permeability after cardiopulmonary bypass. An experimental study. *J Thorac Cardiovasc Surg* 1987;94:225–233.

NEUROLOGIC EFFECTS

DAVID J. COOK

This chapter provides an overview of the neurologic effects of cardiopulmonary bypass (CPB). First, a summary of the extent and nature of bypass-related neurologic injury is presented, with an emphasis on the importance of patient demographics and comorbidities. In this context, etiologic factors are considered. Second, basic cerebral physiology during CPB is reviewed. Third, interventions with the potential to reduce neurologic morbidity are considered, and fourth, neuromonitoring techniques are briefly described.

POPULATION AT RISK, DEMOGRAPHICS, AND COMORBIDITIES

Cardiac operations requiring CPB are some of the most commonly performed surgical procedures in Europe and North America. Studies together describing more than 20,000 cardiac surgical patients indicate that significant morbidity may be experienced by 20% to 25% of patients (1–3). These morbidities consist of cardiac and pulmonary failure, neurologic injury, renal insufficiency, bleeding, and infection. Complications have predictable effects on length of stay and cost of hospitalization (4–7) in addition to patient well-being and functional capacity at discharge (7–9).

It is important to emphasize that the primary risk factors for stroke and cognitive impairment in the general population also define the persons at highest risk for neurologic morbidity in the cardiac surgical patient pool. Surgery itself, whether cardiac or noncardiac, entails neurologic risk. The European study of cognitive outcomes after noncardiac surgery illustrates this superbly (10). In that study, 1,218 elderly patients having major noncardiac surgery underwent neurocognitive assessment preoperatively, before discharge, and at 3 months postoperatively. A large ($n = 321$) nonsurgical control group was also enrolled. That study reported a 26% incidence of cognitive dysfunction 1 week after surgery and a 10% incidence at 3 months. Cardiac surgery

poses greater risks, because cardiac surgical patients experience more neurologic morbidity than age- and health-matched controls undergoing noncardiac surgery (9) (Table 21.1). Nevertheless, it is useful to think of the perioperative period as an acute stress in a subpopulation chronically at risk.

In regard to stroke risk, there is general agreement about preoperative patient-related factors that increase the likelihood of perioperative stroke, but the role of many intraoperative factors remains unclear. Preoperatively, advanced age, history of prior neurologic events, aortic atherosclerosis, states of low cardiac output, atrial dysrhythmias, hypertension, and diabetes are associated with increased risk. The effect of increased age is most dramatic and appears to concentrate the other risk factors.

This emphasis is important because between 1974 and 1991, the number of patients over age 60 undergoing cardiac surgery with CPB doubled, and the percentage over age 70 increased sevenfold (11). Age alone is an independent risk factor for perioperative stroke; patients under age 60 have an incidence of stroke of less than 1% (1,11,12), whereas those over age 70 have a 4% to 9% incidence of stroke or coma following operation (1,11–13) (Fig. 21.1).

As the surgical population has aged, the proportion of patients with multiple risk factors for neurologic injury has increased. Hypertension and diabetes occur in approximately 55% and 25% of cardiac surgical patients, respectively (11,14–18). Fifteen percent demonstrate carotid stenosis of 50% or greater, and up to 13% may have had a transient ischemic attack or prior stroke (14,18). These processes may double the risk for stroke in the cardiac surgical population (11,19).

The Cardiovascular Health Study illustrates preexisting cerebral morbidity and cerebral risk in the general population (20). In that investigation, 3,360 community patients over the age of 65 (who were seeing a cardiologist routinely) underwent magnetic resonance imaging. Of these, 31% had "silent" cerebral infarcts (20). These infarcts were primarily subcortical, lacunar, and so strategically placed or small that clinical signs of stroke were not evident. However, when detailed testing is done, these infarcts can be associated with

D. J. Cook: Department of Anesthesiology, Mayo Clinic and Mayo Foundation, Rochester, Minnesota 55905.

TABLE 21.1. SEVERITY OF POSTOPERATIVE NEUROPSYCHOLOGICAL DETERIORATION IN CORONARY ARTERY BYPASS GRAFT AND SURGICAL CONTROL PATIENTS

Severity of Deterioration	CABG (n = 298)	Control (n = 48)
Mild (deterioration on 1 or 2 tests)	164 (55%)	15 (31%)
Moderate (deterioration on 3 or 4 tests)	57 (19%)	0
Severe (deterioration on ≥5 tests)	14 (4.7%)	0

Only patients completing both preoperative and postoperative test batteries are included. CABG, coronary artery bypass graft group; control, peripheral vascular surgery group.
From Shaw PJ, Bates D, Cartlidge NE, et al. Neurologic and neuropsychological morbidity following major surgery: comparison of coronary artery bypass and peripheral vascular surgery. *Stroke* 1987;18:700–707, with permission.

cognitive and gait changes (20). These lesions are thought to be related to chronic hypertension, which narrows the penetrating vessels supplying deep white matter and renders these regions highly vulnerable to focal ischemia (21,22).

These findings have implications for the cardiac surgical population. Of the 5,888 men and women enrolled in the Cardiovascular Health Study, those who underwent magnetic resonance imaging were "... younger ... and were more likely never to have smoked and less likely to have prior cardiovascular disease, hypertension ... and diabetes than those who did not undergo scanning" (20,23). As such, the cardiac surgical population probably has an incidence of preexisting "silent" cerebral infarction exceeding 31%. One study of 31 neurologically asymptomatic patients

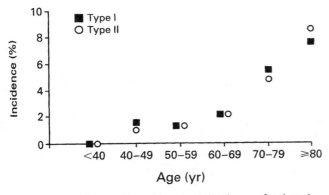

FIG. 21.1. Incidence of type I (cerebral deaths, nonfatal strokes, and new transient ischemic attacks) and type II (new intellectual deterioration at discharge or new seizures) cerebral outcomes according to age. (From Roach GW, Kanchuger M, Mangano CM, et al. Adverse cerebral outcomes after coronary bypass surgery. Multicenter Study of Perioperative Ischemia Research Group and the Ischemia Research and Education Foundation Investigators. *N Engl J Med* 1996;335:1857–1863, with permission.)

undergoing coronary artery bypass graft (CABG) reported a 16% incidence of thromboembolic infarcts and a 58% incidence of lacunar infarcts on preoperative magnetic resonance imaging (24).

Neurologic Complications in Cardiac Surgery

Neurologic injury has been a source of concern since the inception of cardiac surgery, and this injury can be generally divided into frank stroke, encephalopathy, and neurocognitive disorders. The incidence of major neurologic morbidity related to cardiac surgery is 1% to 6% (6,12,15,25–27), although select populations may have a stroke risk as high as 8% to 9% (1,7).

Two recent multicenter studies examined neurologic outcomes and their predictors in patients undergoing CABG (6) or combined CABG and open-ventricle procedures (7). Morbid neurologic outcomes were classified as type I (cerebral deaths, nonfatal strokes, and new transient ischemic attacks) or type II (new intellectual deterioration at discharge or new seizures). Of 2,108 patients in the CABG study, 3.1% had type I and 3% had type II outcomes (6). The predictors of type I outcomes were aortic atherosclerosis, a history of neurologic disease, and older age, whereas the predictors of type II outcomes were age, systolic hypertension, pulmonary disease, and excessive alcohol consumption (Table 21.2). Among 273 patients undergoing combined CABG and open-ventricle procedures, adverse neurologic outcomes occurred in 16% (8.4% type I and 7.3% type II) (7). In that study, predictors of type I outcome were related to aortic atherosclerosis or thrombus, and type II outcomes were predicted by aortic atherosclerosis, a history of endocarditis, postoperative low-output state, a history of alcohol abuse, perioperative dysrhythmias, and elevated systolic blood pressure on admission (7). The latter study also provides critical information on the effects of neurologic morbidity on intensive care unit stay, total hospitalization, and discharge disposition.

In the cardiac surgical population, neurocognitive morbidity is much more frequent than frank neurologic morbidity. The incidence of neurocognitive deficits at discharge ranges from approximately 10% to 60%, with 5% to 20% of deficits still being demonstrated 3 to 6 months after surgery (27–35). Because the results of cognitive testing before discharge may be confounded by pain, drugs, and sleep deprivation, these results may be less important than the assessment 3 to 7 months postoperatively.

The large variations in the reported incidence of neuropsychological impairment result from several factors. First, the incidence may vary twofold depending on whether the examination is retrospective or prospective (36,37). Results also differ depending on the batteries of tests performed and the definition of an abnormal test result. Differences

TABLE 21.2. ADJUSTED ODDS RATIOS FOR TYPE I AND TYPE II CEREBRAL OUTCOMES ASSOCIATED WITH SELECTED RISK FACTORS[a]

Factor	Model for Type I Cerebral Outcome	Model for Type II Cerebral Outcome
	Odds Ratio	
Significant factors (p < 0.05)		
Proximal aortic atherosclerosis	4.52	
History of neurologic disease	3.19	
Use of intraaortic balloon pump	2.60	
Diabetes mellitus	2.59	
History of hypertension	2.31	
History of pulmonary disease	2.09	2.37
History of unstable angina	1.83	
Age (per additional decade)	1.75	2.20
Systolic blood pressure >180 mm Hg at admission		3.47
History of excessive alcohol consumption		2.64
History of CABG		2.18
Dysrhythmia on day of surgery		1.97
Antihypertensive therapy		1.78
Other factors (p not significant)[b]		
Perioperative hypotension	1.92	1.88
Ventricular venting	1.83	
Congestive heart failure on day of surgery		2.46
History of peripheral vascular disease		1.64

[a] Odds ratios are for the risk for a type I or II outcome in patients with the risk factor in question in comparison with those without the risk factor. Odds ratios have been adjusted for all the factors listed for each model. Excessive alcohol consumption indicates hospitalization because of alcohol consumption or alcohol withdrawal. Perioperative hypotension indicates a systolic blood pressure <80 mm Hg (during surgery but before cardiopulmonary bypass or after bypass) or <40 mm Hg (during bypass) for more than 10 minutes.
[b] The following characteristics, studied in unvariable analysis, did not remain in the model: sex, aortic cross-clamping, duration of cardiopulmonary bypass and surgery, and institution.
CABG, coronary artery bypass graft.
From Roach GW, Kanchuger M, Mangano CM, et al. Adverse cerebral outcomes after coronary bypass surgery. Multicenter Study of Perioperative Ischemia Research Group and the Ischemia Research and Education Foundation Investigators. *N Engl J Med* 1996;335:1857–1863, with permission.

may also arise secondary to the timing of test administration and preoperative variables such as preexisting deficit or impaired language skills (38,39). However, a 1995 consensus conference addressed these issues, and better agreement now exists over appropriate test batteries, test timing, and the definition of an abnormal result (40–42).

Despite methodologic differences, specific patterns of deficits are generally described. These include deficits in psychomotor speed, attention and concentration, new learning ability, and short-term memory (9,34,35,42–44) (Table 21.3). Ophthalmologic abnormalities have also been described in 25% of patients, and primitive reflexes may develop in 39% (27). Although a significant proportion of deficits are clinically silent and become evident only on testing, Shaw et al. (9) reported a 38% incidence of significant intellectual impairment and a 10% incidence of overt disability in 235 patients showing postoperative neuropsychological test score deterioration. The pattern of neurologic injury in children undergoing cardiac surgery differs from that of adults and more often includes seizures, move-

ment disorders, and developmental delays (45,46). The need for deep hypothermic circulatory arrest, and its duration when it is used, influences these events in children (47,48).

Even conservative estimates indicate that tens of thousands of patients experience cardiac surgery-related neurologic morbidity annually. The cost of this morbidity to the patient is immeasurable, and the social costs of cognitive impairment and disability are enormous. The increased costs of medical care for patients suffering a neurologic event during cardiac surgery are more easily calculated. Clinically evident neurologic events may increase mortality fourfold and more than double intensive care unit time and the duration of hospitalization (4,6,7,49). The authors of the 1996 multicenter study on adverse cerebral outcomes following CABG estimated the in-hospital cost of neurologic complications at approximately $400 million annually, and out-of-hospital medical and rehabilitative costs may be as high as $2 billion to $4 billion annually in the United States alone (6).

TABLE 21.3. OUTCOME CHANGES WITHIN EACH COGNITIVE DOMAIN[a]

Cognitive Domain	No Decline[b] (%)	Decline and Improvement[c] (%)	Persistent Decline[d] (%)	Late Decline[e] (%)
Visual construction	50	15	11	24
Language	56	26	5	13
Verbal memory	63	21	10	6
Attention	71	8	9	12
Executive function	82	4	3	11
Visual memory	85	2	9	4
Motor speed	85	6	4	5
Psychomotor speed	90	1	4	5

[a] Each cognitive domain is considered as a separate entity, and so an individual patient will have different outcomes in different domains.
[b] No decline: Score does not decline by more than 0.5 standard deviation (SD) from preoperative score.
[c] Decline and improvement: Score declines by more than 0.5 SD at 1 month and then increases by more than 0.5 SD at 1 year.
[d] Persistent decline: Score decline reaches -0.5 SD at 1 year.
[e] Late decline: Score declines 0.5 SD or more from 1 month to 1 year.
From McKhann GM, Goldsborough MA, Borowicz LM Jr, et al. Cognitive outcome after coronary artery bypass: a one-year prospective study. *Ann Thorac Surg* 1997;63:510–515, with permission.

SURGICAL STRESS AND NEUROLOGIC RISK

Although the perioperative period may be associated with increased atheroembolic risk, hypotension and hypertension, anemia, dysrhythmias, dehydration, and disorders of coagulation, it is difficult to determine the contribution of perioperative factors to neurologic risk and outcome. First, the incidence of frank neurologic injury is relatively low, making the role of individual physiologic factors in neurologic risk difficult to determine. Neurocognitive studies are more revealing because of the high incidence of these disorders, but few institutions have the resources to conduct such studies. Because several preoperative risk factors for adverse neurologic or neuropsychologic outcomes tend to coexist in patients undergoing cardiac surgery with CPB, it becomes difficult to determine which ones are most important. Neurologic morbidity might best be conceptualized as the cumulative effect of a patient chronically at risk and a variety of surgically related insults that exceed the compensatory capacities of the cerebral vasculature and the brain.

In the absence of hypoxia, neurologic morbidity results from inadequate tissue perfusion. In its simplest form, ischemia may result from embolic obstruction of a large or small vessel, from inadequate flow through a fixed stenosis, or from failure of collateral circulation. At the level of the microvasculature, inflammation and endothelial dysfunction can also compromise oxygen delivery and neuronal functional integrity (50–53).

Embolization

Probably all patients experience cerebral embolization during CPB (44,49,54,55). Transcranial Doppler, echocardiographic (44,54,56), retinal angiographic (57,58), patho-logic, and radiographic information (59–64) indicate that cerebral embolization during CPB is the primary cause of cardiac surgery-related brain injury (Table 21.4). These embolic events are associated with aortic atheromas (65,66), platelet–fibrin and leukocyte aggregates (57,67,68), and possibly bubbles generated in the CPB circuit or in the surgical field (44,69). The central nervous system is exposed to hundreds to thousands of particulate and nonparticulate embolic events, and the periods of embolic risk are usually associated with specific surgical events (44,54,56,70) (Fig. 21.2). These events can result in transient or permanent regional ischemia.

Hypoperfusion

Although there are no compelling data to indicate that mean arterial pressure (MAP) during CPB is a primary determi-

TABLE 21.4. NEUROPSYCHOLOGICAL DEFICIT RELATED TO HIGH-INTENSITY TRANSCRANIAL SIGNAL COUNT DURING CARDIOPULMONARY BYPASS

HITS Count during CPB	No. of Patients	No. with Deficit	Percentage with Deficit
≤200	58	5	8.6
201–500	13	3	23.1
501–1,000	16	5	31.3
>1,000	7	3	43

HITS, high-intensity transcranial signal; CPB, cardiopulmonary bypass.
From Pugsley W, Klinger L, Paschalis C, et al. The impact of microemboli during cardiopulmonary bypass on neuropsychological functioning. *Stroke* 1994;25:1393–1399, with permission.

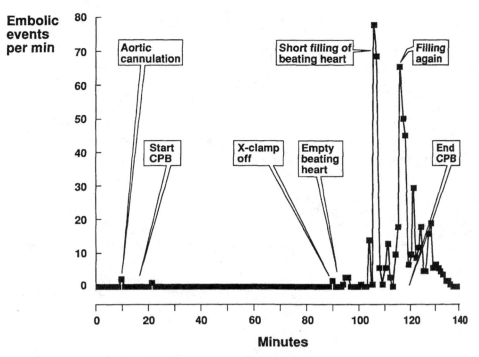

FIG. 21.2. Number of embolic events per minute in a representative patient from before insertion of the aortic cannula to after the end of cardiopulmonary bypass (*CPB*). (*X-clamp*, cross-clamp). (From van der Linden J, Casimir-Ahn H. When do cerebral emboli appear during open heart operations? A transcranial Doppler study. *Ann Thorac Surg* 1991;51:237–241, with permission.)

nant of neurologic outcome, regional cerebral hypoperfusion during CPB probably occurs as a result of hypertensive, diabetic, or senile atherosclerotic disease. Both hypertension and diabetes are independent risk factors for neurologic complications following cardiac surgery (6,18,71,72), and one or more of these forms of vascular disease exist in at least 50% of adult cardiac surgical patients. In addition to the rightward shift of the autoregulatory curve (73,74), chronic hypertension may narrow penetrating arteries, decrease collateral blood flow, and reduce ischemic tolerance (22,75,76). Similarly, diabetes results in macroangiopathies and degenerative changes in cerebral penetrating arteries, increases the likelihood of embolization (77,78), and alters cerebral autoregulatory capacity (79,80). Therefore, the increased neurologic risk associated with hypertension and diabetes may result from either increased embolization or regional hypoperfusion. However, it is reasonable to assume that increased neurologic morbidity in these patients derives from the interaction of these two processes.

Therefore, even without compelling evidence that perioperative MAP is a primary determinant of neurologic outcome, regional hypoperfusion, manifesting either as a direct result of vascular disease or as the inability to compensate for regional ischemia induced by microembolization, probably contributes importantly to perioperative cerebral ischemia.

Inflammation

Our thinking about ischemic injury is rapidly moving beyond discussions of vascular obstruction and hypoperfusion. During CPB, a variety of pathophysiologic mechanisms affect the vascular lining, and these events may be critical to post-CPB encephalopathy and neurocognitive disorders. Because the endothelium regulates vasomotor tone, thrombosis, fluid transport, and the inflammatory response, alterations in endothelial function may be integral to post-bypass integrity of the central nervous system. The interaction of inflammation, ischemia, and the endothelium is just being defined.

Ischemia and reperfusion of the heart and lung, in addition to a generalized inflammatory response, occur during CPB. Ischemia and reperfusion potently activate leukocytes and lead to leukocyte–endothelium or leukocyte–platelet–endothelium binding (53,81,82) (Fig. 21.3). Vascular integrity may then be impaired either through capillary plugging (83–85) or by the liberation of free radicals, hydrogen peroxide, and proteolytic enzymes during leukocyte degranulation (53,81,86). Endothelial dysfunction has been demonstrated in pulmonary and coronary vessels following CPB reperfusion (87–89). CPB may also alter endothelial function in nonischemic tissues through a variety of other mechanisms (90–92).

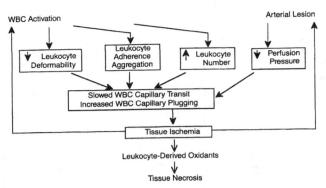

FIG. 21.3. White blood cells (*WBCs*) and ischemia. WBCs, especially neutrophils, may cause or aggravate ischemic lesions by several mechanisms that can interact with and amplify one another. (From Ernst E, Hammerschmidt DE, Bagge U, et al. Leukocytes and risk of ischemic diseases. *JAMA* 1987;257:2318–2324, with permission.)

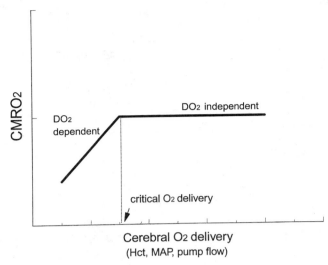

FIG. 21.4. Schematic representing the relationship of cerebral oxygen consumption (*CMR*O_2) to cerebral oxygen delivery (*D*O_2) or its determinants.

In addition to the localized inflammation that occurs during CPB, exposure of blood to the bypass circuit activates platelets, monocytes, and neutrophils (68,93–97). The endothelium normally inhibits platelet aggregation and also leukocyte activation and binding (53,81,98,99). However, contact activation, complement production, and the release of a variety of cytokines (100) stimulate the endothelium to bind circulating blood elements actively (101). Therefore, activation of blood elements and the endothelium during CPB may overwhelm the homeostasis normally achieved in the regulation of inflammation.

It remains to be seen whether CPB-related inflammation is sufficient to alter endothelial function in the absence of an ischemic substrate. Possibly, the inflammatory response triggered by CPB is sufficient to transform otherwise insignificant insults into clinically important pathology.

CEREBRAL PHYSIOLOGY DURING CARDIOPULMONARY BYPASS

In the course of clinical practice, it becomes easy for clinicians to take CPB for granted, yet its physiology is unique. Only during bypass would one acutely undergo up to a 20°C change in body temperature, a rapid reduction in hematocrit (Hct), and a loss of pulsatile flow. We subject patients to these physiologic disturbances daily, and it becomes difficult to define what is "normal" under these conditions.

During bypass, cerebral oxygen demand (CMRO_2) is determined primarily by temperature, such that normal values at different temperatures have been established. However, the same cannot be said of cerebral blood flow (CBF). Cerebral blood flow is determined by CMRO_2, P$_a$CO$_2$, Hct, and MAP. Each of these variables may act independently or

together to increase or decrease CBF. As such, asking what is "normal" CBF during bypass may be counterproductive. Fundamentally, cerebral oxygen delivery (CDO_2) must be sufficient to support metabolic demand. So if we are trying to determine the minimum MAP, Hct, or pump flow required at a given temperature, it is best to examine the effect of these variables on CDO_2.

Under non-bypass conditions, CDO_2 far exceeds CMRO_2, such that CMRO_2 is independent of CDO_2 over a broad range. When CDO_2 is progressively reduced, CMRO_2 can be maintained by an increase in oxygen extraction, but when that capacity is exhausted, further decreases in delivery will cause cerebral ischemia and CMRO_2 will decrease. Figure 21.4 schematically represents these relationships.

Because CDO_2 equals the product of CBF and arterial oxygen content (CaO$_2$), the individual determinants of CBF or CaO$_2$ each contribute to the abscissa in Fig. 21.4. Temperature change may shift the curve describing the CDO_2–CMRO_2 relationship upward or downward. The minimum oxygen delivery supporting oxygen demand is the "critical oxygen delivery" (102–104). Similarly, during CPB, the critical Hct (Hct$_{crit}$) or critical perfusion pressure for brain can be defined as the minimum Hct or perfusion pressure maintaining CMRO_2 at a given temperature (105,106).

Determinants of Cerebral Blood Flow

Cardiopulmonary bypass is typically associated with changes in body temperature and Hct. Significant alterations in PaCO$_2$ and MAP may also be experienced. Although it is common for these variables to change simultaneously, each has a predictable effect on cerebral perfusion.

Temperature

Temperature is the primary determinant of CBF during CPB, having both direct and indirect effects. Generally, the brain regulates its flow in response to its oxygen demand such that increases or decreases in CMRO$_2$ are associated with proportional changes in CBF. This relationship has been termed "flow–metabolism coupling" (107).

The Q$_{10}$ describes the change in CMRO$_2$ per 10°C change in temperature. Between 37° and 27°C, this value is approximately 2.4 to 3.0 mL/100 g per minute. Therefore, a 10°C temperature reduction decreases metabolic rate by more than 50%, and, all other things being equal, CBF is reduced proportionally. The Q$_{10}$ is nonlinear, such that at more profound levels of hypothermia (15° to 27°C) the Q$_{10}$ rises significantly to 4 to 5 mL/100 g per minute (107,108).

As temperature decreases progressively, the effects of hypothermia on CBF become more complex. In addition to the change in metabolic rate, there is a change in blood rheologic character, and probably in cerebral vascular responsiveness. Below approximately 22° to 23°C, CBF and metabolism appear to become uncoupled, so that CBF does not fall in proportion to CMRO$_2$ (Fig. 21.5); rather, a cerebral "vasoparesis" has been described (109,110). This can be especially important in children undergoing cardiac repairs

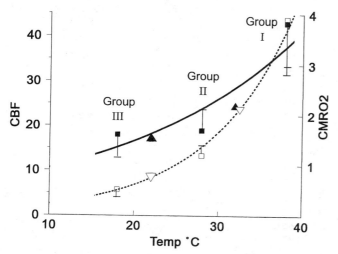

FIG. 21.5. Cerebral blood flow (*CBF*) (■) and metabolic rate for oxygen (*CMRO$_2$*) (□) (both in mL/100 g per minute) versus temperature during CPB (group I, 38°C; group II, 28°C; group III, 18°C; *n* = 8 per group). Mean values for CBF (▲) and CMRO$_2$ (▽) in 10 additional animals at 33°C (*n* = 5) and 22°C (*n* = 5) are also shown. (From Cook DJ, Orszulak TA, Daly RC. Minimum hematocrit at differing cardiopulmonary bypass temperatures in dogs. *Circulation* 1998;98:II-170–II-175, with permission.)

with CPB, because deep hypothermia (<20°C) is often employed in that patient population. The physiologic or biophysical reasons for this phenomenon are unknown.

Mean Arterial Pressure

Under non-bypass conditions, the healthy brain maintains CBF to a MAP of approximately 50 to 55 mm Hg. Significant autoregulatory capacity can also be preserved during CPB, but this is in large part a function of how other CPB variables are managed.

Because the determinants of cerebral perfusion are the same under bypass and non-bypass conditions, one would anticipate that MAP during CPB would determine cerebral perfusion. However, clinical studies in the 1980s deemphasized the role of MAP and reported that CBF is maintained with alpha-stat management (see Chap. 12) to MAPs as low as 20 to 35 mm Hg under hypothermic conditions (111–113). These results were interpreted to mean that the cerebral autoregulatory curve shifts leftward during hypothermia (111,114). However, clinical studies indicating a leftward autoregulatory shift must be viewed with caution because those studies pooled measurements of MAP and CBF from multiple patients under differing conditions of temperature, carbon dioxide, and Hct. Because of large between-patient variations in the physiologic determinants of CBF, the resulting high variability in CBF virtually precludes finding a correlation between MAP and CBF when single data points are pooled.

These limitations are overcome in animal models, in which multiple cerebral physiologic measurements can be made at differing MAPs with extremely tight physiologic control. The lower limits of autoregulation can also be evaluated in animal models. In contrast to the clinical studies of the 1980s, laboratory reports have not indicated a leftward shift of the autoregulatory curve during hypothermic CPB (106,115–117).

Because CPB is now commonly conducted with mild ("tepid") hypothermia, Plöchl et al. (106) examined critical cerebral perfusion pressure at 33°C in dogs. The relationships between MAP, CBF, CDO$_2$, and CMRO$_2$ were described as having two parts, a pressure-independent portion and a pressure-dependent portion. CBF and CDO$_2$ were preserved at MAPs of 60 mm Hg and higher, whereas at pressures of 50 mm Hg or less, CBF and, more importantly, CDO$_2$ became pressure-dependent (Fig. 21.6). However, cerebral ischemia was not observed at 50 mm Hg because the reduction in CDO$_2$ was compensated for by an increased cerebral oxygen extraction. Although cerebral ischemia was first statistically significant at an MAP of 40 mm Hg, the authors suggest that an MAP of 45 mm Hg may be inadequate at 33°C because some animals showed evidence of cerebral ischemia at that level.

Laboratory studies in healthy animals indicate that rela-

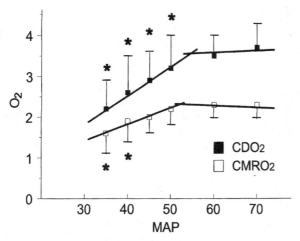

FIG. 21.6. Cerebral oxygen delivery (*CD*O₂) and cerebral oxygen consumption (*CMR*O₂) versus mean arterial pressure (*MAP*) during cardiopulmonary bypass (*CPB*) at 33°C. Values for oxygen (on ordinate in mL/100 g per minute) are the mean ± standard deviation (*p* <0.05 versus MAP of 60 mm Hg by repeated-measure analysis of variance followed by Student-Neuman-Keuls test). (From Plöchl W, Cook DJ, Orszulak TA, et al. Critical cerebral perfusion pressure during tepid heart surgery in dogs. *Ann Thorac Surg* 1998;66: 118–124, with permission.)

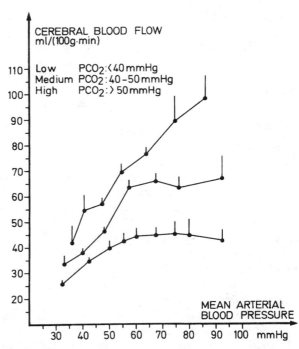

FIG. 21.7. Response of cerebral blood flow to changes in mean arterial blood pressure at three different levels of P_aCO_2. The mean $PaCO_2$ values were 33 (*bottom curve*), 45 (*middle curve*), and 57 (*top curve*) mm Hg. (From Henriksen L. Brain luxury perfusion during cardiopulmonary bypass in humans. A study of the cerebral blood flow response to changes in CO₂, O₂, and blood pressure. *J Cereb Blood Flow Metab* 1986;6:366–378, with permission.)

tively normal MAPs should be maintained during CPB between 27° and 37°C (106,115,117). Physiologically, an MAP of at least 50 mm Hg appears desirable because at this pressure some safety margin for the brain (increased oxygen extraction) will exist.

Carbon Dioxide

Although hypothermia increases ischemic tolerance, it also introduces unique physiologic questions. One of the most practical has been the appropriate management of carbon dioxide. Carbon dioxide can be managed with pH-stat or alpha-stat techniques (see Chap. 12), but discussions of which approach is more "physiologic" are not productive because body temperatures between 15° and 30°C do not normally occur in humans. Consequently, rather than attempting to determine which carbon dioxide strategy is "correct," it would seem more appropriate to determine which carbon dioxide management strategy best achieves certain physiologic goals.

Carbon dioxide is one of the most potent determinants of CBF, and most (118–121), but not all (122), studies indicate that carbon dioxide reactivity is preserved during bypass. Depending on carbon dioxide strategy, CBF may vary by more than 50% in either direction. Changes in P_aCO_2 alter CBF largely independently of CMRO₂, so like hemodilution, changes in P_aCO_2 may alter the ratio of CBF to CMRO₂ without being pathologic.

Henriksen (118) clearly demonstrated the effect of carbon dioxide on CBF and the effect of P_aCO_2 on cerebral

autoregulation during clinical CPB. Figure 21.7 shows that during bypass an elevated P_aCO_2 (*upper curve*) is associated with a higher CBF for any given MAP. Additionally, Henriksen's data show that autoregulation is preserved with an alpha-stat strategy between MAPs of 55 to 95 mm Hg (Fig. 21.7, *lower curve*), whereas CBF becomes largely pressure-passive with elevated P_aCO_2 (Fig. 21.7, *upper curve*). Subsequent clinical and animal studies have confirmed these findings (120,122–125). This effect of carbon dioxide is seen across different values of MAP, CMRO₂, and Hct.

Hematocrit

In adults, CPB hemodilution typically reduces the hemoglobin concentration by a third. This reduces blood viscosity and vascular resistance and increases CBF (105,118, 126,127). These increases in CBF support CDO₂ as the Hct is reduced, so CMRO₂ is independent of Hct over a broad range. However, with progressive hemodilution, CDO₂ and then oxygen consumption become compromised when the capacity of CBF and oxygen extraction to compensate for the reduction in arterial oxygen are exhausted. At this point the Hct$_{crit}$ is reached (105) (Fig. 21.4).

During hypothermic CPB, the increase in CBF occurring with hemodilution may be offset by the decrease in CBF associated with the reduction in CMR_{O_2} (126). As such, during hypothermia CBF may increase, decrease, or remain largely unchanged. The net change in CBF is a function of the magnitudes of both temperature change and Hct reduction (126).

Hemodilution practice during CPB is relatively unique, and this can lead to a misunderstanding of CBF responses. Under non-CPB conditions, the ratio between CBF and CMR_{O_2} (14–18) is relatively fixed (107). Investigators have described increases in this ratio (uncoupling) during normothermic or moderately hypothermic CPB (111,128,129), and it has been suggested that this is pathophysiologic. Although $CBF–CMR_{O_2}$ uncoupling may occur with profound hypothermia, a change in this ratio should be expected with hemodilution. The effect of hemodilution on the ratio of CBF to CMR_{O_2} can be isolated during normothermic CPB, at which time this ratio is elevated in proportion to the reduction in Hct. This leaves CD_{O_2} unchanged from that in the pre-bypass state (126). For this reason, during CPB, discussions of the $CBF–CMR_{O_2}$ ratio can be misleading.

Although experience dictates that very low Hcts can be tolerated during CPB (130,131), until recently these limits have not been examined. To determine temperature-dependent limits on hemodilution, our group placed dogs on bypass at either 38°, 28°, or 18°C, and the cerebral effects of progressive hemodilution were determined (105). We predicted that the Hct_{crit} would be reduced in proportion to the reduction in CMR_{O_2}; however, this was not seen. Between 38° and 18°C, appropriate reductions in metabolic rate were demonstrated; however, the Hct_{crit} at 28°C was 15% only slightly lower than that at 38°C (18–19%). Similarly, at 18°C, the CMR_{O_2} was less than half that at 28°C, but the Hct_{crit} at 18°C was 11% and only slightly lower than that at 28°C (Fig. 21.8). Therefore, the leftward shift in the Hct_{crit} is quite small and disproportionate to the decrease in CMR_{O_2}. This occurs because the CBF response to hemodilution is attenuated with progressive hypothermia (105).

Finally, there is an impression that hemodilution increases tolerance for hypotension because it increases organ blood flow. Although hemodilution increases CBF, this is not equivalent to saying that tolerance to hypotension is increased. CBF may be "normal" at a lower MAP, but CD_{O_2} will be reduced. Autoregulatory curves can be constructed to demonstrate that although the absolute levels of CBF are shifted upward with hemodilution, the curve "breaks" at about the same MAP as in the nonhemodiluted state (118).

Cardiopulmonary Bypass Flow and Brain Perfusion

To a large extent, asking whether pump flow or MAP is of greater importance during bypass is an artificial distinction.

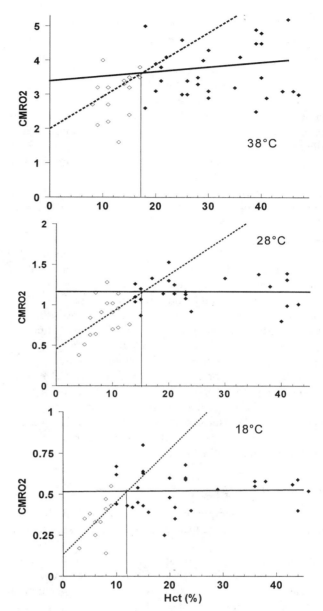

FIG. 21.8. Relationship of hematocrit to cerebral oxygen consumption (*CMR*$_{O_2}$) at 38°, 28°, and 18°C. There are 40 value pairs per group (*n* = 8 per group). Linear regression curves were drawn for data points above and below a range of hematocrits below which the transition from hematocrit independence to hematocrit dependence occurs. (From Cook DJ, Orszulak TA, Daly RC. Minimum hematocrit at differing cardiopulmonary bypass temperatures in dogs. *Circulation* 1998;98:II-170–II-175, with permission.)

As in the intact circulation, changes in pump flow during CPB are usually associated with changes in MAP. However, this relationship may not be linear. At higher flows, changes in vascular resistance may dampen the effect of pump flow changes on MAP, whereas at low flows, MAP may be reduced in direct proportion to a change in pump flow

(117,132). A focus on the low-flow range, where cerebral physiologic variables show pump flow dependence (110,133,134), may lead to the conclusion that pump flow is a primary determinant of cerebral perfusion. However, the effect of pump flow on cerebral perfusion is indirect.

These relationships were well demonstrated by Sadahiro et al. (117), who described the effect of stepwise CPB flow reductions on MAP and CBF in dogs. In that report, pump flow did not alter CBF until the MAP decreased below 50 mm Hg. At that point, pump flow, MAP, and cerebral perfusion were related in a nearly linear fashion. Scrutiny of other reports examining the effects of pump flow on cerebral physiologic variables reveals a similar CBF dependency on pump flow when reduced flows cause reduced MAPs (110,135–139).

The primacy of perfusion pressure has been demonstrated under conditions in which MAP was normal (61 mm Hg) and pump flow was low (0.75 L/m^2 per minute) and also in which pump flow was normal (2.2 L/m^2 per minute) and MAP was low (24 mm Hg) (136,140,141). These studies showed that when MAP was maintained, pump flow rate had no effect on CBF; however, reduced perfusion pressure reduced CBF even if pump flow rate was normal. Data from both animal models (116,138,139,142) and clinical CPB (110,143–145) support those conclusions. These results indicate that CPB flow is important to cerebral perfusion insofar as it generates an MAP, and that maintenance of CPB flow is not sufficient to guarantee cerebral perfusion if MAP is reduced.

Pulsatility

Like the acute changes in temperature and Hct that may occur during CPB, the loss of pulsatile flow is a physiologic condition unique to CPB. As such, the effect of pulse pressure on organ perfusion during CPB has been of sustained interest. Nonpulsatile perfusion has been reported to result in arteriolar closure (146) and a disturbance in the coupling of blood flow and metabolism (129). Conversely, pulsatile flow has been reported to improve CBF, microcirculatory perfusion, and tissue oxygen consumption, and to facilitate the recovery of CBF following ischemia, low-flow CPB, and circulatory arrest (147–149).

At least an equal number of reports have documented no significant physiologic effect of pulsatility during CPB. Hindman and colleagues found no difference in CBF or CMRO$_2$ between pulsatile and nonpulsatile CPB in rabbits under normothermic (150) or hypothermic (151) conditions. Sadahiro et al. (117) reported similar results in dogs, as did Cook and colleagues (142) under three temperature and CPB flow conditions. Conflicting reports about the effects of pulsatile CPB exist for essentially every variable examined. Because convincing evidence of benefit is lacking and because of the technical complexity and difficulty of generating a meaningful pulse pressure in the systemic circu-

lation, pulsatile CPB systems have not become part of standard practice.

Cardiopulmonary Bypass Time

Two clinical reports have indicated that CBF decreases with bypass time (152,153). In one study, two CBF measurements were obtained 20 to 30 minutes apart during hypothermia, and although nasopharyngeal temperature, P$_a$CO$_2$, and MAP were stable, a decrease in CBF of 0.7% to 1% per minute was observed (153). A second study from the same group concluded that CBF declines with time based on alterations in carbon dioxide responsiveness (152). Although decreases in CBF with time were shown in these studies, there is evidence to suggest that these decreases in CBF may have been related to other factors.

Hindman et al. (154) were unable to document an effect of CPB time on CBF in a rabbit model in which brain temperature was directly measured. They speculated that the previous clinical findings were a function of brain cooling not reflected in nasopharyngeal temperature. A study in baboons also failed to show an effect of CPB time on CBF (141). The canine study by Johnston et al. (122) is particularly notable. During CPB, blood flow to cerebral cortex and cerebellum were measured, and although some decrease was seen following rewarming, three measurements taken during 120 minutes of stable hypothermia demonstrated no decline in CBF under either alpha-stat or pH-stat conditions. Subsequent clinical studies have also failed to show a decrease in CBF with bypass time (126,155).

INTRAOPERATIVE MANAGEMENT AND NEUROLOGIC OUTCOME

Mean Arterial Pressure

A variety of early reports (59,156–158) in addition to a few from the 1980s (159–161) identified a relationship between intraoperative MAP and neurologic outcome. This relationship has not been identified in other clinical studies (6,8,37,43,162). However, it should be emphasized that no investigation before 1995 was specifically designed to examine the role of MAP in neurologic outcome. The studies lacked a control group and were often retrospective or designed to examine the neurologic effects of other interventions (37,158,162–164), and the effect of MAP on outcome was examined secondarily. Additionally, neurologic follow-up was typically only short-term, and the patients were younger and had fewer comorbidities than our current surgical population. These studies also used both alpha-stat and pH-stat management (163,164) and bubble and membrane oxygenators (8,162,163), and they may not have used arterial line filtration (8,37). Therefore, the applicability of all these studies to our current surgical population must be considered with some caution.

TABLE 21.5. EFFECT OF MEAN ARTERIAL PRESSURE ON NEUROLOGICAL CARDIAC OUTCOMES IN PATIENTS RANDOMIZED TO LOWER OR HIGHER MEAN ARTERIAL PRESSURE DURING BYPASS

	MAP 50–60 mm Hg (%) (n = 124)	MAP 80–100 mm Hg (%) (n = 124)	p^a
Stroke	7.2	2.4	0.076
Minor neurodeficits	3.2	0.8	—
Cardiac complications	4.8	2.4	0.3
Six-month cognitive deficit	12	11	—
Overall major cardiac and neurologic outcomes	12.9	4.8	0.026
Total mortality	4	1.6	0.25

[a] The authors do not provide *p* values for each variable.
From Gold JP, Charlson ME, Williams-Russo P, et al. Improvement of outcomes after coronary artery bypass. A randomized trial comparing intraoperative high versus low mean arterial pressure. *J Thorac Cardiovasc Surg* 1995;110:1302–1311.

A more recent multicenter study on cerebral outcomes following CABG described a 6% incidence of neurologic deficit at discharge and reflects our current surgical population (6). Although perioperative hypotension was not identified as a risk factor for adverse neurologic outcome, as in earlier studies, patients were not randomized to differing MAPs. To date, only one prospective, randomized study has evaluated this. Gold et al. (165) randomized 248 patients to either lower (50 to 60 mm Hg) or higher (80 to 100 mm Hg) MAP during hypothermic (28° to 30°C) CPB and examined outcomes at 6 months. Patient characteristics and CPB management were otherwise equivalent and reflect current perfusion practice and patient risk profiles. Although statistical differences were not shown for individual outcomes, the overall incidence of cardiac and neurologic morbidity at 6 months was significantly reduced in the high-MAP group, and a trend to better results for every variable except neurocognitive outcome was noted in the group with the higher MAP (Table 21.5). The authors speculate that their study size may have been underpowered for relatively low-frequency events. Also of note were the fact that the "high-MAP" group achieved a mean MAP of only 70 mm Hg during CPB, as opposed to the targeted levels of 80 to 100 mm Hg, and the retrospective observation that when mean MAPs were broken down into deciles, the "break point" for overall morbidity appeared to occur at an MAP of 60 mm Hg.

Within the range of temperatures at which most adult CPB is practiced, physiologic data indicate that CDo_2 may become compromised at an MAP of approximately 50 mm Hg. Although physiologic measurements do not translate directly into clinical outcomes, the clinical report by Gold and colleagues (165) is highly suggestive, and that report is the best one conducted to date on the relationship between MAP and outcome. Finally, our current surgical population is older and their risk factors for stroke are more numerous than when many prior studies with "negative" outcomes were performed. Thus, although not all data agree, it seems prudent to be conservative and assume that our patients will benefit from MAPs in the usual autoregulatory range during CPB (i.e., 50 mm Hg or higher).

Temperature and Outcomes

The role of CPB temperature in neurologic outcome came to the forefront in 1994 when two large, randomized outcome studies were published. The Warm Heart Investigators reported on 1,732 patients who underwent CPB at either 33° to 37°C or 25° to 30°C (166). In that study, the incidence of stroke at discharge was equivalent between temperature groups (Table 21.6). However, in the same year, Martin et al. (167) reported a trial of 1,001 patients undergoing CPB at either 35°C or higher (*n* = 493) or 28°C or lower (*n* = 508). The study of Martin et al. reported a threefold greater incidence of neurologic morbidity in the "warm" group.

Reports during the next year (168,169) identified a variety of demographic and intraoperative management issues that may have accounted for the outcome differences be-

TABLE 21.6. NEUROLOGIC OUTCOME AND CARDIOPULMONARY BYPASS TEMPERATURE

		Cold (%)	Warm (%)
Martin TD, Craver JM, Gott JP, et al. (n = 1,001) (167)	Stroke	1.2	4.1
	Encephalopathy	0.2	0.4
	Total	1.4	4.5
The Warm Heart Investigators (n = 1,732) (166)	Stroke	1.6	1.5

tween the two studies. They pointed out that the Toronto (Warm Heart Investigators) population had fewer female patients, a smaller proportion of patients older than 70 (16% vs. 38%), and fewer repeated operations. Differences in cardioplegia and aortic cross-clamp management may also have placed the Emory (Martin et al.) patients at greater risk for cerebral embolism (66,170–172). Finally, the "warm" group at Toronto was 2° to 4°C cooler than the "warm" group at Emory (169). The potential importance of this difference was underscored by a follow-up nonrandomized study from the Emory group in which 379 CABG patients underwent CPB with systemic temperatures between 29° and 33°C. The incidence of stroke in that study (1.8%) compared favorably with the incidence in their previous group that was perfused at 28°C or less (1.4%), and was less than that observed in their previously normothermic (≥35°C) group (4.5%) (168).

Neurocognitive outcomes for part of these study populations have also been provided. Complete test results were reported for 89 of the 1,001 patients enrolled at Emory (32). Although CPB resulted in deficits in both temperature groups, there was no difference in neurocognitive outcome between the warm and cold populations (32). Neurocognitive outcomes were also reported for 153 patients from the Toronto study. As in the Emory report, temperature was not found to be a determinant of neurocognitive injury 3 months postoperatively (33,173).

A variety of other investigations have commented on neurologic outcomes with CPB temperature. Plourde et al. (174) randomized 62 patients to CPB at either 34° to 35°C or 28°C and could not identify neuropsychological differences between groups at postoperative day 7. Hvass et al. (175) reported 100 patients operated on with a warm body (37°C)–cold heart technique and documented a 1% incidence of stroke, and Birdi et al. (176) documented a 0% to 1% incidence of stroke in 300 patients randomized to CPB at either 37°, 32°, or 28°C. Singh et al. (177) compared 2,585 consecutive patients undergoing CPB at 37°C with a historical cohort of 1,605 patients operated on with systemic hypothermia (25° to 30°C). In that study, the stroke incidences were 1% and 1.3% in the warm and cold groups, respectively. Regragui and colleagues (178) conducted neurocognitive testing on 96 patients randomized to CPB at either 37°, 32°, or 28°C and found that the neurocognitive score was worst in the 37°C group ($n = 31$), better in the 32°C group ($n = 36$), and equivalent between the 28°C ($n = 29$) and 32°C groups. From these results, the authors argued for mild hypothermia. However, their article was followed by a commentary that faulted the study's statistical power, neurocognitive testing methods, and data analysis.

Overall, the evidence indicates that mildly hypothermic ("tepid") CPB, defined as CPB at a nasopharyngeal temperature of 33° to 35°C, as opposed to CPB at strict normothermia, does not significantly increase neurologic risk in a relatively healthy patient population. There is at least the suggestion from the Emory study that strict maintenance of normothermia may increase neurologic risk.

Glucose Management

Another difference between the Toronto and Emory populations was a significantly higher glucose in the warm CPB group at Emory (168). This is of interest because elevations in blood glucose aggravate neurologic ischemic injury in experimental models (179–181). However, no study to date has documented an independent effect of glucose on neurologic outcome in clinical CPB (32,168,182,183). Although the mean blood glucose in the "warm" Emory group may have exceeded 275 mg/dL (32), a multivariate analysis did not identify blood glucose as a predictor of neurologic or neurocognitive status in that study (32,168).

It appears that neurologic injury arises from the combination of preexisting patient conditions and surgical factors. Therefore, as with MAP, it is difficult to demonstrate that management of an isolated physiologic variable determines patient outcome. Nevertheless, there are good physiologic data to support keeping glucose levels below 200 to 250 mg/dL intraoperatively, and in the absence of well-demonstrated disadvantages, this approach is probably prudent.

Carbon Dioxide Management and Outcome

In the 1990s, studies from four countries examined the effects of P_aCO_2 management on neurologic outcome in adults (120,164,184,185). In 1990, Bashein et al. (164) randomized 86 patients to undergo hypothermic (30°C) CPB with either alpha-stat or pH-stat management and examined neurologic and neurocognitive outcomes at discharge and 7 months postoperatively. Neurologic impairment was unrelated to P_aCO_2 at either short-term or long-term follow-up. Stephan et al. (120) randomized 65 patients at 26°C and conducted a neurologic examination on the seventh postoperative day. The pH-stat and alpha-stat groups had a 29% and 7% incidence of neurologic sequelae, respectively, and multivariate analysis identified only P_aCO_2 as an etiologic factor in adverse neurologic outcome. In 1996, Patel and colleagues (185) randomized 70 patients undergoing CPB at 28°C to pH-stat or alpha-stat management and performed neuropsychological testing preoperatively and 6 weeks postoperatively. When deterioration in the results of three or more tests was used as the threshold for abnormality, a greater proportion of patients in the pH-stat group had an adverse outcome. In 1996, Murkin et al. (184) reported on the neurologic effects of carbon dioxide management in 316 patients undergoing CABG randomized to alpha-stat or pH-stat carbon dioxide strategy and pulsatile or nonpulsatile flow. Overall, the stroke rate in the two carbon dioxide groups did not differ (2.5%), nor did the incidence of neurologic or neurocognitive dysfunction at 7 days. Approximately half of the patients had CPB times longer than 90 minutes, and in those patients cognitive dysfunction was less prevalent with alpha-stat (27%) than with pH-stat (44%) at 2-month follow-up. However, an effect of carbon dioxide was not seen in patients with shorter CPB times.

All these studies have limitations, but there is a suggestion that pH-stat management may be associated with a worsened neurologic outcome and that carbon dioxide management may be more important in populations at higher risk. The underlying hypothesis is that reductions in carbon dioxide should reduce cerebral embolization, but this effect may be clinically evident only when embolic risk is greater. The hypothesis relating increased carbon dioxide to embolization has been expressed since the early 1980s (186) but was only recently confirmed in an animal model (187).

The pediatric literature has identified a different effect of carbon dioxide on neurologic outcome. The Boston Children's group retrospectively reviewed their outcome data in children who had undergone cardiac surgery with profound hypothermia and found that the introduction of alpha-stat management worsened neurologic outcome (46). They speculated that the increased CBF associated with pH-stat management improved cerebral cooling and neuroprotection in the precirculatory arrest period. Subsequent clinical studies measuring jugular bulb saturation (188,189) and animal studies measuring brain temperature, intracellular pH, and high-energy phosphates (190–192) have confirmed their hypothesis. These studies have indicated that in the context of profound hypothermia and circulatory arrest, pH-stat management may have important metabolic advantages in addition to facilitating brain cooling.

From all these results, it appears that the effect of P_aCO_2 on outcome is likely to be a function of the type of cerebral stress introduced by the operation. In adults experiencing moderate levels of hypothermia, alpha-stat management is probably primarily important in reducing atheroembolic risk. In children undergoing deep hypothermic circulatory arrest, who lack atherosclerosis, the primary neurologic stress is hypoperfusion, so pH-stat management should be beneficial. The appropriate P_aCO_2 management in adults undergoing deep hypothermic circulatory arrest remains uncertain.

Other Cardiopulmonary Bypass Variables

The effects of pulsatility, Hct, or flow rate on neurologic outcome have received less attention. Two studies have failed to show an effect of pulsatility on neurocognitive outcome (184,193). The effect of Hct on neurologic outcome has been addressed only secondarily. The study of Shaw et al. (9) related a drop in hemoglobin during the operation to worsened outcome, but this was in relation to a vascular surgery control group that did not undergo hemodilution. Short-term neurologic outcome has also been related to perioperative blood loss, but not to CPB Hct (161). Finally,

well-designed trials relating CPB flow rate to outcomes have been conducted only in children. With profound hypothermia, low flow is associated with a better outcome than is circulatory arrest (47,137), but in the adult literature, there is no evidence to indicate that CPB flow rate *per se* influences neurologic outcome.

INTERVENTIONS

Efforts to reduce cardiac surgery-related neurologic morbidity are proceeding in multiple directions. Broadly, these can be described as surgical and technical changes, pharmacologic interventions, and physiologic management strategies.

Surgical and Technical Interventions

A greater understanding of surgically related causes of neurologic morbidity has changed clinical practice. In the surgical literature, the role of atheroembolism in brain injury is appreciated, and techniques to reduce this problem are emphasized. Greater attention to the atherosclerotic aorta has led to the application of epiaortic ultrasonography in the assessment and management of aortic cannulation (16,66,194) (Fig. 21.9) and also to the use of single cross-clamp and "no touch" techniques (195–197). In addition, surgeons are aware of the relationship between CPB and neurocognitive injury, and this is providing additional impetus for off-bypass CABG (198–200). Echocardiographic assessment of ventricular "de-airing" has become a greater part of operating room practice as this technology has become more widely available (201,202). CPB circuit modifications such as hollow fiber oxygenators and arterial line filters may also affect neurologic morbidity

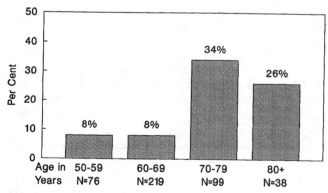

FIG. 21.9. Frequency of moderate or severe atherosclerosis of the ascending aorta necessitating modifications in operative technique according to age. (From Wareing TH, Davila-Roman VG, Barzilai B, et al. Management of the severely atherosclerotic ascending aorta during cardiac operations. A strategy for detection and treatment. *J Thorac Cardiovasc Surg* 1992;103:453–462, with permission.)

(44,69,203,204). Another technical modification of the CPB circuit, with the potential to influence outcomes, is biocompatibility. If the CPB surface can mimic the endothelial glycocalyx, the generalized inflammatory response to CPB may be reduced. Surface heparinization has been the first step; given the regulatory role of the glycoproteins in neutrophil, platelet, and endothelial interactions (53,81,98,205), biocompatibility may evolve into more specific glycoprotein surfaces (see Chap. 9).

Pharmacologic Interventions

In addition to surgical and technical interventions to reduce embolic risk, pharmacologic neuroprotection represents a second line of investigation. Broadly, at least three forms of pharmacologic neuroprotection can be considered. These include metabolic depressants, agents that inhibit different steps in the cellular ischemic pathway, and anti-adhesive strategies.

Metabolic Suppression

The most basic understanding of ischemia as a state of CDo_2 insufficient to meet demand immediately leads to considerations of metabolic suppression as a means of neuroprotection. Although this inference is obvious, agents such as barbiturates have not become a routine part of our practice. The experimental literature indicates that barbiturate therapy improves outcome in models of incomplete ischemia (206,207), but the usefulness of barbiturate therapy for brain protection during CPB has been difficult to demonstrate.

The 1982 study by Slogoff et al. (37) randomized 204 cardiac surgical patients to a thiopental (15 mg/kg) or a control group and evaluated neurologic outcome on the first and fourth postoperative days. Although the data suggested neuroprotection in the thiopental group, the result was not statistically significant. A subsequent study from the Texas Heart Institute randomized 182 patients undergoing open-ventricle procedures to a control group or to a group that received burst suppression doses of thiopental throughout CPB (208). As in the earlier study, patients approximated normothermia (>34°C); a bubble oxygenator and no arterial line filter were used. Neurologic evaluation on the tenth postoperative day demonstrated a 7.5% incidence of neurologic defects in the control group and no defects in the treatment group. This was the first demonstration of barbiturate cerebral protection in humans (209).

To address the side effects associated with the high-dose thiopental infusion (the requirements for greater inotropic and longer-lasting ventilatory support), Metz and Slogoff (210) conducted a subsequent study in which neurologic outcomes were compared in groups receiving bolus thiopental before aortic declamping or thiopental throughout CPB. Neurologic outcome was equivalent between groups, and

the authors concluded that bolus thiopental administration without electroencephalographic (EEG) monitoring offered the same neuroprotection as the infusion technique. However, an accompanying editorial (211) pointed out that the lack of a control group required comparison of the bolus thiopental group with a historical control group, and that several practice changes occurring between the study of Nussmeier et al. (208) and that of Metz and Slogoff might have made the use of Nussmeier's group as a control invalid.

A major study of barbiturate neuroprotection was also published by Zaidan et al. in 1991 (212). In that investigation, 300 patients undergoing CABG at 28°C with a membrane oxygenator and an arterial line filter were randomly assigned to placebo or to thiopental infusion sufficient to achieve an isoelectric EEG throughout CPB. A neurologic examination was performed on the second and fifth postoperative days. As in the previous studies, patients receiving thiopental required more inotropic support (208), but significant neuroprotection was not provided. An accompanying editorial speculated about reasons why the Nussmeier and Zaidan results differed (213).

The primary differences between the two studies were CPB temperature (28° vs. 34°C), closed versus open ventricles, and the presence or absence of a membrane oxygenator and arterial line filter. It is difficult to determine the relative importance of these factors. Open-ventricle procedures are usually associated with poorer outcomes and more air embolism, but the relationship between air embolism and neurophysiologic or neurologic outcome has not been clearly defined (214–217). Additionally, if atheroembolism is the primary cause of neurologic injury in cardiac surgery, then the use of arterial filters and membrane oxygenators would not be expected to explain the study differences. Whether CPB temperature differences are sufficient to explain the outcome differences is also not discernible. Regardless, the results of this combination of studies led the editors to conclude that ". . . routine thiopental therapy has no place in the management of patients undergoing CABG." Furthermore, they note, ". . . demonstration of barbiturate protection in normothermic, unfiltered, bubble oxygenator bypass is not a reasonable argument for barbiturate use during alternative bypass circumstances unless the appropriate trials are performed" (213).

The introduction of propofol led to some interest in its applicability for neuroprotection in cardiac surgery, but studies similar to those of Nussmeier et al. or Zaidan et al. have not been performed. The effect of burst suppression doses of propofol on CBF and $CMRo_2$ was evaluated, and the authors speculated that propofol may have a role in reducing cerebral embolism during CPB by reducing CBF (218). Other investigators have evaluated the effect of propofol on CBF velocity (219), and Souter et al. found that propofol-induced burst suppression does ameliorate cerebral venous oxygen desaturation during rewarming (220). Given the body of work on thiopental in cardiac surgery, it is unlikely that large outcome studies testing the effects of other cerebral metabolic depressants will be conducted in the near future.

Calcium Antagonists

Of a variety of neuroprotectant agents showing efficacy in animal models, only calcium channel blockers have found their way into clinical trials in cardiac surgery. Intracellular accumulation of Ca^{2+} is one of the key factors leading to cell death in cerebral ischemia. In non-bypass models, calcium channel blockers limit ischemic injury (221,222). These agents have also improved neurologic outcome in human stroke trials (223). In cardiac surgery, the effect of nimodipine on neurologic outcome was assessed in a small trial by Forsman et al. (224). Thirty-nine patients undergoing cardiac surgery were randomized to receive nimodipine or placebo, and neurocognitive outcome was determined at 6 months. Six of 28 patients (21%) showed deficits at 6 months. Nimodipine-treated patients were described as having a slightly better outcome in verbal fluency and visual retention, but the authors emphasize that the small study size prevented any definitive conclusions from being drawn (224).

A critical trial of calcium channel blockers in cardiac surgery was reported in 1996 (225). Nimodipine neuroprotection was to be tested in a double-blind, randomized trial of 400 patients undergoing valve replacement, but the trial was interrupted at 150 patients because of greater morbidity and mortality in the nimodipine treatment group. At termination there was a 10.7% incidence of death in the nimodipine group and a 1.3% incidence in the control group. Major bleeding occurred in 13.3% of nimodipine patients versus 4.1% of control patients. Additionally, there were no differences in neurocognitive outcomes between the two groups at 1 week, 1 month, and 6 months.

The authors attributed the morbidity and mortality with nimodipine treatment to bleeding and speculate that this might have resulted from a combination of vasodilation and the antiplatelet effects of the drug (225). The authors do not extend their observations to other calcium antagonists, but based on these results, it would be difficult to justify another large trial of calcium channel blockers as neuroprotectants in cardiac surgery.

Leukocyte Inhibition and Endothelial Protection: Anti-adhesion Therapies

A variety of other pharmacologic agents with the potential to inhibit ischemic pathways have not reached clinical trials in cardiac surgery. These agents include aminosteroid compounds (226), excitatory amino acid receptor antagonists (227), and agents directed at the nitric oxide pathway (228–230). Another class of investigational agents, anti-adhesion therapies, also warrants comment.

Investigation in the last 5 years has shown that multiple inflammatory mediators contribute to the progression of ischemic injury (52,82,231). In particular, neutrophils aggregate in the capillary beds of ischemic tissues and may contribute to plugging, endothelial dysfunction, and tissue damage. Characterization of the receptors responsible for neutrophil–endothelium binding is leading to the development of specific monoclonal antibodies against these receptors and of nonspecific inhibitors of neutrophil–endothelium binding (232–234).

Monoclonal antibodies to the adhesion molecules mediating neutrophil–endothelium binding have shown promise in laboratory models of transient focal ischemia (51,235,236). Additionally, oligosaccharides and oligopeptides structurally related to endothelial binding sites competitively inhibit neutrophil binding to the endothelium (205,237–240). Application of these oligosaccharides can reduce lung injury and myocardial reperfusion injury (238,240) and block lymphocyte adhesion to cardiac endothelium in animal models (239). More specific glycoproteins, representing the selectin binding sites for leukocytes, have also been shown to decrease ischemic injury and increase CBF after transient focal ischemia (237). These observations are interesting because the inhibitory oligosaccharide fragments are structurally related to, and can be generated from, multiple fractionations of heparin (241–244), and there is some evidence that heparin itself may reduce cerebral ischemic injury by acting as an anti-adhesion molecule (245). These new therapeutic agents may hold promise, and preliminary trials with them are just being considered in cardiac surgery.

Physiologic Interventions

Temperature

Reductions in cerebral oxygen requirements with hypothermia provide for flexibility in surgical and perfusion practice. Cerebral hypothermia attenuates the physiologic impact of reductions in perfusion pressure and Hct and extends the "safe" period of low-flow CPB and circulatory arrest. Hypothermia reduces cerebral injury in both regional and global models of cerebral ischemia; however, the magnitude of neuroprotection is not directly related to the reduction in $CMRO_2$ (107,246–248).

There is a convincing body of evidence in the experimental stroke literature that even small temperature differences have important effects on neurochemical, neuropathologic, and neurophysiologic outcomes in ischemia (246, 248–250). As little as 2°C of hypothermia significantly attenuates brain injury (246,247). These effects are probably related to a reduction in the cascade of injury precipitated by an ischemic insult and so are independent of the effect of temperature on metabolism (246,247). Mild hypothermia attenuates the depletion of cerebral adenosine triphosphate following ischemia and decreases the production of the excitatory neurotransmitter glutamate (248,251); infarct volume is reduced, particularly in the neocortex, and neurologic outcome may be improved (246–248).

The effects of small temperature differences on the EEG, cerebral metabolism, excitatory amino acids, and cellular high-energy phosphates were recently evaluated in a swine model of CPB (251). When pigs were subjected to 20 minutes of global ischemia at 37°, 34°, 31°, or 28°C, Conroy and colleagues (251) found that hypothermia to 28° and 31°C facilitated recovery from ischemia, but that cooling to 28°C did not provide greater protection than cooling to 31°C. At 34°C, metabolic and EEG recovery, release of excitatory amino acids, and levels of S100 were intermediate between those observed at the colder temperatures and at 37°C.

In this context, the avoidance of cerebral hyperthermia deserves comment (252). As 2° to 3°C of hypothermia may offer significant brain protection in ischemia models, 2°C of hyperthermia significantly worsens outcome. Minamisawa et al. (246) demonstrated the effect of mild hyperthermia on neuronal necrosis following 10 minutes of ischemia in a rat model. As ischemic temperature was increased from 35°C to 39°C, the percentage of neurons damaged increased from approximately 15% to 80% (Fig. 21.10). This is clinically relevant because cerebral temperatures above 39°C have been documented in patients during rewarming (253), and these high temperatures may occur when cerebral embolic risk is greatest. From these reports, rewarming practice is being changed to avoid high brain temperatures. Additionally, when CPB is to be conducted "warm," systemic temperatures have been shifted toward mild hypothermia (33° to 34°C) from strict normothermia (254).

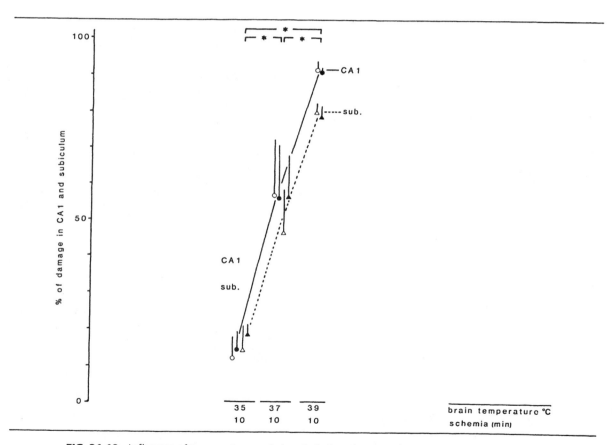

FIG. 21.10. Influence of temperature on ischemia-induced neuronal necrosis in the hippocampus (CAI sector and subiculum). Quantitative calculation of percentage of damaged neurons was performed bilaterally in each animal. There was no statistically significant difference between right and left hemispheres. Values are the mean ± standard error. Statistics were analyzed by analysis of variance, followed by Scheffé F test. *l s*, right hemisphere; *m Δ*, left hemisphere; **p* < 0.05. (Modified from Minamisawa H, Smith ML, Siesjo BK. The effect of mild hyperthermia and hypothermia on brain damage following 10 minutes of forebrain ischemia. *Ann Neurol* 1990;28:26–33, with permission.)

Physiologic Interventions to Reduce Embolization: Carbon Dioxide, Temperature, and Cardiopulmonary Bypass Flow

Surgical attention to embolic risk and technologic changes in the CPB circuit decrease cerebral embolization. Physiologic interventions may also be relevant. It has been suggested that increases in CBF, such as occur with pH-stat management or normothermic CPB, may result in a higher incidence of cerebral embolization. Similarly, acute reductions in CBF during periods of embolic risk might reduce cerebral embolization. This was recently tested in a swine CPB model. The effect of P_aCO_2 on total and regional cerebral embolization of microspheres was determined during normothermic CPB (187). The study demonstrated that a change of 25 mm Hg in P_aCO_2 during a 5-minute period of embolic risk could reduce total cerebral embolization by more than 50% (Fig. 21.11). These results indicate that during periods of embolic risk, such as clamping and unclamping of the aorta and the initial phases of ventricular ejection, a moderate reduction in P_aCO_2 may significantly decrease cerebral embolization.

The same model has been used to examine the effect of temperature and bypass flow on cerebral embolization. The investigators found that 10°C of hypothermia also effectively reduced embolization, but that the combination of hypothermia and hypocarbia did not reduce cerebral embolization more than hypocarbia alone. The relationship between CPB flow rate and cerebral embolization has also been examined (255). At a stable MAP, an inverse relationship between cerebral embolization and pump flow was described in dogs. Essentially, at lower pump flows, a greater proportion of that flow is delivered to the brain. Therefore, if a fixed number of emboli enter the aortic root, more emboli will be delivered to the brain if CPB flow is lower. The authors suggest that elevating pump flow during periods of embolic risk may also reduce cerebral embolization during clinical CPB.

Hypocarbia, hypothermia, and a high flow rate all effectively reduce cerebral embolization in an animal model. A combination of these physiologic interventions during periods of embolic risk may reduce neurologic morbidity. A clinical outcome study applying these physiologic interventions has yet to be conducted.

Paco₂ and Facilitated Cooling

Although there is clinical evidence that pH-stat management may be associated with worsened neurologic outcomes in adults, the opposite may be true in certain pediatric populations. A series of reports from the Boston Children's Hospital suggests that elevation of P_aCO_2 during cooling may improve neurologic outcome in children undergoing circulatory arrest (46,48). Elevation of CBF during the cooling phase may result in improved cerebral protection (46,48). Second, the rightward shift of the oxyhemoglobin dissociation curve with the more acidotic strategy might facilitate transfer of oxygen from hemoglobin. These hypotheses have largely been confirmed in a series of laboratory and clinical studies (48,190–192). Given these results, elevating P_aCO_2 may serve as a useful physiologic intervention to improve neuroprotection in select patient populations.

NEUROMONITORING

Given the unusual physiologic conditions of CPB and the incidence of neurologic injury, persistent efforts have been made to assess the adequacy of CDO_2 during CPB. Some current techniques include (a) measurement of venous oxyhemoglobin saturation at the jugular bulb ($S_{jv}O_2$), (b) near-infrared optical spectroscopy (NIRS), (c) transcranial Doppler (TCD), and (d) electrophysiologic monitors—EEG and evoked potentials.

Jugular Bulb Oxyhemoglobin Saturation

The measurement of cerebral venous oxygen saturation is clinically appealing because under non-bypass conditions, the $S_{jv}O_2$ provides an index of the adequacy of global cerebral oxygenation, for which normal values have been established (256,257). Additionally, fiberoptic oximetry allows for continuous measurement, placement of a jugular bulb catheter is simple, and the measurement is immediately familiar. Nevertheless, the role of $S_{jv}O_2$ monitoring in cardiac

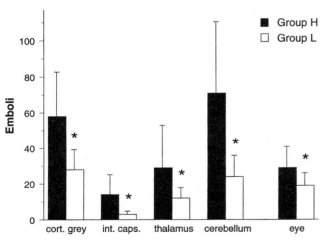

FIG. 21.11. The regional distribution of cerebral emboli in pigs with a mean P_aCO_2 of 52 mm Hg (■) or 27 mm Hg (□). Values are the mean number (± standard deviation) of emboli per gram (n = 10 in each group). *p <0.05. (Modified from Plöchl W, Cook, DJ. Quantification and distribution of cerebral emboli during cardiopulmonary bypass in the swine: the impact of P_aCO_2. *Anesthesiology* 1999;90:183–190, with permission.)

surgery is limited. Although $S_{jv}O_2$ can provide useful trends in cerebral oxygenation, the technique is limited by the fact that it is a measure of global oxygenation, so that focal events may be undetected. The $S_{jv}O_2$ value is also potentially difficult to interpret during progressive hypothermia, when changes in the P-50 (oxygen half-saturation pressure of hemoglobin) become important.

One of the first reports of $S_{jv}O_2$ during clinical CPB was by Croughwell et al. (258), who documented an $S_{jv}O_2$ of 50% or less or a P_vO_2 of 25 mm Hg or less in 23% of 133 patients. In the same year, Nakajima and colleagues (259) reported continuous recording of $S_{jv}O_2$ in 12 patients and described an inverse relationship between CPB temperature and $S_{jv}O_2$ in addition to a relationship between desaturation and rewarming speed. The effect of CPB temperature on $S_{jv}O_2$ was further examined in a randomized comparison of normothermic and hypothermic CPB (260), with the finding that desaturation tended to occur in normothermic patients at the onset of CPB, whereas in hypothermic patients it tended to occur during rewarming.

Perhaps the most prominent work on $S_{jv}O_2$ identified a relationship between $S_{jv}O_2$ and post-CPB cognitive dysfunction (261). In that report, intraoperative $S_{jv}O_2$ and neurocognitive outcome at discharge were evaluated in 255 patients. Desaturation during CPB was demonstrated in 17% of patients, whereas 38% demonstrated neurocognitive impairment at discharge. Neurocognitive impairment was related to the patients' baseline scores, educational level, and $S_{jv}O_2$ during CPB.

Studies have continued to examine the determinants of cerebral venous desaturation or have used $S_{jv}O_2$ as a monitor of cerebral oxygen balance. Enomoto and colleagues (262) reported that cerebral venous desaturation during rapid rewarming was a function of $CMRO_2$ and increased more quickly than CBF. Sapire and colleagues (263) examined $S_{jv}O_2$ during rewarming and found it to be a function of Hct, rewarming speed, and mean arterial pressure. Grubhofer et al. (264) also identified a dependency of $S_{jv}O_2$ on MAP during CPB. Von Knobelsdorff et al. (265) could not identify a relationship between rewarming speed and $S_{jv}O_2$, but patients in that study were rewarmed from 27° to 36°C in either 7 or 15 minutes.

Dexter and Hindman (266) published a provocative theoretical analysis of $S_{jv}O_2$ during hypothermia. They pointed out that the decrease in the hemoglobin P-50 with progressive hypothermia requires that the lower limit of normal for $S_{jv}O_2$ be increased as temperature decreases. The most interesting physiologic question posed by this discussion is whether the decreased P-50 at low temperatures compromises oxygen delivery to tissues. This question has not been answered, but another new technology may offer insight.

Near-infrared Spectroscopy

Hemoglobin undergoes a characteristic near-infrared absorption shift with oxygen binding, so NIRS has the poten-

tial to provide a continuous, noninvasive assessment of regional brain oxygenation (267,268). The hemoglobin emission spectrum is a function of the aggregate of arterial, venous, and capillary blood, so it is not surprising that there is no clear correlation between NIRS output and either arterial or venous oxyhemoglobin saturation during CPB (267,269,270). However, trends provided by NIRS are of interest. It has been reported that NIRS is sensitive to changes in temperature, carbon dioxide, and Hct and also to the cessation and reestablishment of CPB flow (269,271–273) (Fig. 21.12). Additionally, the rate of NIRS desaturation during circulatory arrest has been reported to be a function of temperature at arrest (273) and patient age (272).

Other studies have reported that during hypothermia, NIRS tissue saturation and $S_{jv}O_2$ may move in opposite directions (269,270,274). This might be interpreted as impaired off-loading of oxygen by hemoglobin, but at present the technology is not sufficiently advanced to determine whether a high P-50 could result in cerebral hypoxia.

Although NIRS technology has great potential, its development is ongoing. Currently, (a) quantitative measurements of oxyhemoglobin are not possible (268); (b) the region of interrogation is not clearly defined; (c) there is no external standard against which NIRS can be calibrated; (d) scalp blood and skull may contaminate the output of the devices, particularly in adults (275); and, perhaps most importantly, (e) hemoglobin saturation in the brain, whether venous, arterial, or capillary, may not reflect tissue oxygen utilization because of the high hemoglobin P-50. Measurement of the redox state of intracellular cytochrome oxidase

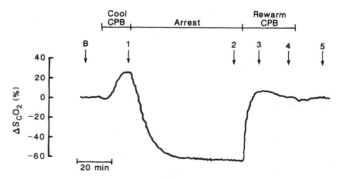

FIG. 21.12. Near-infrared spectroscopy (*NIRS*) record of the changes in cerebrovascular hemoglobin oxygen saturation (ΔS_cO_2) illustrating the points at which ΔS_cO_2 was captured and the deoxygenation curve during circulatory arrest. The 9-month-old patient underwent a hemi-Fontan operation. *B*, baseline at normothermia; *1*, on deep hypothermic cardiopulmonary bypass (*cool CPB*); *2*, at the end of circulatory arrest (*arrest*); *3*, on recirculation 3 minutes after resumption of CPB (*rCPB*); *4*, normothermic CPB (*wCPB*); *5*, after CPB (*end*). By definition, $+S_cO_2$ equals 0 at baseline. (From Kurth CD, Steven JM, Nicolson SC. Cerebral oxygenation during pediatric cardiac surgery using deep hypothermic circulatory arrest. *Anesthesiology* 1995;82:74–82, with permission.)

(aa_3) may be the solution to the latter problem because the aa_3 signal may be intimately related to intracellular concentrations of high-energy phosphate (276–278). However, at present, analysis of the aa_3 signal is highly complex. This technology is exciting and noninvasive, but the potential clinical implications of NIRS remain unclear.

Transcranial Doppler

Under non-CPB conditions, TCD measurements of blood flow velocity in the middle cerebral artery may correlate with measured CBF (279). The technique is noninvasive and provides continuous measurements, so it has been evaluated as a monitor of cerebral perfusion during CPB. Blood flow velocity may be sensitive to temperature change, MAP, and pump flow in addition to carbon dioxide and Hct, but for flow velocity to be a reliable measure of CBF, the diameter of the insonated vessel must not change (280,281). This condition may not be met during CPB, so the correlation of TCD flow velocity with measured CBF is relatively poor (282–284). Nevertheless, TCD can provide trends, and the relative changes in flow velocity show a better correlation than do absolute flow measurements (283,285,286).

Although strict quantitative measurements of CBF are not possible, the applicability of TCD may be greater in pediatric CPB. Obtaining the temporal window is easier in infants and children, and this population may be subjected to profound reductions in CPB flows at stable temperatures and Hcts. Under these conditions, TCD monitoring may be useful to determine whether these reduced CPB flows and MAPs are sufficient to maintain cerebral perfusion (287). The response of the cerebral circulation when flow is reestablished following circulatory arrest can also be evaluated (288).

In adult cardiac surgery, TCD has been found to be of much greater use in the detection of emboli than in the assessment of cerebral perfusion. Although not a cerebral monitor *per se*, detection of TCD emboli can be used to evaluate surgical technique (54,56) and CPB circuit modifications (58,69,204,289) indirectly, and it may serve as an independent predictor of neurologic outcome (44,49,172).

Although it is becoming popular, the limits of emboli detection must also be considered (290,291). The resolution limit for embolus size depends on the physical character of the embolus. Microthrombi are difficult to detect against the blood background signal, whereas air or plaque emboli may provide an adequate signal even if significantly smaller. In this regard, another limit of the current technology is the inability to determine embolus composition. Finally, the "gating" used to separate signal from background will in large part determine the results. However, automated signal detection and a recent technical consensus on microembolus detection (292) will help limit this source of variability.

Electroencephalogram and Evoked Potentials

In theory, electrophysiologic monitors should provide one of the best means for determining the adequacy of cerebral oxygenation. Although intraoperative EEG is familiar from carotid surgery, and although its use during CPB has been periodically advocated, for the most part it has not found its way into the operating room. This remains true although the technology has become simpler to use and advances have been made in data acquisition, processing, and display.

During the last 40 years, EEG during cardiac surgery has been evaluated in numerous studies, and certain EEG changes, such as slowing at the onset of CPB, have been demonstrated with consistency (293–295). However, establishing a clear relationship between EEG output and intraoperative physiology or clinical outcome has proved elusive. Both Arom et al. (296) and Edmonds et al. (297) found that neurologic outcome might be improved by the institution of physiologic interventions in response to an abnormal EEG. However, these studies were not randomized and lacked concurrent control groups. Furthermore, much of the evidence indicates that intraoperative EEG lacks both sensitivity and specificity. Patients may show an abnormal EEG during CPB and recover without neurologic deficit, whereas others may have a normal intraoperative EEG examination and experience stroke. This is not surprising, as advances in data processing cannot address the primary limitation of EEG, which is that it records only superficial cortical electrical activity. If most neurologic injury is embolic in origin, the EEG cannot be expected to detect focal ischemia occurring in small areas deep in the brain (298). Secondarily, the background anesthetic and hypothermia may alter both the power and frequency spectra of the EEG, as can CPB-related artifact (295).

In the study by Bashein and colleagues (299), 78 patients underwent CPB at 28° to 32°C with EEG recording; neurocognitive status was determined preoperatively and at 8 days and 7 months postoperatively (297). Electrical noise contaminated the EEG in 40% of patients despite extensive computational modeling, and there was no clear relationship between EEG power or frequency and outcome.

Evoked potentials provide another means of assessing functional neurologic integrity during CPB (300). Most common is the somatosensory evoked potential (SSEP), in which a stimulus is delivered peripherally and the integrity of its transmission from the peripheral nerve through the spinal cord and to the sensory cortex is recorded (301). As in EEG, a decrease in potential amplitude may represent ischemia, as can an increase in signal latency. In the experimental setting, evoked potentials have been successfully used as monitors for ischemia (134,302), and they have been used clinically for detecting brachial plexus injury (303). Like EEG, evoked potential amplitude and latency are sensitive to hypothermia (304–306). Proper signals may

TABLE 21.7. IMPACT OF RECORDED VARIABLES ON S100 PROTEIN RELEASE AT DIFFERENT SAMPLING INTERVALS[a]

Variable	No. of Patients	Sampling Times (p value)			
		T0	T5	T15	T48
Age	515	<0.0001	<0.0001	<0.001	NS
Perfusion time	515	<0.0001	NS	NS	NS
History of CVI/TIA	42	<0.01	NS	NS	NS
Diseased ascending aorta	53	<0.001	<0.005	NS	<0.005
Renal insufficiency	12	NS	<0.05	NS	NS
Perioperative stroke	13	NS	NS	NS	<0.0001
Encephalopathy	17	NS	NS	NS	NS
Delayed awakening	12	NS	NS	NS	<0.05

[a] Multiple linear regression analysis showing the variables significantly influencing the S100 protein levels after cardiac operation with extracorporeal circulation in the 515 patients studied. The presence of a diseased ascending aorta was confirmed with palpation intraoperatively. Renal insufficiency was defined as a preoperative serum creatinine level >2.2 mg/dL. Cerebrovascular accident/transient ischemic attack (CVI/TIA) relates to a history of stroke or transient ischemic attack. Age and perfusion time were continuous variables, whereas the other variables were analyzed as dichotomous variables. All correlations found were positive.
NS, not significant; T0, immediately after termination of extracorporeal circulation; T5, 5 hours; T15, 15 hours; T48, 48 hours afer T0.
From Jönsson H, Johnsson P, Alling C, et al. Significance of serum S100 release after coronary artery bypass grafting. *Ann Thorac Surg* 1998;65:1639–1644, with permission.

also be difficult to obtain, and hundreds of potentials must be averaged to separate signal from noise (298,307). Finally, the definition of what constitutes an abnormality has not been decided. In clear cases of brachial plexus injury, a change of 3 standard deviations from the pre-CPB measurement was required to identify neurologic injury (303). As such, the sensitivity and specificity of evoked potential monitoring may be at least as limited as those of EEG monitoring.

Protein S100

Although not a technique for cerebral monitoring, astroglial and Schwann cell protein S100 release is of interest because serum and cerebrospinal fluid levels of S100 increase following brain damage from stroke, trauma, and subarachnoid hemorrhage (308). Therefore, the relationship between S100 levels and CPB-related cerebral injury is being evaluated (309). Observational studies describing the time course of S100 release have shown that the protein is not detected before CPB and that peak levels occur intraoperatively between the end of rewarming and the end of CPB (308–311). These levels appear to be related to CPB time (311–314) and patient age (314,315). Intracardiac operations have been reported to result in higher levels than do CABG procedures (316). Arterial line filtration may reduce S100 levels (310), and there appears to be some correlation between embolization and S100 levels (315). Patients undergoing non-CPB CABG have undetectable or fractionally elevated levels (311).

The sensitivity or specificity of S100 as a marker for cerebral injury has not been established, although it is clear that levels measured at the end of CPB are not specific (Table 21.7). In a study by Jönsson et al. (314), 93% of 515 consecutive patients had detectable S100 at the end of surgery, but stroke, encephalopathy, or delayed awakening was noted in fewer than 10%. In a study of 40 patients, 58% showed elevated S100 levels 1 hour postoperatively, but no patient demonstrated overt cerebral injury (310). Elevation of S100 48 hours postoperatively may be more sensitive or specific than early postoperative levels (314). However, what therapeutic intervention could be based on a 48-hour measurement is not clear.

CONCLUSIONS

In adults, postcardiac surgical brain injury occurs because the cardiac surgical population concentrates a variety of neurologic risk factors. Surgery precipitates those risks and imposes additional ischemic, physiologic, and inflammatory stresses for which the patient is unable to compensate. Because neurologic morbidity is a function of the interaction between patient and surgery, the greatest reductions in morbidity will come from the application of risk stratification to decide who is best served by surgery and who is not. Although technical and pharmacologic innovations such as off-bypass surgery, anti-adhesion therapies, and near-infrared monitoring are seductive, they cannot be used as the basis for a decision not to take certain patients to the operating room.

For the patients who go to surgery, we must be comprehensive and practical in our thinking. Because neurologic injury is largely a function of patient factors, multivariate analysis indicates that age and atherosclerotic disease determine outcome. Although patient factors may determine outcome in multivariate analysis, this is not equivalent to saying that surgical, physiologic, and pharmacologic management is unimportant. We have acquired a great deal of understanding about hypertensive cerebral vascular disease, regional blood flow in focal ischemia, and the potent effect of temperature on the cascade of injury. This allows us to make well-informed choices about physiologic management. Similarly, the principles of gas physiology can be applied to facilitate absorption of bubbles or change the distribution of blood flow during periods of embolic risk. Echocardiography can tell us when it is appropriate to remove an aortic vent, and we know that administering a barbiturate may be advantageous if circulatory arrest must take place before adequate cooling.

We help our patients by understanding their risk factors and by putting them in a physiologic condition that can minimize the impact of specific surgical stressors and maximize the mechanisms that facilitate compensation. Exquisite control of these variables is possible during CPB and in the perioperative period; application of this knowledge will affect outcomes.

KEY POINTS

- Operations requiring CPB carry a significant risk for stroke (1% to 9%) and are associated with a higher (10% to 60%) incidence of neurocognitive deficits at hospital discharge, with 5% to 20% of patients retaining neurocognitive deficits 3 to 6 months postoperatively. Deficits in psychomotor speed, attention and concentration, learning ability, and short-term memory are most commonly found. Etiologic factors include embolization, hypoperfusion, and inflammation.
- Factors influencing CBF during CPB include $CMRO_2$, P_aCO_2, Hct, and MAP. Once MAP drops below a critical threshold, CBF becomes pressure-passive regardless of pump flow in animal models. Human studies also suggest that CDO_2 may be compromised at MAPs below 50 mm Hg during CPB.
- Recent studies focusing on temperature management suggest that mild hypothermia (32° to 35°C) during CPB ("tepid" CPB) protects the central nervous system as well as lower temperatures (25° to 30°C) during CPB, and that maintaining strict normothermia (36° to 37°C) increases the risk for stroke and possibly neurocognitive deterioration. Experimental evidence strongly suggests that the CPB rewarming process should be conducted in a manner that avoids cerebral hyperthermia.

- For moderately hypothermic CPB, the preponderance of neurologic outcome evidence supports alpha-stat acid–base management during CPB, but at profound hypothermia (<20°C), recent evidence favors pH-stat management.
- Management of the surgical field has become increasingly important in preventing embolic events, with particular emphasis on epiaortic ultrasound scanning to avoid manipulation of atherosclerotic plaques in the ascending aorta, single aortic clamping techniques, and improved ventricular de-airing maneuvers.
- Under prevailing conditions (e.g., moderate hypothermia, membrane oxygenator, and arterial filtration) for CPB, pharmacologic neuroprotective interventions have not been shown to improve outcomes.
- A variety of central nervous system monitors have been investigated for use during CPB.
  - Jugular bulb oximetry offers intuitive appeal, and one study shows an inverse correlation between $S_{jv}O_2$ and neurocognitive impairment.
  - The clinical utility of NIRS, a noninvasive tool that measures some aggregate of arterial, venous, and capillary blood oxygen saturation, remains uncertain.
  - TCD can measure flow velocity in the middle cerebral artery and detect microemboli, but its utility in judging cerebral blood flow is predicated on the assumption that the diameter of the middle cerebral artery is constant, which has not been adequately established.
  - EEG (processed or unprocessed) and evoked potentials thus far lack the sensitivity and specificity to be clinically useful during CPB, and electrical interference in the cardiac surgical milieu is a significant limitation to their use.

REFERENCES

1. Tuman KJ, McCarthy RJ, Najafi H, et al. Differential effects of advanced age on neurologic and cardiac risks of coronary artery operations. *J Thorac Cardiovasc Surg* 1992;104:1510–1517.
2. Tu JV, Jaglal SB, Naylor CD. Multicenter validation of a risk index for mortality, intensive care unit stay, and overall hospital length of stay after cardiac surgery. (Steering Committee of the Provincial Adult Cardiac Care Network of Ontario.) *Circulation* 1995;91:677–685.
3. Hammermeister KE, Burchfiel C, Johnson R, et al. Identification of patients at greatest risk for developing major complications at cardiac surgery. *Circulation* 1990;82:IV-380–IV-389.
4. Weintraub WS, Jones EL, Craver J, et al. Determinants of prolonged length of hospital stay after coronary bypass surgery. *Circulation* 1989;80:276–284.
5. Tu JV, Mazer CD, Levinton C, et al. A predictive index for length of stay in the intensive care unit following cardiac surgery. *Can Med Assoc J* 1994;151:177–185.
6. Roach GW, Kanchuger M, Mangano CM, et al. Adverse cere-

bral outcomes after coronary bypass surgery. Multicenter Study of Perioperative Ischemia Research Group and the Ischemia Research and Education Foundation Investigators. *N Engl J Med* 1996;335:1857–1863.

7. Wolman RL, Nussmeier NA, Aggarwal A, et al. Cerebral injury after cardiac surgery. Identification of a group of extraordinary risk. The Multicenter Study of Perioperative Ischemia (McSPI) Research Group and the Ischemia Research and Education Foundation (IREF) Investigators. *Stroke* 1999;30:514–522.

8. Gardner TJ, Horneffer PJ, Manolio TA, et al. Stroke following coronary artery bypass grafting: a ten-year study. *Ann Thorac Surg* 1985;40:574–581.

9. Shaw PJ, Bates D, Cartlidge NE, et al. Neurologic and neuropsychological morbidity following major surgery: comparison of coronary artery bypass and peripheral vascular surgery. *Stroke* 1987;18:700–707.

10. Moller JT, Cluitmans P, Rasmussen LS, et al. Long-term postoperative cognitive dysfunction in the elderly ISPOCD1 study. (ISPOCD Investigators. International Study of Post-Operative Cognitive Dysfunction.) *Lancet* 1998;351:857–861.

11. Weintraub WS, Wenger NK, Jones EL, et al. Changing clinical characteristics of coronary surgery patients. Differences between men and women. *Circulation* 1993;88:79–86.

12. Jones EL, Weintraub WS, Craver JM, et al. Coronary bypass surgery: is the operation different today? *J Thorac Cardiovasc Surg* 1991;101:108–115.

13. He GW, Acuff TE, Ryan WH, et al. Determinants of operative mortality in elderly patients undergoing coronary artery bypass grafting. Emphasis on the influence of internal mammary artery grafting on mortality and morbidity. *J Thorac Cardiovasc Surg* 1994;108:73–81.

14. Berens ES, Kouchoukos NT, Murphy SF, et al. Preoperative carotid artery screening in elderly patients undergoing cardiac surgery. *J Vasc Surg* 1992;15:313–323.

15. Mickleborough LL, Takagi Y, Maruyama H, et al. Is sex a factor in determining operative risk for aortocoronary bypass graft surgery? *Circulation* 1995;92:II-80–II-84.

16. Wareing TH, Davila-Roman VG, Daily BB, et al. Strategy for the reduction of stroke incidence in cardiac surgical patients. *Ann Thorac Surg* 1993;55:1400–1408.

17. Ricotta JJ, Faggioli GL, Castilone A, et al. Risk factors for stroke after cardiac surgery: Buffalo cardiac–cerebral study group. *J Vasc Surg* 1995;21:359–364.

18. Rao V, Christakis GT, Weisel RD, et al. Risk factors for stroke following coronary bypass surgery. *J Card Surg* 1995;10:468–474.

19. McKhann GM, Goldsborough MA, Borowicz LM Jr, et al. Predictors of stroke risk in coronary artery bypass patients. *Ann Thorac Surg* 1997;63:516–521.

20. Price TR, Manolio TA, Kronmal RA, et al. Silent brain infarction on magnetic resonance imaging and neurological abnormalities in community-dwelling older adults. The Cardiovascular Health Study. *Stroke* 1997;28:1158–1164.

21. Skoog I. A review on blood pressure and ischaemic white matter lesions. *Dement Geriatr Cogn Disord* 1998;9:13–19.

22. Matsushita K, Kuriyama Y, Nagatsuka K, et al. Periventricular white matter lucency and cerebral blood flow autoregulation in hypertensive patients. *Hypertension* 1994;23:565–568.

23. Longstreth WT Jr, Manolio TA, Arnold A, et al. Clinical correlates of white matter findings on cranial magnetic resonance imaging of 3301 elderly people. The Cardiovascular Health Study. *Stroke* 1996;27:1274–1282.

24. Schmidt R, Fazekas F, Offenbacher H, et al. Brain magnetic resonance imaging in coronary artery bypass grafts: a pre- and postoperative assessment. *Neurology* 1993;43:775–778.

25. Breuer AC, Furlan AJ, Hanson MR, et al. Central nervous system complications of coronary artery bypass graft surgery: prospective analysis of 421 patients. *Stroke* 1983;14:682–687.

26. Redmond JM, Greene PS, Goldsborough MA, et al. Neurologic injury in cardiac surgical patients with a history of stroke. *Ann Thorac Surg* 1996;61:42–47.

27. Shaw PJ, Bates D, Cartlidge NEF, et al. Early neurological complications of coronary artery bypass surgery. *BMJ* 1985;291:1384–1387.

28. Aberg T, Ronquist G, Tyden H. Cerebral damage during open-heart surgery. *Scand J Thorac Cardiovasc Surg* 1987;21:159–163.

29. Sotaniemi KA, Mononen H, Hokkanen TE. Long-term cerebral outcome after open-heart surgery. A five-year neuropsychological follow-up study. *Stroke* 1986;17:410–416.

30. Savageau JA, Stanton BA, Jenkins CD, et al. Neuropsychological dysfunction following elective cardiac operation. II. A six-month reassessment. *J Thorac Cardiovasc Surg* 1982;84:595–600.

31. Newman MF, Croughwell ND, Blumenthal JA, et al. Predictors of cognitive decline after cardiac operation. *Ann Thorac Surg* 1995;59:1326–1330.

32. Mora CT, Henson MB, Weintraub WS, et al. The effect of temperature management during cardiopulmonary bypass on neurologic and neuropsychologic outcomes in patients undergoing coronary revascularization. *J Thorac Cardiovasc Surg* 1996;112:514–522.

33. McLean RF, Wong BI, Naylor D, et al. Cardiopulmonary bypass, temperature, and central nervous system dysfunction. *Circulation* 1994;90:II-250–II-255.

34. Vingerhoets G, Van Nooten G, Vermassen F, et al. Short-term and long-term neuropsychological consequences of cardiac surgery with extracorporeal circulation. *Eur J Cardiothorac Surg* 1997;11:424–431.

35. McKhann GM, Goldsborough MA, Borowicz LM Jr, et al. Cognitive outcome after coronary artery bypass: a one-year prospective study. *Ann Thorac Surg* 1997;63:510–515.

36. Sotaniemi KA. Cerebral outcome after extracorporeal circulation. Comparison between prospective and retrospective evaluations. *Arch Neurol* 1983;40:75–77.

37. Slogoff S, Girgis KZ, Keats AS. Etiologic factors in neuropsychiatric complications associated with cardiopulmonary bypass. *Anesth Analg* 1982;61:903–911.

38. Borowicz LM, Goldsborough MA, Selnes OA, et al. Neuropsychologic change after cardiac surgery: a critical review. *Cardiothorac Vasc Anesth* 1996;10:105–111; quiz 111–112.

39. Blumenthal JA, Mahanna EP, Madden DJ, et al. Methodological issues in the assessment of neuropsychologic function after cardiac surgery. *Ann Thorac Surg* 1995;59:1345–1350.

40. Newman SP. Analysis and interpretation of neuropsychologic tests in cardiac surgery. *Ann Thorac Surg* 1995;59:1351–1355.

41. Murkin JM, Newman SP, Stump DA, et al. Statement of consensus on assessment of neurobehavioral outcomes after cardiac surgery. *Ann Thorac Surg* 1995;59:1289–1295.

42. Stump DA. Selection and clinical significance of neuropsychologic tests. *Ann Thorac Surg* 1995;59:1340–1344.

43. Townes BD, Bashein G, Hornbein TF, et al. Neurobehavioral outcomes in cardiac operations. A prospective controlled study. *J Thorac Cardiovasc Surg* 1989;98:774–782.

44. Pugsley W, Klinger L, Paschalis C, et al. The impact of microemboli during cardiopulmonary bypass on neuropsychological functioning. *Stroke* 1994;25:1393–1399.

45. Ferry PC. Neurologic sequelae of cardiac surgery in children. *Am J Dis Child* 1987;141:309–312.

46. Jonas RA, Bellinger DC, Rappaport LA, et al. Relation of pH strategy and development outcome after hypothermic circulatory arrest. *J Thorac Cardiovasc Surg* 1993;106:362–368.

47. Newburger JW, Jonas RA, Wernovsky G, et al. A comparison of the perioperative neurologic effects of hypothermic circulatory arrest versus low-flow cardiopulmonary bypass in infant heart surgery. *N Engl J Med* 1993;329:1057–1064.

48. Jonas RA. Review of current research at Boston Children's Hospital. *Ann Thorac Surg* 1993;56:1467–1472.

49. Barbut D, Lo YW, Gold JP, et al. Impact of embolization during coronary artery bypass grafting on outcome and length of stay. *Ann Thorac Surg* 1997;63:998–1002.

50. Wagerle LC, Russo P, Dahdah NS, et al. Endothelial dysfunction in cerebral microcirculation during hypothermic cardiopulmonary bypass in newborn lambs. *J Thorac Cardiovasc Surg* 1998;115:1047–1054.

51. Verrier ED, Shen I. Potential role of neutrophil anti-adhesion therapy in myocardial stunning, myocardial infarction, and organ dysfunction after cardiopulmonary bypass. *J Card Surg* 1993;8:309–312.

52. Hallenbeck JM. Significance of the inflammatory response in brain ischemia. *Acta Neurochir Suppl* 1996;66:27–31.

53. Elliott MJ, Finn AHR. Interaction between neutrophils and endothelium. *Ann Thorac Surg* 1993;56:1503–1508.

54. Barbut D, Yao FSF, Lo YW, et al. Determination of size of aortic emboli and embolic load during coronary artery bypass grafting. *Ann Thorac Surg* 1997;63:1262–1267.

55. Stump DA, Rogers AT, Hammon JW, Newman SP. Cerebral emboli and cognitive outcome after cardiac surgery. *J Cardiothorac Vasc Anesth* 1996;10:113–118; quiz 118–119.

56. van der Linden J, Casimir-Ahn H. When do cerebral emboli appear during open heart operations? A transcranial Doppler study. *Ann Thorac Surg* 1991;51:237–241.

57. Blauth CI, Arnold JV, Schulenberg WE, et al. Cerebral microembolism during cardiopulmonary bypass. Retinal microvascular studies *in vivo* with fluorescein angiography. *J Thorac Cardiovasc Surg* 1988;95:668–676.

58. Blauth C, Smith P, Newman S, et al. Retinal microembolism and neuropsychological deficit following clinical cardiopulmonary bypass: comparison of a membrane and a bubble oxygenator. A preliminary communication. *Eur J Cardiothorac Surg* 1989;3:135–139.

59. Javid H, Tufo HM, Najafi H, et al. Neurological abnormalities following open-heart surgery. *J Thorac Cardiovasc Surg* 1969; 58:502–509.

60. Steinberg GK, De La Paz R, Mitchell RS, et al. MR and cerebrospinal fluid enzymes as sensitive indicators of subclinical cerebral injury after open-heart valve replacement surgery. *Am J Neuroradiol* 1996;17:205–212; discussion 213–215.

61. Hise JH, Nipper ML, Schnitker JC. Stroke associated with coronary artery bypass surgery. *Am J Neuroradiol* 1991;12:811–814.

62. Blossom GB, Fietsam R Jr, Bassett JS, et al. Characteristics of cerebrovascular accidents after coronary artery bypass grafting. *Am Surg* 1992;58:584–589.

63. Howard G, Trend P, Russell WR. Clinical features of ischemia in cerebral arterial border zones after periods of reduced cerebral blood flow. *Arch Neurol* 1987;44:934–940.

64. Moody DM, Brown WR, Challa VR, et al. Brain microemboli associated with cardiopulmonary bypass: a histologic and magnetic resonance imaging study. *Ann Thorac Surg* 1995;59: 1304–1307.

65. Blauth CI, Cosgrove DM, Webb BW, et al. Atheroembolism from the ascending aorta. An emerging problem in cardiac surgery. *J Thorac Cardiovasc Surg* 1992;103:1104–1112.

66. Wareing TH, Davila-Roman VG, Barzilai B, et al. Management of the severely atherosclerotic ascending aorta during cardiac operations. A strategy for detection and treatment. *J Thorac Cardiovasc Surg* 1992;103:453–462.

67. Blauth CI. Macroemboli and microemboli during cardiopulmonary bypass. *Ann Thorac Surg* 1995;59:1300–1303.

68. Dewanjee MK, Wu SM, De D, et al. Reduction of neutrophil margination by L-arginine during hypothermic cardiopulmonary bypass in a pig model. *ASAIO J* 1996;42:M661–M666.

69. Padayachee TS, Parsons S, Theobold R, et al. The effect of arterial filtration on reduction of gaseous microemboli in the middle cerebral artery during cardiopulmonary bypass. *Ann Thorac Surg* 1988;45:647–649.

70. Barbut D, Yao FS, Hager DN, et al. Comparison of transcranial Doppler ultrasonography and transesophageal echocardiography to monitor emboli during coronary artery bypass surgery. *Stroke* 1996;27:87–90.

71. Lynn GM, Stefanko K, Reed JF III, et al. Risk factors for stroke after coronary artery bypass. *J Thorac Cardiovasc Surg* 1992; 104:1518–1523.

72. Herlitz J, Brandrup-Wognsen G, Haglid M, et al. Mortality and morbidity during a period of 2 years after coronary artery bypass surgery in patients with and without a history of hypertension. *J Hypertens* 1996;14:309–314.

73. Strandgaard S, Olesen J, Skinhoj E, et al. Autoregulation of brain circulation in severe arterial hypertension. *BMJ* 1973;1: 507–510.

74. Baumbach GL, Heistad DD. Cerebral circulation in chronic arterial hypertension. *Hypertension* 1988;12:89–95.

75. Coyle P. Outcomes to middle cerebral artery occlusion in hypertensive and normotensive rats. *Hypertension* 1984;6:I-69–I-74.

76. Coyle P, Heistad DD. Blood flow through cerebral collateral vessels in hypertensive and normotensive rats. *Hypertension* 1986;8:II-67–II-71.

77. Aronow WS, Gutstein H, Lee NH, et al. Three-year follow-up of risk factors correlated with new atherothrombotic brain infarction in 708 elderly patients. *Angiology* 1988;39:563–566.

78. Caplan LR. Diabetes and brain ischemia. *Diabetes* 1996;45: S95–S97.

79. Croughwell N, Lyth M, Quill TJ, et al. Diabetic patients have abnormal cerebral autoregulation during cardiopulmonary bypass. *Circulation* 1990;82:IV-407–IV-412.

80. Bentsen N, Larsen B, Lassen NA. Chronically impaired autoregulation of cerebral blood flow in long-term diabetics. *Stroke* 1975;6:497–502.

81. Granger DN, Kubes P. The microcirculation and inflammation: modulation of leukocyte–endothelial cell adhesion. *J Leukoc Biol* 1994;55:662–675.

82. del Zoppo GJ. Microvascular responses to cerebral ischemia/inflammation. *Ann N Y Acad Sci* 1997;823:132–147.

83. del Zoppo GJ, Schmid-Schonbein GW, Mori E, et al. Polymorphonuclear leukocytes occlude capillaries following middle cerebral artery occlusion and reperfusion in baboons. *Stroke* 1991; 22:1276–1283.

84. Okada Y, Copeland BR, Fitridge R, et al. Fibrin contributes to microvascular obstructions and parenchymal changes during early focal cerebral ischemia and reperfusion. *Stroke* 1994;25: 1847–1853; discussion 1853–1854.

85. Obrenovitch TP, Hallenbeck JM. Platelet accumulation in regions of low blood flow during the postischemic period. *Stroke* 1985;16:224–234.

86. Hall RI, Smith MS, Rocker G. The systemic inflammatory response to cardiopulmonary bypass: pathophysiological, therapeutic, and pharmacological considerations. *Anesth Analg* 1997; 85:766–782.

87. Shafique T, Johnson RG, Dai HB, et al. Altered pulmonary microvascular reactivity after total cardiopulmonary bypass. *J Thorac Cardiovasc Surg* 1993;106:479–486.

88. Friedman M, Johnson RG, Wang SY, et al. Pulmonary micro-

vascular responses to protamine and histamine. *J Thorac Cardiovasc Surg* 1994;108:1092–1099.

89. Seccombe JF, Schaff HV. Coronary artery endothelial function after myocardial ischemia and reperfusion. *Ann Thorac Surg* 1995;60:778–788.

90. Feerick AE, Johnston WE, Steinsland O, et al. Cardiopulmonary bypass impairs vascular endothelial relaxation: effects of gaseous microemboli in dogs. *Am J Physiol* 1994;267: H1174–H1182.

91. Schmeling DJ, Caty MG, Oldham KT, et al. Evidence for neutrophil-related acute lung injury after intestinal ischemia–reperfusion. *Surgery* 1989;106:195–202.

92. Poggetti RS, Moore EE, Moore FA, et al. Liver injury is a reversible neutrophil-mediated event following gut ischemia. *Arch Surg* 1992;127:175–179.

93. Bhujle R, Li J, Shastri P, et al. Influence of cardiopulmonary bypass on platelet and neutrophil accumulations in internal organs. *ASAIO J* 1997;43:M739–M744.

94. Chandler W. The effects of cardiopulmonary bypass on fibrin formation and lysis: is a normal fibrinolytic response essential? *J Cardiovasc Pharmacol* 1996;27:S63–S68.

95. Body SC. Platelet activation and interactions with the microvasculature. *J Cardiovasc Pharmacol* 1996;27:S13–S25.

96. Rinder C, Fitch J. Amplification of the inflammatory response: adhesion molecules associated with platelet/white cell responses. *J Cardiovasc Pharmacol* 1996;27:S6–S12.

97. Cameron D. Initiation of white cell activation during cardiopulmonary bypass: cytokines and receptors. *J Cardiovasc Pharmacol* 1996;27:S1–S5.

98. Korthuis RJ, Anderson DC, Granger DN. Role of neutrophil–endothelial cell adhesion in inflammatory disorders. *J Crit Care* 1994;9:47–71.

99. Said S, Rosenblum WI, Povlishock JT, et al. Correlations between morphological changes in platelet aggregates and underlying endothelial damage in cerebral microcirculation of mice. *Stroke* 1993;24:1968–1976.

100. Nandate K, Vuylsteke A, Crosbie AE, et al. Cerebrovascular cytokine responses during coronary artery bypass surgery: specific production of interleukin-8 and its attenuation by hypothermic cardiopulmonary bypass. *Anesth Analg* 1999;89(4): 823–828.

101. Boyle EM Jr, Pohlman TH, Johnson MC, et al. Endothelial cell injury in cardiovascular surgery: the systemic inflammatory response. *Ann Thorac Surg* 1997;63:277–284.

102. Gutierrez G, Warley AR, Dantzker DR. Oxygen delivery and utilization in hypothermic dogs. *J Appl Physiol* 1986;60: 751–757.

103. Schumacker PT, Rowland J, Saltz S, et al. Effects of hyperthermia and hypothermia on oxygen extraction by tissues during hypovolemia. *J Appl Physiol* 1987;63:1246–1252.

104. Adams RP, Dieleman LA, Cain SM. A critical value for O_2 transport in the rat. *J Appl Physiol* 1982;53:660–664.

105. Cook DJ, Orszulak TA, Daly RC. Minimum hematocrit at differing cardiopulmonary bypass temperatures in dogs. *Circulation* 1998;98:II-170–II-175.

106. Plöchl W, Cook DJ, Orszulak TA, et al. Critical cerebral perfusion pressure during tepid heart surgery in dogs. *Ann Thorac Surg* 1998;66:118–124.

107. Michenfelder JD. *Anesthesia and the brain.* New York: Churchill Livingstone, 1988.

108. Michenfelder JD, Milde JH. The relationship among canine brain temperature, metabolism, and function during hypothermia. *Anesthesiology* 1991;75:130–136.

109. Greeley WJ, Kern FH, Ungerleider RM, et al. The effect of hypothermic cardiopulmonary bypass and total circulatory arrest on cerebral metabolism in neonates, infants, and children. *J Thorac Cardiovasc Surg* 1991;101:783–794.

110. Kern FH, Ungerleider RM, Reves JG, et al. Effect of altering pump flow rate on cerebral blood flow and metabolism in infants and children. *Ann Thorac Surg* 1993;56:1366–1372.

111. Murkin JM, Farrar JK, Tweed WA, et al. Cerebral autoregulation and flow/metabolism coupling during cardiopulmonary bypass: the influence of $PaCO_2$. *Anesth Analg* 1987;66:825–832.

112. Govier AV, Reves JG, McKay RD, et al. Factors and their influence on regional cerebral blood flow during nonpulsatile cardiopulmonary bypass. *Ann Thorac Surg* 1984;38:592–600.

113. Brusino FG, Reves JG, Smith LR, et al. The effect of age on cerebral blood flow during hypothermic cardiopulmonary bypass. *J Thorac Cardiovasc Surg* 1989;97:541–547.

114. Davis RF, Dobbs JL, Casson H. Conduct and monitoring of cardiopulmonary bypass. In: Gravlee GP, Davis RF, Utley JR, eds. *Cardiopulmonary bypass: principles and practice.* Baltimore: Williams & Wilkins, 1993:578–602.

115. Mutch WAC, Sutton IR, Teskey JM, et al. Cerebral pressure–flow relationship during cardiopulmonary bypass in the dog at normothermia and moderate hypothermia. *J Cereb Blood Flow Metab* 1994;14:510–518.

116. Tanaka J, Shiki K, Asou T, et al. Cerebral autoregulation during deep hypothermic nonpulsatile cardiopulmonary bypass with selective cerebral perfusion in dogs. *J Thorac Cardiovasc Surg* 1988;95:124–132.

117. Sadahiro M, Haneda K, Mohri H. Experimental study of cerebral autoregulation during cardiopulmonary bypass with or without pulsatile perfusion. *J Thorac Cardiovasc Surg* 1994;108: 446–454.

118. Henriksen L. Brain luxury perfusion during cardiopulmonary bypass in humans. A study of the cerebral blood flow response to changes in CO_2, O_2, and blood pressure. *J Cereb Blood Flow Metab* 1986;6:366–378.

119. Johnsson P, Messeter K, Ryding E, et al. Cerebral vasoreactivity to carbon dioxide during cardiopulmonary perfusion at normothermia and hypothermia. *Ann Thorac Surg* 1989;48:769–775.

120. Stephan H, Weyland A, Kazmaier S, et al. Acid–base management during hypothermic cardiopulmonary bypass does not affect cerebral metabolism but does affect blood flow and neurological outcome. *Br J Anaesth* 1992;69:51–57.

121. Cheng W, Hartmann JF, Cameron DE, et al. Cerebral blood flow during cardiopulmonary bypass: influence of temperature and pH management strategy. *Ann Thorac Surg* 1995;59: 880–886.

122. Johnston WE, Vinten-Johansen J, DeWitt DS, et al. Cerebral perfusion during canine hypothermic cardiopulmonary bypass: effect of arterial carbon dioxide tension. *Ann Thorac Surg* 1991; 52:479–489.

123. Hindman BJ, Dexter F, Cutkomp J, et al. Hypothermic acid–base management does not affect cerebral metabolic rate for oxygen at 27°C. A study during cardiopulmonary bypass in rabbits. *Anesthesiology* 1993;79:580–587.

124. Patel RL, Turtle MR, Chambers DJ, et al. Hyperperfusion and cerebral dysfunction. Effect of differing acid–base management during cardiopulmonary bypass. *Eur J Cardiothorac Surg* 1993; 7:457–463; discussion 464.

125. Prough DS, Rogers AT, Stump DA, et al. Hypercarbia depresses cerebral oxygen consumption during cardiopulmonary bypass. *Stroke* 1990;21:1162–1166.

126. Cook DJ, Oliver WC Jr, Orszulak TA, et al. Cardiopulmonary bypass temperature, hematocrit, and cerebral oxygen delivery in humans. *Ann Thorac Surg* 1995;60:1671–1677.

127. Todd MM, Wu B, Maktabi M, et al. Cerebral blood flow and oxygen delivery during hypoxemia and hemodilution: role of arterial oxygen content. *Am J Physiol* 1994;267:H2025–H2031.

128. Croughwell N, Smith LR, Quill T, et al. The effect of temperature on cerebral metabolism and blood flow in adults during

cardiopulmonary bypass. *J Thorac Cardiovasc Surg* 1992;103: 549–554.

129. Andersen K, Waaben J, Husum B, et al. Nonpulsatile cardiopulmonary bypass disrupts the flow–metabolism couple in the brain. *J Thorac Cardiovasc Surg* 1985;90:570–579.

130. Henling CE, Carmichael MJ, Keats AS, et al. Cardiac operation for congenital heart disease in children of Jehovah's Witnesses. *J Thorac Cardiovasc Surg* 1985;89:914–920.

131. Eke CC, Gundry SR, Baum MF, et al. Neurologic sequelae of deep hypothermic circulatory arrest in cardiac transplant infants. *Ann Thorac Surg* 1996;61:783–788.

132. Read RC, Kuida H, Johnson JA. Effect of alterations in vasomotor tone on pressure–flow relationships in the totally perfused dog. *Circ Res* 1957;5:676–682.

133. Swain JA, McDonald TJ Jr, Griffith PK, et al. Low-flow hypothermic cardiopulmonary bypass protects the brain. *J Thorac Cardiovasc Surg* 1991;102:76–83; discussion 83–84.

134. Rebeyka IM, Coles JG, Wilson GJ, et al. The effect of low-flow cardiopulmonary bypass on cerebral function: an experimental and clinical study. *Ann Thorac Surg* 1987;43:391–396.

135. Fox LS, Blackstone EH, Kirklin JW, et al. Relationship of whole body oxygen consumption to perfusion flow rate during hypothermic cardiopulmonary bypass. *J Thorac Cardiovasc Surg* 1982;83:239–248.

136. Schwartz AE, Sandhu AA, Kaplon RJ, et al. Cerebral blood flow is determined by arterial pressure and not cardiopulmonary bypass flow rate. *Ann Thorac Surg* 1995;60:165–169.

137. Swain JA, Anderson RV, Siegman MG. Low-flow cardiopulmonary bypass and cerebral protection: a summary of investigations. *Ann Thorac Surg* 1993;56:1490–1492.

138. Hindman BJ, Funatsu N, Harrington J, et al. Differences in cerebral blood flow between alpha-stat and pH-stat management are eliminated during periods of decreased systemic flow and pressure. A study during cardiopulmonary bypass in rabbits. *Anesthesiology* 1991;74:1096–1102.

139. Fox LS, Blackstone EH, Kirklin JW, et al. Relationship of brain blood flow and oxygen consumption to perfusion flow rate during profoundly hypothermic cardiopulmonary bypass. An experimental study. *J Thorac Cardiovasc Surg* 1984;87:658–664.

140. Michler RE, Sandhu AA, Young WL, et al. Low-flow cardiopulmonary bypass: importance of blood pressure in maintaining cerebral blood flow. *Ann Thorac Surg* 1995;60:S525–S528.

141. Schwartz AE, Kaplon RJ, Young WL, et al. Cerebral blood flow during low-flow hypothermic cardiopulmonary bypass in baboons. *Anesthesiology* 1994;81:959–964.

142. Cook DJ, Orszulak TA, Daly RC. The effects of pulsatile cardiopulmonary bypass on cerebral and renal blood flow in dogs. *J Cardiothorac Vasc Anesth* 1997;11:420–427.

143. Johnsson P, Messeter K, Ryding E, et al. Cerebral blood flow and autoregulation during hypothermic cardiopulmonary bypass. *Ann Thorac Surg* 1987;43:386–390.

144. Cook DJ, Proper JA, Orszulak TA, et al. Effect of pump flow rate on cerebral blood flow during hypothermic cardiopulmonary bypass in adults. *J Cardiothorac Vasc Anesth* 1997;11: 415–419.

145. Rogers AT, Prough DS, Roy RC, et al. Cerebrovascular and cerebral metabolic effects of alterations in perfusion flow rate during hypothermic cardiopulmonary bypass in man. *J Thorac Cardiovasc Surg* 1992;103:363–368.

146. Sanderson JM, Wright G, Sims FW. Brain damage in dogs immediately following pulsatile and non-pulsatile blood flows in extracorporeal circulation. *Thorax* 1972;27:275–286.

147. Tranmer BI, Gross CE, Kindt GW, et al. Pulsatile versus nonpulsatile blood flow in the treatment of acute cerebral ischemia. *Neurosurgery* 1986;19:724–731.

148. Anstadt MP, Tedder M, Hegde SS, et al. Pulsatile versus non-

149. Watanabe T, Orita H, Kobayashi M, et al. Brain tissue pH, oxygen tension, and carbon dioxide tension in profoundly hypothermic cardiopulmonary bypass. *J Thorac Cardiovasc Surg* 1989;97:396–401.

pulsatile reperfusion improves cerebral blood flow after cardiac arrest. *Ann Thorac Surg* 1993;56:453–461.

150. Hindman BJ, Dexter F, Smith T, et al. Pulsatile versus nonpulsatile flow. No difference in cerebral blood flow or metabolism during normothermic cardiopulmonary bypass in rabbits. *Anesthesiology* 1995;82:241–250.

151. Hindman BJ, Dexter F, Ryu KH, et al. Pulsatile versus nonpulsatile cardiopulmonary bypass. No difference in brain blood flow or metabolism at 27°C. *Anesthesiology* 1994;80: 1137–1147.

152. Prough DS, Rogers AT, Stump DA, et al. Cerebral blood flow decreases with time whereas cerebral oxygen consumption remains stable during hypothermic cardiopulmonary bypass in humans. *Anesth Analg* 1991;72:161–168.

153. Rogers AT, Stump DA, Gravlee GP, et al. Response of cerebral blood flow to phenylephrine infusion during hypothermic cardiopulmonary bypass: influence of $PaCO_2$ management. *Anesthesiology* 1988;69:547–551.

154. Hindman BJ, Dexter F, Cutkomp J, et al. Brain blood flow and metabolism do not decrease at stable brain temperature during cardiopulmonary bypass in rabbits. *Anesthesiology* 1992; 77:342–350.

155. Croughwell ND, Reves JG, White WD, et al. Cardiopulmonary bypass time does not affect cerebral blood flow. *Ann Thorac Surg* 1998;65:1226–1230.

156. Gilman S. Cerebral disorders after open-heart operations. *N Engl J Med* 1965;272:489–498.

157. Tufo HM, Ostfeld AM, Shekelle R. Central nervous system dysfunction following open-heart surgery. *JAMA* 1970;212: 1333–1340.

158. Stockard JJ, Bickford RG, Schauble JF. Pressure-dependent cerebral ischemia during cardiopulmonary bypass. *Neurology* 1973;23:521–529.

159. Shaw PJ, Bates D, Cartlidge NEF, et al. An analysis of factors predisposing to neurological injury in patients undergoing coronary bypass operations. *Q J Med* 1989;72:633–646.

160. Rorick MB, Furlan AJ. Risk of cardiac surgery in patients with prior stroke. *Neurology* 1990;40:835–837.

161. Savageau JA, Stanton BA, Jenkins CD, et al. Neuropsychological dysfunction following elective cardiac operation. I. Early assessment. *J Thorac Cardiovasc Surg* 1982;84:585–594.

162. Kolkka R, Hilberman M. Neurologic dysfunction following cardiac operation with low-flow, low-pressure cardiopulmonary bypass. *J Thorac Cardiovasc Surg* 1980;79:432–437.

163. Slogoff S, Reul GJ, Keats AS, et al. Role of perfusion pressure and flow in major organ dysfunction after cardiopulmonary bypass. *Ann Thorac Surg* 1990;50:911–918.

164. Bashien G, Townes BD, Nessly ML, et al. A randomized study of carbon dioxide management during hypothermic cardiopulmonary bypass. *Anesthesiology* 1990;72:7–15.

165. Gold JP, Charlson ME, Williams-Russo P, et al. Improvement of outcomes after coronary artery bypass. A randomized trial comparing intraoperative high versus low mean arterial pressure. *J Thorac Cardiovasc Surg* 1995;110:1302–1311.

166. Anonymous. Randomised trial of normothermic versus hypothermic coronary bypass surgery. The Warm Heart Investigators. *Lancet* 1994;343:559–563.

167. Martin TD, Craver JM, Gott JP, et al. Prospective, randomized trial of retrograde warm blood cardioplegia: myocardial benefit and neurologic threat. *Ann Thorac Surg* 1994;57:298–304.

168. Craver JM, Bufkin BL, Weintraub WS, et al. Neurologic events

after coronary bypass grafting: further observations with warm cardioplegia. *Ann Thorac Surg* 1995;59:1429–1434.

169. Guyton RA, Mellitt RJ, Weintraub WS. A critical assessment of neurological risk during warm heart surgery. *J Card Surg* 1995;10:488–492.

170. Baker AJ, Naser B, Benaroia M, et al. Cerebral microemboli during coronary artery bypass using different cardioplegia techniques. *Ann Thorac Surg* 1995;59:1187–1191.

171. Ikonomidis JS, Rao V, Weisel RD, et al. Myocardial protection for coronary bypass grafting: the Toronto Hospital perspective. *Ann Thorac Surg* 1995;60:824–832.

172. Clark RE, Brillman J, Davis DA, et al. Microemboli during coronary artery bypass grafting. Genesis and effect on outcome. *J Thorac Cardiovasc Surg* 1995;109:249–258.

173. Wong BI, McLean RF, Naylor CD, et al. Central-nervous-system dysfunction after warm or hypothermic cardiopulmonary bypass. *Lancet* 1992;339:1383–1384.

174. Plourde G, Leduc AS, Morin JE, et al. Temperature during cardiopulmonary bypass for coronary artery operations does not influence postoperative cognitive function: a prospective, randomized trial. *J Thorac Cardiovasc Surg* 1997;114:123–128.

175. Hvass U, Depoix JP. Clinical study of normothermic cardiopulmonary bypass in 100 patients with coronary artery disease. *Ann Thorac Surg* 1995;59:46–51.

176. Birdi I, Regragui I, Izzat MB, et al. Influence of normothermic systemic perfusion during coronary artery bypass operations: a randomized prospective study. *J Thorac Cardiovasc Surg* 1997;114:475–481.

177. Singh AK, Bert AA, Feng WC, et al. Stroke during coronary artery bypass grafting using hypothermic versus normothermic perfusion. *Ann Thorac Surg* 1995;59:84–89.

178. Regragui IA, Izzat MB, Birdi I, et al. Cardiopulmonary bypass perfusion temperature does not influence perioperative renal function. *Ann Thorac Surg* 1995;60:160–164.

179. Pulsinelli WA, Levy DE, Sigsbee B, et al. Increased damage after ischemic stroke in patients with hyperglycemia with or without established diabetes mellitus. *Am J Med* 1983;74:540–544.

180. Dietrich WD, Alonso O, Busto R. Moderate hyperglycemia worsens acute blood–brain barrier injury after forebrain ischemia in rats. *Stroke* 1993;24:111–116.

181. Chopp M, Welch KM, Tidwell CD, et al. Global cerebral ischemia and intracellular pH during hyperglycemia and hypoglycemia in cats. *Stroke* 1988;19:1383–1387.

182. Frasco P, Croughwell N, Blumenthal J, et al. Association between blood glucose level during cardiopulmonary bypass and neuropsychiatric outcome. *Anesthesiology* 1991;75:A55(abst).

183. Metz S, Keats AS. Benefits of a glucose-containing priming solution for cardiopulmonary bypass. *Anesth Analg* 1991;72:428–434.

184. Murkin JM, Martzke JS, Buchan AM, et al. A randomized study of the influence of perfusion technique and pH management strategy in 316 patients undergoing coronary artery bypass surgery. II. Neurologic and cognitive outcomes. *J Thorac Cardiovasc Surg* 1995;110:349–362.

185. Patel RL, Turtle MR, Chambers DJ, et al. Alpha-stat acid–base regulation during cardiopulmonary bypass improves neuropsychologic outcome in patients undergoing coronary artery bypass grafting. *J Thorac Cardiovasc Surg* 1996;111:1267–1279.

186. Henriksen L, Hjelms E, Lindeburgh T. Brain hyperperfusion during cardiac operations. Cerebral blood flow measured in man by intra-arterial injection of xenon 133: evidence suggestive of intraoperative microembolism. *J Thorac Cardiovasc Surg* 1983;86:202–208.

187. Plöchl W, Cook DJ. Quantification and distribution of cerebral

emboli during cardiopulmonary bypass in the swine: the impact of PaCO$_2$. *Anesthesiology* 1999;90:183–190.

188. Kern FH, Jonas RA, Mayer JE Jr, et al. Temperature monitoring during CPB in infants: does it predict efficient brain cooling? *Ann Thorac Surg* 1992;54:749–754.

189. Kern FH, Ungerleider RM, Schulman SR, et al. Comparing two strategies of cardiopulmonary bypass cooling on jugular venous oxygen saturation in neonates and infants. *Ann Thorac Surg* 1995;60:1198–2002.

190. Aoki M, Nomura F, Stromski ME, et al. Effects on pH on brain energetics after hypothermic circulatory arrest. *Ann Thorac Surg* 1993;55:1093–1103.

191. Kurth CD, O'Rourke MM, O'Hara IB, et al. Brain cooling efficiency with pH-stat and α-stat cardiopulmonary bypass in newborn pigs. *Circulation* 1997;96:II-358–II-363.

192. Hiramatsu T, Miura T, Forbess JM, et al. pH Strategies and cerebral energetics before and after circulatory arrest. *J Thorac Cardiovasc Surg* 1995;109:948–958.

193. Henze T, Stephan H, Sonntag H. Cerebral dysfunction following extracorporeal circulation for aortocoronary bypass surgery: no differences in neuropsychological outcome after pulsatile versus nonpulsatile flow. *Thorac Cardiovasc Surg* 1990;38:65–68.

194. Barzilai B, Marshall WG Jr, Saffitz JE, et al. Avoidance of embolic complications by ultrasonic characterization of the ascending aorta. *Circulation* 1989;80:I275–I279.

195. Akpinar B, Guden M, Sanisoglu I, et al. A no-touch technique for calcified ascending aorta during coronary artery surgery. *Tex Heart Inst J* 1998;25:120–123.

196. Mills NL, Everson CT. Atherosclerosis of the ascending aorta and coronary artery bypass. Pathology, clinical correlates, and operative management. *J Thorac Cardiovasc Surg* 1991;102:546–553.

197. Ribakove GH, Katz ES, Galloway AC, et al. Surgical implications of transesophageal echocardiography to grade the atheromatous aortic arch. *Ann Thorac Surg* 1992;53:758–761; discussion 762–763.

198. Buffolo E, de Andrade CS, Branco JN, et al. Coronary artery bypass grafting without cardiopulmonary bypass. *Ann Thorac Surg* 1996;61:63–66.

199. Riess FC, Schofer J, Kremer P, et al. Beating heart operations including hybrid revascularization: initial experiences. *Ann Thorac Surg* 1998;66:1076–1081.

200. Zenati M, Cohen HA, Holubkov R, et al. Preoperative risk models for minimally invasive coronary bypass: a preliminary study. *J Thorac Cardiovasc Surg* 1998;116:584–589.

201. Oka Y, Inoue T, Hong Y, et al. Retained intracardiac air. Transesophageal echocardiography for definition of incidence and monitoring removal by improved techniques. *J Thorac Cardiovasc Surg* 1986;91:329–338.

202. Hartman GS, Yao FS, Bruefach M III, et al. Severity of aortic atheromatous disease diagnosed by transesophageal echocardiography predicts stroke and other outcomes associated with coronary artery surgery: a prospective study. *Anesth Analg* 1996;83:701–708.

203. Blauth CI, Smith PL, Arnold JV, et al. Influence of oxygenator type on the prevalence and extent of microembolic retinal ischemia during cardiopulmonary bypass. Assessment by digital image analysis. *J Thorac Cardiovasc Surg* 1990;99:61–69.

204. Pugsley WB, Klinger L, Paschalis C, et al. Does arterial line filtration affect the bypass-related cerebral impairment in patients undergoing coronary artery surgery. *Clin Sci* 1988;76:30–31.

205. Cecconi O, Nelson RM, Roberts WG, et al. Inositol polyanions. Noncarbohydrate inhibitors of L- and P-selectin that block inflammation. *J Biol Chem* 1994;269:15060–15066.

206. Michenfelder JD, Milde JH, Sundt TM Jr. Cerebral protection

by barbiturate anesthesia. Use after middle cerebral artery occlusion in Java monkeys. *Arch Neurol* 1976;33:345–350.

207. Smith AL, Hoff JT, Nielsen SL, et al. Barbiturate protection in acute focal cerebral ischemia. *Stroke* 1974;5:1–7.

208. Nussmeier NA, Arlund C, Slogoff S. Neuropsychiatric complications after cardiopulmonary bypass: cerebral protection by a barbiturate. *Anesthesiology* 1986;64:165–170.

209. Michenfelder JD. A valid demonstration of barbiturate-induced brain protection in man—at last. *Anesthesiology* 1986;64:140–142.

210. Metz S, Slogoff S. Thiopental sodium by single bolus dose compared to infusion for cerebral protection during cardiopulmonary bypass. *J Clin Anesth* 1990;2:226–231.

211. Prough DS, Mills SA. Should thiopental sodium administration be a standard of care for open cardiac procedures? *J Clin Anesth* 1990;2:221–225.

212. Zaidan JR, Klochany A, Martin WM, et al. Effect of thiopental on neurologic outcome following coronary artery bypass grafting. *Anesthesiology* 1991;74:406–411.

213. Todd MM, Hindman BJ, Warner DS. Barbiturate protection and cardiac surgery: a different result. *Anesthesiology* 1991;74:402–405.

214. Warren BA, Philp RB, Inwood MJ. The ultrastructural morphology of air embolism: platelet adhesion to the interface and endothelial damage. *Br J Exp Pathol* 1973;54:163–172.

215. Johnston WE, Stump DA, DeWitt DS, et al. Significance of gaseous microemboli in the cerebral circulation during cardiopulmonary bypass in dogs. *Circulation* 1993;88:319–329.

216. Hindman BJ, Dexter F, Enomoto S, et al. Recovery of evoked potential amplitude after cerebral arterial air embolism in the rabbit. A comparison of the effect of cardiopulmonary bypass with normal circulation. *Anesthesiology* 1998;88:696–707.

217. Helps SC, Parsons DW, Reilly PL, et al. The effect of gas emboli on rabbit cerebral blood flow. *Stroke* 1990;21:94–99.

218. Newman MF, Murkin JM, Roach G, et al. Cerebral physiologic effects of burst suppression doses of propofol during nonpulsatile cardiopulmonary bypass. CNS Subgroup of McSPI. *Anesth Analg* 1995;81:452–457.

219. Ederberg S, Westerlind A, Houltz E, et al. The effects of propofol on cerebral blood flow velocity and cerebral oxygen extraction during cardiopulmonary bypass. *Anesth Analg* 1998;86:1201–1206.

220. Souter MJ, Andrews PJ, Alston RP. Propofol does not ameliorate cerebral venous oxyhemoglobin desaturation during hypothermic cardiopulmonary bypass. *Anesth Analg* 1998;86:926–931.

221. Bielenberg GW, Burniol M, Rosen R, et al. Effects of nimodipine on infarct size and cerebral acidosis after middle cerebral artery occlusion in the rat. *Stroke* 1990;21:IV90–IV92.

222. Hara H, Nagasawa H, Kogure K. Nimodipine prevents postischemic brain damage in the early phase of focal cerebral ischemia. *Stroke* 1990;21:IV102–IV104.

223. Gelmers HJ, Hennerici M. Effect of nimodipine on acute ischemic stroke. Pooled results from five randomized trials. *Stroke* 1990;21:IV81–IV84.

224. Forsman M, Olsnes BT, Semb G, et al. Effects of nimodipine on cerebral blood flow and neuropsychological outcome after cardiac surgery. *Br J Anaesth* 1990;65:514–520.

225. Legault C, Furberg CD, Wagenknecht LE, et al. Nimodipine neuroprotection in cardiac valve replacement: report of an early terminated trial. *Stroke* 1996;27:593–598.

226. Hall ED. Inhibition of lipid peroxidation in central nervous system trauma and ischemia. *J Neurol Sci* 1995;134:79–83.

227. Baumgartner WA, Redmond M, Brock M, et al. Pathophysiology of cerebral injury and future management. *J Card Surg* 1997;12:300–310; discussion 310–311.

228. Tseng EE, Brock MV, Lange MS, et al. Neuronal nitric oxide synthase inhibition reduces neuronal apoptosis after hypothermic circulatory arrest. *Ann Thorac Surg* 1997;64:1639–1647.

229. Tsui SS, Kirshbom PM, Davies MJ, et al. Nitric oxide production affects cerebral perfusion and metabolism after deep hypothermic circulatory arrest. *Ann Thorac Surg* 1996;61:1699–1707.

230. Engelman DT, Watanabe M, Maulik N, et al. L-Arginine reduces endothelial inflammation and myocardial stunning during ischemia/reperfusion. *Ann Thorac Surg* 1995;60:1275–1281.

231. Becker KJ. Inflammation and acute stroke. *Curr Opin Neurol* 1998;11:45–49.

232. Pantoni L, Sarti C, Inzitari D. Cytokines and cell adhesion molecules in cerebral ischemia: experimental bases and therapeutic perspectives. *Arterioscler Thromb Vasc Biol* 1998;18:503–513.

233. Gillinov AM, Redmond JM, Zehr KJ et al. Inhibition of neutrophil adhesion during cardiopulmonary bypass. *Ann Thorac Surg* 1994;57:126–133.

234. Chopp M, Zhang ZG. Anti-adhesion molecule and nitric oxide protection strategies in ischemic stroke. *Curr Opin Neurol* 1996;9:68–72.

235. Chopp M, Li Y, Jiang N, et al. Antibodies against adhesion molecules reduce apoptosis after transient middle cerebral artery occlusion in rat brain. *J Cereb Blood Flow Metab* 1996;16:578–584.

236. Murohara T, Buerke M, Lefer AM. Polymorphonuclear leukocyte-induced vasocontraction and endothelial dysfunction. Role of selectins. *Arterioscler Thromb* 1994;14:1509–1519.

237. Morikawa E, Zhang SM, Seko Y, et al. Treatment of focal cerebral ischemia with synthetic oligopeptide corresponding to lectin domain of selectin. *Stroke* 1996;27:951–955; discussion 956.

238. Buerke M, Weyrich AS, Zheng Z, et al. Sialyl Lewis^x-containing oligosaccharide attenuates myocardial reperfusion injury in cats. *J Clin Invest* 1994;93:1140–1148.

239. Turunen JP, Majuri ML, Seppo A, et al. *De novo* expression of endothelial sialyl Lewis(a) and sialyl Lewis(x) during cardiac transplant rejection: superior capacity of a tetravalent sialyl Lewis(x) oligosaccharide in inhibiting L-select–independent lymphocyte adhesion. *J Exp Med* 1995;182:1133–1141.

240. Mulligan MS, Lowe JB, Larsen RD, et al. Protective effects of sialylated oligosaccharides in immune complex-induced acute lung injury. *J Exp Med* 1993;178:623–631.

241. Nelson RM, Cecconi O, Roberts WG, et al. Heparin oligosaccharides bind L- and P-selectin and inhibit acute inflammation. *Blood* 1993;82:3253–3258.

242. Ishai-Michaeli R, Svahn CM, Weber M, et al. Importance of size and sulfation of heparin in release of basic fibroblast growth factor from the vascular endothelium and extracellular matrix. *Biochemistry* 1992;31:2080–2088.

243. Sternbergh WC III, Sobel M, Makhoul RG. Heparinoids with low anticoagulant potency attenuate postischemic endothelial cell dysfunction. *J Vasc Surg* 1995;21:477–483.

244. Ishihara M, Tyrrell DJ, Stauber GB, et al. Preparation of affinity-fractionated, heparin-derived oligosaccharides and their effects on selected biological activities mediated by basic fibroblast growth factor. *J Biol Chem* 1993;268:4675–4683.

245. Ryu KH, Hindman BJ, Reasoner DK, et al. Heparin reduces neurological impairment after cerebral arterial air embolism in the rabbit. *Stroke* 1996;27:303–309; discussion 310.

246. Minamisawa H, Smith ML, Siesjo BK. The effect of mild hyperthermia and hypothermia on brain damage following 5, 10, and 15 minutes of forebrain ischemia. *Ann Neurol* 1990;28:26–33.

247. Busto R, Dietrich WD, Globus MY, et al. Small differences in

intraischemic brain temperature critically determine the extent of ischemic neuronal injury. *J Cereb Blood Flow Metab* 1987; 7:729–738.

248. Ginsberg MD, Sternau LL, Globus MY, et al. Therapeutic modulation of brain temperature: relevance to ischemic brain injury. *Cerebrovasc Brain Metab Rev* 1992;4:189–225.

249. Morikawa E, Ginsberg MD, Dietrich WD, et al. The significance of brain temperature in focal cerebral ischemia: histopathological consequences of middle cerebral artery occlusion in the rat. *J Cereb Blood Flow Metab* 1992;12:380–389.

250. Minamisawa H, Nordstrom CH, Smith ML, et al. The influence of mild body and brain hypothermia on ischemic brain damage. *J Cereb Blood Flow Metab* 1990;10:365–374.

251. Conroy BP, Lin CY, Jenkins LW, et al. Hypothermic modulation of cerebral ischemic injury during cardiopulmonary bypass in pigs. *Anesthesiology* 1998;88:390–402.

252. Ginsberg MD, Busto R. Combating hyperthermia in acute stroke. A significant clinical concern. *Stroke* 1998;29:529–534.

253. Cook DJ, Orszulak TA, Daly RC, et al. Cerebral hyperthermia during cardiopulmonary bypass in adults. *J Thorac Cardiovasc Surg* 1996;111:268–269.

254. Cook DJ. Changing temperature management for cardiopulmonary bypass [Review Article]. *Anesth Analg* 1999;88: 1254–1271.

255. Sungurtekin H, Plöchl W, Cook DJ. Relationship between CPB flow rate and cerebral embolization. *Anesthesiology* 1999;91: 1387–1393.

256. Clauss RH, Hass WK, Ransohoff J. Simplified method for monitoring adequacy of brain oxygenation during carotid artery surgery. *N Engl J Med* 1965;273:1127–1131.

257. Meyer JS, Gotoh F, Ebihara S, et al. Effects of anoxia on cerebral metabolism and electrolytes in man. *Neurology* 1965;15: 892–901.

258. Croughwell ND, Frasco P, Blumenthal JA, et al. Warming during cardiopulmonary bypass is associated with jugular bulb desaturation. *Ann Thorac Surg* 1992;53:827–832.

259. Nakajima T, Kuro M, Hayashi Y, et al. Clinical evaluation of cerebral oxygen balance during cardiopulmonary bypass: on-line continuous monitoring of jugular venous oxyhemoglobin saturation. *Anesth Analg* 1992;74:630–635.

260. Cook DJ, Oliver WC Jr, Orszulak TA, et al. A prospective, randomized comparison of cerebral venous oxygen saturation during normothermic and hypothermic cardiopulmonary bypass. *J Thorac Cardiovasc Surg* 1994;107:1020–1029.

261. Croughwell ND, Newman MF, Blumenthal JA, et al. Jugular bulb saturation and cognitive dysfunction after cardiopulmonary bypass. *Ann Thorac Surg* 1994;58:1702–1708.

262. Enomoto S, Hindman BJ, Dexter F, et al. Rapid rewarming causes an increase in the cerebral metabolic rate for oxygen that is temporarily unmatched by cerebral blood flow. A study during cardiopulmonary bypass in rabbits. *Anesthesiology* 1996;84: 1392–1400.

263. Sapire KJ, Gopinath SP, Farhat G, et al. Cerebral oxygenation during warming after cardiopulmonary bypass. *Crit Care Med* 1997;25:1655–1662.

264. Grubhofer G, Lassnigg AM, Schneider B, et al. Jugular venous bulb oxygen saturation depends on blood pressure during cardiopulmonary bypass. *Ann Thorac Surg* 1998;65:653–657; discussion 658.

265. von Knobelsdorff G, Tonner PH, Hanel F, et al. Prolonged rewarming after hypothermic cardiopulmonary bypass does not attenuate reduction of jugular bulb oxygen saturation. *J Cardiothorac Vasc Anesth* 1997;11:689–693.

266. Dexter F, Hindman BJ. Theoretical analysis of cerebral venous blood hemoglobin oxygen saturation as an index of cerebral oxygenation during hypothermic cardiopulmonary bypass. A

counterproposal to the "luxury perfusion" hypothesis. *Anesthesiology* 1995;83:405–412.

267. Brown R, Wright G, Royston D. A comparison of two systems for assessing cerebral venous oxyhaemoglobin saturation during cardiopulmonary bypass in humans. *Anaesthesia* 1993;48: 697–700.

268. McCormick PW, Stewart M, Goetting MG, et al. Regional cerebrovascular oxygen saturation measured by optical spectroscopy in humans. *Stroke* 1991;22:596–602.

269. Nollert G, Mohnle P, Tassani-Prell P, et al. Determinants of cerebral oxygenation during cardiac surgery. *Circulation* 1995; 92:II-327–II-333.

270. Daubeney PE, Pilkington SN, Janke E, et al. Cerebral oxygenation measured by near-infrared spectroscopy: comparison with jugular bulb oximetry. *Ann Thorac Surg* 1996;61:930–934.

271. Kurth CD, Steven JM, Nicolson SC, et al. Kinetics of cerebral deoxygenation during deep hypothermic circulatory arrest in neonates. *Anesthesiology* 1992;77:656–661.

272. Kurth CD, Steven JM, Nicolson SC. Cerebral oxygenation during pediatric cardiac surgery using deep hypothermic circulatory arrest. *Anesthesiology* 1995;82:74–82.

273. Daubeney PE, Smith DC, Pilkington SN, et al. Cerebral oxygenation during paediatric cardiac surgery: identification of vulnerable periods using near-infrared spectroscopy. *Eur J Cardiothorac Surg* 1998;13:370–377.

274. du Plesis AJ, Newburger J, Jonas RA, et al. Cerebral oxygen supply and utilization during infant cardiac surgery. *Ann Neurol* 1995;37:488–497.

275. Germon TJ, Kane NM, Manara AR, et al. Near-infrared spectroscopy in adults: effects of extracranial ischaemia and intracranial hypoxia on estimation of cerebral oxygenation. *Br J Anaesth* 1994;73:503–506.

276. Nollert G, Shin'oka T, Jonas RA. Near-infrared spectrophotometry of the brain in cardiovascular surgery. *Thorac Cardiovasc Surg* 1998;46:167–175.

277. Nomura F, Naruse H, duPlessis A, et al. Cerebral oxygenation measured by near-infrared spectroscopy during cardiopulmonary bypass and deep hypothermic circulatory arrest in piglets. *Pediatr Res* 1996;40:790–796.

278. Wardle SP, Yoxall CW, Weindling AM. Cerebral oxygenation during cardiopulmonary bypass. *Arch Dis Child* 1998;78: 26–32.

279. Spencer MP, Thomas GI, Moehring MA. Relation between middle cerebral artery blood flow velocity and stump pressure during carotid endarterectomy. *Stroke* 1992;23:1439–1445.

280. Bishop CC, Powell S, Rutt D, et al. Transcranial Doppler measurement of middle cerebral artery blood flow velocity: a validation study. *Stroke* 1986;17:913–915.

281. Kontos HA. Validity of cerebral arterial blood flow calculations from velocity measurements. *Stroke* 1989;20:1–3.

282. Weyland A, Stephan H, Kazmaier S, et al. Flow velocity measurements as an index of cerebral blood flow. *Anesthesiology* 1994;81:1401–1410.

283. Nuttall GA, Cook DJ, Fulgham JR, et al. The relationship between cerebral blood flow and transcranial Doppler blood flow velocity during hypothermic cardiopulmonary bypass in adults. *Anesth Analg* 1996;82:1146–1151.

284. Grocott HP, Amory DW, Lowry E, et al. Transcranial Doppler blood flow velocity versus ^{133}Xe clearance cerebral blood flow during mild hypothermic cardiopulmonary bypass. *J Clin Monit Comput* 1998;14:35–39.

285. Endoh H, Shimoji K. Changes in blood flow velocity in the middle cerebral artery during nonpulsatile hypothermic cardiopulmonary bypass. *Stroke* 1994;25:403–407.

286. Trivedi UH, Patel RL, Turtle MR, et al. Relative changes in cerebral blood flow during cardiac operations using xenon-133

clearance versus transcranial Doppler sonography. *Ann Thorac Surg* 1997;63:167–174.

287. Zimmerman AA, Burrows FA, Jonas RA, et al. The limits of detectable cerebral perfusion by transcranial Doppler sonography in neonates undergoing deep hypothermic low-flow cardiopulmonary bypass. *J Thorac Cardiovasc Surg* 1997;114: 594–600.

288. Jonassen AE, Quaegebeur JM, Young WL. Cerebral blood flow velocity in pediatric patients is reduced after cardiopulmonary bypass with profound hypothermia. *J Thorac Cardiovasc Surg* 1995;110:934–943.

289. Padayachee TS, Parsons S, Theobold R, et al. The detection of microemboli in the middle cerebral artery during cardiopulmonary bypass: a transcranial Doppler ultrasound investigation using membrane and bubble oxygenators. *Ann Thorac Surg* 1987;44:298–302.

290. Spencer MP. Detection of cerebral arterial emboli. In: Newell DW, Aaslid R, eds. *Transcranial Doppler.* New York: Raven Press, 1992;215–230.

291. Markus HS, Tegeler CH. Experimental aspects of high-intensity transient signals in the detection of emboli. *J Clin Ultrasound* 1995;23:81–87.

292. Ringelstein EB, Droste DW, Babikian VL, et al. Consensus on microembolus detection by TCD (International Consensus Group on Microembolus Detection). *Stroke* 1998;29:725–729.

293. Theye RA, Patrick RT, Kirklin JW. The electroencephalogram in patients undergoing open intracardiac operations with the aid of extracorporeal circulation. *J Thorac Surg* 1957;34:709–716.

294. Lundar T, Lindegaard KF, Froysaker T, et al. Cerebral perfusion during nonpulsatile cardiopulmonary bypass. *Ann Thorac Surg* 1985;40:144–150.

295. Levy WJ. Quantitative analysis of EEG changes during hypothermia. *Anesthesiology* 1984;60:291–297.

296. Arom KV, Cohen DE, Strobl FT. Effect of intraoperative intervention on neurological outcome based on electroencephalographic monitoring during cardiopulmonary bypass. *Ann Thorac Surg* 1989;48:476–483.

297. Edmonds HL Jr, Griffiths LK, van der Laken J, et al. Quantitative electroencephalographic monitoring during myocardial revascularization predicts postoperative disorientation and improves outcome. *J Thorac Cardiovasc Surg* 1992;103:555–563.

298. Levy WJ. Monitoring of the electroencephalogram during cardiopulmonary bypass. Know when to say when. *Anesthesiology* 1992;76:876–877.

299. Bashein G, Nessly ML, Bledsoe SW, et al. Electroencephalography during surgery with cardiopulmonary bypass and hypothermia. *Anesthesiology* 1992;76:878–891.

300. Stecker MM, Cheung AT, Patterson T, et al. Detection of stroke during cardiac operations with somatosensory evoked responses. *J Thorac Cardiovasc Surg* 1996;112:962–972.

301. Lopez JR. Intraoperative neurophysiological monitoring. *Int Anesthesiol Clin* 1996;34:33–54.

302. Wilson GJ, Rebeyka IM, Coles JG, et al. Loss of the somatosensory evoked response as an indicator of reversible cerebral ischemia during hypothermic, low-flow cardiopulmonary bypass. *Ann Thorac Surg* 1988;45:206–209.

303. Hickey C, Gugino LD, Aglio LS, et al. Intraoperative somatosensory evoked potential monitoring predicts peripheral nerve injury during cardiac surgery. *Anesthesiology* 1993;78:29–35.

304. Lam AM, Manninen PH, Contreras J, et al. Monitoring of somatosensory evoked responses during cardiopulmonary bypass—the influence of temperature. *Anesth Analg* 1986;65:S85.

305. Hett DA, Smith DC, Pilkington SN, et al. Effect of temperature and cardiopulmonary bypass on the auditory evoked response. *Br J Anaesth* 1995;75:293–296.

306. Yang LC, Jawan B, Chang KA, et al. Effects of temperature on somatosensory evoked potentials during open heart surgery. *Acta Anaesthesiol Scand* 1995;39:956–959.

307. Lam AM, Manninen PH, Ferguson GG, et al. Monitoring electrophysiologic function during carotid endarterectomy: a comparison of somatosensory evoked potentials and conventional electroencephalogram. *Anesthesiology* 1991;75:15–21.

308. Persson L, Hardemark HG, Gustafsson J, et al. S-100 protein and neuron-specific enolase in cerebrospinal fluid and serum: markers of cell damage in human central nervous system. *Stroke* 1987;18:911–918.

309. Johnsson P. Markers of cerebral ischemia after cardiac surgery. *J Cardiothorac Vasc Anesth* 1996;10:120–126.

310. Taggart DP, Bhattacharya K, Meston N, et al. Serum S-100 protein concentration after cardiac surgery: a randomized trial of arterial line filtration. *Eur J Cardiothorac Surg* 1997;11: 645–649.

311. Westaby S, Johnsson P, Parry AJ, et al. Serum S100 protein: a potential marker for cerebral events during cardiopulmonary bypass. *Ann Thorac Surg* 1996;61:88–92.

312. Gao F, Harris DNF, Sapsed-Byrne S. Time course of neurone-specific enolase and S-100 protein release during and after coronary artery bypass grafting. *Br J Anaesth* 1999;82:266–267.

313. Blomquist S, Johnsson P, Luhrs C, et al. The appearance of S-100 protein in serum during and immediately after cardiopulmonary bypass surgery: a possible marker for cerebral injury. *J Cardiothorac Vasc Anesth* 1997;11:699–703.

314. Jönsson H, Johnsson P, Alling C, et al. Significance of serum S100 release after coronary artery bypass grafting. *Ann Thorac Surg* 1998;65:1639–1644.

315. Grocott HP, Croughwell ND, Amory DW, et al. Cerebral emboli and serum S100-beta during cardiac operations. *Ann Thorac Surg* 1998;65:1645–1649; discussion 1649–1650.

316. Taggart DP, Mazel JW, Bhattacharya K, et al. Comparison of serum S-100 beta levels during CABG and intracardiac operations. *Ann Thorac Surg* 1997;63:492–496.

HEMATOLOGY

ANTICOAGULATION FOR CARDIOPULMONARY BYPASS

LINDA SHORE-LESSERSON
GLENN P. GRAVLEE

HISTORY

Numerous events led to the first performance of surgical procedures with cardiopulmonary bypass (CPB) in Philadelphia in 1953 (1). Development of an effective and reversible method to prevent blood clotting in an extracorporeal circuit impeded this development. Heparin was discovered accidentally in 1916 by an ambitious young medical student named Jay McLean, who had been assigned to experiment with cephalin, a thromboplastic substance. McLean investigated extracts of heart and liver to determine if the thromboplastic substance found in the brain extracts might be something other than cephalin. Using similar extraction procedures, he discovered an extract that retarded plasma coagulation from both the heart (named *cuorin*) and the liver (named *heparphosphatide* initially, then changed to *heparin*) (2,3). Although McLean had made an important scientific discovery at a young age, he subsequently selected a clinically oriented career that apparently precluded his participation in the development of heparin as a drug (4).

The purification of heparin proceeded in the 1920s, and a fairly crude preparation was first used to anticoagulate blood for transfusion in 1924. Febrile reactions curbed this application, and it took another 12 years to attain a heparin preparation that appeared safe for intravenous administration. During that interval, the discovery that heparin could be obtained from bovine lung less expensively than from bovine liver proved practical in the commercial development of heparin. Clinical trials in thrombotic disorders were initiated in 1935, and it was evident even then that heparin could prevent clot formation or extension, although it possessed minimal ability to dissolve existing clots. Chargaff and Olson (5) discovered in 1937 that the peptide prot-

amine dramatically neutralizes the anticoagulant effects of heparin. Gibbon (6) reported heparin-induced anticoagulation for CPB in animals in 1939. These events led to the selection of heparin for anticoagulation and protamine for its subsequent neutralization in the first human operation in which CPB was used, in 1953. Although most other aspects of CPB practice have changed markedly since that time, the use of heparin and protamine has continued for nearly 40 years. This longevity serves as a testimonial to the astute judgment of Gibbon and his colleagues at Jefferson Medical College. Consequently, this chapter primarily discusses the pharmacology and clinical use of heparin for this purpose. Strategies for monitoring the anticoagulant effects of heparin and of other heparin alternatives are also presented. The final portion of the chapter is devoted to discussion of heparin-induced thrombocytopenia (HIT) and HIT with thrombosis (HITT) syndromes.

HEPARIN PHARMACOLOGY

Structural Characteristics and Biologic Function

Heparin, more specifically described as a glycosaminoglycan, is a polysaccharide that resides almost exclusively in mast cells (7). Its physiologic purpose, however, remains uncertain. Clearly, endogenous heparin plays no significant role in maintaining the fluidity of circulating blood. Heparan, a related glycosaminoglycan having a substantially lower sulfur content, dangles tantalizingly from endothelial cell membranes to attract circulating antithrombin III (AT III) irresistibly and potentiate thrombin inhibition. Physiologic anticoagulation at the blood–tissue interface thus derives not from heparin but from heparan. The primary physiologic purpose of heparin may be to participate in nonimmunologic defense against bacterial infections, with other roles likely in capillary angiogenesis and lipid metabolism (8,9).

Most heparin preparations can be described as unfrac-

L. Shore-Lesserson: Department of Anesthesiology, Mount Sinai Medical Center, New York, New York 10029.

G. P. Gravlee: Department of Anesthesiology, Ohio State University Medical Center, Columbus, Ohio 43210.

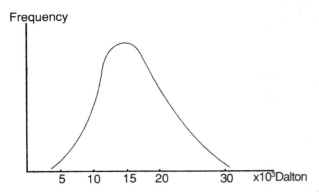

FIG. 22.1. Molecular weight distribution pattern of a typical commercial preparation of unfractionated heparin. (From Stiekema JCJ. Heparin and its biocompatibility. *Clin Nephrol* 1986; 26[Suppl 1]:S3–S8, with permission.)

tionated, which means that the heparin compound isolated from animal tissues contains heparin molecules of various lengths, with molecular weights ranging from 3,000 to more than 40,000 Da. The mean molecular mass approximates 15,000 Da (10,11) (Fig. 22.1). The molecular weight distribution varies somewhat with the tissue source, animal source, and method of purification (12,13). This variability has some clinical relevance because the spectrum of clinical actions of heparin derives in part from the molecular weight distribution of a heparin compound (14). As a result, each unfractionated commercial heparin preparation might best be described as a family of drugs with actions and potency that may vary from batch to batch (15–17).

Heparin can be distinguished from other polysaccharides by its acid nature. It is the strongest macromolecular acid in the body, a characteristic that derives from abundant sulfation of its saccharide units. The basic subunit consists of a repeating disaccharide that contains a uronic acid residue linked to a glucosamine residue (18) (Fig. 22.2). Both the uronic acid and glucosamine residues can assume many different forms based on the side groups attached to these hexose units. Sulfate groups may attach to the hexose ring via an oxygen, amino, aminoacetyl, or methane link. The result is a large molecule that bears a highly negative charge within the physiologic pH range, and that therefore attracts positively charged molecules. Specific saccharide sequences along the heparin chain determine binding sites to other macromolecules for which it has high affinity, such as AT III, thrombin, and lipoprotein lipase. In the case of AT III, a specific pentasaccharide sequence binds consistently to a specific amino acid sequence on the AT III molecule (18,19).

Tissue Source and Commercial Preparation

Heparin can be purified from several tissues and from several mammalian species. Although the name *heparin* was

selected because the substance was originally isolated from liver extracts, intestinal mucosa and lung tissue represent the most common commercial sources. Mucosal heparin tends to have a lower mean molecular weight, a more cross-linked polysaccharide structure, and a lower cost than lung heparin (15). Differences in the tissue source from which heparin is extracted influence molecular structure and activity more than differences in the animal source (20,21). However, nuclear magnetic resonance spectroscopy has enabled the identification of differences between porcine and bovine mucosal heparin in sulfation of various subunits. Nuclear magnetic resonance spectroscopy has also demonstrated a higher content of 3-*O*-sulfated glucosamine units (active site for AT III binding) in porcine than in bovine mucosal heparin (22). Heparin manufacturers most often extract mucosal heparin from pigs (porcine mucosal heparin) and lung heparin from cattle (bovine lung heparin).

Both porcine mucosal heparin and bovine lung heparin have been widely used as anticoagulants for CPB. Both provide effective anticoagulation and prevent thrombosis in experimental models (23,24) and in adult volunteers (25). Investigating standardized needle punctures in exposed carotid arteries in dogs, Abbott et al. (26) found a higher incidence of delayed hemorrhage in animals anticoagulated with mucosal heparin than with lung heparin. This difference remained significant even when the anticoagulation was neutralized with protamine. Two studies prospectively compared mucosal and lung heparin for CPB in humans. Stewart and Gaich (27) found that higher doses of mucosal heparin than of lung heparin were needed to reach the desired prolongation of the activated clotting time (ACT), a finding that might be attributable to batch variability. Fiser et al. (28) observed greater postoperative blood loss in patients randomly assigned to receive mucosal heparin than in those who received lung heparin. Both animal and human studies indicate that mucosal heparin can be neutralized with 25% to 30% less protamine than can lung heparin (21,29). These studies used standard tests of plasma coagulation such as clotting time and activated partial thromboplastin time (APTT), which might not detect residual unneutralized inhibition of factor Xa. Because of its lower mean molecular weight, mucosal heparin, in concert with AT III, more effectively inhibits factor Xa than does lung heparin (30), and protamine only partially neutralizes this effect. The higher mean molecular weight of lung heparin enables this molecule to inhibit factor IIa more effectively, via AT III. The anti-IIa activity is more susceptible to protamine antagonism, which may explain the greater propensity for delayed bleeding found after anticoagulation with mucosal heparin (25,27). Fairly limited prospective comparisons and some theoretical considerations thus suggest a slight advantage of lung heparin for CPB anticoagulation.

Because of the acid nature of heparin, a ligand must be bound to it when the compound is prepared for commercial use. Sodium and calcium have been used for this purpose.

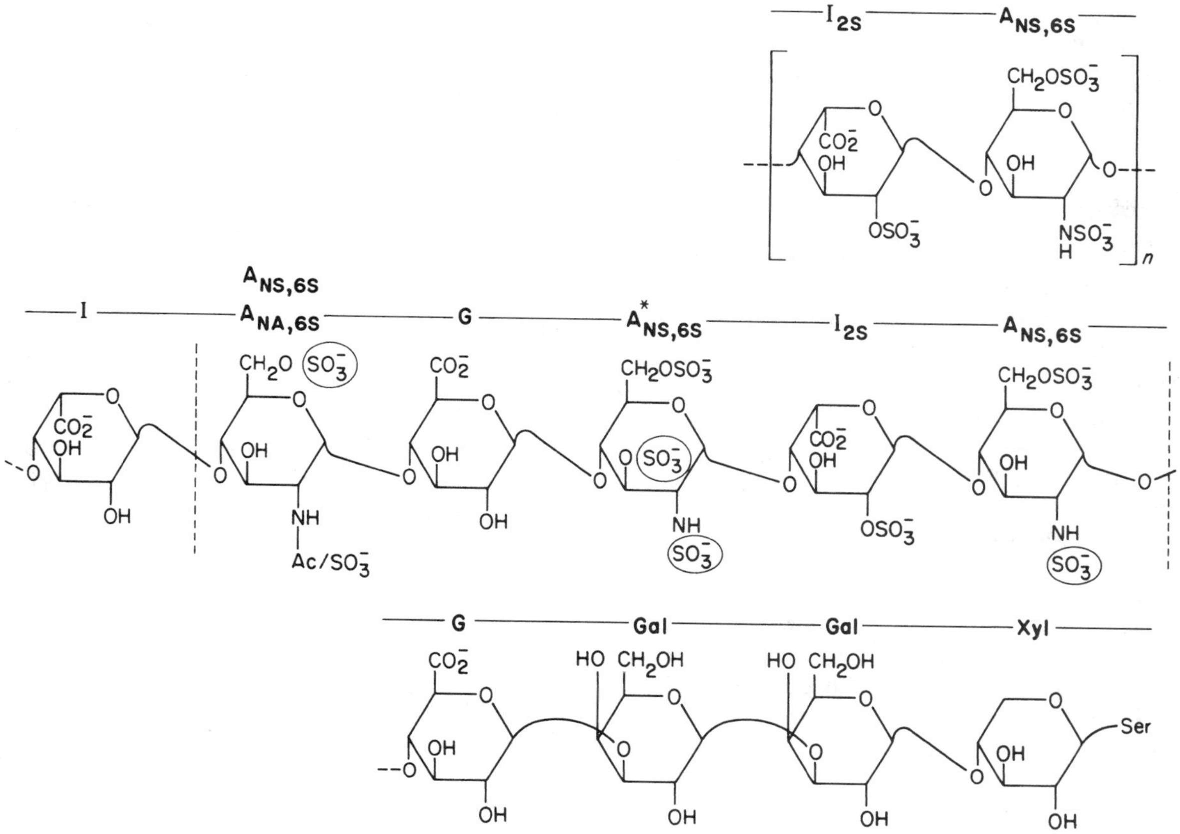

FIG. 22.2. Molecular structure of different parts of the heparin polysaccharide chain. The top row demonstrates a common repeating disaccharide subunit consisting of L-iduronic acid 2-sulfate (I_2^S) and N-sulfo-α-D-glucosamine 6-sulfate ($A_{NS,6S}$), which represents up to 90% of beef lung heparin and 70% of porcine mucosal heparin. In the middle row, the five saccharide units between the *vertical dotted lines* comprise the pentasaccharide sequence required for binding antithrombin III ($A_{NA,6S}$ substitutes an N-acetyl for the N-sulfo group on $A_{NS,6S}$, G represents β-D-glucuronic acid, and I represents β-L-iduronic acid). This sequence occurs in about 33% of the chains of mucosal heparin and about 20% of the chains of lung heparin. The *circled sulfate groups* are believed essential for high-affinity binding. The bottom row shows the typical terminal sequence of a heparin molecule (*Gal*, galactose; *Xyl*, xylose) linking to a serine amino acid residue. (From Casu B. Methods of structural analysis. In: Lane DA, Lindahl U, eds. *Heparin. Chemical and biological properties, clinical applications.* Boca Raton, FL: CRC Press, 1989:25–49, with permission.)

The two salts are indistinguishable with intravenous heparin administration, but the calcium salt retards the uptake of subcutaneously administered heparin (12,31) and may reduce local hematoma formation with subcutaneously administered heparin (32).

Potency Standardization

Four assays have been used in recent years to determine the potency of unfractionated heparin (23,33), including international, United States, British, and European standards. The International Standard represents the mean of the pharmacopoeial methods, which results in some variation in potency between international units (IU) and United States Pharmacopoiea (USP) units (32). The USP assay de-fines 1 USP unit as the amount of heparin that maintains the fluidity of 1 mL of citrated sheep plasma for 1 hour after recalcification. The British Pharmacopoiea (BP) method uses sulfated ox blood activated with thromboplastin. The BP method has been superseded by a European Pharmacopoiea (EP) method, which recalcifies sheep plasma in the presence of kaolin and cephalin incubated for 2 minutes, thus constituting an APTT for sheep plasma. The EP method rigorously standardizes the collection of sheep plasma, which might diminish the assay variability previously reported between batches of sheep plasma substrate (20). Although speculation exists about the clinical significance of batch-to-batch variability in heparin potency, it seems more likely that pharmacodynamic differences account for most of the observed variations in the clinical anticoagulation response to heparin (see Heparin Resistance). Because the relationship between mass (milligrams) and potency (units) varies among heparin preparations, it appears more sensible to record heparin doses in units than in milligrams.

Pharmacokinetics

Because heparin administration for CPB is exclusively intravenous, this discussion is limited to that route of administration. After central venous injection of a heparin bolus, the onset of maximal ACT prolongation in the radial artery occurs within 1 minute. Previous work (34) suggested that heparin action peaks 10 to 20 minutes after administration in cardiac surgical patients, but this finding probably was an artifact representing prolongation of the ACT by other factors, such as hemodilution and hypothermia. Controlling for these factors, another study clearly demonstrated that the onset of action of heparin is much faster, and maximal ACT prolongation probably occurs in less than 5 minutes (35). A rapid redistribution effect probably accounts for a modest reduction in the anticoagulant effect of heparin that occurs 3 to 13 minutes after the peak effect (Fig. 22.3). It remains possible that the onset of action would be slightly delayed in states of low cardiac output or with peripheral venous injection.

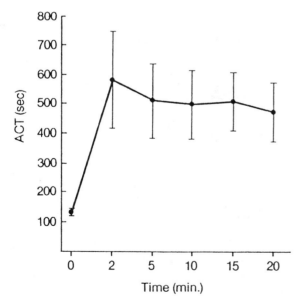

FIG. 22.3. The activated clotting time (*ACT*) measured via radial artery blood sampling at five different intervals after the injection of 300 U of heparin per kilogram into the right atrium. Maximum ACT prolongation occurred within 2 minutes in most patients, with subsequent moderate ACT reduction, likely reflecting a rapid redistribution effect. (From Gravlee GP, Angert KC, Tucker WY, et al. Early anticoagulation peak and rapid distribution after intravenous heparin. *Anesthesiology* 1988;68:126–129, with permission.)

Distribution

Heparin is macromolecular and highly polarized, so one would expect minimal distribution beyond the bloodstream. These principles and the results of bioassay studies of heparin kinetics were the basis for the former belief that the distribution of heparin is virtually confined to the plasma compartment of the bloodstream (36,37). Substantial *in vitro* evidence now points to the redistribution of heparin into the endothelial cells (38–41), although this redistribution appears small in comparison with that of most other drugs. Some uptake into extracellular fluid, alveolar macrophages, splenic and hepatic reticuloendothelial cells, and vascular smooth muscle may also occur (42–44). Some or all of these tissues create a relatively small reservoir for heparin that probably contributes to the delayed recurrence of heparin-induced anticoagulation (heparin rebound) after protamine neutralization of the heparin residing in the bloodstream. Defining an apparent volume of distribution for heparin remains elusive because pharmacokinetic studies in humans have used some measure of heparin effect (i.e., a bioassay) rather than direct measurement of plasma heparin concentration. Bioassays represent the most practical approach to the clinical evaluation of heparin pharmacodynamics, but these assays can only indirectly and crudely assess pharmacokinetics.

Elimination and Excretion

Heparin elimination has been studied by using various clotting times as bioassays, so the available information largely defines the time course of its clinical activity. The clotting times differ in their sensitivities to heparin, so differences reported in heparin "elimination" kinetics under similar conditions are not necessarily inconsistent. Despite these unavoidable limitations, several aspects of heparin pharmacokinetics can be explained by existing studies. Very small doses of heparin produce minimal or no effect, suggesting a rapid initial clearance, possibly the result of the affinity of heparin for endothelial membranes (45,46). The doses used for CPB anticoagulation are very large, and the biologic elimination half-life of heparin is dose-dependent (47,48). In the only volunteer study in which doses sufficient for CPB were used, Olsson et al. (47) found a half-life of 126 ± 24 minutes with a heparin dose of 400 U/kg. The half-lives for doses one-fourth and one-half that large were 61 ± 9 and 93 ± 6 minutes, respectively. Because CPB distorts the bioassay methods via hypothermia and hemodilution, attempts to define heparin pharmacokinetics in patients undergoing CPB are largely impractical. Hypothermia delays heparin elimination, with virtually constant heparin concentrations shown during 40 to 100 minutes of CPB at 25°C (49). Wright et al. (50) found a progressive decline in heparin concentrations at all temperatures, but the rate of decline was delayed in proportion to

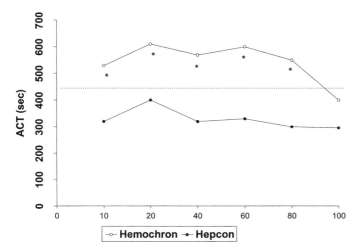

FIG. 22.4. The Hemochron and HemoTec (Hepcon) activated clotting time (*ACT*) values in 22 pediatric patients at six time points during cardiopulmonary bypass. Hemochron ACT was significantly higher than HemoTec ACT at five time points, and HemoTec ACT was below the threshold value of 400 seconds at all time points. *$p < 0.01$. (Modified from Horkay F, Martin P, Rajah M, et al. Response to heparinization in adults and children undergoing cardiac operations. *Ann Thorac Surg* 1992;53: 822–826, with permission.)

the hypothermia. Bull et al. (51) found a small decrease in the rate of ACT decline at 30°C (in comparison with normothermia), although the independent prolongation of ACT by hypothermia had not been discovered at the time of that study. Mabry et al. (52) found the consumption of heparin to vary from 0.01 to 3.86 U/kg per minute during CPB. In addition, there is little correlation between the initial ACT-based sensitivity to heparin and the rate of heparin decay (53). In children, the variability in ACT response is greater than that in adults and is highly dependent on the test mechanism and activators used (54) (Fig. 22.4).

Severe renal impairment may also prolong heparin action, although available studies yield conflicting results. Liver disease apparently has little effect on heparin elimination (45). The primary mechanism for heparin elimination remains uncertain, but metabolism in the reticuloendothelial system and renal elimination both occur (42,44,46).

Pharmacodynamics

Inhibition of Fibrin Formation

Heparin induces anticoagulation primarily by potentiating the activity of AT III, a plasma glycoprotein with a molecular weight of 58,000 Da. Heparin attaches to a lysine residue on AT III, thereby altering the AT III configuration and rendering it much more attractive to thrombin (19,55). Heparin thus increases the thrombin-inhibitory potency of circulating AT III by a factor of 1,000 or more. In addition to converting fibrinogen to fibrin enzymatically, thrombin

activates cofactors VIII and V, thus greatly increasing the rate of fibrin clot formation via the intrinsic and common pathways, respectively. Figure 22.5 shows the plasma coagulation cascade, which can be somewhat crudely divided into intrinsic, extrinsic, and common pathways. AT III also inhibits factors IXa, Xa, XIa, and XIIa (56,57), kallikrein, and plasmin. Plasma coagulation factors vary in their sensitivity to AT III and to different chain lengths of heparin. Unfractionated heparin inhibits thrombin most quickly, then inactivates Xa, IXa, XIa, and XIIa with progressively decreasing rate constants (57). Thrombin inhibition involves transient simultaneous heparin binding to AT III and to thrombin, which requires a relatively long oligosaccharide chain. This is the reason why shorter heparin chains are relatively ineffective in thrombin inhibition, even if they contain the pentasaccharide sequence required for AT III binding (58) (Fig. 22.6). Factor Xa inhibition involves heparin binding to AT III, which in turn binds to factor Xa molecules that need not bind separately to heparin, as depicted in Fig. 22.6. Two-thirds or more of the heparin molecules present in commercially available preparations have no anticoagulant effect (14), which probably results from an absence of the specific pentasaccharide sequence that binds to AT III.

Heparin also binds to cofactor II, a glycoprotein of 65,000 Da that inactivates thrombin independently of AT III (59). This reaction occurs more slowly and requires higher heparin concentrations than does thrombin inhibition via the heparin–AT III complex. The thrombin–heparin–cofactor II interaction is significantly catalyzed *in vitro* by plasma heparin concentrations between 0.1 and 0.4 U/mL, which is well below the heparin concentrations used for CPB. This mechanism might therefore contribute routinely to the anticoagulant effect of heparin during CPB, and might assume particular importance in patients with AT III deficiency.

Variability of Patient Response

Whether heparin concentration or a clotting time is measured, the response to a fixed-dose heparin bolus varies substantially from patient to patient (34,51,60–67). The variability of clotting time responses usually exceeds the variability of blood or plasma heparin concentrations observed, as demonstrated by Monkhouse et al. (61) as early as 1953 (62,63,68). Bull et al. (51,69) showed a threefold variation in ACT response to a heparin bolus of 200 U/kg, and Esposito et al. (62) found a fourfold ACT range (62 to 267 seconds) at that dose and a sixfold range (128 to 755 seconds) after an intravenous bolus of 400 U/kg. Bull et al. (51,69) reported equally impressive ranges of heparin elimination rates during CPB when using ACT as an indirect heparin assay.

Side Effects

Plasma coagulation, the formation of a platelet plug, and fibrinolysis constitute the three major components of blood

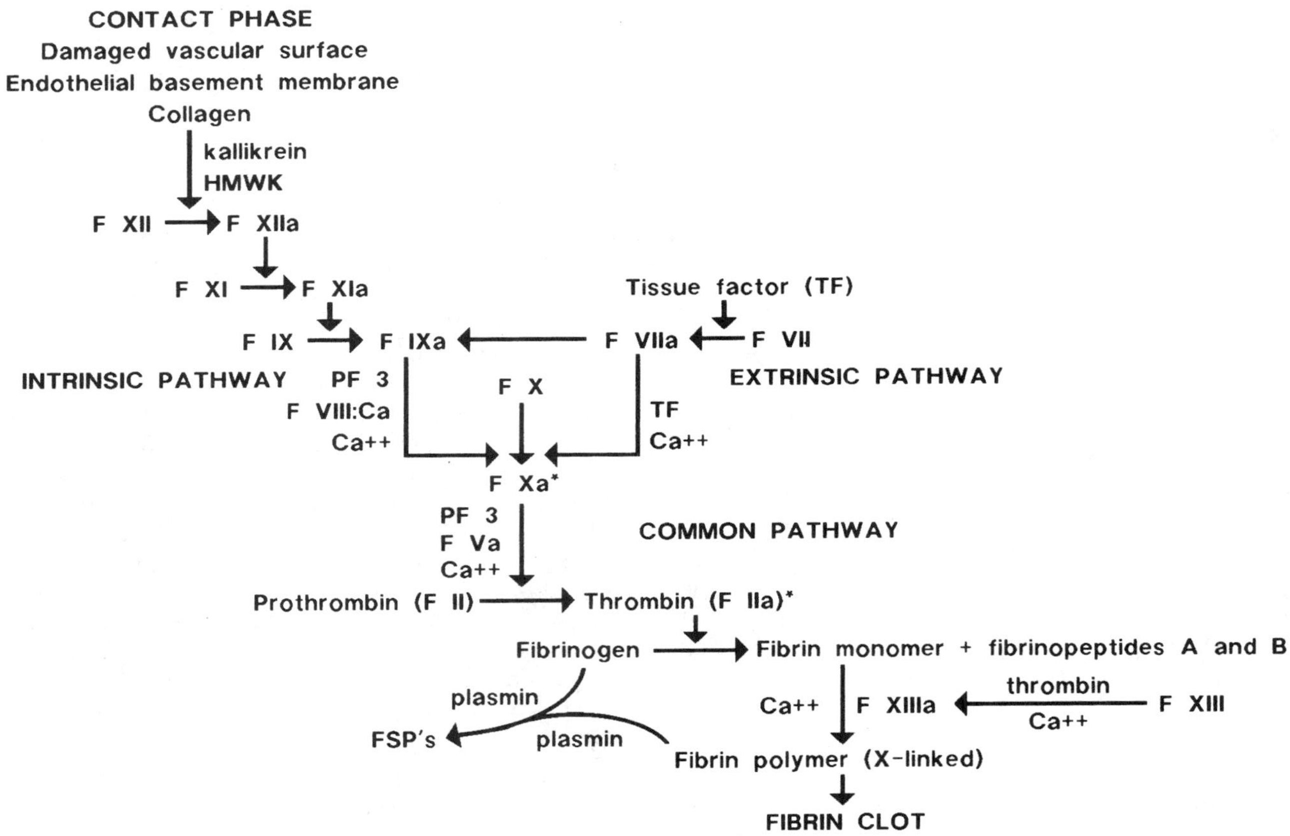

CONTACT PHASE
Damaged vascular surface
Endothelial basement membrane
Collagen

kallikrein
HMWK

F XII ➝ F XIIa

F XI ➝ F XIa   Tissue factor (TF)

F IX ➝ F IXa ⟵   F VIIa ⟵ F VII

INTRINSIC PATHWAY   PF 3   **EXTRINSIC PATHWAY**
                        F VIII:Ca   F X   TF
                        Ca++   Ca++

                                F Xa*

PF 3   **COMMON PATHWAY**
F Va
Ca++

Prothrombin (F II) ➝ Thrombin (F IIa)*

                        Fibrinogen ➝ Fibrin monomer + fibrinopeptides A and B

            plasmin   thrombin
                            Ca++ | F XIIIa ⟵ F XIII
        FSP's ⟵ plasmin   Ca++
                        Fibrin polymer (X-linked)

                                FIBRIN CLOT

FIG. 22.5. Schematic diagram of the plasma coagulation pathway, divided into intrinsic, extrinsic, and common component pathways. *F*, factor; *roman numerals*, different coagulation factors by number; *a*, activated coagulation factor; *Ca⁺⁺*, ionized calcium; *HMWK*, high-molecular-weight kininogen; *PF3*, platelet factor 3.

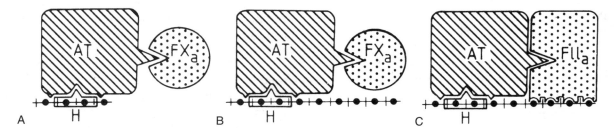

FIG. 22.6. Schematic representation of the interaction between heparin (*H*) and activated factors X (*FX*ₐ) and II (thrombin, *FII*ₐ). Inhibition of factor IIa requires a heparin chain containing at least 18 saccharide units (shown in B and C) in addition to the critical pentasaccharide sequence for antithrombin III (*AT III*) binding (shown as the framed portion of H bound to AT). This occurs because the heparin molecule must simultaneously bind AT III and thrombin. Factor Xa inhibition is also accomplished with polysaccharide chains long enough to inhibit factor IIa (shown in B), but shorter chains can also inhibit factor Xa (shown in A with an octasaccharide chain) because simultaneous binding of heparin, AT III, and factor Xa is not required for Xa inhibition. (From Holmer E. Low molecular weight heparin. In: Lane DA, Lindahl U, eds. *Heparin. Chemical and biological properties, clinical applications.* Boca Raton, FL: CRC Press, 1989:575–595, with permission.)

TABLE 22.1. ACUTE EFFECTS OF HEPARIN ON PLATELETS

Action
Serotonin release (330)
Increased adenosine diphosphate-induced aggregation (331–333)
Decreased thrombin-induced aggregation (334)
Opposes prostacyclin-mediated platelet inhibition (335,336)
Increased collagen-induced aggregation (333)
Dose-dependent increase in bleeding time (337,338)
Increased platelet factor 4 release (333)
Increased epinephrine-induced platelet aggregation (331)
Decreased platelet count (339)
P-selectin expression (79)
Suppresses α-granule release (high-dose heparin only) (80)

clot formation and dissolution. The therapeutic effects of heparin derive primarily its effects on plasma coagulation, described above, but heparin also affects the other two components.

Heparin-induced activation of fibrinolysis has been identified in a primate model (70). During simulated CPB in a baboon model, heparin administration led to activation of fibrinolysis as measured by plasmin activity, immunoreactive plasmin light chain, and immunoreactive fibrinogen fragment E (71). The mechanism whereby heparin facilitates fibrinolysis may involve the direct stimulation of plasminogen activator release from endothelial cells and monocytes. Additional modes of activation include indirect stimulation of plasminogen activator by release of protein C, inhibition of fibrin polymerization (72), modulation of antiplasmin effects, and enhancement of the effects of tissue factor pathway inhibitor (TFPI). Activation of the fibrinolytic pathway does occur during anticoagulation associated with CPB, so heparin might participate in this activation.

Heparin also has numerous effects on platelets, many of which occur acutely, and these would therefore be relevant in patients undergoing CPB. Table 22.1 lists the aggregatory effects of heparin on platelets, which most often represent laboratory findings obtained in human platelet-rich plasma. The clinical significance of these findings is uncertain, but clearly heparin binds avidly to platelets. With the use of specific chemical and enzymatic treatments to produce heparin-derived glycosaminoglycans, the platelet-binding properties of heparin have been elucidated (73). Although specific receptors for heparin on the platelet surface have not been identified, heparin binding relates directly to molecular weight and sulfation and is unrelated to AT III affinity (74–77). Heparin binding decreases with the decreasing size of the heparin fragment and is therefore clinically negligible in the low-molecular-weight heparin (LMWH) preparations. Small quantities of heparin may bind to the glycopro-

tein (GP)IIb/IIIa platelet receptor, but this is not the major locus for heparin binding. At clinical doses, heparin induces a platelet release reaction characterized by release of platelet factor 4 (PF4), GPIIb/IIIa activation, P-selectin expression, and increased aggregation that is not seen with LMWH derivatives (78,79). At plasma levels as high as 100 U/mL, heparin suppresses degranulation and P-selectin expression, a finding that indicates the future possibility of separation of the anticoagulant and the antiplatelet properties of heparin (80,81). Moderate prolongation of bleeding time and transient decreases in platelet count have been present in some investigations and absent in others (76). Both predictable and idiosyncratic effects of heparin on platelets have been reviewed by Warkentin and Kelton (76). The idiosyncratic syndrome of HIT is discussed later in a separate section (see Heparin-induced Thrombocytopenia).

In clinical settings other than CPB, bleeding complications comprise the most common side effect of heparin, with reported incidences varying from 1% to 37% (82–85). The profound anticoagulation present during CPB probably increases surgical bleeding, but blood salvage via the cardiotomy suction usually renders this unimportant. Large doses of heparin induce fibrinolysis and activate platelet activation to contribute to abnormalities of hemostasis (86). Conversely, insufficient heparin anticoagulation during CPB causes consumption of coagulation factors, which may also result in a bleeding diathesis (87). Excessive postoperative bleeding from residual unneutralized heparin or from heparin rebound can occur after CPB and should be closely monitored (see Chap. 25).

The intravenous heparin bolus dose administered before CPB decreases arterial pressure and systemic vascular resistance approximately 10% to 20% without affecting cardiac output or heart rate (88,89). Urban et al. (89) related this change to a decrease in ionized calcium levels, and they were able to prevent them by prophylactically administering 125 mg of calcium chloride.

Heparin can induce a variety of metabolic and immunologic effects (90) that might contribute to the array of abnormalities known to occur in those systems during CPB. Heparin dramatically increases plasma levels of lipoprotein lipase by releasing this enzyme from vascular endothelium. This activity bears no relation to AT III affinity, and it results in triglyceride degradation and increased circulating levels of free fatty acids (9). Although the clinical significance of these effects remains unclear, they could potentially affect myocardial metabolism and the plasma free fraction of lipid-soluble drugs.

Rare acute reactions attributed to heparin include anaphylaxis, pulmonary edema (91–97), and disseminated intravascular coagulation (98). Some of these reactions have been traced to the preservatives chlorocresol and chlorbutol (93,94). Harada et al. (91) reported the uneventful use of bovine lung heparin for CPB in a child who had previously experienced anaphylaxis from porcine mucosal heparin, and Schey (99) reported resolution of a localized skin reaction to subcutaneous heparin injections when LMWH was substituted for unfractionated heparin. Interactions with antibiotics have also been reported, notably with gentamicin and erythromycin (100,101), although these appear unlikely to have clinical significance. Administration of heparin for weeks to months has been associated with osteoporosis, alopecia, hyperaldosteronism, and benign elevation of serum glutamic oxaloacetic transaminase levels (102–105).

HEPARIN DOSING AND MONITORING

During more than two decades of cardiac surgery with CPB, heparin dosing was accomplished empirically, with initial doses usually ranging from 200 to 400 U/kg and maintenance doses of 50 to 100 U/kg given as often as every 30 minutes or as infrequently as every 2 hours (51). The priming fluid used for the extracorporeal circuit usually contained 10,000 to 20,000 U of heparin. Heparin monitoring, defined as laboratory testing for the adequacy of blood heparin concentration or of a heparin-induced anticoagulant effect, was limited by the absence of an easily applicable test. This situation changed with the introduction of two coagulation tests that could be performed practically at the bedside on whole blood. The activated coagulation time (more appropriately called the activated clotting time in later publications) was introduced by Hattersley in 1966 (106), and the blood-activated recalcification time (BART), also termed the recalcified whole blood partial thromboplastin time, was introduced by Blakely in 1968 (107). Both of these tests were first reported for CPB heparin monitoring in 1974, BART for cardiac surgery and ACT for long-term respiratory support (65,108). The two classic papers by Bull et al. in 1975 (51,69) pointed out the apparent inadequacy of empiric heparin and protamine dosing protocols and recommended a structured approach using the ACT. This served as a turning point for heparin management during CPB, and the application of ACT monitoring to CPB

evolved from virtually nonexistent to widespread during the ensuing 5 years.

Laboratory Tests for Heparin Monitoring

These tests fall into two categories, clotting times and measurements of blood or plasma heparin concentration. Those who advocate clotting time measurement cite the importance of assessing a clinical effect of heparin, recognizing that measuring heparin concentration alone may fail to detect patients who are markedly resistant to heparin-induced anticoagulation (62). Advocates of heparin concentration monitoring note the changing relationship between ACT and blood heparin concentration induced by CPB, especially during hypothermia (109). Jobes et al. (110) outlined ideal characteristics for a CPB anticoagulation monitor. Desirable characteristics include low cost, the use of whole blood, bedside testing capability with minimal equipment and operator attention, reproducible results that are quickly available, and the use of shelf-stable reagents.

Clotting Times

Most plasma and whole blood tests of the intrinsic or extrinsic coagulation pathways involve measurement of the time taken to form a clot in the presence of selected coagulation stimulants. Because heparin exerts its anticoagulation effects at multiple sites along the coagulation cascade, incremental heparin doses will ultimately prolong any of these clotting times. The responsiveness of each test to heparin depends on the reagents chosen (111–113) and on the heparin sensitivity of that part of the coagulation cascade being tested by a particular clotting time. Table 22.2 lists several clotting times in decreasing order of heparin sensitivity. Thrombin time (TT) isolates the thrombin-mediated conversion of fibrinogen to fibrin, and the exquisite sensitivity of TT to heparin derives from the sensitivity of thrombin to heparin-enhanced AT III (114). The partial thromboplastin time (PTT) and the APTT are similarly very sensitive to low concentrations of heparin. These two tests are most often

TABLE 22.2. CLOTTING TIMES PROLONGED BY HEPARIN

Heparin Sensitivity	Text	Pathway Tested
Very sensitive	Thrombin time	Common
	Activated partial thromboplastin time	Intrinsic and common
	Whole blood clotting time	Intrinsic and common
Moderately sensitive	Saline clotting time	Intrinsic and common
	Activated clotting time	Intrinsic and common
	Blood activated recalcification time	Intrinsic and common
	BaSon clotting time	Intrinsic and common
Slightly sensitive	Prothrombin time	Extrinsic and common

performed on plasma, in which case they require blood collection in a citrated test tube, centrifugation to isolate plasma, then activation with an appropriate reagent followed by automated or manual measurement of the time to plasma coagulation. The TT and APTT are so sensitive to heparin-induced anticoagulation that blood becomes unclottable, within the time frame of the test, at heparin concentrations below those considered acceptable for CPB (65,115–117). This disadvantageous feature with respect to establishing the adequacy of CPB anticoagulation converts to an advantage for detecting small residual amounts of unneutralized heparin after protamine administration (118). On balance, however, TT, PTT, and APTT are inconvenient and impractical as routine monitors for heparin therapy during cardiac surgery.

The whole blood clotting time was the first clotting time used to measure the anticoagulant effect of heparin (60,119). A common form of this test is sometimes termed the *Lee-White clotting time*, which simply requires the collection of a blood sample, placement of an equal volume in each of three test tubes, and manual tilting of the tubes one at a time in succession until clotting occurs in each one. Although it offers bedside simplicity, low cost, and slightly less sensitivity to heparin than the APTT (53,117), this test requires nearly undivided attention from the operator for periods often exceeding 30 minutes in heparinized patients, especially at the heparin doses used for CPB. Jaberi et al. (65) found this test and the APTT similarly impractical, with blood becoming unclottable within an acceptable period of time after the administration of 400 U of heparin

per kilogram. The ACT, BART, and BaSon tests are activated whole blood coagulation tests, a primary purpose of which is to automate and hasten the whole blood clotting time (65,106,115,120,121). The ACT and BART have heparin sensitivities appropriate for CPB heparin monitoring (51,65,66,69). The prothrombin time (PT) is least sensitive to heparin-induced anticoagulation because heparin does not inhibit factor VII, and because cephalin is such a potent coagulation activator that even small amounts of unneutralized thrombin permit a normal or near-normal PT (122) (Fig. 22.5).

Activated Clotting Time

Since the late 1970s, the ACT has served as the primary workhorse for monitoring CPB anticoagulation. Like those of the APTT, the normal range and responsiveness of the ACT to heparin depend on the equipment used and the reagents selected. The three most common types of ACT are the manual ACT, the Hemochron ACT (International Technidyne, Edison, NJ) (Fig. 22.7), and the HemoTec ACT (HemoTec, Englewood, CO) (Fig. 22.8). When Bull et al. (51) introduced the ACT to cardiac surgery, they recommended the manual ACT as described by Hattersley (106), which uses diatomaceous earth (celite) as an activator. Hattersley described previously withdrawing and discarding 1 mL or more of blood by venipuncture, then removing the tourniquet and allowing blood to flow into an evacuated and prewarmed (37°C) tube. A timer was started when blood appeared in the tube, then the tube was inverted a

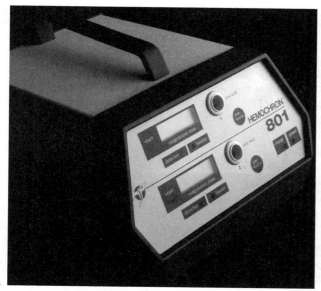
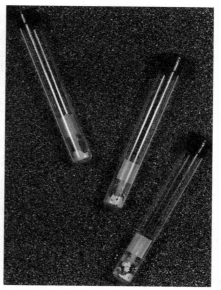

FIG. 22.7. The Hemochron activated clotting time (*ACT*) device (**A**) and three examples of the celite-containing test tube (**B**), which is placed into one of the testing wells shown in A after vigorous agitation. (Photographs courtesy of International Technidyne, Edison, NJ.)

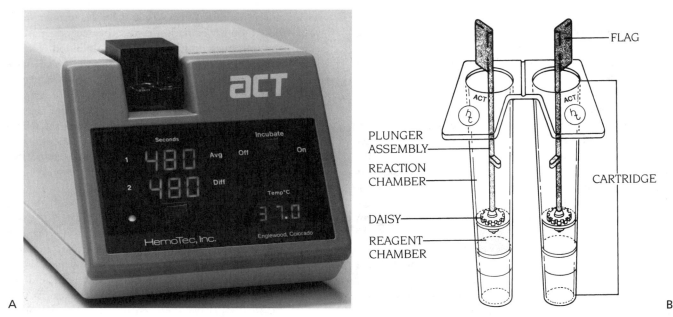

FIG. 22.8. The HemoTec ACT device (**A**) and a diagram (**B**) of the dual cartridge containing the kaolin activant (initially isolated in the reagent chamber), which is placed in the well located at the top center of the ACT device. (Photograph and diagram courtesy of Medtronic-HemoTec, Englewood, CO.)

few times for mixing and placed in a water bath at 37°C or heat block. At 1-minute and at 5-second intervals thereafter, the tube was withdrawn from the bath and tilted, and the timer was stopped at the appearance of the first unmistakable clot. Bull et al. used 2 mL of blood withdrawn from an indwelling venous catheter, inverted the tube once per second for 30 seconds, placed the glass tube in a heat block warmed by a 40-watt light bulb (temperature unspecified), and rocked the tube slowly until clotting occurred. These authors used a stopwatch that was started when the blood first entered the tube and stopped when the first clearly defined clot was visible. Hattersley (106) reported a mean ACT of 107 ± 13 seconds (range, 81 to 133 seconds), whereas Bull et al. (51) reported a mean ACT of 84 ± 13 seconds (range, 65 to 115 seconds). The different means and ranges reported in these two investigations could be explained by differences in technique (fresh venipuncture vs. indwelling catheter, different mixing technique, water bath vs. heat block) or by differences between the patient populations (5,000 surgical patients screened preoperatively by Hattersley, 50 cardiac surgical patients screened preoperatively by Bull). Variations in baseline ACT values reported in different studies probably derive from factors like these as well as from instrument-, operator-, and patient-related factors (123).

The ACT decreases slightly even with surgical incision and increases if the tubes are not prewarmed (123,124).

Prewarming the tubes may also improve ACT reproducibility. Using a manual ACT technique, Kase and Dearing (125) showed that performing the ACT without a heat block prolonged the control ACT by 50% and the CPB ACT by 100% to 150%. Such factors as the catheter material and the technique used for clearing residual heparin flush solution may also influence the results of ACT (126–128). Two reports indicate that one should withdraw and discard at least two times the sampling system dead space, defined as the volume contained within the system between the point of sampling and the intravascular end of the indwelling catheter (127,129).

The ACT was designed as a bedside test to be initiated immediately after blood sample withdrawal (106), although the effect of delayed test initiation on ACT results has not been reported. Because the blood sample is drawn without anticoagulant, performing the ACT at a location remote from the patient's bedside cannot be recommended. Cugno et al. (130) reported collecting whole blood in citrate, then recalcifying the sample to perform an ACT. This technique would accommodate modest delays between blood sample collection and test initiation. Because seemingly minor variations in ACT technique can significantly influence results, it appears reasonable to define a normal range for each testing site, with the assumption that operator-related factors can be fairly well controlled within a particular operating suite, critical care unit, angiography suite, or dialysis unit. Results might not be interchangeable, even between the operating room and the postoperative critical care unit. In an evaluation of 683 ACT values in 100 cardiac surgical patients, a heparin management strategy other than what would have been used after the single test method was chosen after duplicate testing in 16% of samples (131). Because of the dangers of inadequate anticoagulation or the risk for excessive administration of heparin because of ACT variability, duplicate testing for each ACT determination seems advisable (132).

Manual ACT techniques have been largely replaced by automated ACT techniques, probably because automated techniques require less training and distract the operator for a shorter period, especially when the clotting times are prolonged by heparin. One report apparently links a water bath used for manual ACTs to a cluster of sternal wound infections (133). An easily overlooked aspect of automated ACT instruments is that they should undergo regularly scheduled cleaning, calibration, and quality control testing (134). At least three automated ACT devices are commonly used in North America.

The International Technidyne Hemochron ACT (Fig. 22.7A) uses a 2-mL volume of whole blood activated by celite. A timer is started as the blood sample is placed in a test tube (Fig. 22.7B) that contains a small magnet and a plastic baffle. After vigorous manual mixing, the test tube is placed in a tilted well within a heat block and rotated continuously. The formation of a solid clot engages the magnet and causes it to leave the most dependent part of the test tube as rotation continues. This interrupts a magnetic field and automatically stops the timer. The coefficient of variation [(standard deviation ÷ mean) × 100] of the Hemochron ACT is 4% under control conditions (130,132) but rises to 8% in the presence of blood heparin concentrations used for CPB (132).

International Technidyne also offers glass tubes that contain kaolin as an activator. These tubes can be used specifically in patients receiving aprotinin therapy; the celite ACT in heparinized patients is prolonged in the presence of aprotinin (135). This prolongation may be artifactual, or it may represent a true anticoagulant effect. However, this should not be interpreted as enhanced anticoagulation, and the heparin dose should not be reduced. A potential explanation for the prolonged clotting time is that aprotinin inhibits kallikrein and may delay activation of the intrinsic coagulation pathway by XIIa. The kaolin ACT is less affected by aprotinin therapy than is the celite ACT, perhaps because kaolin, unlike celite, activates the intrinsic pathway by stimulation of factor XI directly (136). Others have suggested that kaolin binds to aprotinin and reduces the anticoagulant effect of aprotinin *in vitro* (137). However, the heparinized kaolin ACT is still somewhat prolonged in the presence of aprotinin (138). Additional ACT glass tubes that lack a particular activator and contain saline solution are available.

These tubes can be used in the same fashion, and they produce a longer clotting time and a test that is slightly more sensitive to low concentrations of heparin.

The HemoTec ACT uses 0.4 mL of whole blood injected into each of two plastic cartridges, which are then placed in a heat block (Fig. 22.8). Each cartridge contains a plunger that is engaged by a mechanical lifting device when the test is initiated. The initial plunger movement mixes the whole blood with a kaolin activator, and the continuous rise and fall of the plunger then gently agitates each sample until clot formation retards the passive fall of the plunger after its active elevation. The absence of plunger fall, detected photo-optically, stops the timer to yield the ACT. At the relatively moderate heparin doses used with extracorporeal membrane oxygenation for pulmonary support (mean ACT 152 ± 26 seconds), Green et al. (139) found a mean coefficient of variation of 9.2% with the HemoTec ACT. The HemoTec ACT cartridges are also available with three different concentrations of kaolin to produce different sensitivities and dose–response relationships to heparin. The low-range ACT cartridge provides heparin dose–response characteristics similar to those of the APTT (140).

Few direct comparisons of manual or automated ACT techniques have been reported. Mabry and colleagues (141) compared manual ACT with Hemochron ACT in patients undergoing vascular surgery and found a slightly lower control ACT with the manual technique (100 ± 12 seconds) than with the Hemochron technique (117 ± 18 seconds), which is similar to the findings of Kurec et al. (117) (manual ACT 91 ± 7 seconds, Hemochron ACT 129 ± 10 seconds). These differences were not subjected to statistical analysis, and values from the two ACT techniques were indistinguishable 5 and 30 minutes after heparin administration in the study of Mabry et al. Kurec and colleagues found manual ACT more sensitive than Hemochron ACT to low concentrations of heparin (0.2 U/mL). Zahl and Ellison (142) compared the Hemochron and HemoTec ACT methods and found similar baseline ACTs, but the HemoTec ACT was much more sensitive to heparin. When the Hemochron ACT rose into the 400- to 500-second range, 10 of 12 HemoTec ACTs exceeded 1,000 seconds. When Reich at al. (143) compared Hemochron ACT with the high-range HemoTec ACT, the least heparin-sensitive of the HemoTec ACT cartridges, they found no differences at baseline and at high heparin concentrations (ACT >500 seconds, cumulative heparin dose 300 U/kg), but significantly lower HemoTec ACTs at moderate heparin concentrations (HemoTec 263 ± 51 seconds, Hemochron 338 ± 63 seconds after 120 U of heparin per kilogram). Stead (144) found significantly lower control ACTs with Hemo-Tec (103 ± 5 seconds, presumably mean ± 1 standard error) than with Hemochron (147 ± 4 seconds), no difference after the initial heparin dose before starting CPB, and a significant tendency for Hemochron ACT to increase into

TABLE 22.3. CLINICAL CONDITIONS INFLUENCING ACTIVATED CLOTTING TIME

Condition	Effect on ACT
Hypothermia	Increase (340,341)
Hemodilution	Increase or NE (146,148,341,342)
Thrombocytopenia	Increase or NE (106,147,148,342)
Inhibition of platelet function	Increase (148,149)
Lysed platelets	Decrease (151)
Protamine	Increase (152,153)
Aprotinin	Increase (154,155)
Surgical incision	Decrease (123)

NE, no effect; ACT, activated clotting time.

the >700-second range while HemoTec ACT remained stable in the 500- to 600-second range. The HemoTec ACT technique used by Stead differed from the HemoTec ACT methods reported above, so that at least three different HemoTec ACT methods (differences in kaolin concentration or in blood agitation and clot detection techniques) are represented by these comparisons between Hemochron and HemoTec. One can conclude that results differ among different ACT methods, whereas the clinical significance of these differences remains uncertain.

A third ACT monitor is predicated on the Hemochron ACT principle but utilizes a dual endpoint detection system to signal termination of the test, thus enhancing the sensitivity of the ACT. This ACT (Actalyke, Array Medical, Somerville, NJ) has tests and tubes that are compatible with the Hemochron system and offers additional features, including a built-in bar code reader and improved labeling of individual tubes. Actalyke and Hemochron tubes can be used interchangeably in the Actalyke or the Hemochron system. Actalyke ACT tubes are available with celite, kaolin, or glass bead activator.

Table 22.3 lists some clinical conditions or interventions other than heparin that can affect ACT. The largest and most consistent effect is hypothermia-induced ACT prolongation, an effect that is proportional to the level of hypothermia. One study suggests that experimental hypothermia in dogs releases a heparin-like factor that inhibits factor Xa, a mechanism that could potentially explain this effect (145). Hemodilution has a relatively small effect within the hematocrit range most often present during cardiac surgery (15% to 40%). Ottesen and Froysaker (146) performed *in vitro* hemodilution on nonanticoagulated blood from six patients and found no convincing ACT increase in five patients until the sample contained more than 70% Ringer's acetate. It has been shown by Culliford et al. (68) that although hemodilution and hypothermia significantly increase the ACT of a heparinized blood sample, similar increases do not occur in the absence of added heparin. Results with thrombocyto-

penia have varied, but ACTs have been either unchanged or slightly increased with platelet counts in the range of 30,000 to 70,000/μL. The initial report of Hattersley (106) included one patient with a platelet count of 18,000/μL whose ACT was prolonged (190 seconds), and another patient with a platelet count of 10,000/μL whose ACT was normal (120 seconds). In a series of normal volunteers, *in vitro* thrombocytopenia was induced to a platelet count of 49,000 $\pm$ 8,000/μL. This level of moderate thrombocytopenia did not affect ACT in either heparinized or unheparinized samples. However, in thrombocytopenic patients with platelet counts of less than 20,000/μL, the ACT was prolonged (147). Kesteven et al. (148) found a significant but relatively modest inverse correlation ($r = 0.51$) between platelet count and ACT during CPB anticoagulation. Substantial platelet functional impairment induced by prostacyclin or by platelet activation with adenosine diphosphate increases the mean ACT by 50% to 60% (149). The latter study suggests that when heparin levels exceed 4 U/mL, further ACT increases depend almost entirely on platelet functional impairment.

A synergistic enhancement of the heparinized ACT has been noted in patients receiving GPIIb/IIIa platelet membrane inhibitor therapy. The ACT of nonheparinized blood is not prolonged in the presence of these platelet inhibitors. A small *in vitro* study by Ammar et al. (150), utilizing differential platelet membrane receptor blockade, suggests that this ACT prolongation is a direct result of GPIIb/IIIa inhibition and is not the result of decreased PF4 release. (PF4 is a heparin-neutralizing agent stored in platelet α-granules.) The clotting time of blood anticoagulated with direct thrombin inhibitors was also prolonged by GPIIb/IIIa inhibition. Similarly, the platelet membrane fraction created by platelet lysis significantly decreases ACT in an *in vitro* model, an effect that seems unlikely to be mediated by PF4 release (151). Gravlee et al. (123) showed that anesthesia and surgery decrease the ACT to suggest a hypercoagulable state, possibly by creating a thromboplastic response or by activation of platelets. Excessive protamine increases the ACT (152,153), as does the nonspecific protease inhibitor aprotinin (154,155).

Monitoring heparin therapy with clotting times assumes a predictable relationship between the blood heparin concentration and the clotting time response within an individual patient. Clotting times sensitive to low heparin concentrations (e.g., whole blood clotting time, APTT, TT) demonstrate a concave dose–response relationship, which converts to a straight line when heparin concentration is plotted against the log of the clotting time (47,112, 115,119). Congdon et al. (115) demonstrated a linear dose–response relationship between heparin and ACT in dogs at the heparin doses required for CPB. The heparin management protocol recommended by Bull et al. in 1975 (51,69) thus assumed a linear relationship between heparin

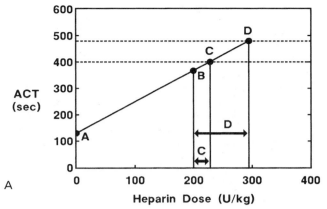

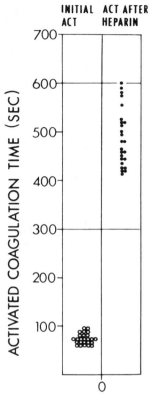

FIG. 22.9. A: Graph of the heparin dosing algorithm proposed by Bull et al. in 1975 (69). The control activated clotting time (*ACT*) is shown as *point A*, and the ACT resulting from an initial heparin bolus of 200 U/kg is shown as *point B*. The line connecting A and B is then extrapolated, and a desired ACT is selected. *Point C* represents the intersection between this line and an ACT of 400 seconds, which theoretically requires an additional heparin dose represented by the difference between points C and B on the horizontal axis (*arrow C*). Similarly, to achieve an ACT of 480 seconds (*higher horizontal dotted line* intersecting the ACT vs. heparin dose line at *point D*), one would administer the additional heparin dose represented by *arrow D*. **B:** The column on the left shows ACT values before heparin administration, and the column on the right shows ACT values obtained after application of a two-stage heparin administration protocol designed to produce an ACT value of 480 seconds. (From Bull BS, Huse WM, Brauer FS, et al. Heparin therapy during extracorporeal circulation. II. The use of a dose–response curve to individualize heparin and protamine dosage. *J Thorac Cardiovasc Surg* 1975;69:685–689, with permission.)

dose and ACT. Bull and colleagues recommended measuring a control ACT level before surgery, administering an initial heparin dose of 200 U/kg, measuring ACT 5 minutes later, then constructing a graph with heparin dose administered on one axis and ACT on the other (Fig. 9A). Those authors sought an initial ACT of 480 seconds, but a graphic depiction of their results suggests that the ACTs obtained from this algorithm were fairly evenly distributed between 400 and 600 seconds (Fig. 9B). In a similar study from the same group, ACT prolongation produced by this algorithm appeared to range from 380% to more than 1,000% (156). The predictive accuracy of this algorithm thus falls considerably short of pinpoint. Bull et al. (51) also reported that the ACT endpoint becomes unreliable at ACTs exceeding 600 seconds, a finding that was confirmed by Stenbjerg and colleagues (64). Stenbjerg et al. found coefficients of correlation between 0.80 and 0.97 between plasma heparin concentration and ACT at ACT values below 600 seconds. Cohen (157) updated the dose–response relationship after each heparin dose by using least-squares regression and showed good predictive accuracy (mean error, 5.6 ±

14.3%) and linear correlation ($r = 0.98$) with this technique when ACTs longer than 500 seconds and any ACTs measured within the first hour of CPB were excluded.

The studies of Stenbjerg et al. and of Cohen assess the linear correlation between heparin concentration (or dose) within an ACT range spanning from normal to markedly prolonged. This large range lends itself to high correlation coefficients even if the relationship between blood heparin concentration and ACT breaks down somewhat within the heparin concentration range used for CPB. Accordingly, scrutiny of the data of Stenbjerg et al. during CPB suggests a much less predictable CPB relationship between heparin concentration and ACT than their correlation coefficients suggest, although ACT prolongation by hypothermia might have caused this breakdown. Investigating the predictability of the heparin dose response in 157 patients divided into two groups with respective pre-CPB target ACTs of 480 and 600 seconds, Gravlee et al. (158) found a significantly reduced slope in the heparin dose–response relationship in the latter group (Fig. 22.10A). Because the groups were demographically comparable and differed only in the size

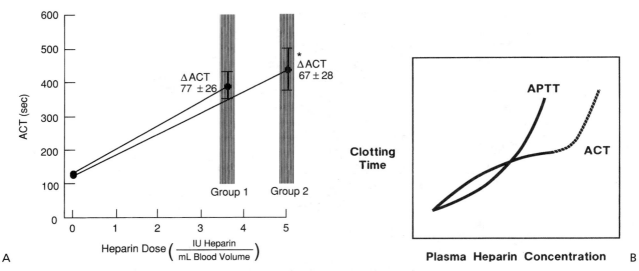

FIG. 22.10. A: Slope of the activated clotting time (*ACT*) vs. heparin dose line in two groups of 75 patients, each prospectively assigned to receive heparin doses designed to produce ACT values of 480 seconds (group 1) or 600 seconds (group 2) by application of an *ex vivo* algorithm to predict heparin dose requirements. The groups differed only in initial heparin dose, yet the slope of the ACT vs. heparin dose line was significantly lower in group 2. (From Gravlee GP, Brauer SD, Roy RC, et al. Predicting the pharmacodynamics of heparin: a clinical evaluation of the Hepcon System 4. *J Cardiothorac Anesth* 1987;1:379–387, with permission.) **B:** The proven relationship between activated partial thromboplastin time (*APTT*) and plasma heparin concentration and a hypothesized relationship between ACT and plasma heparin concentration. The *solid portion* of the ACT curve shows the relationship suggested in Fig. 22.9A and by unpublished work of Gravlee et al. The *interrupted portion* of the ACT curve suggests the clinical observation that infinite ACT prolongation can eventually be reached with sufficient heparin concentrations.

of the initial heparin bolus, this suggested a convex relationship between heparin concentration and ACT. This observation has been confirmed by the author in unpublished work with *ex vivo* heparinization of whole blood. Figure 22.10B contrasts this relationship with the well-established concave dose–response relationship between heparin and APTT. The *dotted line* continuation of the proposed heparin-ACT dose response relationship shown in Fig. 22.10B suggests the common (but not formally documented) clinical observation that the ACT response eventually becomes concave, which might derive from platelet inhibition at high heparin concentrations (149). The relationship between blood heparin concentration and ACT thus appears more complex than early studies indicated. Factors such as intrinsic variability of the test in the anticoagulated state, platelet activation and lysis, depression of platelet function, and hypothermia probably combine to limit greatly the predictability of the ACT response to heparin during CPB. The relatively crude nature of the ACT and its response to heparin should not cause concern, however, because, except when aprotinin is used, the cumulative mechanisms leading to ACT prolongation during CPB apparently have little importance as long as sufficiently high ACTs are maintained (155,159).

The Thrombolytic Assessment System, or TAS (Cardio-

vascular Diagnostics, Raleigh, NC) is a point-of-care coagulation system monitor that is capable of measuring PT, APTT, and a heparin management test (HMT) (Fig. 22.11). The HMT is designed to measure the high concentrations of heparin used during CPB. This system is able to perform testing on citrated plasma or whole blood and utilizes disposable cards that contain the reagents used in the specific test. In the case of the HMT, the card contains calcium chloride and celite activator. The card contains iron oxide particles that move in response to an oscillating magnetic field within the device. When clot formation is detected, movement of the iron oxide particles decreases. The HMT result correlates with anti-Xa activity in CPB patients and is less variable (160). In a comparison with ACT, the coefficients of variation were similar for the tests at baseline but were three times higher for the ACT during heparinization. The HMT result was prolonged by the presence of aprotinin (200 kallikrein inhibition units (KIU)/mL) at heparin concentrations of 0, 1, 2, and 5 IU/mL (161); however, this prolongation was more pronounced at higher heparin concentrations.

Monitoring of Heparin Concentration

Because CPB changes the sensitivity of ACT to heparin (68,162) (Fig. 22.12), some have advocated monitoring

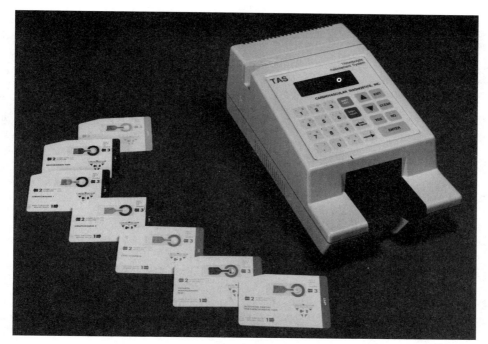

FIG. 22.11. The Thrombolytic Assessment System (Cardiovascular Diagnostics) utilizes disposable cards containing iron oxide particles that move in response to a magnetic field. This movement ceases when clot is formed. Cards are available to perform the heparin management test and to measure the prothrombin time, activated partial thromboplastin time, and thrombolysis. (Photograph courtesy of Cardiovascular Diagnostics, Raleigh, NC.)

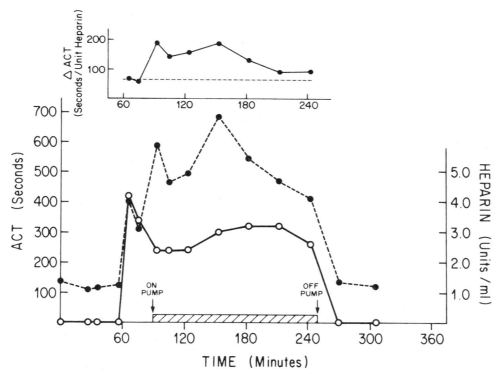

FIG. 22.12. The activated clotting time (*ACT*) and heparin concentration values from a single patient during the course of a cardiac surgical procedure. Once cardiopulmonary bypass had begun, ACT (*dotted line connecting solid circles*) increased while heparin concentration (*solid line connecting open circles*) decreased. The inset shows the changing relationship between ACT and heparin concentration over time plotted as the change in ACT from the control value divided by blood heparin concentration. (From Culliford AT, Gitel SN, Starr N, et al. Lack of correlation between activated clotting time and plasma heparin during cardiopulmonary bypass. *Ann Surg* 1981; 193:105–111, with permission.)

TABLE 22.4. HEPARIN CONCENTRATION MEASUREMENT TECHNIQUES

Protamine titration (manual or automated)
Polybrene titration
Factor Xa inhibition
Chromogenic assay (manual or automated)
Fluorogenic assay
Colorimetric assay (azure A or toluidine blue)

heparin concentration directly (109,163,164). Table 22.4 lists several laboratory techniques that measure whole blood or plasma heparin concentration. Protamine and polybrene titrations measure heparin concentration by identifying the reagent concentration that optimally neutralizes heparin, judged by the fastest clot formation under standardized conditions (110,156,165,166). This information can be converted to a plasma or blood heparin concentration if the neutralization ratio of protamine to heparin is known (usually 1.0 to 1.2 mg of protamine to 100 U of heparin). Excesses of protamine and polybrene inhibit clot formation, so the tube or cartridge with the shortest clotting time represents the closest match between heparin and its neutralizing agent. These titrations are performed on whole blood, which offers a practical advantage over most other nonclotting time heparin assays. HemoTec offers automated techniques that greatly simplify the bedside measurement of blood heparin concentration and have therefore become second in popularity only to ACT measurement in heparin monitoring. The maintenance of a stable heparin concentration (Hepcon, Medtronic Hemotec Inc., Parker, CO) usually results in the administration of larger doses of heparin than those given with ACT monitoring because hemodilution and hypothermia during CPB increase the sensitivity of the ACT to heparin. Additionally, use of the Hepcon system may result in the administration of larger heparin doses because this particular ACT uses kaolin as the activator, which has a lower response to heparin at ACTs of less than 500 seconds (167). Automated protamine titration more closely correlates with measurements of antifactor Xa activity than with ACT during CPB (168), although the reproducibility of these devices has not been systematically confirmed (169) (Fig. 22.13). This factor may pose a significant unexplored problem because a decisive endpoint for the automated heparin–protamine titration is sometimes difficult to determine.

Hepcon heparin concentrations have been shown to reflect anti-Xa and anti-IIa heparin activity accurately when

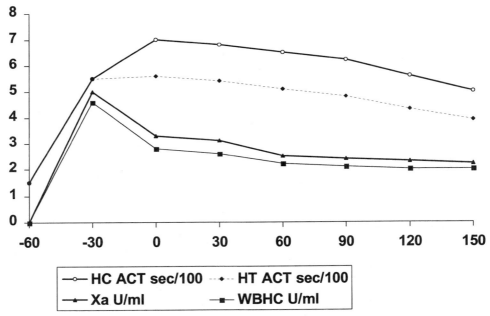

FIG. 22.13. A strong linear relationship exists between whole blood heparin concentration (*WB HC*), measured by the Hepcon (Medtronic-HemoTec, Parker, CO) protamine titration assay, and plasma anti-Xa heparin activity (*Xa U/ml*). Values for whole blood heparin concentration were corrected for the hematocrit. The Xa heparin concentration was measured in plasma with a substrate assay. Note the poor relationship between activated clotting time (*ACT*) and anti-Xa heparin activity. *HC*, Hemochron (International Technidyne, Edison, NJ). *HT*, HemoTec (Medtronic-HemoTec, Englewood, CO). (From Despotis GJ, Summerfield AL, Joist JH. Comparison of activated coagulation time and whole blood heparin measurements with laboratory plasma anti-Xa heparin concentration in patients having cardiac operations. *J Thorac Cardiovasc Surg* 1994;108:1076–1082, with permission.)

the effects of hemofiltration are measured during CPB. The increases in heparin activity that result from hemofiltration are directly related to the removal of filtrate and are directly proportional to filtered volume and hematocrit (170). The careful monitoring of heparin concentrations during hemofiltration may obviate the need to administer additional heparin doses.

In a fluorogenic heparin assay, plasma or diluted whole blood is mixed with pooled normal plasma, then incubated for a fixed period with a known amount of thrombin (109,163,171–174). This mixture is then added to a fibrin analogue that is cleaved predictably by any residual thrombin (i.e., thrombin not bound by heparin or AT III) to form a quantifiably fluorescent product. Most applications of this technique require plasma, which makes the procedure impractical for the bedside. Nevertheless, some operating room laboratories have found an automated version of this test (Protopath, Dade, Miami, FL) to be feasible for CPB heparin monitoring, in part because results can be quickly obtained once the plasma has been separated (109,173). Saleem et al. (163) showed reasonable correlation ($r = 0.7$) between Protopath and automated protamine titration.

High-dose Thrombin Time

The high-dose thrombin time (HiTT) (International Technidyne, Edison, NJ) is a functional test of heparin-induced anticoagulation that overcomes some of the inadequacies of the ACT. This test correlates well with heparin levels because the clotting time for the conversion of fibrinogen to fibrin by active thrombin is a direct reflection of the antithrombin activities of heparin. Fewer confounding factors are present at this late point in the common pathway of the coagulation cascade. Unlike the ACT, the HiTT is not altered by hemodilution and hypothermia and correlates better with heparin concentration than does the ACT during CPB (175) (Fig. 22.14). The standard TT is so sensitive a measure of heparin activity that it is not clinically useful at the high levels of heparin employed during CPB. Conversely, the unheparinized or "baseline" HiTT values are often unmeasurable because the large dose of thrombin in the test tube causes clot to form earlier than can be temporally detected by the test. The HiTT incorporates a large dose of thrombin into the test tube to bind a significant proportion of the heparin–AT III complexes that are present during heparinization. The remaining unbound heparin prolongs the time to fibrin formation, measured as the HiTT. The test result is measured in a standard Hemochron machine; whole blood is added to a prewarmed, prehydrated test tube that contains a lyophilized thrombin preparation. After addition of 1.5 mL of blood, the tube is inserted into a Hemochron well and the time to clot formation is measured. *In vitro* assays indicate that HiTT is equivalent to the ACT in evaluation of the anticoagulant effects of heparin at concentrations in the range 0 to 4.8 U/mL. During CPB,

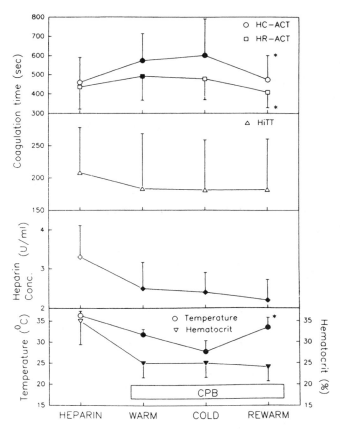

FIG. 22.14. Hemochron activated clotting time (*HC-ACT*), Hepcon ACT (*HR-ACT*), high-dose thrombin time (*HiTT*), and heparin concentration were measured at initiation of cardiopulmonary bypass. Note that with hemodilution and hypothermia, Hemochron ACT and Hepcon ACT increased while HiTT and heparin concentration decreased. *Solid mark* indicates $p < 0.05$ vs. first time point (heparin). *Asterisk* (*) denotes $p < 0.05$ vs. immediately preceding time point. (From Wang J-S, Lin C-Y, Karp RB. Comparison of high-dose thrombin time with activated clotting time for monitoring of anticoagulant effects of heparin in cardiac surgical patients. *Anesth Analg* 1994;79:9–13, with permission.)

heparin concentration and HiTT decrease while Hemochron and Hepcon ACT values increase. HiTT monitoring may be advantageous for patients receiving aprotinin therapy (176) because the HiTT is not affected by aprotinin therapy (celite ACT is prolonged by aprotinin). However, the HiTT was found to be less accurate than the Hepcon protamine titration assay in predicting heparin concentrations below 4.8 U/mL in patients receiving aprotinin (177). The HiTT is being investigated as a monitor of the heparin dose response in patients on preoperative heparin infusions who have a diminished ACT response to heparin (178).

High-dose Thromboplastin Time

The high-dose thromboplastin time, also unaffected by aprotinin therapy, is a whole blood clotting time in which celite is replaced by rabbit brain thromboplastin. The coagulation time via activation of the extrinsic pathway is measured. The rich thromboplastin environment of the pericardial cavity also stimulates this pathway during pericardiotomy.

Other types of heparin assays rely exclusively on plasma samples and would not be practical for routine use during CPB. These tests are based on a color change induced by binding to heparin (azure A, toluidine, and chromogenic tests) or on the ability of heparin to inhibit factor Xa (179–182).

Clinical Assessments and Comparisons of Heparin Monitoring Techniques

Once Bull et al. (51) had outlined the potential problems in heparin management during CPB with the use of standardized dosing schemes that varied widely among institutions, numerous investigators followed up on their work by comparing clinical outcomes of ACT monitoring with those of standardized unmonitored heparin management (Table 22.5). Blood loss, blood transfusion comparisons, or both were compared in the clinical investigations shown in Table 22.5. Six of 10 studies showed decreased blood loss with ACT monitoring, and five of seven showed decreased homologous blood transfusion requirements. Unfortunately, only one of these studies appeared to be completely prospec-

tive (183), and that study did not specify the method of patient assignment to the two study groups, nor was statistical analysis performed on the observed differences. Ottesen et al. (184) found no difference in postoperative blood loss between two groups that differed only in precise versus crude application of the Bull protocol for determining maintenance doses of heparin during CPB. The studies comparing transfusion requirements did not list the criteria for blood transfusion, which can vary substantially among physicians and institutions (185). From these studies, it appears likely that ACT-based CPB heparin management does not increase postoperative bleeding or transfusion requirement; thus, its effect on these parameters is either neutral or favorable. Furthermore, Metz and Keats (186) found no relationship between lower CPB ACTs and postoperative bleeding when empiric heparin management was used. Although limitations in experimental designs, notably the use of historical control groups, preclude a more ambitious conclusion favoring ACT, unmonitored heparin management is rarely practiced. Because protamine dosing can also influence postoperative bleeding (187), differences in protamine dosing might also have influenced the results of most of these studies.

Table 22.5 also lists clinical outcome studies comparing heparin concentration monitoring with no monitoring, and ACT monitoring with heparin concentration monitoring.

TABLE 22.5. CLINICAL OUTCOME COMPARISON OF DIFFERENT TYPES OF HEPARIN MONITORING FOR CARDIOPULMONARY BYPASS

Investigators and Year	No. of Patients	Blood Loss	Transfusion	Experimental Method
A. ACT vs. no monitoring				
Babka et al. 1977 (183)	20	ACT<NM[a]	NE	Prospective, randomized?
Verska 1977 (343)	114	ACT<NM	ACT<NM	Historical control group
Roth et al. 1979 (344)	56	ND	ND	Historical control group
Akl et al. 1980 (67)	120	ND	ACT<NM	Historical control group
Papaconstantinou and Rådegran 1981 (345)	126	ACT<NM[b]	ACT<NM[b]	Historical control group
Jumean and Sudah 1983 (346)	77[c]	ACT<NM	NE	Historical control group
Dearing et al. 1983 (347)	648	ACT<NM	ACT<NM	Retrospective, sequential grouping
Niinikoski et al. 1984 (348)	100	ACT<NM	ND	Retrospective, sequential grouping
Lefemine and Lewis 1985 (349)	61	ND	NE	Not specified[d]
Preiss et al. 1985 (350)	350	ND	ACT<NM	Retrospective, not randomized
B. Heparin concentration vs. no monitoring				
Jobes et al. 1981 (110)	46	ND	NE	Prospective, randomized
Bowie and Kemna 1985 (188)	150	HC<NM[a]	HC<NM[a]	Prospective, randomized
C. ACT vs. heparin concentration monitoring				
Gravlee et al. 1990 (159)	21	ACT<HC[e]	NE	Prospective, randomized
Urban et al. 1991 (351)	38	ND	ND	Prospective, randomized
Gravlee et al. 1992 (189)	163	ND[f]	ND	Prospective, randomized
Despotis et al. 1995 (190)	254	ND	HC<ACT	Prospective, randomized

[a] No statistical analysis.
[b] Intraoperative only, no difference in postoperative period.
[c] Pediatric patients.
[d] Forty-three ACT patients, 18 NM patients.
[e] No systematic assessment of heparin rebound postoperatively.
[f] Heparin rebound systematically assessed and treated. HC >ACT for incidence of heparin rebound.
ACT, activated clotting time; HC, heparin concentration; ND, no difference; NE, not evaluated; NM, no monitoring.

One of two studies shows that heparin concentration monitoring decreases blood loss in comparison with no monitoring (188). This study appears to be prospective and randomized, although the method of randomization was not specified and the unmonitored (control) group may have been historical. Three published studies have compared ACT monitoring with heparin concentration monitoring (Table 22.5, part C). The two studies by Gravlee et al. (159,189) showed conflicting results with regard to postoperative blood loss. This discrepancy might be explained by aggressive diagnosis and treatment of heparin rebound in the second study. Despotis et al. (190) prospectively compared heparin concentration monitoring with ACT monitoring in conjunction with a point-of-care transfusion algorithm for post-CPB bleeding. In the course of maintaining a threshold heparin concentration, determined before CPB for each patient, the authors' study group received nearly twice the dose of heparin of the ACT group. In addition, the study group had a small reduction in the volume of mediastinal tube drainage and received significantly fewer transfusions of non-red blood cell allogeneic blood products. The transfusion-sparing result was attributed to better suppression of intravascular coagulation during CPB.

Is there an optimal range for ACT or heparin concentration during CPB? Bull et al. (51) reported clinical experience that a clot does not form in the oxygenator circuit with an ACT exceeding 300 seconds. Those authors further stated the opinions that (a) ACTs below 180 seconds should be considered so inadequate as to be life-threatening, (b) ACTs between 180 and 300 seconds should be considered highly questionable, and (c) maintaining ACTs exceeding 600 seconds would seem unwise. They noted that a minimum ACT of 180 seconds had been suggested for patients undergoing long-term extracorporeal oxygenation for pulmonary support, and that the higher minimum ACT recommended for cardiac surgery requiring CPB was needed because of the greater amounts of tissue fluid gaining access to the circulation in that setting. Although this hypothesis holds some appeal, it remains unproven. Bull et al. also recommended attaining an ACT of 480 seconds before initiating CPB, suggesting that this particular ACT value provides a safety margin over the believed minimum safe ACT of 300 seconds. It appears that many practitioners have misinterpreted their recommendation by assuming that an ACT of 480 seconds represents the minimum safe level for CPB anticoagulation, when the authors were simply offering a suggestion without scientific validation. In 1978, Young et al. (191) raised the minimum recommended ACT level of Bull et al. (300 seconds) by demonstrating fibrin formation and depletion of clotting factors, AT III, and platelets in monkeys sustaining ACTs below 400 seconds during CPB. They then applied this information to five pediatric patients undergoing CPB, finding no untoward events when ACTs above 400 seconds were maintained. They did not, however, investigate the possibility that ACTs below 400 seconds might also be safe in humans. At least six studies have re-

ported ACT values below 400 seconds for CPB without complications (68,110,116,159,162,186). Five of these studies reported some CPB maintenance ACTs below 300 seconds (68,110,116,162,186), and Dauchot et al. (116) reported a mean ACT of 296 ± 51 seconds (range, 230 to 437 seconds) after rewarming during CPB in 22 adults.

Metz and Keats (186) assessed the utility of ACT monitoring by administering heparin (300 U/kg) to 193 patients undergoing CPB, then blindly measuring ACT at predetermined intervals. Fifty-one of their patients had ACTs below 400 seconds during CPB, with four patients having ACT values below 300 seconds. No clots were visible in the extracorporeal circuits during or after CPB, and no relationship was found between lower CPB ACTs and postoperative bleeding. Cardoso et al. (192) recently reported no differences in coagulation factors, platelet counts, or membrane oxygenator performance between two groups of six pigs assigned to an ACT range of 250 to 300 seconds or of more than 450 seconds for 2 hours of hypothermic CPB.

Several reports suggest the safety of ACTs either in the 170- to 250-second range or twice normal for prolonged respiratory support with extracorporeal membrane oxygenators (108,193–197). Defining ideal anticoagulation in that clinical setting proves difficult, however, because the patients' disease processes predispose to both thromboembolic events and disseminated intravascular coagulation, and even the relatively modest level of anticoagulation used appears to increase bleeding complications (193–195).

Two studies measuring plasma levels of fibrinopeptide A (FpA), a sensitive marker of fibrin formation, found higher-than-normal levels during CPB for cardiac surgery, but these levels were still considerably lower than those measured after surgical incision alone. Davies et al. (198) noted that 54 of their 73 CPB ACT measurements in 15 patients were below 400 seconds, and they concluded (without assessing a clinical outcome) that the anticoagulation of these patients had been inadequate. Investigating 21 patients with two different heparin-monitoring protocols, Gravlee et al. (159) found that higher heparin concentrations better suppressed FpA levels early in CPB, but that this difference was not sustained during rewarming (Fig. 22.15). Those authors found no correlation between CPB FpA levels and postoperative bleeding, although five patients exhibited CPB FpA levels more than 10 times the upper limit of normal. It thus appears that plasma FpA levels are not reliable indicators of inadequate CPB anticoagulation in humans unless the threshold for morbidity exceeds the levels reported thus far.

Is there a *maximum* safe level of anticoagulation for CPB? Exaggerating the hemorrhagic diathesis during CPB poses little difficulty so long as the blood losses are scavenged effectively into the extracorporeal circuit. One study suggests that higher blood heparin concentrations (>4 U/mL) and ACTs (>600 seconds) during CPB predispose to increased postoperative blood loss (159), although a follow-up study from the same group of investigators failed to

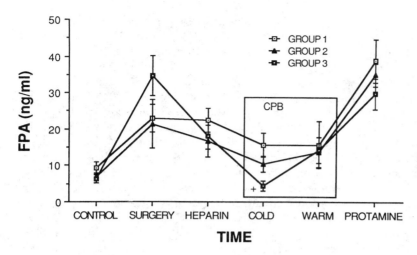

FIG. 22.15. Fibrinopeptide A (*FpA*) levels in three groups of patients during cardiac surgery. Patients in groups 1 and 2 received an initial heparin dose of 200 or 300 U/kg and additional heparin during cardiopulmonary bypass whenever the activated clotting time was below 400 seconds. Group 3 patients received an initial heparin dose of 400 U/kg and additional heparin whenever the whole blood heparin concentration was below 4.0 U/kg. The FpA levels peaked before heparin and after protamine and were significantly different between the groups during hypothermic bypass (group 3 vs. group 1 only). (From Gravlee GP, Haddon WS, Rothberger HK, et al. Heparin dosing and monitoring for cardiopulmonary bypass. A comparison of techniques with measurement of subclinical plasma coagulation. *J Thorac Cardiovasc Surg* 1990;99:518–527, with permission.)

confirm this (189). In the latter study, higher CPB heparin concentrations predisposed to postoperative heparin rebound, which required treatment with protamine. In addition to the need for higher initial protamine doses and a higher incidence of heparin rebound, heparin doses exceeding the presumed minimum safe requirement for CPB may be associated with a greater degree of platelet dysfunction as measured by aggregometry (199). The use of high-dose aprotinin seems to counter the platelet-inhibiting capacity of large doses of heparin. It remains unclear whether large doses of heparin are detrimental as a result of the aforementioned complications, or whether they confer an advantage by better suppression of coagulation activity. The maintenance of stable heparin concentrations does suppress coagulant activity during CPB, as evidenced by lower levels of FpA and lower levels of D-dimers in the period before protamine (87). However, after protamine administration, markers of fibrin formation and thrombin activation increase in all patients and are likely to be indistinguishable between patients who have experienced ACT monitoring and those who have undergone heparin concentration monitoring. There is no consistent substantiation for the hypothesis that lower levels of fibrin formation or thrombin activation predict improved clinical outcomes; however, it would seem prudent to suppress thrombin activation as much as possible. Despotis advocates doing so by administering larger doses of heparin (87). Because heparin does not inhibit clot-bound thrombin, total inhibition is not possible. Ideally, further thrombin inhibition could be achieved through the use of a direct thrombin inhibitor or through the use of an anticoagulant that works at a different point in the coagulation cascade (i.e., extrinsic pathway).

More studies purport to evaluate safe ACT levels for CPB than safe blood or plasma heparin concentrations. Jobes et al. (110) found no adverse effects with whole blood heparin concentrations exceeding 2 U/mL. The findings of Kesteven (162) were similar, except that he measured *plasma* heparin concentrations, which should be higher than whole blood

heparin concentrations in proportion to the relative volumes of the two compartments. Possibly, Kesteven corrected his heparin concentrations to represent whole blood levels because his patients otherwise would have sustained CPB whole blood heparin concentrations between 1.0 and 1.5 U/mL, which would likely represent inadequate anticoagulation.

In summary, the optimal ACT or heparin concentration range for CPB has not been definitively established. The ACT minimum of 300 seconds originally recommended by Bull et al. (51) has withstood the test of time, but it appears that lower ACTs may also be acceptable with heparin-coated circuits (200–202). It has not been clearly established whether it is better to monitor heparin concentration or heparin effect, but Nielsen et al. (203) reported one case of clots in both the surgical field and the extracorporeal circuit despite maintenance of whole blood heparin concentrations of 4.0 U/mL or higher. The ACTs were not reported for that patient, who had a previously undiagnosed familial deficiency of AT III. It seems likely that this clinical scenario could have been avoided by monitoring heparin effect (i.e., ACT) rather than heparin concentration, as there have been no reports of clots (although the authors have received verbal reports from colleagues) in the extracorporeal circuit with ACTs above 300 seconds.

Because there is no apparent advantage to maintaining ACTs below 400 seconds, the simplest clinical guideline is to exceed that value during CPB for cardiac surgery. Metz and Keats (186) appropriately questioned the need for any heparin monitoring, although the rare occurrences of marked heparin resistance (203) or accidental injection of a substance other than heparin suggest some virtue in doing so. There is no proven need to compensate for hypothermia-induced ACT prolongation by maintaining the blood heparin concentration that was present before hypothermia so long as one anticipates the expected decrease in ACT on rewarming (157). However, some suggest that the ACT may prove inadequate as a sole heparin monitor with deeper levels of hypothermia (<24°C) and with profound hemodilution (as often occurs with neonates and infants). Others suggest that the ACT should be used in conjunction with heparin concentration monitoring during moderate levels of hypothermia or with CPB of prolonged duration (204). In most situations, the authors see no clinical advantage to heparin concentration monitoring and have selected the following CPB heparin management protocol for adults, while recognizing that other protocols may be equally acceptable:

1. Administer 300 U of heparin per kilogram intravenously.
2. Draw an arterial sample for ACT in 3 to 5 minutes.
3. Give additional heparin as needed to achieve an ACT above 400 seconds before initiating CPB and to maintain an ACT above 400 seconds during normothermic CPB and above 480 seconds during hypothermia between 24° and 30°C.
4. Prime the extracorporeal circuit with approximately 3 U of heparin per milliliter (e.g., 5,000 U for a 1,600-mL clear priming solution).
5. Monitor the ACT every 30 minutes during CPB, or more frequently if the patient proves resistant to heparin-induced prolongation of the ACT.

Although some prefer to select supplemental heparin doses precisely with the aid of a manual or computer-generated graphic plot, as recommended by Bull et al. (69), the authors believe that the relative imprecision of the ACT, the unpredictability and likely nonlinearity of the ACT-to-heparin dose–response relationship, and the lack of any proven benefit to a narrowly defined ACT endpoint render such maneuvers unnecessary. If ACT decreases below the desired minimum value, supplemental heparin doses of 50 to 100 U/kg most often prolong the ACT sufficiently without the aid of precise calculations.

In vitro techniques have been introduced that measure individual patient dose–response relationships between heparin and either blood heparin concentration (HemoTec, Englewood, CO) or ACT (International Technidyne, Edison, NJ) (158,205). These assays are patient-specific in that they measure a patient's heparin sensitivity and incorporate the patient's estimated blood volume into a formula that calculates the heparin dose required to achieve a target ACT or heparin concentration. The Hemochron RxDx (International Technidyne) system is an ACT-based heparin dose–response assay. The heparin response test is an ACT with a known quantity of *in vitro* heparin (3 IU/mL); along with a baseline ACT, it allows generation of a dose–response curve that enables calculation of the heparin dose required to attain the target ACT. The RxDx system also provides a protamine response test. This is an ACT with one of two specific quantities of protamine, depending on the amount of circulating heparin suspected (2 U/mL or 3 U/mL). By using the patient's heparinized ACT, the protamine response test, and an estimate of the patient's blood volume,

the protamine dose needed to return the ACT to baseline can be calculated based on a protamine-response curve. Jobes et al. (206) randomly assigned patients to receive standard ACT-based management or individualized heparin management with the RxDx system. They were able to lower their protamine doses significantly by using the protamine titration assay, and they reported significantly reduced transfusions and chest tube drainage in the group that received individualized dosing. A follow-up study, however, was unable to confirm that transfusions or chest tube drainage is significantly affected by the RxDx intervention (207). Both studies revealed that the RxDx system results in administration of a reduced protamine dose, but differences in transfusion outcomes may have resulted from different total heparin doses or different management strategies for heparin rebound.

Another *in vitro* individualized heparin dose–response assay is the Hepcon (Medtronic) Heparin Dose Response, which constructs a three-point dose–response curve based on baseline, 1.5-U/mL, and 2.5-U/mL concentrations of heparin. From this curve, extrapolation to the desired ACT or heparin concentration yields the indicated dose of heparin to be given.

If a true emergency dictates the need to institute immediate CPB, it would seem reasonable to administer a large systemic dose of heparin (400 U/kg) because there may be insufficient time to confirm the effect of heparin with an ACT. Under these circumstances, it also seems reasonable to place a larger-than-usual heparin dose in the extracorporeal circuit (e.g., 10,000 U for a usual adult priming volume of 1,500 to 2,000 mL).

HEPARIN RESISTANCE

Heparin resistance can be loosely defined as the need for higher-than-normal heparin doses to induce sufficient anticoagulation for the safe conduct of CPB. Many factors have been reported to alter the anticoagulation response to heparin (Table 22.6). Usually, these effects are clinically insignificant (208), but they may cumulatively account for the consistent demonstration of marked interpatient variability in the anticoagulation response to a fixed heparin dose (expressed in units per kilogram). In most cases, heparin resistance can be adequately treated with increased doses of heparin. In some reports, the magnitude of the increased heparin dose and the necessity for other interventions have been exaggerated by misconceptions about the safe minimum ACT required for CPB (209–211). Clinical situations sometimes inducing noteworthy heparin resistance have included familial AT III deficiency (212), ongoing heparin therapy (208,213), extreme thrombocytosis (platelet count >700,000/μL) (214), septicemia (52,210), and hypereosinophilic syndrome (215). It is also well accepted that histidine-rich glycoprotein in the plasma binds to heparin and modulates its anticoagulant activity to a degree that may be clinically relevant (216,217). Young et al. (218) studied patients with venous thromboembolism who received a

TABLE 22.6. FACTORS REPORTED TO DECREASE THE ANTICOAGULANT RESPONSE TO HEPARIN

Factor	Human Studies	Case Reports	Animal or *in vitro* Models
1. AT III deficiency			
A. Familial		Nielsen 1987 (203)	
		Soloway 1980 (209)	
		Marciniak 1974 (212)	
B. Acquired		Chung 1981 (210)	Reuter 1978 (244)
2. Platelets			
A. Thrombocytosis	Gravlee 1987 (158)	Wilds 1982 (214)	Conley 1948 (352)
B. Heparin-induced thrombocytopenia		Olinger 1984 (317)	
3. Age			
A. Pediatrics/newborns	Doty 1979 (63)		
	Dauchot 1983 (116)		
B. Increased adult age	Gravlee 1987 (158)		
4. Circadian rhythm	Schved 1985 (353)		
	Decousus 1985 (354)		
	Decousus 1985 (355)		
5. Hemoglobin concentration			
Decreased	Kase 1985 (125)		
Increased			Whitfield 1980 (356)
6. Preheparin ACT or PTT			
Decreased	Esposito 1983 (62)		Bjornsson 1986 (111)
Increased			Whitfield 1980 (356)
7. Drugs			
A. Several medications			Nelson 1958 (357)
B. Ongoing heparin therapy	Esposito 1983 (62)	Hicks 1983 (359)	
	Dietrich 1991 (213)		
	Cloyd 1986 (358)		
C. Nitroglycerin	Habbab 1987 (223)		
	Becker 1990 (224)		
8. pH and protein effects			
A. Increased acid glycoprotein			Godal 1961 (360)
B. Decreased pH	Kase 1985 (125)		Jaques 1967 (361)
C. Antiheparin immunoglobulin		Glueck 1972 (362)	
		Pogliani 1975 (363)	
D. Neutrophil elastase			Jordan 1987 (364)
E. Increased lipoprotein levels			Bleyl 1975 (365)
F. Increased HRG	Lijnen 1983 (216)		
G. Protein binding	Young 1992 (218)		
9. Pregnancy	Whitfield 1983 (366)		
10. Hypereosinophilic syndrome		Hanowell 1981 (215)	
11. Sepsis/endocarditis		Mabry 1979 (52)	
		Chung 1981 (210)	
12. Autologous blood withdrawal	Mummaneni 1983 (367)		
13. Hypercoagulable states	de Takats 1943 (60)	Reuter 1978 (244)	
14. Male sex			Whitfield 1980 (356)

AT III, antithrombin III; HRG, histidine-rich glycoprotein.

fixed dose of intravenous heparin therapy. Using low-affinity heparin to effect reversible heparin neutralization, the authors demonstrated that protein binding is a significant factor in the neutralization of the anticoagulant effect of heparin. Reversible heparin neutralization refers to the fact that low-affinity heparin is devoid of anticoagulant anti-Xa activity yet competes with and displaces protein-bound heparin, thus making anti-Xa measurements a relative measure of the protein-binding capacity of heparin. However, the authors did not find significant individual relationships between reversible heparin neutralization and concentrations of specific proteins such as AT III, histidine-rich glycoprotein, or PF4. They suggest that heparin binding to endothelium, macrophages, and potentially other plasma proteins contributes to the variable clinical response to intravenous heparin. Furthermore, protein-bound heparin persists after protamine neutralization of heparin (219). The dissociation of these protein–heparin complexes after CPB may contribute to the phenomenon known as *heparin rebound*. The variable response to heparin in states of acute illness also results from increased protein binding rather than decreased clearance. This was demonstrated with radiolabeled heparin and reversible heparin neutralization in rabbits made experimentally endotoxemic (220). Dermatan sulfate also binds to plasma proteins, although the clinical significance of this is not clear. LMWHs do not bind plasma proteins as avidly as does unfractionated heparin; therefore, their relative anticoagulant activity should be little affected by plasma protein concentrations (221,222). Generally, heparin fractions larger than 6000 Da bind nonspecifically to plasma proteins. The molecular weight of most LMWH fragments falls below this threshold. Several groups have reported an interaction between heparin and nitroglycerin in the coronary care unit setting (223,224), but Reich et al. (225) could not confirm this interaction in the cardiac surgical setting, and Amin and Horrow (226) did not find a significant *in vitro* interaction with AT III.

Antithrombin III deficiency can be inherited or acquired. Congenital AT III deficiency follows an autosomal dominant transmission pattern and has an estimated prevalence of 1 in every 2,000 to 20,000 people (227,228). A reduced amount of normal AT III constitutes the most common form (228). Affected persons usually have AT III levels below 50% of normal, and they most often present between the ages of 15 and 30 years with lower limb venous thrombosis or pulmonary embolism. Factors precipitating this occurrence include pregnancy, infection, and surgery, so the primary clinical presentation may be either thrombosis after surgery or difficulty achieving adequate anticoagulation for CPB (211,212,227–229). The early institution of lifelong antithrombotic therapy after diagnosis decreases the incidence of thromboembolic phenomena by 65%.

Newborns and infants normally have AT III levels averaging 60% to 80% of adult levels, yet they do not exhibit the thrombotic events that adults do at these levels. AT III levels reach or exceed 90% of adult levels at approximately 3 months of age (230), which probably explains the relative heparin resistance of newborns in comparison with adults (Table 22.6).

Some investigators suggest that ACT is not an appropriate monitor for heparin-induced anticoagulation because of the extremes of hemodilution experienced in newborns and infants (54). Support for this opinion lies in the fact that both Hemochron and HemoTec ACT values increase at institution of CPB, whereas whole blood heparin concentrations decrease (231). Thus, the heparin administration protocol for pediatric patients undergoing CPB should account for a large volume of distribution, increased consumption, and a shorter elimination half-life. In a controlled trial, Turner-Gomes et al. (232) compared markers of thrombin generation and fibrinolysis in pediatric patients receiving either 1 U or 3 U of heparin per milliliter in the CPB circuit priming volume. The higher-dose heparin group did not demonstrate improved bleeding outcomes, but there was a trend toward lower D-dimer levels in this group. In monitoring the effects of heparin in pediatric patients, the mini-

mum acceptable ACT value should be increased or an additional monitor, such as heparin concentration, should be employed (233). For this reason, some might choose to increase the initial heparin dose (e.g., 400 U/kg) in newborns and small infants.

Heparin resistance can occur even if therapeutic plasma heparin concentrations are attained. In conjunction with measurable circulating heparin levels, heparin resistance is marked by the inability of heparin to suppress thrombin activity, a reaction that may be mediated through AT III. Acquired AT III deficiency is probably more common than inherited AT III deficiency. The multiple conditions associated with acquired AT III deficiency are listed in Table 22.7 (234–239). Certain other conditions, listed in Table 22.6, may also be related to acquired AT III deficiency (e.g., septicemia, endocarditis, hypercoagulable states). The most likely causes of AT III deficiency in patients requiring cardiac surgery are preoperative heparin treatment and disseminated intravascular coagulation. Heparin treatment decreases AT III levels (238), but the decrease usually plateaus at levels exceeding 60% of normal. The moderate heparin resistance often observed in patients receiving preoperative heparin therapy has not consistently been associated with decreased AT III levels (62,240,241). Moreover, AT III levels above 60% apparently do not predispose to thrombotic events in the nonsurgical setting (242). AT III levels can be measured preoperatively, although a critical AT III level has not been established for the cardiac surgical patient, and the absence of outcome data supporting this practice makes it most often seem inappropriate.

Antithrombin III deficiency in patients about to undergo CPB is largely a presumptive diagnosis based on substantial heparin resistance (e.g., failure to attain an ACT >300 seconds after administration of >600 U of heparin per kilogram). This condition has been shown both *in vivo* and *in vitro* to respond to fresh-frozen plasma, which contains normal concentrations of AT III (213,241,243,244), or to AT III concentrate (245). Heparin resistance resulting from

TABLE 22.7. CONDITIONS ASSOCIATED WITH ACQUIRED ANTITHROMBIN DEFICIENCY

Decreased synthesis from liver cirrhosis
Drug-induced
  L-Asparaginase
  Estrogens
  Heparin
Increased excretion
  Protein-losing enteropathy
  Inflammatory bowel disease
  Nephrotic syndrome
Accelerated consumption
  Disseminated intravascular coagulation
  Surgery
Dilutional
  Cardiopulmonary bypass
  Autologous blood withdrawal

AT III deficiency would be unlikely to respond to changing the biologic source of heparin from beef lung to porcine mucosa or vice versa. No guidelines or clinical studies formally establish an appropriate intervention threshold for fresh-frozen plasma or AT III concentrate. Because of the potential risks associated with fresh-frozen plasma (246), the authors prefer to persist with additional heparin under most circumstances, perhaps administering an AT III concentrate if an ACT above 400 seconds cannot be achieved after administration of 600 U of heparin per kilogram. Fresh-frozen plasma constitutes a less expensive source of AT III, but it is less specific and inconvenient, and it carries the risk for infectious complications. However, very high doses of heparin to overcome heparin resistance must be given with caution because a bleeding diathesis can result from fibrinolysis, platelet dysfunction, or heparin rebound. The volume of AT III or fresh-frozen plasma needed to raise AT III levels sufficiently to induce safe anticoagulation depends on the magnitude of the deficiency, but 500 to 1,000 U of AT III or 2 to 3 U of fresh-frozen plasma is sufficient for most adults. The ACT prolongation after administration of AT III or fresh-frozen plasma does not establish that AT III deficiency has caused the heparin resistance, because increasing plasma AT III levels should increase heparin-induced anticoagulation whether or not initial AT III levels are inadequate (241,247). This might be important if the cause of heparin resistance is HIT or marked thrombocytosis. In both instances, ACT may respond to AT III administration; however, other therapeutic modalities, such as plasmapheresis, would more specifically treat the mechanism of heparin resistance.

We believe that the use of fresh-frozen plasma to replace AT III deficiencies has become obsolete with the introduction of a human AT III concentrate (248). The AT III concentrate preparation is a stable, lyophilized product derived from pooled normal human plasma. It is heat-treated at $60° \pm 0.5°C$ for at least 10 hours and should therefore be relatively free of infectious agents. This concentrate has been used successfully to treat pregnancy-induced heparin resistance and other manifestations of AT III deficiency (249). In cardiac surgical procedures, Hashimoto et al. (250) evaluated the effect of AT III on markers of thrombin activity in adults and children. Although this was a descriptive study, the authors reported the use of lower heparin doses in patients receiving AT III. AT III therapy resulted in unchanged FpA levels during and after CPB, which suggests a reduction in thrombin activity, whereas control patients had large increases in FpA levels. In pediatric patients, the AT III level was most predictive of FpA production, whereas in adults, heparin concentration had the strongest correlation (250). Another study measuring AT III levels and a battery of coagulation tests in patients undergoing complex cardiac surgery demonstrated an inverse relationship between the production of FpA and AT III levels (246). The use of AT III therapy during heparinization for extracorporeal circulation enhances anticoagulation and may

theoretically prevent thrombosis by increasing heparin sensitivity and preserving platelets. The recommended dose (in units) to increase AT III activity from zero to 100% is 100 times the body weight (in kilograms), and the half-life is approximately 22 hours (249). The AT III level of an average adult would be raised approximately 30% with 1,000 U, which would probably equal the rise in AT III level accruing from 4 to 5 U of fresh-frozen plasma. Consequently, AT III concentrate constitutes the theoretical treatment of choice for severe heparin resistance for which the presumptive cause is AT III deficiency (e.g., active endocarditis with low-grade disseminated intravascular coagulation). Despite the apparently low risk and elimination of the waiting time required for thawing fresh-frozen plasma, before selecting this therapy one should consider the high cost of AT III concentrate and the rare occurrence of heparin resistance requiring therapy other than increased heparin doses. The cost of 1,000 U of AT III concentrate is approximately $650. Currently, the production of recombinant AT III is under investigation and holds promise for development of a product with an even lower risk profile than that of the currently available AT III concentrates. Clinical investigations with the recombinant product are currently underway.

ALTERNATIVES TO UNFRACTIONATED HEPARIN

Clinical situations that might call for avoidance of heparin include protamine allergy, HIT, or heparin allergy. Until recently, no viable alternatives existed, but at least three intravenous alternatives to unfractionated heparin are presently available. None of these drugs has yet been approved by the Food and Drug Administration for use in cardiac surgery in the United States.

Low-molecular-weight Heparin and Heparinoids

The discovery that different components of unfractionated heparin possess differing affinities for platelets and for AT III suggested a potential advantage to fractionating heparin into different compounds to be used for different indications (58,251–253). These heparin fractions are produced by either chemical or enzymatic depolymerization of conventional heparins or by *de novo* synthesis (254,255). At least six commercially prepared LMWH compounds have been studied for their ability to reduce venous thrombosis. These include enoxaparin sodium (Lovenox, Rhône-Poulenc Rorer); dalteparin sodium (Fragmin, Pharmacia & Upjohn); Fraxiparin (Sanofi); Logiparin (Novo Nordisk); RD Heparin (Wyeth-Ayerst); and danaparoid sodium (Lomoparan, Orgaran, manufactured by Organon). Enoxaparin and danaparoid have been approved by the United States Food and Drug Administration for prophylaxis against deep vein thrombosis. Methods used to depolymerize unfractionated heparin include nitrous acid (Fraxiparin, Fragmin), peroxidative depolymerization (RD Heparin), alkaline depolymerization (enoxaparin), gamma irradiation, and heparinase digestion (Logiparin). Lomoparan is a synthetic heparinoid compound prepared from a porcine intestinal source.

Shorter heparin chains have a lower affinity for platelets, bind less avidly to plasma proteins (256), and do not bind at all to endothelial cells in culture (257). The reduced protein binding may enhance the bioavailability of LMWH molecules and allow a more consistent dose–response relationship in comparison with that for unfractionated heparin. It is protein binding that facilitates digestion, elimination, and neutralization of anticoagulant effects. Thus, LMWH has a longer plasma half-life than unfractionated heparin. The half-lives of the different compounds range from 110 to 200 minutes (except for Lomoparan), and renal excretion is the principal route of elimination. As a result of their small size, LMWHs have a reduced ability to inhibit thrombin (factor IIa) but are potent inhibitors of factor Xa (58,258). Typically, only 25% to 50% of LMWH molecules contain the chain length necessary for binding factor IIa. The anti-Xa to anti-IIa ratios of LMWHs range from 2:1 to 4:1, with mean molecular weights of 4,000 to 6,500 Da (259); however, the distribution of molecular weights may differ among preparations, rendering mean molecular weight an inaccurate way to assess anti-IIa efficacy (260). Moderate inhibition of factor Xa appears to inhibit thrombus formation without impairing hemostasis as intensely as simultaneous inhibition of Xa and IIa; therefore, effective prophylaxis against deep vein thrombosis might occur with a lower incidence of bleeding complications (261). This potential benefit has fueled the development of many different LMWH compounds. Some evidence supports the antithrombotic efficacy of Xa inhibition, but other reports support the need for IIa inhibition to achieve the same goal (262–264).

The lower platelet binding capacity of LMWHs provides potential benefit in a number of clinical scenarios. LMWHs are less likely to cause HIT because they elicit less immune response than does unfractionated heparin (265). When platelet activity is measured with hemostatometry, the force of platelet retraction is minimally reduced by LMWH but is dramatically reduced by unfractionated heparin (266). When flow cytometric techniques are used to identify P-selectin, a marker for platelet activation, LMWH induces less platelet activation than does unfractionated heparin (80) (Fig. 22.16). In an *in vitro* study designed to test the proinflammatory and antiinflammatory responses to 2.5 U of unfractionated heparin per milliliter versus LMWH, the addition of these drugs to monocyte cell cultures induced similar increases in cytokine levels. Increases in interleukin-1β levels reached statistical significance only with unfractionated heparin (267).

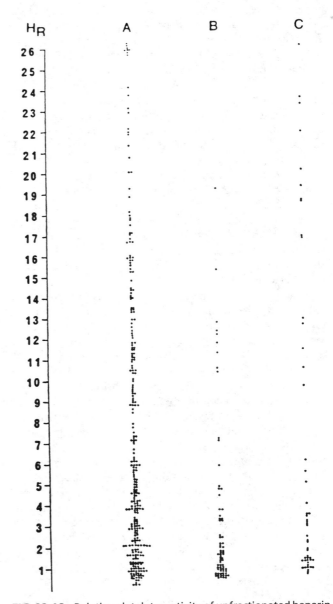

FIG. 22.16. Relative platelet reactivity of unfractionated heparin (**A**), low-molecular weight heparin (*LMWH*) (**B**), and hirudin (**C**), measured by hemostatometry, which yields values inversely related to platelet function. *HR* is a ratio of the hemostatometry measurement with anticoagulant to a baseline measurement with no anticoagulant. HR values of less than 1 indicate enhanced platelet reactivity, values between 1 and 10 indicate mild to moderate platelet inhibition, and values greater than 10 indicate severe platelet inhibition. Note that a significantly greater proportion of samples exposed to LMWH had preservation of platelet reactivity and a smaller number had platelet inhibition in comparison with samples exposed to unfractionated heparin. (From John LCH, Rees GM, Kovacs IB. Different anticoagulants and platelet reactivity in cardiac surgical patients. *Ann Thorac Surg* 1993;56: 899–902, with permission.)

Low-molecular-weight heparin therapy complicates heparin monitoring because APTT (and presumably ACT) are much less sensitive to Xa inhibition than to IIa (thrombin) inhibition (268). Factor Xa inhibition can be measured, but not with a simple bedside test (269–271). The difficulties of measuring Xa inhibition have complicated the potency standardization of LMWH compounds (45). The recent development of a standard based on potency of Xa inhibition should assist future comparisons of different LMWH compounds (24).

Intravenously administered LMWH has a half-life at least twice as long as that of unfractionated heparin, and the half-life of some LMWH compounds is possibly several times as long (45,252,281). The half-life poses a potential problem with LMWH use for CPB because Xa inhibition is much less responsive to protamine neutralization than is IIa inhibition, and the hemodynamic toxicity of protamine is still evident (272,273).

Some experience with LMWH for CPB has accrued. In 1983, Gouault-Heilmann et al. (274) reported LMWH use for a pulmonary embolectomy in a 66-year-old man suffering from HITT. Apparently no attempt was made to neutralize the LMWH after CPB, and postoperative blood loss figures were not reported. This patient survived in a situation in which, in theory, the administration of a large dose of unfractionated heparin might have induced severe morbidity via further intravascular clotting. After determining that LMWH could be used safely to anticoagulate sheep for CPB, Massonnet-Castel et al. (275) used LMWH to anticoagulate six adults undergoing elective procedures requiring CPB, decreasing the dose with each successive patient. Although no clots developed in the extracorporeal circuit, all patients bled excessively in the 6 hours following CPB. Although protamine was initially avoided, its use was deemed necessary in five patients, and the authors viewed heparin neutralization as only partially effective. Three of the six patients required reoperation for bleeding. One patient died 3 days later of a myocardial infarction, and autopsy revealed several "spots of subperitoneal hemorrhage." The same group subsequently reported anticoagulation in 15 patients undergoing CPB with LMWH doses smaller than the lowest dose administered in the previous report (276). Protamine was successfully avoided in nine patients, although three of those patients bled excessively. Three different patients received protamine as treatment for excessive bleeding, and this was again considered only partially effective because bleeding in two of these patients via their mediastinal tubes amounted to more than 2,000 mL in the first 24 hours. *In vitro* evidence supports a possible role for aminocaproic acid in this situation (272). Three patients received protamine prophylactically, and they did not bleed excessively despite the lack of effective reduction in anti-Xa activity by protamine. Touchot et al. (277) successfully anticoagulated nine dogs (one died of postoperative hemorrhage) and four patients with LMWH. No clots were seen during CPB, but no postoperative data were provided. Subsequently, a randomized prospective study of an extracorporeal CPB model in dogs compared unfractionated heparin (250 IU/kg) with the LMWH enoxaparin (250 anti-Xa U/kg) and measured hematologic variables up to 24 hours postoperatively. Protamine was used to reverse anticoagulation in both groups. These authors found no differences between the groups in postoperative blood loss or fibrin deposition on the arterial filters of the circuits, and they suggest that this anticoagulation regimen may be safe (278). Prospective randomized clinical studies in humans are still lacking.

Two glycosaminoglycans with heparin-like properties are available for clinical use: dermatan sulfate and danaparoid (Org 10172). These glycosaminoglycans are also referred to as *heparinoids* because they represent a class of synthetic or naturally occurring heparin analogues. Henny et al. (279) compared unfractionated heparin with danaparoid [a natural composite of heparan sulfate (80%), dermatan sulfate (20%), and chondroitin sulfates] for CPB in dogs and found that both produced satisfactory anticoagulation. The group receiving danaparoid experienced less postoperative bleeding despite the absence of protamine, which was administered to the dogs receiving heparin. Danaparoid has been shown to have a lower cross-reactivity with HIT antibodies than does LMWH (10% to 18%) and has been used successfully to anticoagulate patients with HIT for CPB. Monitoring the plasma level and the anti-Xa activity is strongly recommended because there is no known antidote for danaparoid excess, and bleeding complications have been demonstrated (280). Danaparoid was used successfully for CPB in one patient with HIT in whom a therapeutic APTT was maintained; however, macroscopic clots were noted in the circuit filters after CPB (281). Typically, danaparoid levels are maintained by a bolus dose aimed at achieving a plasma level of 1.0 to 1.5 U/mL. As expected, plasma danaparoid levels correlate poorly with the ACT and APTT (282). Many questions remain unanswered about LMWH and heparinoids for CPB, so this therapy must currently be viewed as experimental. Emergency CPB in a patient experiencing HIT is the only compelling indication, and other options may be preferred even in that setting.

Defibrinogenating Agents

Zulys et al. (283) prospectively reported the successful use of ancrod for CPB anticoagulation in 20 patients. Derived from Malayan pit viper venom, this agent lyses fibrinogen in a manner that precludes the formation of fibrin polymers. The unstable fibrin formed is removed from the circulation by fibrinolysis and reticuloendothelial sequestration. Ancrod also stimulates the release of tissue plasminogen activator (t-PA) from the vascular endothelium. The rapid elimination half-life of ancrod is 3 to 5 hours; however, achieving a sufficient fibrinogen depletion for safe CPB anticoagulation (plasma fibrinogen concentration of 0.4 to 0.8 g/L made APTT and ACT infinite) takes at least 12 hours.

Restoration of plasma coagulation after CPB requires fresh-frozen plasma and cryoprecipitate. When compared with 20 control patients receiving heparin-induced anticoagulation, the ancrod patients experienced no difference in blood loss but received more packed red blood cells, fresh-frozen plasma, and cryoprecipitate. A case report describes the successful use of ancrod anticoagulation in a patient in whom HITT was diagnosed and in whom LMWH failed to prevent the formation of thrombi in the extracorporeal circuit (284). Another patient in whom HIT was diagnosed underwent successful CPB anticoagulation with the combination of ancrod and danaparoid sodium (Orgaran). In this case, ancrod alone was ineffective in suppressing thrombin formation for CPB, but the combination allowed for safe CPB (285). The delayed onset and the increased need for homologous blood products represent clear disadvantages to the clinical use of ancrod. An antivenom is available, but it would not assist in the regeneration of fibrinogen, which is determined by the synthetic capacity of the liver.

Defibrinogenation can also be achieved with thrombolytic agents such as streptokinase and its derivatives urokinase and recombinant t-PA (286). This would be at the expense of increased plasmin formation and commensurate hyperfibrinolysis, which would set the stage for a potentially severe post-CPB coagulopathy. Consequently, thrombolytic agents would serve as undesirable heparin substitutes and probably should not be considered except in an emergency when heparin is relatively contraindicated (e.g., ongoing HITT) and other heparin substitutes are unavailable.

Hirudin and Congeners

Hirudin

A coagulation inhibitor isolated from the salivary glands of the medicinal leech (*Hirudo medicinalis*), hirudin is a potent inhibitor of thrombin that, unlike heparin, acts independently of AT III and inhibits clot-bound in addition to fluid-phase thrombin (287,288). Currently available via recombinant genetics, this substance is a polypeptide (molecular weight of approximately 7,000 Da) that has been used in patients with chronic disseminated intravascular coagulation (287). Pharmacokinetic studies in healthy volunteers show a plasma elimination half-life of approximately 1 hour and a urinary excretion half-life of 2 1/2 hours (288). After an intravenous bolus, the APTT is prolonged markedly but transiently, returning to normal in 15 minutes, whereas the TT remains markedly prolonged for 2 to 3 hours. The APTT prolongation correlates well with plasma hirudin levels but does not correlate well with chromogenic antifactor II levels. For this reason, a surrogate PTT with the snake venom ecarin for activation has been described. This whole blood test yields excellent linear correlation with *in vitro* hirudin concentrations between 0.5 and 4 μg/mL, with coefficients of variation of 2% to 5% (289). Walenga et al. (290) prospectively compared two hirudin dosing protocols

with traditional heparin anticoagulation in 30 dogs and found that hirudin induced satisfactory anticoagulation that appears measurable with ACT. The relatively short-lived effect of a single intravenous bolus suggests the advisability of bolus administration followed by a continuous infusion. The authors report that all clotting times returned to normal within 30 minutes of hirudin discontinuation, but one of their figures suggests moderate ACT prolongation for as much as 2 hours. The hirudin groups displayed a trend toward increased blood loss in the 150-minute observation period after CPB, but this did not reach statistical significance. In a pig model, heparin (400 IU/kg) was compared with hirudin (1 mg/kg) during 60 minutes of extracorporeal circulation. There were no gross thrombotic episodes noted in either group. Moreover, pigs in the heparin group exhibited a higher incidence of fibrin deposition on the arterial line filters, detected by electron microscopy, and a higher incidence of tissue bleeding. Platelet aggregation was also better preserved in the hirudin group than in the heparin group (291). Although human studies are lacking, recombinant hirudin shows greater promise than LMWH or ancrod as a substitute for heparin-induced anticoagulation.

Hirudin may demonstrate an additional benefit as an anticoagulant for CPB in that it has been shown to inhibit the platelet activation induced by non-ionic contrast media (292). The mechanism of this has not been investigated; however, one could speculate that hirudin inhibits platelet activation induced by CPB.

Bivalirudin (Hirulog)

The synthetic peptide bivalirudin, formerly hirulog, is a bivalent thrombin inhibitor consisting of a moiety that binds to the active-site cleft of thrombin, and a hirudin-like C-terminal region that binds to the positively charged surface groove of thrombin known as the anion-binding exosite. Bivalirudin has advantages in regard to both safety and potential efficacy over hirudin. Bivalirudin appears to have a wider therapeutic window, possibly because it only transiently inhibits the active site of thrombin. The better safety profile of bivalirudin permits administration of higher doses, which may give it an efficacy advantage. Hirudin prevents thrombin from activating protein C, thereby suppressing an anticoagulant pathway. In contrast, bivalirudin may promote protein C activation by transiently inhibiting thrombin until it can be bound by thrombomodulin. Differences between bivalirudin, hirudin, and other direct thrombin inhibitors illustrate that all direct thrombin inhibitors do not have equivalent risk–benefit profiles. The safe use of bivalirudin as an anticoagulant for CPB has not been determined.

Platelet Inhibitors

Pharmacologic platelet inhibition has been used to supplement or replace heparin for CPB anticoagulation. This technique is discussed in Chapter 24.

Coated Surfaces

This topic is discussed in Chapter 29.

Factor Inhibitors

The development of factor IXa inhibitor (factor IXai) represents a novel approach to designing the optimal anticoagulant for CPB. This molecule was developed by modifying the active site of the enzyme. Factor IXai competitively blocks active factor IX and replaces it in the intrinsic coagulation cascade, thereby preventing activation of factor X and thrombin formation via this pathway. It leaves the extrinsic coagulation pathway intact, allowing for normal coagulation in response to tissue factor release. Twenty mongrel dogs undergoing CPB were studied, 15 receiving factor IXai (300 to 600 μg/kg) and five receiving standard heparin and protamine. The group receiving IXai experienced no fibrin deposition in the circuit and less bleeding than did the heparin group (293). A case is described in which a patient on ventricular assist device received factor IXai, with subsequent reductions in markers of thrombin activation and activity; however, these results are difficult to interpret as the patient proceeded to have a massive hemorrhagic death (294). Trials with a specific factor Xa inhibitor have not been able to demonstrate reduced thrombin formation and in fact have shown increased fibrin formation in comparison with heparin and LMWH anticoagulation (295).

HEPARIN-INDUCED THROMBOCYTOPENIA

The syndrome known as HIT develops in anywhere from 5% to 28% of patients receiving heparin and is commonly divided into two subtypes. Type I HIT, characterized by a mild decrease in platelet count, results from the proaggregatory effects of heparin on platelets (77). Type II HIT is considerably more severe, most often occurs after more than 5 days of heparin administration (average onset time of 9 days), and is most likely immune-mediated. Antibody binding directly to the heparin molecule was sought initially but was not consistently demonstrated. It has subsequently been shown that antibody binds to the complex formed between heparin and PF4 to cause the syndrome, so the heparin–PF4 complex acts as an antigenic stimulus (296,297). These heparin–PF4 complexes bind to platelets and endothelial cells, which become activated when antibody binds. Associated immune-mediated endothelial injury and complement activation may set the stage for the activated platelets to adhere, aggregate, and form platelet clots (298,299). When carried to an extreme, this syndrome can cause severe morbidity or fatal intravascular thromboembolic phenomena (300,301). Among the patients in whom HIT develops, the incidence of thrombotic complications approximates 20%, which in turn may carry a mortality rate as high as 35% (302). Both of these figures may be overestimated as a result of reporting

bias, although some prospective investigations support the 20% incidence of thrombosis (76,302). Demonstration of heparin-induced aggregation of platelets confirms the diagnosis of HIT type II (303). This can be accomplished with a heparin-induced serotonin release assay (304) or a specific heparin-induced platelet activation assay (305). A highly specific enzyme-linked immunosorbent assay for the heparin–PF4 complex has been developed and used to delineate the course of immunoglobulin G and immunoglobulin M antibody responses in patients exposed to unfractionated heparin during cardiac surgery (306).

This syndrome differs from other immune-mediated, drug-induced thrombocytopenias in the following ways: (a) The antibodies associated with heparin-induced thrombocytopenia often become undetectable several weeks after the drug is discontinued, (b) the clinical syndrome does not always recur on reexposure to the drug and sometimes resolves despite continued drug therapy, (c) the *in vitro* platelet aggregation reaction is sometimes patient-specific, and (d) thrombosis and disseminated intravascular coagulation develop only in some patients (76,302). Most studies have found a fivefold higher incidence with bovine lung heparin than with porcine mucosal heparin (76,77,302,307–310).

How does the occurrence of this syndrome influence anticoagulation for CPB? Prophylactic continuous intravenous heparin therapy decreases the incidence of thrombotic complications of anterior myocardial infarction, of recurrent thrombosis after percutaneous transluminal coronary angioplasty for acute coronary thrombosis, and of myocardial infarction in patients with unstable angina pectoris (84,311–313). Because some of these patients may need subsequent surgical myocardial revascularization, the possibility exists that patients could present for urgent surgery with unrecognized HIT. In clinical settings other than CPB, initiating therapeutic heparin doses in patients with unrecognized HIT has been associated with life-threatening complications (76). A report of two cases documents HIT in which the sole exposure to heparin was intermittent flushing of a single intraarterial catheter used only for intraoperative monitoring. One of these cases proved fatal (314). Would the larger heparin doses administered for CPB induce profound thrombocytopenia or acute intravascular thrombosis in patients with unrecognized or incipient HIT? Reports of such events could not be found, but thrombocytopenia disproportionate to hemodilution has been reported in such situations, even in the protective presence of antiplatelet drugs (315,316). Heparin resistance commonly occurs in patients receiving heparin infusions in whom thrombocytopenia has not developed, but it has also been temporally associated with HIT (76,317,318). Consequently, unrecognized HIT should be considered in the differential diagnosis of intraoperative heparin resistance in patients receiving preoperative heparin therapy.

Patients with existing HIT or a history of HIT pose special therapeutic difficulties. In essence, a patient for whom heparin is contraindicated is placed in a clinical situation that requires the use of heparin. Several approaches to this dilemma have been taken. Olinger et al. (317) reported three patients in whom discontinuation of heparin for 4 to 8 weeks resulted in resolution of the antiplatelet antibody reaction. Those patients then tolerated the brief period of heparinization for CPB without complication and without development of thrombocytopenia beyond that expected from hemodilution. Because HIT often requires 2 to 6 days to recur once the antibodies have cleared, this approach seems reasonable for patients whose need for cardiac surgery is not urgent. The antibody response might not always resolve within 8 weeks, however.

Changing the tissue source of heparin might circumvent the reaction (319), although cross-reactivity often exists, so this approach should be taken only if it can be proved safe by testing the patient's platelet-rich plasma *in vitro* with the alternative heparin. Some types of LMWH have proved effective in heparin-induced thrombocytopenia (see above), but their use presents another set of problems, and nonreactivity with the patient's platelets should be confirmed *in vitro* before this option is selected (320). Low-molecular-weight heparinoids appear safer than LMWHs in this setting (321). Supplementation of heparin administration with pharmacologic platelet inhibition via prostacyclin, iloprost, aspirin, or aspirin and dipyridamole has been reported (315,316,322,324), all with favorable outcomes. The use of iloprost titrated to a documented level of platelet functional suppression permitted heparin use without undue thrombocytopenia (322,324), whereas aspirin or aspirin plus dipyridamole may less consistently protect against thrombocytopenia (315,316). It seems logical that prostaglandin E_1 would also serve effectively in this role (325,326), although this agent shares the vasodilator side effect of prostacyclin. Plasmapheresis acutely reduced heparin-induced platelet aggregation in two cases (327,328). All of the above options involve maneuvers designed to reduce or eliminate the harmful effects of heparin while accepting the unavoidability of heparin-induced anticoagulation for CPB. The use of heparin could be avoided altogether by anticoagulating with ancrod or hirudin.

Hirudin has specific advantages in the treatment of patients with HIT because, unlike heparin, hirudin does not require a cofactor, is capable of inhibiting "clot-bound" thrombin, and is not susceptible to neutralization by PF4. This would seem beneficial in patients in whom platelet activation and thrombosis are a hallmark of disease. In a prospective study, recombinant hirudin was given successfully for CPB as a bolus of 0.25 mg/kg, followed by administration of a 5-mg bolus whenever the hirudin concentration fell below 2,500 ng/mL, determined by the ecarin clotting time (329). This study also treated noncardiac surgical patients experiencing HIT or HITT with recombinant hirudin and compared their outcomes with those of a historical control group. They found that patients treated with recombinant hirudin sustained increases in their platelet counts and maintained stable hemoglobin levels with very few

bleeding complications. Median plasma hirudin levels in the noncardiac surgical patients with thrombosis ranged from 1,149 to 1,698 ng/mL. The incidence of death, new limb amputations, or thromboembolic complications was lower in the hirudin group, with a risk-adjusted hazard ratio of 0.508 (95% CI, 0.290 to 0.892; $p = 0.014$).

CONCLUSION

Advances in our understanding of coagulation and our ability to monitor for appropriate levels of anticoagulation during CPB allow us to employ extracorporeal circulation safely in a variety of clinical settings. Inhibition of microvascular coagulation is important for minimization of the inflammatory response to CPB, and reversal of this effect is important in postoperative hemostasis. The aforementioned devices, tests, and pharmaceuticals are important components in the blood conservation armamentarium for patients undergoing cardiac surgery.

KEY POINTS

- *Heparin* is a heterogeneous, heavily sulfated polysaccharide compound derived from pig intestinal mucosa or bovine lung. Some of the polysaccharide chains possess a specific pentasaccharide sequence that binds AT III, profoundly facilitating its native ability to inhibit plasma coagulation, most prominently through inhibition of factors IIa (thrombin) and Xa. Longer polysaccharide chains effectively inhibit IIa and Xa, whereas shorter chains preferentially inhibit Xa. Heparin offers the advantages of a rapid onset of action, clinical efficacy as an anticoagulant for CPB, and rapid neutralization by protamine.
- Common or routine *side effects of heparin* include facilitation of fibrinolysis, stimulation of tissue factor pathway inhibitor, platelet binding and activation, activation of lipoprotein lipase, and a decrease in systemic vascular resistance. HITT represents an immune and potentially life-threatening reaction that occurs in 5% to 28% of patients, who most often have been receiving heparin for a period of several days. Heparin administration has rarely been associated with immediate anaphylaxis or pulmonary edema.
- Anticoagulation with heparin for CPB can be monitored by measuring clotting times or whole blood heparin concentrations. Of the many tests available, those most commonly used for CPB are the *ACT* and *heparin concentration* as determined by an automated protamine titration method. The ACT shows that anticoagulation has occurred, but it is imprecise, results vary among different commonly used ACT techniques, and it is prolonged by hypothermia and hemodilution. Au-

tomated heparin concentrations generally remain stable with hypothermia and hemodilution but do not measure the degree of anticoagulation. Newer clotting tests showing some promise for heparin monitoring include the heparin management test and the high-dose thrombin time.

- *Clinical outcome studies* do not clearly demonstrate the superiority of any specific heparin monitoring or dosing technique, but they do show that anticoagulation with heparin is incomplete (as judged by markers of thrombin activity) regardless of dose. For most clinical situations requiring CPB, the authors recommend monitoring ACT and maintaining levels above 400 seconds. Some exceptions (e.g., aprotinin use) are detailed in the text.

- *Heparin resistance*, defined as the need for higher-than-normal doses of heparin to achieve the desired level of anticoagulation for CPB, has a variety of potential causes and may be multifactorial in any specific patient. When excessive doses of heparin are required to achieve a desired ACT, the authors recommend administering an AT III concentrate, although fresh-frozen plasma will also suffice.

- Several *alternatives to heparin* have undergone investigation in animal models, humans, or both. LMWHs and low-molecular-weight heparinoids appear unsatisfactory for CPB because of limited thrombin inhibition, long clinical half-lives, difficulty in monitoring anticoagulation, and incomplete reversal with protamine. Other possibilities include ancrod, hirudin and its congeners, and factor IXa inhibitor.

- When patients with *HIT* present for cardiac surgery requiring CPB, several clinical approaches have been used successfully. The approach should probably vary according to the presence or absence of active disease (as judged by diagnostic assays), the severity of disease, and the urgency of surgery. Depending on these factors, approaches may include delaying surgery to allow "business as usual" with heparin, preoperative pharmacologic inactivation of platelets in preparation for intraoperative anticoagulation with heparin, or selection of an anticoagulant other than heparin.

REFERENCES

1. Gibbon JH Jr. Application of a mechanical heart and lung apparatus to cardiac surgery. *Minn Med* 1954;37:171–185.
2. McLean J. The discovery of heparin. *Circulation* 1959;19:75–78.
3. Howell WH, Holt E. Two new factors in blood coagulation—heparin and pro-antithrombin. *Am J Physiol* 1918;viii:328–341.
4. Best CH. Preparation of heparin and its use in the first clinical cases. *Circulation* 1959;19:79–86.
5. Chargaff E, Olson KB. Studies on the chemistry of blood coagulation. VI. Studies on the action of heparin and other anticoagulants. The influence of protamine on the anticoagulant effect *in vivo. J Biol Chem* 1938;125:671–676.
6. Gibbon JH Jr. The maintenance of life during experimental occlusion of the pulmonary artery followed by survival. *Surg Gynecol Obstet* 1939;69:602–614.
7. Nader HB, Dietrich CP. Natural occurrence and possible biological role of heparin. In: Lane DA, Lindahl U, eds. *Heparin. Chemical and biological properties, clinical applications.* Boca Raton, FL: CRC Press, 1989:81–96.
8. Folkman J, Ingber DE. Angiogenesis: regulatory role of heparin and related molecules. In: Lane DA, Lindahl U, eds. *Heparin. Chemical and biological properties, clinical applications.* Boca Raton, FL: CRC Press, 1989:317–333.
9. Olivecrona T, Bengtsson-Olivecrona G. Heparin and lipases. In: Lane DA, Lindahl U, eds. *Heparin. Chemical and biological properties, clinical applications.* Boca Raton, FL: CRC Press, 1989:335–361.
10. Stiekema JCJ. Heparin and its biocompatibility. *Clin Nephrol* 1986;26[Suppl 1]:S3–S8.
11. Hirsh J. Heparin. *N Engl J Med* 1991;324:1565–1574.
12. Thomas DP, Barrowcliffe TW, Johnson EA. The influence of tissue source, salt and molecular weight on heparin activity. *Scand J Haematol* 1980;25[Suppl 36]:40–48.
13. Walton PL, Ricketts CR, Bangham DR. Heterogeneity of heparin. *Br J Haematol* 1966;12:310–325.
14. Jaques LB, McDuffie NM. The chemical and anticoagulant nature of heparin. *Semin Thromb Hemost* 1978;4:277–297.
15. Rodriguez HJ, Vanderwielen AJ. Molecular weight determination of commercial heparin sodium USP and its sterile solutions. *J Pharm Sci* 1979;68:588–591.
16. Lasker SE. The heterogeneity of heparins. *Fed Proc* 1977;36:92–97.
17. Eika C. The platelet aggregating effect of eight commercial heparins. *Scand J Haematol* 1972;9:480–482.
18. Casu B. Methods of structural analysis. In: Lane DA, Lindahl U, eds. *Heparin. Chemical and biological properties, clinical applications.* Boca Raton, FL: CRC Press, 1989:25–49.
19. Rosenberg RD. Biochemistry of heparin antithrombin interactions, and the physiologic role of this natural anticoagulant mechanism. *Am J Med* 1989;87[Suppl 3B]:2S–9S.
20. Bangham DR, Woodward PM. A collaborative study of heparins from different sources. *Bull World Health Organ* 1970;42:129–149.
21. Novak E, Sekhar NC, Dunham NW, et al. A comparative study of the effect of lung and gut heparins on platelet aggregation and protamine neutralization in man. *Clin Med* 1972;79:22–27.
22. Casu B, Guerrini M, Naggi A, et al. Characterization of sulfation patterns of beef and pig mucosal heparins by nuclear magnetic resonance spectroscopy. *Arzneimittelforschung* 1996;46:472–477.
23. Silverglade A. Biological equivalence of beef lung and hog mucosal heparins. *Curr Ther Res* 1975;18:91–103.
24. Barrowcliffe TW. Heparin assays and standardization. In: Lane DA, Lindahl U, eds. *Heparin. Chemical and biological properties, clinical applications.* Boca Raton, FL: CRC Press, 1989:393–415.
25. Baltes BJ, Diamond S, D'Agostino RJ. Comparison of anticoagulant activity of two preparations of purified heparin. *Clin Pharmacol Ther* 1973;14:287–290.
26. Abbott WM, Warnock DF, Austen WG. The relationship of heparin source to the incidence of delayed hemorrhage. *J Surg Res* 1977;22:593–597.
27. Stewart SR, Gaich PA. Clinical comparison of two brands of heparin for use in cardiopulmonary bypass. *J Extracorp Technol* 1980;12:29–33.
28. Fiser WP, Read RC, Wright FE, et al. A randomized study of

beef lung and pork mucosal heparin in cardiac surgery. *Ann Thorac Surg* 1983;35:615–620.

29. Lowary LR, Smith FA, Coyne E, et al. Comparative neutralization of lung- and mucosal-derived heparin by protamine sulfate using *in vitro* and *in vivo* methods. *J Pharm Sci* 1971;60:638–640.

30. Barrowcliffe TW, Johnson EA, Eggleton CA, et al. Anticoagulant activities of lung and mucous heparins. *Thromb Res* 1977;12:27–36.

31. Thomas DP, Sagar S, Stamatakis JD, et al. Plasma heparin levels after administration of calcium and sodium salts of heparin. *Thromb Res* 1976;9:241–248.

32. Whitehead MI, McCarthy TG. A comparative trial of subcutaneous sodium and calcium heparin as assessed by local haematoma formation and pain. In: Kakkar VV, Thomas DP, eds. *Heparin: chemistry and clinical usage.* London: Academic Press, 1976:361–366.

33. Merton RE, Curtis AD, Thomas DP. A comparison of heparin potency estimates obtained by activated partial thromboplastin time and British pharmacopoeial assays. *Thromb Haemost* 1985;53:116–117.

34. Effeney DJ, Goldstone J, Chin D, et al. Intraoperative anticoagulation in cardiovascular surgery. *Surgery* 1981;90:1068–1074.

35. Gravlee GP, Angert KC, Tucker WY, et al. Early anticoagulation peak and rapid distribution after intravenous heparin. *Anesthesiology* 1988;68:126–129.

36. Estes JW. The fate of heparin in the body. *Curr Ther Res* 1975;18:45–57.

37. Estes JW. Clinical pharmacokinetics of heparin. *Clin Pharmacokinet* 1980;5:204–220.

38. Hiebert LM, Jaques LB. The observation of heparin on endothelium after injection. *Thromb Res* 1976;8:195–204.

39. Glimelius B, Busch C, Hook M. Binding of heparin on the surface of cultured human endothelial cells. *Thromb Res* 1978;12:773–782.

40. Bârzu T, Molho P, Tobelem G, et al. Binding and endocytosis of heparin by human endothelial cells in culture. *Biochim Biophys Acta* 1985;845:196–203.

41. Mahadoo J, Heibert L, Jaques LB. Vascular sequestration of heparin. *Thromb Res* 1977;12:79–90.

42. Jaques LB, Mahadoo J. Pharmacodynamics and clinical effectiveness of heparin. *Semin Thromb Hemost* 1978;4:298–325.

43. Castellot JJ Jr, Wong K, Herman B, et al. Binding and internalization of heparin by vascular smooth muscle cells. *J Cell Physiol* 1985;124:13–20.

44. Dawes J, Pepper DS. Catabolism of low-dose heparin in man. *Thromb Res* 1979;14:845–860.

45. Albada J, Nieuwenhuis HK, Sixma JJ. Pharmacokinetics of standard and low molecular weight heparin. In: Lane DA, Lindahl U, eds. *Heparin. Chemical and biological properties, clinical applications.* Boca Raton, FL: CRC Press, 1989:417–431.

46. de Swart CAM, Nijmeyer B, Roelofs JMM, et al. Kinetics of intravenously administered heparin in normal humans. *Blood* 1982;60:1251–1258.

47. Olsson P, Lagergren H, Ek S. The elimination from plasma of intravenous heparin. An experimental study on dogs and humans. *Acta Med Scand* 1963;173:619–630.

48. Bjornsson TD, Wolfram KM, Kitchell BB. Heparin kinetics determined by three assay methods. *Clin Pharmacol Ther* 1982;31:104–113.

49. Cohen JA, Frederickson EL, Kaplan JA. Plasma heparin activity and antagonism during cardiopulmonary bypass with hypothermia. *Anesth Analg* 1977;56:564–570.

50. Wright JS, Osborn JJ, Perkins HA, et al. Heparin levels during and after hypothermic perfusion. *J Cardiovasc Surg* 1964;5:244–250.

51. Bull BS, Korpman RA, Huse WM, et al. Heparin therapy during extracorporeal circulation. I. Problems inherent in existing heparin protocols. *J Thorac Cardiovasc Surg* 1975;69:674–684.

52. Mabry CD, Read RC, Thompson BW, et al. Identification of heparin resistance during cardiac and vascular surgery. *Arch Surg* 1979;114:129–134.

53. Estes JW. Kinetics of the anticoagulant effect of heparin. *JAMA* 1970;212:1492–1495.

54. Horkay F, Martin P, Rajah M, et al. Response to heparinization in adults and children undergoing cardiac operations. *Ann Thorac Surg* 1992;53:822–826.

55. Villanueva GB, Danishefsky I. Evidence for a heparin-induced conformational change on antithrombin III. *Biochem Biophys Res Commun* 1977;74:803–809.

56. Björk I, Olson ST, Shore JD. Molecular mechanisms of the accelerating effect of heparin on the reactions between antithrombin and clotting proteinases. In: Lane DA, Lindahl U, eds. *Heparin. Chemical and biological properties, clinical applications.* Boca Raton, FL: CRC Press, 1989:229–255.

57. Pixley RA, Colman RW. Effect of heparin on the inactivation rate of human activated factor XII by antithrombin III. *Blood* 1985;66:198–203.

58. Holmer E. Low molecular weight heparin. In: Lane DA, Lindahl U, eds. *Heparin. Chemical and biological properties, clinical applications.* Boca Raton, FL: CRC Press, 1989:575–595.

59. Ofosu FA, Fernandez F, Gauthier D, et al. Heparin cofactor II and other endogenous factors in the mediation of the antithrombotic and anticoagulant effects of heparin and dermatan sulfate. *Semin Thromb Hemost* 1985;11:133–137.

60. de Takats G. Heparin tolerance. A test of the clotting mechanism. *Surg Gynecol Obstet* 1943;77:31–39.

61. Monkhouse FC, MacMillan RL, Brown KWG. The relation between heparin blood levels and blood coagulation times. *J Lab Clin Med* 1953;42:92–97.

62. Esposito RA, Culliford AT, Colvin SB, et al. Heparin resistance during cardiopulmonary bypass. The role of heparin pretreatment. *J Thorac Cardiovasc Surg* 1983;85:346–353.

63. Doty DB, Knott HW, Hoyt JL, et al. Heparin dose for accurate anticoagulation in cardiac surgery. *J Cardiovasc Surg* 1979;20:597–604.

64. Stenbjerg S, Berg E, Albrechtsen OK. Heparin levels and activated clotting time (ACT) during open heart surgery. *Scand J Haematol* 1981;26:281–284.

65. Jaberi M, Bell WR, Benson DW. Control of heparin therapy in open-heart surgery. *J Thorac Cardiovasc Surg* 1974;67:133–141.

66. Friesen RH, Clement AJ. Individual responses to heparinization for extracorporeal circulation. *J Thorac Cardiovasc Surg* 1976;72:875–879.

67. Akl BF, Vargas GM, Neal J, et al. Clinical experience with the activated clotting time for the control of heparin and protamine therapy during cardiopulmonary bypass. *J Thorac Cardiovasc Surg* 1980;79:97–102.

68. Culliford AT, Gitel SN, Starr N, et al. Lack of correlation between activated clotting time and plasma heparin during cardiopulmonary bypass. *Ann Surg* 1981;193:105–111.

69. Bull BS, Huse WM, Brauer FS, et al. Heparin therapy during extracorporeal circulation. II. The use of a dose–response curve to individualize heparin and protamine dosage. *J Thorac Cardiovasc Surg* 1975;69:685–689.

70. Fareed J, Walenga JM, Hoppensteadt DA, et al. Studies on the profibrinolytic actions of heparin and its fractions. *Semin Thromb Hemost* 1985;11:199–207.

71. Upchurch GR, Valeri CR, Khuri SF, et al. Effect of heparin on fibrinolytic activity and platelet function *in vivo. Am J Physiol* 1996;271:H528–H534.

72. Carr ME, Carr SL, Greilich PE. Heparin ablates force development during platelet-mediated clot retraction. *Thromb Haemost* 1996;75:674–678.

73. Suda Y, Marques D, Kermode JC, et al. Structural characterization of heparin's binding domain for human platelets. *Thromb Res* 1993;69:501–508.

74. Holmer E, Lindahl U, Bäckström G, et al. Anticoagulant activities and effects on platelets of a heparin fragment with high affinity for antithrombin. *Thromb Res* 1980;18:861–869.

75. Cella G, Scattolo N, Luzzatto G, et al. Effects of low-molecular-weight heparin on platelets as compared with commercial heparin. *Res Exp Med* 1984;184:227–229.

76. Warkentin TE, Kelton JG. Heparin and platelets. *Hematol Oncol Clin North Am* 1990;4:243–264.

77. Salzman EW, Rosenberg RD, Smith MH, et al. Effect of heparin and heparin fractions on platelet aggregation. *J Clin Invest* 1980;65:64–73.

78. Bode AP, Castellani WJ, Hodges ED, et al. The effect of lysed platelets on neutralization of heparin *in vitro* with protamine as measured by the activated coagulation time (ACT). *Thromb Haemost* 1991;66:213–271.

79. Xiao Z, Theroux P. Platelet activation with unfractionated heparin at therapeutic concentrations and comparisons with a low-molecular-weight heparin and with a direct thrombin inhibitor. *Circulation* 1998;97:251–256.

80. Rohrer MJ, Kestin AS, Ellis PA, et al. High-dose heparin suppresses platelet alpha granule secretion. *J Vasc Surg* 1992;15:1000–1008.

81. Carr ME, Carr SL. At high heparin concentrations, protamine concentrations which reverse heparin anticoagulant effects are insufficient to reverse heparin anti-platelet effects. *Thromb Res* 1994;75:617–630.

82. Cines DB. Heparin: do we understand its antithrombotic actions? *Chest* 1986;89:420–426.

83. Myers TM, Hull RD, Weg JG. Antithrombotic therapy for venous thromboembolic disease. *Chest* 1986;89[Suppl]:26S–35S.

84. Kaplan K. Prophylactic anticoagulation following acute myocardial infarction. *Arch Intern Med* 1986;146:593–597.

85. Levine MN. Nonhemorrhagic complications of anticoagulant therapy. *Semin Thromb Hemost* 1986;12:63–66.

86. Khuri SF, Valeri CR, Loscalzo J, et al. Heparin causes platelet dysfunction and induces fibrinolysis before cardiopulmonary bypass. *Ann Thorac Surg* 1995;60:1008–1014.

87. Despotis GJ, Joist JH, Hogue CW, et al. More effective suppression of hemostatic system activation in patients undergoing cardiac surgery by heparin dosing based on heparin blood concentrations rather than ACT. *Thromb Haemost* 1996;76:902–908.

88. Seltzer JL, Gerson JI. Decrease in arterial pressure following heparin injection prior to cardiopulmonary bypass. *Acta Anaesthesiol Scand* 1979;23:575–578.

89. Urban P, Scheidegger D, Buchmann B, et al. The hemodynamic effects of heparin and their relation to ionized calcium levels. *J Thorac Cardiovasc Surg* 1986;91:303–306.

90. Jaques LB. Heparin: an old drug with a new paradigm. Current discoveries are establishing the nature, action, and biological significance of this valuable drug. *Science* 1979;206:528–533.

91. Harada A, Tatsuno K, Kikuchi T, et al. Use of bovine lung heparin to obviate anaphylactic shock caused by porcine gut heparin. *Ann Thorac Surg* 1990;49:826–827.

92. Ahmed SS, Nussbaum M. Development of pulmonary edema related to heparin administration. *J Clin Pharmacol* 1981;21:126–128.

93. Dux S, Pitlik S, Perry G, et al. Hypersensitivity reaction to chlorbutol-preserved heparin [Letter]. *Lancet* 1981;1:149.

94. Hancock BW, Naysmith A. Hypersensitivity to chlorocresol-preserved heparin. *BMJ* 1975;3:746–747.

95. Ansell JE, Clark WP Jr, Compton CC. Fatal reactions associated with intravenous heparin. *Drug Intell Clin Pharm* 1986;20:74–75.

96. Rosenzweig P, Gary NE, Gocke DJ, et al. Heparin allergy accompanying acute renal failure. *Artif Organs* 1979;3:78–79.

97. Bernstein IL. Anaphylaxis to heparin sodium. Report of a case, with immunologic studies. *JAMA* 1956;161:1379–1380.

98. Klein HG, Bell WR. Disseminated intravascular coagulation during heparin therapy. *Ann Intern Med* 1974;80:477–481.

99. Schey SA. Hypersensitivity reactions to heparin and the use of new low molecular weight heparins. *Eur J Haematol* 1989;42:107.

100. Yourassowsky E, de Broe ME, Wieme RJ. Effect of heparin on gentamicin concentration in blood. *Clin Chim Acta* 1972;42:189–191.

101. Colburn WA. Pharmacologic implications of heparin interactions with other drugs. *Drug Metab Rev* 1976;5:281–293.

102. Levine MN, Hirsh J. Hemorrhagic complications of anticoagulant therapy. *Semin Thromb Hemost* 1986;12:39–57.

103. Leehey D, Gantt C, Lim V. Heparin-induced hypoaldosteronism. Report of a case. *JAMA* 1981;246:2189–2190.

104. Majerus PW, Broze GJ, Miletich JP, et al. Anticoagulant thrombolytic and anti-platelet drugs. In: Gilman AG, Rall TW, Nies AS, et al., eds. *Goodman and Gilman's pharmacological basis of therapeutics,* 8th ed. New York: Pergamon Press, 1990:1311–1331.

105. Salomon F, Schmid M. Heparin [Letter]. *N Engl J Med* 1991;325:1585.

106. Hattersley PG. Activated coagulation time of whole blood. *JAMA* 1966;196:436–440.

107. Blakely JA. A rapid bedside method for the control of heparin therapy. *Can Med Assoc J* 1968;99:1072–1076.

108. Hill JD, Dontigny L, de Leval M, et al. A simple method of heparin management during prolonged extracorporeal circulation. *Ann Thorac Surg* 1974;17:129–134.

109. Umlas J, Gauvin G, Taff R. Heparin monitoring and neutralization during cardiopulmonary bypass using a rapid plasma separator and a fluorometric assay. *Ann Thorac Surg* 1984;37:301–303.

110. Jobes DR, Schwartz AJ, Ellison N, et al. Monitoring heparin anticoagulation and its neutralization. *Ann Thorac Surg* 1981;31:161–166.

111. Bjornsson TD, Nash PV. Variability in heparin sensitivity of APTT reagents. *Am J Clin Pathol* 1986;86:199–204.

112. Brandt JT, Triplett DA. Laboratory monitoring of heparin. Effect of reagents and instruments on the activated partial thromboplastin time. *Am J Clin Pathol* 1981;76:530–537.

113. Ts'ao CH, Galluzzo TS, Lo R, et al. Whole-blood clotting time, activated partial thromboplastin time, and whole-blood recalcification time as heparin monitoring tests. *Am J Clin Pathol* 1979;71:17–21.

114. Delorme MA, Inwood MJ, O'Keefe B. Sensitivity of the thrombin clotting time and activated partial thromboplastin time to low level of antithrombin III during heparin therapy. *Clin Lab Haematol* 1990;12:433–436.

115. Congdon JE, Kardinal CG, Wallin JD. Monitoring heparin therapy in hemodialysis. A report on the activated whole blood coagulation time tests. *JAMA* 1973;226:1529–1533.

116. Dauchot PJ, Berzina-Moettus L, Rabinovitch A, et al. Activated coagulation and activated partial thromboplastin times in assessment and reversal of heparin-induced anticoagulation for cardiopulmonary bypass. *Anesth Analg* 1983;62:710–719.

117. Kurec AS, Morris MW, Davey FR. Clotting, activated partial thromboplastin and coagulation times in monitoring heparin therapy. *Ann Clin Lab Sci* 1979;9:494–500.

118. Hooper TL, Conroy J, McArdle B, et al. The use of the Hemochron in assessment of heparin reversal after cardiopulmonary bypass. *Perfusion* 1988;3:295–300.

119. Jaques LB, Ricker AG. The relationship between heparin dosage and clotting time. *Blood* 1948;3:1197–1212.

120. Hattersley PG. Progress report: the activated coagulation time of whole blood (ACT). *Am J Clin Pathol* 1976;66:899–904.

121. Reno WJ, Rotman M, Grumbine FC, et al. Evaluation of the BART test (a modification of the whole-blood activated recalcification time test) as a means of monitoring heparin therapy. *Am J Clin Pathol* 1974;61:78–84.

122. Fareed J. Heparin, its fractions, fragments and derivatives. Some newer perspectives. *Semin Thromb Hemost* 1985;11:1–9.

123. Gravlee GP, Whitaker CL, Mark LJ, et al. Baseline activated coagulation time should be measured after surgical incision. *Anesth Analg* 1990;71:549–553.

124. Mammen EF, Koets MH, Washington BC, et al. Hemostasis changes during cardiopulmonary bypass surgery. *Semin Thromb Hemost* 1985;11:281–292.

125. Kase PB, Dearing JP. Factors affecting the activated clotting time. *J Extracorp Technol* 1985;17:27–30.

126. Nichols AB, Owen J, Grossman BA, et al. Effect of heparin bonding on catheter-induced fibrin formation and platelet activation. *Circulation* 1984;70:843–850.

127. Palermo LM, Andrews RW, Ellison N. Avoidance of heparin contamination in coagulation studies drawn from indwelling lines. *Anesth Analg* 1980;59:222–224.

128. Harper J. Use of heparinized intraarterial lines to obtain coagulation samples. *Focus Crit Care* 1988;15:51–55.

129. Clapham MCC, Willis N, Mapleson WW. Minimum volume of discard for valid blood sampling from indwelling arterial cannulae. *Br J Anaesth* 1987;59:232–235.

130. Cugno M, Colombo A, Cacciabue E, et al. Statistical evaluation of commonly used tests for heparin monitoring. *Life Support Systems* 1986;4:120–128.

131. Bennett JA, Horrow JC. Activated coagulation time: one tube or two? *J Cardiothorac Vasc Anesth* 1996;10:471–473.

132. Gravlee GP, Case LD, Angert KC, et al. Variability of the activated coagulation time. *Anesth Analg* 1988;67:469–472.

133. Richet HM, Craven PC, Brown JM, et al. A cluster of *Rhodococcus* (*Gordona*) *bronchialis* sternal-wound infections after coronary-artery bypass surgery. *N Engl J Med* 1991;324:104–109.

134. Sedor FA, Mayo E, Kirvan KE. A quality-control system for the "activated clotting time" test. *Clin Chem* 1987;33:1261.

135. Wang J-S, Lin C-Y, Hung W-T, et al. Monitoring of heparin-induced anticoagulation with kaolin-activated clotting time in cardiac surgical patients treated with aprotinin. *Anesthesiology* 1992;77:1080–1084.

136. Heimark RL, Kotoku K, Fujikawa K, et al. Surface activation of blood coagulation, fibrinolysis and kinin formation. *Nature* 1980;286:456–460.

137. Dietrich W, Jochum M. Effect of celite and kaolin on activated clotting time in the presence of aprotinin: activated clotting time is reduced by binding of aprotinin to kaolin [Brief Correspondence]. *J Thorac Cardiovasc Surg* 1995;109:177–178.

138. Huyzen RJ, Harder MP, Huet RCGG, et al. Alternative perioperative anticoagulation monitoring during cardiopulmonary bypass in aprotinin-treated patients. *J Cardiothorac Vasc Anesth* 1994;8:153–156.

139. Green TP, Isham-Schopf B, Steinhorn RH, et al. Whole blood activated clotting time in infants during extracorporeal membrane oxygenation. *Crit Care Med* 1990;18:494–498.

140. Varah N, Smith J, Baugh RF. Heparin monitoring in the coronary care unit after percutaneous transluminal coronary angioplasty. *Heart Lung* 1990;19:265–270.

141. Mabry CD, Thompson BW, Read RC, et al. Activated clotting time monitoring of intraoperative heparinization: our experience and comparison of two techniques. *Surgery* 1981;90:889–895.

142. Zahl K, Ellison N. An evaluation of three different ACT monitors. In: *Proceedings of the Society of Cardiovascular Anesthesiologists*, 10th Annual Meeting, 1988:158.

143. Reich DL, Zahl K, Perucho MH, et al. An evaluation of two activated clotting time monitors during cardiac surgery. *J Clin Monit* 1992;8:33–36.

144. Stead SW. Comparison of two methods for heparin monitoring: a semi-automated heparin monitoring device and activated clotting time during extracorporeal circulation. *Int J Clin Monit Comput* 1989;6:247–254.

145. Paul J, Cornillon B, Baguet J, et al. *In vivo* release of a heparin-like factor in dogs during profound hypothermia. *J Thorac Cardiovasc Surg* 1981;82:45–48.

146. Ottesen S, Froysaker T. Use of haemonetics cell saver for autotransfusion in cardiovascular surgery. *Scand J Thorac Cardiovasc Surg* 1982;16:263–268.

147. Ammar T, Fisher CF, Sarier K, et al. The effects of thrombocytopenia on the activated coagulation time. *Anesth Analg* 1996;83:1185–1188.

148. Kesteven PJ, Pasaoglu I, Williams BT, et al. Significance of the whole blood activated clotting time in cardiopulmonary bypass. *J Cardiovasc Surg* 1986;27:85–89.

149. Moorehead MT, Westengard JC, Bull BS. Platelet involvement in the activated coagulation time of heparinized blood. *Anesth Analg* 1984;63:394–398.

150. Ammar T, Scudder LE, Coller BS. *In vitro* effects of the platelet glycoprotein IIb/IIIa receptor antagonist c7E3 Fab on the activated clotting time. *Circulation* 1997;95:614–617.

151. Bode AP, Eick L. Lysed platelets shorten the activated coagulation time (ACT) of heparinized blood. *Am J Clin Pathol* 1989;91:430–434.

152. Kresowik TF, Wakefield TW, Fessler RD II, et al. Anticoagulant effects of protamine sulfate in a canine model. *J Surg Res* 1988;45:8–14.

153. Dutton DA, Hothersall AP, McLaren AD, et al. Protamine titration after cardiopulmonary bypass. *Anaesthesia* 1983;38:264–268.

154. Dietrich W, Spannagl M, Jochum M, et al. Influence of high-dose aprotinin treatment on blood loss and coagulation patterns in patients undergoing myocardial revascularization. *Anesthesiology* 1990;73:1119–1126.

155. de Smet AAEA, Joen MCN, van Oeveren W, et al. Increased anticoagulation during cardiopulmonary bypass by aprotinin. *J Thorac Cardiovasc Surg* 1990;100:520–527.

156. Bull MH, Huse WM, Bull BS. Evaluation of tests used to monitor heparin therapy during extra-corporeal circulation. *Anesthesiology* 1975;43:346–353.

157. Cohen JA. Activated coagulation time method for control of heparin is reliable during cardiopulmonary bypass. *Anesthesiology* 1984;60:121–124.

158. Gravlee GP, Brauer SD, Roy RC, et al. Predicting the pharmacodynamics of heparin: a clinical evaluation of the Hepcon System 4. *J Cardiothorac Anesth* 1987;1:379–387.

159. Gravlee GP, Haddon WS, Rothberger HK, et al. Heparin dosing and monitoring for cardiopulmonary bypass. A comparison of techniques with measurement of subclinical plasma coagulation. *J Thorac Cardiovasc Surg* 1990;99:518–527.

160. Fitch JCK, Geary KLB, Mirto GP, et al. Heparin management test (HMT) versus activated clotting time (ACT) in cardiovascular surgery: correlation with anti-Xa activity. *Anesth Analg* 1998;86:SCA96(abst).

161. Gibbs NM, Weightman WM, Thackray NM, et al. Evaluation of the TAS coagulation analyzer for monitoring heparin effect in cardiac surgical patients. *J Cardiothorac Vasc Anesth* 1998;12:536–541.

162. Kesteven PJL. *Blood coagulation studies during open-heart surgery* [Thesis]. London: St. Thomas' Hospital, 1985.

163. Saleem A, Shenaq SS, Yawn DH, et al. Heparin monitoring during cardiopulmonary bypass. *Ann Clin Lab Sci* 1984;14:474–479.

164. Fox DJ, Gaines J, Reed G. Vehicles of heparin management: a comparison. *J Extracorp Technol* 1979;11:137–142.

165. Gomperts ED, Bethlehem B, Hockley J. The monitoring of heparin activity during extracorporeal circulation. *S Afr Med J* 1977;51:973–976.

166. Baugh RF. Detection of whole blood coagulation. *Am Clin Products Rev* 1984;45:38–45.

167. Despotis GJ, Alsoufiev AL, Spitznagel E, et al. Response of kaolin ACT to heparin: evaluation with an automated assay and higher heparin doses. *Ann Thorac Surg* 1996;61:795–799.

168. Despotis GJ, Summerfield AL, Joist JH. Comparison of activated coagulation time and whole blood heparin measurements with laboratory plasma anti-Xa heparin concentration in patients having cardiac operations. *J Thorac Cardiovasc Surg* 1994;108:1076–1082.

169. Hardy J-F, Belisle S, Robitaille D, et al. Measurement of heparin concentration in whole blood with the Hepcon/HMS device does not agree with laboratory determination of plasma heparin concentration using a chromogenic substrate for activated factor X. *J Thorac Cardiovasc Surg* 1996;112:154–161.

170. Despotis GJ, Levine V, Filos KS, et al. Hemofiltration during cardiopulmonary bypass: the effect on anti-Xa and anti-IIa heparin activity. *Anesth Analg* 1997;84:479–483.

171. Anido G, Freeman DJ. Heparin assay and protamine titration. *Am J Clin Pathol* 1981;76:410–415.

172. Choo IHF, Didisheim P, Doerge ML, et al. Evaluation of a heparin assay method using a fluorogenic synthetic peptide substrate for thrombin. *Thromb Res* 1982;25:115–123.

173. Gauvin G, Umlas J, Chin N. Measurement of plasma heparin levels using a fluorometric assay. *Med Instrum* 1983;17:165–168.

174. Savidge GF, Kesteven PJ, Al-Hasani SF, et al. Rapid quantitation of plasma heparin and antithrombin III levels for cardiopulmonary bypass monitoring, using fluorometric substrate assays. *Thromb Haemost* 1983;50:745–748.

175. Wang J-S, Lin C-Y, Karp RB. Comparison of high-dose thrombin time with activated clotting time for monitoring of anticoagulant effects of heparin in cardiac surgical patients. *Anesth Analg* 1994;79:9–13.

176. Tabuchi N, Njo TL, Tigchelaar I, et al. Monitoring of anticoagulation in aprotinin-treated patients during heart operation. *Ann Thorac Surg* 1994;58:774–777.

177. Chan KK, Stover EP, Hood PA, et al. Heparin concentration measured by protamine titration versus high-dose thrombin time in the presence of aprotinin. *Anesth Analg* 1998;86:SCA56(abst).

178. Shore-Lesserson L, Alfarone J, DePerio M. High-dose thrombin time (HiTT) is a better monitor of anticoagulation in heparin-resistant patients. *Anesth Analg* 1996;82:SCA7(abst).

179. van Putten J, van de Ruit M, Beunis M, et al. Automated spectrophotometric heparin assays. Comparison of methods. *Haemostasis* 1984;14:195–204.

180. Gundry SR, Klein MD, Drongowski RA, et al. Clinical evaluation of a new rapid heparin assay using the dye azure A. *Am J Surg* 1984;148:191–194.

181. Klein MD, Drongowski RA, Linhardt RJ, et al. A colorimetric assay for chemical heparin in plasma. *Anal Biochem* 1982;124:59–64.

182. Yin ET, Wessler S, Butler JV. Plasma heparin: a unique, practical, submicrogram-sensitive assay. *J Lab Clin Med* 1973;81:298–310.

183. Babka R, Colby C, El-Etr A, et al. Monitoring of intraoperative heparinization and blood loss following cardiopulmonary bypass surgery. *J Thorac Cardiovasc Surg* 1977;73:780–782.

184. Ottesen S, Stormorken H, Hatteland K. The value of activated coagulation time in monitoring heparin therapy during extracorporeal circulation. *Scand J Thorac Cardiovasc Surg* 1984;18:123–128.

185. Goodnough LT, Johnston MFM, Toy PTCY. The variability of transfusion practice in coronary artery bypass surgery. *JAMA* 1991;265:86–90.

186. Metz S, Keats AS. Low activated coagulation time during cardiopulmonary bypass does not increase postoperative bleeding. *Ann Thorac Surg* 1990;49:440–444.

187. Guffin AV, Dunbar RW, Kaplan JA, et al. Successful use of a reduced dose of protamine after cardiopulmonary bypass. *Anesth Analg* 1976;55:110–113.

188. Bowie JE, Kemna GD. Automated management of heparin anticoagulation in cardiovascular surgery. *Proc Am Acad Cardiovasc Perfusion* 1985;6:1–10.

189. Gravlee GP, Rogers AT, Dudas LM, et al. Heparin management protocol for cardiopulmonary bypass influences postoperative heparin rebound but not bleeding. *Anesthesiology* 1992;76:393–401.

190. Despotis GJ, Joist JH, Hogue CW, et al. The impact of heparin concentration and activated clotting time monitoring on blood conservation. *J Thorac Cardiovasc Surg* 1995;110:46–54.

191. Young JA, Kisker CT, Doty DB. Adequate anticoagulation during cardiopulmonary bypass determined by activated clotting time and the appearance of fibrin monomer. *Ann Thorac Surg* 1978;26:231–240.

192. Cardoso PFG, Yamazaki F, Keshavjee S, et al. A reevaluation of heparin requirements for cardiopulmonary bypass. *J Thorac Cardiovasc Surg* 1991;101:153–160.

193. Hickling KG. Extracorporeal CO_2 removal in severe adult respiratory distress syndrome. *Anaesth Intensive Care* 1986;14:46–53.

194. Kanter KR, Pennington DG, Weber TR, et al. Extracorporeal membrane oxygenation for postoperative cardiac support in children. *J Thorac Cardiovasc Surg* 1987;93:27–35.

195. Uziel L, Agostoni A, Pirovano E, et al. Hematologic survey during low-frequency positive pressure ventilation with extracorporeal CO_2 removal. *ASAIO Trans* 1982;28:359–364.

196. Heiden D, Mielke CH Jr, Rodvien R, et al. Platelets, hemostasis, and thromboembolism during treatment of acute respiratory insufficiency with extracorporeal membrane oxygenation. Experience with 28 clinical perfusions. *J Thorac Cardiovasc Surg* 1975;70:644–655.

197. Uziel L, Cugno M, Fabrizi I, et al. Physiopathology and management of coagulation during long-term extracorporeal respiratory assistance. *Int J Artif Organs* 1990;13:280–287.

198. Davies GC, Sobel M, Salzman EW. Elevated plasma fibrinopeptide A and thromboxane B_2 levels during cardiopulmonary bypass. *Circulation* 1980;61:808–814.

199. Boldt J, Schindler E, Osmer C, et al. Influence of different anticoagulation regimens on platelet function during cardiac surgery. *Br J Anaesth* 1994;73:639–644.

200. Ovrum E, Holen EA, Tangen G, et al. Completely heparinized cardiopulmonary bypass and reduced systemic heparin: clinical and hemostatic effects. *Ann Thorac Surg* 1995;60:365–371.

201. Aldea GS, Doursounian M, O'Gara P, et al. Heparin-bonded circuits with a reduced anticoagulation protocol in primary CABG: a prospective, randomized study. *Ann Thorac Surg* 1996;62:410–417.

202. Von Segesser LK, Weiss BM, Pasic M, et al. Risk and benefit of low systemic heparinization during open heart operations. *Ann Thorac Surg* 1994;58:391–398.

203. Nielsen LE, Bell WR, Borkon AM, Neill CA. Extensive thrombus formation with heparin resistance during extracorporeal circulation. A new presentation of familial antithrombin III deficiency. *Arch Intern Med* 1987;147:149–152.

204. Jobes DR. Safety issues in heparin and protamine administration for extracorporeal circulation. *J Cardiothorac Vasc Anesth* 1998;12[2 Suppl 1]:17–20.

205. Cipolle RJ, Uden DL, Gruber SA, et al. Evaluation of a rapid monitoring system to study heparin pharmacokinetics and pharmacodynamics. *Pharmacotherapy* 1990;10:367–372.

206. Jobes DR, Aitken GL, Shaffer GW. Increased accuracy and precision of heparin and protamine dosing reduces blood loss and transfusion in patients undergoing primary cardiac operations. *J Thorac Cardiovasc Surg* 1995;110:36–45.

207. Shore-Lesserson L, Reich DL, DePerio M. Individual heparin and protamine dose titration does not improve haemostasis parameters in cardiac surgical patients. *Can J Anaesth* 1998;45:10–18.

208. Hodby ED, Hirsh J, Adeniyi-Jones C. The influence of drugs upon the anticoagulant activity of heparin. *Can Med Assoc J* 1972;106:562–564.

209. Soloway HB, Christiansen TW. Heparin anticoagulation during cardiopulmonary bypass in an antithrombin-III deficient patient. Implications relative to the etiology of heparin rebound. *Am J Clin Pathol* 1980;73:723–725.

210. Chung F, David TE, Watt J. Excessive requirement for heparin during cardiac surgery. *Can Anaesth Soc J* 1981;28:280–282.

211. Anderson EF. Heparin resistance prior to cardiopulmonary bypass. *Anesthesiology* 1986;64:504–507.

212. Marciniak E, Farley CH, DeSimone PA. Familial thrombosis due to antithrombin III deficiency. *Blood* 1974;43:219–231.

213. Dietrich W, Spannagl M, Schramm W, et al. The influence of preoperative anticoagulation on heparin response during cardiopulmonary bypass. *J Thorac Cardiovasc Surg* 1991;102:505–514.

214. Wilds SL, Camerlengo LJ, Dearing JP. Activated clotting time and cardiopulmonary bypass, III. Effect of high platelet count on heparin management. *J Extracorp Technol* 1982;14:322–324.

215. Hanowell ST, Kim YD, Rattan V, et al. Increased heparin requirement with hypereosinophilic syndrome. *Anesthesiology* 1981;55:450–452.

216. Lijnen HR, Van Hoef B, Collen D. Interaction of heparin with histidine-rich glycoprotein and with antithrombin III. *Thromb Haemost* 1983;50:560–562.

217. Lijnen HR, Van Hoef B, Collen D. Histidine-rich glycoprotein modulates the anticoagulant activity of heparin in human plasma. *Thromb Haemost* 1984;51:266–268.

218. Young E, Prins M, Levine MN, et al. Heparin binding to plasma proteins, an important mechanism for heparin resistance. *Thromb Haemost* 1992;67:639–643.

219. Teoh KH, Young E, Bradley CA, et al. Heparin binding proteins. Contribution to heparin rebound after cardiopulmonary bypass. *Circulation* 1993;88:II420–II425.

220. Manson L, Weitz JI, Podor TJ, et al. The variable anticoagulant response to unfractionated heparin *in vivo* reflects binding to plasma proteins rather than clearance. *J Lab Clin Med* 1997;130:649–655.

221. Young E, Wells P, Holloway S, et al. *Ex-vivo* and *in-vitro* evidence that low molecular weight heparins exhibit less binding to plasma proteins than unfractionated heparin. *Thromb Haemost* 1994;71:300–304.

222. Cosmi B, Fredenburgh JC, Rischke J, et al. Effect of nonspecific binding to plasma proteins on the antithrombin activities of unfractionated heparin, low-molecular-weight heparin, and dermatan sulfate. *Circulation* 1997;95:118–124.

223. Habbab MA, Haft JI. Heparin resistance induced by intravenous nitroglycerin. A word of caution when both drugs are used concomitantly. *Arch Intern Med* 1987;147:857–860.

224. Becker RC, Corrao JM, Bovill EG, et al. Intravenous nitroglycerin-induced heparin resistance: a qualitative antithrombin III abnormality. *Am Heart J* 1990;119:1254–1261.

225. Reich DL, Hammerschlag BC, Rand JH, et al. Modest doses of nitroglycerin do not interfere with beef lung heparin anticoag-

ulation in patients taking nitrates. *J Cardiothorac Vasc Anesth* 1992;6:677–679.

226. Amin F, Horrow S. Nitroglycerin antagonism of heparin [Letter]. *Anesthesiology* 1990;73:193–194.

227. Hirsh J, Piovella F, Pini M. Congenital antithrombin III deficiency. Incidence and clinical features. *Am J Med* 1989;87[Suppl 3B]:34S–38S.

228. Thaler E, Lechner K. Antithrombin III deficiency and thromboembolism. *Clin Haematol* 1981;10:369–390.

229. Towne JB, Bernhard VM, Hussey C, et al. Antithrombin deficiency—a cause of unexplained thrombosis in vascular surgery. *Surgery* 1981;89:735–742.

230. Andrew M, Paes B, Milner R, et al. Development of the human coagulation system in the full-term infant. *Blood* 1987;70:165–172.

231. Martindale SJ, Shayevitz JR, D'Errico C. The activated coagulation time: suitability for monitoring heparin effect and neutralization during pediatric cardiac surgery. *J Cardiothorac Vasc Anesth* 1998;10:458–463.

232. Turner-Gomes SO, Nitschmann EP, Norman GR, et al. Effect of heparin loading during congenital heart operation on thrombin generation and blood loss. *Ann Thorac Surg* 1997;63:482–488.

233. Andrew M, MacIntyre B, MacMillan J, et al. Heparin therapy during cardiopulmonary bypass in children requires ongoing quality control. *Thromb Haemost* 1993;70:937–941.

234. Büller HR, ten Cate JW. Acquired antithrombin III deficiency: laboratory diagnosis, incidence, clinical implications, and treatment with antithrombin III concentrate. *Am J Med* 1989;87[Suppl 3B]:44S–48S.

235. Arai H, Miyakawa T, Ozaki K, et al. Changes of the levels of antithrombin III in patients with cerebrovascular diseases. *Thromb Res* 1983;31:197–202.

236. Duckert F. Behaviour of antithrombin III in liver disease. *Scand J Gastroenterol* 1973;19[Suppl]:109–112.

237. Bick RL, Bick MD, Fekete LF. Antithrombin III patterns in disseminated intravascular coagulation. *Am J Clin Pathol* 1980;73:577–583.

238. Marciniak E, Gockerman JP. Heparin-induced decrease in circulating antithrombin-III. *Lancet* 1977;2:581–584.

239. Pickering NJ, Brody JI, Fink GB, et al. The behavior of antithrombin III, alpha$_2$-macroglobulin, and alpha$_1$-antitrypsin during cardiopulmonary bypass. *Am J Clin Pathol* 1983;80:459–464.

240. von Blohn G, Hellstern P, Köhler M, et al. Clinical aspects of acquired antithrombin III deficiency. *Behring Inst Mitt* 1986;79:200–215.

241. Barnette RE, Shupak RC, Pontius J, et al. *In vitro* effect of fresh frozen plasma on the activated coagulation time in patients undergoing cardiopulmonary bypass. *Anesth Analg* 1988;67:57–60.

242. Cosgriff TM, Bishop DT, Hershgold EJ, et al. Familial antithrombin III deficiency: its natural history, genetics, diagnosis and treatment. *Medicine* 1983;62:209–220.

243. Sabbagh AH, Chung GKT, Shuttleworth P, et al. Fresh frozen plasma: a solution to heparin resistance during cardiopulmonary bypass. *Ann Thorac Surg* 1984;37:466–468.

244. Reuter NF. Heparin insensitivity responding to fresh frozen plasma. *Minn Med* 1978;61:79–81.

245. Despotis GJ, Levine V, Joist JH, et al. Antithrombin III during cardiac surgery: effect on response of activated clotting time to heparin and relationship to markers of hemostatic activation. *Anesth Analg* 1997;85:498–506.

246. Practice guidelines for blood component therapy: a report by the American Society of Anesthesiologists Task Force on Blood Component Therapy. *Anesthesiology* 1996;84:732–747.

247. Dietrich W, Schroll A, Göb E, et al. Improved heparin response by substitution of antithrombin III concentrate during extracorporeal circulation. *Anaesthesist* 1984;33:422–427.

248. Hoffman DL. Purification and large-scale preparation of antithrombin III. *Am J Med* 1989;87[Suppl 3B]:23S–26S.

249. Schwartz RS, Bauer KA, Rosenberg RD, et al. Clinical experience with antithrombin III concentrate in treatment of congenital and acquired deficiency of antithrombin. *Am J Med* 1989;87[Suppl 3B]:53S–60S.

250. Hashimoto K, Yamagishi M, Sasaki T, et al. Heparin and antithrombin III levels during cardiopulmonary bypass: correlation with subclinical plasma coagulation. *Ann Thorac Surg* 1994;58:799–804.

251. Hirsh J, Ofosu FA, Levine M. The development of low molecular weight heparins for clinical use. In: Verstraete M, Vermylen J, Lijnen HR, et al., eds. *Thrombosis and haemostasis.* Leuven, The Netherlands: International Society on Thrombosis and Haemostasis and Leuven University Press, 1987:325–346.

252. Horner AA. The nature of two components of pig mucosal heparin, separated by electrophoresis in agarose gel. *Can J Biochem* 1967;45:1015–1020.

253. Jordan RE, Oosta GM, Gardner WT, et al. The kinetics of hemostatic enzyme–antithrombin interactions in the presence of low molecular weight heparin. *J Biol Chem* 1980;255:10081–10090.

254. Fareed J, Kumar A, Rock A, et al. A primate model (*Macaca mulatta*) to study the pharmacokinetics of heparin and its fractions. *Semin Thromb Hemost* 1985;11:138–154.

255. Jordan RE, Favreau LV, Braswell EH, et al. Heparin with two binding sites for antithrombin or platelet factor 4. *J Biol Chem* 1982;257:400–406.

256. Lane DA, Pejler G, Flynn AM, et al. Neutralization of heparin-related saccharides by histidine-rich glycoprotein and platelet factor 4. *J Biol Chem* 1986;261:3980–3986.

257. Barzu T, Van Rijn JL, Petitou M, et al. Endothelial binding sites for heparin. Specificity and role in heparin neutralization. *Biochem J* 1986;238:847–854.

258. Hirsh J, Ofosu F, Buchanan M. Rationale behind the development of low molecular weight heparin derivatives. *Semin Thromb Hemost* 1985;11:13–16.

259. Fareed J, Hoppensteadt D, Jeske W, et al. Low molecular weight heparins: are they different? *Can J Cardiol* 1998; 14 [Suppl E]:28E–34E.

260. Lane DA, Ryan K. The importance of anti-factor Xa and antithrombin activities of low molecular weight heparins. *J Lab Clin Med* 1990;116:269–270.

261. Salzman EW. Low-molecular-weight heparin. Is small beautiful [Editorial]? *N Engl J Med* 1986;315:957–959.

262. Messmore HL. Clinical efficacy of heparin fractions: issues and answers. *Crit Rev Clin Lab Sci* 1986;23:77–94.

263. Ofosu FA, Blajchman MA, Modi GJ, et al. The importance of thrombin inhibition for the expression of the anticoagulant activities of heparin, dermatan sulphate, low molecular weight heparin and pentosan polysulphate. *Br J Haematol* 1985;60:695–704.

264. Turpie AGG, Levine MN, Hirsh J, et al. A randomized controlled trial of a low-molecular-weight heparin (enoxaparin) to prevent deep-vein thrombosis in patients undergoing elective hip surgery. *N Engl J Med* 1986;315:925–929.

265. Warkentin TE, Levine MN, Hirsh J, et al. Heparin-induced thrombocytopenia in patients treated with low-molecular-weight heparin or unfractionated heparin. *N Engl J Med* 1995;332:1330–1335.

266. John LCH, Rees GM, Kovacs IB. Different anticoagulants and platelet reactivity in cardiac surgical patients. *Ann Thorac Surg* 1993;56:899–902.

267. McBride WT, Armstrong MA, McMurray TJ. An investigation of the effects of heparin, low molecular weight heparin, prot-

amine, and fentanyl on the balance of pro- and anti-inflammatory cytokines in in-vitro monocyte cultures. *Anaesthesia* 1996;51:634–640.

268. Gitlin SD, Deeb GM, Yann C, et al. Intraoperative monitoring of danaparoid sodium anticoagulation during cardiovascular operations. *J Vasc Surg* 1998;27:568–575.

269. Abildgaard U, Norrheim L, Larsen AE, et al. Monitoring therapy with LMW heparin: a comparison of three chromogenic substrate assays and the Heptest clotting assay. *Haemostasis* 1990;20:193–203.

270. Mammen EF. Why low molecular weight heparin? *Semin Thromb Hemost* 1990;16:1–4.

271. Bara L, Billaud E, Kher A, Samama M. Increased anti-Xa bioavailability for a low molecular weight heparin (PK 10169) compared with unfractionated heparin. *Semin Thromb Hemost* 1985;11:316–317.

272. Fareed J. Development of heparin fractions: some overlooked considerations. *Semin Thromb Hemost* 1985;11:227–236.

273. Racanelli A, Fareed J, Walenga JM, et al. Biochemical and pharmacologic studies on the protamine interactions with heparin, its fractions and fragments. *Semin Thromb Hemost* 1985;11:176–189.

274. Gouault-Heilmann M, Huet Y, Contant G, et al. Cardiopulmonary bypass with a low-molecular-weight heparin fraction [Letter]. *Lancet* 1983;2:1374.

275. Massonnet-Castel S, Pelissier E, Dreyfus G, et al. Low-molecular-weight heparin in extracorporeal circulation [Letter]. *Lancet* 1984;1:1182–1183.

276. Massonnet-Castel S, Pelissier E, Bara L, et al. Partial reversal of low molecular weight heparin (PK 10169) anti-Xa activity by protamine sulfate: *in vitro* and *in vivo* study during cardiac surgery with extracorporeal circulation. *Haemostasis* 1986;16:139–146.

277. Touchot B, Laborde F, Dum F, et al. Use of low molecular weight heparin CY 222 during cardiopulmonary bypass. Experimental study and clinical application. *Perfusion* 1986;1:99–102.

278. Koza MJ, Messmore HL, Wallock ME, et al. Evaluation of a low molecular weight heparin as an anticoagulant in a model of cardiopulmonary bypass surgery. *Thromb Res* 1993;70:67–76.

279. Henny CP, ten Cate H, ten Cate JW, et al. A randomized blind study comparing standard heparin and a new low molecular weight heparinoid in cardiopulmonary bypass surgery in dogs. *J Lab Clin Med* 1985;106:187–196.

280. Doherty DC, Ortel TL, De Bruijn N, et al. "Heparin-free" cardiopulmonary bypass: first reported use of heparinoid (Org 10172) to provide anticoagulation for cardiopulmonary bypass. *Anesthesiology* 1990;73:562–565.

281. Marshall LR, Cannell PK, Herrmann RP. Successful use of the APTT in monitoring of the anti-factor-Xa activity of the heparinoid organon 10172 in a case of HITS requiring open heart surgery [Letter]. *Thromb Haemost* 1992;67:587.

282. Wilhelm MJ, Schmid C, Kececioglu D, et al. Cardiopulmonary bypass in patients with heparin-induced thrombocytopenia using Org 10172. *Ann Thorac Surg* 1996;61:920–924.

283. Zulys VJ, Teasdale SJ, Michel ER, et al. Ancrod (Arvin^R) as an alternative to heparin anticoagulation for cardiopulmonary bypass. *Anesthesiology* 1989;71:870–877.

284. Teasdale SJ, Zulys VJ, Mycyk T, et al. Ancrod anticoagulation for cardiopulmonary bypass in heparin-induced thrombocytopenia and thrombosis. *Ann Thorac Surg* 1989;48:712–713.

285. Kanagasabay RR, Unsworth-White MJ, Robinson G, et al. Cardiopulmonary bypass with danaparoid sodium and ancrod in heparin-induced thrombocytopenia. *Ann Thorac Surg* 1998;66:567–569.

286. Marder VJ. Comparison of thrombolytic agents: selected hematologic, vascular and clinical events. *Am J Cardiol* 1989;64:2A–7A.

287. Markwardt F. Pharmacology of selective thrombin inhibitors. *Nouv Rev Fr Hematol* 1988;30:161–165.

288. Bichler J, Fichtl B, Siebeck M, et al. Pharmacokinetics and pharmacodynamics of hirudin in man after single subcutaneous and intravenous bolus administration. *Arzneimittelforschung* 1988;38:704–710.

289. Potzsch B, Madlener K, Seelig C, et al. Monitoring of r-hirudin anticoagulation during cardiopulmonary bypass—assessment of the whole blood ecarin clotting time. *Thromb Haemost* 1997; 77:920–925.

290. Walenga JM, Bakhos M, Messmore HL, et al. Potential use of recombinant hirudin as an anticoagulant in a cardiopulmonary bypass model. *Ann Thorac Surg* 1991;51:271–277.

291. Riess FC, Potzsch B, Behr I, et al. Recombinant hirudin as an anticoagulant during cardiac operations: experiments in a pig model. *Eur J Cardiothorac Surg* 1997;11:739–745.

292. Koza MJ, Shankey TC, Walenga JM, et al. Flow cytometric evaluation of platelet activation by ionic or nonionic contrast media and modulation by heparin and recombinant hirudin. *Invest Radiol* 1995;30:90–97.

293. Spanier TB, Oz MC, Minanov OP, et al. Heparinless cardiopulmonary bypass with active-site blocked factor IXa: a preliminary study on the dog. *J Thorac Cardiovasc Surg* 1998;115: 1179–1188.

294. Smith CR. Management of bleeding complications in redo cardiac operations. *Ann Thorac Surg* 1998;65:S2–S8.

295. Gikakis N, Khan MMH, Hiramatsu Y, et al. Effect of factor Xa inhibitors on thrombin formation and complement and neutrophil activation during *in vitro* extracorporeal circulation. *Circulation* 1996;94:II341–II346.

296. Visentin GP, Ford SE, Scott JP, et al. Antibodies from patients with heparin-induced thrombocytopenia/thrombosis are specific for platelet factor 4 complexed with heparin or bound to endothelial cells. *J Clin Invest* 1994;93:81–88.

297. Greinacher A, Potzsch B, Amiral J, et al. Heparin-associated thrombocytopenia: isolation of the antibody and characterization of a multimolecular PF4–heparin complex as the major antigen. *Thromb Haemost* 1994;71:247–251.

298. Cines DB, Kaywin P, Bina M, et al. Heparin-associated thrombocytopenia. *N Engl J Med* 1980;303:788–795.

299. Cines DB, Tomaski A, Tannenbaum S. Immune endothelial-cell injury in heparin-associated thrombocytopenia. *N Engl J Med* 1987;316:581–589.

300. White PW, Sadd JR, Nensel RE. Thrombotic complications of heparin therapy. Including six cases of heparin-induced skin necrosis. *Ann Surg* 1979;190:595–608.

301. Kappa JR, Fisher CA, Berkowitz HD, et al. Heparin-induced platelet activation in sixteen surgical patients: diagnosis and management. *J Vasc Surg* 1987;5:101–109.

302. Godal HC. Heparin-induced thrombocytopenia. In: Lane DA, Lindahl U, eds. *Heparin. Chemical and biological properties, clinical applications.* Boca Raton, FL: CRC Press, 1989:533–548.

303. Chong BH, Burgess J, Ismail F. The clinical usefulness of the platelet aggregation test for the diagnosis of heparin-induced thrombocytopenia. *Thromb Haemost* 1993;69:344–350.

304. Sheridan D, Carter C, Kelton JG. A diagnostic test for heparin-induced thrombocytopenia. *Blood* 1986;67:27–30.

305. Greinacher A, Michels I, Kiefel V, et al. A rapid and sensitive test for diagnosing heparin-associated thrombocytopenia. *Thromb Haemost* 1991;66:734–736.

306. Visentin GP, Malik M, Cyganiak KA, et al. Patients treated with unfractionated heparin during open heart surgery are at high risk to form antibodies reactive with heparin: platelet factor 4 complexes. *J Lab Clin Med* 1996;128:376–383.

307. Cipolle RJ, Rodvold KA, Seifert R, et al. Heparin-associated thrombocytopenia: a prospective evaluation of 211 patients. *Ther Drug Monit* 1983;5:205–211.

308. Ansell J, Slepchuk N Jr, Kumar R, et al. Heparin-induced thrombocytopenia: a prospective study. *Thromb Haemost* 1980; 43:61–65.

309. Bell WR, Royall RM. Heparin-associated thrombocytopenia: a comparison of three heparin preparations. *N Engl J Med* 1980; 303:902–907.

310. Bailey RT, Ursick JA, Heim KL, et al. Heparin-associated thrombocytopenia: a prospective comparison of bovine lung heparin manufactured by a new process, and porcine intestinal heparin. *Drug Intell Clin Pharm* 1986;20:374–378.

311. Laskey MAL, Deutsch E, Hirshfeld JW Jr, et al. Influence of heparin therapy on percutaneous transluminal coronary angioplasty outcome in patients with coronary arterial thrombus. *Am J Cardiol* 1990;65:179–182.

312. Resnekov L, Chediak J, Hirsh J, et al. Antithrombotic agents in coronary artery disease. *Chest* 1986;2[Suppl]:54S–67S.

313. Kander NH, Holland KJ, Pitt B, et al. A randomized pilot trial of brief versus prolonged heparin after successful reperfusion in acute myocardial infarction. *Am J Cardiol* 1990;65:139–142.

314. Ling E, Warkentin TE. Intraoperative heparin flushes and subsequent acute heparin-induced thrombocytopenia. *Anesthesiology* 1998;89:1567–1569.

315. Makhoul RG, McCann RL, Austin EH, et al. Management of patients with heparin-associated thrombocytopenia and thrombosis requiring cardiac surgery. *Ann Thorac Surg* 1987;43: 617–621.

316. Smith JP, Walls JT, Muscato MS, et al. Extracorporeal circulation in a patient with heparin-induced thrombocytopenia. *Anesthesiology* 1985;62:363–365.

317. Olinger GN, Hussey CV, Olive JA, et al. Cardiopulmonary bypass for patients with previously documented heparin-induced platelet aggregation. *J Thorac Cardiovasc Surg* 1984;87: 673–677.

318. Rhodes GR, Dixon RH, Silver D. Heparin-induced thrombocytopenia: eight cases with thrombotic-hemorrhagic complications. *Ann Surg* 1977;186:752–758.

319. Guay DRP, Richard A. Heparin-induced thrombocytopenia—association with a platelet aggregating factor and cross-sensitivity to bovine and porcine heparin. *Drug Intell Clin Pharm* 1984;18:398–401.

320. Horellou MH, Conard J, Lecrubier C, et al. Persistent heparin-induced thrombocytopenia despite therapy with low molecular weight heparin [Letter]. *Thromb Haemost* 1984;51:134.

321. Harenberg J, Zimmermann R, Schwarz F, et al. Treatment of heparin-induced thrombocytopenia with thrombosis by new heparinoid [Letter]. *Lancet* 1983;1:986–987.

322. Kappa JR, Horn MK III, Fisher CA, et al. Efficacy of iloprost (ZK36374) versus aspirin in preventing heparin-induced platelet activation during cardiac operations. *J Thorac Cardiovasc Surg* 1987;94:405–413.

323. Kappa JR, Fisher CA, Todd B, et al. Intraoperative management of patients with heparin-induced thrombocytopenia. *Ann Thorac Surg* 1990;49:714–723.

324. Kraenzler EJ, Starr NJ. Heparin-associated thrombocytopenia: management of patients for open heart surgery. Case reports describing the use of iloprost. *Anesthesiology* 1988;69:964–967.

325. Addonizio VP Jr, Macarak EJ, Niewiarowski S, et al. Preservation of human platelets with prostaglandin E_1 during *in vitro* simulation of cardiopulmonary bypass. *Circ Res* 1979;44: 350–357.

326. Kappa JR, Musial J, Fisher KA, et al. Quantitation of platelet preservation with prostanoids during simulated bypass. *J Surg Res* 1987;42:10–18.

327. Vender JS, Matthew EB, Silverman IM, et al. Heparin-associated thrombocytopenia: alternative managements. *Anesth Analg* 1986;65:520–522.

328. Brady J, Riccio JA, Yumen OH, et al. Plasmapheresis. A therapeutic option in the management of heparin-associated thrombocytopenia with thrombosis. *Am J Clin Pathol* 1991;96: 394–397.

329. Greinacher A, Volpel H, Janssens U, et al. Recombinant hirudin (lepirudin) provides safe and effective anticoagulation in patients with heparin-induced thrombocytopenia. A prospective study. *Circulation* 1999;99:73–80.

330. Zucker MB. Effect of heparin on platelet function. *Thromb Diath Haemorrh* 1974;33:63–65.

331. Thomson C, Forbes CD, Prentice CRM. The potentiation of platelet aggregation and adhesion by heparin *in vitro* and *in vivo*. *Clin Sci Mol Med* 1973;45:485–494.

332. Abela M, McArdle B, Qureshi M, Pearson DT. Heparin-enhanced ADP-induced platelet aggregation in patients undergoing cardiopulmonary bypass surgery. *Perfusion* 1986;1: 175–178.

333. Cella G, Menardo A, Girolami A. Effect of heparin on *in vivo* platelet factor 4 (PF4) release and platelet aggregation after aspirin administration. *Clin Lab Haematol* 1980;2:333–338.

334. Michalski R, Lane DA, Kakkar VV. Comparison of heparin and a semi-synthetic heparin analogue. A73025. *Br J Haematol* 1977;37:247–256.

335. Bertelé V, Roncaglioni MC, Donati MB, de Gaetano G. Heparin counteracts the antiaggregating effect of prostacyclin by potentiating platelet aggregation. *Thromb Haemost* 1983;49: 81–83.

336. Eldor A, Weksler BB. Heparin and dextran sulfate antagonize PGI₂ inhibition of platelet aggregation. *Thromb Res* 1979;16: 617–628.

337. Heiden D, Mielke CH Jr, Rodvien R. Impairment by heparin of primary haemostasis and platelet [^{14}C]5-hydroxytryptamine release. *Br J Haematol* 1977;36:427–436.

338. O'Brien JR, Path FRC. Heparin and platelets. *Curr Ther Res* 1975;18:79–90.

339. Davey MG, Lander H. Effect of injected heparin on platelet levels in man. *J Clin Pathol* 1968;21:55–59.

340. Kopriva CJ, Sreenivasan N, Stafansson S, Farrell DT, Shaffer WB Jr, Geha AS. Hypothermia can cause errors in activated coagulation time [Abstract]. *Anesthesiology* 1980;33:S85.

341. Cohen EJ, Camerlengo LJ, Dearing JP. Activated clotting times and cardiopulmonary bypass I: The effect of hemodilution and hypothermia upon activated clotting time. *J Extra-Corp Technol* 1980;12:139–141.

342. Berg E, Stenbjerg S, Albrechtsen OK. Monitoring heparin and protamine therapy during cardiopulmonary bypass by activated clotting time. *J Extra-Corp Technol* 1979;11:229–235.

343. Verska JJ. Control of heparinization by activated clotting time during bypass with improved postoperative hemostasis. *Ann Thorac Surg* 1977;24:170–173.

344. Roth JA, Cukingnan RA, Scott CR. Use of activated coagulation time to monitor heparin during cardiac surgery. *Ann Thorac Surg* 1979;28:69–72.

345. Papaconstantinou C, Rådegran K. Use of the activated coagulation time in cardiac surgery. Effects on heparin-protamine dosages and bleeding. *Scand J Cardiovasc Surg* 1981;15:213–215.

346. Jumean HG, Sudah F. Monitoring of anticoagulant therapy during open-heart surgery in children with congenital heart disease. *Acta Haematol (Basel)* 1983;70:392–395.

347. Dearing JP, Bartles DM, Stroud MR, Sade RM. Activated clotting times versus protocol anticoagulation management. *J Extra-Corp Technol* 1983;15:17–19.

348. Niinikoski J, Laato M, Laaksonen V, Jalonen J, Inberg MV. Use of activated clotting time to monitor anticoagulation during cardiac surgery. *Scand J Thorac Cardiovasc Surg* 1984;18:57–61.

349. Lefemine AA, Lewis M. Activated clotting time for control of anticoagulation during surgery. *Am Surg* 1985;51:274–278.

350. Preiss DU, Schmidt-Bleibtreu H, Berguson P, Metz G. Blood transfusion requirements in coronary artery surgery with and without the activated clotting time (ACT) technique. *Klin Wochenschr* 1985;63:252–256.

351. Urban MK, Gordon M, Farrell DT, Shaffer WB. The management of anticoagulation during cardiopulmonary bypass (CPB) [abstract]. *Anesthesiology* 1991;75(suppl 3A):A437.

352. Conley CL, Hartmann RC, Lalley JS. The relationship of heparin activity to platelet concentration. *Proc Soc Exp Biol Med* 1948;69:284–287.

353. Schved JF, Gris JC, Eledjam JJ. Circadian changes in anticoagulant effect of heparin infused at a constant rate. *Br Med J* 1985; 290:1286.

354. Decousus HA, Croze M, Levi FA, et al. Circadian changes in anticoagulant effect of heparin infused at a constant rate. *Br Med J* 1985;290:341–344.

355. Decousus M, Gremillet E, Decousus H, et al. Nycthemeral variations of ^{99}Tc^m-labelled heparin pharmacokinetic parameters. *Nuclear Med Comm* 1985;6:633–640.

356. Whitfield LR, Levy G. Relationship between concentration and anticoagulant effect of heparin in plasma of normal subjects: magnitude and predictability of interindividual differences. *Clin Pharmacol Ther* 1980;28:509–516.

357. Nelson RM, Frank CG, Mason JO. The antiheparin properties of the antihistamines, tranquilizers, and certain antibiotics. *Surg Forum* 1958;9:146–150.

358. Cloyd G, D'Ambra M, Koski G, Akins C. Heparin resistance in coronary artery bypass graft patients: the role of preoperative heparin therapy vs intraaortic balloon pumps. *Proceedings of the Society of Cardiovascular Anesthesiologists 8th annual meeting.* 1986:71.

359. Hicks GL Jr. Heparin resistance during cardiopulmonary bypass [letter]. *J Thorac Cardiovasc Surg* 1983;86:633.

360. Godal HC. Heparin tolerance and the plasma proteins. *Scand J Clin Lab Invest* 1961;13:314–325.

361. Jaques LB. The pharmacology of heparin and heparinoids. *Prog Med Chem* 1967;6:139–198.

362. Glueck HI, MacKenzie MR, Glueck CJ. Crystalline IgG protein in multiple myeloma: identification effects on coagulation and on lipoprotein metabolism. *J Lab Clin Med* 1972;79:731–744.

363. Pogliani E, Cofrancesco E, Praga C. Anti-heparin activity of a macroglobulin from a patient with breast adenocarcinoma. *Acta Haematol (Basel)* 1975;53:249–255.

364. Jordan RE, Kilpatrick J, Nelson RM. Heparin promotes the inactivation of antithrombin by neutrophil elastase. *Science* 1987;237:777–779.

365. Bleyl H, Addo O, Roka L. Heparin neutralizing effect of lipoproteins. *Thromb Diath Haemorrh* 1975;34:549–555.

366. Whitfield LR, Lele AS, Levy G. Effect of pregnancy on the relationship between concentration and anticoagulant action of heparin. *Clin Pharmacol Ther* 1983;34:23–28.

367. Mummaneni N, Istanbouli M, Pifarré R, El-Etr AA. Increased heparin requirements with autotransfusion. *J Thorac Cardiovasc Surg* 1983;66:446–447.

HEPARIN NEUTRALIZATION

VENKAT PATLA
MARK E. COMUNALE
EDWARD LOWENSTEIN

Heparin remains the anticoagulant of choice for cardiopulmonary bypass (CPB). The action of heparin is well understood, and one of its principal advantages is the ease with which it can be neutralized. Protamine remains the mainstay of this process.

This chapter discusses the process of protamine neutralization of heparin-induced anticoagulation and its side effects, including life-threatening and sometimes fatal reactions. Further, we present recent work examining alternatives to protamine.

CHEMISTRY OF PROTAMINE

Heparin acts by enhancing the activity of antithrombin III (AT III), a circulating proteinase inhibitor that acts on serine proteases (1). AT III inhibits (activated) factors XIIa, XIa, IXa, Xa, thrombin (IIa), and XIIIa. Heparin-modified AT III especially accelerates inactivation of factors Xa and thrombin (1).

Protamine, a polycationic protein derived from salmon sperm, is strongly alkaline because its amino acid composition is 67% arginine (2). The numerous positive charges on the protamine molecule in its natural state bind with the negatively charged phosphate groups of the nucleoprotein material of salmon sperm. Heparin, a polyanion, binds ionically to protamine to produce a stable precipitate. Protamine contains two active sites, one that neutralizes heparin and another that exerts a mild anticoagulant effect independently of heparin.

Other clinical uses of protamine include complexing it with insulin to produce NPH (neutral protamine Hagedorn) insulin. This renders insulin relatively insoluble at neutral pH, extending the duration of action to approxi-

mately 24 hours. Similarly, complexing protamine with zinc forms protamine–zinc insulin, which has a duration of 36 hours. Protamine also inhibits angiogenesis (3), a property which led to its previous unsuccessful evaluation as an antineoplastic agent (4).

The anticoagulant effect of protamine has been demonstrated *in vitro* (5). Debate exists as to whether this effect is clinically important and at what doses it occurs. It has been suggested that the anticoagulant effect of protamine becomes important only at doses approximately three times those required for neutralization of residual heparin (6). However, Ellison et al. (7) subsequently demonstrated only a mild, transient (30-minute) increase in the Lee-White whole blood coagulation time, with no effect on the partial thromboplastin time, despite a large excess of protamine (Table 23.1). These effects occurred at intravenous doses of up to 800 mg for a 70-kg adult. These authors initially proposed that the anticoagulant effect of protamine appears to become clinically important only if exceedingly large amounts are infused. This relatively large therapeutic window for protamine has been confirmed by more recent studies (8), which also examined the effects of protamine on partial thromboplastin time without examining platelet function.

Ellison's group and others have suggested that the anticoagulant effect of protamine may be attributable to inhibition of platelet-induced aggregation. More recent work by Ellison et al. (9) showed a decrease in *in vitro* platelet sensitivity to adenosine diphosphate (ADP) and collagen in the presence of the heparin–protamine complex. Protamine alone has no effect on platelet aggregation. Mammen et al. (10) showed decreased platelet aggregation in response to ADP and ristocetin when protamine was administered to patients at the conclusion of CPB. They also demonstrated a decrease in platelet volume and suggested that a change in platelet surface membranes could be responsible for this altered platelet function. A human trial that compared administration of protamine equal to the total heparin dose versus protamine at a reduced dose based on a heparin half-life of 2 hours resulted in markedly decreased chest tube

---

V. Patla and M. E. Comunale: Department of Anesthesia, Beth Israel Deaconess Medical Center, Boston, Massachusetts 02215.

E. Lowenstein: Department of Anesthesia and Critical Care, Massachusetts General Hospital, Boston, Massachusetts 02114.

TABLE 23.1. EFFECTS OF PROTAMINE ON LEE-WHITE COAGULATION AND PARTIAL THROMBOPLASTIN TIMES AFTER SINGLE DOSES OF 600 MG/KG IN VOLUNTEERS

	Control	Time after Injection (min)		
		5	30	60
Lee-White, three-tube (min)				
Mean	6.58	8.89[a]	6.83	6.58
SE	0.25	0.48	0.53	0.53
PTT (sc)				
Mean	41.5	40.7	41.8	40.7
SE	1.3	1.6	1.8	1.4

[a] Mean differs significantly from control mean, $p < 0.05$, with two-dimensional analysis of variance.
PTT, partial thromboplastin time; SE, standard error.
From Ellison N, Ominsky AJ, Wollman H. Is protamine a clinically significant anticoagulant? A negative answer, *Anesthesiology* 1971; 35:621–629, with permission.

drainage, higher platelet counts, and postoperative clotting times closer to control values in those patients receiving the smaller protamine doses (11).

Dutton et al. (12) showed that smaller protamine doses (derived by protamine titration just before the discontinuation of CPB) resulted in acceptable values for activated clotting time (ACT) at the conclusion of bypass with no subsequent evidence of heparin rebound. A recent study administering different doses of protamine (1.5, 3.0, 6.0, and 15.0 mg/kg) to heparinized and unheparinized animals showed decreasing platelet aggregation in response to ADP with increasing protamine doses. Significant effects on coagulation (expressed as ACT, prothrombin time, and partial thromboplastin time) became evident at excess protamine doses of 6.0 and 15.0 mg/kg in both heparinized and unheparinized animals (13). Based on these studies, most patients will probably tolerate an excess protamine dose of 1 to 2 mg/kg without adverse effects on hemostasis. The clinician should be aware, however, that protamine overdose can result in platelet dysfunction lasting several hours into the post-bypass period.

ASSESSMENT OF REVERSAL OF ANTICOAGULATION

Monitoring the level of anticoagulation during and following CPB is a widely accepted practice. Tests evaluating anticoagulation should yield quick results and be easily performed in the operating room. ACT, a variation of the whole blood clotting time, has been the test most commonly utilized for this purpose and is described in detail in Chapter 22.

Calculation of Protamine Dose

The anticoagulant effects of a given dose of heparin vary considerably between patients. Bull et al. (14) demonstrated that simple weight-based dosing without monitoring of the anticoagulant effects can lead to underdosing or overdosing in some patients (Fig. 23.1). It has recently been shown that the effects of protamine also vary between patients (15). Accurate calculation of the protamine dose is thus important because unneutralized heparin can increase postoperative bleeding. Several inherent problems in calculating protamine dosage have been pointed out by Hurt et al. (16). These include the following: (a) The dose of protamine

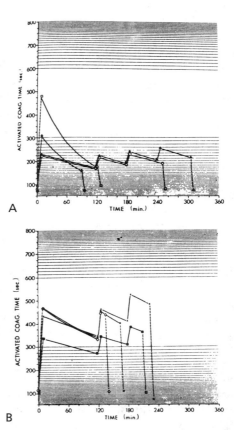

FIG. 23.1. Before the initiation of cardiopulmonary bypass, a heparin dose of 300 U/kg was given, with 100 U/kg given after 2 hours and each hour thereafter. Neutralization was accomplished with protamine at 1.5 times the total dose of heparin. For each procedure, **A** shows patients (*darkened triangles* and *open circles*) who had the least sensitivity to heparin and the shortest half-life of heparin (*closed diamonds* and *open squares*). **B** shows the course of anticoagulant therapy for patients who were the most sensitive to heparin (*open diamonds* and *closed circles*) and patients who had the longest half-life of heparin (*darkened squares* and *x*). *Solid lines* depict the coagulation times during bypass, and *broken lines* indicate the institution and termination of anticoagulation. (From Bull BS, Korpman RA, Huse WM, et al. Heparin therapy during extracorporeal circulation, I. Problems inherent in existing heparin protocols. *J Thorac Cardiovasc Surg* 1975;69: 674–684, with permission.)

TABLE 23.2. COMPARISON OF METHODS FOR CALCULATING PROTAMINE DOSAGE

Method	Advantages	Disadvantages
Fixed dose	Simple Not reliant on ACT	Inadequate or excessive protamine Potential for increased coagulation times with standard doses
ACT/heparin dose-response curves	Rapid, easy to use in the operating room More accurate protamine administration Decreased blood product requirements	No correlation between ACT and heparin levels Relies on ACT Dependence on plasma volume
Heparin levels	Less protamine given Not reliant on ACT	Requires peripheral laboratory Time-consuming Assumes point on static curve Dependence on plasma volume
Protamine titration	Less protamine required than with fixed dose Decreased postoperative bleeding (suggested by some studies) Suggested that no rebound effect seen with small protamine doses	Variability between heparin–protamine preparations Dependence on blood volume estimate Several steps for potential error Assumes point on static curve

ACT, activated clotting time.

necessary to neutralize heparin is not the same *in vivo* as *in vitro*; (b) heparin and protamine preparations vary in their potency; and (c) because heparin undergoes continuous metabolism, the dose of protamine needed decreases with time.

Many different dose regimens for protamine neutralization of heparin anticoagulant are employed. Inappropriate protamine dosage may result in inadequate reversal, protamine anticoagulation, or adverse side effects. Table 23.2 highlights the advantages and disadvantages of the different techniques.

Fixed Protamine Dose Regimen

The easiest method for calculating a protamine dose is a fixed-dose ratio of protamine to heparin. This method involves giving 1.0 to 1.3 mg of protamine for each 100 U of heparin. Either the total dose of heparin administered for the case or the heparin dose given initially defines the amount of heparin to be neutralized (17,18). Simplicity constitutes the main advantage of this method, as no assays are required at the end of bypass and there is no need to measure the ACT. The disadvantage is the considerable variability in the half-life of heparin, which makes it difficult to predict the status of the coagulation system immediately preceding heparin neutralization (17).

Heparin–Activated Clotting Time Dose–Response Curves

This technique uses the method described by Bull et al. (19) and involves determining three ACT values and plotting them on a graph versus the heparin dose (Figs. 23.2,

23.3). The calculated amount of heparin is then neutralized by giving 1.3 mg of protamine per 100 U of heparin at the conclusion of CPB. This method is rapid and easy to use. Other advantages of this method include the following: (a) The protamine dose can be calculated more accurately than with the fixed regimen; (b) a reduced quantity of protamine is administered; and (c) infusion of blood, platelets, and fresh-frozen plasma is possibly decreased (20). One disadvantage is the reliance on the ACT, which is affected by numerous factors. Culliford et al. (21) demonstrated that CPB distorts the relationship between ACT and heparin levels, with the ACT becoming prolonged beyond what could be explained by the plasma heparin concentration. The authors also noted that protamine doses calculated by this method exceeded those calculated by measuring plasma heparin concentration, and the amount calculated by measuring plasma heparin concentration was usually sufficient to neutralize heparin-induced anticoagulation.

Heparin Concentration

Precise determination of the plasma heparin concentration remaining at the conclusion of bypass is infrequently utilized. One method incubates the plasma to be analyzed for heparin with factor Xa in the presence of an excess of its inhibitor (Xai). Heparin accelerates factor Xa inhibition, and residual factor X remaining after 2 minutes is measured and converted to a heparin concentration, expressed in units per milliliter (22).

Culliford et al. (21) demonstrated the use of decreased protamine doses after calculation by this method as opposed to heparin–ACT dose–response curves. The major disadvantage of this method is the delayed acquisition of test results. Thus, the values may not be accurate when received because the patient's heparin concentration decreases at an

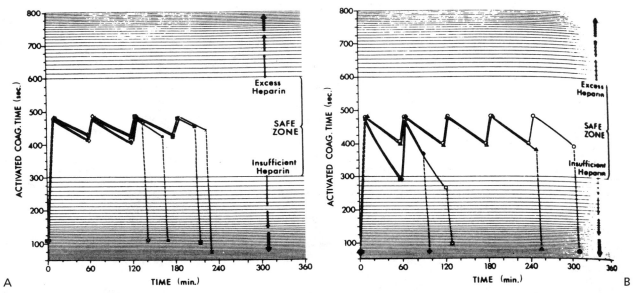

FIG. 23.2. The descriptions for **A** and **B** are the same as in Fig. 23.1. Monitoring approach (computer simulation). The activated coagulation time was raised to 8 minutes initially and was returned to that level every 60 minutes during the operation. Protamine was administered in a ratio of 1.3 mg for every 100 U of heparin remaining in the circulation at the conclusion of bypass. (From Bull BS, Korpman RA, Huse WM, et al. Heparin therapy during extracorporeal circulation, I. Problems inherent in existing heparin protocols. *J Thorac Cardiovasc Surg* 1975;69:674–684, with permission.)

unknown rate while the blood specimen is being analyzed. Furthermore, the conversion of plasma heparin concentrations into a protamine dose requires an estimation of plasma volume, which is difficult to assess at the completion of bypass (19). Additionally, there is not always good correlation between heparin levels and clotting times (23).

Recently, Wahr et al. (24) have developed an improved electrode for monitoring heparin concentrations in whole blood. The sensor can serve as a single endpoint detector for the determination of heparin via potentiometric titration with protamine. In addition to correlating well with the currently available methods of measuring heparin concentration, it offers the possibility of fully automating these titrations, thus providing a simple, inexpensive, and accurate method for monitoring heparin concentration in whole blood. Schlueter et al. (25) compared a factor Xa inhibition assay with a new low-level heparin–protamine titration (LLHPT) assay to measure the concentration of heparin *in vitro*. Both assays have comparable precision over a wide range of heparin concentrations. In addition, the LLHPT assay is rapid and has the potential to become a bedside monitor of heparin concentration.

Protamine Titration

Calculation of protamine dose by protamine titration was initially described by Allen and co-workers (26), and several variations of this method have been described (6,12,14,27). All methods employ tubes with several dilutions of a standard protamine solution, to which a fixed volume of whole heparinized blood is added. The lowest protamine concentration resulting in the shortest clotting time represents the optimal neutralization of heparin. The protamine dose is then calculated based on an assumed neutralization ratio (e.g., 1.1 mg of protamine per 100 U of heparin) and on estimated blood volume. Therefore, this method is actually an indirect way of estimating heparin concentrations. Advantages claimed for this method include administration of a lower protamine dose than with a fixed-dose regimen (28), absence of excessive postoperative bleeding response (28), and absence of heparin rebound despite reduced protamine doses (12). Disadvantages include the following: (a) It is necessary to calculate blood volume (27,28); (b) potency varies between different heparin and protamine preparations (although this can be compensated for by using the same source of protamine for dilutions as for reversal) (12); (c) manual versions of this method can be time-consuming, so that when the protamine value has been defined, the patient's heparin level may have dropped or the patient may have received an additional dose; and (d) numerous steps are involved, each incurring some error (23).

In a prospective, randomized trial, Shore-Lesserson et al. (29) compared the titration method with their standard management using 1 mg protamine for every 100 U of the

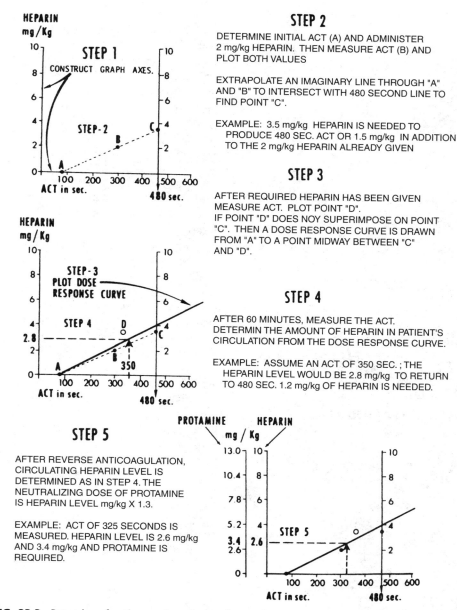

STEP 1
CONSTRUCT GRAPH AXES.

STEP-2

STEP 2
DETERMINE INITIAL ACT (A) AND ADMINISTER 2 mg/kg HEPARIN. THEN MEASURE ACT (B) AND PLOT BOTH VALUES

EXTRAPOLATE AN IMAGINARY LINE THROUGH "A" AND "B" TO INTERSECT WITH 480 SECOND LINE TO FIND POINT "C".

EXAMPLE: 3.5 mg/kg HEPARIN IS NEEDED TO PRODUCE 480 SEC. ACT OR 1.5 mg/kg IN ADDITION TO THE 2 mg/kg HEPARIN ALREADY GIVEN

STEP 3
AFTER REQUIRED HEPARIN HAS BEEN GIVEN MEASURE ACT. PLOT POINT "D".
IF POINT "D" DOES NOY SUPERIMPOSE ON POINT "C". THEN A DOSE RESPONSE CURVE IS DRAWN FROM "A" TO A POINT MIDWAY BETWEEN "C" AND "D".

STEP-3 PLOT DOSE RESPONSE CURVE

STEP 4

STEP 4
AFTER 60 MINUTES, MEASURE THE ACT. DETERMIN THE AMOUNT OF HEPARIN IN PATIENT'S CIRCULATION FROM THE DOSE RESPONSE CURVE.

EXAMPLE: ASSUME AN ACT OF 350 SEC.; THE HEPARIN LEVEL WOULD BE 2.8 mg/kg TO RETURN TO 480 SEC. 1.2 mg/kg OF HEPARIN IS NEEDED.

STEP 5
AFTER REVERSE ANTICOAGULATION, CIRCULATING HEPARIN LEVEL IS DETERMINED AS IN STEP 4. THE NEUTRALIZING DOSE OF PROTAMINE IS HEPARIN LEVEL mg/kg X 1.3.

EXAMPLE: ACT OF 325 SECONDS IS MEASURED. HEPARIN LEVEL IS 2.6 mg/kg AND 3.4 mg/kg AND PROTAMINE IS REQUIRED.

STEP 5

FIG. 23.3. Procedure for the construction and use of the dose–response curve. (From Bull BS, Huse WM, Brauer FS, et al. Heparin therapy during extracorporeal circulation, II. The use of a dose–response curve to individualize heparin and protamine dosage. *J Thorac Cardiovasc Surg* 1975;69:685–689, with permission.)

total heparin dose. They found that the protamine titration method significantly decreased the total protamine dose needed to reverse heparin; however, the protamine titration method did not offer advantages with regard to transfusion requirements, mediastinal chest tube drainage, heparin rebound, or incomplete heparin neutralization. Thus, the simple, weight-based method of neutralizing heparin was as good as the heparin–protamine titration method.

In contrast, Jobes et al. (30) found that basing heparin and protamine dosing on *in vitro* heparin and protamine titration reduces postoperative chest tube drainage. Additionally, fewer patients received blood transfusions, and there were fewer donor exposures. Control patients in this study were managed according to the authors' standard practice (300 U of heparin per kilogram, with repeated boluses as needed to achieve and maintain an ACT >400

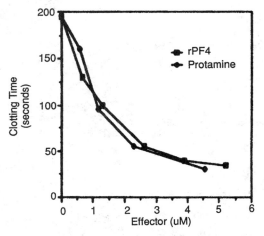

FIG. 23.4. Neutralization of heparin elongation of activated partial thromboplastin time (*APTT*). [From Hunt AJ, Gray GS, Myers JA, et al. Heparin neutralization by recombinant human PF4 *in vitro. FASEB J* 1990;4:A1991(abst), with permission.]

seconds; 1 mg of protamine per 100 U of the total heparin dose for CPB, with additional protamine as needed to return ACT to control values).

OTHER DRUGS USED TO NEUTRALIZE HEPARIN

The reported incidence of severe reactions to protamine, including respiratory compromise, hypotension, and shock,

varies from 0.2% to 3% in the general population to as high as 27% in patients who are allergic to fish or have received NPH insulin (31). This has led to an ongoing search for alternative agents to neutralize heparin-induced anticoagulation and also alternatives to heparin. Most of these substitutes have thus far met with limited success and are discussed below, with the exception of hexadimethrine toxicity.

Platelet Factor 4

The α-granules of human platelets contain platelet factor 4 (PF4), which binds and neutralizes heparin when released during platelet aggregation (1). PF4 is released at the site of vascular injury, binding heparin and facilitating thrombin accumulation and clot formation (26). The PF4 in platelet concentrates and fresh-frozen plasma was presumed to have been responsible for heparin reversal following CPB in two diabetic patients with a history of previous anaphylactic reactions to protamine (32). However, it should be noted that these patients still had significant post-bypass bleeding and that actual documentation of heparin reversal versus normal heparin decay was lacking.

Recombinant PF4 cloned in *Escherichia coli* neutralizes heparin as effectively as protamine *in vitro* (Fig. 23.4). Recombinant PF4 and protamine both neutralize heparin inhibition of factor Xa and thrombin. Recombinant PF4 restored factor Xa levels more effectively than protamine (by approximately 50% to 60%) and was equipotent with human PF4 (26) (Fig. 23.5). In a rat model, recombinant PF4 was as effective as protamine in reversing heparin anti-

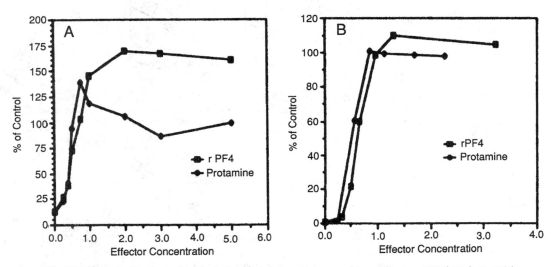

FIG. 23.5. Neutralization of heparin by protamine and recombinant human PF4 (*rPF4*). **A:** With factor Xa, rPF4 and protamine were both effective, although 1 μm of rPF4 could restore factor Xa activity to higher levels than could protamine. **B:** Both rPF4 and protamine were equally effective (on a molar basis) in preventing inhibition of thrombin. [From Hunt AJ, Gray GS, Myers JA, et al. Heparin neutralization by recombinant human PF4 *in vitro. FASEB J* 1990;4:A1991(abst), with permission.]

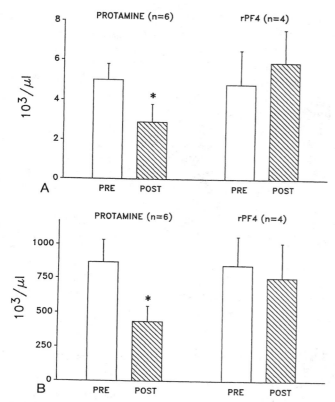

FIG. 23.6. Effect of injection of protamine sulfate or recombinant PF4 (*rPF4*) on the number of circulating white blood cells (**A**) and platelets (**B**). Number of experiments in parentheses. *p < 0.01, significantly different from platelet count before heparin. The values correspond to the mean ± standard error of the mean. (From Cook JJ, Niewiarowski S, Yan Z, et al. Platelet factor 4 efficiently reverses heparin anticoagulation in the rat without adverse effects of heparin–protamine complexes. *Circulation* 1992; 85:1102–1109, with permission.)

coagulation. The PF4 injection produced normal platelet counts in this model (33).

Human or recombinant PF4 administered to Sprague-Dawley rats after heparinization had no effect on white blood cell count, platelet count, or complement levels (34) (Fig. 23.6). In contrast, protamine administered after heparin (0.1 mg/100 g) caused decreases of these same parameters. Furthermore, heparin neutralization by recombinant or human PF4 caused no decrease in mean arterial blood pressure or pathologic pulmonary changes, whereas protamine neutralization produced these adverse effects (32).

Dehmer et al. (35) compared PF4 with protamine in a prospective, double-blind fashion in patients undergoing cardiac catheterization. In this study, the administration of PF4 to patients was both safe and effective in the doses used. In addition, PF4 had the advantage of rapid administration, within 2 minutes, in comparison with 10 minutes for protamine. The number of patients is small and clinical experience in humans is limited. PF4 is expensive, and its cost

effectiveness remains to be established. The advantages of rapid administration and lack of serious side effects merit a larger study in patients undergoing CPB.

Kurrek and colleagues (36) showed that PF4 produces acute pulmonary hypertension in lambs. The magnitude of pulmonary hypertension was similar to that seen with protamine. However, PF4 did not cause hypoxemia and neutropenia, indicating that complement was not activated by PF4. In contrast, Cook et al. (34) studied reversal of heparin anticoagulation with PF4 in the rat and concluded that PF4 is both effective and devoid of serious side effects. Similarly, Bernabei et al. (37) demonstrated the safety and efficacy of PF4 in baboons. The effectiveness of PF4 has been established *in vitro*; heparinized blood obtained from patients undergoing CPB was reversed with PF4. PF4 merits further studies as a replacement to protamine.

Protamine Variants

Wakefield et al. (38) have been working on a protamine variant, a so-called "designer protamine," to neutralize the anticoagulant effect of heparin. Two such variants are currently under investigation. The first, +18BE (standard protamine being +21), has a +18 charge with acetyl and amide groups on the ends and glutamic acid replacing prolene in the background structure. The second molecule has a side group, RGD (arginine–glycine–aspartate), that is a known recognition site for platelet adhesion protein.

In a dog model (39), the reversal of anticoagulation (measured by the reversal of antifactor Xa activity) achieved with the RGD compound was superior to that achieved with standard protamine. As measured by changes in oxygen consumption, blood pressure, and cardiac output, side effects were significantly reduced by the RGD variant. Platelet clumping and prolongation of bleeding times were not observed with the RGD variant. This area of research holds exciting prospects for decreasing the toxicity of protamine.

Heparinase

Heparinase, derived from the bacterium *Flavobactum heparinum*, neutralizes heparin by enzymatic cleavage of α-glycoside linkages at the AT III binding site. Heparinase is an effective antagonist of heparin as measured by ACT and heparin concentrations. Michelson et al. (40) found that heparinase did not produce any significant hemodynamic changes when administered as an intravenous bolus to anesthetized heparinized dogs. In an *in vitro* study of the blood of healthy volunteers, Ammar and Fisher (41) demonstrated that heparinase has minimal effects on platelets, whereas protamine markedly inhibits platelet responsiveness. In these studies, heparinase was as effective as protamine in neutralizing heparin-induced anticoagulation, and it appears to be a promising potential alternative to protamine. Human trials are ongoing.

Heparin-removal Devices

A heparin-removal device is a separate extracorporeal circuit used at the end of CPB. The principle of plasmapheresis is applied in the heparin-removal device system to expose heparinized plasma from the patient to poly-L-lysine. The negatively charged heparin molecules bind irreversibly with the positively charged poly-L-lysine and are removed from plasma. Hendrikx et al. (42) used this system to neutralize heparin-induced anticoagulation in dogs undergoing CPB and concluded that the heparin-removal device was as efficient as systemic administration of protamine. Thrombocytopenia and complement activation were less than with protamine. Although this method is unique, simple, and effective, the time taken to reverse heparin activity (30 minutes or longer) is currently unacceptable for routine clinical practice.

The use of immobilized protamine during extracorporeal circulation has been reported by Yang et al. (43). Their method utilizes a "protamine bioreactor" in the bypass circuit that is composed of protamine bonded to the cellulose fibers of a hemodialyzer. This protamine bioreactor is placed directly into the bypass circuit to remove and neutralize heparin *in vitro*. Because heparin-bonded tubing is used downstream from these devices, clot formation and embolic phenomena do not appear to be a concern. Use of this device was associated with decreased complement activation in comparison with the systemic administration of protamine. This device provides an interesting avenue for future investigations.

PROTAMINE REACTIONS

Adverse cardiopulmonary responses to protamine have been observed during the entire history of clinical cardiac surgery. The complexity of the clinical situation has made this adverse drug reaction very difficult to define. In 1983, a specific clinical syndrome of catastrophic pulmonary vasoconstriction was described. Within 1 month, Lowenstein and co-workers (44) observed three severe protamine reactions, and in another 3 months they had collected a total of five such incidents. They observed profound increases in pulmonary arterial and central venous pressures with concurrent dramatic decreases in left atrial and systemic arterial pressures. These five patients shared certain characteristics: valvular heart disease, bolus administration of protamine, low total dose of protamine (<0.5 mg/kg), tolerance to further protamine infusions without adverse effects, and no adverse sequelae. Since then, substantial clinical and basic science investigation has led to the recognition of three mechanisms producing adverse protamine reactions (Table 23.3).

It now appears that catastrophic pulmonary vasoconstriction after protamine occurs in about 0.6% of adult cardiac surgical patients or fewer (45,46). Numerous risk factors have been suggested, including valvular heart disease (particularly mitral), preexisting pulmonary hypertension, bolus protamine administration, infusion rates greater than 5 mg/min, diabetes with prior NPH insulin exposure, specific brands of protamine, sterilization via ligation of the vas deferens, site of administration, and rate of administration. To date, none of these predisposing risk factors has been verified, but some deserve mention and are discussed below (see Pulmonary Vasoconstrictive Reactions) (47).

Classification of Protamine Reactions

Two classifications of protamine reactions have been proposed (Table 23.3). The classification of Horrow (50) differentiates protamine reactions into types I, II, and III. Type I reactions result in transient systemic hypotension secondary to rapid administration. Type II reactions consist of anaphylactic and anaphylactoid reactions, which are further divided into types IIa, IIb, and IIc. Type IIa comprises true anaphylactic reactions. Immediate anaphylactoid reactions characterize type IIb, and delayed anaphylactoid reactions (e.g., noncardiogenic pulmonary edema) are considered type IIc reactions. Type III reactions consist of catastrophic pulmonary vasoconstriction (48).

We propose an alternative classification, as follows: (a) pharmacologic histamine release, (b) true anaphylaxis mediated by a specific antiprotamine immunoglobulin E (IgE) antibody, and (c) anaphylactoid thromboxane release leading to pulmonary vasoconstriction and bronchoconstriction. Thus, Horrow's type I reactions, which are characterized by systemic hypotension secondary to rapid administration, correspond in our classification to pharma-

TABLE 23.3. CLASSIFICATION OF PROTAMINE REACTIONS

Type	Horrow	Moorman, Zapol, Lowenstein
I.	Hypotension resulting from rapid administration	Pharmacologic histamine release
IIa.	Anaphylactic reactions	True anaphylaxis (IgE-mediated)
IIb.	Immediate anaphylactoid reactions	
IIc.	Delayed anaphylactoid reactions	Anaphylactoid reactions
III.	Catastrophic pulmonary vasoconstriction	Pulmonary vasoconstriction (IgG/complement-mediated)
		Noncardiogenic pulmonary edema

cologic histamine release. Whereas Horrow includes true anaphylactic and anaphylactoid reactions in his type II, we consider them as two different types because true anaphylaxis is mediated by a specific antiprotamine IgE antibody that can be produced by protamine in the absence of heparin. The role of antiprotamine IgG antibodies is not clear. The anaphylactoid reaction is independent of a specific IgE antibody, is associated with the heparin–protamine complex, and does not occur in the absence of heparin. Catastrophic pulmonary vasoconstriction is the most common example of the anaphylactoid reaction in our categorization, whereas Horrow classifies it separately. The rare occurrences of delayed pulmonary edema and adult respiratory distress syndrome appear to represent different manifestations of anaphylactoid responses, so we classify them that way. In this chapter, we employ the latter classification system.

Pharmacologic Release

Alkaline drugs, such as morphine sulfate and D-tubocurare, cause histamine release with rapid infusion (49). Protamine, also a basic drug, was believed to induce hypotension by this mechanism, and it was demonstrated to release histamine by degranulating isolated mast cells (50). We classify protamine-induced hypotension resulting from this mechanism as pharmacologic release. Pharmacologic release of histamine does not depend on the formation of heparin–protamine complexes, but it can occur after the infusion of protamine alone. Its occurrence appears to depend on the rate of infusion (51).

Stoelting et al. (51) demonstrated that the rapid administration of 4.7 mg of protamine per kilogram within 5 minutes in heparinized humans and 4.5 mg/kg at the same rate in unheparinized dogs did not change hemodynamics or histamine levels at the conclusion of CPB. The administration of 4.5 mg of protamine per kilogram (1) as a rapid infusion caused decreases in blood pressure with parallel increases of histamine levels in unheparinized dogs (49).

Parsons and Mohandas (52) gave 1 mg of protamine per 1 mg of remaining heparin at a rate of 2.5 mg/s to patients pretreated with histamine₁ (10 mg of chlorpheniramine) and histamine₂ (400 mg of cimetidine) receptor blockers. These patients experienced a 23% decrease in mean arterial pressure, versus a 34% decrease in patients not given pretreatment. These data again suggest a possible role of histamine in this type of reaction (52).

A greater degree of hypotension and greater increases in plasma histamine levels have been observed after rapid right-sided protamine injections than after rapid left-sided administration in humans (47). These same observations have been made in animal models, which suggests a pulmonary source of the histamine released in this response (40).

Some human studies have demonstrated only a very mild and transient decrease of blood pressure and systemic vascular resistance after rapid protamine administration (53), but clinical experience has demonstrated that rapid protamine administration can result in hypotension in humans. The variable degree of hypotension produced in many of these studies may also reflect the variability of myocardial contractile reserve. Perhaps patients with good myocardial reserve can compensate for the decreased systemic vascular resistance with a sufficient increase of cardiac index to avoid a major decline in blood pressure (51).

A direct myocardial depressant effect of protamine has been proposed as being partially responsible for this hypotension (54,55). It is difficult to determine whether depressed myocardial function is the consequence of a reduced reserve or of direct effects of the drug on the heart (52,56). The data on myocardial depression are far from conclusive because others have shown no changes in global myocardial metabolism or hemodynamic parameters (including cardiac index) in patients with normal left ventricular function after rapid protamine administration (57).

In summary, it appears that protamine can induce hypotension independently of the heparin–protamine complex in a fashion dependent on the rate of administration. Thus, hypotension appears to be partly mediated by histamine release. The degree of histamine release may be greater when a right-sided injection route is utilized, possibly reflecting pulmonary histamine release, although this is controversial. This type of protamine-induced hypotension is accompanied by increased histamine levels, whereas increased plasma thromboxane and C5a levels and pulmonary hypertension are absent.

True Anaphylactic Protamine Reactions

True anaphylaxis to protamine (Horrow's type IIa) does not require the heparin–protamine complex and is mediated by a specific antiprotamine IgE antibody. This reaction is perhaps the most dreaded adverse effect of protamine. True anaphylaxis requires prior protamine exposure to sensitize and produce IgE antibodies, which then bind to mast cells on reexposure to the challenging antigen, protamine. These reactions, although uncommon, have to date been convincingly documented exclusively in diabetics receiving NPH or protamine–zinc insulin. Patients with prior protamine exposure, or patients with a fish allergy, have been suspected as candidates for these reactions, but documentation is lacking. Physiologically, they are characterized by decreased systemic arterial, pulmonary arterial, left atrial, and right atrial pressures; bronchospasm is variably present.

Using an enzyme-linked immunosorbent assay, Sharath et al. (58) showed that 53% of diabetics taking NPH insulin had elevated protamine-specific IgE antibodies. They also noted that IgE levels were highest in patients taking protamine for long periods and in those who had begun protamine before age 20. Nondiabetics and diabetics not using a protamine-containing form of insulin had no IgE reacting with protamine. Levy et al. (59) prospectively studied blood samples from 50 diabetic patients taking NPH insulin. They found only one sample that demonstrated an *in vitro* leukocyte histamine release in response to protamine challenge.

Weiss et al. (60), in a case–control study, examined 27 diabetic and nondiabetic patients who had adverse protamine reactions. Of these 27 patients, only diabetics who received protamine-containing insulin preparations had antiprotamine IgE antibodies (Fig. 23.7). Their reactions were characterized primarily by a decreased blood pressure, with the variable occurrence of bronchospasm. Some diabetics receiving protamine-containing insulin injections had

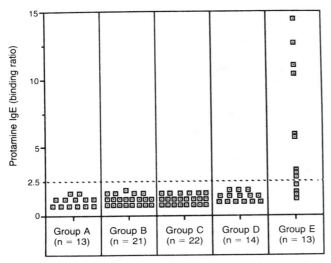

FIG. 23.7. The immunoglobulin E (*IgE*) antibody to protamine. Serum levels of IgE antibody to protamine were measured with the use of the radioallergosorbent test in five patient populations. Normal subjects (group A) had never been exposed to protamine in any form and included three atopic subjects with total serum IgE levels of more than 1,000 ng/mL. Group B consisted of diabetic patients who had not received subcutaneous protamine insulin injections but who had received intravenous protamine after coronary artery bypass surgery without a reaction. Group C consisted of diabetic patients who were receiving daily subcutaneous injections of protamine and insulin and who had no reaction to intravenous protamine after bypass surgery. Group D consisted of 13 nondiabetic patients and one diabetic patient who had adverse reactions to intravenous protamine but had had no previous exposure to protamine insulin preparations. Group E was composed of diabetic patients receiving daily subcutaneous injections of protamine and insulin who had had adverse reactions when given intravenous protamine. The response was reported as a binding ratio (counts per minute of an unknown serum sample per counts per minute of a negative serum sample). A ratio of 2.5 or higher indicated a positive response. Nine of the 13 patients in group E had IgE antibodies to protamine, in comparison with none of the 70 patients in the other four groups. Soluble protamine inhibited the binding of IgE antibody to the protamine–agarose complex in all nine positive serum samples. The inhibition of direct binding ranged from 60.7% to 99.5% (mean, 85.8%; data not shown). (From Weiss ME, Nyhan D, Peng Z, et al. Association of protamine IgE and IgG antibodies with life-threatening reactions to intravenous protamine. *N Engl J Med* 1989;320:886–892, with permission.)

adverse drug reactions but lacked this IgE antibody. These patients exhibited a different clinical picture, characterized by increased pulmonary artery pressures, decreased systemic arterial pressure, and often by the presence of antiprotamine IgG antibody. Patients not receiving protamine insulin had reactions characterized by pulmonary vasoconstriction. These differing clinical presentations suggest two different mechanisms, one being anaphylactic and mediated by IgE antibody and the other being anaphylactoid and associated with IgG antibody. Patients may not exhibit positive skin test reactions to dilute protamine insulin preparations because of desensitization; thus, the absence of a positive skin test reaction does not reliably exclude an IgE- or IgG-mediated protamine reaction.

There have been three reports of patients with true fish allergies experiencing adverse cardiopulmonary protamine reactions, including one patient who experienced cardiovascular collapse following protamine administration at the conclusion of CPB (61). This patient subsequently was shown to have elevated levels of IgE antibody specific for codfish antigen, peripheral eosinophilia, and a positive protamine skin test reaction, as well as IgG, IgM, and IgE specific antibodies directed against protamine sulfate. Vertebrate fish protamines exhibit a similar nucleoprotein structure to that found in humans, and it has been suggested that patients with a true fish allergy have antibodies that can cross-react with the protamine derived from salmon sperm, or with antigenic contaminants accompanying the protamine (62). Because shellfish and true fish are phylogenetically different, a shellfish allergy should not predispose a patient to a protamine reaction.

Vasectomized men have been suggested as having an increased risk for protamine reactions because of the development of antisperm antibodies and antibodies to protamine (63). Men with a positive complement fixation test to human protamine also fix complement in the presence of salmon protamine. It has been speculated that cross-reactivity could cause problems on exposure to protamine (64). Because human and fish protamines are similar, some cross-reactivity is possible. This possibility remains only theoretical, however, because to date there is no documentation that protamine reactions occur more frequently in vasectomized men. Levy et al. (45) prospectively observed cardiac surgical patients with prior vasectomies and fish allergies and also retrospectively evaluated a cohort of 3,245 consecutive cardiac surgical patients requiring CPB in search of adverse reactions to protamine. There were no adverse reactions to protamine in six patients with fish allergies nor in 16 patients with vasectomies. Recognizing that their study did not have sufficient power to exclude fish allergy and vasectomy as risk factors for protamine allergy, they appropriately concluded that a history of fish allergy or prior vasectomy does not contraindicate protamine administration.

Anaphylactoid Reactions

These reactions include those classified as types IIb, IIc, and III by Horrow. Mediators of anaphylaxis can be liberated by pathways other than classic antigen–antibody interactions (Fig. 23.8). Certain types of adverse responses to protamine are believed to be anaphylactoid in nature and mediated by complement activation with secondary release of histamine, thromboxane, or other vasoactive substances (65).

Protamine itself is incapable of activating complement. However, the interaction of heparin with protamine has been shown to deplete plasma C1, suggesting classic activation of the complement cascade, as in the depletion produced by antibody–antigen interactions (66).

Complement activation by the alternate pathway with increased C3a levels has been demonstrated following CPB in humans (67,68). A second peak in C3a and C4a levels, indicating activation of the classic pathway, has also been demonstrated following protamine neutralization of heparin. The anaphylatoxins C3a and C5a can produce systemic inflammatory-type reactions with histamine release, increased capillary permeability, leukosequestration, and hemodynamic derangements (69) manifesting as edema of the skin and mucosa, decreased systemic vascular resistance, bronchospasm, and flushing (47). Protamine has been shown to inhibit human plasma carboxypeptidase semicompetitively *in vitro*. This enzyme is responsible for the inactivation of anaphylatoxins and kinins. It appears therefore that protamine can cause activation of the complement cascade and then block the hydrolysis of the various mediators produced by that process (70). It is believed that certain types of adverse protamine reactions are caused by these mechanisms.

Adverse reactions to protamine in nondiabetic patients with prior protamine exposure have not been proved to be mediated by IgE antibodies. Our own data suggest that these reactions are anaphylactoid in nature. Levy et al. (59) reported a 2% incidence of protamine reactions in a series of more than 1,500 nondiabetic patients undergoing cardiac surgery with CPB, but subsequent studies show an incidence of <1% (46). The mediator profile and antigen or antibody status of these patients were not defined. Presumably, most of these patients had previously received protamine following cardiac catheterization.

Stewart and co-workers (71), in a series of 866 patients undergoing cardiac catheterization, noted two major reactions in patients with prior protamine exposure as the only apparent risk factor. Again, their antibody status was undefined. Weiss and co-workers (60) showed that patients with antiprotamine IgG antibody had an increased risk for protamine reactions and speculated that this was a consequence of prior exposure during cardiac catheterization. The ability of IgG antibodies to cause anaphylactoid reactions to protamine was suspected by others (72).

Pulmonary Vasoconstrictive Reactions

The most extensively studied protamine reactions are anaphylactoid in nature and manifested by intense pulmonary vasoconstriction. Because most types of protamine reactions are heralded by the onset of systemic hypotension, it is only in recent years that the widespread use of pulmonary artery catheters, continuous hemodynamic recording, and meticu-

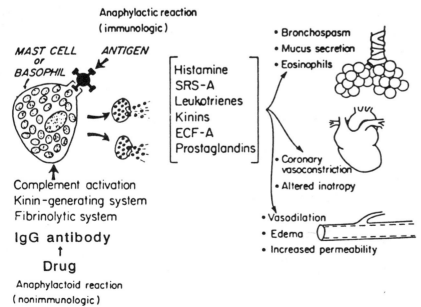

FIG. 23.8. Both true anaphylactic and anaphylactoid reactions can cause similar pathophysiologic responses, including the release of many of the same mediators and end-organ responses. The only reliable way of differentiating mechanisms is by measuring specific antibody levels. The presence of IgG antibody is not specific. SRS-A, slow release substance of anaphylaxis; ECF-A, eosinophil chemotactic factor A. (Modified from Levy JH. *Anaphylactic reactions in anesthesia and intensive care.* Boston: Butterworth–Heineman, 1986:40, with permission.)

lous review of these records has permitted this type of protamine reaction to be recognized. As their name implies, pulmonary vasoconstrictive protamine reactions are characterized by an increased pulmonary artery pressure secondary to pulmonary vasoconstriction, which leads in turn to right ventricular failure, systemic hypotension, and decreased left atrial pressures during protamine administration (Fig. 23.9). This syndrome has occurred after minute doses of protamine, often less than 0.5 mg/kg and as little as 0.14 mg/kg (73).

Heparin–protamine interactions have been extensively studied in animal models to elucidate the possible mechanisms in humans. Much recent research has focused on anaphylactoid reactions, which can be catastrophic and are considered idiosyncratic and thus unpredictable. Compounding the idiosyncratic nature of anaphylactoid reactions is a lack of clear risk factors. This makes pulmonary vasoconstrictive reactions especially frustrating to the clinician.

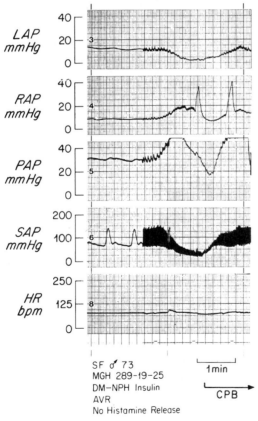

FIG. 23.9. An example of a pulmonary vasoconstrictive (anaphylactoid) protamine reaction. *LAP,* left atrial pressure; *RAP,* right atrial pressure; *PAP,* mean pulmonary artery pressure; *SAP,* systemic arterial pressure; *HR bpm,* heart rate, beats per minute. The two spikes on the right atrial pressure trace represent artifact from central venous sampling. *MGH,* Massachusetts General Hospital number; *DM,* diabetes mellitus on NPH (neutral protamine Hagedorn) insulin; *AVR,* aortic valve replacement.

The expression of heparin–protamine reactions in animals has been very species-dependent (Table 23.4). However, recent studies have established their presence in an increasing number of mammals. The sheep model has been most extensively utilized because the ovine pulmonary vasculature is very prone to vasoconstriction. Morel et al. (74) consistently elicited pulmonary hypertension accompanied by an increased pulmonary vascular resistance, pulmonary capillary occlusion pressure, and thromboxane B_2 levels and a decreased cardiac output and stroke volume in awake sheep given 200 U of heparin per kilogram as a bolus followed by 2 mg of protamine per kilogram administered during 10 seconds through the right atrial catheter. This response was not seen in animals given protamine without prior heparin, nor was it observed in animals pretreated with indomethacin (a cyclooxygenase inhibitor) or a thromboxane synthetase inhibitor. Animals pretreated with dimethylsulfoxide (a hydroxide scavenger) experienced increased pulmonary artery pressures, whereas dimethylthiourea (a hydrogen peroxide scavenger) pretreatment prevented the response (Fig. 23.10). Sheep were also found to have a profound leukopenia with the heparin–protamine interaction. Analysis of complement and histamine levels revealed a consistent increase in C3a levels but no change in plasma histamine levels during heparin–protamine interactions (74). Montalescot et al. (75) were able to prevent this reaction by pretreatment with a thromboxane receptor blocker despite unchanged levels of the plasma thromboxane metabolite. Leukopenia was not prevented by pretreatment with this agent. In pigs, the heparin–protamine complex consistently induced pulmonary hypertension with increased thromboxane B_2 levels (76–79).

Degges et al. (79) showed that increased thromboxane B_2 release and pulmonary hypertension could be blocked by pretreating pigs with aspirin but not antihistamines. They also demonstrated the pulmonary vasoconstrictor response in isolated lungs by using an acellular dextran perfusion medium. Thus, platelet aggregation, leukocyte sequestration, and plasma complement activation are not required. Recently, in a prospective, randomized study involving 1,501 patients, Comunale et al. (46) reported that none of the 10 patients who had pulmonary hypertension were taking aspirin preoperatively. Preoperative use of aspirin seems to confer protection against pulmonary hypertension during protamine neutralization of heparin.

Thromboxane A_2, a short-lived vasoconstrictor, is rapidly hydrolyzed to thromboxane B_2, which is inactive and long-lived. Thromboxane A_2 is known to be a potent pulmonary vasoconstrictor. Pretreatment with thromboxane antagonists would seem to offer one solution to pulmonary vasoconstrictive reactions, at least in the animal model. However, thromboxane receptor antagonists can cause platelet dysfunction, which could lead to increased hemorrhage following CPB. Thus, an extremely short-acting antagonist would be required for clinical utility.

TABLE 23.4. HEPARIN–PROTAMINE INTERACTIONS IN ANIMAL MODELS

Author	Species	Hemodynamics	TX Levels	Antagonist	Reaction	Coagulation
Morel 1988 (74)	Sheep	PAP,PVR,SVR,PW increased	Increased	TX synthetase	Attenuated	Not studied
		CO,SV decreased		Indomethacin	Blocked	
		BP,HR no change		DMTU	Blocked	
				DMSO	Present	
Montalescot 1990 (75)	Sheep	PAP increased	Increased	TXA$_2$ receptor	Blocked	BT no change
		CO,SV no change				
Degges 1987 (79)	Pigs	PAP increased	Increased	Diphenhydramine	Present	Not studied
				Cromolyn sodium	Present	
				ASA	Blocked	
Schumacher 1988 (78)	Pigs	PAP,PVR increased		TX receptor	Blocked	Not studied
Conzen 1989 (77)	Pigs	PAP,PVR increased	Increased	TX receptor	Blocked	Not studied
		MABP decreased		Indomethacin	Blocked	
		HR no change				
Nuttall 1991 (76)	Pigs	PAP increased	Increased	TXA$_2$ receptor (given 2 min after protamine)	Decreased duration	BT increased in 50%, platelet aggregation inhibited

TX, thromboxane; PAP, pulmonary artery pressure; PVR, pulmonary vascular resistance; PW, pulmonary capillary wedge pressure; SVR, systemic vascular resistance; SV, stroke volume; CO, cardiac output; MABP, mean arterial blood pressure; HR, heart rate; BP, blood pressure; ASA, aspirin (acetylsalicylic acid); BT, bleeding time; DMTU, dimethylthiourea; DMSO, dimethylsulfoxide; TXA$_2$, thromboxane A$_2$.

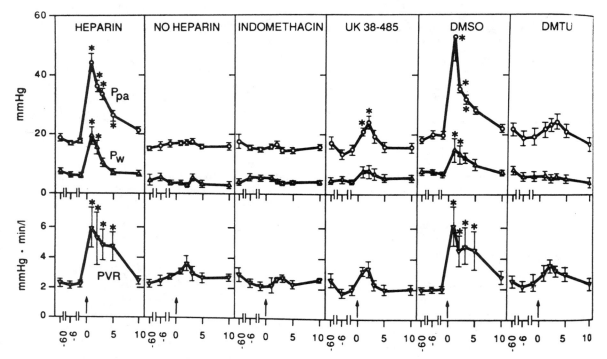

FIG. 23.10. Effect of bolus injection of protamine (*arrow*) on mean pulmonary arterial pressure (*Ppa*), pulmonary capillary wedge pressure (*Pw*), and pulmonary vascular resistance (*PVR*) in the six treatment groups. Heparinized controls, $n = 4$; unheparinized controls (no heparin), $n = 10$ (except for times $+1$ and $+2$ minutes for PVR values, where $n = 6$ and $n = 7$, respectively); indomethacin-pretreated heparinized sheep, $n = 3$; UK 38-485–pretreated heparinized sheep, $n = 5$; DMSO-pretreated heparinized sheep, $n = 4$; DMTU-pretreated heparinized sheep, $n = 6$. Values are the mean ± standard error of the mean. *$p = 0.05$ value differs from before protamine injection. *DMSO*, dimethylsulfoxide hydroxide scavenger; *DMTU*, dimethylthiourea hydrogen peroxide scavenger; *UK 38-485*, thromboxane synthetase inhibitor. (From Morel DR, Lowenstein E, Nguyenduy T, et al. Acute pulmonary vasoconstriction and thromboxane release during protamine reversal of heparin anticoagulation in awake sheep. *Circ Res* 1988;62:905–915, with permission.)

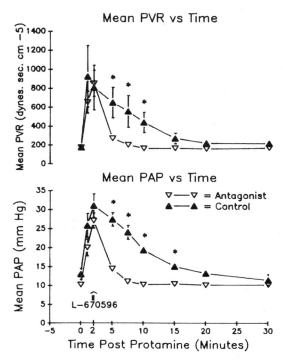

FIG. 23.11. The increase in mean pulmonary vascular resistance (*PVR*) and mean pulmonary arterial pressure (*PAP*) after protamine administration at time *t* = 0 for control and antagonist-treated pigs. The thromboxane receptor antagonist (L-670596) was administered 2 minutes after protamine administration. Data plotted as mean ± standard error of the mean. At lower PAP and PVR, error bars are hidden by figure points. *$p \geq 0.05$. (From Nuttall GA, Murray MJ, Bowie JW. Protamine–heparin-induced pulmonary hypertension in pigs; effects of treatment with a thromboxane receptor antagonist on hemodynamics and coagulation. *Anesthesiology* 1991;74:138–145, with permission.)

Some thromboxane receptor antagonists are known to inhibit platelet aggregation to collagen and arachidonic acid stimulation and cause a brief prolongation of bleeding times (76,80), whereas other antagonists cause no increase in bleeding times, even at the highest dosages used (75). Nuttall et al. (76) showed that thromboxane A_2 receptor blockade initiated 2 minutes after protamine administration shortened the duration of the pulmonary hypertensive response in pigs despite similar elevations in pulmonary artery pressures and plasma thromboxane B_2 levels (Fig. 23.11).

Although thromboxane release appears to be a central factor in pulmonary vasoconstriction induced by heparin–protamine, the source of thromboxane is unclear. A blood source seems doubtful, as the reaction can be produced in isolated lungs perfused with acellular media (77) and in platelet-depleted animals (81). Endothelial cells or more likely pulmonary intravascular macrophages (PIMs) may be the source of the thromboxane.

It has been speculated that PIMs may be the source of the thromboxane generated in pulmonary vasoconstrictive reactions (82). These lung macrophages have been described

in sheep (83) and pigs (84) and occur less commonly in rats (85,86) and dogs (87). They are five times more numerous than neutrophils in sheep lung (88) and occupy 15% of intracapillary volume (81). These macrophages respond to the infusion of various foreign particles by releasing vasoactive eicosanoids, particularly thromboxane (89). Infusion of radioactively labeled protamine into rats and sheep showed uptake primarily by the lungs in sheep with rapid development of pulmonary vasoconstriction, in comparison with uptake primarily by the liver in rats. Based on these data, it has been hypothesized that the uptake of heparin–protamine complexes by PIMs causes the release of mediators, namely thromboxane, with resultant pulmonary vasoconstriction. Humans have a lesser population of these macrophages than do sheep, which may partially explain the variable development of this syndrome in humans (80).

Platelet-depleted sheep still exhibit increased thromboxane B_2 levels, pulmonary vascular resistance, and leukopenia when protamine is administered after heparin (79). These studies suggest that platelets do not cause this adverse response.

Rate of Administration

Morel et al. (90) determined the rate of protamine administration to be an important factor leading to pulmonary vasoconstriction in sheep. In their study, sheep given protamine during 3 seconds consistently demonstrated thromboxane release, pulmonary vasoconstriction, increased pulmonary artery pressure, increased systemic vascular resistance, and decreased cardiac output, whereas those given protamine during 30 minutes exhibited no change. The intermediate infusion rates were associated with variable and attenuated reactions.

Site of Administration

The site of protamine administration has been considered and studied as a triggering factor for protamine reactions. Canine studies (91,92) suggest that detrimental vasoactive substances are released on exposure of the pulmonary vasculature to protamine. Giving the drug on the left side of the circulation or via a peripheral vein with subsequent dilution was hypothesized to limit the first-pass pulmonary exposure. Casthely and co-workers (92) confirmed this hypothesis in a canine model in which protamine delivered during 4 minutes via a peripheral vein or the left atrium proved benign, whereas delivery via central venous injection decreased systemic blood pressure and systemic vascular resistance and increased pulmonary vascular resistance and pulmonary artery pressure. These results were not confirmed by others (93,94).

Frater et al. (94) demonstrated decreased systolic blood pressure and increased plasma histamine levels in patients given protamine via the right atrium, changes that were not observed when protamine was administered via the left atrium. However, the majority of human studies to date have not demonstrated any advantage to left-sided versus right-sided protamine administration (95,96). The rate of infusion, and not the infusion site, appears to be the more important variable to control. Lastly, because of the risk for air embolization when a left atrial or aortic route is used, protamine is probably best administered on the right side of the circulation.

Summary of Pulmonary Vasoconstrictive Reactions

In summary, pulmonary vasoconstrictive protamine reactions in certain animal models result from uptake or activation in the lung, perhaps by PIMs, of the heparin–protamine complex. This interaction causes nonimmunologic activation of the classic complement pathway with increased levels of C3a and C5a, which can release vasoconstrictor substances, most importantly thromboxane. The question of whether complement activation is merely associated with the formation of heparin–protamine complexes or is a prerequisite for thromboxane generation is still unsettled. Leukocytes do not appear to play a crucial role, as evidenced by work with acellular perfusates. Histamine and platelets also do not appear to be involved. Certain drugs can block the development of this syndrome at various points of the reaction, but because of interference with coagulation or other problems, these agents are not yet feasible for clinical use after CPB.

Patients in whom pulmonary vasoconstriction and bronchoconstriction developed following protamine administration at the conclusion of CPB had markedly elevated levels of plasma thromboxane B_2 and C5a in comparison with controls in whom adverse responses to protamine administration did not develop. The time of peak thromboxane B_2 levels corresponded to the maximum pulmonary artery pressures. These data suggest that the activation of complement fraction C5a is associated with thromboxane generation. It was also documented that (consistent with the animal model) leukopenia and increased C3a and C4a plasma levels were universal after protamine administration, although only patients in whom pulmonary vasoconstrictive reactions developed had elevated levels of thromboxane and C5a (97).

One difference between the animal and human studies has been that catastrophic pulmonary vasoconstriction is demonstrated consistently in animal models, whereas the incidence in humans is relatively low (1% to 2%). This fact suggests that different factors may play a role in humans. Hobbhahn and co-workers (98) examined the effects of protamine neutralization of heparin in 14 noncardiac surgical patients undergoing transurethral surgery. Nine of these 14 (64%) patients responded with increases in mean pulmonary artery pressures, mean arterial pressure, pulmonary vascular resistance, and increased thromboxane B_2 and C3a levels. This work confirms the relevance of the animal model to the human reaction.

One interesting aspect of this syndrome is that although initial mediator release can cause catastrophic hemodynamic changes, there is usually no long-lasting tissue damage or sequelae if the patient can be supported through the initial event.

Diagnosis

Diagnosis of the type of protamine reaction in a patient experiencing one is based on the clinical hemodynamic presentation, the mediators that are present, and the presence or absence of specific IgE or IgG antibodies. Screening for antibodies in insulin-dependent diabetics may be a useful way to identify patients at risk for anaphylaxis to protamine.

Skin testing is available but requires a strict protocol to yield reproducible results, is unreliable in diabetics, and can cause an adverse systemic response when an antigen is reintroduced (99). Additionally, as stated earlier, the absence of a positive skin test reaction does not ensure the lack of an IgE-mediated protamine reaction. The leukocyte histamine response is an *in vitro* test that has been used to detect protamine allergy in NPH insulin-dependent diabetics and protect them from adverse reactions (57). A positive response to this standard technique in *in vitro* allergy studies indicates specific IgE antibodies (100). However, there is little documented evidence of the usefulness of this test in screening for patients at risk for adverse protamine reactions. Serum levels of IgG or complement can be measured but are nonspecific indicators of a potential allergic reaction, and they are difficult to interpret *post hoc* because of consumption during the reaction and dilution by volume therapy during an adverse reaction (95).

The radioimmunosorbent assay is a semiquantitative assay of a specific antibody described by Weiss et al. (58), who used it to determine the presence of antiprotamine IgE. The enzyme-linked immunosorbent assay involves anti-IgE tagged with an enzyme that catalyzes a photochemical reaction, and a modification was employed to determine IgG specific for protamine. Both tests described by Weiss and co-workers are probably the best currently available for the diagnosis of protamine allergy.

Prevention and Therapy

Prevention of the heparin–protamine reaction would be the best strategy. Until a reliable screening test for antiprotamine antibodies becomes available, a history of a proven anaphylactic reaction can be helpful. We have administered hexadimethrine for successful protamine reversal in three protamine insulin-dependent diabetics who had experienced a prior protamine reaction. A compassionate use Investigational New Drug application from the Food and Drug Administration is required to gain permission to administer hexadimethrine bromide in the United States.

Protamine should be administered slowly. The protamine package insert suggests that infusion be no faster than

5 mg/min, although in practice, a rate of 15 mg/min seems to be well tolerated. Administration should be terminated at the first sign of any adverse reaction. Pharmacologic release reactions are rate-dependent, so that slow administration prevents them. Protamine anaphylaxis is treated like any classic anaphylactic reaction with oxygen, fluids, and epinephrine/norepinephrine. Excessive protamine doses should be avoided because protamine has been shown to inhibit the enzyme responsible for the inactivation of anaphylatoxins and kinins, as mentioned earlier in this chapter. Also, because protamine does not inhibit angiotensin I, which can also break down these compounds, patients on angiotensin-converting enzyme inhibitors may be at some increased risk for pulmonary hypertensive reactions to protamine (68).

Prophylactic histamine$_1$ and histamine$_2$ blockers and corticosteroids have not reduced the incidence of pulmonary vasoconstrictor reactions. Histamine blockers are known to decrease the severity of hypotension with rapid protamine administration (50), which suggests a role in IgE-mediated reactions, but there is no evidence to support their routine use for this purpose. Therefore, we do not recommend this strategy.

Various supportive strategies have been used to treat acute pulmonary vasoconstriction and hypotension, including such pulmonary vasodilators as nitroglycerin and isoproterenol and virtually all vasoactive/inotropic drugs. The comparative efficacy of different regimens for these short-lived reactions has not been documented. Reinstitution of bypass may be required. *It is crucial to heparinize effectively before the reinstitution of bypass to avoid gross clotting and the consumption of components of coagulation, which can lead to disseminated intravascular coagulation.* Case reports suggest that the reinstitution of bypass with heparin administration causes the reaction to abate (101); however, it is likely that this represents merely the conclusion of a transient reaction. The role of thromboxane receptor blockade for treatment has not been studied in patients.

Inhaled nitric oxide has recently been reported as a therapy for the pulmonary vasoconstrictor reactions induced by heparin–protamine complexes in lambs (102). Nitric oxide selectively produces profound relaxation of the pulmonary vascular smooth muscle without systemic vasodilation. In this animal model, breathing nitric oxide at 180 parts per million has been shown to attenuate the pulmonary vasoconstrictor response markedly following heparin neutralization by protamine. Nitric oxide is short-lived, easily administered, and effective for treating certain types of reversible pulmonary hypertension. The value of nitric oxide inhalation for treating protamine-induced pulmonary vasoconstriction in patients has yet to be determined.

The initial pulmonary vasoconstrictive episode usually abates after a few minutes (3). Once this occurs, continued inotropic infusion can result in a hyperdynamic heart, and it may need to be withdrawn. Protamine administration may be reinstituted at a rate of 5 mg/min following resolution of the episode and after resumption of hemodynamic stability.

FUTURE MANAGEMENT

To date there is no well-proven substitute for heparin anticoagulation and its reversal with protamine for the management of CPB. Research is ongoing in such areas as total elimination of systemic heparinization through the use of heparin-bonded bypass circuitry (103). Also, different forms of heparin, such as low-molecular-weight heparins and heparinoids, are under investigation (see Chap. 22). Reversal of heparin by PF4 and by heparinase, which was discussed earlier in this chapter, is also currently under investigation.

KEY POINTS

- *Protamine*, a strongly alkaline polycationic protein, attracts the polyanionic heparin sufficiently to separate it from its binding site on AT III and reverse its anticoagulant effect.
- *Inhibition of plasma coagulation and platelet function* is one of the side effects of protamine, so it appears prudent to avoid administering protamine doses beyond the amount needed to neutralize heparin.
- Methods for *calculating the protamine dose* include the following:
  - Use a *fixed ratio* of protamine to the total or initial dose of heparin.
  - Use the *heparin–ACT dose–response* to determine the amount of circulating heparin, then assume a protamine-to-heparin neutralization ratio of approximately 1.3 mg to 100 U of heparin.
  - Measure *whole blood* or *plasma heparin concentration*, assume a protamine-to-heparin neutralization ratio, and estimate blood or plasma volume.
- A variety of methods exist for methods 2 and 3, some of which are automated. Each method has advantages and disadvantages, and there is no widely accepted "gold standard" for calculating the protamine dose.
- Aside from commercially available protamine, other possible approaches to heparin neutralization include the administration of hexadimethrine, PF4, heparinase, or protamine variants ("designer protamine"), and the use of heparin-removal devices. Although some of these alternative methods are under investigation, none is currently generally available.

- *Protamine reactions* can be classified as pharmacologic histamine release, true anaphylaxis, and anaphylactoid reactions.
  - *Pharmacologic histamine release* is principally related to overly rapid administration of protamine and can result in vasodilation and possibly myocardial depression.
  - *True anaphylaxis* requires previous exposure to protamine, which has been conclusively demonstrated only in diabetics taking intermediate-duration insulin preparations that contain protamine. Even in that group of patients, the incidence of anaphylaxis after protamine administration is low ($<3\%$ in most studies).
- The interaction of protamine with heparin activates complement, which has been associated with the release of thromboxane A_2. Thromboxane A_2 (in sufficient amounts) causes *intense pulmonary vasoconstriction*. Factors predisposing some patients to the development of this rare, life-threatening reaction, which is predictable in some animal species, remain ill-defined.
- Antibody screening techniques may be useful for identifying insulin-dependent diabetic patients at risk for protamine-induced anaphylaxis.
- The treatment of protamine reactions is largely supportive. It is possible that inhaled nitric oxide can rapidly and effectively terminate a life-threatening pulmonary hypertensive response.

REFERENCES

1. Hunt AJ, Gray GS, Myers JA, et al. Heparin neutralization by recombinant human PF4 *in vitro. FASEB J* 1990;4:A1991(abst).
2. Ando T, Yamasaki M, Suzuki K. Protamines. In: Kleinzeller A, Springer GF, Wittman HG, eds. *Molecular biology, biochemistry, and biophysics.* Berlin: Springer-Verlag, 1973;12:1–30.
3. Taylor S, Folkman J. Protamine as an inhibitor of angiogenesis. *Nature* 1982;297:307–312.
4. Wright JEC. Clinical trial of protamine in the treatment of malignant diseases. *Br J Cancer* 1968;22:415–421.
5. Chargaff E, Olson KB. Studies on the chemistry of blood coagulation. *J Biol Chem* 1937–38;122:153–167.
6. Perkins HA, Osborn JJ, Hurt R, et al. Neutralization of heparin *in vivo* with protamine: a simple method of estimating the required dose. *J Lab Clin Med* 1956;48:223–226.
7. Ellison N, Ominsky AJ, Wollman H. Is protamine a clinically significant anticoagulant? A negative answer. *Anesthesiology* 1971;35:621–629.
8. Inagaki M, Goto K, Katayama H, et al. Activated partial thromboplastin time-protamine dose in the presence and absence of heparin. *J Cardiothorac Anesth* 1989;3:734–736.
9. Ellison N, Edmunds LH, Colman RW. Platelet aggregation following heparin and protamine administration. *Anesthesiology* 1978;48:65–68.
10. Mammen EF, Koets MH, Washington BC, et al. Hemostasis changes during cardiopulmonary bypass surgery. *Semin Thromb Hemost* 1985;11:281–292.
11. Guffin AV, Dunbar RW, Kaplan JA, et al. Successful use of a reduced dose of protamine after cardiopulmonary bypass. *Anesth Analg* 1976;55:110–113.
12. Dutton DA, Hothersall AP, McLaren AD, et al. Protamine titration after cardiopulmonary bypass. *Anesthesiology* 1983;38:264–268.
13. Kresowik TF, Wakefield TW, Fessler RD, et al. Anticoagulant effects of protamine sulfate in the canine model. *J Surg Res* 1988;45:8–14.
14. Bull BS, Korpman RA, Huse WM, et al. Heparin therapy during extracorporeal circulation, I. Problems inherent in existing heparin protocols. *J Thorac Cardiovasc Surg* 1975;69:674–684.
15. Kimmel SE, Sekeres MA, Berlin JA, et al. Adverse events after protamine administration in patients undergoing cardiopulmonary bypass: risks and predictors of underreporting. *J Clin Epidemiol* 1998;51:1–10.
16. Hurt R, Perkins HA, Osborn JJ, et al. The neutralization of heparin by protamine in extracorporeal circulation. *J Thorac Surg* 1956;32:612–619.
17. Hattersley PG. Activated coagulation time of whole blood. *JAMA* 1966;196:150–154.
18. Akl BF, Vargas GM, Neal J, et al. Clinical experience with the activated clotting time for the control of heparin and protamine therapy during cardiopulmonary bypass. *J Thorac Cardiovasc Surg* 1980;79:97–102.
19. Bull BS, Huse WM, Brauer FS, et al. Heparin therapy during extracorporeal circulation, II. The use of a dose–response curve to individualize heparin and protamine dosage. *J Thorac Cardiovasc Surg* 1975;69:685–689.
20. Ellison N, Beatty CP, Blake DR, et al. Heparin rebound, studies in patients and volunteers. *J Thorac Cardiovasc Surg* 1974;67:723–729.
21. Culliford AT, Gitel SN, Starr N, et al. Lack of correlation between activated clotting time and plasma heparin during cardiopulmonary bypass. *Ann Surg* 1981;193:105–111.
22. Yin ET, Wessler S, Butler JV. Plasma heparin: a unique, practical, submicrogram-sensitive assay. *J Lab Clin Med* 1973;81:298–310.
23. Senning A. Plasma heparin concentration in extracorporeal circulation. *Acta Chir Scand* 1959;117:55–59.
24. Wahr JA, Yun JH, Yang VC, et al. A new method of measuring heparin levels in whole blood by protamine titration using a heparin-responsive electrochemical sensor. *J Cardiothorac Vasc Anesth* 1996;10:447–450.
25. Schleuter AJ, Pennell BJ, Olson JD. Evaluation of a new protamine titration method to assay heparin in whole blood and plasma. *Am J Clin Pathol* 1997;107:511–520.
26. Allen JG, Moulder PV, Elghammer RM, et al. A protamine titration as an indication of a clotting defect in certain hemorrhagic states. *J Lab Clin Med* 1949;34:473–476.
27. Hawksley M. De-heparinisation of blood after cardiopulmonary bypass. *Lancet* 1966;1:563–565.
28. Bull BS, Korpman RA, Huse WM, et al. Heparin therapy during extracorporeal circulation, I. Problems inherent in existing heparin protocols. *J Thorac Cardiovasc Surg* 1975;69:674–684.
29. Shore-Lesserson L, Reich DL, DePerio M. Heparin and protamine titration do not improve hemostasis in cardiac surgical patients. *Can J Anaesth* 1998;45:10–18.
30. Jobes DR, Aitken GL, Shaffer GW. Increased accuracy and precision of heparin and protamine dosing reduces blood loss and transfusion in patients undergoing primary cardiac operations. *J Thorac Cardiovasc Surg* 1995;110:36–45.
31. Kanbak M, Kahraman S, Celebioglu B, et al. Prophylactic administration of histamine 1 and/or histamine 2 receptor blockers in the prevention of heparin- and protamine-related hemodynamic effects. *Anaesth Intensive Care* 1996;15:559–563.

32. Walker WS, Reid KG, Hider CF, et al. Successful cardiopulmonary bypass in diabetics with anaphylactoid reactions to protamine. *Br Heart J* 1984;52:112–114.

33. Cook JJ, Schaffer LH, Niewiarowski S, et al. Heparin neutralization by protamine and platelet factor 4 in the rat. *FASEB J* 1990;4:A1234(abst).

34. Cook JJ, Niewiarowski S, Yan Z, et al. Platelet factor 4 efficiently reverses heparin anticoagulation in the rat without the adverse effects of heparin–protamine complexes. *Circulation* 1992;85:1102–1109.

35. Dehmer GJ, Lange RA, Tate DA, et al. Randomized trial of recombinant platelet factor 4 versus protamine for the reversal of heparin anticoagulation in humans. *Circulation* 1996; 94[Suppl]:II347–II352.

36. Kurrek M, Winkler M, Robinson DR, et al. Platelet factor 4 injection produces acute pulmonary hypertension in the awake lamb. *Anesthesiology* 1995;82:183–188.

37. Bernabei A, Gikakis N, Maione TE, et al. Reversal of heparin anticoagulation by recombinant platelet factor 4 and protamine sulfate in baboons during cardiopulmonary bypass. *J Thorac Cardiovasc Surg* 1995;109:765–771.

38. Wakefield TW, Andrews PC, Wrobleski SK, et al. Effective and less toxic reversal of low-molecular-weight heparin anticoagulation by a designer variant of protamine. *J Vasc Surg* 1995;21: 839–849.

39. Wakefield TW, Andrews PC, Wrobleski SK, et al. A [+18RGD] protamine variant for nontoxic and effective reversal of conventional heparin and low-molecular-weight heparin anticoagulation. *J Surg Res* 1996;63:280–286.

40. Michelson LG, Kikura M, Levy JH, et al. Heparinase I (neutralase) reversal of systemic anticoagulation. *Anesthesiology* 1996; 85:339–346.

41. Ammar T, Fisher CF. The effects of heparinase 1 and protamine on platelet reactivity. *Anesthesiology* 1997;6:1382–1386.

42. Hendrikx M, Leuvens V, Vandezarde E, et al. The use of heparin removal devices: a valid alternative to protamine. *Int J Artif Organs* 1997;20:166–174.

43. Yang VC, Port FK, Kim JS, et al. The use of immobilized protamine in removing heparin and preventing protamine-induced complications during extracorporeal blood circulation. *Anesthesiology* 1991;75:288–297.

44. Lowenstein E, Johnston WE, Lappas DG, et al. Catastrophic pulmonary vasoconstriction associated with protamine reversal of heparin. *Anesthesiology* 1983;59:470–473.

45. Levy JH, Schwieger IM, Zaidan JR, et al. Evaluation of patients at risk for protamine reactions. *J Thorac Cardiovasc Surg* 1989; 98:200–220.

46. Comunale ME, Haering JM, Robertson LK, et al. Aspirin prevents protamine-induced pulmonary hypertension. *Anesth Analg* 1997;84:S66.

47. Schapira M, Christman BW. Neutralization of heparin by protamine, time for a change? *Circulation* 1990;82:1887–1879.

48. Horrow JC. Protamine allergy. *J Cardiothorac Anesth* 1988;2: 225–252.

49. Rosow CE, Moss J, Philbin DM, et al. Histamine release during morphine and fentanyl anesthesia. *Anesthesiology* 1982;56: 93–96.

50. Keller R. Interrelation between different types of cells. II. Histamine release for the mast cells of various species by cationic polypeptides of polymorphonuclear leukocytes, lysosomes and other cationic compounds. *Int Arch Allergy Appl Immunol* 1968; 34:139–144.

51. Stoelting RK, Henry DP, Verbur KM, et al. Haemodynamic changes and circulating histamine concentrations following protamine administration to patients and dogs. *Can Anaesth Soc J* 1984;31:534–540.

52. Parsons RS, Mohandas K. The effect of histamine-receptor blockade on the hemodynamic responses to protamine. *J Cardiothorac Anesth* 1989;3:37–43.

53. Shapira N, Schaff HV, Piehler JM, et al. Cardiovascular effects of protamine sulfate in man. *J Thorac Cardiovasc Surg* 1982; 84:505–514.

54. Sethna D, Gray R, Bussell J, et al. Further studies on the myocardial metabolic effect of protamine sulfate following cardiopulmonary bypass. *Anesth Analg* 1982;61:476–477.

55. Goldman BS, Joison J, Austen WG. Cardiovascular effects of protamine sulfate. *Ann Thorac Surg* 1969;7:459–471.

56. Michaels IAL, Barash PG. Hemodynamic changes during protamine administration. *Anesth Analg* 1983;62:831–835.

57. Sethna DH, Moffitt E, Gray RJ, et al. Effects of protamine sulfate on myocardial oxygen supply and demand in patients following cardiopulmonary bypass. *Anesth Analg* 1982;61: 157–251.

58. Sharath MD, Metzger WJ, Richerson HB, et al. Protamine-induced fatal anaphylaxis, prevalence of antiprotamine immunoglobin E antibody. *J Thorac Cardiovasc Surg* 1985;90:86–90.

59. Levy JH, Zaidan JR, Faraj B. Prospective evaluation of risk of protamine reactions in patients with NPH insulin-dependent diabetes. *Anesth Analg* 1986;65:739–742.

60. Weiss ME, Nyhan D, Peng Z, et al. Association of protamine IgE and IgG antibodies with life-threatening reactions to intravenous protamine. *N Engl J Med* 1989;320:886–892.

61. Knape JTA, Schuller JL, De Haan P, et al. An anaphylactic reaction to protamine in a patient allergic to fish. *Anesthesiology* 1981;55:315–325.

62. Caplan SN, Berkman EM. Protamine sulfate and fish allergy [Letter]. *N Engl J Med* 1976;295:172.

63. Samuel T, Kolk AHJ, Rumke P, et al. Auto-immunity to sperm antigens in vasectomized men. *Clin Exp Immunol* 1975;21: 65–74.

64. Samuel T, Kolk A. Auto-antigenicity of human protamines. In: Lepow IH, Crozier R, eds. *Vasectomy: immunological and pathophysiologic effect in animal and man.* New York: Academic Press, 1979:203–220.

65. Best N, Teisner B, Grudzinkas JG, et al. Classical pathway activation during an adverse response to protamine sulfate. *Br J Anaesth* 1983;55:1149–1153.

66. Rent R, Ertel N, Eisenstein R, et al. Complement activation by interaction of polyanions and polycations, I. Heparin–protamine induced consumption of complement. *J Immunol* 1975; 114:120–115.

67. Kirklin JK, Chenoweth DE, Naftel DC, et al. Effects of protamine administration after cardiopulmonary bypass on complement, blood elements, and the hemodynamic state. *Ann Thorac Surg* 1986;41:193–199.

68. Cavarocchi NC, Schaff HV, Orszulak TA, et al. Evidence for complement activation by protamine–heparin interaction after cardiopulmonary bypass. *Surgery* 1985;98:525–530.

69. Grant JA, Dupree E, Goldman AS, et al. Complement-mediated release of histamine from human leukocytes. *J Immunol* 1975; 114:1101–1106.

70. Tan F, Jackman H, Skidgel RA, et al. Protamine inhibits plasma carboxypeptidase N, the inactivator of anaphylatoxins and kinins. *Anesthesiology* 1989;70:267–275.

71. Stewart WJ, McSweeney SM, Kellett MA, et al. Increased risk of severe protamine reactions in NPH insulin-dependent diabetics undergoing cardiac catheterization. *Circulation* 1984;5: 788–792.

72. Lakin JD, Blocker TJ, Strong DM, et al. Anaphylaxis to protamine sulfate mediated by a complement-dependent IgG antibody. *J Allergy Clin Immunol* 1978;61:102–107.

73. Lowenstein E. Lessons from studying an infrequent event: ad-

verse hemodynamic responses associated with protamine reversal of heparin anticoagulation. *J Cardiothorac Anesth* 1989;3: 99–107.

74. Morel DR, Lowenstein E, Nguyenduy T, et al. Acute pulmonary vasoconstriction and thromboxane release during protamine reversal of heparin anticoagulation in awake sheep. *Circ Res* 1988;62:905–915.

75. Montalescot G, Lowenstein E, Ogletree ML, et al. Thromboxane receptor blockade prevents pulmonary hypertension induced by heparin–protamine reactions in awake sheep. *Circulation* 1990;82:1765–1777.

76. Nuttall GA, Murray MJ, Bowie JW. Protamine–heparin-induced pulmonary hypertension in pigs: effects of treatment with a thromboxane receptor antagonist on hemodynamics and coagulation. *Anesthesiology* 1991;74:138–145.

77. Conzen PF, Habazettl H, Gutman R, et al. Thromboxane mediation of pulmonary hemodynamic responses after neutralization of heparin by protamine in pigs. *Anesth Analg* 1989;68: 25–31.

78. Schumacher WA, Heran CL, Ogletree ML. Effect of thromboxane receptor antagonism on pulmonary hypertension caused by protamine–heparin interaction in pigs. *Circulation* 1988; 78[suppl]:II-207.

79. Degges RD, Foster ME, Dang AQ, et al. Pulmonary hypertensive effect of heparin and protamine interaction: evidence for thromboxane B2 release from the lung. *Am J Surg* 1987;154: 696–699.

80. Friedhoff LT, Manning J, Funke PT, et al. Quantitation of drug levels and platelet receptor blockade caused by a thromboxane antagonist. *Clin Pharmacol Ther* 1986;40:634–642.

81. Montalescot G, Kreil E, Lynch K, et al. Effect of platelet depletion on lung vasoconstriction in heparin–protamine reactions. *J Appl Physiol* 1989;66:2344–2350.

82. Kreil E, Montalescot G, Robinson DR, et al. Adverse heparin–protamine neutralization interactions and the lung. In: Zapol WM, Lemarie F, eds. *Adult respiratory distress sydrome*. New York: Marcel Dekker Inc, 1991:451–490.

83. Warner AE, Barry BE, Brain JD. Pulmonary intravascular macrophages in sheep: morphology and function of a novel constituent of the mononuclear phagocyte system. *Lab Invest* 1986;55:276–288.

84. Bertram TA, Overby LH, Danilowicz R, et al. Pulmonary intravascular macrophages metabolize arachidonic acid *in vitro*. *Am Rev Respir Dis* 1988;138:936–944.

85. Warner AE, DeCamp MM, Molina RM, et al. Pulmonary removal of circulating endotoxin results in acute lung injury in sheep. *Lab Invest* 1988;59:219–230.

86. Warner A, Molina A, Brain JD. Uptake of blood-borne bacteria by pulmonary intravascular macrophages and consequent inflammatory responses in sheep. *Am Rev Respir Dis* 1987;136: 683–690.

87. Crocker SH, Eddy DO, Obenauf RN, et al. Bacteremia: host-specific lung clearance and pulmonary failure. *J Trauma* 1981; 21:215–220.

88. Albertine KH, Decker SA, Schultz EL, et al. Clearance of monastral blue by intravascular macrophages in pulmonary microvessels of sheep, goat, and pig. *Anat Rec* 1987;218:6A(abst).

89. Bertram TA, Thigpen J, Eling TE, et al. Bacterial phagocytosis and consequent arachidonic acid metabolism by pulmonary intravascular and alveolar macrophages *in vitro*. *Am Rev Respir Dis* 1989;139:A159.

90. Morel DR, Costabella PM, Pittet JF. Adverse cardiopulmonary effects and increased thromboxane concentrations following the neutralization of heparin with protamine in awake sheep are infusion rate-dependent. *Anesthesiology* 1990;73:415–424.

91. Goldman BS, Joison J, Austen WG. Cardiovascular effects of protamine sulfate. *Ann Thorac Surg* 1969;7:459–471.

92. Casthely PA, Goodman K, Fryman PN, et al. Hemodynamic changes after the administration of protamine. *Anesth Analg* 1986;65:78–80.

93. Taylor RL, Little WC, Freeman GL, et al. Comparison of the cardiovascular effects of intravenous and intraaortic protamine in the conscious and anesthetized dog. *Ann Thorac Surg* 1986; 42:22–26.

94. Frater RWM, Oka Y, Hong Y, et al. Protamine-induced circulatory changes. *J Thorac Cardiovasc Surg* 1984;87:687–692.

95. Milne B, Rogers K, Cervenko F, et al. The hemodynamic effects of intaaortic versus intravenous administration of protamine for reversal of heparin in man. *Can Anaesth Soc J* 1983;30:347–351.

96. Cherry DA, Chiu CJ, Wynands JE, et al. Intraaortic vs. intravenous administration of protamine: a prospective randomized clinical study. *Surg Forum* 1985;36:238–250.

97. Morel DR, Zapol WM, Thomas SJ, et al. C5a and thromboxane generation associated with pulmonary vaso- and bronchoconstriction during protamine reversal of heparin. *Anesthesiology* 1987;66:597–604.

98. Hobbhahn J, Conzen P, Habazettl H, et al. Heparin reversal by protamine in humans—complement, prostaglandins, leukocytes, platelets, and hemodynamics. *J Appl Physiol* 1991;71: 1415–1421.

99. Fisher M. Intradermal testing after anaphylactoid reaction to anaesthetic drugs: practical aspects of performance and interpretation. *Anaesth Intensive Care* 1984;12:115–120.

100. May CD, Lyman M, Alberto R, et al. Procedures for immunochemical study of histamine release from leukocytes with small volumes of blood. *J Allergy* 1970;46:12–20.

101. Loch R, Hessel EA. Probable reversal of protamine reactions by heparin administration. *J Cardiothorac Anesth* 1990;4:604–608.

102. Fratacci MD, Frostell CG, Chen TY, et al. Inhaled nitric oxide. A selective pulmonary vasodilator of heparin protamine vasoconstriction in sheep. *Anesthesiology* 1991;75:990–999.

103. Von Segesser LK, Turina M. Cardiopulmonary bypass without systemic heparinization. *J Thorac Cardiovasc Surg* 1989;98: 386–396.

24

HEMATOLOGIC EFFECTS OF CARDIOPULMONARY BYPASS

CHRISTINE S. RINDER

Normal blood circulation maintains prothrombotic and antithrombotic factors, all carefully balanced in number and function, to preserve blood fluidity, and yet, this balance can instantly alter to seal off any site of bleeding. The importance of this homeostasis is underscored by the redundancy built into all aspects of clotting and endogenous anticoagulation, such that most heterozygous defects can be tolerated if they occur in isolation. The first half of this chapter discusses the procoagulant and anticoagulant factors that make up the system of checks and balances critical to the maintenance of normal blood circulation. The second part explores the ways in which cardiopulmonary bypass (CPB) challenges this hemostatic system, simultaneously activating coagulant and inflammatory processes and creating hemostatic impairment that can lead to excessive bleeding and transfusion requirements.

HEMOSTASIS IN THE ARTERIAL AND VENOUS CIRCULATIONS

The arterial and venous circulations, with their widely disparate flow conditions, impose very different needs on the coagulation system. In the pressurized arteries, a relatively small degree of vascular damage can rapidly cause significant blood loss and hematoma formation, so that a system is needed that can rapidly and securely seal off sites of bleeding. As is described in detail later in this chapter, platelets dominate this "rapid response team," initially containing blood loss and then providing a surface for localization and acceleration of the fibrin formation that ultimately consolidates hemostasis. In the venous circulation, by contrast, the more leisurely flow rates diminish the need for speed, so that platelets are less critical; indeed, the pivotal reaction controlling venous hemostasis is the rate of *thrombin* generation. The differences between the arterial and venous circu-

lations are underscored by the anticoagulant agents that are effective for prophylaxis in these two settings (i.e., antiplatelet agents such as aspirin to prevent coronary thrombosis (1) and antithrombin-based interventions such as warfarin for the treatment of deep venous thrombosis). Much of the discussion that follows focuses on coagulation in the arterial circulation and microcirculation, as these areas present the greatest challenge for postsurgical hemostasis.

Platelet Adhesion in the Presence of High Shear

Significant mechanical stresses are created by the high-flow velocities present in arterial systems. The interaction between a vessel wall and rapidly flowing blood, as shown in Fig. 24.1, creates parallel planes of blood moving at different velocities, with blood near the wall moving more slowly than blood at the center of the vessel (2). The different velocities of these moving layers of blood create shear stress that is greatest at the vessel wall and diminishes toward the center (Fig. 24.1). This fluid shear stress, expressed in inverse seconds (s^{-1}), is greatest in the arterial circulation, with levels estimated to vary between 500 s^{-1} in the larger arteries and 5,000 s^{-1} in the smallest arterioles. Shear rates at the interface with arteriosclerotic plaques when stenosis is a modest 50% may reach 3,000 to 10,000 s^{-1}, with even greater shear stress in "tight" stenoses. The high shear created by the arterial circulation strongly opposes any tendency of the flowing blood to clot by (a) limiting the time available for procoagulant reactions to occur and (b) disrupting cells or proteins not tightly adherent to the vessel wall. However, when the vessel wall is damaged and bleeding occurs, these forces trigger a series of hemostatic events designed to respond rapidly and decisively to the loss of endothelial integrity and simultaneously resist the tendency to be swept downstream by high shear stress. One of the forces enhancing the state of hemostatic readiness in the arterial circulation is radial dispersion, or the tendency of larger cells (e.g., erythrocytes and leukocytes) to migrate to the center of the vessel. Such coaxial migration effectively

C. S. Rinder: Department of Anesthesiology, Yale University School of Medicine, New Haven, Connecticut 06520.

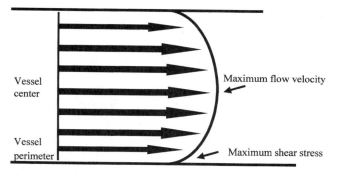

FIG. 24.1. Schematic representation of velocity and shear rate as a function of radial distance from the vessel wall. The velocity is parabolic, and the maximum velocity (v_{max}), at the vessel center, is twice the mass average velocity. The shear rate is maximal at the vessel wall and approaches zero at the vessel center.

mation dictate the balance of procoagulant and anticoagulant forces.

The constraints imposed by arterial dynamic flow stresses make a sequence of interrelated platelet receptor–ligand interactions critical for initiating arterial hemostasis. These interactions include (a) platelet adhesion to subendothelial proteins, (b) platelet activation and formation of stable platelet–platelet bonds, and ultimately (c) platelet–coagulation factor interactions culminating in the formation of fibrin. Given the velocity of blood flow at an arterial bleeding site, the platelets must activate and adhere to the injured vessel nearly instantaneously. Two molecules present in the subendothelium are critical for this process: von Willebrand's factor (vWf) and collagen. Control of bleeding in vessels under very high shear stress depends on the presence of vWf (4). The large, multimeric forms of this molecule, immobilized by binding to subendothelial collagen, are able to bind to a receptor on the platelet surface known as glycoprotein Ib (GPIb) despite the high shear stress present at the vessel wall (Fig. 24.2). This extremely rapid but low-affinity interaction markedly slows platelets but does not firmly anchor them to the subendothelium. With platelets no longer streaming by, but instead tumbling over the subendothelium, the high shear stress coupled with transmembrane signaling caused by the GPIb–vWf interaction (5) produces platelet activation and loss of discoid shape (platelet shape change). One consequence of platelet activation is conformational change in GPIIb/IIIa, the platelet receptor that is the target of a number of the newer antiplatelet agents (6). This conformational change in GPIIb/IIIa allows it to bind to the larger vWf multimers at a site distinct from the

pushes the smaller platelets to the vessel perimeter, optimally positioning them to respond to hemostatic challenges. This size-dependent cellular flow pattern may also explain the seemingly paradoxical tendency of arterial bleeding accompanied by anemia to decrease with red cell transfusions (3). This effect also underscores the importance of platelets in arterial hemostasis; reductions in platelet number or function may be associated with catastrophic arterial hemorrhage. By contrast, the lesser shear forces experienced in the venous circulation permit more random cell movement, making the minimum requirements for platelet number and function correspondingly less stringent. As such, the venous circulation is much more sensitive to defects in the soluble coagulation cascade, in which the kinetics of thrombin formation

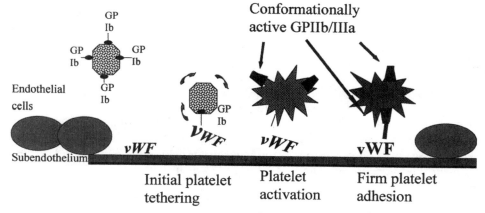

FIG. 24.2. Schematic representation of the mechanisms responsible for platelet adhesion to subendothelium under conditions of high shear stress. The first contact tethers the platelet to immobilized von Willebrand's factor (*vWf*) via platelet glycoprotein Ib (*GPIb*). This bond must be formed rapidly and have high resistance to shear stress, yet also have a high dissociation rate. Thus, GPIb rapidly forms attachments to vWf at the leading edge of the platelet while detaching at the tailing edge, which creates a rolling behavior. This vWf–GPIb bond generates a transmembrane signaling event that causes the platelet to become activated, inducing a conformational change in GPIIb/IIIa. The conformationally altered GPIIb/IIIa is then able to bind to the arginine–glycine–aspartate (*RGD*) sequence in the vWf molecule, producing stable, irreversible adhesion to the subendothelium.

GPIb-binding epitope. This secondary adhesion to vWf via GPIIb/IIIa is a higher-affinity interaction than that occurring with GPIb, and it causes platelets to become securely adherent to the subendothelium. A separate binding mechanism occurs via subendothelial collagen, another adhesive moiety that, at more moderate shear, is also capable of arresting the platelet via binding to GPIa/IIa (7). Thus, subendothelial vWf and collagen act cooperatively to initiate platelet adhesion, with the former predominating at higher shear. Collagen is unique in that it can act both to anchor platelets by binding to platelet GPIa/IIa at one locus, and to induce platelet activation by binding to platelet GPVI at a second locus (8), thereby allowing platelets simultaneously to bind to and be activated by subendothelial collagen. The combined actions of vWf and collagen exposed in the subendothelium to produce platelet adhesion and activation are pivotal to arresting blood loss through defects in arterial vessel wall integrity.

Formation of the Platelet Plug: Activation

Once a layer of adherent platelets is securely bound to the site of bleeding, the bound platelets must next coordinate an array of interdependent processes that together are referred to as *activation*. Ultimately, platelet activation has five major goals: (a) recruitment of additional platelets, (b) vasoconstriction of smaller arteries to slow bleeding, (c) local release of ligands essential to a stable platelet–platelet matrix, (d) localization and acceleration of platelet-associated fibrin formation, and (e) protection of clot from fibrinolysis.

Additional platelets are recruited to the platelet plug by the release of platelet stimulants, or agonists, into the local microenvironment. One of these agonists is thromboxane A_2, formed in the platelet cytosol following cyclooxygenase cleavage of arachidonic acid and released into the clot milieu on platelet activation (9). Thromboxane A_2 is both a platelet agonist and a vasoconstrictor and is rapidly degraded to its inert by-product, thromboxane B_2. Cyclooxygenase activity is *irreversibly* inhibited by aspirin, so that thromboxane A_2 formation is blocked. Platelet activation releases other platelet agonists located in the dense granules of the resting platelets. These are liberated by the fusion of dense granules with the platelet canalicular membrane, followed by extrusion of the granule contents. One of these dense granule constituents, serotonin, is both an agonist and a vasoconstrictor (10). The other constituent, adenosine diphosphate (ADP), is a platelet agonist with no known vasoactive properties. Having these agonists in the immediate vicinity of the damaged vessel activates passing platelets, which then join the growing platelet plug. The importance of the vasoconstrictive effects of thromboxane A_2 and serotonin to hemostasis is not entirely clear. Vasoconstriction, by acting distally to the site of bleeding, may slow the flow of blood past the platelet plug and simultaneously decrease shear stress, thereby facilitating recruitment of platelets to the injured

site. The severe bleeding diathesis expressed in patients with a congenital deficiency of dense granules (e.g. Hermansky-Pudlak syndrome and storage pool disease) demonstrates the importance of dense granule release to the maintenance of arterial hemostasis (11).

The basic building block of the platelet aggregate is a platelet–ligand–platelet matrix in which fibrinogen or vWf serves as the bridging ligand. Both fibrinogen and vWf are stored in platelet α-granules and are released with activation; both are capable of binding to GPIIb/IIIa on each of two platelets, thereby linking them. GPIIb/IIIa is maintained in an inactive form on the resting platelet. On activation, it undergoes a calcium-dependent conformational change that allows it to bind to either fibrinogen or vWf at a locus containing the amino acid sequence arginine–glycine–aspartate (RGD). Each fibrinogen molecule has two RGD sites on its polar ends, and the larger vWf multimers have several RGD sites, all capable of binding to conformationally altered GPIIb/IIIa to create the platelet–ligand–platelet matrix (12). GPIIb/IIIa is the most abundant glycoprotein on the platelet surface, with approximately 50,000 receptors on the *resting* platelet and additional receptors within a cytoplasmic pool that can be mobilized to the surface during activation.

Soluble Coagulation Cascade in Arterial and Venous Hemostasis

In isolation, activation and coordinated assembly of the soluble coagulation cascade proceeds relatively slowly, with a high probability of its being diluted at or displaced beyond the site of bleeding. However, when platelets are bound to sites of injury, they serve both to localize and to accelerate the soluble coagulation process. In addition to providing an essential negative phospholipid surface for coagulation reactions, activated platelets provide specific receptors for factors Xa, IXa, and Va (13); the latter factor also is released from the α-granule of the activated platelet. Membrane binding of coagulation factors and phospholipid optimally positions the factors to accelerate procoagulant enzymatic reactions that culminate in thrombin generation (14) (Fig. 24.3). Current models of coagulation suggest that the initiation of clotting requires the exposure of tissue factor (also known as *thromboplastin*) (15), whereas older models give equal weight to the intrinsic and extrinsic pathways. Growing evidence points to a primary role for tissue factor.

Cells not normally in contact with blood that may be exposed by vessel damage (e.g., fibroblasts and myocytes) express tissue factor even "at rest" (16). By contrast, cells constantly in contact with blood (e.g., endothelial cells and monocytes) synthesize and express tissue factor on their surface only after appropriate stimulation by factors such as endotoxin. Tissue factor binds to circulating factor VIIa to convert factors X and IX to their active forms (Xa and IXa), both of which bind to receptors on the activated platelet

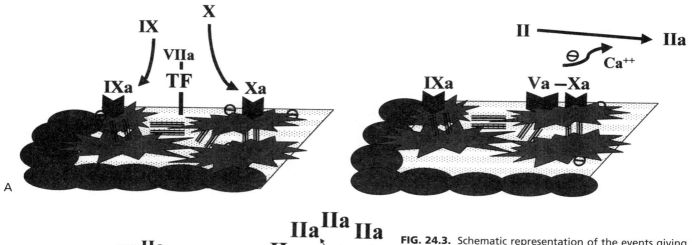

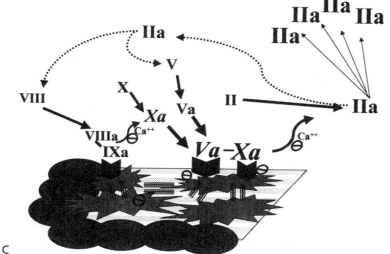

FIG. 24.3. Schematic representation of the events giving rise to thrombin formation under high shear. **A:** Activated platelets have formed a platelet plug (starburst-shaped), bound together by fibrinogen (*bridgelike triple lines*). Tissue factor (*TF*), constitutively expressed on extravascular surfaces and exposed following vascular damage, binds to low levels of circulating factor VIIa. The TF–VIIa extrinsic Xase complex generates active factors Xa and IXa, and these serine proteases bind to receptors on the activated platelet surface. **B:** Platelet-bound Xa associates with platelet-bound Va to form the prothrombinase complex, which, with membrane-derived phosphatidylserine (θ) and Ca^{2+}, generates relatively small amounts of thrombin (IIa) from prothrombin. **C:** Formed thrombin cleaves cofactors VIII and V to their active forms, VIIIa and Va. VIIIa complexes with platelet-bound factor IXa to form the "intrinsic Xase" complex. Intrinsic Xase is kinetically superior to extrinsic Xase, and intrinsic Xase markedly accelerates the generation of Xa. Abundant Xa and Va now amplify thrombin generation, producing sufficient fibrin for clot stabilization.

membrane (Fig. 24.3A). The platelet Xa receptor closely associates with platelet-bound factor Va. These factors, together with free Ca^{2+} and platelet membrane-associated phosphatidylserine (Fig. 24.3B), form the prothrombinase complex to generate thrombin, albeit in relatively small amounts. This thrombin formed initially is then able to activate factor VIII to factor VIIIa, which binds to membrane-bound factor IXa (Fig. 24.3C). Until this point in the cascade, the rate of Xa and thrombin generation formed via the tissue factor–VIIa complex is relatively slow. However, once an initial amount of thrombin can subsequently generate appreciable quantities of cofactors Va and VIIIa, the rate of both factor Xa and thrombin generation ratchets up exponentially (17) (Fig. 24.3C). With explosive thrombin generation, a fibrin matrix is formed that integrates with the surfaces of the platelet plug. Factor XIIIa, produced by the action of thrombin on either plasma or platelet-released factor XIII, then cross-links the fibrin chains and binds α_2-antiplasmin to the fibrin to protect it from plasmin-mediated dissolution (18). Finally, the platelet plug undergoes clot retraction, which also protects the platelet–fibrino-

gen–platelet unit from lysis by plasmin (19). These antilysis mechanisms, largely linked to platelet activation, may in part explain the relative resistance of platelet-rich clots to pharmacologic thrombolysis following myocardial infarction.

In the venous circulation, although negatively charged phospholipid surfaces serve as essential coagulation cofactors, the role of platelets in the membrane assembly of the coagulation cascade appears to be less critical. For this reason, thrombocytopenia rarely causes spontaneous venous bleeding, and in fact, prophylaxis against venous thrombosis with antiplatelet agents has had only limited success. Instead, antithrombin agents, often with anti-Xa activity as a supplement, are the mainstay of anticoagulation to prevent venous thrombosis (20).

Endogenous Anticoagulants: Striking a Balance

In the resting state, a number of endogenous mechanisms operate to prevent clotting and maintain blood in a liquid form. These tonic anticoagulant influences take different forms in the arterial and venous circulations, with, for reasons outlined above, antiplatelet activity predominating in the former and antithrombin activity in the latter. However, both mechanisms require an intact endothelial cell barrier. In the arterial circulation, total occlusion by thrombus is opposed by a number of mechanisms that operate to control the size of the thrombus. As described above, high-velocity blood flow itself, by locally diluting coagulation factors, has anticoagulant effects. Several antiplatelet factors also contribute to the function of a healthy endothelial cell lining to limit growth of the platelet plug past the area of damage. The endothelial cell surface carries a net negative surface charge, repelling similarly charged platelets. Endothelial cells constitutively release nitric oxide (also termed *endothelium-derived relaxant factor*) and prostacylin (PGI$_2$), both of which inhibit platelet adhesion and aggregation. Healthy endothelial cells also synthesize ADPase, which is capable of inactivating platelet-released ADP, thereby limiting the ability of activated platelets to recruit and activate other platelets (21). These naturally occurring antiplatelet mechanisms, in addition to the hemodynamic forces present in the arterial circulation, work to maintain vessel patency and active blood flow simultaneously with clot formation and vessel repair as needed.

Once the platelet plug and associated fibrin deposition have halted the bleeding and covered the exposed endothelium, systems that rein in the coagulation system become dominant. Many of these factors are bound to extracellular matrix associated with neighboring intact endothelium, and like the analogous antiplatelet agents, they act to prevent the clot from encroaching on areas of normal endothelium. Endothelial cells synthesize an endogenous heparin congener, heparan sulfate, which is secreted but remains associated with the extracellular matrix; heparan sulfate forms complexes with blood antithrombin and neutralizes locally developed thrombin. Thrombomodulin similarly associates with endothelial cell surfaces. When thrombin escapes the neutralization efforts described above, it binds to thrombomodulin, subsequently activating protein C. Activated protein C then cleaves factors Va and VIIIa, thereby downregulating thrombin formation. Healthy endothelial cells, stimulated by a number of coagulation-generated factors, also release tissue plasminogen activator (t-PA) as part of the effort to contain the clot and maintain vessel patency. Because t-PA is able to generate plasmin from plasminogen effectively only when it is bound to formed fibrin (22), it cannot cause fibrinogenolysis; however, excess t-PA can produce a bleeding diathesis by disrupting formed clots, particularly in a postsurgical setting, such as after CPB.

Summary

Prothrombotic and antithrombotic factors are carefully regulated under conditions of normal blood flow, with tonic

anticoagulation balanced by the presence of platelets and coagulation zymogens ready to be activated. Perturbations in the vessel wall that expose subendothelium uncover highly prothombotic factors that rapidly initiate clot formation. Blood exiting the wound, although capable of disrupting any clot material that is not tightly adherent, also *stimulates* platelet activation to begin formation of the plug designed to seal the wound. Modulation of clot formation occurs simultaneously, as the formation of highly procoagulant moieties, such as thrombin, activates anticoagulant systems aimed at limiting clot growth. At the same time, fibrinolysis, which dominates after bleeding ceases, is opposed by mechanisms that prevent excessive clot lysis and thus decrease the risk for rebleeding. This system of checks and balances generally restores homeostasis following mild-to-moderate hemostatic insults. CPB, with its profound heparin-induced anticoagulation, variable hypothermia, exposure to foreign biomaterials, and wide variations in flow conditions, may activate these processes in the extreme. In addition, significant patient-to-patient variability occurs in many of the pathways described above. Such variability may be clinically inapparent in the face of mild hemostatic challenges, which are most often effectively counteracted by the redundancy of the hemostatic process. When taxed by the extreme conditions of CPB, however, this biologic variability may predispose some patients to excess bleeding or even pathologic thrombosis.

CARDIOPULMONARY BYPASS: UPSETTING THE BALANCE

Cardiopulmonary bypass imposes extremes on the hemostatic system. Despite efforts aimed at improving biocompatibility, the CPB surface is generally perceived as foreign by circulating blood elements, which attempt to "clot it off" and reject it by mounting an inflammatory attack. During this systemic response to the bypass circuit, the host also appears to be attacked as an "innocent bystander." Table 24.1 lists some of the vascular constituents activated by CPB, together with the mediators they generate that amplify their own or related activation pathways. Ideally, complete arrest of coagulation and inflammation would be maintained throughout the bypass period; then separation from CPB would be accompanied by the full return of coagulation and immunologic function. Some limits on both coagulation and inflammation might be desirable after CPB, the former to aid in graft patency and the latter to prevent tissue injury. In reality, the coagulation "arrest" achieved by current anticoagulation techniques is partial at best, and the subsequent restoration of coagulation is frequently suboptimal and occasionally profoundly impaired, resulting in excessive blood loss and the need for transfusion. Likewise, stimulation of the immune system by the bypass circuit produces a deleterious inflammatory response persisting

TABLE 24.1. HEMATOLOGIC FACTORS ACTIVATED BY CARDIOPULMONARY BYPASS

Activation Pathways	Active Mediators Generated
Soluble factors	
Coagulation cascade	Kallikrein, HMWK, thrombin
Complement cascade	C3a, C5a, C5b–9
Fibrinolytic system	Plasmin
Cellular factors	
Platelets	TXA₂, Serotonin
Neutrophils	Oxygen radicals, elastase
Monocytes	Oxygen radicals, cytokines
Lymphocytes	Cytokines
Endothelial cells	t-PA, cytokines

HMWK, high-molecular-weight kininogen; TXA$_2$, thromboxane A$_2$; t-PA, tissue plasminogen activator.

TABLE 24.2. POSSIBLE CONTRIBUTORS TO BLEEDING AFTER CARDIOPULMONARY BYPASS

Non–platelet-related causes

Hyperfibrinolysis
Hypothermia
Heparin excess (inadequate neutralization, rebound)
Protamine excess
Consumption of soluble coagulation factor(s)
Decreased vWF, especially high-molecular-weight multimers

Platelet-related causes

Thrombocytopenia
Aspirin-induced platelet dysfunction
Impaired aggregation response to agonists (epinephrine, collagen, ADP, thrombin)
Selective loss of youngest (most functional) platelets
Platelet fragmentation/loss of membrane receptors
Impaired platelet-mediated clot retraction
Plasmin-induced platelet activation/dysfunction
Platelet activation/dysfunction induced by C5b–9

VWF; von Willebrand's factor; ADP, adenosine diphosphate.

into the post-CPB period, possibly with its own adverse hemostatic effects.

The Coagulation Challenge

Aggressive blood conservation techniques and the use of algorithms to standardize transfusion practices have reduced the average number of allogeneic transfusions to two to three red cell units per CPB patient, although the variation among cardiac surgical centers is impressive (23). Nonetheless, in a recent study, more than 35% of patients having a surgical procedure requiring CPB bled more than 1 L in the first 24 postoperative hours (24). Although some factors, such as female sex, preoperative aspirin use, and lower total heparin dose, correlated with bleeding, no preoperative hematologic variable reliably identified patients at risk for bleeding. Likewise, treatment of bleeding frequently is not based on demonstrated laboratory abnormalities, but rather is largely empiric and highly institution-specific (25). Our inability to find a single, unifying explanation for most cases of post-CPB bleeding has contributed to these shortcomings.

Table 24.2 lists a number of potential contributors to post-CPB bleeding. Many of the defects listed are, on average, not very severe, and they would not by themselves be expected to result in major bleeding. However, individual patients differ in their baseline hemostatic function and additionally exhibit significant variability in their response to CPB. Some patients after CPB manifest one particular coagulation defect to a sufficient degree that it alone induces severe bleeding. Alternatively, some patients may exceed some critical *number* of defects, or else experience a specific *combination* of defects that act synergistically to create a bleeding diathesis. It is likely that each of these possibilities occurs, which could explain why no single abnormality has been found that uniformly or even dominantly accounts for post-CPB bleeding. For that reason, the CPB-associated hematologic alterations discussed below are presented roughly in order of clinical appearance, with the purpose of illustrating the way in which these processes potentially interact to produce bleeding defects.

Intrinsic Requirements of Cardiopulmonary Bypass: Heparinization, Hemodilution, and Hypothermia

Intact endothelial cells, as outlined above, actively secrete antithrombotic agents to maintain blood fluidity. All synthetic surfaces, the CPB circuit included, activate the coagulation cascade to varying degrees (26). Therefore, an essential component of CPB is the establishment of profound anticoagulation before blood contact with the CPB circuit. Heparin binds to circulating antithrombin and causes a conformational change that accelerates its binding to and inactivation of three critical coagulation factors: thrombin, factor Xa, and factor IXa. Thus, heparinization represents the first major alteration in coagulation imposed by CPB. Heparin also has both direct and indirect antiplatelet effects, and despite post-CPB neutralization, residual heparin may contribute to post-CPB bleeding; this phenomenon is comprehensively covered in Chapter 23. Among its antiplatelet actions, heparin binds to vWf at a site critical for binding to platelet GPIb (27,28); this effectively blocks vWf–platelet interaction and can impair initial platelet rolling and adhesion to the subendothelium. This effect is seen only at high heparin concentrations (≥2 U/mL) and does not appear to inhibit GPIIb/IIIa-dependent platelet–vWf interactions. However, the impairment in vWf- and GPIb-dependent adhesion is likely responsible for the increased bleeding time noted during CPB when heparinization is maximal. Whether this heparin–vWf interaction plays any role in

TABLE 24.3. LEVELS OF COAGULATION FACTORS NECESSARY FOR HEMOSTASIS

Factor	Common Names	Percentage of Normal Concentration Needed for Coagulation
	Intrinsic system only	
XII	Hageman factor	None
XI	Plasma thromboplastin antecedent	20
IX	Christmas factor	40
VIII	Antihemophilic factor	30
	Extrinsic system only	
VII	Proconvertin, serum prothrombin conversion accelerator	25
	Common pathway	
X	Stuart factor	40
V	Proaccelerin, labile factor	40
II	Prothrombin	40
I	Fibrinogen	100 mg/dL

bleeding following heparin reversal, especially in the setting of heparin rebound, is not known at this time.

Once adequacy of anticoagulation by heparin is certain, typically determined by prolongation of the activated clotting time, the passage of blood through the CPB circuit is initiated. Owing to the large volume of the circuit, which must be primed with blood-compatible fluid, hemodilution is the next challenge imposed on the hemostatic system. The degree of hemodilution varies with the institution, type of CPB circuit, and size of the patient. In a typical adult, the onset of CPB decreases hematocrit from 40% to approximately 25%. For specific coagulation factors, this degree of hemodilution is generally well tolerated, although patients with low hematocrits initially may need a red cell transfusion to maintain oxygen-carrying capacity. Soluble coagulation factors can be diluted to 20% to 40% of normal values before symptoms of bleeding are manifested or clotting times are prolonged (Table 24.3). Similarly, most normal platelet counts can be halved without an increase in tendency to bleed. Therefore, the intrinsic anticoagulant effect of hemodilution is generally mild, and hemodilution may actually augment the coagulation "arrest" imposed by heparinization. Following CPB, however, any tendency to bleed may be aggravated by the borderline coagulation factor concentrations and decreased platelet numbers brought on by hemodilution.

The next systemic alteration frequently imposed early during CPB is hypothermia. The degree of systemic hypothermia achieved at different institutions varies highly, with a trend in recent years to more moderate hypothermia, accomplished by allowing the temperature to drift downward passively. Hypothermia in the range of 22°C inhibits platelet activation and the platelet aggregation response to thrombin (29). In addition, hypothermia may adversely af-

fect the kinetics of the coagulation cascade and may even impair the ability of local vasculature to constrict in response to bleeding. Furthermore, whether hypothermia decreases or only delays the inflammatory response to CPB remains controversial.

Platelet Defect(s) Resulting from Cardiopulmonary Bypass

Cardiopulmonary bypass produces a number of changes in circulating platelets. One of the most common features is a rapid, early decrease in platelet number that exceeds the decrease explainable by hemodilution alone (Fig. 24.4). This relative thrombocytopenia only occasionally dips below 50,000/μL, a level generally accepted as the threshold for platelet transfusion in surgical patients. By contrast, CPB-induced functional platelet defects may produce bleeding that requires platelet transfusion despite seemingly adequate platelet counts (30).

Several alterations in platelet function can occur in the peri-CPB patient, with no single functional defect accounting for the preponderance of bleeding. In general, most patients exhibit blunted platelet responses to stimulation by most agonists, without a clear cause for this dysfunction. Accordingly, after CPB, higher concentrations of ADP, collagen, thrombin, and other platelet agonists are required than before CPB to achieve irreversible platelet aggregation (31). The combination of a decrease in platelet number and global platelet function may be responsible for a major proportion of blood loss associated with CPB (32,33). These observations raise some important questions: Why are platelets often lost out of proportion to hemodilution? What is the nature of the platelet defect(s)? Is the process

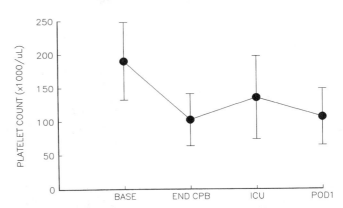

FIG. 24.4. Platelet counts during and after cardiopulmonary bypass (*CPB*). Platelet counts (mean ± standard error of the mean) are shown for 85 patients who underwent nonemergent surgery and required CPB. On average, platelet counts remained ≥ 100,000/μL throughout CPB and into the post-CPB period. Base, baseline conditions; ICU, after arrival in intensive care unit; PODI, postoperative day 1. (From Mathew JP. Unpublished observations.)

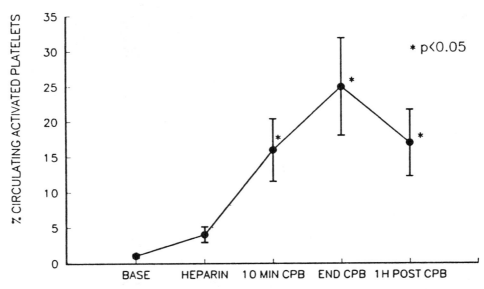

FIG. 24.5. Platelet activation during cardiopulmonary bypass (*CPB*). Percentage of circulating platelets expressing CD62P (GMP-140) over time on CPB and into the post-CPB period. *H*, hour; *Min*, minute. Base, baseline conditions; heparin, after heparinization for CPB; 10 min CPB, 10 minutes into CPB; H, hour; * p<0.05 compared to base. (Reprinted from Rinder C, Gaal D, Student L, et al. Platelet–leukocyte activation and modulation of adhesion receptors in pediatric patients with congenital heart disease undergoing cardiopulmonary bypass. *J Thorac Cardiovasc Surg* 1994; 107:280–288, with permission.)

leading to platelet loss also responsible for the impaired platelet function?

Studies have demonstrated that CPB activates large numbers of platelets, manifested and measured by release of the contents of internal granules (34,35) (Fig. 24.5). These activated platelets may then bind to exposed subendothelium, to the CPB circuit (36), or to circulating monocytes and neutrophils (37), potentially causing platelet numbers to decrease beyond what would be expected from hemodilution alone. Furthermore, the activation response of still-circulating platelets is impaired. *In vitro* studies have demonstrated that stimulated platelets become refractory to repeated stimulation by the same agonist (38). It is possible that the activation stimulus might, by "preactivating" platelets, produce a pool of granule-depleted, spent platelets, incapable of contributing their granule contents to the platelet plug. Indeed, electron microscopic examination of platelets during CPB demonstrates a heterogeneous mixture of discoid and shape-changed platelets, in addition to partially and completely degranulated platelets (39). Investigators have attempted to "anesthetize" platelets better during CPB, hypothesizing that by rendering them transiently inert to activation stimuli, their function might be better preserved postoperatively (40). Indeed, administration of the reversible platelet inhibitor prostacyclin (41) and its analogue iloprost (42) has been associated with some success in reducing bleeding and preserving platelet activity after CPB. The hypotensive side effects of these agents, however, precludes their widespread use. Investigators in pursuit of

a more hemodynamically inert "platelet anesthetic" are now turning to a class of agents known as *disintegrins* (43), which compete with fibrinogen and vWf for binding sites on platelet GPIIb/IIIa receptors. However, evidence linking the activating stimulus to subsequent defects in the aggregation response remains indirect. Furthermore, patients exhibiting the highest percentages of circulating activated platelets are not necessarily the ones most affected by platelet aggregation dysfunction (44) (Fig. 24.6). It may be that platelet activation and the acquisition of the aggregation defect are distinct entities produced simultaneously by CPB.

The normal circulating platelet population is extremely heterogeneous in age and function, with platelets recently released from the marrow exhibiting a more robust response to stimulation than senescent ones (45,46). A sustained, low-grade platelet-activating stimulus like CPB may over time activate the most vigorous young platelets and cause them to be culled from the circulation, thereby passively increasing the proportion of "hyporesponders" among the remaining circulating platelets (47). This effect would be particularly noticeable with longer bypass times, given the increased platelet activation seen with time. Eventually, this loss would be compensated for by increased release of fresh young platelets from the marrow, but this negative selection process would still produce temporary platelet dysfunction in the early hours after bypass, a time when coagulation function is critical. Evidence that a reduction in the average platelet volume, signaling loss of younger platelets, is associ-

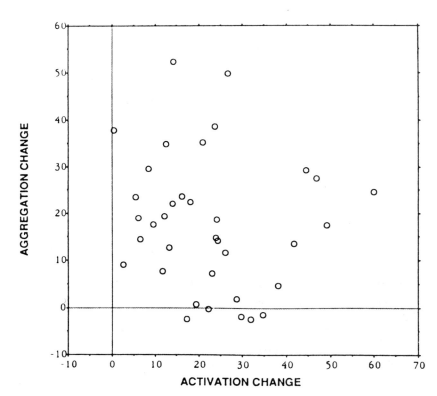

FIG. 24.6. Correlation between changes in platelet activation and platelet aggregation within the time period extending from the start of surgery to the end of cardiopulmonary bypass (*CPB*). Platelet activation was the percentage of circulating CD62P-positive platelets, and platelet aggregation was the percentage of platelet aggregates following incubation with adenosine diphosphate (*ADP*). No correlation was observed ($r = 0.03$). (Reprinted from Rinder CS, Bohnert J, Rinder HM, et al. Platelet activation and aggregation during cardiopulmonary bypass. *Anesthesiology* 1991;75:388–393, with permission.)

ated with increased post-CPB bleeding supports this hypothesis (48).

Catecholamines are generated in large quantities during CPB despite aggressive efforts to provide a stress-free anesthetic. Both epinephrine and norepinephrine are relatively weak platelet agonists *in vivo*. However, by binding to α-adrenergic receptors on platelets, epinephrine and norepinephrine prime platelets for a more exuberant response to other agonists (49), which may contribute importantly to postsurgical hemostasis. It is possible that during CPB the catecholamine-induced hyperresponsiveness contributes to early platelet activation and associated decreases in platelet number. with time on CPB, however, circulating platelets lose their α-adrenergic receptors and likewise their responsiveness to catecholamine stimulation (50). Although this effect is unlikely to constitute "the post-CPB platelet defect" by itself, impaired adrenergic responsiveness does appear to contribute to the overall platelet dysfunction occurring in the post-bypass period.

Fibrinogen is known to bind to extracorporeal surfaces within minutes of blood passage through the CPB circuit. This bound fibrinogen is conformationally altered such that it is capable of binding to the resting GPIIb/IIIa receptor on platelets (51), and this tethering action is likely responsible for some of the excess decrease in platelet number associated with CPB. In addition, with time, the bound platelets break free of the circuit, leaving portions of their receptors still bound to the circuit. This may be responsible for the

modest decrease (in the range of 40% to 50%) in surface expression of the fibrinogen receptor, GPIIb/IIIa, on circulating platelets (52,53). Recent experience with blocking monoclonal antibodies has demonstrated that well over 50% of GPIIb/IIIa receptors must be blocked to produce significant aggregation impairment (54), so that bypass-induced decreases in GPIIb/IIIa likely contribute little to post-CPB bleeding.

Clot strength, particularly platelet-mediated clot retraction, is also impaired following CPB, and this reduction has been correlated with increased chest tube drainage (55) (Fig. 24.7). Clot retraction may affect the ability of the clot to hold securely against high shear forces. In addition, platelet-mediated clot retraction is thought to make the platelet–fibrin–platelet unit more resistant to fibrinolysis (19). Thus, any decrease in clot strength after CPB, in addition to diminishing shear resistance, may also cause the platelet-rich clot to be more vulnerable to fibrinolysis by plasmin.

Endothelial Cell Activation and Impaired Clotting

Activation of endothelial cells during CPB has been demonstrated in animal models of bypass (56). In humans, increased release of t-PA during bypass provides indirect evidence of endothelial cell activation (57). Plasmin, formed by the activity of t-PA, has been shown *in vitro* to produce

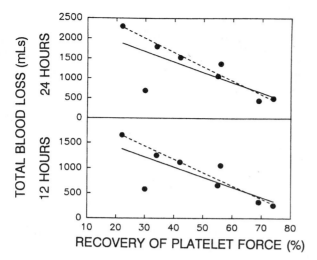

FIG. 24.7. Correlation between the percentage recovery of platelet force development after protamine sulfate administration and total mediastinal tube drainage. *Solid lines* depict the best line of correlation for all study patients at 12 (*lower panel*) and 24 hours (*upper panel*) after bypass (r_s = -0.74, p = 0.036 and r_s = -0.71, p = 0.048, respectively; n = 8). *Dotted lines* represent the best line of correlation when patient 6 is excluded because of incomplete heparin reversal (r_s = -0.96, p = 0.0006 and r_s = -0.93, p = 0.0024, respectively; n = 7). (Reprinted from Greilich PE, Carr ME Jr, Carr SL, et al. Reductions in platelet force development by CPB are associated with hemorrhage. *Anesth Analg* 1995;80:459–464, with permission.)

platelet activation (58) and platelet dysfunction simultaneously; the mechanism for this is not well understood (59). However, this antiplatelet action of plasmin is unlikely to contribute importantly to the dysfunction demonstrable in freely circulating platelets during CPB, given that active t-PA is localized to formed fibrin. Indeed, the literature has been somewhat mixed with respect to the abilities of plasmin inhibitors such as ϵ-aminocaproic acid (EACA) and aprotinin to preserve platelet number and function following CPB (60,61).

Plasmin *in vitro* has also been shown to cause internalization of platelet GPIb (62), the vWf receptor critical for adhesion under flow conditions. On average, CPB is associated with a modest decrease, in the range of 20% to 30%, in platelet GPIb (63), and aprotinin has been shown to preserve platelet GPIb levels (64). In Bernard-Soulier syndrome, a congenital deficiency of GPIb, the critical number of GPIb receptors necessary for surgical hemostasis is unclear, but heterozygotes with approximately 50% receptor density show no predisposition to bleeding (65). With the possible exception of children with cyanotic congenital heart disease (66) (Fig. 24.8), very few CPB patients exhibit a decrease in GPIb into the range that would, by itself, be a major cause of post-CPB bleeding. In association with modest thrombocytopenia and impaired platelet aggregation, however, this GPIb-based adhesion defect may contribute to poor platelet function overall.

Activation of the Soluble Coagulation Cascade

Despite profound anticoagulation with heparin, coagulation factors are still activated by the CPB circuit, even to the point of producing some thrombin. The contact activation system, historically known as the *intrinsic coagulation system*, is activated by the bypass surface (67), which mimics naturally occurring contact activators like extracellular matrices and bacterial lipopolysaccharides. Contact activation is initiated by the cleavage of factor XII to XIIa, a serine protease that initiates the intrinsic pathway of coagulation but also converts prekallikrein into kallikrein and high-molecular-weight kininogen into bradykinin. Kallikrein and bradykinin amplify both the coagulation and inflammatory systems; kallikrein is a neutrophil activator, and bradykinin is a potent vasoactive peptide that additionally has platelet inhibitory activity. Factor XIIa also activates complement via the classic pathway.

The tissue factor pathway of coagulation, known as the *extrinsic system*, is also activated during CPB. Indeed, there is evidence that most of the thrombin that escapes heparin inhibition during CPB is generated via the tissue factor pathway (68). Tissue factor is exposed in part by surgical disruption of the endothelium, so that coagulation is activated. Although activation of the soluble coagulation cascade only rarely produces a consumptive coagulopathy after CPB, formed thrombin, likely protected from heparin–antithrombin neutralization by being clot-bound (69), undoubtedly contributes to the activation of platelets and endothelial cells during CPB.

Complement Activation

The complement system constitutes one of the more primitive biologic systems activated by blood contact with foreign elements. Although traditionally considered a proinflammatory system (70), activated complement (71) components also exhibit activity in hemostatic pathways, and increased markers of complement activation have in some studies (48) correlated with post-CPB bleeding. The alternative pathway of this system is principally activated initially during CPB, resulting in formation of the opsonin C3b, the common pathway anaphylatoxins C3a and C5a, and finally the membrane attack complex, C5b-9 (72,73). After CPB, the administration of protamine induces an additional surge of complement activation, presumably stemming from activation of the classic pathway by the heparin–protamine complex (74). The formation of these bioactive elements amplifies both hemostatic and inflammatory pathways that are initially activated by exposure to the circuit. The by-products of this inflammatory cascade in turn activate leukocytes, platelets, and endothelial cells (75,76). Studies have suggested that the terminal complement components, C5a and beyond, are principally responsible for the activation

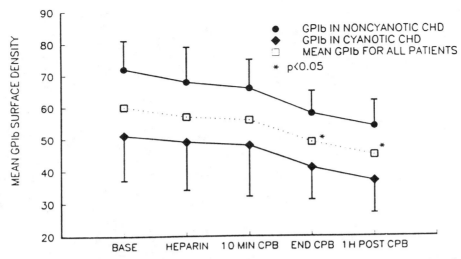

FIG. 24.8. Changes in platelet surface glycoprotein Ib (*GPIb*) in pediatric patients on cardiopulmonary bypass (*CPB*). GPIb is measured as mean platelet fluorescence with an anti-GPIb antibody. Platelets were examined before the start of the operation (*BASE*), 5 minutes after heparinization (*HEPARIN*), 10 minutes after the start of CPB (*10 MIN CPB*), shortly before separation from CPB (*END CPB*), and 1 to 2 hours after termination of CPB (*1 H POST CPB*). Values are mean ± standard deviation. Noncyanotic pediatric patients are represented by *black circles*, cyanotic pediatric patients by *black diamonds*, and means for all patients by *open squares*. GPIb decreased significantly at the end of CPB and 1 to 2 hours after CPB in comparison with baseline values for all patients. In addition, surface expression of GPIb in cyanotic children was significantly lower than in noncyanotic patients (*p* = 0.01) for all time points. * p<0.05, compared to base. (Reprinted from Rinder C, Gaal D, Student L, et al. Platelet–leukocyte activation and modulation of adhesion receptors in pediatric patients with congenital heart disease undergoing cardiopulmonary bypass. *J Thorac Cardiovasc Surg* 1994;107:280–288, with permission.)

of neutrophils and platelets (77), whereas monocytes can be stimulated by the C3a fragment also (78). The membrane attack complex, C5b-9, is a potent activator of platelets, inducing α-granule release, formation of procoagulant microparticles, and surface exposure of the negatively charged phosphatidylserine residues essential to the coagulation cascade (79). *In vitro*, platelets activated by C5b-9 are unable to bind fibrinogen to their GPIIb/IIIa receptors, so that an aggregation defect similar to that induced *in vitro* by CPB is created (80). Clearly, the generation of complement components plays a role in platelet activation during CPB; whether this is responsible for some of the CPB-associated platelet dysfunction remains unknown.

Leukocyte Activation

A number of the pathways described above, including both the complement cascade and the contact system, contribute to the activation of immune cells during CPB. Circulating monocytes and neutrophils become activated, which primes them to cause tissue damage when they enter organs (37). Leukocyte adhesion receptors CD11b/CD18 are upregulated, so that they can bind to endothelial cells and migrate into extravascular tissues. Leukocytes also release their granules on activation, liberating destructive elements including

oxygen radicals, elastase, and cathepsin G (81). In addition to having proinflammatory activity, mediators such as elastase and cathepsin G are capable of degrading fibrin, potentially contributing to the instability of newly formed clots. Such cell-mediated fibrinolysis may be facilitated by CD11b/CD18-dependent adhesion to fibrin for the purpose of promoting neutrophil egress out of the circulation (82). The contribution of cell-mediated fibrinolysis to clot instability after CPB is difficult to ascertain. However, recent work has demonstrated that patients who exhibit the greatest increase in white blood cell count during the course of CPB are most likely to bleed during the first 24 postoperative hours (83) (Fig. 24.9). Whether these increased numbers of white blood cells actively participate in the bleeding diathesis or simply signal an exaggerated inflammatory response is presently unknown. The links between inflammatory and hemorrhagic processes represent an important emerging field of investigation.

In summary, no single entity has been identified as the source of post-CPB bleeding. Indeed, the list of potential hemorrhagic contributors is so impressive that it makes the degree of hemostasis presently achieved after CPB seem remarkable. A better understanding of the underlying pathophysiology of both CPB and hemostasis, which is likely to result in better control of CPB-induced hemorrhage, will

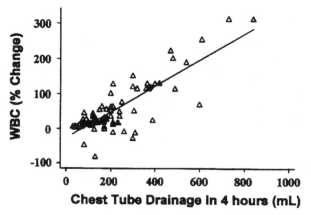

FIG. 24.9. Linear relationship ($n = 85$) between white blood cell (*WBC*) values (percentage change) and cumulative mediastinal chest tube drainage in the first 4 postoperative hours. WBC percentage change was calculated with the following formula: [(WBC before end CPB − WBC before start CPB)/WBC before start CPB] × 100. The linear equation for this relationship is as follows: cumulative mediastinal chest tube drainage in the first 4 postoperative hours = (1.9 × WBC) + 112; $r^2 = 0.71$. (Reprinted from Despotis GJ, Levine V, Goodnough LT. Relationship between leukocyte count and patient risk for excessive blood loss after cardiac surgery. *Crit Care Med* 1997;25:1338–1346, with permission.)

involve advances on multiple fronts, including (a) improving the biocompatibility of circuits, (b) improving the "arrest" of coagulation and inflammation during CPB, (c) developing diagnostic tests to treat bleeding more rapidly and specifically, and (d) developing more effective pharmacologic treatments for bleeding.

KEY POINTS

- The *initial hemostatic response* to a vascular disruption involves the "margination" of platelets to the periphery of the axially directed blood stream to adhere to subendothelial proteins (especially collagen and vWf). These platelets are then metabolically activated to attract other platelets and form platelet-to-platelet bonds, thereby creating the *primary platelet plug*. This process is more difficult to initiate in arteries than in veins because faster flows and higher pressures limit the time available for platelets to bind to subendothelial proteins.
- In *platelet activation*, products are released from platelet granules that serve to recruit additional platelets, constrict small arteries to slow bleeding, form ligands needed to develop a stable platelet-to-platelet matrix, localize and accelerate fibrin formation, and protect clots from fibrinolysis.
- Vascular disruption also exposes tissue factor to stimulate the *soluble coagulation cascade*, which in turn stabilizes and solidifies the platelet plug by depositing fibrin

into the interstices of the platelet-to-platelet matrix. Subsequently, clot retraction confers protection from lysis by plasmin.

- Various checks and balances keep blood clots from spreading to the point at which they would obstruct intact blood vessels. These include plasmin, heparan, antithrombin III, and protein C.
- Despite improvements in the materials used for extracorporeal circuits, the bloodstream still perceives these surfaces as foreign, and an inflammatory and procoagulant response is provoked that can be pathologic even in the presence of massive anticoagulation with heparin.
- A variety of factors can contribute to *inadequate clotting function after CPB*. Hypothermia, unneutralized heparin, excessive protamine doses, dilution or consumption of platelets and coagulation factors, platelet dysfunction, and fibrinolysis are some of the most important contributors to this condition. Variability in the baseline clotting function (which can be influenced by medications) of individual patients and in the response of the hemostatic system to CPB contribute to the wide variation in hemostatic competence observed after heparin neutralization.
- As evidenced by impaired aggregation responses to agonists such as epinephrine, collagen, and ADP, *platelet dysfunction* commonly occurs after CPB; causes include platelet activation by plasmin or complement to result in loss of platelet secretory products, loss of platelet membranes and GPIIb/IIIa receptors to the extracorporeal circuit, and impaired platelet-mediated clot retraction.
- Despite profound anticoagulation with heparin, the soluble coagulation cascade produces *thrombin* during CPB, and heparin possesses little capacity to inactivate thrombin inside clots. *Tissue factor* generated by surgery, probably facilitated by extracorporeal circulation, plays a major role in coagulation activation during CPB.
- Associations have recently been demonstrated between post-CPB bleeding and both complement activation and leukocytosis. Whether these are coincidental or causative remains to be determined. Links between inflammatory and hemorrhagic/hemostatic responses constitute an emerging field of investigation.

REFERENCES

1. Almony GT, Lefkovits JK, Topol EJ. Antiplatelet and anticoagulant use after myocardial infarction. *Clin Cardiol* 1996;19:357–365.
2. Ruggeri ZM. Mechanisms initiating platelet thrombus formation. *Thromb Haemost* 1997;78:611–616.
3. Livio M, Gotti E, Marchesi D, et al. Uraemic bleeding: role of

anaemia and beneficial effect of red cell transfusions. *Lancet* 1982; 2:1013–1015.

4. Ruggeri ZM. Von Willebrand factor. *J Clin Invest* 1997;99: 559–564.

5. Kroll MH, Harris TS, Moake HL, et al. von Willebrand factor binding to platelet GPIb initiates signals for platelet activation. *J Clin Invest* 1991;88:1568–1573.

6. Ferguson JJ, Waly HM, Wilson JM. Fundamentals of coagulation and glycoprotein IIb/IIIa receptor inhibition. *Eur Heart J* 1998;19[Suppl D]:D3–D9.

7. Saelman EUM, Niewenhuis HK, Hese KM, et al. Platelet adhesion to collagen types I through VIII under conditions of stasis and flow is mediated by GPIa/IIa. *Blood* 1994;83:1244–1250.

8. Kehrel B, Wierwille S Clemetson KJ, et al. *Blood* 1998;91: 491–499.

9. Zucker MB, Nachmias VT. Platelet activation. *Arteriosclerosis* 1985;5:2–18.

10. Anderson GM, Hall LM, Yang JX, et al. Platelet dense granule release reaction monitored by HPLC-fluorometric determination of endogenous serotonin. *Anal Biochem* 1992;206:64–67.

11. Dephino RA, Kaplan K. The Hermansky-Pudlak syndrome: report of three cases and review of pathophysiologic and management considerations. *Medicine* 1985;64:192–202.

12. Lefkovits J, Plow EF, Topol EJ. Platelet glycoprotein IIb/IIIa receptors in cardiovascular medicine. *N Engl J Med* 1995;332: 1553–1559.

13. Scandura JM, Walsh PN. Factor X bound to the surface of activated human platelets is preferentially activated by platelet-bound factor IXa. *Biochemistry* 1996;35:8890–8901.

14. Swords NA, Mann KG. The assembly of the prothrombinase complex on adherent platelets. *Arterioscler Thromb* 1993;13: 1602–1612.

15. Banner EW. The factor VIIa/tissue factor complex. *Thromb Haemost* 1997;78:512–515.

16. Weiss HJ, Turitto VT, Baumgartner HR, et al. Evidence for the presence of tissue factor activity on subendothelium. *Blood* 1989; 73:968–975.

17. Ofosu FA, Longbin L, Freedman J. Control mechanisms in thrombin generation. *Semin Thromb Hemost* 1996;22:303–308.

18. Muszbek L, Pogar J, Boda Z. Platelet factor XIII becomes active without the release of activation peptide during platelet activation. *Thromb Haemost* 1993;69:282–285.

19. Braaten JV, Jerome WG, Hantgan RR. Uncoupling fibrin from integrin receptors hastens fibrinolysis at the platelet–fibrin interface. *Blood* 1994;83:982–993.

20. Hirsch J, Fuster V. Guide to anticoagulant therapy part I: heparin. *Circulation* 1994;1449–1468.

21. Marcus AJ, Safier SV, Hajjar KA, et al. Inhibition of platelet function by an aspirin-insensitive endothelial cell ADPase: thromboregulation by endothelial cells. *J Clin Invest* 1991;88: 1690–1696.

22. Coller BS. Platelets and thrombolytic therapy. *N Engl J Med* 1990;322:33–42.

23. Goodnough LT, Despotis GJ, Hogue CW, et al. On the need for improved transfusion indictors in cardiac surgery. *Ann Thorac Surg* 1995;60:473–480.

24. Despotis GJ, Filos KS, Zoys TN, et al. Factors associated with excessive postoperative blood loss and hemostatic transfusion requirements: a multivariate analysis in cardiac surgical patients. *Anesth Analg* 1996;82:13–21.

25. Stover EP, Siegel LC, Parks R, et al. Variability in transfusion practice for coronary artery bypass surgery persists despite national consensus guidelines. *Anesthesiology* 1998;8:327–333.

26. Courtney JM, Forbes CD. Thrombosis on foreign surfaces. *Br Med Bull* 1994;50:966–981.

27. Fujimura Y, Titani K, Holland L, et al. A heparin-binding domain of human von Willebrand factor. *J Biol Chem* 1987;262; 1734–1739.

28. Sobel M, McNeill PM, Carslon PL, et al. Heparin inhibition of von Willebrand factor-dependent platelet function *in vitro* and *in vivo*. *J Clin Invest* 1991;87:1878–1893.

29. Michelson AD, MacGregor H, Barnard MR, et al. Reversible inhibition of human platelet activation by hypothermia *in vivo* and *in vitro*. *Thromb Haemost* 1994;71:633–640.

30. Beurling-Harbury C, Galvan CA. Acquired decrease in platelet secretory ADP associated with increased bleeding in post-cardiopulmonary bypass patients and patients with severe valvular heart disease. *Blood* 1978;52:13–23.

31. Friedenberg WR, Myers WO, Plotka ED, et al. Platelet dysfunction associated with cardiopulmonary bypass. *Ann Thorac Surg* 1978;25:298–305.

32. McKenna T, Bachman F, Whittaker B, et al. The hemostatic mechanism after open-heart surgery. II. Frequency of abnormal platelet functions during and after extracorporeal circulation. *J Thorac Cardiovasc Surg* 1975;70:298–307.

33. Holloway DS, Summarie L, Sandesara J, et al. Decreased platelet number and function and increased fibrinolysis contribute to postoperative bleeding in cardiopulmonary bypass patients. *Thromb Haemost* 1988;59:62–67.

34. Harker LA, Malpass TW, Branson HE, et al. Mechanism of abnormal bleeding in patients undergoing CPB: acquired transient platelet dysfunction associated with selective alpha-granule release. *Blood* 1980;56:824–834.

35. Addonizio VP Jr, Strauss JF III, Colman RW, et al. Thromboxane synthesis and platelet secretion during cardiopulmonary bypass with a bubble oxygenator. *J Thorac Cardiovasc Surg* 1980; 79:91–96.

36. Addoniziio VP Jr, Strauss FJ III, Colman RW, et al. Effects of prostaglandin E$_1$ on platelet loss during *in vivo* and *in vitro* extracorporeal circulation with a bubble oxygenator. *J Thorac Cardiovasc Surg* 1979;77:119–126.

37. Rinder CS, Bonan JL, Rinder HM, et al. Cardiopulmonary bypass induces leukocyte–platelet adhesion. *Blood* 1992;79: 1201–1205.

38. Rao GHR, White JG. *Am J Hematol* 1998;11:355–366.

39. Zill P, Fasol R, Broscurth P, et al. Blood platelets in CPB operations. Recovery occurs after initial stimulation rather than continual activation. *J Thorac Cardiovasc Surg* 1989;97:379.

40. Addonizio VP. Platelet function in cardiopulmonary bypass and artificial organs. *Hematol Oncol Clin North Am* 1990;4:145–155.

41. Addonizio VP, Macarak J, Nicolaou KC, et al. Effects of prostacyclin and albumin on platelet loss during *in vitro* simulation of extracorporeal circulation. *J Lab Clin Med* 1985;105:514–522.

42. Addonizio VP Jr, Fisher CA, Jenkin BK, et al. Iloprost, a stable analogue of prostacyclin, preserves platelets during simulated extracorporeal circulation. *J Thorac Cardiovasc Surg* 1985;89: 926–933.

43. Musial J, Rucinski B, Williams JA, et al. Inhibition of platelet adhesion to surfaces of extracorporeal circuit by disintegrins: RGD-containing peptides from viper venoms. *Circulation* 1990; 82: 261–273.

44. Rinder CS, Bohnert J, Rinder HM, et al. Platelet activation and aggregation during cardiopulmonary bypass. *Anesthesiology* 1991; 75:388–393.

45. Thompson CB, Eaton KA, Princiotta SM, et al. Size-dependent platelet subpopulations: relationship of platelet volume to ultrastructure, enzymatic activity, and function. *Br J Haematol* 1982; 50:509–519.

46. Rinder HM, Tracey JB, Techt M, et al. Differences in platelet granule release between normals and immune thrombocytopenic patients and between young and old platelets. *Thromb Haemost* 1998;80:457–462.

47. Laufer N, Merin G, Grover NB, et al. The influence of cardiopulmonary bypass on the size of human platelets. *J Thorac Cardiovasc Surg* 1975;70:727–731.

48. Khuri SF, Wolfe JA, Josa M, et al. Hematologic changes during and after CPB and their relationship to bleeding time and nonsurgical blood loss. *J Thorac Cardiovasc Surg* 1992;104:94–107.

49. Gant JA, Scrutton MC. Positive interactions between agonists in the aggregation response of human blood platelets: interaction between ADP, adrenaline and vasopressin. *Br J Haematol* 1980: 44:109–115.

50. Wachtfogel YT, Musial J, Jenkin V, et al. Loss of platelet alpha 2-adrenergic receptors during simulated extracorporeal circulation: prevention with prostaglandin E₁. *J Lab Clin Med* 1985;105: 601–607.

51. Musial J, Niewiarowski S, Hershock D, et al. Loss of fibrinogen receptors from the platelet surface during simulated circulation. *J Lab Clin Med* 1985;105:514–522.

52. Wenger RK, Lukasiewicz H, Mikuta BS, et al. Loss of platelet fibrinogen receptors during clinical cardiopulmonary bypass. *J Thorac Cardiovasc Surg* 1989;97:235–239.

53. Rinder CS, Mathew JP, Rinder HM, et al. Modulation of platelet surface adhesion receptors during CPB. *Anesthesiology* 1991;75: 563–570.

54. Mascelli MA, Worley S, Veriabo N, et al. Rapid assessment of platelet function with a modified whole-blood aggregometer in percutaneous transluminal coronary angioplasty patients receiving anti-GPIIb/IIIa therapy. *Circulation* 1997;96:3860–3866.

55. Greilich PE, Carr ME Jr, Carr SL, et al. Reductions in platelet force development by CPB are associated with hemorrhage. *Anesth Analg* 1995;80:459–464.

56. Boyle EM Jr, Pohlman TH, Johnson MC, et al. Endothelial cell injury in cardiovascular surgery; the systemic inflammatory response. *Ann Thorac Surg* 1997;63:277–284.

57. Stibbe J, Kluft C, Brommer E, et al. Enhanced fibrinolytic activity during CPB in open-heart surgery in man is caused by extrinsic (tissue-type) plasminogen activator. *Eur J Clin Invest* 1984:14: 375–382.

58. Niewiarowski S, Senui AF, Gillies P. Plasmin-induced platelet aggregation and platelet release reaction. *J Clin Invest* 1973;51: 1647–1659.

59. Schafer AI, Adelman B. Plasmin inhibition of platelet function and arachidonic acid metabolism. *J Clin Invest* 1985;75: 456–461.

60. Marx G, Pokar H, Reuter H, et al. The effects of aprotinin on hemostatic function during cardiac surgery. *J Cardiothorac Vasc Anesth* 1991;5:467–470.

61. Boldt J, Knothe C, Zickmann B, et al. Aprotinin in pediatric cardiac operations: platelet function, blood loss, and use of homologous blood. *Ann Thorac Surg* 1993;55:1460–1466.

62. Adelman B, Michelson AD, Loscalzo J, et al. Plasmin effect on platelet glycoprotein Ib–von Willebrand factor interactions. *Blood* 1985;65:32–40.

63. George JN, Pickett EB, Saucerman S, et al. Platelet surface glycoproteins: studies on resting and activated platelets and platelet membrane microparticles in normal subjects, and observations in patients during adult respiratory distress syndrome and cardiac surgery. *J Clin Invest* 1986;78:340–348.

64. Van Oeveren W, Harder MP, Roozendaal KJ, et al. Aprotinin protects platelets against the initial effect of cardiopulmonary bypass. *J Thorac Cardiovasc Surg* 1990;99;788–797.

65. Dunlop LC, Andrews TK, Lopez J, et al. Congenital platelet adhesion defects: Bernard-Soulier syndrome. In: Loscalzo J, Schafer AI, eds. *Thrombosis and hemorrhage.* Baltimore: Williams & Wilkins, 1998:685–689.

66. Rinder C, Gaal D, Student L, et al. Platelet–leukocyte activation and modulation of adhesion receptors in pediatric patients with congenital heart disease undergoing cardiopulmonary bypass. *J Thorac Cardiovasc Surg* 1994;107:280–288.

67. Wachtfogel YT, Harpel PC, Edmunds LH Jr, et al. Formation of C1s-C1 inhibitor, kallikrein-C1 inhibitor, and plasmin-alpha-2–plasmin inhibitor complexes during CPB. *Blood* 1989;73: 468–471.

68. Boisclair MD, Lane DA, Phillippou H, et al. Mechanisms of thrombin generation during surgery and CPB. *Blood* 1993:82: 3350–3357.

69. Mirshahi M, Soria J, Soria C, et al. Evaluation of the inhibition of heparin and hirudin on coagulation activation during r-tPA-induced thrombolysis. *Blood* 1989;74:1025–1030.

70. Morgan BP. Complement membrane attack on nucleated cells: resistance, recovery and non-lethal effects. *Biochem J* 1989;264: 1–14.

71. Wiedmer T, Esmon CT, Sims PJ. Complement proteins C5b-9 stimulate procoagulant activity through the platelet prothrombinase. *Blood* 1986;68:875–880.

72. Chenowith DE, Cooper SW, Hugli TE, et.al. Complement activation during cardiopulmonary bypass: evidence for generation of C3a and C5a anaphylatoxins. *N Engl J Med* 1981;81:370–377.

73. Haslam P, Townsend P, Branthwaite M. Complement activation during cardiopulmonary bypass. *Anaesthesia* 1980;25:22–26.

74. Cavarocchi NC, Schaff HV, Orszulak TA, et al. Evidence for complement activation by protamine–heparin interaction after CPB. *Surgery* 1985;98:525–530.

75. Fletcher MP, Stahl G, Longhurst J. C5a-induced myocardial ischemia: role for CD18-dependent PMN localization and PMN-platelet interactions. *Am J Physiol* 1993;265[*Heart Circ Physiol* 34]:H1750–H1761.

76. Hattori R, Hamilton KK, Fugate RD, et al. Complement proteins C5b-9 induce secretion of high-molecular-weight multimers of endothelial von Willebrand factor and translocation of granule membrane protein GMP-140 to the cell surface. *J Biol Chem* 1989;264:9053–9060.

77. Rinder CS, Rinder HM, Smith BR, et.al. Blockade of C5a and C5b-9 generation inhibits leukocyte and platelet activation during extracorporeal circulation. *J Clin Invest* 1995;96:1564–1572.

78. Rinder CS, Rinder HM, Johnson K, et al. Role of C3 cleavage in monocyte activation during extracorporeal circulation. *Circulation* 1999;100:553–558.

79. Wiedmer T, Esmon CT, Sims PJ. Complement proteins C5b-9 stimulate procoagulant activity through the platelet prothrombinase. *Blood* 1986;68:875–880.

80. Ando B, Wiedmer T, Sims PJ. The secretory release reaction initiated by complement proteins C5b-9 occurs without platelet aggregation through glycoprotein IIb-IIIa. *Blood* 1989;73: 462–467.

81. Butler J, Rocker GM, Westaby S. Inflammatory response to cardiopulmonary bypass. *Ann Thorac Surg* 1993;55:552–559.

82. Plow EF. The major fibrinolytic proteases of human leukocytes. *Biochim Biophys Acta* 1980;630:47–56.

83. Despotis GJ, Levine V, Goodnough LT. Relationship between leukocyte count and patient risk for excessive blood loss after cardiac surgery. *Crit Care Med* 1997;25:1338–1346.

25

MANAGEMENT OF COAGULOPATHY ASSOCIATED WITH CARDIOPULMONARY BYPASS

JAN C. HORROW
JANE C.K. FITCH

COMPONENTS OF HEMOSTASIS

Blood must remain fluid in the vessels but congeal upon vascular disruption to prevent exsanguination. Hemostasis requires participation of platelets, coagulation proteins, and the vascular endothelium. Vessel patency depends on both hemostasis and fibrinolysis, which governs clot remodeling and breakdown. Chapter 24 dealt with aspects of platelet physiology and dysfunction and the interaction with vascular endothelium. This chapter covers the impact of cardiopulmonary bypass (CPB) on coagulation proteins and fibrinolysis and the management of bleeding associated with bypass.

Definition of a few terms fosters an appreciation and understanding of the complexity of hemostasis. *Coagulation* refers to the formation of a clot *in vitro*, as occurs in the performance of routine laboratory tests. *Thrombosis* refers to formation of clot *in vivo*, as occurs pathologically in veins of the lower extremity or pelvis after some operations. *Hemostasis* refers to cessation of bleeding following injury (1). Thus, the ideal anticoagulant is also antithrombotic, but not antihemostatic. Although all components of hemostasis are essential and the platelet response occurs first, the most fundamental part is the formation of fibrin.

FIBRIN FORMATION

Clotting Factors and their Activation

The liver synthesizes a series of inactive glycoproteins that circulate in the blood and lead to the production of fibrin. Activation of one of these clotting factors sequentially activates another in a series of reactions, ultimately yielding cross-linked fibrin. Fibrin formation in cellular material produces clot; when red cells and platelets are absent, it is termed gel. The sequentially activating glycoproteins earn the name "serine proteases" because their active sites, serine amino acid residues, cleave the next protein in sequence. Thus, in inactive ("zymogen") form, these substances serve as substrate in one reaction and in active form as enzyme in the next reaction in sequence (2). The endothelial system, not the liver, synthesizes factor VIII. Table 25.1 summarizes important information about the clotting factors.

Roman numerals I through XIII identify the clotting factors, with an appended "a" denoting the activated form. The activation sequences do not follow numerical order, for several reasons. First, discovery of the clotting factors, which governed the numeric assignments, did not proceed in order of their activation; second, the factors interact among themselves in complex ways, rendering a strict order difficult; and third, new knowledge changes the clotting factor identities and revises their relationships. As examples, factor IV was subsequently identified as calcium ion and is now referred to as such, whereas a postulated factor VI was subsequently discovered not to exist. This text refers to the factors by their Roman numerals. However, factor I will be identified as fibrinogen, factor II as prothrombin, factor IIa as thrombin, and factor III as tissue factor, except where numerical notation is expedient.

Figure 25.1 displays a simplified version of the activation sequence of the clotting factors. Factor X occupies a central position in this scheme. Events preceding formation of factor Xa are termed either "intrinsic" or "extrinsic" based on whether the initiating stimulus arises from within or outside of the vasculature. Events subsequent to factor Xa form a "common pathway" leading to fibrin generation. Each component is considered in turn.

Intrinsic Events

Circulating factor XII binds to negatively charged surfaces such as glass, resulting in its activation. Factor XI also binds

J.C. Horrow: Department of Anesthesiology, MCP-Hahnemann University, Philadelphia, Pennsylvania 19102.

J.C.K. Fitch: Department of Anesthesiology, Baylor College of Medicine, 6550 Fannin, Suite 1003, Houston, Texas 77030.

TABLE 25.1. CLOTTING FACTORS

Factor	Activated By	Acts On	Surgical Level (min)	Replacement Source	Half-Life	Vitamin K Dependent?	Natural Source	Comments
I	IIa		1 g/L	CRYO, FFP	3–6 days	No	Liver	Fibrinogen
II	Xa	I	20–40%	FFP, Pcx	3 days	Yes	Liver	Prothrombin
III		X				No	Tissue	Tissue Factor
IV							Plasma	Calcium ion
V	IIa	II	15% or less	FFP	12 hr	No	Liver	Cofactor
VII	Xa	X	10–20%	FFP, Pcx	3 hr	Yes	Liver	
VIII	IIa	X	>30%	CRYO, 8C, FFP	8–12 hr	No	RES	Cofactor
IX	VIIa, XIa	X	25–30%	FFP, 9C, Pcx	12–14 hr	Yes	Liver	
X	VIIa, IXa	II	10–20%	FFP, Pcx	30–50 hr	Yes	Liver	
XI	XIIa	IX	15–25%	FFP	48–77 hr	No	Liver	
XII	Endothelium	XI	None	Not needed	48–52 hr	No	Liver	
XIII	IIa	Fibrin	5% or less	FFP, CRYO	3–12 days	No	Liver	
vWF		VIII	See footnote	FFP, CRYO		No	Endothelium	
ProtC	IIa	Va, VIIIa			3 hr	Yes	Liver	Needs ProtS

CRYO, cryoprecipitate; FFP, fresh frozen plasma; Pcx, prothrombinase complex concentrate; 9C, factor 9 concentrate; 8C, factor 8 concentrate; RES, reticuloendothelial system; min, minimum; ProtC, protein C; ProtS, protein S; vWF, von Willebrand factor. Note there is no factor VI. For von Willebrand factor, cryoprecipitate or FFP administration will obtain a factor VIII coagulant activity > 30%.

with assistance from high-molecular-weight kininogen (HMWK). Factor XIIa then cleaves a peptide fragment from factor XI to form factor XIa. In similar fashion, HMWK binds prekallikrein to the surface so that factor XIIa may split it to form kallikrein. Kallikrein accelerates the process by enhancing prekallikrein cleavage by factor XIIa. Factor XIa, however, inactivates HMWK, thus limiting this process. The term "surface activation" describes these reactions, all of which form a subset of the intrinsic events (2). Factor XIa then splits factor IX to form factor IXa. Calcium ion must be present for this process. The intrinsic pathway may have minimal biologic significance and may represent *ex vivo* phenomena only.

Factor IXa then cleaves factor X to form factor Xa. Splitting of factor X by factor IXa, a complex process, requires a phospholipid surface, calcium ion, and an accelerating

cofactor, factor VIIIa. The phospholipid surface, contributed by platelets and sometimes termed platelet factor 3, facilitates the molecular interactions. Calcium ions tether the substrates in this reaction to the phospholipid surface. Placement of carboxyl groups on glutamic acid residues of the substrate factors by vitamin K supplies negative charges by which the positively charged calcium ions link the factors to the phospholipid surface. Factors II, VII, IX, and X depend on vitamin K to insert these negative charges, without which factor activation does not proceed (3).

With calcium and phospholipid, factor IXa will cleave factor X slowly. In the presence of the accelerating cofactor, factor VIIIa, factor X activation proceeds rapidly. Figure 25.2 depicts this final intrinsic event, leading to formation of factor Xa. The entity formed by these interacting molecules is termed the tenase ("ten-ase") complex.

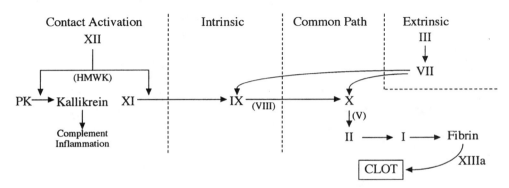

FIG. 25.1. Simplified schematic of the sequence of coagulation protein activation. The high-molecular weight kininogen (*HMWK*) fosters binding of prekallikrein (*PK*) and factor XI to an activating surface. Parentheses indicate cofactors.

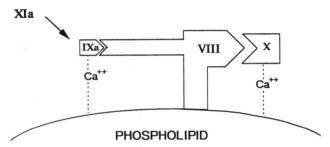

PHOSPHOLIPID

FIG. 25.2. The role of factor VIII in activation of factor X. Calcium tethers factors IXa and X to the phospholipid surface (usually the platelet membrane). Although factor IXa alone can activate factor X, factor VIII greatly facilitates this process. (From Horrow JC. Desmopressin and antifibrinolytics. *Int Anesth Clin* 1990;28: 216–222, with permission.)

Extrinsic Events

Tissue factor (factor III) consists of a 219-amino acid transmembrane peptide chain of which 21 amino acids reside in the cell. When exposed to the interior of the vasculature by endothelial cell damage, tissue factor activates factor IX, thus linking the extrinsic and intrinsic pathways. Factor IXa is then transported from endothelial cell surface to platelet surface to participate in common pathway reactions. Tissue factor also facilitates initial activation of factor X by factor VII. In a double positive feedback arrangement (Fig. 25.3), factor Xa then cleaves small amounts of factor VII to form factor VIIa. Thus activated, factor VIIa rapidly splits factor X, using phospholipid and calcium ions (4).

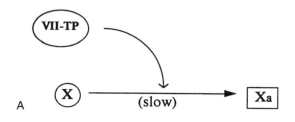

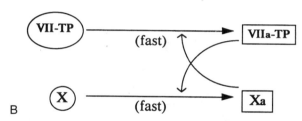

FIG. 25.3. A: Initial extrinsic-mediated activation of factor X. **B:** A double-positive feedback loop then activates factors X and VII. *TP,* (thromboplastin tissue factor).

Common Pathway

Factor Xa splits prothrombin (factor IIa) to form thrombin (factor II), requiring a phospholipid surface and calcium ion. In analogous fashion to the role of factor VIII, a cofactor, factor Va, accelerates this "prothrombinase complex" reaction. Thrombin splits fibrinogen to form fibrin monomer.

Modulators of Coagulation

Thrombin

Thrombin has an impact on every aspect of hemostasis. Its procoagulant activities include splitting fibrinogen to fibrin; activation of factors V and VIII to accelerate fibrin formation; activation of factor XIII, which cross-links soluble fibrin; and stimulation of platelet recruitment. Actions limiting clot formation include release from endothelial cells of tissue plasminogen activator (t-PA), which activates plasmin, and activation of protein C, which inactivates factors Va and VIIIa (2).

Feedback

Both positive and negative feedback modulation exert a powerful influence on coagulation protein activation sequences. Positive feedback amplifies a minor molecular event to create a dramatic result. For example, the weak formation of factor Xa by factor VII and tissue factor becomes amplified by activation of factor VII by factor Xa, which then strongly activates factor X. This positive feedback permits circulating factor VII to remain harmless until tissue factor enters the vasculature. Another example is potentiation of prekallikrein cleavage by its end-product, kallikrein. Negative feedback mechanisms prevent runaway coagulation factor consumption, as exemplified by factor XIa inactivation of HMWK. Note that thrombin exhibits both positive feedback (activation of factors V and VIII) and negative feedback (protein C activation) activity.

Protein C

Endothelial cells express thrombomodulin, a regulatory protein that accelerates thrombin activation of protein C. Protein C, labeled such because it was the third protein eluted in an ion exchange chromatogram, functions as an anticoagulant by inactivating factor Va and factor VIIIa and by stimulating fibrinolysis. Like other coagulation proteins, it circulates as an inactive zymogen. Thrombin cleaves a polypeptide fragment of protein C, creating the active serine protease. A cofactor, protein S, accelerates inactivation of factors Va and VIIIa by protein C. Both protein C and protein S require vitamin K for incorporation of γ-carboxyglutamate, similar to factors II, VII, IX, and X. Deficiency of protein C, an autosomal dominant trait, results in fatal neonatal thrombosis or in recurrent venous thromboses and pulmonary embolism (5).

Antithrombin

Serine protease inhibitors, or "serpins," also control fibrin formation. Antithrombin, the most important serpin, inhibits thrombin, kallikrein, and factors XIIa, XIa, Xa, and IXa by binding to their active sites at a serine residue. Antithrombin primarily inhibits propagation of coagulation, as opposed to its initiation. Antithrombin also inhibits plasmin, a mediator of fibrinolysis (6).

von Willebrand Factor

von Willebrand factor (vWF) protects factor VIII from enzymatic degradation, thus prolonging its half-life. It also tethers the platelet membrane glycoprotein Ib to exposed subendothelial matrix, thus promoting platelet adhesion (7). A massive heterogeneous molecule, vWF consists of different numbers of linked glycosylated peptides. Some of these multimers are large enough to be imaged with electron microscopy.

Tissue Factor Pathway Inhibitor

Secreted by hepatocytes and endothelium, this lipid-associated inhibitor of the tissue factor pathway requires factor Xa to exert its anticoagulant effect (8). Tissue factor pathway inhibitor influences the initiation but not the propagation phase of thrombin generation (9), complementing the profile of antithrombin. Heparin releases tissue factor pathway inhibitor from endothelium binding sites (10).

Fibrinogen and Fibrin

Molecular Structure

Figure 25.4 depicts the six polypeptide chains that form the fibrinogen molecule—two each of α, β, and γ subunits.

Disulfide bonds link them in antiparallel fashion. Fibrinogen's three-dimensional structure features a central globular domain with twisted coils extending in opposite directions terminating in hydrophilic regions. Nonhelical protease-sensitive regions interrupt the coiled-coils about midway in their length. The central "E" domain and peripheral hydrophilic "D" domains participate in fibrin polymerization (11).

Normal plasma fibrinogen concentration is 1.5 to 4.5 g/L. An "acute phase reactant," fibrinogen increases in concentration during infection, inflammation, and stress. Thus, a low normal fibrinogen concentration in a septic patient reflects fibrinogen consumption. Fibrinogen resists degradation during storage of banked whole blood and is present in fresh frozen plasma. Cryoprecipitate replaces fibrinogen best because each 10- to 15-mL unit contains about 20% of the fibrinogen present in one 200- to 250-mL unit of fresh frozen plasma or one 400- to 450-mL unit of whole blood (12).

Formation and Polymerization of Fibrin

Thrombin cleaves peptide fragment A from the Aα subunit and fragment B from the Bβ subunit of fibrinogen to form fibrin. The peptide fragments, termed fibrinopeptides, serve as markers of thrombin activity. The resulting soluble fibrin monomers associate in end-to-end and staggered fashions. End-to-end linking occurs via long contact of D domains, whereas stacking of molecules arises from D-E staggered contacts. Figure 25.5 demonstrates formation of fibrin protofibrils via these associations. These weak molecular interactions alone do not produce an insoluble clot, however.

Factor XIII

In activated form, this coagulation factor cross-links associated fibrin monomers by covalent bonds between the α-chains and between the γ-chains. The only coagulation en-

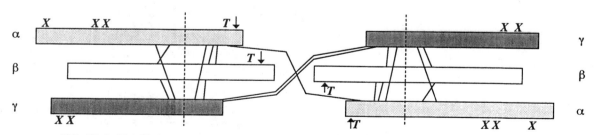

FIG. 25.4. The fibrinogen molecule, composed of six polypeptide chains, one pair each of α, β, and γ. Thrombin cleaves the fibrinopeptides at sites indicated by an *arrow* and *T*. The *vertical dashed line* indicates where plasmin, formed from bound plasminogen by tissue plasminogen activator, or other activators, cleaves the molecule. Factor XIII cross-links one fibrin molecule to another at sites designated with an *X*. *Solid lines* indicate placement of disulfide cross-linkages within the fibrinogen molecule. (Modified from Hantgan RR, Francis CW, Marder VJ. Fibrinogen structure and physiology. In: Colman RW, Hirsch J, Marder VJ, et al., eds. *Hemostasis and thrombosis,* 3rd ed. Philadelphia: J.B. Lippincott, 1994:277–300, with permission.)

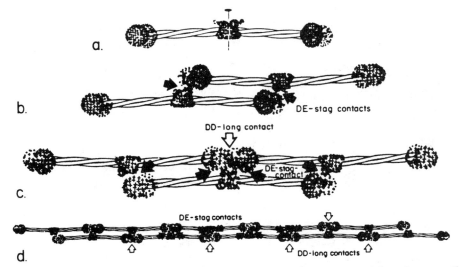

FIG. 25.5. Sequence of fibrin polymerization. **A:** Fibrin molecule as a central domain connecting with two peripheral domains via a coiled coil. **B:** Two fibrin monomers associate in staggered fashion (DE contact). **C:** A third molecule joins end-to-end with the second molecule (DD contact) and in staggered fashion with the first molecule (DE contact). **D:** A protofibril formed by addition of several more monomers. (From Hermans J, McDonagh J. Fibrin: structure and interactions. *Semin Thromb Hemost* 1982;8:11–24, with permission.)

zyme not a serine protease, factor XIIIa contains a cysteine active site that functions as a transamidase. Thrombin exposes the active cysteine sites of factor XIII. Calcium then separates the active enzyme, factor XIIIa, from a carrier protein moiety (13). The insoluble cross-linked fibrin so formed thickens the blood or plasma in which it is contained.

FIBRINOLYSIS

Physiologic fibrin breakdown occurs in the vicinity of clot, remodeling and dissolving clot during repair of the underlying endothelium. Pathologic fibrinolysis occurs when newly formed fibrin clots lyse prematurely, exposing damaged vessels and causing renewed bleeding. In similar fashion to fibrin formation, its breakdown proceeds by several paths. Figure 25.6 summarizes the fibrinolytic pathway.

Plasminogen and Plasmin

Lysis of fibrin depends on activation of a cleaving enzyme, plasminogen. Hepatic synthesis results in circulating plasminogen concentrations of 21 mg/dL in plasma or serum. The enzyme circulates as the inactive zymogen. Figure 25.7 demonstrates its molecular structure, which features five outpouchings termed "kringles," each of which contains a binding site for lysine residues of fibrinogen. Cleavage of the arginine 561—valine 562 bond transforms the single-chain plasminogen to the two-chained plasmin molecule (14). Figure 25.4 denotes the sites at which plasminogen

binds to fibrinogen. Conversion of fibrinogen to fibrin encrypts the bound plasminogen, where it awaits activation.

Formation and Fate of Plasmin

Tissue Plasminogen Activator

The physiologic activator of plasminogen is t-PA, a 530-residue serine protease synthesized in endothelial cells and released by exercise, stress, venous occlusion, and certain drugs, including desmopressin and heparin. The activity of

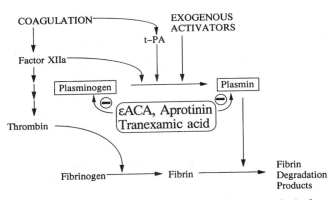

FIG. 25.6. The fibrinolytic pathway. Coagulation results in formation of thrombin, which yields fibrin, and of tissue plasminogen activator and factor XIIa, which convert plasminogen to plasmin in the vicinity of clot. Plasmin splits fibrin. Antifibrinolytic drugs inhibit plasminogen and plasmin. Exogenous activators of fibrinolysis, such as streptokinase, may also convert plasminogen to plasmin. *εACA, ε-aminocaproic acid.*

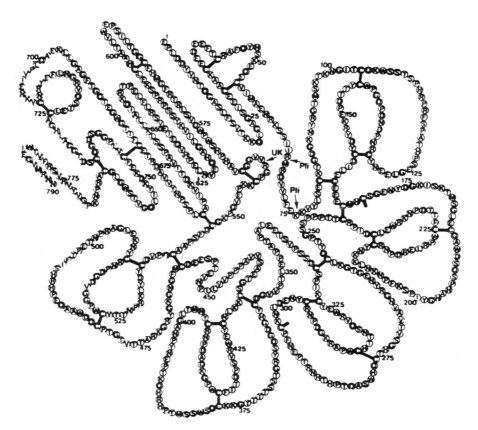

FIG. 25.7. The structure of human plasminogen. The five outpouchings of this macromolecule are called "kringles," after a Scandinavian pastry of the same name. (From Collen D. On the regulation and control of fibrinolysis. *Thromb Haemost* 1980;43:77–89, with permission.)

t-PA enhances 1,000-fold in the presence of fibrin, essentially restricting its effect to the vicinity of clot and protecting circulating plasminogen from activation. Normally, small amounts of t-PA remodel and dissolve clots dynamically, resulting in a low level of fibrinolysis (14). Bypass may release t-PA from endothelium (15-17), resulting in decreased concentrations after bypass (17).

Plasminogen activator inhibitor 1 (PAI-1, pronounced "pie-one"), the naturally occurring inhibitor of t-PA, increases during bypass (17), binding to t-PA to form t-PA–PAI complexes and decreased free PAI-1 concentrations (16). Heparin facilitates PAI-1 inhibition of thrombin (10). Platelets secrete large amounts of PAI-1 (18).

Factor XII

The surface activation coagulation proteins (factor XII, prekallikrein, and HMWK) appear to initiate fibrinolysis by a path independent of t-PA. Conversion of prourokinase, another circulating fibrinolytic protein, to a potent plasminogen activator by kallikrein mediates this minor pathway, which accounts for less than half of plasma fibrinolytic activity (19).

Once plasmin is formed, it splits fibrin at parallel locations on all six peptide chains. If plasmin reaches the systemic circulation, it can also hydrolyze fibrinogen, factor V, factor VIII, complement, and some hormones. A scavenging protease, α_2-antiplasmin, binds and destroys any plasmin that circulates. If α_2-antiplasmin becomes saturated, α_1-macroglobulin will perform the same function (19).

Thrombolytic Therapy

Plasminogen activators may be exogenously administered to dissolve pathologically formed intravascular clots (20). The first generation of these agents included streptokinase, an antigenic protein derived from group C β-hemolytic streptococci, and urokinase, a 411-residue nonantigenic proteolytic enzyme derived from purified human urine. Streptokinase forms a complex with plasminogen, exposing the active site, thus facilitating its conversion to plasmin. Activation occurs systemically without benefit of fibrin specificity (i.e., restriction to clot location), which is important because circulating plasmin can lyse fibrinogen and fibrin. Systemic effects combined with a long half-life (30 minutes) make bleeding complications common. Allergy

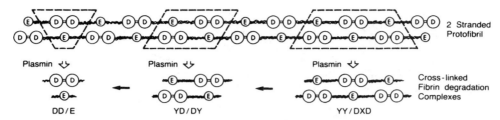

FIG. 25.8. Formation of fibrin degradation products from cross-linked fibrin. Plasmin cleaves fibrin between its D and E domains at the *dashed lines* to yield D-dimer (DD), fragment Y (DE), fragment X (DED), and larger combinations (DY, YY, DXD, and others not shown). D-dimer serves as a specific marker for lysis of cross-linked fibrin. (From Francis CW, Marder VJ. Physiologic regulation and pathologic disorders of fibrinolysis. In: Colman RW, Hirsh J, Marder VJ, et al., eds. *Hemostasis and Thrombosis*, 3rd ed. Philadelphia: J.B. Lippincott, 1994:1076–1103, with permission.)

and anaphylaxis may occur. Urokinase converts plasminogen to plasmin directly but still without fibrin specificity. Its half-life in plasma is 16 minutes. Limited availability and high cost preclude its widespread clinical use.

The second generation of thrombolytic agents include anisoylated plasminogen-streptokinase activator, single-chain urokinase plasminogen activator, and recombinant t-PA. The chemically modified streptokinase, anisoylated plasminogen-streptokinase activator, retains antigenicity and produces a sustained lytic effect because of a prolonged half-life (≈ 3 hours), with fibrin specificity between that of t-PA and streptokinase. Recombinant t-PA (alteplase) enjoys wide clinical use for treatment of thrombosis. Large doses must be administered to deliver enough drug to the site of thrombosis, thus compromising fibrin specificity somewhat. Rapid elimination (3- to 5-minute half-life) requires continuous infusions for efficacy. The lack of antigenicity makes this alternative attractive, despite its expense. Recombinant single-chain urokinase plasminogen activator (saruplase), like t-PA, exhibits fibrin specificity, nonreactivity in plasma, and a short half-life. It is still investigational. Second-generation agents demonstrate efficacy in reversing acute coronary thromboses (21).

The third generation of these compounds includes modifications to facilitate dosing and improve efficacy. For example, TNK-tPA consists of t-PA strategically substituted at several amino acid locations to yield biphasic pharmacokinetics with prolonged persistence in plasma (22), enhanced fibrin specificity, and increased resistance to the inhibitor PAI-1. A single 40-mg dose of TNK-tPA demonstrated equivalent efficacy to t-PA bolus and infusion (23). For a review, see the article by Gersh (18).

Products of Fibrinolysis

Breakdown of fibrin yields numerous products, best understood by first considering lysis of a fibrin monomer. The product formed after plasmin cleavage of the Aα appendage and the remaining part of the Bβ chain (residues 15 through 42) is termed fragment X. Further activity at sites midway

along the coiled coils yields three kinds of products: a peripheral domain with attached polypeptide strand (fragment D), a central domain with polypeptide strands (fragment E), and the product of incomplete digestion (central domain with one peripheral domain intact, labeled fragment Y) (19). Figure 25.8 displays a two-stranded protofibril, formed after cross-linking by factor XIIIa, and its degradation products, which include a fragment containing two D domains, termed D-dimer. Tests for these various degradation products permit detection of a fibrinolytic state.

Fibrin degradation products intercalate into the forming fibrin protofibrils, preventing proper alignment of fibrin monomers for correct cross-linking by factor XIIIa. As a result, intense fibrinolysis impairs formation of subsequent clot.

Local versus Systemic Fibrinolysis

Lysis of circulating fibrinogen is not physiologic. Plasmin degradation of the fibrinogen molecule (i.e., before separation of the fibrinopeptides Aα(1–16) and Bβ(1–14)) yields fragments X; Y, D, and E; the Aα appendage, and the Bβ(1–42) peptide fragment. This last product serves as a marker specific for fibrinogenolysis. Fibrinogenolysis occurs with administration of nonselective plasminogen activators, from therapeutic doses of second-generation thrombolytic drugs, or more rarely when release of plasminogen activator from tissues overwhelms the circulating plasmin scavengers.

Localized fibrinolysis occurring in response to intense bursts of coagulation may flood the circulation with fibrin degradation products, causing hemorrhage. In this case, fibrinogen remains intact and no plasmin circulates. In consumptive coagulopathy, formation and breakdown of fibrin in the microcirculation deplete coagulation factors and platelets and form fibrin degradation products, yielding hemorrhage.

LABORATORY TESTS OF COAGULATION

No laboratory coagulation test can duplicate the complex milieu present at an injured vessel. Merely placing a needle or catheter in a vessel initiates a host of hemostatic responses that alter measurements on the sample removed. Surface activation begins when blood leaves the protective environment of the endothelial cell and enters into collection tubes. For these reasons, one must view the results of any coagulation test as only an approximation of actual events. This section presents tests performed at central laboratory facilities followed by near-patient (also called point-of-care) tests.

Centralized Coagulation Laboratory Tests

Devices using formation of a clot as an endpoint usually use electrical or optical detection methods. The classic instrument, the Fibrometer (BBL Microbiological Systems, Cockeysville, MD), places a stationary and a moving probe in the sample. When fibrin strands bridge the two electrodes, conductivity increases and a timer halts (24). Laboratory prothrombin time (PT), activated partial thromboplastin time (aPTT), fibrinogen, and thrombin time determinations use this technology.

Prothrombin Time and Activated Partial Thromboplastin Time

Figure 25.9 illustrates the steps in performing these tests. Each test involves centrifuging a citrated specimen of blood. Citrate complexes calcium, preventing coagulation factor

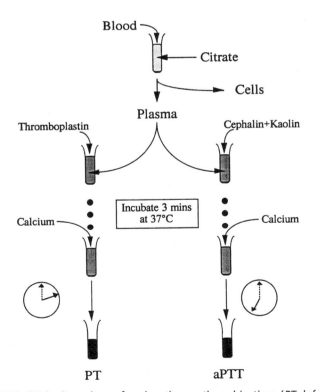

FIG. 25.9. Steps in performing the prothrombin time (*PT*, left side) and the activated partial thromboplastin time (*aPTT*, right side). See text for details.

activation. The supernatant obtained by centrifugation, plasma, is incubated for 3 minutes with an additive that differs for the two tests. After addition of excess calcium, the time to formation of gel is clocked.

The PT, which would be labeled better as the complete thromboplastin time, incubates plasma with tissue extract (thromboplastin). As a tissue product, thromboplastin supplies its own phospholipid. If the plasma sample contains sufficient factor VII and factors in the common pathway, it will gel in about 12 seconds. Variations in the potency and quality of thromboplastin reagents require simultaneous determination of a control sample and comparison of the patient's result with the control result. Each batch of thromboplastin reagent is graded in potency. This grade permits calculation of the international normalized ratio (INR), which essentially standardizes PT results regardless of thromboplastin potency. See Point-of-Care Coagulation Tests, below, for more information on the INR. Ratios over 1.5 indicate a coagulation factor abnormality.

The PTT incubates plasma with an extract of thromboplastin that contains the phospholipid but not the tissue factor, thus preventing activation of factor VII. When dependent on surface activation alone, gel forms slowly (73 ± 11 [SD] seconds) (25). The *activated* PTT (aPTT) uses a surface activation accelerator such as kaolin, ellagic acid, silica, bentonite, or celite (24). Gel formation then occurs in about 32 seconds. As with the PT, simultaneous controls are required, with abnormal patient results at 1.5 or more times control.

Coumadin therapy prolongs the PT without affecting the aPTT because factor VII is most vulnerable to lack of vitamin K. Large doses of coumadin will elevate the aPTT also. Heparin primarily affects the aPTT and not the PT because the inhibition of factors Xa and thrombin from doses of heparin commonly used to treat venous thrombosis is easily overwhelmed by the potent procoagulant action of thromboplastin. The less potent partial thromboplastin reagent, however, does not mask heparin's anticoagulant effects. Large doses of heparin will prolong the PT also.

Thrombin Time

Adding thrombin to a plasma sample will form fibrin within 10 seconds if functionally active fibrinogen is present, heparin is absent, and fibrin degradation products are absent (26). Sensitivity of the thrombin time to small amounts of heparin occurs because small amounts of thrombin are added. The traditional thrombin time is relatively insensitive to fibrinogen deficiency and to fibrin degradation products: Detectable prolongation requires less than 0.75 g/L fibrinogen (27) or more than 200 μg/mL fibrin degradation products. Sensitivity to fibrin degradation products increases if fibrinogen concentrations are low. Also, diluted plasma increases sensitivity of the thrombin test to fibrinogen deficiency.

Reptilase Time

The reptilase time measures the interval between addition to plasma of venom from the South American pit viper *Bothrops jararaca* and formation of fibrin. Because this snake venom does not require thrombin to split fibrinogen, an elevated reptilase time implicates reduced plasma fibrinogen concentration rather than the presence of heparin as the cause of a prolonged thrombin time (28). The reptilase time is severalfold more insensitive to fibrin degradation products than even the thrombin time.

Fibrinogen

Most laboratories use the Claus method for fibrinogen determination, in which a thrombin time is performed on diluted plasma. With diluted samples, fibrinogen becomes the factor limiting clot formation, so that the clotting time varies inversely with fibrinogen activity (24). Antibody-based tests for fibrinogen can distinguish among the dysfibrinogenemias.

Fibrin Degradation Products

Immunologic tests provide a semiquantitative determination of the various fragments resulting from fibrin and fibrinogen degradation. The most common test for fibrin degradation products (FDP), uses latex agglutination of serum. It provides results as either negative (<10 μg/mL) or positive (≥10 μg/mL) for antigens, which are the breakdown products of either fibrin or fibrinogen. Serial dilutions of plasma yield more specific information when the undiluted sample is positive. More expensive quantitative analysis reveals normal serum levels of 2.1 to 2.7 μg/mL for fibrin degradation products in the absence of exercise or stress (24). This test does not differentiate the breakdown products of fibrinogen from those of fibrin.

D-Dimer

Molecules of two linked "D" domains, a specific degradation product of cross-linked fibrin, can be detected either semiquantitatively with a latex agglutination technique or in a fully quantitative manner with an ELISA. Many hospital coagulation laboratories offer this test on a batched basis. The D-dimer is more specific for fibrinolysis than the FDP test. Like the FDP test, D-dimer results appear as fibrinogen equivalent units (i.e., the quantity of fibrinogen initially present that leads to the observed level of breakdown product). Normally, D-dimer is less than 0.5 μg/mL (fibrinogen equivalent units).

Platelet Count

The central role of platelets in coagulation and the impact of bypass on platelet function (see Chapter 24) augment the importance of monitoring platelets during surgery. Because bypass affects both platelet function and count, measurement of platelet count is necessary but not sufficient to assess platelet role in coagulation. Although cell counters can and have been made mobile (29), measurement of platelet count has remained a central laboratory function at nearly all centers.

Point-of-Care Coagulation Tests

For clinicians, the ability to obtain coagulation results in a timely fashion has a critical impact on the diagnosis and treatment of specific hemostatic derangements. In fact, laboratory performance, as judged by clinicians, depends as much on the timeliness of results as on their accuracy. Prompt turnaround also offers a potential advantage for point-of-care testing in clinical situations where saving time translates into financial savings. Thus, the need for accurate and prompt coagulation information has created an interest in point-of-care testing (30).

Point-of-care coagulation monitoring performs tests on whole blood samples within close proximity to the patient. "On-site," "alternate site," and "bedside testing" refer to the same process. In comparison, standard laboratory coagulation testing is performed on a plasma sample for analysis in a more remote hospital laboratory. Standard laboratory coagulation testing involves several stages: obtaining the whole blood sample from the patient, transporting it to the coagulation laboratory, centrifugation of the sample, extraction of plasma, and testing the plasma, often in batches. These stages add time to the standard laboratory testing procedure (30).

Timeliness of reporting constitutes an important, though sometimes overlooked, component of any laboratory service. For clinicians, turnaround time begins when they order a test and ends when they have reviewed the results. For laboratory medicine physicians, turnaround time begins with specimen receipt and ends with result reporting. When tests fail to have an impact on patient care because of result unavailability, the question often remains unanswered as to whether clinician expectations are unrealistic or whether laboratory performance is inadequate (30).

Point-of-care tests clearly perform better than standard laboratory tests with regard to turnaround time: PT, INR, aPTT results are returned in 90 minutes compared to 2.23 minutes (range, 20 to 418 seconds) for point-of-care testing. In one study, the quickest standard laboratory coagulation result (21 minutes) was three times longer than the most tardy point-of-care result (6.97 minutes) (30).

Point-of-care testing is not without criticism. These tests are limited in scope and are often performed by personnel without formal laboratory training. The tests are expensive; cost-to-benefit ratios remain unanalyzed. Associated patient charges, already addressed for standard laboratory testing, have not yet been addressed for point-of-care testing. Also, point-of-care testing in the United States must meet the requirements of the Clinical Laboratory Improvement Amendment, College of American Pathologists, Health Care Finance Administration, and the Joint Commission on Accreditation of Healthcare Organizations (31).

The endpoints for these near-patient tests take slightly longer than in the traditional laboratory-based aPTT. Manual or automatic conversion to values obtained from the laboratory is easily accomplished. With the near-patient tests, each sample does not have a coincident control sample. Thus, periodic quality control assumes great importance to provide reproducible tests. Hospital credentials depend on adequate quality control of all patient tests. Thus, clinicians must ensure routine quality control of near-patient tests they perform. Because near-patient testing technology undergoes rapid development, the reader should seek additional current information when implementing it in the operating room.

With these strengths and limitations in mind, this chapter now presents information on the utility of several point-of-care tests in evaluating the coagulation status of patients during and after CPB. Chapter 22 addresses the most widely known point-of-care coagulation test, the activated coagulation time (ACT). This section does not deal with heparin monitoring tests, including the ACT; its predecessors, the whole blood clotting time and protamine titration (see Chapter 22); and the heparin management test.

Prothrombin Time and Activated Partial Thromboplastin time

Point-of-care PT and aPTT tests use whole blood rather than plasma. Even though platelets remain and provide phospholipid, a phospholipid reagent is added to ensure an excess. The Hemochron-based tests (International Technidyne Corp., Edison, NJ), as performed on model 801 or 8000 machines, use citrated tubes and a true 3-minute incubation period in the Hemochron 37°C chamber, after which calcium is added and the sample timed until the magnetic detector becomes trapped in clot. For the Hemochron aPTT test, yellow-stoppered tubes containing citrate, phospholipid, and diatomaceous earth (which activates factor XII) receive 1.5 mL of blood to yield a normal range of 55 to 85 seconds. Figure 25.10 demonstrates heparin sensitivity of the ACT, bedside aPTT, and laboratory aPTT tests. Note that the whole blood aPTT lies intermediate in sensitivity between the laboratory aPTT and the ACT. For the Hemochron PT test, burgundy-stoppered tubes containing rabbit brain thromboplastin receive 2 mL of blood (normal, 45 to 65 seconds). Medtronic, HemoTec, Inc. (Englewood, CO) also supplies cartridges for bedside determination of PT and aPTT using a stir-bar based monitor.

The Biotrack 512 coagulation monitor performs point-of-care PT and aPTT tests. Cards containing reagents and a capillary tube path for blood receive one large drop of

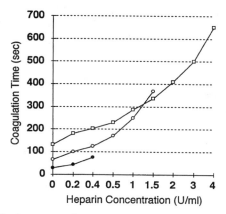

FIG. 25.10. Response of three coagulation tests to heparin. Data are the mean of results from 30 volunteers. □, Hemochron-activated coagulation time (ACT); ○, Hemochron whole blood activated partial thromboplastin time (aPTT); ●, plasma aPTT. The plasma aPTT becomes unmeasurable with heparin concentrations > 0.4 U/mL. Note that whole blood aPTT is linear up to ≈1.0 U/mL and the ACT linear up to ≈3 U/mL. Heparin concentrations are estimated from dose administered and estimated blood volume. (Data from F. LaDuca, PhD, and International Technidyne Corporation, with permission.)

blood (about 0.1 mL). Blood moves by capillary action into a well where it picks up the reagents and then continues to move along the path. A laser detects tardy flow resulting from fibrin formation. The device then converts the actual time measured to one equivalent to that obtained from the hospital laboratory and supplies the ratio of the patient's value to a historical control. The aPTT card uses soybean phosphatide as phospholipid and a sulfatide activator. The PT cards contain thromboplastin. Although a true 3-minute incubation does not occur with this device, the technology is extremely easy to use. In one comparison of devices in a diverse population of anticoagulated and normal patients, the Hemochron aPTT, Biotrack coagulation monitor, and the HemoTec aPTT tests all correlated well with the laboratory-based standard ($r = 0.849$ to 0.963; $n = 50$) (32). All instruments proved adequate to test for reversal of heparin therapy. However, the Biotrack failed to reach an endpoint for samples with reference aPTT more than 70 seconds and the HemoTec aPTT failed to reach an endpoint in six samples.

The Hemochron Jr., a microcoagulation device, uses fresh whole blood to perform the PT and aPTT and provides a calculation of INR (30). With this device, one places a whole blood sample in the well of a test cuvette from which a precise volume is automatically measured and moved into the test channel. The Hemochron Jr. detects a mechanical endpoint for clotting by optical means. It displays the results of the whole blood test as a clotting time in seconds and the extrapolated plasma equivalent clotting time, based on previous simultaneous measurements of whole blood and plasma analyzed by linear regression.

The PT cuvette uses a highly sensitive lyophilized preparation of rabbit brain thromboplastin. The INR calculation allows for comparison of PT results from different commercial thromboplastin reagents: $INR = PCR^{ISI}$, where PCR is the ratio of patient sample to control sample PT results and ISI is the international sensitivity index, a measure of responsiveness to decreased concentrations of vitamin K-dependent factors. The higher a thromboplastin's ISI, the less responsive the clotting time to changes in coagulation factors when using that thromboplastin. Thus a less responsive thromboplastin, which yields a smaller PCR, carries a larger ISI, yielding a similar calculated INR. Thromboplastin reagent manufacturers determine the ISI by comparing the reactivity of each specific lot of thromboplastin with an international reference preparation (33).

The aPTT cuvette uses a lyophilized activator plus a phospholipid derived from either brain or lung tissue. Phospholipid and activator preparations for all aPTT tests vary considerably between manufacturers and even between lots from the same manufacturer (30).

Thrombin Time

This test (Hemochron, International Technidyne Corporation, Edison, NJ) contains lyophilized thrombin sensitive to small concentrations of heparin, to decreased or dysfunctional fibrinogen, and to the presence of fibrin degradation products. It is prolonged in the presence of heparin.

High-dose Thrombin Time

Based on the thrombin time, this whole blood assay uses a higher thrombin concentration so that results can correlate with high heparin concentrations. Unlike the celite ACT, the high-dose thrombin time is unaffected by aprotinin and relatively unaffected by hemodilution or hypothermia. Therefore, the high-dose thrombin time tests both heparin effect and heparin concentration (34).

Heparin-neutralized Thrombin Time

The reagent tubes for this test contain lyophilized thrombin and protamine. Protamine removes heparin as a potential cause of a prolonged test result, allowing the heparin-neutralized thrombin time to be specific to fibrinogen and FDP presence. Simultaneous measurement of the thrombin time and the heparin-neutralized thrombin time may verify complete heparin neutralization or identify heparin rebound. Both tests are sensitive to fibrinogen concentration, prolonging with decreased fibrinogen concentration (35).

Thromboelastography

This viscoelastic test on whole blood rotates a specimen in a cuvette through a small arc (9.5 degrees) every 10 seconds.

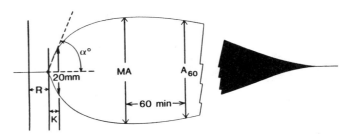

FIG. 25.11. Idealized thromboelastogram, with commonly measured parameters. See text and Table 25.2 for definition and normal ranges of these measurements. (From Spiess BD, Tuman RJ, McCarthy RJ, et al. Thromboelastography as an indicator of postcardiopulmonary bypass coagulopathies. *J Clin Monit* 1987;3: 25–30, with permission.)

A central piston, positioned to provide a 1-mm rim of blood (0.35 mL) between it and the cuvette, remains immobile until fibrin strands couple it to the cuvette's rotatory motion. Torsion on the piston results in movement of a recording heat stylus across sensitive paper advancing at 2 mm/min. The width of the resultant tracing relates to the shear modulus (elasticity) of the specimen (36).

Figure 25.11 and Table 25.2 display the measurements obtained from the thromboelastogram (TEG) and their normal ranges. Appreciation of the overall shape of the TEG purportedly provides more information than these component measures. For example, a tear-drop shape caused by loss of clot strength may denote high fibrinolytic activity (37,38). In fact, TEG tracings cannot diagnose specific hematologic abnormalities because they reflect a global physical property of clot formation. The TEG parameters correlate poorly with routine laboratory coagulation tests (39–42). An abnormal TEG tracing does, however, suggest further investigation.

Sonoclot

This viscoelastic test performed on whole blood uses a probe vibrating in a small sample (0.4 mL) of whole blood at 200 Hz. Although the TEG displays clot shear modulus, the Sonoclot charts impedance to probe motion, which increases as coagulation events proceed. This outcome variable is not calibrated in physical units, appearing instead in units of "percent." The curve obtained divides into several parts, termed "waves," based on the rate of increase of impedance with time (43). The manufacturer (Sienco, Inc., Morrison, CO) identifies a component analogous to the ACT ("SonAct") and certain curve shapes reflecting platelet dysfunction, thrombocytopenia, and "hypercoagulability." No independent data verify these associations. In an unblinded study, the Sonoclot predicted that platelet transfusion would correct post-bypass bleeding in 21 of 25 patients

TABLE 25.2. PARAMETERS MEASURED ON THE THROMBOELASTOGRAM

Name	Definition	Normal Range[a]	Significance of Abnormal Values	References
R (reaction time)	Time from sample collection until pen deviation from midline	7.5–15 min	Hypercoagulability Factor deficiency?	?
K (coagulation time)	Time from initial pen deviation from midline to amplitude of 20 mm	3–6 min	?	?
α (speed of clot formation)	Angle formed by midline and tangent of amplitude tracing upslope	45–55 degrees	?	?
MA (maximum amplitude)	Maximum amplitude	50–60 mm	Hypofibrinogenemia, thrombocytopenia, platelet dysfunction	Howland et al. (21) Zuckerman et al. (22)
A_{60} (amplitude)	Tracing amplitude 60 min after MA	$\geq$ (MA − 5) mm	Fibrinolysis or uremia	Howland et al. (21) von Kaulla et al. (23)

[a] Normal values from Spiess et al. (20).

(44). Figure 25.12 displays Sonoclot signatures before and after aspirin administration to 1 of 22 volunteers. The Sonoclot failed to reflect the prolongation in bleeding time associated with aspirin (45). Hematopathologists accept neither the TEG nor the Sonoclot for diagnostic purposes, perhaps because of insufficient data linking test results with independently confirmed pathology.

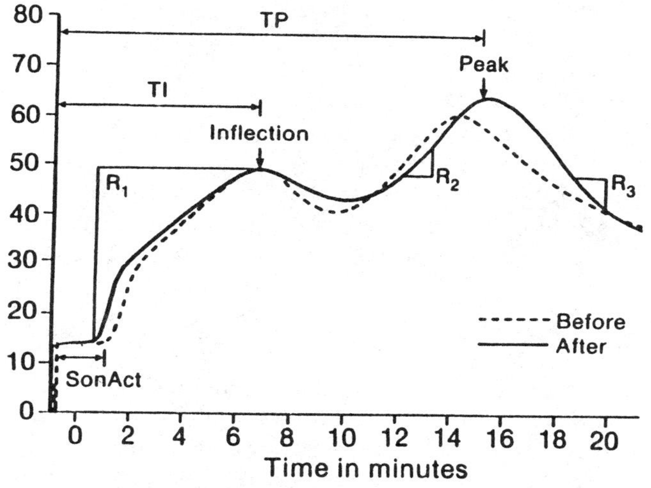

Platelet Function Tests

New point-of-care technologies using whole blood might also evaluate platelet function. The HemoSTATUS (Medtronic, Inc., Parker, CO) is performed on the Hepcon monitoring system. It compares clotting times in a native whole blood sample with those obtained with sample to which platelet activator has been added in several concentrations. Different platelet activators may be chosen. The most common is platelet activating factor.

Another whole blood point-of-care technology, the Platelet Function Analyzer (PFA-100, Dade International, Miami, FL), performs the equivalent of a bleeding time *in vitro*. The PFA was formerly known as the Thrombostat 4000. The Rapid Platelet Function Analyzer (RPFA, Accumetrics, San Diego, CA) performs a computerized whole blood platelet aggregation test. The Clot Signature Analyzer (Xylum Corporation, Scarsdale, NY), formerly known as the Hemostatometer, measures platelet function via shear-induced activation and aggregation in a physiologic flow environment. The Hemodyne (Hemodyne, Inc., Richmond, VA) provides a measure of platelet-mediated force transduction, which relates to quantitative and qualitative platelet function. The above whole blood point-of-care platelet tests await widespread clinical validation.

Sophisticated Hematology Tests

Research laboratories and a few clinical centers specializing in hemostasis and thrombosis offer a host of specialized

FIG. 25.12. A Sonoclot signature in a patient before (*dashed line*) and after (*solid line*) receiving four doses of 325 mg aspirin over 2 days. The initial flat portion (SonAct) is normally 60 to 130 seconds. R_1, R_2, and R_3, slopes of the curves, measure the rate of change in viscosity of the sample. *TI*, time to the first inflection point; *TP*, time to peak viscosity. Normally R_1 is 15% to 30% per minute and TP 5 to 10 minutes. The vertical axis, called "percent," lacks calibration against a standard. (From Samra SK, Harrison RL, Bee DE, et al. A study of aspirin induced changes in bleeding time, platelet aggregation, and Sonoclot coagulation analysis in humans. *Ann Clin Lab Sci* 1991;21:315–327, with permission.)

coagulation tests. Chromogenic technology, in which a color-absorbing molecule is linked to a component of the reaction to be measured, permits quantitation of the activity of many hemostatic elements, such as antithrombin, t-PA, heparin, and anti-IIa, and anti-Xa activities. Tests based on antibody technology include quantitation of fibrinopeptides A and B, the latter available for the fibrinogen split product Bβ1–42 and for the fibrin split product Bβ15–42; t-PA antigen; thrombin–antithrombin complex; plasmin–anti-plasmin complex; PAI-1; and t-PA–PAI complex.

Predictive Value of Laboratory Tests for Bleeding

The literature yields conflicting results regarding the absolute and relative abilities of various coagulation tests to predict hemostasis after CPB. Routine laboratory tests succeed in some studies (46–49) and fail in others (50,51). Likewise, the TEG predicts post-bypass hemorrhage in one study (47), demonstrates superiority to laboratory tests in three others (39,52,53) and to the HemoSTATUS (53), yet fails to identify patients at risk in a different investigation (48). More sophisticated tests such as D-dimer concentration and glycoprotein Ib expression correlate with blood loss after surgery but are cumbersome and expensive to measure (54). Single reports each tout the usefulness of specific devices, viz., the Hemostatometer (55) and the Hemodyne (56).

When evaluating the literature on coagulation test utility, clinicians must temper enthusiasm for new technologies with the need for properly designed and properly analyzed comparisons with available tests. Large variation in patient populations and in blood loss after bypass even in well-defined populations further complicate these judgments.

BYPASS-INDUCED COAGULATION ABNORMALITIES

In the earlier days of CPB, the cellular and molecular elements of blood sustained significant mechanical trauma during perfusion, resulting in destruction of red cells and platelets and denaturation of plasma proteins. Although the improved materials now used for bypass incite less damage, an intrinsically nonthrombogenic surface still evades discovery (57). Some heparin-coated surfaces do show promise (see Chapter 9). This section covers hemostatic abnormalities induced by bypass, except for platelet effects, which are covered in Chapter 24.

Coagulation Factors

With rare exception, normal levels for the coagulation factors range from 0.5 to 1.5 activity units/mL, corresponding to 50% to 150% of population means. (In contrast, the inhibitory proteins, such as antithrombin and protein C,

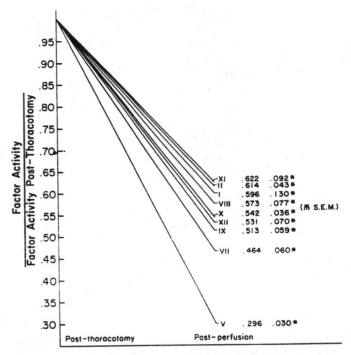

FIG. 25.13. Decline in factor activity in 11 patients during bypass with a bubble oxygenator. Although factor V activity declines to only 30 ± 3% of normal, surgical hemostasis requires 15% to 25% at most. (From Kalter RD, Saul CM, Wetstein L, et al. Cardiopulmonary bypass. Associated hemostatic abnormalities. *J Thorac Cardiovasc Surg* 1979;77:425–435, with permission.)

adhere to a more restricted range.) When factor replacement is indicated for major surgery, the usual target, 1.0 units/mL, incorporates a threefold safety factor, because only levels below 0.3 units/mL impair the sequential enzyme activation ending with fibrin formation. The exception, factor V, retains sufficient activity at levels of 0.1 to 0.15 units/mL. Coagulation factor abnormalities induced by bypass include dilution, denaturation, deposition on extracorporeal surfaces, and hypothermia.

Dilution

Hemodilution, a process now synonymous with CPB, reduces the concentrations of all coagulation factors. For adult surgery, factor levels rarely fall below 0.3 units/mL (58). Figure 25.13 displays the effect of bypass on factor concentrations. With neonates, even heroic efforts to reduce the priming volume of the extracorporeal circuit fail to prevent significant coagulation factor dilution.

Denaturation

The air–blood interface modifies coagulation factors. Bubble oxygenators and cardiotomy suction each involve significant mechanical perturbation of blood elements. Their prolonged use may contribute to a coagulation factor defect (59).

Deposition on Extracorporeal Surfaces

Platelets and coagulation proteins, notably fibrinogen, deposit on the extracorporeal circuit surface. Blood proteins adsorb onto its solid surfaces (60,61). Platelets then adhere to the adsorbed proteins.

Hypothermia

In most centers, hypothermia contributes to organ preservation during bypass. Temperature-dependent enzymatic processes determine sequential activation of the coagulation factors. Because many enzymatic reactions attenuate 7% for each decrease of 1°C, fibrin formation may likewise be retarded (62). The prolongation of ACTs with cold samples represents this phenomenon *ex vivo* (63). This anticoagulant effect of hypothermia, desirable during bypass, probably has an impact on coagulation when inadequate rewarming produces post-bypass core temperatures below 35°C.

Fibrinolysis

CPB activates the fibrinolytic pathways. In the past, inadequate anticoagulation during bypass accounted for a high incidence and severity of fibrinolysis (64). With the advent of routine intraoperative coagulation testing by protamine titration or ACT, "inadequate" heparin levels (as currently defined) occur more rarely (65). Does bypass-induced fibrinolysis no longer occur or have less impact on hemostasis?

Despite a therapeutic ACT and clinically acceptable heparin levels, thrombin formation and activity both continue during bypass, as demonstrated by relentless appearance of fibrinopeptides and thrombin–antithrombin complexes (Fig. 25.14) (16,66–69). The foreign extracorporeal circuit provides a surface with adsorbed proteins upon which thrombin can act. Products of thrombin activity *ex vivo* may then be carried *in vivo*, where endothelium responds with release of t-PA.

Usually, bypass-induced fibrinolysis does not achieve clinically significant proportions, with fibrin breakdown products clearing within an hour of bypass (70–72). An occasional patient, however, exhibits more marked fibrinolysis and its hemostatic consequences—renewed capillary bleeding from clot lysis and interference with polymerization of newly formed fibrin. The success of antifibrinolytic drugs in decreasing bleeding in patients undergoing cardiac surgery (see Pharmacologic Measures, below) suggests that fibrinolytic mechanisms contribute to bypass-induced alterations in hemostasis.

Consumptive Coagulopathy

Disseminated intravascular coagulation, or consumptive coagulopathy, occurs rarely after CPB despite ongoing thrombin activity. This feared disorder involves activation of coagulation factors within the vasculature. Fibrin formation during bypass occurs outside the vasculature (i.e., in the extracorporeal circuit) and thus is not disseminated. Circulating α_2-antiplasmin readily scavenges plasmin that reenters the body. Thus, systemic fibrinogenolysis does not occur unless heparin is seriously lacking (73). Of course, bypass does not protect patients from subsequent consumptive coagulopathy, which may occur should sepsis, shock, or a large retained clot occur (74).

TREATMENT OF COAGULOPATHY AFTER BYPASS

Identify the Cause

The diagnostic approach to hemostatic deficiency, like that of other disorders in medicine, benefits from a detailed consideration of the physiology of each component: vascular integrity, coagulation factors, platelets, and fibrinolysis.

Vascular Integrity

Although properly functioning platelets and coagulation factors will successfully address capillary and small vessel trespass, more egregious vascular damage requires mechanical attention with suture or its equivalent. This "surgical" bleeding is strongly suggested by any sudden increase of 300 mL/hr or more after minimal initial chest tube drainage or by more than 10 mL/kg in the first hour or 20 mL/kg total over the first 3 hours after operation (75). For patients weighing less than 10 kg, more liberal criteria apply. Unfortunately, no noninvasive maneuver can indicate that sustained chest tube drainage occurs from an unattended mechanical vascular defect. Because only mediastinal exploration provides this information, one must be prepared for this intervention by providing proper depth of anesthesia, a secure airway for positive pressure ventilation, appropriate monitoring of systemic and venous pressures, continuation of any mechanical and inotropic support, and replacement of intravascular volume.

Coagulation Factors

Bleeding from coagulation factor deficiency can arise from preexisting disease, excessive hemodilution, factor consumption, or unneutralized heparin. A post-bypass PT or aPTT up to 1.5 times control is common. Bleeding patients with values in excess of that level should be treated with banked plasma products.

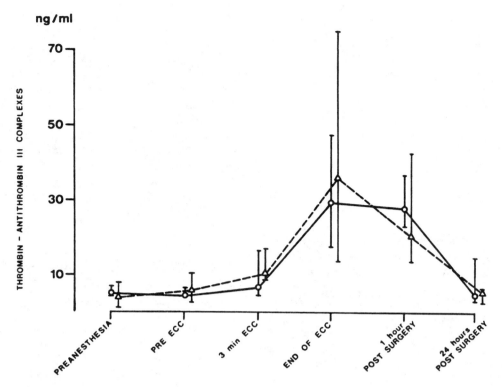

FIG. 25.14. Formation of thrombin–antithrombin complex (TAT) during cardiac surgery. The TAT levels did not differ between a control group (*triangles*) and one receiving aprotinin (*circles*). Note the effect of cardiopulmonary bypass (*ECC*). (From Havel M, Teufelsbauer H, Knöbl P, et al. Effect of intraoperative aprotonin administration on postoperative bleeding in patients undergoing cardiopulmonary bypass operation. *J Thorac Cardiovasc Surg* 1991;101:968–972, with permission.)

Platelets

Both thrombocytopenia and platelet dysfunction occur after bypass. Chapter 26 presents a treatment plan for these hemostatic disorders. Maintenance of normothermia after operation contributes to proper platelet number and function. This aspect of hemostasis should not be overlooked, particularly during rapid infusion of refrigerated banked blood products to replace lost intravascular volume. A "core" temperature of at least 35°C represents a suitable goal.

Fibrinolysis

Fibrinolysis causes bleeding not only by clot breakdown, but also by fibrin degradation products preventing proper association of fibrin monomers. Its treatment thus includes three aspects: halting the lytic process, removing its cause, and allowing time for reticuloendothelial clearance of fibrin degradation products. Because patients rarely suffer from an active lytic process in the post-bypass period, initiation of treatment at that time with antifibrinolytic drug proves useful only in extreme cases. Treatment of fibrinolysis-in-

duced bleeding remains of questionable efficacy, in contrast to prevention of clot lysis.

Laboratory Tests

Investigation should be initiated with the response as focused as possible given the limitations of time; the "shotgun" approach to therapy obfuscates final resolution of bleeding. Initial tests include platelet count, PT, aPTT, plasma fibrinogen, and fibrin degradation products. Figure 25.15 presents a first approach to the diagnosis of bleeding after bypass.

Maintain Blood Volume and Composition

Replenishment of lost intravascular volume with clear fluids, albumin, and packed red cells progressively decreases the concentrations of platelets and coagulation factors. Thus, the etiology of bleeding quickly becomes multifactorial. Nevertheless, intravascular volume must be maintained before identifying the cause of bleeding. Postponement of intravascular volume restoration not only compromises car-

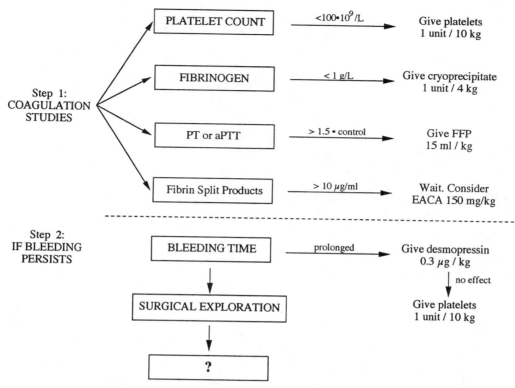

FIG. 25.15. Idealized strategy for diagnosis and treatment of postoperative bleeding. The initial tests of hemostasis include platelet count, fibrinogen, prothrombin time, and activated partial thromboplastin time. Bleeding that persists despite normal results of these tests suggests performance of a bleeding time. Marked prolongation in the bleeding time (over 16 minutes) may respond to desmopressin. Otherwise, surgical exploration may reveal an anatomic source. Increased fibrin degradation products suggests antifibrinolytic therapy, although some would withhold that therapy until a consumptive coagulopathy is ruled out. As indicated in the text, therapy must sometimes precede definitive diagnosis. FFP, fresh frozen plasma; EACA, epsilon amino caproic acid; PT, prothrombin time; aPTT, activated partial thromboplastin time.

diac output and the major organ systems but may also create bleeding itself as a result of protracted shock initiating consumptive coagulopathy.

Banked Plasma Products

Dilution of coagulation factors by bypass alone to levels below which hemostasis becomes impaired (usually less than 30% of normal) occurs rarely in patients who are not neonates. Routine administration of coagulation factors via fresh frozen plasma or cryoprecipitate after bypass constitutes not only needless waste of a valuable resource but also unnecessary exposure of the patient to potentially infectious material (76). Continued depletion and dilution that occurs with bleeding after bypass, however, validates replenishment of coagulation factors with these banked blood products. As replacement therapy for hemorrhage, platelet concentrates may suffice by themselves, because six units of platelets contain more than one unit of plasma (albeit lacking

somewhat in factors V and VIII) (76). For a discussion of treatment of bleeding due to unneutralized heparin, see Chapter 23. Regardless of laboratory results, patients not actively bleeding should not receive banked plasma products or platelets.

Red Cells and Platelets

Adequate delivery of oxygen to tissues determines the need to administer red cells. Replacement of rapid blood loss with factor-poor platelet-poor packed red cells does not permit enough time to verify factor and platelet deficiencies with coagulation tests. In noncardiac surgery, many clinicians administer platelets after 10 to 15 units of red cells. Coagulation factor dilution and partial activation of platelets by bypass demand earlier replacement in patients bleeding soon after bypass. See Chapter 26 regarding transfusion practice.

Hypertension

When an aortotomy has been performed, as for aortic valve replacement, avoidance of hypertension is an essential part of the treatment of postoperative hemorrhage. However, the clinician should wait until intravascular volume has been replenished and ensure adequate sedation and analgesia before administering vasodilators to treat hypertension.

Pharmaceuticals

Desmopressin

Figure 25.16 displays the chemical structure of this drug, modified from the nonapeptide arginine vasopressin (antidiuretic hormone [ADH]). Receptors for ADH occur on vascular smooth muscle (V_1 receptors) and the renal distal tubule (V_2 receptors). Removal of an amine group from the

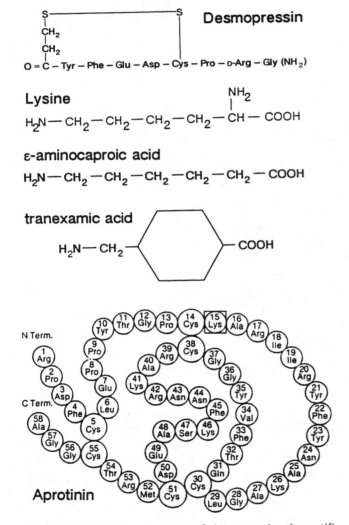

FIG. 25.16. Molecular structures of desmopressin, the antifibrinolytic molecules, and lysine. (Modified from Fritz H, Wunderer G. Biochemistry and applications of aprotinin, the kallikrein inhibitor from bovine organs. *Drug Res* 1983;33:479–494, with permission; and from Horrow JC. Desmopressin and antifibrinolytics. *Int Anesth Clin* 1990;28:216–222, with permission.)

carboxy terminal cysteine residue of ADH protects the molecule from degradation by circulating peptidases. Replacement of D-arginine for L-arginine in the eighth position removes pressor activity. Rapid administration of desmopressin actually decreases blood pressure and systemic vascular resistance, possibly by stimulation of extrarenal V_2 receptors (77,78).

Like ADH, epinephrine, and insulin, desmopressin releases a variety of hemostatically active substances from vascular endothelium: factor VIII, prostacyclin, t-PA, and vWF (79). Factor VIII coagulant activity increases to levels about fourfold (range, 2- to 20-fold) those of baseline within 30 to 90 minutes of desmopressin injection (80). Release of large multimers of vWF results in persistence of factor VIII activity long after desmopressin has been eliminated. Prostacyclin, by preventing platelet activation, and t-PA, by inciting fibrinolysis, both thwart hemostasis. However, the overall effect of desmopressin favors hemostasis. Conceivably, rapid administration may release sufficient prostacyclin to explain desmopressin's transient hypotension.

Desmopressin is administered in 0.3 μg/kg doses by intravenous, intranasal, or subcutaneous routes. The biologic half-life of 55 minutes belies its clinical effects, which last at least 6 hours (80). However, tachyphylaxis often occurs within 4 to 5 days, probably because of depletion of endothelial stores of vWF. In rare instances, water intoxication may occur from inappropriate fluid therapy during repeated desmopressin administration (81). Anecdotal reports of coronary thromboses temporally associated with desmopressin administration led to concern that the drug engenders a prothrombotic state in patients with ischemic heart disease (82–84).

In several disorders characterized by a prolonged bleeding time, desmopressin demonstrates hemostatic efficacy, viz., uremia (85), cirrhosis (80), and rare platelet disorders (86). Limited data from 2 patients and 10 volunteers indicate that desmopressin may also correct aspirin-induced prolongation of the bleeding time (87). Patients with mild or moderate hemophilia A or von Willebrand's disease respond to desmopressin with increases in factor VIII and shortening of prolonged bleeding times, respectively (80). In severe factor deficiency, however, there is little endogenous factor to release, so desmopressin proves of no value. When depending on desmopressin, individual responsiveness should be determined before the anticipated need.

Can desmopressin treat excessive bleeding after bypass? Although many investigations address the prophylactic role of desmopressin (see Prevention of Coagulopathy, below), few data assess its ability to halt established bleeding. Czer et al. (88) administered desmopressin 20 μg intravenously to 23 patients who demonstrated a chest tube drainage greater than 100 mL/hr for at least 2 hours after bypass. These patients received fewer blood products (15 ± 13 versus 29 ± 19 units) than a historical comparison group of 16 patients who received no drug. All patients received dipyridamole before surgery and bubble oxygenators during bypass and demonstrated a bleeding time greater than 10 minutes when bleeding. Lack of both randomization and blinding and presence of methodologic bias (transfusion was not permitted for 1 hour after infusion of desmopressin) cast doubt on those results. A subsequent double-blind, prospective, randomized investigation disclosed that desmopressin provided no hemostatic effect when administered to patients with substantial mediastinal bleeding and prolonged bleeding times after cardiac surgery (89). Mongan and Hosking (140) administered desmopressin randomly to cardiac surgical patients and later correlated the results of concomitant TEG results with chest tube drainage, revealing a hemostatic effect of desmopressin to those patients with decreased maximum amplitude (MA) as a TEG result. These results challenge clinicians to obtain TEG results soon enough to administer desmopressin immediately after protamine administration.

LoCicero et al. (90) retrospectively compared 74 patients who received desmopressin after bypass because of excessive bleeding as perceived by the operating surgeon with 91 matched historical control subjects. Although the desmopressin group bled more and received more blood products than the control group, this result should be expected because they were selected because of excessive bleeding.

Antifibrinolytics

These therapeutic agents include the synthetic lysine analogues ε-aminocaproic acid (EACA) and tranexamic acid (TA) and the naturally occurring protease inhibitor aprotinin (Fig. 25.16). The antifibrinolytics bind to plasminogen and plasmin, blocking the ability of the fibrinolytic enzymes to bind at lysine residues of fibrinogen. Excretion occurs renally, with urinary concentrations 75- to 100-fold those of plasma. Plasma half-life is 80 minutes. Loading doses (150 mg/kg EACA or 10 to 20 mg/kg TA) should be followed by continuous infusions (10 mg/kg EACA or 1 to 2 mg/kg TA), adjusted for creatinine clearance (91).

Antifibrinolytics have a postive impact on surgical hemostasis in hemophiliacs, in patients with von Willebrand's disease and other blood dyscrasias, and after chemotherapy (92–96). Additional applications include prevention of rebleeding after subarachnoid hemorrhage, liver transplantation, and prostate surgery (37,97–99).

Often bleeding after bypass is treated with a single 5-g dose of intravenous EACA along with a host of blood products and other modalities. Although studies indicate that prophylactic administration of EACA or TA after bypass decreases bleeding approximately 15% (100–102), no data permit extension of these results to a population of bleeding patients. Similarly, aprotinin has no well-defined role as a hemostatic agent in the patient already bleeding after bypass. In contrast, antifibrinolytic drugs do decrease bleeding and blood transfusion requirements when given prophylactically. The next section addresses this aspect.

PREVENTION OF COAGULOPATHY

Compared with efforts to treat established bleeding, efforts to prevent bleeding after CPB are less costly and better rewarded. Knowledge of the mechanisms of bypass-induced coagulopathy guides the approach to its prevention. Accordingly, the following discussion focuses on coagulation factors and fibrinolysis. For aspects relating to platelet function, see Chapter 24.

Prevention includes eliminating or reducing preoperative factors that incite bleeding. Preexisting disorders of hemostasis should be effectively addressed. These include factor deficiencies, uremia, hepatic compromise, and exposure to platelet-inhibiting drugs.

Antiplatelet Drugs

Attempts to restore perfusion to thrombotic vessels have created three series of novel pharmacologic agents: thrombolytics, direct thrombin inhibitors, and platelet glycoprotein receptor antagonists. See elsewhere in this chapter regarding thrombolytic agents and Chapter 22 regarding direct thrombin inhibitors.

Aspirin

Platelet function depends on thromboxane, which cannot form when aspirin irreversibly acetylates the active site of cyclooxygenase, the enzyme responsible for its formation. Between 30% and 50% of patients presenting for elective coronary artery surgery take aspirin up to the day of surgery to prevent occlusive coronary syndromes. Increased bleeding accompanies aspirin therapy (103–105) as does increased frequency of reoperation for bleeding (106). However, not all well-conducted studies demonstrate increased bleeding in patients receiving aspirin (107–110).

Dipyridamole

This vasodilator blocks cyclic nucleotide phosphodiesterase, thus increasing intracellular concentrations of cyclic AMP, which then act to impair platelet function. Because dipyridamole alone carries little or no antithrombotic activity, other agents such as aspirin or coumadin usually accompany its administration. Thus, the bleeding patient who had received dipyridamole deserves therapy to establish functional circulating platelets, but prophylaxis remains inappropriate.

Adenosine Diphosphate Receptor Blockers

Platelet aggregation depends on membrane recognition of the ADP released upon activation. Ticlopidine and clopidogrel are thienopyridines that bind to platelet surface ADP receptors. Clinical trials suggest these agents exert more efficacious blockade of platelet function compared with aspirin

(111,112). Ticlopidine features a prolonged terminal half-life of 20 to 50 hours. Ticlopidine's prolonged plasma presence and irreversible inhibition of aggregation suggest a 2-week drug-free period before surgery (113).

Platelet Integrin Antagonists

Platelet–platelet interactions via glycoprotein IIb/IIIa receptors constitute the final common pathway for platelet function. A monoclonal antibody, abciximab (Reopro), first accomplished blockade of these integrin receptors. Subsequent inhibitor development yielded peptide and nonpeptide molecules. These substances, eptifibatide (Integrelin), tirofiban (Aggrastat), and lamifiban, exhibit various plasma half-lives and are in various stages of clinical development (114). Abciximab, given during percutaneous coronary interventions, will interfere with platelet function following a potential surgical procedure, whereas tirofiban's and eptifibatide's half-lives are sufficiently short to most often preclude this concern.

Physical Measures

Coagulation Factors

Two potential contributors to coagulation factor dysfunction are hypothermia and dilution, both essential elements of bypass in most centers. Slower enzyme kinetics may account for part of the impaired coagulation seen at temperatures below 35°C. Prevention of post-bypass hypothermia requires rewarming sufficient not only to restore core temperature to 37°C or more but also to raise a more peripherally measured temperature, such as urinary bladder, to at least 34°C (115). Because core temperature at the end of surgery usually equals the average of the core and intermediate zone (urinary bladder or rectal) temperatures when active warming is discontinued at the termination of bypass, hypothermia after surgery can be prevented by a suitable warming period during surgery. The speed of surgical closure has a significant impact on hemostasis. Quicker sternal approximation limits convective heat loss, whereas more expedient removal of the exposed patient from the cold operating room reduces heat loss by radiation. However, speed must not compromise reasonable attention to open vessels that must be sealed to stop bleeding. Optimal management results from focused, efficient, and effective surgical attention.

Restricting the priming volume will limit hemodilution. Other methods for preserving factor levels include restriction of both intravenous fluids and cardioplegia volume, administration of diuretics when oliguria occurs, and hemoconcentration during bypass via filtration devices. Acute preoperative plasmapheresis withdraws platelet-rich plasma for infusion after bypass. Should it be shown to have a hemostatic benefit, the mechanism will more likely be platelet, rather than coagulation factor, preservation (116).

Fibrinolysis

Membrane, rather than bubble, oxygenators should be chosen when prolonged bypass is anticipated, because this will limit platelet destruction and fibrinolysis (117). Sufficient heparin doses limit thrombin activity during bypass. Because thrombin acts directly on endothelium to release plasminogen activators, inadequate thrombin inhibition fosters fibrinolysis. Prevention of bleeding thus requires frequent bedside verification of heparin activity via ACT or heparin concentration (via protamine titration) coupled with prompt effective treatment when coagulation times are not sufficiently prolonged.

Pharmacologic Measures

Heparin Rebound

Chapter 23 addresses the adequacy of heparin neutralization with protamine. This section considers "heparin rebound," a term denoting the reappearance of clinical bleeding and prolonged coagulation times after complete heparin neutralization. Direct evidence supports the generally accepted notion that heparin rebound occurs from reappearance of circulating heparin (118). Explanations for this phenomenon include more rapid clearance of protamine relative to that of heparin, lymphatic-delayed return of heparin to blood, clearance of a postulated heparin antagonist, and late release of heparin sequestered in tissues (119–121). Heparin binds to endothelium; the currently favored theory involves late release of bound heparin from endothelium. Theoretically, transfusion of blood components containing antithrombin III, including fresh frozen plasma, platelet concentrates, and whole blood, may attract heparin away from protamine, thus reactivating heparin.

Prolonged coagulation times occur as soon as 1 hour after neutralization and may persist as long as 6 hours (122–124). If clinical bleeding does not accompany a prolonged coagulation time, no intervention is necessary. Otherwise, additional 0.5- to 1-mg/kg doses of protamine usually suffice.

Clinical practice varies widely in the selection of an initial neutralizing dose of protamine, from less than 1 mg for every 100 units of remaining heparin, as determined by protamine titration, to as much as 4 mg for every 100 units of total heparin administered (125). Surveys in North America indicate the most common initial dose to be 1 mg protamine per 100 units of total heparin administered. Does a particular protamine dose scheme prevent heparin rebound? Data in the literature provide conflicting answers. Table 25.3 presents results of representative studies, which indicate no best dosing scheme to prevent heparin rebound (122,123,126,127). The initial heparin dose affects the development of heparin rebound, albeit without a difference in bleeding after operation (128).

Whether initially unneutralized or appearing as "re-

TABLE 25.3. VARIATIONS IN PROTAMINE DOSE TO PREVENT HEPARIN REBOUND[a]

Authors	Study Group	Control Group	Results
Ellison et al. (1974) (122)	1:100 of remaining heparin by protamine titration (n = 6)	1:100 of total heparin given (n = 6)	All six study patients had heparin rebound vs. none of six control patients
Guffin et al. (1976) (126)	1:100 of remaining heparin by assuming 2-hr half-life (n = 30)	1:100 of total heparin given (n = 30)	Study group had higher platelet count, less prolonged PT and aPTT, and less bleeding
Kaul et al. (1979) (123)	Ratio = ?; protamine according to blood heparin level (n = 27)	Heparin: 300 U/kg then 150 U/kg hourly; protamine: 6 mg/kg (n = 44)	No heparin rebound in study group vs. 10/44 patients in control group
Kesteven et al. (1986) (127)	3 mg/kg protamine in divided doses; heparin levels measured at end of CPB (n = 35)	None	29% had heparin present 2 hr later (all had ratios less than 1.6:100)

[a] All ratios are milligram per kilogram of protamine to units per kilogram of heparin.
CPB, cardiopulmonary bypass; PT; prothrombin time; aPTT, activated partial thromboplastin time.

bound," heparin can cause bleeding after surgery. Thus, administration of protamine to neutralize remaining heparin constitutes the first pharmaceutical intervention in the treatment of a bleeding patient. Reasonable clinicians infuse protamine doses of 1 mg/kg or less over a few minutes to patients bleeding after CPB, even in the absence of coagulation tests. However, residual antiplatelet effects of protamine suggest an increasing role for a suitable protamine alternative, although none is currently available (129).

Desmopressin

Can desmopressin prevent bleeding after bypass when given prophylactically? A small group of adolescents who received desmopressin during Harrington rod placement bled less and received less blanked blood compared with a control group (130). Interest in prophylactic desmopressin's hemostatic potential in cardiac surgery stems from the known acquired platelet abnormalities (see Chapter 24) and theo-

retic salutary effects of released vWF on platelet adhesion and in shortening prolonged bleeding times (131). Salzman et al. (132) initially reported a marked reduction in bleeding after bypass in patients undergoing cardiac procedures known for excess postoperative bleeding (i.e., reoperations and valve replacements). Subsequent investigations have not reproduced those results (133–139). Table 25.4 summarizes those studies.

Of course, prophylactic desmopressin finds utility for the cardiac surgical patient with a hematologic abnormality known to respond to desmopressin, such as uremia, hemophilia, or von Willebrand's disease. Intraoperative thromboelastography may identify subsets of patients who may benefit from administration of prophylactic desmopressin immediately after bypass (140). Timely drug delivery in this scenario presents a challenge to the clinician. For other cardiac surgical patients, however, prophylactic desmopressin does not impart a hemostatic advantage. Lack of desmopressin's effect extends to other surgical scenarios as well.

TABLE 25.4. PROSPECTIVE STUDIES OF DESMOPRESSIN IN CARDIAC SURGERY

Year	Authors	N[a]	Blood Loss	Structure	Population Studied
1986	Salzman et al. (132)	35/35	41% Reduced	Blinded; randomized	Reoperation or valve replacement
1988	Rocha et al. (134)	50/50	No difference	Blinded; randomized	Valve replacement; atrial septal defect
1989	Seear et al. (133)	30/30	No difference	Blinded; randomized	Children (30 of 60 cyanotic)
1989	Hackmann et al. (135)	74/76	No difference	Blinded; randomized	Elective cardiac surgery
1990	Andersson et al. (136)	10/9	No difference	Blinded; randomized	Elective coronary surgery
1990	Lazenby et al. (137)	30/30	No difference	Unblinded; consecutive	Primary coronary surgery
1991	Reich et al. (138)	14/13	No difference	Blinded; randomized	Elective cardiac surgery
1991	Horrow et al. (139)	78/81	No difference	Blinded; randomized	Elective cardiac surgery
1992	de Prost et al. (89)	47/47	No difference	Blinded; randomized	Patients bleeding after cardiac surgery

[a] Number of patients in the treated group/number in the control group.

TABLE 25.5. RANDOMIZED AND BLINDED STUDIES OF SYNTHETIC ANTIFIBRINOLYTIC GIVEN PROPHYLACTICALLY BEFORE BYPASS

Year	Authors	N[a]	Bloss Loss	Structure	Dose of Drug[a]	Timing of Dose
1971	Midell et al. (146)	48/25	58% reduced	Prospective	(125) EACA	Before bypass
1974	McClure and Izsak (147)	12/18	42% reduced	Blinded; randomized	(75) EACA	At sternotomy
1989	DelRossi et al. (142)	170/180	30% reduced	Blinded; randomized	(5 g) EACA	Before incision
1990	Horrow et al. (143)	18/20	34% reduced	Blinded; randomized	(10) [1] TA	Before incision
1991	Horrow et al. (139)	77/82	30% reduced	Blinded; randomized	(10) [1] TA	Before incision
1993	Karski et al. (145)	300/91	25–35% reduced	Retrospective	(6 or 10g) TA or (10 or 15g) EACA	By sternotomy
1995	Karski et al. (148)	98/48	35% reduced	Blinded; randomized	(10 g) [2 g] TA	By sternotomy
1995	Horrow et al. (149)	121/27	35% reduced	Blinded; randomized	(2.5–40) [0.25–4] TA	Before incision
1996	Shore-Lesserson et al (150)	17/13[b]	30% reduced	Blinded; randomized	(20) [2] TA	At skin incision
1996	Zonis et al. (151)[b]	40/42	52% reduced	Blinded; randomized	(50) TA	unspecified
1996	Katsaros et al. (152)	104/106	48% reduced	Randomized	(10 g) TA	Before incision
1996	VanderSalm et al. (153)	51/52	23% reduced	Blinded, randomized	(30 g) EACA	Before incision
1996	Montesano et al. (154)	20/26	20% reduced	Blinded, randomized	(5 g) EACA	Before incision
1997	Brown et al. (155)	30/30	41% reduced	Blinded, randomized	(15) [1] TA	Before bypass
1997	Reid et al. (156)	20/21	24% reduced	Blinded, randomized	(200) [10] ?TA	At skin incision
1997	Dryden et al. (157)[c]	22/19	54% reduced	Blinded, randomized	unspecified	unspecified
1997	Katoh et al. (158)	31/31	48% reduced	Blinded, randomized	(100) TA	Before bypass
1997	Slaughter et al. (159)	20/20	29% reduced	Blinded, randomized	(150) [15] EACA	Before incision

[a] N given as number in the treatment group/number in the control group; Dose given as (bolus mg/kg) [infusion mg/kg/hr].
[b] Children aged 1 day to 14 years; result applies to cyanotic children only.
[c] All patients underwent repeat sternotomy procedures.
EACA, epsilon aminocaproic acid; TA, tranexamic acid.

Of 50 patients undergoing aortoiliac surgery, 25 received desmopressin immediately before surgery without benefit of either decreased bleeding or transfusion requirement (141).

Synthetic Antifibrinolytics

Prophylactic administration of the synthetic antifibrinolytics decreases bleeding after bypass and reduces transfusion of homologous blood products. Table 25.5 summarizes the investigative data supporting the hemostatic efficacy of prophylactic antifibrinolytic therapy. Prophylactic administration of either synthetic or naturally occurring antifibrinolytic has achieved widespread acceptance among clinicians for patients undergoing CPB without circulatory arrest. Either EACA or TA administered before bypass generates approximately a 30% reduction in bleeding (139,142–159). Most studies also demonstrate decreased transfusions compared with placebo (139,142,150–152, 154–158). This salutary hemostatic effect may arise from inhibition of plasmin at platelet plasmin receptors and at fibrinogen (Fig. 25.17) (160,161).

Decades ago, antifibrinolytic therapy fell into disfavor after an anecdotal report of thrombotic complications in patients with prostate carcinoma (162,163). However, prospective studies of prophylactic antifibrinolytics during noncardiac and cardiac surgery do not substantiate fears of thrombotic complications (97,98,139,142,143). The prudent clinician withholds antifibrinolytic therapy from patients with demonstrated consumptive coagulopathy and

from those with upper urinary tract bleeding. Infusion rates should be adjusted for elevated serum creatinine to account for impaired excretion. Plasma concentrations decrease upon institution of bypass and then slowly increase due to impaired excretion presumably from hypothermia (163a).

Pharmacokinetic measurements of plasma EACA concentrations during surgery indicate wide variation. How-

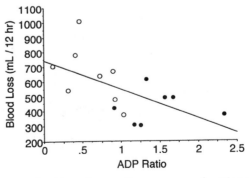

FIG. 25.17. Blood loss after cardiac surgery as a function of platelet adenosine diphosphate (ADP), expressed as the ratio measured 2 hours after surgery to that measured before bypass. Platelet dense granules contain ADP. Each *solid circle* represents a patient who received tranexamic acid beginning before skin incision (prophylactic); each *open circle* represents a patient who received tranexamic acid beginning after protamine neutralization. Note that prophylactic tranexamic acid preserved platelet ADP and decreased bleeding. (From Soslau G, Horrow J, Brodsky I. The effect of tranexamic acid on platelet ADP during extracorporeal circulation. *Am J Hematol* 1991;38:113–119, with permission.)

ever, all but 1 of 26 patients who received 30-mg/kg infusions after a 150-mg/kg loading dose achieved plasma concentrations necessary for fibrinolytic inhibition (164). Do these data suggest that all patients receive more than the recommended 10-mg/kg/hr infusions? They do not because of the absence of pharmacokinetic data at lower concentrations and, more fundamentally, because of the likelihood that the hemostatic benefit of EACA derives from a combination of its platelet protective and its antifibrinolytic effects.

Natural Antifibrinolytic

Aprotinin, the naturally occurring antifibrinolytic, differs from its synthetic congeners with respect to size and spectrum of activity. In contrast to the smaller lysine amino acid analogues, aprotinin is a 58-residue protein derived from bovine lung. As a result, the dose of aprotinin is expressed in activity units, in a fashion similar to that of heparin. Although the variation and shortcomings of heparin activity standards receive appropriate attention, these issues remain unexplored with aprotinin (165,166). Like any foreign protein, aprotinin may cause anaphylaxis, although the incidence is only 1 per 1,000 (167,168). Likewise, fears of renal dysfunction from rapid tubular uptake have not been confirmed in clinical use (169). Also, reports of disseminated platelet thrombi (169a), increased bleeding (169b), and more frequent serious postoperative complications (169c) associated with aprotinin use during deep hypothermic circulatory arrest have resulted in the suggestion that aprotinin should be administered only after perfusion has recommenced after circulatory arrest (169d).

Like the synthetic antifibrinolytics, aprotinin inhibits plasmin and plasminogen. In addition, aprotinin inhibits kallikrein, the contact activation protein that enhances factor XII activation (170–172). The hemostatic effect of an inhibitory action on kallikrein is difficult to predict for two reasons. First, factor XII is known to be unnecessary for clinical hemostasis (173). Second, the extent to which factor XIIa contributes to fibrinolysis is not known (2). In this regard, aprotinin-associated thrombus formation on pulmonary artery catheters remains unexplained (174). The salutary hemostatic effects of aprotinin may, in fact, derive from inhibition of plasmin alone.

Kallikrein inhibition may, however, explain prolongation of the celite-activated ACT by aprotinin (175). This *in vitro* anticoagulant effect may or may not reflect an *in vivo* antithrombotic action (176,177). Kaolin, a more potent activator, remains unaffected by aprotinin (178).

In the past decade, scores of clinical studies have confirmed the initial observations of Royston et al. that large doses of this bovine serine protease produce a remarkably dry surgical field and decrease bleeding after CPB. As with TA, platelet preservation during bypass appears to contribute to aprotinin's beneficial hemostatic effect (69,91,169, 176,179,180).

Antifibrinolytic Comparisons

Several clinical investigations explored the relative efficacy of antifibrinolytic agents. The ideal study includes a contemporaneously randomized placebo group and demonstrates sufficient power to detect a relevant clinical difference in both blood loss and transfusions administered. Although no study available at this writing satisfies all criteria, the available data support the notion that available antifibrinolytic agents do not differ in their relative abilities to decrease blood loss and transfusions after bypass. Comparative data continue to document lack of efficacy of desmopressin. Table 25.6 summarizes some of these results (181–188).

Cost

Any prophylactic therapy entails fixed costs to prevent presumed complications. Factors that will determine the appro-

TABLE 25.6. HEMOSTATIC PHARMACEUTICAL PAIRWISE COMPARISONS

	TA	EACA	DDAVP
Aprotinin	Equivalent (181)[a]	Equivalent (182[b], 183[c]) Less bleeding but RBC transfusions equivalent with aprotinin (184)[d]	Less bleeding and fewer transfusions with aprotinin (185,186)
EACA	Equivalent (187) Less bleeding but transfusions equivalent with TA (188)		No studies performed

[a] Historical control group.
[b] Unrandomized control group.
[c] Meta-analysis.
[d] No control group.
TA, tranexamic acid; EACA, epsilon aminocaproic acid; DDAVP, desmopressin; RBC, red blood cell.

priateness of pharmaceuticals to prevent bleeding include the cost of the drug, the expected savings in terms of blood loss and transfusions prevented, and the estimated adverse outcome from omission of prophylaxis. Bennett-Guerrero et al. (184) accumulated cost data on 204 patients randomized to receive either high-dose aprotinin or EACA. Despite less bleeding and fewer platelet transfusions in the aprotinin group, the aprotinin group incurred substantially greater total bleeding-related costs (U.S.$1813 vs. $1,088, $p = 0.0001$), explained largely by the cost of aprotinin.

Will improved screening techniques and sterilization methods for donated blood provide greater protection from infectious diseases, making trivial the impact of bleeding prevention on patient care (189)? Or will they merely permit elucidation of the immunosuppressive effects of transfusion and identification of yet more bloodborne transmissible diseases? The future, hopefully, will bring antithrombotic bypass techniques that preserve hemostasis and use neither heparin nor protamine. Until these goals materialize, bypass-associated coagulopathy requires prevention and treatment.

KEY POINTS

- Fibrin formation is fundamental to clotting and hemostasis. This can be stimulated by intrinsic and extrinsic pathways and modulated by a number of positive and negative feedback mechanisms.

- Once formed, fibrin can be lysed by plasmin. Formation of plasmin can be initiated by t-PA or by surface activation coagulation proteins, and plasmin's capacity to induce widespread proteolysis is tempered by the natural inhibitor, PAI-1.

- Fibrinolysis can also be initiated exogenously with older drugs such as streptokinase and urokinase or with newer ones such as recombinant t-PA, anisoylated plasminogen-streptokinase activator, and single-chain urokinase plasminogen activator. Whether initiated endogenously or exogenously, hazards of fibrinolysis include unintentional lysis of fibrinogen and the release of fibrin degradation products, which can impair blood clotting.

- A variety of laboratory tests evaluates the functional integrity of blood clotting. These tests can be performed in a centralized location or at the bedside. Common centralized tests include PT, aPTT, thrombin time, fibrinogen, fibrinogen degradation products, D-dimer, and platelet count. Bedside or point-of-care tests include PT, aPTT, thrombin time (also high-dose thrombin time and heparin-neutralized thrombin time), the ACT, TEG, Sonoclot, and some platelet function tests. Although many of these tests can effectively diagnose specific blood-clotting deficits and thereby facilitate therapy (with point-of-care testing

expediting this process), overall the ability of laboratory testing to predict post-CPB clotting disorders has been disappointing.

- Factors that may contribute to coagulation abnormalities (other than platelet-related causes, see Chapter 24) after CPB include hemodilution, protein denaturation and deposition, hypothermia, fibrinolysis, and consumption.

- A variety of pharmacologic strategies has been used to prevent post-CPB coagulopathy. Among these, only synthetic (EACA and TA) and naturally occurring (aprotinin) antifibrinolytic agents have been consistently demonstrated to reduce bleeding and transfusions. Prospective comparisons of these three agents predominantly show equal efficacy and that all three agents are safe to administer during CPB.

REFERENCES

1. Fransson L-A. Heparin sulfate proteoglycans: structure and properties. In: Lane DA, Lindahl U, eds. *Heparin*. Boca Raton, FL: CRC Press, 1989:115–134.
2. Colman RW, Marder VJ, Salzman EW, et al. Overview of hemostasis. In: Colman RW, Hirsh J, Marder VJ, et al., eds. *Hemostasis and thrombosis*, 3rd ed. Philadelphia: J.B. Lippincott, 1994:3–18.
3. Suttie JW. Vitamin K antagonists. In: Colman RW, Hirsh J, Marder VJ, et al., eds. *Hemostasis and thrombosis*, 3rd ed. Philadelphia: J.B. Lippincott, 1994:1562–1566.
4. Nemerson Y. The tissue factor pathway of blood coagulation. In: Colman RW, Hirsh J, Marder VJ, et al., eds. *Hemostasis and thrombosis*, 3rd ed. Philadelphia: J.B. Lippincott, 1994:81–93.
5. Kitchens CS. Thrombophilia and thrombosis in unusual sites. In: Colman RW, Hirsh J, Marder VJ, et al., eds. *Hemostasis and thrombosis*, 3rd ed. Philadelphia: J.B. Lippincott, 1994: 1255–1273.
6. Rosenberg RD, Bauer KA. The heparin antithrombin system: a natural anticoagulant mechanism. In: Colman RW, Hirsh J, Marder VJ, et al., eds. *Hemostasis and thrombosis*, 3rd ed. Philadelphia: J.B. Lippincott, 1994:837–860.
7. George J, Shattil SJ. The clinical importance of acquired abnormalities of platelet function. *N Engl J Med* 1991;324:27–39.
8. Jaffe EA. Biochemistry, immunology, and cell biology of endothelium. In: Colman RW, Hirsh J, Marder VJ, et al., eds. *Hemostasis and thrombosis*, 3rd ed. Philadelphia: J.B. Lippincott, 1994:718–744.
9. Mann KG, van't Veer C, Cawthern K, et al. The role of the tissue factor pathway in initiation of coagulation. *Blood Coagul Fibrinol* 1998;9[Suppl 1]:S3–S7.
10. Majerus PW, Broze Jr GJ, Miletich JP, et al. Anticoagulant, thrombolytic, and antiplatelet drugs. In: Hardman JG, Limbird LE, eds. *Goodman & Gilman's The pharmacological basis of therapeutics*, 9th ed. New York: McGraw-Hill, 1996:1341–1359.
11. Hantgan RR, Francis CW, Marder VJ. Fibrinogen structure and physiology. In: Colman RW, Hirsh J, Marder VJ, et al., eds. *Hemostasis and thrombosis*, 3rd ed. Philadelphia: J.B. Lippincott, 1994:277–300.
12. van Aken WG. Preparation of plasma derivatives. In: Rossi EC, Simon TL, Moss GS, eds. *Principles of transfusion medicine*. Baltimore: Williams & Wilkins, 1991:323–334.
13. McDonagh J. Structure and function of factor XIII. In: Colman

RW, Hirsh J, Marder VJ, et al., eds. *Hemostasis and thrombosis,* 3rd ed. Philadelphia: J.B. Lippincott, 1994:301–313.

14. Bachmann F. The plasminogen-plasmin enzyme system. In: Colman RW, Hirsh J, Marder VJ, et al., eds. *Hemostasis and thrombosis,* 3rd ed. Philadelphia: J.B. Lippincott, 1994: 1592–1622.

15. Chandler WL, Fitch JC, Wall MH, et al. Individual variations in the fibrinolytic response during and after cardiopulmonary bypass. *Thromb Haemost* 1995;74:1293–1297.

16. Valen G, Eriksson E, Risberg B, et al. Fibrinolysis during cardiac surgery. Release of tissue plasminogen activator in arterial and coronary sinus blood. *Eur J Cardiothorac Surg* 1994;8:324–330.

17. Ray MJ, Marsh NA, Hawson GA. Relationship of fibrinolysis and platelet function to bleeding after cardiopulmonary bypass. *Blood Coagul Fibrinol* 1994;5:679–685.

18. Gersh BJ. Current issues in reperfusion therapy. *Am J Cardiol* 1998;82:3P–11P.

19. Francis CW, Marder VJ. Physiologic regulation and pathologic disorders of fibrinolysis. In: Colman RW, Hirsh J, Marder VJ, et al., eds. *Hemostasis and thrombosis,* 3rd ed. Philadelphia: J.B. Lippincott, 1994:1076–1103.

20. Marder VJ, Sherry S. Thrombolytic therapy: current status. *N Engl J Med* 1988;318:1512–1520, 1585–1595.

21. The GUSTO Investigators. An international randomized trial comparing four thrombolytic strategies for acute myocardial infarction. *N Engl J Med* 1993;329:673–682.

22. Modi NB, Eppler S, Breed J, et al. Pharmacokinetics of a slower clearing tissue plasminogen activator variant, TNK-tPA, in patients with acute myocardial infarction. *Thromb Haemost* 1998; 79:134–139.

23. Cannon CP, Gibson CM, McCabe CH, et al. TNK-tissue plasminogen activator compared with front-loaded alteplase in acute myocardial infarction: results of the TIMI 10B trial. Thrombolysis in myocardial infarction (TIMI) 10B investigators. *Circulation* 1998;98:2805–2814.

24. Koepke JA. Coagulation testing systems. In: Koepke JA, ed. *Laboratory hematology.* New York: Churchill Livingstone, 1984: 1113–1140.

25. Miale JB. *Hematology,* 4th ed. St. Louis: Mosby, 1972:1280.

26. Shafer K, Santoro S, Sobel B, et al. Monitoring activity of fibrinolytic agents. *Am J Med* 1984;76:879–886.

27. Schmaier AH. Diagnosis and therapy of disseminated intravascular coagulation and activated coagulation. In: Koepke JA, ed. *Laboratory hematology.* New York: Churchill Livingstone, 1984: 631–658.

28. Bell WR. Defibrinogenating enzymes. In: Colman RW, Hirsh J, Marder VJ, et al., eds. *Hemostasis and thrombosis,* 3rd ed. Philadelphia: J.B. Lippincott, 1994:886–900.

29. Despotis GJ, Santoro SA, Spitznagel E, et al. Prospective evaluation and clinical utility of on-site monitoring of coagulation in patients undergoing cardiac operation. *J Thorac Cardiovasc Surg* 1994;107:271–279.

30. Fitch JCK, Mirto GP, Geary KLB, et al. Point-of-care and standard laboratory coagulation testing during cardiovascular surgery. Balancing reliability and timeliness. *J Clin Monit Comput* 1999;15:197–204.

31. Gilbert HC, Vender JS. The current status of point-of-care monitoring. *Int Anesth Clin* 1996;34:243–261.

32. O'Neill AI, McAllister C, Corke CF, et al. A comparison of five devices for the bedside monitoring of heparin therapy. *Anaesth Intens Care* 1991;19:592–601.

33. van Rijn JLML, Schmidt NA, Rutten WPF. Correction of instrument and reagent-based differences in determination of the international normalized ratio (INR) for monitoring anticoagulant therapy. *Clin Chem* 1989;35:840–843.

34. Huyzen RJ, Harder MP, Gallandat HRCG, et al. Alternative

perioperative anticoagulation monitoring during cardiopulmopnary bypass in aprotinin-treated patients. *J Cardiothorac Vasc Anesth* 1994;8:153–156.

35. Reich DL, Yanakakis MJ, Vela-Cantos FP, et al. Comparison of bedside coagulation monitoring tests with standard laboratory tests in patients after cardiac surgery. *Anesth Analg* 1993; 77:673–679.

36. Bjoraker DG. The thromboelastograph D coagulation analyzer. *Anesthesiol Rev* 1991;18:34–40.

37. Kang Y, Lewis JH, Navalgund A, et al. Epsilon-aminocaproic acid for treatment of fibrinolysis during liver transplantation. *Anesthesiology* 1987;66:766–773.

38. Spiess BD, Logas WG, Tuman KJ, et al. Thromboelastography used for detection of perioperative fibrinolysis: a report of four cases. *J Cardiothorac Vasc Anesth* 1988;2:666–672.

39. Spiess BD, Tuman RJ, McCarthy RJ, et al. Thromboelastography as an indicator of post-cardiopulmonary bypass coagulopathies. *J Clin Monit* 1987;3:25–30.

40. Howland WS, Schweizer O, Goulp P. Comparison of intraoperative measurements of coagulation. *Anesth Analg* 1974;53: 657–663.

41. Zuckerman L, Cohen E, Vagher JP, et al. Comparison of thromboelastography with common coagulation tests. *Thromb Haemost* 1981;46:752–756.

42. von Kaulla K, von Kaulla E, Wasantapruck S, et al. Blood coagulation in uremic patients before and after hemodialysis and transplantation of the kidney. *Arch Surg* 1966;92:184–191.

43. Shenaq SA, Saleem A. Viscoelastic measurement of clot formation: the Sonoclot. In: Ellison E, Jobes DR, eds. *Effective hemostasis in cardiac surgery.* Philadelphia: W.B. Saunders, 1988: 183–193.

44. Saleem A, Blifeld C, Saleh SA, et al. Viscoelastic measurement of clot formation: a new test of platelet function. *Ann Clin Lab Sci* 1983;13:115–124.

45. Samra SK, Harrison RL, Bee DE, et al. A study of aspirin induced changes in bleeding time, platelet aggregation, and Sonoclot coagulation analysis in humans. *Ann Clin Lab Sci* 1991; 21:315–327.

46. Nutall GA, Oliver WC, Ereth MH, et al. Coagulation tests predict bleeding after cardiopulmonary bypass. *J Cardiothorac Vasc Anesth* 1997;11:815–823.

47. Wang JS, Lin CY, Hung WT, et al. Thromboelastogram fails to predict postoperative hemorrhage in cardiac patients. *Ann Thorac Surg* 1992;53:435–439.

48. Dorman BH, Spinale FG, Bailey MK, et al. Identification of patients at risk for excessive blood loss during coronary artery bypass surgery. Thromboelastography versus coagulation screen. *Anesth Analg* 1993;76:694–700.

49. Ereth MH, Nutall GA, Santrach PJ, et al. The relationship between the platelet-activated clotting test (HemoSTATUS) and blood loss after cardiopulmonary bypass. *Anesthesiology* 1998;88:962–969.

50. Ramsey G, Arvan DA, Stewart S, et al. Do preoperative laboratory tests predict blood transfusion needs in cardiac operations? *J Thorac Cardiovasc Surg* 1983;85:564–569.

51. Gravlee GP, Arora S, Lavendar SW, et al. Predictive value of blood clotting tests in cardiac surgical patients. *Ann Thorac Surg* 1994;58:216–221.

52. Tuman KJ, Spiess BD, McCarthy RJ, et al. Comparison of viscoelastic measures of coagulation after cardiopulmonary bypass. *Anesth Analg* 1989;69:69–75.

53. Ereth MH, Nutall GA, Klindworth JT, et al. Does the platelet-activated clotting test (HemoSTATUS) predict blood loss and platelet dysfunction associated with cardiopulmonary bypass? *Anesth Analg* 1997;85:259–264.

54. Wahba A, Rothe G, Lodes H, et al. Predictors of blood loss

after coronary artery bypass grafting. *J Cardiothorac Vasc Anesth* 1997;11:824–827.

55. Ratnatunga CP, Rees GM, Kovacs IB. Preoperative hemostatic activity and excessive bleeding after cardiopulmonary bypass. *Ann Thorac Surg* 1991;52:250–257.

56. Greilich PE, Carr ME, Carr SL, et al. Reductions in platelet force development by cardiopulmonary bypass are associated with hemorrhage. *Anesth Analg* 1995;80:459–465.

57. Edmunds LE Jr. The sangreal. *J Thorac Cardiovasc Surg* 1985; 90:1–6.

58. Gelb AB, Roth RI, Levin J, et al. Changes in blood coagulation during and following cardiopulmonary bypass. Lack of correlation with clinical bleeding. *Am J Clin Pathol* 1996;106:87–99.

59. Thelin S, Bagge L, Hultman J, et al. Heparin-coated cardiopulmonary bypass circuits reduce blood cell trauma. Experiments in the pig. *Eur J Cardiothorac Surg* 1991;5:486–491.

60. Baier RE, Dutton RC. Initial events in interactions of blood with a foreign surface. *J Biomed Mater Res* 1969;3:191–206.

61. Engbers GF, Feijen J. Current techniques to improve the blood compatibility of biomaterial surfaces. *Int J Artif Organs* 1991; 14:199–215.

62. Michenfelder JD, Theye RA. Hypothermia: effects on canine brain and whole-body metabolism. *Anesthesiology* 1968;29: 1107–1112.

63. Jobes DR, Ellison N, Campbell FW. Limitations for ACT [Letter]. *Anesth Analg* 1989;69:142–144.

64. Bick RL. Alterations of hemostasis associated with cardiopulmonary bypass: pathophysiology, prevention, diagnosis, and management. *Semin Thromb Hemost* 1976;3:59–82.

65. Mammen EF, Koets MH, Washington BC, et al. Hemostasis changes during cardiopulmonary bypass surgery. *Semin Thromb Hemost* 1985;11:281–292.

66. Davies GC, Sobel M, Salzman EW. Elevated plasma fibrinopeptide A and thromboxane B$_2$ levels during cardiopulmonary bypass. *Circulation* 1980;61:808–814.

67. Tanaka K, Takao M, Yada I, et al. Alterations in coagulation and fibrinolysis associated with cardiopulmonary bypass during open heart surgery. *J Cardiothorac Vasc Anesth* 1989;3:181–188.

68. Gravlee GP, Haddon WS, Rothberger HK, et al. Heparin dosing and monitoring for cardiopulmonary bypass. *J Thorac Cardiovasc Surg* 1990;99:518–527.

69. Havel M, Teufelsbauer H, Knöbl P, et al. Effect of intraoperative aprotinin administration on postoperative bleeding in patients undergoing cardiopulmonary bypass operation. *J Thorac Cardiovasc Surg* 1991;101:968–972.

70. Harker LA, Malpass TW, Branson HE. Mechanism of abnormal bleeding in patients undergoing cardiopulmonary bypass: acquired transient platelet dysfunction associated with selective α-granule release. *Blood* 1980;56:824–834.

71. Moriau M, Masure R, Hurlet A, et al. Haemostasis disorders in open heart surgery with extracorporeal circulation. *Vox Sang* 1977;32:41–51.

72. Kucuk O, Kwaan HC, Frederickson J, et al. Increased fibrinolytic activity in patients undergoing cardiopulmonary bypass operation. *Am J Hematol* 1986;23:223–229.

73. Ellison N, Campbell FW, Jobes DR. Postoperative hemostasis. *Semin Thorac Cardiovasc Surg* 1991;3:33–38.

74. Marder VJ, Martin SE, Francis CW, et al. Consumptive thrombohemorrhagic disorders. In: Colman RW, Hirsh J, Marder VJ, et al., eds. *Hemostasis and thrombosis*, 3rd ed. Philadelphia: J.B. Lippincott, 1994:975–1015.

75. Kirklin JW, Barratt-Boyes BG. Postoperative care. *Cardiac surgery*. New York: Churchill Livingstone, 1986;139–176.

76. Gravlee GP. Optimal use of blood components. *Int Anesth Clin* 1990;28:216–222.

77. Bichet DG, Razi M, Lonergan M, et al. Hemodynamic and coagulation responses to 1-desamino (8-D-arginine) vasopressin in patients with congenital nephrogenic diabetes insipidus. *N Engl J Med* 1988;318:881–887.

78. Frankville DD, Harper GB, Lake CL, et al. Hemodynamic consequences of desmopressin administration after cardiopulmonary bypass. *Anesthesiology* 1991;74:988–996.

79. MacGregor IR, Roberts EN, Provose CV, et al. Fibrinolytic and haemostatic responses to desamino-D-arginine vasopressin (DDAVP) administered by intravenous and subcutaneous routes in healthy subjects. *Thromb Haemost* 1988;59:34–39.

80. Mannucci PM. Desmopressin: a nontransfusional form of treatment for congenital and acquired bleeding disorders. *Blood* 1988;72:1449–1455.

81. Weinstein RE, Bona RD, Althman AJ, et al. Severe hyponatremia after repeated intravenous administration of desmopressin. *Am J Hematol* 1989;32:258–261.

82. Bond L, Bevan D. Myocardial infarction in a patient with hemophilia treated with DDAVP [Letter]. *N Engl J Med* 1986;314: 1402–1406.

83. Byrnes JJ, Larcada A, Moake JL. Thrombosis following desmopressin for uremic bleeding. *Am J Hematol* 1988;28:63–65.

84. O'Brien JR, Green PJ, Salmon G, et al. Desmopressin and myocardial infarction [Letter]. *Lancet* 1989;1:664.

85. Mannucci PM, Remuzzi G, Pusineri F, et al. Deamino-8-D-arginine vasopressin shortens the bleeding time in uremia. *N Engl J Med* 1983;308:8–12.

86. DiMichele DM, Hathaway WE. Use of DDAVP in inherited and acquired platelet dysfunction. *Am J Hematol* 1990;33: 39–45.

87. Kobrinsky NL, Gerrard JM, Watson CM, et al. Shortening of bleeding time by 1-deamino-8-D-arginine vasopressin in various bleeding disorders. *Lancet* 1984;1:1145–1148.

88. Czer LSC, Bateman TM, Gray RJ, et al. Treatment of severe platelet dysfunction and hemorrhage after cardiopulmonary bypass: reduction in blood product usage with desmopressin. *J Am Coll Cardiol* 1987;9:1139–1147.

89. de Prost D, Barbier-Boehm G, Hazebroucq J, et al. Desmopressin has no beneficial effect on excessive postoperative bleeding or blood product requirements associated with cardiopulmonary bypass. *Thromb Haemost* 1992;68:106–110.

90. LoCicero JL III, Massad M, Matano J. Effect of desmopressin acetate on hemorrhage without identifiable cause in coronary bypass patients. *Am Surg* 1991;57:165–168.

91. Verstraete M. Clinical application of inhibitors of fibrinolysis. *Drugs* 1985;29:236–261.

92. Williamson R, Eggleston DJ. DDAVP and EACA used for minor oral surgery in von Willebrand disease. *Austr Dent J* 1988; 33:32–36.

93. Blombäck M, Johansson G, Johnsson H, et al. Surgery in patients with von Willebrand disease. *Br J Surg* 1989;76:398–400.

94. Sindet-Pedersen S, Ramström G, Bernvil S, Blombäck M. Hemostatic effect of tranexamic acid mouthwash in anticoagulant-treated patients undergoing oral surgery. *N Engl J Med* 1989; 320:840–843.

95. Stern N, Catone GA. Primary fibrinolysis after oral surgery. *J Oral Surg* 1975;33:49–52.

96. Avvisati G, Büller HR, ten Cate JW, et al. Tranexamic acid for control of haemorrhage in acute promyelocytic leukaemia. *Lancet* 1989;2:122–124.

97. Vinnicombe J, Shuttleworth KED. Aminocaproic acid in the control of haemorrhage after prostatectomy. *Lancet* 1966;2: 232–234.

98. Sharifi R, Lee M, Ray P, et al. Safety and efficacy of intravesical aminocaproic acid for bleeding after transurethral resection of prostate. *Urology* 1986;27:214–219.

99. Schisano G. The use of antifibrinolytic drugs in aneurysmal subarachnoid hemorrhage. *Surg Neurol* 1978;10:217–222.

100. Sterns LP, Lillehei CW. Effect of epsilon aminocaproic acid upon blood loss following open-heart surgery: an analysis of 340 patients. *Can J Surg* 1967;10:304–307.

101. Ovrum E, Åm Holen E, Abdelnoor M, et al. Tranexamic acid (Cyklokapron) is not necessary to reduce blood loss after coronary artery bypass operation. *J Thorac Cardiovasc Surg* 1993; 105:78–83.

102. Vander Salm T, Ansell JE, Okike ON, et al. The role of epsilon-aminocaproic acid in reducing bleeding after cardiac operation: a double-blind randomized study. *J Thorac Cardiovasc Surg* 1988;95:538–540.

103. Michaelson EL, Morganroth J, Torosian M, et al. Relation of preoperative use of aspirin to increased mediastinal blood loss after coronary artery bypass graft surgery. *J Thorac Cardiovasc Surg* 1978;76:694–697.

104. Goldman S, Copeland J, Moritz T, et al. Improvement in early saphenous vein graft patency after coronary bypass surgery with antiplatelet therapy. Results of a Veterans Administration co-operative study. *Circulation* 1988;77:1324–1332.

105. Taggart DP, Siddiqui A, Wheatley DJ. Low-dose preoperative aspirin therapy, postoperative blood loss and transfusion requirements. *Ann Thorac Surg* 1990;50:425–428.

106. Bashein G, Nessly ML, Rice AL, et al. Preoperative aspirin therapy and reoperation for bleeding after coronary artery bypass surgery. *Arch Intern Med* 1991;151:89–93.

107. Weksler BB, Pett SM, Aloso D, et al. Differential inhibition by aspirin of vascular and platelet prostaglandin synthesis in atherosclerotic patients. *N Engl J Med* 1983;308:800–805.

108. Rajah SM, Salter MCP, Donaldson DR. Acetylsalicylic acid and dipyridamole improve the early patency of aorta-coronary bypass grafts. *J Thorac Cardiovasc Surg* 1985;90:373–377.

109. Karawande S, Weksler BB, Gay WA, et al. Effect of preoperative antiplatelet drugs on vascular prostacyclin synthesis. *Ann Thorac Surg* 1987;43:318–322.

110. Rawitscher RE, Jones JW, McCoy TA, et al. A prospective study of aspirin effect on red blood cell loss in cardiac surgery. *J Cardiovasc Surg* 1991;32:1–7.

111. White HD, French JK, Ellis CJ. New antiplatelet agents. *Aust NZ J Med* 1998;28:558–564.

112. Sharis PJ, Cannon CP, Loscalzo J. The antiplatelet effects of ticlopidine and clopidogrel. *Ann Intern Med* 1998;129: 394–405.

113. Desager JP. Clinical pharmacokinetics of ticlopidin. *Clin Pharmacokinet* 1994;26:347–355.

114. Kong DF, Califf RM, Miler DP, et al. Clinical outcomes of therapeutic agents that block the platelet glycoprotein IIb/IIIa integrin in ischemic heart disease. *Circulation* 1998;98: 2829–2835.

115. Horrow JC, Rosenberg H. Does urinary catheter temperature reflect core temperature during cardiac surgery? *Anesthesiology* 1988;69:986–989.

116. Boldt J, Von Bormann B, Kling D, et al. Preoperative plasmapheresis in patients undergoing cardiac surgery procedures. *Anesthesiology* 1990;72:282–288.

117. van den Dungen JJ, Karliczek GF, Brenken U, et al. Clinical study of blood trauma during perfusion with membrane and bubble oxygenators. *J Thorac Cardiovasc Surg* 1982;83: 108–116.

118. Kesteven PJ, Ahred A, Aps C, et al. Protamine sulphate and rebound following open-heart surgery. *J Cardiovasc Surg* 1986; 27:600–603.

119. Perkins HA, Osborn JJ, Gerbode E. The management of abnormal bleeding following extracorporeal circulation. *Ann Intern Med* 1959;51:658–667.

120. Perkins HA, Acra DJ, Rolfs MR. Estimation of heparin levels in stored and traumatized blood. *Blood* 1961;18:807–808.

121. Frick PG, Brogli H. The mechanism of heparin rebound after extracorporeal circulation for open cardiac surgery. *Surgery* 1966;59:721–726.

122. Ellison N, Beatty P, Blake DR, et al. Heparin rebound. *J Thorac Cardiovasc Surg* 1974;67:723–729.

123. Kaul TK, Crow MJ, Rajah SM, et al. Heparin administration during extracorporeal circulation. *J Thorac Cardiovasc Surg* 1979;78:95–102.

124. Fiser WP, Read RC, Wright FE, et al. A randomized study of beef lung and pork mucosal heparin in cardiac surgery. *Ann Thorac Surg* 1983;35:615–620.

125. Ellison N, Ominsky AJ, Wollman H. Is protamine a clinically important anticoagulant? *Anesthesiology* 1971;35:621–629.

126. Guffin AV, Dunbar RW, Kaplan JA, et al. Successful use of a reduced dose of protamine after cardiopulmonary bypass. *Anesth Analg* 1976;55:110–113.

127. Kesteven PJ, Ahred A, Aps C, et al. Protamine sulphate and rebound following open-heart surgery. *J Cardiovasc Surg* 1986; 27:600–603.

128. Gravlee GP, Rogers AT, Dudas LM, et al. Heparin management protocol for cardiopulmonary bypass influences postoperative heparin rebound but not bleeding. *Anesthesiology* 1992;76: 393–401.

129. Ammar T, Fisher CF. The effects of heparinase I and protamine on platelet reactivity. *Anesthesiology* 1997;86:1382–1386.

130. Kobrinsky NL, Letts M, Patel LR, et al. 1-Desamino-8-D-arginine vasopressin (desmopressin) decreases operative blood loss in patients having Harrington rod spinal fusion surgery. *Ann Intern Med* 1987;107:446–450.

131. Horrow JC. Desmopressin and antifibrinolytics. *Int Anesth Clin* 1990;28:216–222.

132. Salzman EW, Weinstein MJ, Weintraub RM, et al. Treatment with desmopressin acetate to reduce blood loss after cardiac surgery. *N Engl J Med* 1986;314:1402–1406.

133. Seear MD, Wadsworth LD, Rogers PC, et al. The effect of desmopressin acetate (DDAVP) on postoperative blood loss after cardiac operations in children. *J Thorac Cardiovasc Surg* 1989;98:217–219.

134. Rocha E, Llorens R, Paramo JA, et al. Does desmopressin acetate reduce blood loss after surgery in patients on cardiopulmonary bypass? *Circulation* 1988;77:1319–1323.

135. Hackmann T, Gascoyne RD, Naiman SC, et al. A trial of desmopressin (1-desamino-8-D-arginine vasopressin) to reduce blood loss in uncomplicated cardiac surgery. *N Engl J Med* 1989; 321:1437–1443.

136. Andersson TLG, Solem JO, Tengborn L, et al. Effects of desmopressin acetate on platelet aggregation, von Willebrand factor, and blood loss after cardiac surgery with extracorporeal circulation. *Circulation* 1990;81:872–878.

137. Lazenby WD, Russo I, Zadeh BJ, et al. Treatment with desmopressin acetate in routine coronary artery bypass surgery to improve postoperative hemostasis. *Circulation* 1990;82[Suppl IV]: 413–419.

138. Reich DL, Hammerschlag BC, Rand JH, et al. Desmopressin acetate is a mild vasodilator that does not reduce blood loss in uncomplicated cardiac surgical procedures. *J Cardiothorac Vasc Anesth* 1991;5:142–145.

139. Horrow JC, Van Riper DF, Strong MD, et al. The hemostatic effects of tranexamic acid and desmopressin during cardiac surgery. *Circulation* 1991;84:2063–2070.

140. Mongan PD, Hosking MP. The role of desmopressin acetate in patients undergoing coronary artery bypass surgery. *Anesthesiology* 1992;77:38–46.

141. Lethagen S, Rugarn P, Bergqvist D. Blood loss and safety with

desmopressin or placebo during aortoiliac graft surgery. *Eur J Vasc Surg* 1991;5:173–178.

142. DelRossi AJ, Cernaianu AC, Botros S, et al. Prophylactic treatment of post-perfusion bleeding using EACA. *Chest* 1989;96:27–30.

143. Horrow JC, Hlavacek J, Strong MD, et al. Prophylactic tranexamic acid decreases bleeding after cardiac operations. *J Thorac Cardiovasc Surg* 1990;99:70–74.

144. Isetta C, Samat C, Kotaiche M, et al. Low dose aprotinin or tranexamic acid treatment in cardiac surgery [Abstract]. *Anesthesiology* 1991;75:A80.

145. Karski JM, Teasdale SJ, Normal PH, et al. Prevention of post-bypass bleeding with tranexamic acid and ϵ-aminocaproic acid. *J Cardiothorac Vasc Anesth* 1993;7:431–435.

146. Midell AI, Hallman GL, Bloodwell RD, et al. Epsilon-aminocaproic acid for bleeding after cardiopulmonary bypass. *Ann Thorac Surg* 1971;11:577–582.

147. McClure PD, Izsak J. The use of epsilon-aminocaproic acid to reduce bleeding during cardiac bypass in children with congenital heart disease. *Anesthesiology* 1974;40:604–608.

148. Karski JM, Teasdate SJ, Norman P, et al. Prevention of bleeding after cardiopulmonary bypass with high-dose tranexamic acid. *J Thorac Cardiovasc Surg* 1995;110:835–842.

149. Horrow JC, Van Riper DF, Strong MD, et al. The dose-response relationship of tranexamic acid. *Anesthesiology* 1995;82:383–392.

150. Shore-Lesserson L, Reich DL, Vela-Cantos F, et al. Tranexamic acid reduces transfusions and mediastinal drainage in repeat cardiac surgery. *Anesth Analg* 1996;83:18–26.

151. Zonis Z, Seear M, Reichert C, et al. The effect of preoperative tranexamic acid on blood loss after cardiac operations in children. *J Thorac Cardiovasc Surg* 1996;111:982–987.

152. Katsaros D, Petricevic M, Snow NJ, et al. Tranexamic acid reduces postbypass blood use: a double-blinded, prospective, randomized study of 210 patients. *Ann Thorac Surg* 1996;61:1131–1135.

153. Vander Salm TJ, Kaur S, Lancey RA, et al. Reduction of bleeding after heart operations through the prophylactic use of epsilon-aminocaproic acid. *J Thorac Cardiovasc Surg* 1996;112:1098–1107.

154. Montesano RM, Gustafson PA, Palanzo DA, et al. The effect of low-dose epsilon-aminocaproic acid on patients following coronary artery bypass surgery. *Perfusion* 1996;11:53–56.

155. Brown RS, Thwaites BK, Mongan PD. Tranexamic acid is effective in decreasing bleeding and transfusions in primary coronary artery bypass operations. A double-blind, randomized, placebo-controlled trial. *Anesth Analg* 1997;85:962–970.

156. Reid RW, Zimmerman AA, Laussen PC, et al. The efficacy of tranexamic acid versus placebo in decreasing blood loss in pediatric patients undergoing repeat cardiac surgery. *Anesth Analg* 1997;84:990–996.

157. Dryden PJ, O'Connor JP, Jamieson WRE, et al. Tranexamic acid reduces blood loss and transfusion in reoperative cardiac surgery. *Can J Anaesth* 1997;44:934–941.

158. Katoh J, Tsuchiya K, Sato W, et al. Additional postbypass administration of tranexamic acid reduced blood loss after cardiac operations. *J Thorac Cardiovasc Surg* 1997;113:802–804.

159. Slaughter TF, Faghih F, Greenberg CS, et al. The effects of epsilon-aminocaproic acid on fibrinolysis and thrombin generation during cardiac surgery. *Anesth Analg* 1997;85:1221–1226.

160. Soslau G, Horrow J, Brodsky I. The effect of tranexamic acid on platelet ADP during extracorporeal circulation. *Am J Hematol* 1991;38:113–119.

161. Adelman B, Rizk A, Hanners E. Plasminogen interactions with platelets in plasma. *Blood* 1988;72:1530–1535.

162. Charytan C, Purtilo D. Glomerular capillary thrombosis and acute renal failure after epsilon-amino caproic acid therapy. *N Engl J Med* 1969;280:1102–1104.

163. Ratnoff OD. Epsilon aminocaproic acid—a dangerous weapon. *N Engl J Med* 1969;280:1124–1125.

163a. Butterworth J, James RL, Hudspeth AS. Effects of cardiopulmonary bypass on epsilon aminocaproic acid pharmacokinetics. *Anesthesiology* 1998;89:A533.

164. Bennett-Guerrero E, Sorohan JG, Canada AT, et al. Epsilon-aminocaproic acid plasma levels during cardiopulmonary bypass. *Anesth Analg* 1997;85:248–251.

165. Barrowcliffe TW. Heparin assays and standardization. In: Lane DA, Lindahl U, eds. *Heparin*. Boca Raton, FL: CRC Press, 1989;393–416.

166. Coyne E, Outschoorn AS. Some thoughts on a new USP heparin assay—aren't we ready for an upgrade? *Pharmac Forum* 1991:1492–1495.

167. D'Ambra MN, Risk SC. Aprotinin, erythropoietin, and blood substitutes. *Int Anesth Clin* 1990;28:237–240.

168. Böhrer H, Bach A, Fleischer F, et al. Adverse haemodynamic effects of high-dose aprotinin in a paediatric cardiac surgical patient. *Anaesthesia* 1990;45:853–854.

169. Blauhut B, Gross C, Necek S, et al. Effects of high-dose aprotinin on blood loss, platelet function, fibrinolysis, complement, and renal function after cardiopulmonary bypass. *J Thorac Cardiovasc Surg* 1991;101:958–967.

169a. Sundt TM 3d, Kouchoukos NT, Saffitz JE, et al. Renal dysfunction and intravascular coagulation with aprotinin and hypothermic circulatory arrest. *Ann Thorac Surg* 1993;55:1418–1424.

169b. Westaby S, Forni A, Dunning J, et al. Aprotinin and bleeding in profoundly hypothermic perfusion. *Eur J Cardiothorac Surg* 1994;8:82–86.

169c. Parolari A, Antona C, Alamani F, et al. Aprotinin and deep hypothermic circulatory arrest. There are no benefits even when appropriate amounts of heparin are given. *Eur J Cardiothorac Surg* 1997;11:149–156.

169d. Rooney SJ, Pagano D, Bognolo G, et al. Aprotinin in aortic surgery requiring profound hypothermia and circulatory arrest. *Eur J Cardiothorac Surg* 1997;11:373–378.

170. Mammen EF. Natural proteinase inhibitors in extracorporeal circulation. *Ann NY Acad Sci* 1968;146:754–762.

171. Fritz H, Wunderer G. Biochemistry and applications of aprotinin, the kallikrein inhibitor from bovine organs. *Drug Res* 1983;33:479–494.

172. Royston D. The serine antiprotease aprotinin (trasylol): a novel approach to reducing postoperative bleeding. *Blood Coagul Fibrin* 1990;1:55–69.

173. Schmaier AH, Silverberg M, Kaplan AP, et al. Contact activation and its abnormalities. In: Colman RW, Hirsh J, Marder VJ, et al., eds. *Hemostasis and thrombosis*, 3rd ed. Philadelphia: J.B. Lippincott, 1994:18–38.

174. Böhrer H, Fleischer F, Lang J, et al. Early formation of thrombi on pulmonary artery catheters in cardiac surgical patients receiving high-dose aprotinin. *J Cardiothorac Vasc Anesth* 1990;4:222–225.

175. deSmet AAEA, Joen MCN, van Oeveren W, et al. Increased anticoagulation during cardiopulmonary bypass by aprotinin. *J Thorac Cardiovasc Surg* 1990;100:520–527.

176. Royston D. High dose aprotinin therapy: the first five years' experience. *J Cardiothorac Vasc Anesth* 1992;6:76–100.

177. Dietrich W, Dilthey G, Spannagl M, et al. Influence of high-dose aprotinin on anticoagulation, heparin requirement, and celite- and kaolin-activated clotting time in heparin-pretreated patients undergoing open-heart surgery. A double-blind, placebo-controlled study. *Anesthesiology* 1995;83:679–689.

178. Wang J-S, Lin C-Y, Hung W-T, et al. Monitoring of heparin-

induced anticoagulation with kaolin-activated clotting time in cardiac surgical patients treated with aprotinin. *Anesthesiology* 1992;77:1080–1084.

179. Royston D, Taylor KM, Bidstrup BP, et al. Effect of aprotinin on need for blood transfusion after repeat open-heart surgery. *Lancet* 1987;2:1289–1291.

180. van Oeveren W, Harder MP, Roozendaal KJ, et al. Aprotinin protects platelets against the initial effect of cardiopulmonary bypass. *J Thorac Cardiovasc Surg* 1990;99:788–797.

181. Mongan PD, Brown RS, Thwaites BK. Tranexamic acid and aprotinin reduce postoperative bleeding and transfusions during primary coronary revascularization. *Anesth Analg* 1998;87:258–265.

182. Eberle B, Mayer E, Hafner G, et al. High-dose epsilon-aminocaproic acid versus aprotinin: antifibrinolytic efficacy in first-time coronary operations. *Ann Thorac Surg* 1998;65:667–673.

183. Munoz JJ, Nancy JO, Birkmeyer JD, et al. Is epsilon-aminocaproic acid as effective as aprotinin in reducing bleeding with cardiac surgery? *Circulation* 1999;99:81–89.

184. Bennett-Guerrero E, Sorohan JG, Gurevich ML, et al. Cost-benefit and efficacy of aprotinin compared with epsilon-aminocaproic acid in patients having repeated cardiac operations. *Anesthesiology* 1997;87:1373–1380.

185. Rocha E, Hidalgo F, Llorens R, et al. Randomized study of aprotinin and DDAVP to reduce postoperative bleeding after cardiopulmonary bypass surgery. *Circulation* 1994;90:921–27.

186. Casas JI, Zuazu-Jausoro I, Mateo J, et al. Aprotinin versus desmopressin for patients undergoing operations with cardiopulmonary bypass. *J Thorac Cardiovasc Surg* 1995;110:1107–1117.

187. Hardy J-F, Belisle S, Dupont C, et al. Prophylactic tranexamic acid and epsilon-aminocaproic acid for primary myocardial revascularization. *Ann Thorac Surg* 1998;65:371–376.

188. Pinosky ML, Kenedy DJ, Fishman RL, et al. Tranexamic acid reduces bleeding after cardiopulmonary bypass when compared to epsilon aminocaproic acid and placebo. *J Card Surg* 1997;12:330–338.

189. Corash L. Photochemical decontamination of cellular blood components. *Anaesth Pharmacol Rev* 1995;3(2):138–149.

BLOOD TRANSFUSION AND BLOOD CONSERVATION

LAWRENCE T. GOODNOUGH
GEORGE J. DESPOTIS

Blood transfusion and blood conservation practices have evolved substantially over the last 20 years as a result of changes in blood transfusion practices (1) and the development of new tools for blood conservation (2). In this chapter we present an overview of blood transfusion and blood conservation practices in cardiac surgery patients.

TRANSFUSION PRACTICES

Critical Care Patients

A study of transfusion practices was recently performed in 4,875 consecutive patients admitted to six Canadian tertiary-level intensive care units (3). Overall, 28% of the patients received red cell transfusions. However, the number of transfusions ranged from 0.82 to 1.08 per patient-day among institutions, with a mean of 0.95. The institutional effect on this variability remained significant even after adjusting for age and Apache II score. The authors found that the most frequent reasons for administering red cells were acute bleeding (35%) and the augmentation of oxygen delivery (25%). This observation may explain why, in a recent study (4), altering physicians' transfusion trigger based on hemoglobin levels did not affect the transfusion outcomes in an intensive care setting. In this study, basing transfusions on hemoglobin levels (as low as 7.0 g% for asymptomatic patients) successfully altered blood ordering practices but did not reduce overall blood use (4). The mean hemoglobin level at transfusion decreased from 8.5 to 8.1 g%, but the proportion of patients transfused and the number of units transfused (per patient or patient-day) did not change. As noted by the previous study (3), patients are more likely to

receive blood transfusions that are triggered due to hemorrhage, ischemia, or issues related to oxygen delivery.

In a follow-up multicenter clinical trial, 418 intensive care patients were randomized to receive red cell transfusions when the hemoglobin level dropped below 7.0 g/dL (with hemoglobin levels maintained in the range of 7.0 to 9.0 g/dL) and 420 patients were to receive transfusions when the hemoglobin level dropped below 10.0 g/dL (with hemoglobin levels maintained in the range of 10.0 to 11.0 g/dL) (5). The 30-day mortality rates were similar in the two groups (18.7% versus 23.3%, $p = 0.11$), indicating that a transfusion threshold as low as 7.0 g/dL was as safe as a higher transfusion threshold of 10.0 g/dL in critically ill patients. More data are needed to determine when transfusion might be beneficial in critically ill patients.

Patients Undergoing Cardiac Surgery

Considerable variation in transfusion practice among institutions has been identified. A multicenter audit of 18 institutions demonstrated a wide range in allogeneic red blood cell transfusion use for patients undergoing simple first-time coronary artery bypass grafting (CABG) (6). This variability has been confirmed in two subsequent studies (7,8). Follow-up studies of transfusion outcomes in cardiac surgical patients indicate that a substantial number of blood components in patients are transfused unnecessarily (9); hierarchical institutional-related factors are responsible for the variability in transfusion outcomes (10).

Practice guidelines have been summarized by the National Institutes of Health (NIH) consensus conferences on perioperative transfusion of red blood cells (11). Because these guidelines have suggested hemoglobin thresholds as low as 7.0 g/dL for transfusion in surgical patients, concern has been raised over whether the pendulum has swung too far (12). Patients have been reported to be at risk for perioperative myocardial ischemic injury in the setting of postoperative hematocrit levels in the range of 21% to 24%, associated with a delay in myocardial metabolic recovery (13).

L.T. Goodnough: Departments of Medicine and Pathology, Washington University School of Medicine, and Transfusion Services, Barnes-Jewish Hospital, St. Louis, Missouri 63110.

G.J. Despotis: Department of Anesthesiology and Pathology, Washington University School of Medicine, St. Louis, Missouri 63110.

Hemoglobin levels have been suggested as clinical indicators for transfusion in patients undergoing coronary bypass or other procedures (14):

1. Hemoglobin 6.0 g/dL for well-compensated chronically anemic patients, healthy [American Society of Anesthesiologists (ASA) physical status class I and some class II] patients undergoing intentional hemodilution, and patients undergoing hypothermia. (A criterion that probably would apply to cardiac surgical patients only when undergoing marked hypothermia less than 25°.)
2. Hemoglobin 8.0 g/dL for most postoperative bypass patients except those with left ventricular hypertrophy, incomplete coronary revascularization, low cardiac output, poorly controlled tachycardia, or sustained fever.
3. Hemoglobin 10 g/L for patients unlikely to increase cardiac output, patients with symptomatic cerebrovascular disease, and elderly (older than 65 years) patients.

Others emphasize that it is unlikely that any hemoglobin level can be universally applicable and have proposed a need for more physiologic indicators of the adequacy of oxygen delivery (15). The routine placement of a thermodilution pulmonary artery catheter in CABG patients enables regular assessment of mixed venous oxygen saturation ($S_{\bar{V}}O_2$), along with hemodynamic variables such as cardiac index, heart rate, and blood pressure. $S_{\bar{V}}O_2$ is an indicator of the relative balance between the total body oxygen supply and demand. As a sensitive but nonspecific indicator, $S_{\bar{V}}O_2$ represents a weighted balance from all perfused vascular beds. When arterial oxygen saturation is adequate (arterial blood saturated with oxygen greater than 0.90), the $S_{\bar{V}}O_2$ inversely reflects the oxygen supply and demand balance. $S_{\bar{V}}O_2$ provides continuous quantification of global oxygen extraction, in which a mixed venous oxygen tension greater than 40 mm Hg ($S_{\bar{V}}O_2$ approximately 75%) is believed to indicate adequate tissue oxygenation in most clinical states, whereas mixed venous oxygen tension less than 20 mm Hg ($S_{\bar{V}}O_2$ approximately 30%) suggests inadequate tissue oxygenation (16). Thus, in addition to traditional clinical indicators for red blood cell transfusion (tachycardia, hypotension, oliguria, etc.), physiologic indicators of clinically significant impairment in the balance of oxygen supply and demand are also important. When the hemoglobin level falls below "acceptable" values, these physiologic indicators may indicate a potential benefit from transfusion.

The precise acceptable hemoglobin level, however, is unknown. The NIH consensus conference concluded that most patients with hemoglobin levels more than 10.0 g/dL do not require blood, whereas most patients with hemoglobin less than 7.0 g/dL benefit from blood (11). However, silent perioperative ischemia has been identified as a significant clinical problem in noncardiac (17) and cardiac (18) surgical patients, emphasizing that the heart is an organ with a limited oxygen delivery reserve capacity. A recent case report illustrated that in a surgical patient whose hema-

tocrit level was 27%, silent myocardial ischemia was corrected with the transfusion of two units of red blood cells (19). In high-risk vascular surgery patients, Nelso et al. (20) associated a mean hematocrit level of less than 28% on the first postoperative day with myocardial ischemia in 10 of 13 patients and a morbid cardiac event in 6 of these patients. In a recent study of patients undergoing radical suprapubic prostatectomy, a hematocrit level less than 28% was independently associated with risk for myocardial ischemia during and after surgery, particularly in the presence of tachycardia (21). Avoidance of cardiac complications may require higher transfusion thresholds, closer attention to avoidance of tachycardia, or better monitoring for ischemia. However, overtransfusion may also be associated with poor outcomes; Spiess et al. (22) recently reported that a higher mortality rate was associated with cardiac surgery patients who were discharged from surgery at higher levels of hematocrit (more than 30%). Hemoglobin levels from 7.0 to 10.0 g/dL, a range in which physiologic indicators may identify patients who can benefit (or not benefit) from blood, need to be the most closely scrutinized.

TRANSFUSION ALGORITHMS

Although measuring and analyzing discharge hematocrit level can enhance retrospective understanding of transfusion outcomes (23), transfusion guidelines using concurrent clinical indicators are necessary if physician transfusion behavior is to be altered. One promising decision-making approach for the cardiac surgical patient is to couple transfusion algorithms with readily available clinical information obtained from point-of-care testing rather than laboratory-based assays.

We conducted studies to evaluate the impact of point-of-care testing (24,25), in which intraoperative assays (on-site evaluation of whole blood prothrombin time [PT], activated partial thromboplastin time [aPTT], and platelet count with results available within 4 minutes) were linked to a transfusion algorithm (Fig. 26.1) for plasma and platelet transfusions in cardiac surgical patients. Sixty-six patients with a diagnosis of nonsurgical microvascular bleeding were randomized to either standard therapy ($n = 36$), in which blood products were transfused at the discretion of the physician according to any laboratory-based test results requested, or to an algorithm group ($n = 30$), in which on-site platelet count, PT, and aPTT results were available within 4 minutes. Platelet and plasma therapy were given according to an algorithm (Fig. 26.1), based on on-site results. The three decision pathways of this algorithm were based initially on platelet count, followed by branch pathways determined by PT and aPTT. Both intraoperative and initial postoperative chest tube drainage were less in the algorithm group, indicating that hemostatic therapy was more successful in treating microvascular bleeding. Algo-

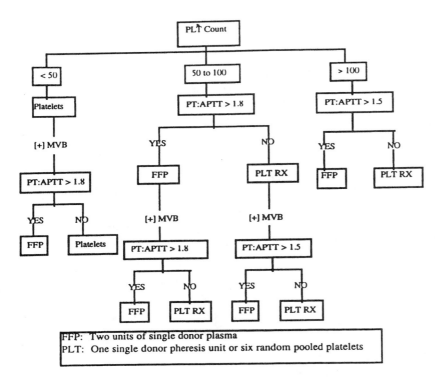

FIG. 26.1. An algorithm approach for hemostatic therapy in cardiac patients determined to have microvascular bleeding (*MVB*) after heparin neutralization. *Platelets*, platelet transfusion (six units of random-donor or apheresis unit equivalent); *PLT RX*, platelet therapy (platelet transfusion and/or desmopressin (DDAVP) therapy at physician's discretion); *FFP*, plasma therapy (two units of fresh frozen plasma); *[+] MVB*, continued MVB; *PT: APTT*, ratio of whole blood prothrombin time and/or activated partial thromboplastin time to control values (values/mean values from a normal reference population); *PLT count*, platelet count ($\times 10^3/mm^3$); *PLT RX*, one single donor pheresis unit or six random pooled platelets. (From Despotis GJ, Grishaber JE, Goodnough LT. The effect of an intraoperative treatment algorithm on physician transfusion behavior in cardiac surgery. *Transfusion* 1994;34:290–296, with permission.)

rithm-treated patients required substantially less plasma therapy intraoperatively and less red cell and platelet therapy postoperatively. Eight of 36 (25%) standard-therapy patients received different blood component therapy from what would have been designated by the algorithm (25). The more effective therapy in the algorithm group was reflected in the lower red blood cell transfusion needs in the algorithm group compared with the standard-therapy group (5.9 ± 3.8 versus 9.8 ± 8.4 units, respectively). The reduced blood transfusions resulted in substantial economic savings as well (24).

Transfusion algorithms have been described as a "powerful engine of change" (26). Other studies have demonstrated that use of point-of-care (27) or laboratory-based (28) coagulation data (i.e., platelet count, PT, aPTT, fibrinogen) coupled with predetermined transfusion criteria can reduce transfusion requirements and blood loss and shorten operative times.

An algorithm that incorporates the balance between oxygen delivery and oxygen consumption, as reflected by changes in SVo_2, may be an effective clinical indicator for red blood cell therapy. Such an approach is illustrated in Figure 26.2 (15). With the recognition that transfusion support depends on both rate of blood loss and hemoglobin level, the decision to transfuse each unit of red blood cells could be based on hemoglobin level, the quantity (rate) of blood lost, and hemodynamic parameters. Each patient would achieve adequate pulmonary capillary wedge pressures filling pressures with crystalloid/colloid therapy before

entering a transfusion algorithm. Controlled clinical trials comparing this approach with current unmonitored transfusion practices are needed.

BLOOD CONSERVATION IN CARDIAC SURGERY

Autologous Blood Donation

Selection of Patients

Several published guidelines identify patients who are not suitable for preoperative autologous donation (PAD) (29–32). Table 26.1 details guidelines recently published by the British Committee for Standards in Hematology (32). The American Association of Blood Banks recommends that patients with evidence of systemic infection or unstable angina are excluded. The first unit collected from a given patient during a 30-day period must have the same testing as allogeneic units for infectious disease markers (35); however, subsequent units need not be tested unless they are to be transferred from the collection facility (33,34). Supplemental iron is ideally prescribed before the first blood collection, because iron availability for erythropoiesis is the limiting factor in the collection of multiple autologous units of blood over a short interval (35,36).

Autologous blood collection can be performed for patients who would not usually be considered for allogeneic donation. With suitable volume modification and parental

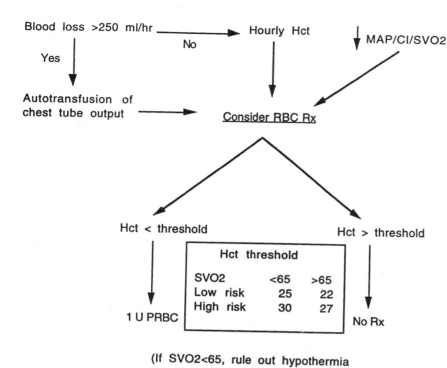

FIG. 26.2. An algorithm approach for postoperative red cell transfusion in cardiac surgical patients. After establishing that the patient's volume status is adequate, decisions to transfuse would be based on hemoglobin/hematocrit level, rate of blood loss, and hemodynamic parameters. Thresholds for transfusion would differ for patients determined to be at "low" risk and "high" risk for perioperative complications. Mixed venous oxygen percent saturation (SVo_2) could serve as a physiologic indicator of the balance between oxygen supply and demand for transfusion decision making. (From Goodnough LT, Despotis GJ, Hogue CW, et al. On the need for improved transfusion indicators in cardiac surgery. *Ann Thorac Surg* 1995;60:473–480, with permission.)

cooperation, pediatric patients can participate in preoperative collection programs (37). Patients with significant cardiac disease are generally considered poor risks for autologous collection. Despite reports demonstrating the safety of PAD in small numbers of patients scheduled for CABG (38), mortality risks associated with autologous blood donation (39) in these patients are probably greater than current estimated mortality risks of allogeneic transfusion (40).

Cost Effectiveness

Blood conservation interventions, such as autologous blood predeposit, need to be held accountable for their costs and benefits. A study (41) of patients undergoing primary elective CABG estimated that PAD costs between $508,000 and $909,000 per quality-adjusted year of life saved, although it was more cost effective (as low as $158,000 per life year saved) when targeted to younger patients undergoing CABG at centers with high transfusion rates (Fig. 26.3). Nevertheless, these estimates compare unfavorably with estimates of cost effectiveness in a variety of medical and surgical procedures, particularly when compared with hemodialysis for chronic renal failure as a generally accepted upper limit for acceptable cost effectiveness at $50,000 per quality-adjusted year of life saved (41). Autologous blood donor programs can potentially reduce costs in several ways, such as limiting the number of unnecessary autologous collections and transfusions and revision of policies regarding donor screening (42). However, the flexibility to limit the costs of autologous blood for donor screening, testing, and handling of these units depends on the recognition that autologous blood procurement is a medical service for these patients (43); this approach runs counter to regulatory agencies that now regard blood as a drug, subject to the standards of good manufacturing practices (44). Cost savings can be achieved only in the setting of hospital-based autologous blood procurement, in which donor screening can be modified and blood testing deferred for autologous blood units drawn within 30 days of the first donation (42).

A recent study of the cost effectiveness of autologous blood donation in cardiac surgical patients estimated that

TABLE 26.1. PATIENTS WHO SHOULD BE DEFERRED FROM AUTOLOGOUS BLOOD DONATION

1. Evidence of infection and risk of bacteremia
2. Scheduled for surgery to correct aortic stenosis
3. Unstable angina
4. Active seizure disorder (seizure within last 3 mo)
5. Myocardial infarction or cerebrovascular accident within 6 mo of donation
6. Patients with significant cardiac or pulmonary disease who have not yet received optimal preoperative medical management
7. High-grade left main coronary artery disease
8. Cyanotic heart disease
9. Uncontrolled hypertension

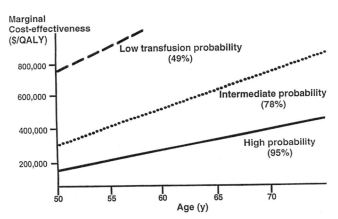

FIG. 26.3. Cost effectiveness of two-unit autologous blood donation in cardiac surgical patients at low, intermediate, and high transfusion medical centers for different age groups. Percentage figures represent the mean percent of patients receiving an allogeneic transfusion perioperatively in the three medical center categories. (From Birkmeyer JD, Aubuchon JP, Littenberg B, et al. The costs and benefits of preoperative autologous blood donation in elective coronary bypass surgery. *Ann Thorac Surg* 1994; 57:161–169, with permission.)

101,000 patients would have to safely undergo autologous blood procurement to save the life of one patient who would otherwise die from the complications of an allogeneic blood transfusion (41). This degree of safety is highly unlikely (45). A recent study of very severe reactions (requiring hospitalization) in autologous blood donors found a reaction rate of 1 per 17,000 donations (46). In view of this, the promotion of autologous blood donation in cardiac surgical patients (47,48) without sufficient evidence of the safety of approach appears to be unwarranted. Additionally, the urgency of coronary revascularization often precludes autologous predonation.

Transfusion of Autologous Blood

Guidelines for autologous blood transfusion are controversial. Some published guidelines recommend that the same utilization review criteria be used for autologous and allogeneic blood units (49). This view is supported by the risks of an immediate transfusion reaction (1:250,000 to 1: 1,000,000), which account for 50% of acute fatalities from transfusion (50); administrative errors and bacterial contamination are the most common etiologies. These risks can occur for autologous blood units and for allogeneic blood units. The alternative view holds that the risk-to-benefit relationship is lower for autologous blood than for allogeneic blood, because the risk for viral disease transmissible by allogeneic blood has been eliminated; this viewpoint argues for different standards for transfusion of autologous than for allogeneic blood, because of increasing evidence that silent myocardial ischemic events occur in patients at risk (19–21).

A randomized trial of two different "transfusion triggers" for autologous blood (one group transfused to achieve a hematocrit level of 32% and a second group transfused for a level of less than 25%) found no difference in outcomes between the two groups (51). This study provides clinical evidence that "liberal" use of autologous blood does not benefit cardiac surgical patients, although the prevalence of ischemic events in the two groups was not studied. Liberal use of autologous blood may be associated with adverse outcomes; data from a study by Spiess et al. (22) suggested that higher postoperative levels of hematocrit (more than 30%) were associated with higher rates of postoperative myocardial infarction. Although transfusion services may choose to establish different guidelines for transfusion of autologous and allogeneic blood, physicians should not retransfuse autologous blood simply because it is available (52).

Acute Perioperative Normovolemic Hemodilution or "Blood Pooling"

Acute isovolemic hemodilution entails the removal of blood from a patient shortly before anticipated significant surgical blood loss while restoring the circulating blood volume with acellular fluid. Blood is collected in standard blood bags containing anticoagulant, stored at room temperature to preserve platelet function, and reinfused after major blood loss has ceased, or sooner if indicated. With hemodilution, the number of units to be withdrawn depends on the expected replacement needs, the initial hematocrit, the patient's blood volume, and cardiovascular status. Recently, the efficacy of moderate hemodilution was questioned (53).

A similar technique has been described in open heart surgery as "blood pooling," in which the removal of one or more autologous blood units at the onset of cardiopulmonary prime has been shown in a recent report to reduce subsequent allogeneic blood requirements (54). However, the potential advantages of fresh whole blood (55,56) procured by this technique are limited by uncertainties regarding its implementation in the large number of patients presenting for surgery who are already anemic, variable or undefined intraoperative clinical transfusion indicators for the retransfusion of this blood in patients who already undergo substantial hemodilution related to the crystalloid/colloid pump prime, and inconsistent demonstration that this practice reduces the need for allogeneic transfusion perioperatively or the incidence of coagulopathy after cardiopulmonary bypass (CPB). A recent European study (57) was able to show that recombinant human erythropoietin (EPO) therapy, coupled with acute preoperative hemodilution, reduced the incidence of allogeneic blood exposure to 11% of patients, compared with 53% in patients undergoing hemodilution without EPO therapy. The controversies over hemodilution have been addressed in a pro and con debate (58,59).

Intraoperative Blood Salvage

The term intraoperative blood salvage describes the technique of salvaging and reinfusing blood lost by a patient during surgery. The oxygen-transport properties of salvaged red blood cells are equal to or better than stored allogeneic red cells, and the survival of salvaged red blood cells appears to be at least comparable with that of transfused allogeneic red cells (60). Cell-washing devices can provide the equivalent of 12 units of banked blood per hour to a massively bleeding patient. Hemolysis of salvaged blood and hemostatic system activation can occur during suctioning from the surface (exterior air–blood interface) rather than from deep pools of shed blood, particularly when blood is aspirated at vacuum settings greater than -100 mm Hg. Although autotransfusion of excessive free hemoglobin (from inadequate cell washing) may result in renal dysfunction, the critical concentration of free hemoglobin to cause this complication has not been established.

Dilutional coagulopathy may occur if large volumes of salvaged blood are administered (61). This is also supported by a recent study demonstrating an association between the volume of blood reinfused and perioperative bleeding (62). Excessive use of these systems can result in a clinically significant loss of platelets and coagulation factors (63,64).

As with PAD, intraoperative autologous blood salvage should undergo scrutiny concerning both safety and cost effectiveness. Although the incidence of adverse effects from blood recovery and reinfusion is unknown, four deaths related to intraoperative blood recovery were reported to the New York Department of Health from 1990 to 1995, for an estimated prevalence of 1 in 35,000 procedures (65). Three controlled studies recently demonstrated that intraoperative salvage did not reduce perioperative allogeneic transfusion requirements in patients undergoing cardiac or vascular surgery (66–68). Although the salvage of a minimum of one blood unit equivalent may be cost effective using less expensive (with unwashed blood) methods, at least two blood unit equivalents need to be salvaged using the cell-saver (with washed blood) to achieve cost effectiveness (69,70).

Hemofiltration was initially described as an effective means of removing free water during CPB in an attempt to raise hematocrit. This maneuver reduced allogeneic red blood cell transfusions, avoided volume overload, and reduced accumulation of tissue water, particularly in the pediatric patient population (71,72). Boldt et al. (64) demonstrated that hemofiltration of intraoperative blood significantly reduced blood loss when compared with routine processing via cell salvage systems. Hemofiltration can also be an effective blood conservation strategy when used to salvage blood from the CPB circuit at the completion of surgery based on its ability to reduce hemostatic and inflammatory derangements related to CPB. Hemofiltration in pediatric patients during CPB has been shown to eliminate mediators of inflammation (73–75), improve perioperative hemostasis, improve early postoperative oxygenation, and reduce ventilatory support requirements (75).

Postoperative Autologous Blood Salvage

The evolution of cardiac surgery has been accompanied by a broad experience in postoperative blood conservation (76) along with identification of preoperative risk factors for subsequent need for blood transfusion (77). Postoperative autologous blood salvage and reinfusion is practiced widely but not uniformly. A recently published survey of tertiary medical centers found that only 5 of 15 institutions salvaged blood postoperatively in cardiac surgery patients; in these five centers, approximately 50% of the blood shed postoperatively into the chest tubes was reinfused in patients undergoing primary elective coronary bypass surgery (6). Prospective and controlled trials have disagreed over the efficacy of postoperative blood salvage in conserving blood in cardiac surgery patients; at least four such studies have demonstrated lack of efficacy (65,78–80), whereas at least two have shown benefit (81,82). In addition, uncontrolled reports of cardiac surgical programs that used a combination of intra- and postoperative salvage techniques have shown a benefit (78,83,84). The disparity of results in these studies may be explained, in part, by differences in transfusion practices. To a greater or lesser extent, the reports cited above incorporated criteria for blood transfusion into their protocols. Additionally, these studies were unblinded, so that modification of physician transfusion practices were uncredited interventions that may have introduced bias into these blood conservation studies (85). These increasingly sophisticated and potentially expensive (Table 26.2) blood conservation techniques may be effective only to the extent that they are accompanied by conservative transfusion practice.

Erythropoietin Therapy to Replace Blood Loss

Current status of approval worldwide for use of recombinant human EPO therapy is shown in Table 26.3. EPO was approved for use in patients undergoing PAD in Japan, the European Union, Canada, and Australia in 1993, 1994, 1996, and 1997, respectively. Approval was granted for perisurgical EPO therapy in major surgical procedures without PAD in Canada in 1996, for orthopedic surgery in the European Union in 1998, and for nonvascular noncardiac procedures in the United States in 1996 (86). EPO (along with iron, B12, and folic acid) therapy "should be used instead of blood transfusion if the clinical condition of the patient permits sufficient time for these agents to promote erythropoiesis" (87).

TABLE 26.2. A COMPARISON OF RED CELL TRANSFUSION AND CONSERVATION COSTS (PER UNIT) AT ONE HOSPITAL

	Allogeneic	Autologous
Blood donated and transfused		
Blood center		
Acquisition	66.75	79.25
Laboratory	12.85	12.85
Administration[a]	13.12	13.12
Overhead[b]	27.80	31.59
Total	120.52	136.81
Hospital		
Acquisition	26.87	23.76
Laboratory	33.13	32.24
Administration	13.12	13.12
Overhead	21.96	20.76
Total	95.08	89.88
Acute preoperative		
Hemodilution (per unit)		
Supplies		12.09
Labor[c]		6.58
Overhead		5.59
Total		24.24
Intraoperative salvaged, washed, and reinfused		
Supplies, administration		175.00
Overhead		52.50
Total		227.50
Postoperative (cardiac) salvaged and reinfused		
Unwashed		
Supplies		45.50
Administration[a]		13.12
Overhead		17.59
Total		76.20
Washed		
Blood Bank		43.83
Overhead		13.15
Total		133.18

[a] Administration calculated at 30 min of registered nurse at $26.24/hr.
[b] Overhead rate calculated at 30% of costs.
[c] Labor calculated at costs of registered nurse for 15 min.
Source: Goodnough LT, Bodner MS, Martin JW. Blood transfusion and blood conservation: cost and utilization issues. Am J Med Qual 1994;9:172–183, with permission.

The safety of EPO therapy in patients undergoing non-cardiac surgery has been demonstrated in over 1,000 patients participating in clinical trials. Thrombotic events attributed to EPO therapy have not been seen in these surgical settings (88). An unresolved question is the issue of safety for EPO therapy in cardiac surgery patients and its use in this setting. In a European trial (89), the authors found no differences in mortality, thrombotic events, or serious adverse events between the EPO-treated and placebo cohorts. However, adverse events and mortalities in a U.S. study (90) indicated that an uneven distribution of these events between the placebo and the EPO-treated groups could not be ruled out to any degree of certainty. Until large safety trials are performed, EPO therapy is currently not recommended for patients undergoing cardiac or vascular surgery in the United States.

Pathophysiology and Epidemiology of Hemostasis Abnormalities

Patients undergoing cardiac surgery with CPB are at risk for excessive perioperative blood loss requiring transfusion of blood products. This risk is influenced by the duration of CPB (91,92). Although excessive perioperative bleeding may occasionally be related to preexisting hemostatic abnormalities (93–96), more often CPB causes hemostatic alterations that predispose to excessive bleeding. Crystalloid or colloid solutions used to prime the CPB circuit (and as a component of cardioplegia) cause significant dilution of coagulation factors and platelets (96). Activation of the hemostatic system during CPB can lead to thrombin and plasmin-mediated consumption of platelets and labile coagulation factors (Fig. 26.4). This activation is related to the interaction of the contact coagulation factors with extracorporeal surfaces (97) and also related to activation of the extrinsic pathway via release of tissue factor by surgical trauma or retransfusion of pericardial blood (98). Fibrinolysis can be triggered by CPB-mediated contact system activation of factor XII (99), the release of tissue plasminogen activator from the pericardial cavity (100), or from surgically injured endothelial cells (101) and through a protamine-mediated mechanism (102). Even after protamine

TABLE 26.3. APPROVAL OF STATUS OF RECOMBINANT HUMAN ERYTHROPOIETIN THERAPY IN SURGICAL ANEMIA

Anemia Related To	United States	Canada	European Union[a]	Australia	Japan
Autologous blood donation	—	1996	1994	1997	1993
Surgery	1996[b]	1996	1998[c]	—	Under review

[a] Approval dates for France, Germany, Italy, and the United Kingdom are the same as for other countries of the European Union.
[b] Noncardiac, nonvascular surgery.
[c] Orthopedic surgery only.

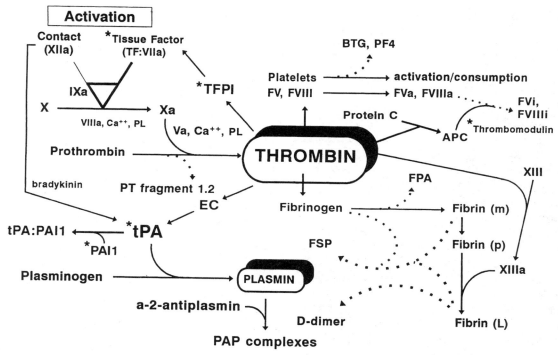

FIG. 26.4. Mechanisms and effects of excessive hemostatic activation with cardiac surgery. Dashed line, release of protein cleavage byproducts. Activated factors are designated using a small "a," whereas inactivated factors are designated using a small "i." *XII*, factor XII; *VII*, factor VII; *X*, factor X; *VIII*, factor VIII; *IX*, factor IX; *V*, factor V; *XIII*, factor XIII; *PT 1.2*, prothrombin fragment 1.2; *Ca⁺⁺*, calcium ions; *FPA*, fibrinopeptide A; *PL*, phospholipid; *PAP*, plasmin–antiplasmin complexes; *EC*, endothelial cells; *tPA:PAI1*, tissue plasminogen activator–plasminogen activator inhibitor 1 complexes; *fibrin (m)*, fibrin monomer; *fibrin (p)*, fibrin polymer; *fibrin (L)*, fibrin cross-linked polymer; *FSP*, fibrinogen/fibrin degradation products; *D-dimers*, polymerized fibrin degradation products; *TFPI*, tissue factor pathway inhibitor; *, endothelial cell related. (From Despotis GJ, Gravlee GP, Levy J, et al. Anticoagulation monitoring during cardiac surgery: a survey of current practice and review of current and emerging technologies. *Anesthesiology* 1999;91:1122–1151.)

neutralization, heparin may potentially inhibit coagulation (103) and platelet function (104); similarly, excess protamine has been shown to inhibit coagulation (105) and affect platelet function (106,107). Finally, release of elastase from polymorphonuclear leukocytes may affect hemostasis (108).

The frequency of severe bleeding with CPB can vary based on the definition used and the institution involved. An incidence of between 13% and 16% can be observed when abnormal bleeding is defined as comprising more than 10 units of blood transfused in the perioperative period, whereas between 5% and 7% of patients can have excessive bleeding when it is defined as greater than 2 L blood loss within the first 24 postoperative hours (62). Using two much larger data sets (*n* = 6,015) (109) and (*n* = 8,586) (110), between 4.2% and 3.6%, respectively, of patients required reexploration for excessive bleeding. Transfusion of allogeneic blood or blood components in cardiac surgical patients with excessive blood loss is potentially associated

with several adverse events, such as bloodborne disease transmission; increased incidence of wound infections; hemolytic and nonhemolytic transfusion reactions; and increased mortality (109,111–113), increased operative time (114), and increased cost. Based on a national annual frequency of 500,000 adult cardiac surgical procedures per year, an average cost of $200/unit of blood and an average transfusion rate of 4 units per patient (3.9 ± 5.9 units), national transfusion-related costs approximate $400 million annually. Not uncommonly, coagulopathic bleeding can lead to reexploration that may also increase perioperative morbidity (i.e., renal failure, sepsis, atrial arrhythmias, prolonged requirement for mechanical ventilatory support, and acute lung injury) and mortality (109,113).

In a series of 487 patients, 14 required reexploration and had a surgical source of bleeding (62). When compared with those not requiring exploration, patients who were reexplored had significantly greater (*p* < 0.001) chest tube drainage in the first 4 (1,161 ± 805 versus 351 ± 281 mL), 8 (1,802 ± 742 versus 529 ± 360 mL), and 24 hours (2,646 ± 1,027 versus 986 ± 581 mL) after surgery (62). The association between reexploration for bleeding and several perioperative risk factors were examined in two large series (109,110). Moulton et al. (109) identified four independent risk factors for reexploration in a large series of patients (4.2% or 253/6,015): increasing patient age ($p <$ 0.001), preoperative renal insufficiency ($p =$ 0.02), noncoronary operation ($p <$ 0.001), and prolonged CPB time (p = 0.03). These authors also demonstrated that reexploration was associated with several negative outcomes such as operative mortality ($p =$ 0.005), renal failure ($p <$ 0.0001), sepsis ($p <$ 0.0001), atrial dysrhythmias ($p =$ 0.006), prolonged requirement for mechanical ventilatory support (p < 0.0001), and acute lung injury ($p =$ 0.03) (109). Dacey et al. (110) also confirmed the association between either older age or prolonged CPB time and reexploration in another large series of patients (3.6% or 305/8,586). These authors also found an association between exploration and the following variables: smaller body surface area, number of distal anastomoses, and the use of thrombolytic therapy within 48 hours of surgery. These authors also found that reexploration was associated with a threefold increase in hospital mortality and a significantly longer length of stay (110). Consequently, pharmacologic interventions that could reduce blood loss or blood transfusion needs merit strong consideration. Many of these blood conservation issues and strategies are covered in Chapter 25.

Topical Agents

Fibrin glue and fibrin gel are blood derivatives rather than pharmacologic agents, but their increasing use as an intervention in surgical hemostasis and blood conservation, along with recent U.S. Food and Drug Administration approval of fibrin glue from commercial pooled plasma, deserves mention. These agents can be applied directly to wounds that display diffuse microvascular bleeding or can be used to seal vascular grafts. Fibrin glue is derived from a source of fibrinogen and factor XIII (fibrin-stabilizing factor), in which a solution of fibrinogen is mixed with a solution of bovine thrombin and applied to a surgical field (115). It is important to note that preparations derived from cryoprecipitate, commercial pooled plasma, or single-donor plasma (115,116) represent additional allogeneic blood donor exposure. Alternatively, the source of fibrinogen and factor XIII can be derived from as little as 40 mL of the patient's autologous blood (117) or prepared from an autologous plasma unit (118).

A review of the potential use of this product has been recently published (119). Patients should be made aware of the potential complications and the potential benefits of its use. To date, there has been one case report of anaphylactic reaction after a total of only 8 mL of fibrin glue administration and one case of human immunodeficiency virus (HIV)

transmission (120,121). The use of autologous donation as a source of fibrinogen would be the safest and therefore preferable approach. A solvent-detergent–treated fibrin glue preparation is currently under evaluation and appears promising; however, this is still under investigation (122). Recent reports of cardiac surgery patients who presented with acquired bovine-thrombin–induced factor V deficiency, each of whom had been previously exposed to bovine thrombin (123,124), caused concern over the potential toxicities associated with the use of both allogeneic and autologous fibrin sealants. Issues of informed consent for administration of these blood products and criteria for utilization review for their use need to be addressed.

Platelet gel consists of platelet-rich plasma mixed with a solution of bovine thrombin and applied to a surgical field. Platelet-rich plasma is provided during the intraoperative period from patients using designated pheresis instruments or combined-function cell-salvage systems. Preliminary evaluations of its use have been reported (125,126). Several other topical hemostatic agents such as hemostatic swabs (calcium alginate) (127); vasoconstricting agents such as oxymetazoline (128), absorbable collagen (INSTAT) (129), topical thrombin (130,131), and topical oxidized cellulose; and porcine collagen have been described to enhance hemostasis (132). However, no study to date has been able to show reduction in allogeneic donor exposure with the use of these products; without these data, these agents cannot be considered true pharmacologic alternatives.

CONCLUSION

In summary, the costs, potential complications, and potential benefits of an increasing variety of blood conservation interventions and the relative costs, risks, and benefits of blood transfusion need to be considered (54), so that a careful balance of the need for blood conservation, along with an acknowledgment of the life-saving properties of blood, can be maintained (55). The generation of new questions regarding the safety, benefit, and costs of autologous blood procurement is a welcome sign of maturity for this field. Emerging pharmacologic agents that conserve blood, including not only recombinant human EPO but also antifibrinolytic agents, hemoglobin solutions, and artificial oxygen carriers, need to be scrutinized and held accountable not only for safety and efficacy but for their costs and cost effectiveness as well. The coordination of the various available options that best suit the individual patient, yet remain cost effective and affordable so that access to these strategies remains available to all patients, remains the challenge for transfusion medicine specialists and their surgical colleagues.

KEY POINTS

- Variation in transfusion practices among different cardiac surgical centers is impressive. Extensive analysis shows that this variation can best be explained by differences among physicians in the criteria used for transfusion therapy decisions, which frequently results in overuse of blood components.

- Transfusion algorithms developed to assist decisions about blood component therapy have been shown to reduce bleeding and blood component use.

- Preoperative autologous donation does not appear to be cost effective in cardiac surgery.

- Pre-bypass intraoperative withdrawal of fresh whole blood may reduce allogeneic transfusion requirements.

- Intraoperative blood salvage with cell-washing and cell-concentrating devices is not routinely cost effective in cardiac surgery but may be worthwhile in cases where large blood loss is anticipated.

- It remains uncertain whether postoperative salvage of mediastinal blood drainage is an effective form of blood conservation.

- EPO therapy in cardiac surgical patients needs further investigation and cannot currently be recommended.

REFERENCES

1. Goodnough LT, Brecher ME, Kanter MH, et al. Blood transfusion. *N Engl J Med* 1999;340:439–447.
2. Goodnough LT, Brecher ME, Kanter MH, et al. Blood conservation. *N Engl J Med* 1999;340:525–533.
3. Herbert PC, Wells G, Marshall J, et al. Transfusion requirements in critical care. *JAMA* 1995;273:1439–1444.
4. Littenberg B, Corwin HL, Gettinger A, et al. A practice guideline and decision aid for blood transfusion. *Immunohematology* 1995;11:88–94.
5. Herbert PC, Wells G, Blajchman MA, et al. Transfusion requirements in critical care. A multicenter randomized controlled clinical trial. *N Engl J Med* 1999;340:409–417
6. Goodnough LT, Johnston MFM, Toy PTCY, et al. The variability of transfusion practice in coronary artery bypass graft surgery. *JAMA* 1991;265:86–90.
7. Surgenor DM, Wallace EL, Churchill WH, et al. Red cell transfusions in coronary artery bypass surgery. *Transfusion* 1992;32:458–464.
8. Stover EP, Siegel LC, Parks R, et al. Variability in transfusion practice for coronary artery bypass surgery persists despite national consensus guidelines. *Anesthesiology* 1998;88:327–333.
9. Goodnough LT, Soegiarso RW, Birkmeyer JD, et al. Economic impact of inappropriate blood transfusions in coronary artery bypass graft surgery. *Am J Med* 1993;94:509–514.
10. Surgenor DM, Churchill WH, Wallace EL. The specific hospital influences red cell and component transfusion in coronary artery bypass graft surgery. A study of five hospitals. *Transfusion* 1998;37:122–134.
11. National Institutes of Health Consensus Conference. Perioperative red cell transfusion. *JAMA* 1988;260:2700–2705.
12. Faust RJ Perioperative indications for red blood cell transfusion - Has the pendulum swung too far? *Mayo Clin Proc* 1993; 68:512–514.
13. Weisel RD, Charlesworth DC, Mickleborough LL, et al. Limitations of blood conservation. *J Thorac Cardiovasc Surg* 1984; 88:26–38.
14. Robertie PG, Gravlee GP. Safe limits of isovolemic hemodilution and recommendations for erythrocyte transfusion. *Int Anesth Clin* 1990;28:197–204.
15. Goodnough LT, Despotis GJ, Hogue CW, et al. On the need for improved transfusion indicators in cardiac surgery. *Ann Thorac Surg* 1995;60:473–480.
16. Bryan-Brown CW, Baek SM, Makabali G, et al. Consumable oxygen: Availability of oxygen in relation to oxyhemoglobin dissociation. *Crit Care Med* 1973;1:17–21.
17. Mangano DT, Browner WS, Hollenberg M, et al. Association of perioperative myocardial ischemia with cardiac morbidity and mortality in men undergoing noncardiac surgery. *N Engl J Med* 1990;323:1781–1788.
18. Rao TLK, Montoya A. Cardiovascular, electrocardiographic and respiratory changes following acute anemia with volume replacement in patients with coronary artery disease. *Anesth Dev* 1985; 12:49–54.
19. Parksloe MRJ, Wuld R, Fox M, et al. Silent myocardial ischemia in a patient with anaemia before operation. *Br J Anaesth* 1990; 64:634–637.
20. Nelson AH, Fleisher LA, Rosenbaum SH. Relationship between postoperative anemia and cardiac morbidity in high-risk vascular patients in the intensive care unit. *Crit Care Med* 1993;21: 860–866.
21. Hogue CW, Goodnough LT, Monk TG. Perioperative myocardial ischemic episodes are related to hematocrit level in patients undergoing radical prostatectomy. *Transfusion* 1998;38: 924–931.
22. Spiess BD, Ley C, Body SC, et al. Hematocrit value on intensive care unit entry influences the frequency of Q-wave myocardial infarction after coronary artery bypass grafting. *J Thorac Cardiovasc Surg* 1998;116:460–467.
23. Goodnough LT, Vizmeg K, Riddell J, et al. Discharge hematocrit as clinical indicator for blood transfusion audit in surgery patients. *Transfus Med* 1994;4:35–44.
24. Despotis GJ, Grishaber JE, Goodnough LT. The effect of an intraoperative treatment algorithm on physician transfusion behavior in cardiac surgery. *Transfusion* 1994;34:290–296.
25. Despotis GJ, Santoro SA, Spitznagel E, et al. Prospective evaluation and clinical utility of on-site coagulation monitoring in cardiac surgical patients. *J Thorac Cardiovasc Surg* 1994;107: 271–279.
26. Reinersten JL. Algorithms, guidelines, and protocols: can they really improve what we do? *Transfusion* 1994;34:281–282.
27. Spiess BD, Gillies BS, Chandler W, et al. Changes in transfusion therapy and reexploration rate after institution of a blood management program in cardiac surgical patients. *J Cardiothorac Vasc Anesth* 1995;9:168–73.
28. Paone G, Spencer T, Silverman NA. Blood conservation in coronary artery surgery. *Surgery* 1994;116:672–677.
29. NHLBI Expert Panel. Transfusion alert: use of autologous blood transfusion. *Transfusion* 1995;35:703–711.
30. National Heart, Lung, and Blood Institute Autologous Transfusion Symposium Working Group. Autologous transfusion: current trends and research issues. *Transfusion* 1995;35:525–531.
31. Consensus Conference on Autologous Transfusion. Final consensus statement. *Transfusion* 1996;36:667.
32. British Committee for Standards in Hematology, Blood Transfusion Task Force. Guidelines for autologous transfusion. *Transfus Med* 1993;3:307–316.
33. Menitov J, ed. *Standards for blood banks and transfusion services,*

19th ed. Bethesda, MD: American Association of Blood Banks, 1999.

34. Food and Drug Administration. *Memorandum: Autologous blood collection and processing procedures* (February 12, 1990). Rockville, MD: Congressional and Consumer Affairs, 1990.

35. Goodnough LT, Price TH, Rudnick S. Iron restricted erythropoiesis as a limitation to autologous blood donation in the erythropoietin-stimulated bone marrow. *J Lab Clin Med* 1991;118:289–296.

36. Goodnough LT, Marcus RE. Erythropoiesis in patients stimulated with erythropoietin: The relevance of storage iron. *Vox Sang* 1998;75:128–133.

37. Silvergleid AJ. Safety and effectiveness of predeposit autologous transfusions in preteen and adolescent children. *JAMA* 1987;257:3403–3404.

38. Mann M, Sacks HJ, Goldfinger D. Safety of autologous blood donation prior to elective surgery for a variety of potentially high risk patients. *Transfusion* 1983;23:229–232.

39. Popovsky MA, Whitaker B, Arnold NL. Severe outcomes of allogeneic and autologous blood donation: frequency and characterization. *Transfusion* 1995;35:734–737.

40. Schreiber GB, Busch MP, Kleinman SH, et al. The risk of transfusion-transmitted viral infections. *N Engl J Med* 1996;334:1685–1690.

41. Birkmeyer JD, Aubuchon JP, Littenberg B, et al. The costs and benefits of preoperative autologous blood donation in elective coronary bypass surgery. *Ann Thorac Surg* 1994;57:161–169.

42. Kruskall MS, Yomtovian R, Dzik WH, et al. On improving the cost-effectiveness of autologous blood transfusion practices. *Transfusion* 1994;34:259–264.

43. Menitove JE. The recent emphasis on good manufacturing practices and the pharmaceutical manufacturing approach damages blood banking and transfusion medicine as medical care activities: con. *Transfusion* 1993;94:439–442.

44. Miller WV. Blood blanks should use good manufacturing practices and the pharmaceutical manufacturing approach: pro. *Transfusion* 1993;94:435–438.

45. Spiess BD, Sassetti R, McCary RJ, et al. Autologous blood donation. Hemodynamics in a high-risk patient population. *Transfusion* 1992;32:17–22.

46. Popovsky MA, Whitaker B, Arnold NL. Severe outcomes of allogeneic and autologous blood donation: frequency and characterization. *Transfusion* 1995;35:734–737.

47. Owings DV, Kruskall MS, Thurer RL, et al. Autologous blood donations prior to elective cardiac surgery. Safety and effect on subsequent blood use. *JAMA* 1989;262:1963–1967.

48. Dzik WH, Fleisher AG, Ciavarella D, et al. Safety and efficacy of autologous blood donation before elective aortic valve operation. *Ann Thorac Surg* 1992;54:1177–1180.

49. National Blood Resource Education Program Expert Panel. The use of autologous blood. *JAMA* 1990;263:414–417.

50. Sazama K. Reports of 355 transfusion-associated deaths: 1976 through 1985. *Transfusion* 1990;30:583–590.

51. Johnson RG, Thurer RL, Kruskall MS, et al. Comparison of two transfusion strategies after elective operations for myocardial revascularization. *J Thorac Cardiovasc Surg* 1992;104:307–314.

52. Welch GH, Meehan K, Goodnough LT. Prudent strategies for elective red cell transfusion. *Ann Intern Med* 1992;116:393–403.

53. Brecher ME, Rosenfeld. Mathematical and computer modeling of acute normovolemic hemodilution. *Transfusion* 1994;34:176–179.

54. Petry AF, Jost T, Sievers H. Reduction of homologous blood requirements by blood pooling at the onset of cardiopulmonary bypass. *J Thorac Cardiovasc Surg* 1994;107:1210–1214.

55. Mohr R, Martinowitz U, Lavee J, et al. The hemostatic effect of transfusing fresh whole blood versus platelet concentrates after cardiac operations. *J Thorac Cardiovasc Surg* 1988;96:530–534.

56. Lavee J, Martinowitz U, Mohr R, et al. The effect of transfusion of fresh whole blood versus platelet concentrates after cardiac operations. *J Thorac Cardiovasc Surg* 1989;97:204–212.

57. Sowade O, Warneke H, Scigalla P, et al. Avoidance of allogeneic blood transfusions by treatment with recombinant human erythropoietin in patients undergoing open heart surgery. *Blood* 1997;89:411–418.

58. Robblee JA. Blood harvested before cardiopulmonary bypass decreased postoperative blood loss. *J Cardiothorac Anesth* 1990;4:519–522.

59. Starr NJ. Con: blood should not be harvested immediately before cardiopulmonary bypass and infused after protamin reversal to decrease blood loss following cardiopulmonary bypass [Comment] [Review]. *J Cardiothorac Anesth* 1990;4:522–525.

60. Ray JM, Flynn JC, Bierman AH. Erythrocyte survival following intraoperative autotransfusion in spinal surgery: an in vivo comparative study and 5-year update. *Spine* 1986;11:879–882.

61. Horst HM, Dlugos S, Fath JJ, et al. Coagulopathy and intraoperative blood salvage. *J Trauma* 1992;32:5:646–653.

62. Despotis GJ, Filos KS, Zoys TN, et al. Factors associated with excessive postoperative blood loss and hemostatic transfusion requirements: a multivariate analysis in cardiac surgical patients. *Anesth Analg* 1996;82:13–21.

63. Horst HM, Dlugos S, Fath JJ, et al. Coagulopathy and intraoperative blood salvage (IBS). *J Trauma* 1992;32:646–653.

64. Boldt J, Zickmann B, Czeke A, et al. Blood conservation techniques and platelet function in cardiac surgery. *Anesthesiology* 1991;75:426–432.

65. Linden JV, Tourault MA, Scribner CL. Decrease in frequency of transfusion fatalities. *Transfusion* 1997;37:243–244.

66. Bell K, Stott K, Sinclair CJ, et al. A controlled trial of intraoperative autologous transfusion in cardiothoracic surgery measuring effect on transfusion requirements and clinical outcome. *Transfus Med* 1992;2:295–300.

67. Claggett GP, Valentine RJ, Jackson MR, et al. A randomized trial of intraoperative transfusion during aortic surgery. *J Vasc Surg* 1999;29:22–31.

68. Body SC, Birmingham J, Parks R, et al. Safety and efficacy of autotransfusion of shed mediastinal blood after cardiac surgery: A multicenter analysis. *J Cardiothorac Vasc Anesth* (in press).

69. Goodnough LT, Monk TG, Sicard G, et al. Intraoperative salvage in patients undergoing elective abdominal aortic aneurysm repair. *J Vasc Surg* 1996;24:213–218.

70. Goodnough LT, Bodner MS, Martin JW. Blood transfusion and blood conservation: Cost and utilization issues. *Am J Med Qual* 1994;9:172–183.

71. Elliott MJ. Ultrafiltration and modified ultrafiltration in pediatric open heart operations. *Ann Thorac Surg* 1993;56:1518–1522.

72. Naik SK, Knight A, Elliott M. A prospective randomized study of a modified technique of ultrafiltration during pediatric open-heart surgery. *Circulation* 1991;84:1181–1189.

73. Andreasson S, Gothberg S, Berggren H, et al. Hemofiltration modifies complement activation after extracorporeal circulation in infants. *Ann Thorac Surg* 1993;56:1515–1517.

74. Millar AB, Armstrong L, van der Linden J, et al. Cytokine production and hemofiltration in children undergoing cardiopulmonary bypass. *Ann Thorac Surg* 1993;56:1499–1502.

75. Journois D, Pouard P, Greeley WJ, et al. Hemofiltration during cardiopulmonary bypass in pediatric cardiac surgery. Effects on hemostasis, cytokines, and complement components. *Anesthesiology* 1994;81:1181–1189.

76. Schaff HY, Hauer J, Gardner TJ, et al. Routine use of autotrans-

fusion following cardiac surgery: experience in 700 patients. *Ann Thorac Surg* 1979;27:493–499.

77. Cosgrove DM, Loop FD, Lytle BW, et al. Determinants of blood utilization during myocardial revascularization. *Ann Thorac Surg* 1985;40:380–384.

78. Ward HB, Smith RA, Candis KP, et al. A prospective, randomized trial of autotransfusion after routine cardiac surgery. *Ann Thorac Surg* 1993;56:137–141.

79. Thurer RL, Lytle BW, Cosgrove DM, et al. Autotransfusion following cardiac operations: a randomized, prospective study. *Ann Thorac Surg* 1979;27:500–506.

80. Roberts SP, Early GL, Brown B, et al. Autotransfusion of unwashed mediastinal shed blood fails to decrease banked blood requirements in patients undergoing aorta coronary bypass surgery. *Am J Surg* 1991;162:477–480.

81. Schaff HV, Hauer JM, Bell WR, et al. Autotransfusion of shed mediastinal blood after cardiac surgery. A prospective study. *J Cardiovasc Thorac Surg* 1978;75:632–641.

82. Eng J, Kay PH, Murday AJ, et al. Post-operative autologous transfusion in cardiac surgery. A prospective, randomized study. *Eur J Cardiothorac Surg* 1990;4:595–600.

83. Tyson GS, Sladen RN, Spainhour V, et al. Blood conservation in cardiac surgery. *Ann Surg* 1989;209:736–742.

84. Jones JW, Witscher RE, McLean TR, et al. Benefit from combining blood conservation measures in cardiac operations. *Ann Thorac Surg* 1991;51:541–546.

85. Goodnough LT. Blood conservation and blood transfusion practices: flip sides of the same coin. *Ann Thorac Surg* 1993; 56:3–4. *Engl J Med* 1991;324:1037–42.

86. Goodnough LT, Monk TG, Andriole GL. Erythropoietin therapy. *N Engl J Med* 1997;336:933–938.

87. Joint Council of the American Red Cross, Council of Community Blood Centers, American Association of Blood Banks. Circular of information for the use of human blood components, March 1994.

88. Goodnough LT, Price TH, EPO Study Group. A phase III trial of recombinant human erythropoietin therapy in non-anemic orthopaedic patients subjected to aggressive autologous blood phlebotomy: dose, response, toxicity, and efficacy. *Transfusion* 1994;34:66–71.

89. Sowade O, Warnke H, Scigalla P, et al. Avoidance of allogeneic blood transfusions by treatment with epoietin beta (recombinant human erythropoietin) in patients undergoing open heart surgery. *Blood* 1997;89:411–418.

90. D'Ambra MN, Gray RJ, Hillman R, et al. The effect of recombinant human erythropoietin on transfusion risk in coronary bypass patients. *Ann Thorac Surg* 1997;64:1686–1693.

91. Khuri SF, Wolfe JA, Josa M, et al. Hematologic changes during and after cardiopulmonary bypass and their relationship to the bleeding time and nonsurgical blood loss. *J Thorac Cardiovasc Surg* 1992;104:94–107.

92. Despotis GJ, Filos KS, Zoys TN, et al. Factors associated with excessive postoperative blood loss and hemostatic transfusion requirements: A multivariate analysis in cardiac surgical patients. *Anesth Analg* 1996;82:13–21.

93. Vander Woude JC, Milam JD, Walker WE, Houchin DP, Weiland AP, Cooley DA. Cardiovascular surgery in patients with congenital plasma coagulopathies. *Ann Thorac Surg* 1988;46: 283–286.

94. Aris A, Pisciotta AV, Hussey CV, et al. Open heart surgery in von-Willebrand's disease. *J Thor Cardio Surg* 1975;69: 183–187.

95. Woodman RC, Harker LA. Bleeding complications associated with cardiopulmonary bypass [Review]. *Blood* 1990;76: 1680–1697.

96. Despotis GJ, Santoro SA, Spitznagel E, et al. Prospective evalua-

97. tion and clinical utility of on-site monitoring of coagulation in patients undergoing cardiac operation. *J Thorac Cardiovasc Surg* 1994;107:271–279.

97. Despotis GJ, Gravlee GP, Levy J, et al. Anticoagulation monitoring during cardiac surgery: a survey of current practice and review of current and emerging technologies. *Anesthesiology* 1999;91:1122–1151.

98. Boisclair MD, Lane DA, Philippou H, et al. Mechanisms of thrombin generation during surgery and cardiopulmonary bypass. *Blood* 1993;82:3350–3357.

99. Holloway DS, Summaria L, Sandesara J, et al. Decreased platelet number and function and increased fibrinolysis contribute to postoperative bleeding in cardiopulmonary bypass patients. *Thromb Haemost* 1988;59:62–67.

100. Tabuchi N, de Haan J, Boonstra PW, et al. Activation of fibrinolysis in the pericardial cavity during cardiopulmonary bypass. *J Thorac Cardiovasc Surg* 1993;106:828–833.

101. Stibbe J, Kluft C, Brommer EJ, et al. Enhanced fibrinolytic activity during cardiopulmonary bypass in open-heart surgery in man is caused by extrinsic (tissue-type) plasminogen activator. *Eur J Clin Invest* 1984;14:375–382.

102. Gram J, Janetzko T, Jespersen J, et al. Enhanced effective fibrinolysis following the neutralization of heparin in open heart surgery increases the risk of post-surgical bleeding. *Thromb Haemost* 1990;63:241–245.

103. Hirsh J. Heparin [Review]. *N Engl J Med* 1991;324: 1565–1574.

104. John LC, Rees GM, Kovacs IB. Inhibition of platelet function by heparin. An etiologic factor in post bypass hemorrhage. *J Thorac Cardiovasc Surg* 1993;105:816–822.

105. Cobel-Geard RJ, Hassouna HI. Interaction of protamine sulfate with thrombin. *Am J Hematol* 1983;14:227–233.

106. Ereth MH, Klindworth JT, Campbell BA, et al. Protamine attenuates agonist induced platelet signaling/adhesion molecule expression [Abstract]. *Anesth Analg* 1996;82:5.

107. Ammar T, Fisher CF. The effects of heparinase 1 and protamine on platelet reactivity. *Anesthesiology* 1997;86:1382–1386.

108. Wachtfogel YT, Kucich U, Greenplate J, et al. Human neutrophil degranulation during extracorporeal circulation. *Blood* 1987;69:324–330.

109. Moulton MJ, Creswell LL, Mackey ME, et al. Reexploration for bleeding is a risk factor for adverse outcomes after cardiac operations. *J Thorac Cardiovasc Surg* 1996;111:1037–1046.

110. Dacey LJ, Munoz JJ, Baribeau YR, et al. Reexploration for hemorrhage following coronary artery bypass grafting: incidence and risk factors. Northern New England Cardiovascular Disease Study Group. *Arch Surg* 1998;133:442–447.

111. Gravlee GP, Haddon WS, Rothberger HK, et al. Heparin dosing and monitoring for cardiopulmonary bypass. A comparison of techniques with measurement of subclinical plasma coagulation. *J Thorac Cardiovasc Surg* 1990;99:518–527.

112. Paone G, Spencer T, Silverman NA. Blood conservation in coronary artery surgery. *Surgery* 1994;116:672–677.

113. van de Watering LM, Hermans J, Houbiers JG, et al. Beneficial effects of leukocyte depletion of transfused blood on postoperative complications in patients undergoing cardiac surgery: a randomized clinical trial. *Circulation* 1998;97:562–568.

114. Despotis GJ, Santoro SA, Spitznagel E, et al. Prospective evaluation and clinical utility of on-site monitoring of coagulation in patients undergoing cardiac operation. *J Thorac Cardiovasc Surg* 1994;107:271–279.

115. Baker JW, Spotnitz WD, Matthew TL, et al. Mediastinal fibrin glue: hemostatic effect and tissue response in calves. *Ann Thorac Surg* 1989;47:450–452.

116. Dresdale A, Bowman FO Jr, Malm JR, et al. Hemostatic effec-

tiveness of fibrin glue derived from single-donor fresh frozen plasma. *Ann Thorac Surg* 1985;40:385–387.

117. Silberstein LE, Williams LJ, Hughlett MA, et al. An autologous fibrinogen-based adhesive for use in otologic surgery. *Transfusion* 1988;28:319–321.

118. Hartman AR, Galanakis DK, Honig MP, et al. Autologous whole plasma fibrin gel. Intraoperative procurement. *Arch Surg* 1992;127:357–359.

119. Gibble JW, Ness PM. Fibrin glue: the perfect operative sealant? *Transfusion* 1990;30:741–747.

120. Milde LN. An anaphylactic reaction to fibrin glue. *Anesth Analg* 1989;69:684–686.

121. Wilson SM, Pell P, Donegan EA. HIV-1 transmission following the use of cryoprecipitated fibrinogen as gel/adhesive [Abstract]. *Transfusion* 1991;31:51S.

122. Burnouf-Radosevich M, Burnouf T, Huart JJ. Biochemical and physical properties of a solvent-detergent-treated fibrin glue. *Vox Sang* 1990;58:77–84.

123. Cmolik BL, Spero JA, Magovern GJ, et al. Redo cardiac surgery: late bleeding complications from topical thrombin-induced factor V deficiency. *J Thorac Cardiovasc Surg* 1993;105:222–227.

124. Banninger H, Hardegger T, Tobler A, et al. Fibrin glue in surgery: frequent development of inhibitors of bovine thrombin and human factor V. *Br J Haematol* 1993;85:528–532.

125. Hood AG, Potter PS, Keating RF, et al. New techniques for the rapid perioperative sequestration of autologous blood components and preparation of platelet gel. *Proc Am Acad Cardiovasc Perfus* 1993;13:191.

126. Tawes RL Jr. Reducing homologous blood use in vascular surgery: the promotion of hemostasis. *Semin Vasc Surg* 1994;7:82–84.

127. Blair SD, Jarvis P, Salmon M, et al. Clinical trial of calcium alginate haemostatic swabs. *Br J Surg* 1990;77:568–570.

128. Riegle EV, Gunter JB, Lusk RP, et al. Comparison of vasoconstrictors for functional endoscopic sinus surgery in children. *Laryngoscope* 1992;102:820–823.

129. Green JG, Durham TM. Application of INSTAT hemostat in the control of gingival hemorrhage in the patient with thrombocytopenia. A case report. *Oral Surg Oral Med Oral Pathol* 1991;71:27–30.

130. Ofodile FA, Sadana MK. The role of topical thrombin in skin grafting. *JAMA* 1991;83:416–418.

131. Decker CJ. An efficient method for the application of Avitene hemostatic agent. *Surg Gynecol Obstet* 1991;172:489.

132. Blair SD, Backhouse CM, Harper R, et al. Comparison of absorbable materials for surgical haemostasis. *Br J Surg* 1988;75:969–971.

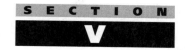

CLINICAL APPLICATIONS

CONDUCT OF CARDIOPULMONARY BYPASS

MARK KURUSZ
RICHARD F. DAVIS
VINCENT R. CONTI

Total body perfusion represents a most exciting hemodynamic experiment, since it offers the unique possibility of controlling blood flows, intravascular pressures and circulating blood volume at will. Because these parameters are interrelated in ways still not fully understood, total body perfusion also presents a difficult challenge to those who attempt it (1).

The preceding thoughts appeared in 1962 when cardiopulmonary bypass (CPB) was still considered by some to be experimental. Although that era and belief have long passed, CPB still represents a challenge because there are aspects primarily involving subtle patient physiologic reactions, and, to a lesser degree, methods of management that are still not fully understood. As a clinical modality practiced many thousands of times daily worldwide, basic principles and practices for the safe conduct of CPB have been mostly empirically determined and refined over the last 40 years, even though a large body of published literature now exists, with several hundred articles appearing each year.

Perfusion as a field of study and practice by professionals has emerged during the last three decades. In the 1950s and 1960s, physicians who had experimented and trained with the technology in the animal research laboratory often performed CPB. Much of the equipment used during that era was fabricated within the institution. Disposable devices were unheard of and polished stainless steel, glass, industrial-grade plastic, and rubber tubing comprised the CPB circuitry.

Today, formal perfusion training programs teach clinical applications of extracorporeal technology for medical situations where it is necessary to support or temporarily replace a patient's circulatory or respiratory function (2). The perfusionist is knowledgeable about applications of the technology and is educated to conduct CPB safely. There is a wide variety of cardiopulmonary equipment and supplies available, and there are many different ways in which these components can be assembled and used. In the last two decades, increased awareness of abnormal events (or the rare perfusion mishap) resulting in adverse clinical outcome has further helped define safe practices and codify institutional protocols and national practice guidelines.

As noted in Galletti and Brecher's classic text (3), "Cardiopulmonary bypass is such a formidable intrusion into the mechanisms of homeostasis that monitoring of a few key parameters is necessary for maintenance of viable conditions." Besides monitoring basic physiologic functions and CPB device and circuit performance, safe conduct also entails activities before and after bypass, including selection of appropriate equipment, assembly and priming of the system, completion of checklists, resumption of normal cardiopulmonary function, disposition of residual perfusate, and initiation and reversal of systemic anticoagulation.

The conduct of CPB involves personnel from different disciplines and backgrounds who must function together as a team (4). These disciplines are surgery, anesthesiology, perfusion, and nursing, none of which individually holds substantially greater importance during CPB. Activities of any team member can affect the performance of other team members, so effective communication is important for successful outcome. The importance of these team members functioning skillfully and in concert during CPB may be without equal in the practice of medicine (5).

This chapter reviews the conduct of CPB including initiation, performance and monitoring, and physiologic response. Generic institutional checklists and protocols are discussed, and guidelines that have been recently promulgated by professional organizations are reviewed and summarized.

CIRCUIT

Chart Review and Selection of Equipment

Before assembling the perfusion circuit, information from the patient's chart is obtained regarding the proposed surgi-

M. Kurusz and V. R. Conti: Department of Surgery, Division of Cardiothoracic Surgery, University of Texas Medical Branch, Galveston, Texas 77555-0528.
R. F. Davis: Portland VA Medical Center and Department of Anesthesiology, Oregon Health Sciences University, Portland, Oregon 97207.

:edure and relevant history. Equipment is then se-
:hat is appropriate to surgical and patient needs. The
circuit consists of reusable equipment and disposable components available from commercial sources (see Chapter 5).
For most adult cardiac surgical procedures, the circuit is
standardized, but for pediatric cases, smaller adults, or special or infrequently performed procedures such as thoracic
aortic surgery, the circuitry is often modified to accommodate patient size or surgical needs specific to the procedure.

Disposable components are supplied sterile and individually wrapped. In a few settings, reusable devices such as
stainless steel connectors or suction tips are used. Reusable
equipment such as the CPB console or cooler–heater are
cleaned after each case and maintained in good working
order with regularly scheduled preventive maintenance (6).
Hospital biomedical personnel or equipment manufacturer
representatives can perform this preventive maintenance
(7).

Assembly

After checking sterile packaging for integrity, the perfusionist assembles the circuit, usually while the patient is
being prepared for surgery by nursing and anesthesia personnel. In some hospitals, a circuit is assembled (but not
primed) and kept available at all times in the event CPB is
needed urgently. These circuits must be kept in a secure
area with sealed ports and vents to maintain sterility of the
blood-contacting surfaces. Such preassembled circuits may
be used for regularly scheduled procedures so that an extended period of time does not elapse before the circuit is
used (8).

The exact sequence of circuit assembly varies among perfusionists but should be done in a consistent manner to
facilitate the occasional need for urgent circuit assembly.
Components routinely include the oxygenator (with or
without integral venous and/or cardiotomy reservoir) and
arterial filter and often also include an external cardiotomy
reservoir, centrifugal pumphead, cardioplegia delivery set,
and hemoconcentrator. The selected components are connected together with precut sterile tubing most commonly
supplied in an institution-specific customized tubing pack.
The tubing or device manufacturer may preconnect some
components for more rapid assembly and convenience. For
tubing that must be cut at the time of assembly, sterile
scissors or a scalpel blade should be used after wiping the
tubing with a betadine-soaked or other antiseptic pad to
avoid potential contamination of the blood-contacting surfaces.

Once the connected devices are mounted on the CPB
console, the water source to the heat exchanger and cardioplegia delivery system should be turned on and tested to
verify adequate flow. These components are then observed
for integrity and absence of water leaks into the blood-
contacting sections. The circuit may be briefly flushed with

filtered 100% carbon dioxide to displace room air. This
technique was originally used as an aid for arterial filter
priming (9) but is also advantageous with membrane oxygenators (10) because carbon dioxide is approximately 30
times more soluble than the nitrogen in room air (11),
thereby facilitating debubbling the circuit when it is primed
with fluid. For most effective displacement of room air,
tubing clamps should be placed in a manner that directs
carbon dioxide flow through all the CPB blood-contacting
components.

Priming

Balanced electrolyte solution and additives, excluding blood
products, are then added to the CPB circuit (usually via the
cardiotomy or venous reservoir) and recirculated through a
pre-bypass filter (0.2 to 5 μm pore size). The pre-bypass
filter is often positioned as a connection between the arterial
and venous lines and is part of the sterile tubing placed on
the surgical field. Its purpose is to remove any potential
small debris that may be present from the manufacture or
assembly of devices or tubing (12). After an appropriate
period of recirculation, the pre-bypass filter is removed,
most often when separating the arterial and venous lines
just before cannulation, in a way that avoids reintroduction
of any captured debris into the circuit. Except for small
adults with a low starting hematocrit or some pediatric patients, bank blood is infrequently used in the CPB priming
solution; if it is required, it should be added after removal
of the pre-bypass filter and recirculated to ensure adequate
mixing with the crystalloid solution and any drug additives.
Recirculation of perfusate also allows the circuit to be
"stressed" at flows and pressures at or exceeding those expected to be used during CPB to ensure circuit integrity.
Recirculation also allows for adjustment of the perfusate
pH, P_{CO_2}, P_{O_2}, and electrolyte composition.

Setting Occlusion and Verifying Accuracy of Pump Flow

To ensure accurate delivery of systemic blood flow, roller
pump occlusion should be set before bypass, but first the
proper blood flow direction must be verified by tracing the
tubing from the operative field to the CPB circuit and back
to ensure proper tubing assembly. A small gap (1/8 to 1/16
inch) should exist between the tubing and the roller pump
backing plate, and the tubing should be aligned so that it
does not ride up or down within the pump housing with
normal rotation. Properly assembled roller pump tubing
resembles a "U" shape maintained by securing it at the inlet
and outlet with correctly sized tubing inserts or holders.

The traditional method for setting occlusion is to allow
a 30- to 40-inch vertical column of fluid in the outlet side
of the tubing to drop slightly (at a rate less than 1 inch/min)
by adjusting roller occlusion against the backing plate (13).

The occlusion should be set by moving the rollers toward the pump backing plate to accommodate any free play in the occlusion adjustment mechanism; if the occlusion is set by moving the rollers away from the backing plate, underocclusion may result. Each roller should be checked in three positions (typically, at 8, 6, and 4 o'clock where 11 and 1 o'clock approximate the positions of the inlet and outlet, respectively). In the event that the two rollers in the pump head do not yield the same rate of fluid drop, the occlusion should be set to the roller that is tightest.

A second method for setting roller pump occlusion (14) is to fill the systemic flow tubing (subsequently referred to herein as a "line" by convention) with priming fluid and then pressurize the line by applying a tubing clamp beyond a pressure-monitoring port and slightly advancing and then stopping the roller pump. The occlusion can be assessed by observing a slow decline in pressure.

A third method (15) for setting roller pump head occlusion is the so-called dynamic method whereby the occlusion is adjusted while the roller pump rotates. A pressure monitor is required, as is a pressure-activated, valved shunt between the outlet and inlet tubing to prevent overpressurization. Like the second method, a tubing clamp is applied to the fluid-filled arterial line downstream of the pump head. With the pump rotating at 6 to 10 revolutions per minute (rpm), the occlusion is adjusted to maintain a pressure above that anticipated during CPB. Using this method, fluid displaced will flow across the valved shunt while the desired pressure is maintained.

Because a centrifugal pump is afterload sensitive in flow output and functions differently from a roller pump, occlusion setting is not required. However, like the roller pump, the inlet and outlet lines must be correctly identified and connected to ensure proper flow. When a centrifugal pump is used for systemic blood flow, a flow probe must also be calibrated and zeroed before CPB to ensure accurate flow readings. A centrifugal pump cannot be used for suction or venting because possible air entrainment will effectively deprime the pump and stop its suction effect and forward flow.

The occlusion of suction and vent roller pumps is set when the tubing is fluid free by clamping the inlet tubing, starting the roller pump at moderate rpm and adjusting the degree of occlusion until the tubing in the roller pump just collapses. This is assessed visually or by hearing a "smacking" sound as the tubing in the pump repeatedly collapses as negative pressure is created and then released with rotation of the rollers. After setting the occlusion but before removing the inlet clamp, each roller should be stopped at three positions to verify that the tubing remains collapsed, thus ensuring occlusion. The response will depend on tubing wall thickness and type (polyvinyl chloride or silicone rubber). Suction pumps should then also be tested with water. If a suction or vent pump is nonocclusive, there is

a risk of air embolism should the cardiotomy reservoir become pressurized (16).

A conventional blood cardioplegia delivery pump contains two segments of tubing, one for blood and the other for the crystalloid component of cardioplegic solution. Because those tubes often have different diameters, setting the occlusion for this pump is more complex. The two segments of tubing are Y-ed together after the roller pump to deliver the mixed cardioplegic solution in the appropriate ratio (typically 4:1 blood to crystalloid). A shunt connecting both sets of tubing may be located before the pump to allow delivery of blood alone. The occlusion must be set to the segment of tubing with the smaller diameter, which necessitates that the larger blood-containing segment is just occlusive. Setting the appropriate occlusion can be accomplished by observing a slow drop and then cessation of fluid drop from a spiked bag of crystalloid solution when the delivery system is initially primed. This should be performed while recirculating fluid through the arterial/venous loop with the systemic flow pump so that the cardioplegia pump is under pressure. Like the method outlined earlier, each roller should be checked in three positions. Alternatively, the cardioplegia pump occlusion can be set by clamping the delivery line after the cardioplegia heat exchanger/bubble trap and slowly rotating the rollers to pressurize the system and then stopping the pump. If the occlusion is properly set, there will be no decline in pressure measured between the pump assembly and clamp.

Regardless of how the occlusion is set on the cardioplegia pump, a second way to assess proper occlusion is to verify that no fluid leaks past the roller pump and begins to fill the crystalloid bag when the systemic pump is rotating and the cardioplegia pump is stopped. When two tubing segments are placed in a single roller pump, it is important that both segments are approximately equal in length to avoid kinking, excessive stretching, or overriding of one segment upon the other, all of which can interfere with effective pump function.

Positioning the Pump and Arrangement of Lines

When the surgeon is ready to begin CPB, the heart–lung machine console is positioned near the operating table. Some surgeons prefer that the pump is placed opposite them, most often parallel to the table and on the patient's left side, whereas others prefer to have the pump positioned on the patient's right side directly behind the primary surgeon. Depending on other equipment in the room or institutional preference, the pump may also be positioned at an angle to the patient or at the foot of the table. Whatever the chosen position, the pump should be placed to minimize tubing lengths to the cannulation sites to decrease the required crystalloid priming volume and its commensurate hemodilution upon initiation of bypass.

Sterile pump lines are most often passed from the sterile surgical field to the perfusionist for connection to the CPB circuit, but alternatively the perfusionist may wear a sterile gown and gloves and pass the sterile lines to personnel at the operative field. The console position and line arrangement also should permit easy line identification and visualization and allow surgical personnel to move during the procedure without compromising operative field sterility or kinking the CPB lines. Sufficient lengths of tubing should be provided between the oxygenator, venous reservoir, and systemic blood pump to enable CPB component change-out or hand-cranking if they are required.

Pre-Cardiopulmonary Bypass Checklist

Between the times of pump assembly and cannulation for CPB, the primary perfusionist completes a pre-bypass checklist to verify proper assembly and function (17). Checklist formats include memorized, written, and automated types (18). The written type is most common and consists of items that are checked off a list sequentially. This exercise can be conducted as a "do-list" format in which the checklist item triggers a response as a series of tasks are performed or as a "done-list" whereby the task is either verified to have been completed or it is repeated. The redundancy incorporated into the second method increases the chance of the task being completed. The checklist procedure may be conducted either "silent," in which one person performs both the checklist and tasks, or it may be carried out as a "challenge and response" where either two people or one person and a computer prompt and then record task performance.

Checklists can be abbreviated or all inclusive. All-inclusive checklists tend to be long and are subject to misuse because of the demands of checking each item on a long list. Checklists are most effective if they contain only those items, which if omitted, would have a direct and adverse effect on the safe conduct of CPB. In aviation checklists, such items are referred to as "killer" items. Examples of such items in perfusion practice would be failure to securely connect the ventilating gas delivery line to the oxygenator, failure to properly set the occlusion on a roller pump, or assembly of vent tubing in a roller pump in the incorrect direction. Generic checklists have been published and promoted by the American Society of Extra-Corporeal Technology (AmSECT) (19) (Fig. 27.1), but in practice checklists are most often customized for specific hospital or surgeon protocol.

The sections of a checklist should include items related to: patient and procedure; sterility of CPB components; proper pump assembly and function; adequacy of electrical connections; adequacy of oxygenator ventilating gas supply; arrangement and integrity of CPB lines; composition of cardioplegic solution; testing and engagement of alarms; calibration and placement of monitors and probes; opera-

tional capacity of water supply system; verification of anticoagulation; and availability of backup supplies and equipment.

INITIATION OF BYPASS

Connection of Patient to Circuit

After administration of systemic heparin and verification that the patient is adequately anticoagulated, perfusate is recirculated through the CPB circuit one final time while the lines are tapped and inspected by the surgeon or an assistant to verify absence of any visible gas bubbles. Recirculation is stopped and the arterial and venous lines are then clamped at the pump and table. The surgeon or assistant divides the arterial/venous recirculation loop. Most often, the surgeon connects the arterial cannula first after securing it in the ascending aorta with purse-string sutures. After the cannula is filled retrograde with the patient's blood, an air-free connection is made between the CPB arterial flow line and the arterial cannula. Having the perfusionist slowly advance the perfusate by activating the systemic flow pump will facilitate an air-free connection; alternatively, an assistant can add sterile fluid from a syringe as the CPB line and cannula are joined. If the latter technique is used, the arterial flow line must be identified and distinguished from the venous drainage line to avoid the risk of reversed lines.

After removal of the arterial line clamp at the field, the perfusionist should manually palpate or observe pulsation on an arterial flow line pressure monitor. The pressure transmitted from the aortic cannula through the arterial flow line will reasonably ensure that the cannula has been placed in the lumen of the aorta (or other arterial site). Absence of adequate pulsation may indicate malposition or insertion of the cannula into the vessel wall that could lead to arterial wall hematoma or dissection upon initiation of CPB.

Fluid Balance and Circuit Priming Volume

It is often prudent to obtain an estimation of the patient's fluid balance from their time of arrival in the operating room by checking and recording the estimated blood loss, urine output, and volume of fluids administered by anesthesia personnel. Knowing the patient's estimated blood volume and hematocrit allows calculation of an estimated hematocrit after initiation of CPB. This will give the perfusionist and anesthesiologist some indication of CPB fluid or blood requirements.

To reduce circuit priming volume and the resultant hemodilution upon starting CPB, a technique called retrograde autologous priming has been introduced (20). After connecting the arterial line and cannula but before starting bypass, priming fluid can be removed from the circuit via a stopcock on the arterial filter or arterial sampling manifold

SUGGESTED PRE-BYPASS PERFUSION CHECKLIST

PLEASE NOTE: This pre-bypass checklist, or a reasonable equivalent, should be used before initiating cardiopulmonary bypass. This is a guideline which perfusionists are encouraged to modify to accommodate differences in circuit design and variations in institutional clinical practice. Users should refer to manufacturers' information for specific procedures and/or precautions. AmSECT disclaims any and all liability and responsibility for injury and damages resulting from following this suggested checklist.

Check when completed. Mark N/A where not applicable. Patient ID may be stamped in upper corner.

PATIENT
_____ Chart reviewed
_____ Procedure verified

STERILITY
_____ Components checked for package integrity/expiration date
_____ Heat exchanger(s) leak tested

PUMP
_____ Speed controls operational
_____ Roller heads smooth and quiet
_____ Occlusion(s) set
_____ Flow meter in correct direction and calibrated
_____ Flow rate indicator correct for patient and/or tubing size
_____ Holders secure

ELECTRICAL
_____ Power cord(s) securely connected

GAS SUPPLY
_____ Gas line securely connected
_____ Flow meter/blender functional
_____ Hoses leak-free
_____ Gas exhaust unobstructed

LINES/PUMP TUBING
_____ Connections secure
_____ Tubing direction traced and correct
_____ No kinks noted
_____ One-way valve(s) in correct direction
_____ Debubbled/leak free
_____ Patency of arterial line/cannula verified

CARDIOPLEGIA
_____ Solution checked
_____ System debubbled/leak free

SAFETY MECHANISMS
_____ Alarms operational and engaged
_____ Arterial filter/bubble trap debubbled
_____ Cardiotomy reservoir vented

MONITORING
_____ Temperature probes in place and calibrated
_____ Pump pressure monitors calibrated
_____ In-line and/or on-line sensors calibrated
_____ Oxygen analyzer calibrated

TEMPERATURE CONTROL
_____ Water source connected and functional

SUPPLIES
_____ Tubing clamps available
_____ Drugs available and properly labeled
_____ Solutions available
_____ Blood available
_____ Sampling syringes/laboratory tubes available

ANTI-COAGULATION
_____ Heparin time and dose verified
_____ Anticoagulation tested and reported

BACKUP
_____ Hand cranks available
_____ Emergency lighting available
_____ Duplicate circuit components available

COMMENTS:
_____
_____
_____
_____

SIGNED:_____

DATE:_____ TIME:_____

FIG. 27.1. Suggested pre-bypass perfusion checklist. (Courtesy American Society of Extra-Corporeal Technology, Herndon, VA.)

by allowing the patient's arterial blood to displace the crystalloid priming solution. This procedure can be accomplished relatively quickly while carefully monitoring the patient's hemodynamics. The volume of priming solution displaced in this manner is 200 to 600 mL.

Another method for reducing priming volume relies on vacuum-assisted venous drainage (21). After final pre-CPB recirculation, priming fluid in the venous line can be discarded or sequestered in a sterile intravenous bag for later administration on CPB, leaving the venous line devoid of fluid and containing only room air. When this technique is used, a clamp must remain in place on the venous cannula until immediately before starting bypass. Because the technique of vacuum-assisted venous drainage does not rely on gravity siphon drainage but instead on a regulated vacuum applied to a hard-shell venous reservoir, removal of the venous line clamp will allow the negative pressure created in the reservoir to actively withdraw venous blood from the patient upon initiation of CPB. This approach eliminates 400 to 1,000 mL of priming solution.

The anticipated result of these circuit prime reduction techniques is a higher hematocrit during CPB and a possible reduced need for administration of homologous blood after bypass (22). This exercise will fail to achieve this goal if the patient's blood volume is marginal before CPB, because ultimately this will present as a reduced blood level in the venous reservoir mandating the addition of crystalloid or blood. Reduction of the hyperdynamic response often seen after CPB has been reported when using minimal CPB priming volumes (23).

Establishing Extracorporeal Blood Flow

Upon instruction from the surgeon, CPB begins by removing the clamp(s) on the arterial line and activating the systemic pump speed control. If a centrifugal pump is used, the pump speed control should be increased to sufficient rpm to avoid retrograde flow before unclamping the arterial line because such retrograde flow has been associated with air entry into the arterial flow line from the aortic cannulation site (24).

The rationale for starting flow in the systemic pump before releasing the venous line clamp is to avoid exsanguinating the patient into the CPB circuit in the event of a pump malfunction. As the volume of perfusate in the CPB reservoir decreases, the venous line clamp or occluder is released (partially or totally depending on whether the surgeon wishes to maintain some cardiac ejection or have the heart immediately decompressed), allowing venous blood to flow into the CPB reservoir. Full CPB flow can be established in most cases within 30 seconds. Systemic flow is most often indexed to the patient body surface area (in m^2) or weight (in kg). Generally accepted indices are 2.2 to 2.4 L/min/m^2 or 50 to 65 mL/kg when normothermic or when cooling. Higher indices often are used in pediatric patients

or when rewarming the adult patient. Once the patient is hypothermic, these indices may be reduced proportionate to the degree of hypothermia because of decreased oxygen consumption (25) (see Blood Flow and Perfusion Pressure, below, and Chapters 12 and 30).

The arterial filter purge line stopcock is opened to provide a low-pressure vent for removal of any potential gas emboli in the systemic flow line. The volume of arterial blood shunted back into the venous reservoir or cardiotomy reservoir through such a purge is generally 150 to 300 mL/min but can be greater than 500 mL/min depending on purge line diameter and length and the arterial line pressure. By connecting the purge line to the cardiotomy reservoir, the volume flow per minute can be measured by clamping the cardiotomy drain line for 10 seconds, noting the volume rise in the reservoir, and then multiplying by 6 to get mL/min shunt flow. Although the effect of this shunt volume is generally insignificant in adults, it can be clinically important in infants or small children, potentially leading to hypoperfusion (26). Consequently, in the latter clinical scenario, the purge line is kept closed or only partially open with brief intermittent periods of unrestricted flow for purging.

Management of Gas Flow

Oxygenators from various manufacturers have different operating characteristics and the instructions for use should be followed for initial gas settings. The ventilating gas flow to the oxygenator is started just before or simultaneously with initiation of CPB. Once adequate oxygenation is verified by observing bright red blood or satisfactory in-line arterial PO_2 or S_vO_2 values, adjustments in gas flow and mixture are made. A useful technique for managing and assessing oxygenator ventilating gas flow settings is to express it in a ratio to the systemic blood flow. Typical gas-to-blood flow ratios with current membrane oxygenators are in the range 0.5 to 1.0:1, depending on patient size and temperature, S_vO_2, and desired arterial PCO_2 values.

Inhalational anesthetics may be delivered to the patient via the oxygenator ventilating gas if a vaporizer is mounted on the CPB console and placed in-line with the oxygenator ventilating gas, which can facilitate systemic blood pressure control in addition to maintaining anesthesia. It is important to mount vaporizers away from disposable circuit components because spilled volatile anesthetic fluid can structurally degrade plastics (27–29). Because incorporation of a vaporizer in the oxygenator ventilating gas line requires additional tubing connections, the integrity of the entire gas line should be verified before starting bypass by clamping the gas line just proximal to its junction with the oxygenator and running a gas flow sufficient to generate a measured gas line pressure of 40 cm H_2O, thus ensuring that this pressure can be maintained at minimal (e.g., less than 200 mL/min) gas flow (30). The controversial issue of blood gas management techniques (alpha-stat and pH-stat) during hypothermia is more fully discussed in Chapters 4 and Chapter 12.

Placement and Use of Vents and Cardioplegia Cannulae

The site of placement and use of vents is discussed more thoroughly in Chapter 6. All vents should be tested before use by briefly immersing the tip of the vent in a basin of saline or pool of blood at the operative site to verify its suctioning effect (Fig. 27.2). It is important to avoid excessive negative pressures, which can cause hemolysis. This may be accomplished by use of a one-way negative pressure relief valve in the vent line. Personnel at the operative field should also verify the direction of flow for correct placement of such valves. Sometimes a small-gauge needle is inserted in the vent line to relieve pressure; the necessity for placement of the needle in the proper (vent) line is extremely important.

Ideally, the perfusionist should be notified when vents are placed, and the surgeon should announce when they are needed for use. This is particularly important if the vent is placed in a nonroutine manner. Discontinuation and/or removal of the vent(s) also should be communicated to the perfusionist, because a significant portion of blood return to the CPB reservoir may be through a vent; thus, its removal may be accompanied by an abrupt decrease in the CPB reservoir level.

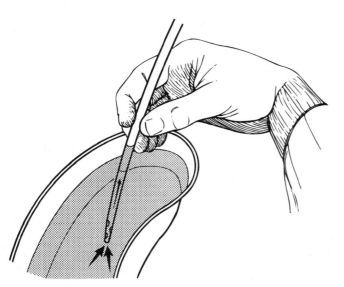

FIG. 27.2. Method for testing the vent before use. Alternatively, the vent tip may be placed in a pool of blood by the surgeon or assistant to verify proper suctioning before its insertion in the heart or vessels.

Operator Safety

Health risks to all open heart team members include percutaneous needle sticks, blade cuts or other exposures to blood, and back injuries. Of these, exposure to bloodborne pathogens represents the most serious risk. Cardiac surgery and CPB pose a high risk of blood exposure, and so-called universal precautions have been developed and promulgated (31) to decrease the risk of acquiring HIV and hepatitis B and C viruses. However, health care worker awareness and compliance with such precautions appears to be highly variable (32–36). According to a recent multicenter study involving surgeons (37), the lifetime risk of acquiring hepatitis B or C is far greater than that of acquiring HIV (30% to 40% versus 0.5%). The HIV seroconversion rate from a percutaneous needle stick is 0.2% to 0.5% (38). Because preoperative universal testing of patients is controversial and more expensive than practicing universal precautions (39), it is prudent for all who have patient contact during open heart surgery to adhere to universal precautions (40). These include the use of personal protective equipment (gloves, gowns, face masks, and eyeshields), avoidance of procedures such as recapping used needles, and proper disposal or cleaning of blood contaminated equipment after the CPB procedure.

MONITORING DURING BYPASS

Physiologic Variables

Because the CPB circuit and the patient's circulation are contiguous during bypass, circuit performance must be monitored and managed continuously to maintain adequate perfusion and organ system viability. Kirklin and Barratt-Boyes (41) distinguished between those physiologic variables under direct external control and other variables determined primarily by patient response. The first type include: total systemic blood flow; input pressure waveform; systemic venous pressure; hematocrit and composition of priming fluid; arterial blood oxygen, carbon dioxide, and nitrogen levels; and temperature of the perfusate and patient. The patient determines other variables, some of which are still, in part, determined by external control: systemic vascular resistance; total body oxygen consumption; mixed venous blood oxygen levels; lactic acidemia and pH; regional and organ blood flow; and organ function.

Monitoring physiologic function during CPB differs little in principle from normal intraoperative monitoring practices for surgical procedures of similar magnitude without CPB. Because CPB occupies only a portion of the total operative interval, management of patients for surgical procedures requiring CPB must include physiologic monitoring appropriate to the patient's condition in addition to the routine monitoring associated with all anesthetic procedures. For example, the pre- and post-CPB course for a patient undergoing a second aortocoronary bypass surgery with a left ventricular aneurysmectomy would be expected to be more complex than that for an otherwise healthy child undergoing closure of a secundum atrial septal defect. Accordingly, the intensity of physiologic monitoring should be based on patient condition, procedural requirements, and expected problems.

From a practical standpoint, in addition to monitoring patient blood pressures (including central venous [CVP], pulmonary artery [PA], and/or left atrial [LA]) and temperatures (including myocardium), the perfusionist and anesthesiologist should monitor the electrocardiogram (ECG) and, if used, the electroencephalogram (EEG). Both can warn of abnormal or unexpected conditions. For example, the development of cardiac electrical activity manifested by a slow but regular wide QRS waveform may indicate myocardial rewarming and inadequate cardioplegia and the need for another infusion of cardioplegic solution. Urine output should be monitored periodically during bypass as a relative indication of adequate perfusion. Blood coagulation status is also monitored throughout bypass (see Chapter 22). Most often a simple activated coagulation test is performed periodically depending on previous test results, patient temperature, or elapsed time. A less specific assessment should be made of patient neuromuscular blockade or anesthetic depth. Decreasing mixed $S_{\bar{v}}O_2$ or overt patient movement may indicate that additional anesthetic drugs are required.

Circuit Variables

Circuit parameters that should be continuously monitored by the perfusionist include the systemic blood flow by calibrated roller pump or by electronic flowmeter when using a centrifugal pump. Venous blood drainage to the CPB circuit is assessed indirectly by monitoring the volume of perfusate in the reservoir. The perfusionist should always be aware whether this blood volume is increasing (indicating venous or other blood return in excess of systemic blood flow), decreasing (indicating the reverse situation), or relatively stable. Awareness of the rate of rise or fall of volume in the reservoir should be anticipated so that appropriate changes in systemic blood flow can be made in a timely manner before a dangerously low volume situation occurs. It has been suggested that the venous reservoir volume should be equal to 25% of the systemic blood flow (L/min) to allow for a 15-second reaction time (42). Recommendations from device manufacturers on minimum blood levels for safe operation to avoid entrainment of air should be considered as well. Figure 27.3 shows reaction times for various reservoir blood volumes at different blood flow rates.

The perfusionist should try to anticipate the surgeon's needs during bypass (43) not only by being aware of CPB circuit function and the various monitored patient parameters, but also by the progression of the operation and activity and movements of personnel at the sterile field. It is

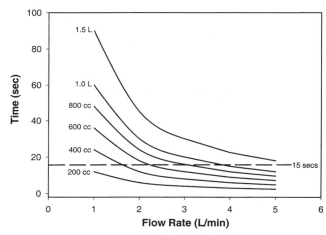

FIG. 27.3. Reaction times with various CPB reservoir volumes. Each curve depicts decreasing reservoir volume plotted as a function of flow rate and time (in seconds) in the event there is a cessation in venous drainage. As the flow rate is increased, the perfusionist's time to make an appropriate reduction in CPB systemic flow is reduced. The *dashed horizontal line* shows the flow rate that should not be exceeded for a given reservoir volume to maintain 15 seconds' reaction time.

useful to establish a pattern of continuous scanning of CPB functions and monitors and the activities of other personnel in the operating room. Distractions and interruptions extraneous to patient management during CPB can lead to errors. In this regard, the perfusionist would be well advised to adopt a "curious and suspicious" attitude any time CPB is being used. This is a philosophy practiced by many airplane pilots to anticipate and avoid potential problems (44) (see Chapter 28).

The perfusionist adjusts the flow and composition of ventilating gas to the oxygenator in response to changing patient temperature and blood gas results. This gas flow is monitored by an in-line flowmeter and oxygen monitor, which should have adjustable upper and lower alarm settings. Inhalational anesthetics, if used, should be scavenged via suction from the oxygenator exhaust port, and the degree of suction applied should be regulated to avoid problems with oxygenator gas transfer (45,46) or air embolism (47). Pressure transducers or aneroid gauges on the systemic blood flow line can warn of arterial cannula malposition or kinks in the arterial line. Some CPB consoles are servoregulated to stop designated roller pumps if a preset line pressure is exceeded. Measuring pre- and postmembrane oxygenator blood pressures allows calculation of pressure drop and may warn of oxygenator failure (48).

Control over patient cooling and warming rates requires the perfusionist to monitor a variety of temperatures, including arterial blood, venous blood, and water sources for the oxygenator and cardioplegia delivery system. Induction and reversal of hypothermia should be guided by maintenance of an 8 to 12°C gradient between the arterial blood and patient temperature when cooling and between the venous blood and heat exchanger water source when rewarming to avoid the potential for free gas to come out of solution (49). It is advisable to monitor at least two patient temperatures (e.g., bladder, nasopharyngeal, tympanic, rectal, and/or esophageal) in the event there is a probe failure or malposition (50). There also should be some periodic assessment of the adequacy of water flow to the oxygenator's heat exchanger and cardioplegia delivery system, which can be assessed by listening to the flow and monitoring the water temperature. Cerebral hyperthermia (51,52) should be avoided by careful monitoring of patient and blood temperatures and by not allowing the perfusate temperature to exceed 37.5°C when on total CPB and 38°C when on partial CPB with reestablishment of pulmonary blood flow.

Suction pump speed should be regulated to achieve adequate blood and/or air removal without excessive pump speed that can cause the lines to "chatter" or obstruct, potentially resulting in hemolysis. Likewise, when a roller pump is used for a vent, its speed must be regulated to prevent possible air embolism, which can occur with high negative pulmonary venous pressures that can pull air across the alveolar membranes (16)

The next section presents a more detailed discussion of physiologic aspects of patient monitoring commonly used to assess abnormalities produced specifically by CPB.

PHYSIOLOGIC RESPONSE

Cardiovascular Monitoring

Systemic Blood Flow and Perfusion Pressure

Maintenance of cardiovascular stability during CPB requires the obvious interplay of machine (CPB) function for blood flow and patient factors such as systemic vascular resistance and venous compliance. Yet despite the ease of blood flow control and the sophisticated pharmacologic agents available for manipulation of vascular smooth muscle tone, there is no uniformly accepted standard for either CPB systemic blood flow rate or perfusion pressure. Any discussion of optimum flow rates and perfusion pressure during CPB should be based on an understanding of oxygen consumption, blood flow distribution, and intrinsic autoregulatory capability of specific vascular beds.

Fortunately, in some of these areas a reasonable body of knowledge has developed over the nearly 50-year history of clinical CPB. Unfortunately, there are large gaps in the data. For example, clinically the regional distribution of blood flow during hypothermic CPB and the regional vascular autoregulatory capability remain relatively poorly understood, with some notable exceptions as discussed below.

Oxygen Consumption

Minute oxygen consumption ($\dot{V}O_2$) is the major determinant of blood flow requirement normally and during CPB.

The well-known Fick equation describes $\dot{V}O_2$ in the readily understandable and clinically measurable terms of cardiac output and arteriovenous oxygen content difference.

$$\dot{V}O_2 = \dot{Q} \, (C_{a-\bar{v}})O_2$$

where $C_{(a-\bar{v})}O_2$ (1.34) (Hb) + $(P_{(a-\bar{v})}O_2)$ (0.0031) and $\dot{V}O_2$ = minute oxygen consumption (ml·min^{-1}), $\dot{Q}$ = cardiac output (liter·min^{-1}). Also, Hb is the hemoglobin concentration (g·liter^{-1}), 1.34 = hemoglobin oxygen content (ml O_2·gm^{-1}) at 100% saturation (ml·g^{-1}), $S_{(a-\bar{v})}O_2$ = arteriovenous hemoglobin oxygen saturation difference (ml·liter^{-1}), $P_{(a-\bar{v})}O_2$ = arteriovenous oxygen partial pressure difference (mm Hg), and 0.0031 = solubility of oxygen in blood (ml O_2·mm Hg^{-1}·100 ml blood^{-1}, at 37°C) increased by hypothermia.

Thus, knowledge of $\dot{V}O_2$ allows reasonable prediction of effective blood flow requirement during CPB for any given level of hemoglobin concentration (hemodilution) and arteriovenous oxygen content difference (oxygen extraction). Two important caveats apply to this simplistic approach. First, there is a requirement for accurate knowledge of $\dot{V}O_2$ and second, the key phrase is "effective flow."

Determinants of $\dot{V}O_2$

Total systemic $\dot{V}O_2$ is primarily a function of age, size (body surface area or lean body mass), and temperature. In the newborn infant, $\dot{V}O_2$ in proportion to body weight is approximately twice that of the average adult (8 versus 4 mL/kg/min). This proportion rises over the first 2 months of life to a peak of 9 to 10 mL/kg/min. Thereafter, there is an exponential decline in $\dot{V}O_2$ per unit mass, as age increases, which parallels the change in cardiac index with age. The relationship between $\dot{V}O_2$ and size is similar to that for $\dot{V}O_2$ and age in that as body mass increases (beyond an age of approximately 6 months), the $\dot{V}O_2$ per unit mass actually decreases. The influence of temperature on $\dot{V}O_2$ is

---

* The precise value for the hemoglobin oxygen content of whole blood at 100% saturation is not definitely known and may not be a constant. Pure hemoglobin in solution (molecular weight 64,458) can combine with 1.39 mL of O_2 per gram, but whole blood contains other hemoglobin subtypes such as methemoglobin, carboxyhemoglobin, and so forth that decrease the net oxygen-carrying capacity (53,54). The value of 1.34 is commonly cited, but in fact one study has shown that 1.306 mL O_2 per gram hemoglobin was the most applicable number clinically (55).

** There is disagreement regarding the declining cardiac output with increasing age that may also apply to the relationship of $\dot{V}O_2$ to increasing age. Early studies demonstrated a clear inverse relationship between increasing age and cardiac output (56). However, the study populations were unselected and the increasing prevalence of cardiovascular disease with advancing age makes the interpretation of the data unclear. More recent studies have confirmed the earlier data for sedentary individuals but show well-preserved cardiac function, including cardiac output, in physically fit elderly persons free of overt cardiovascular disease (57,58).

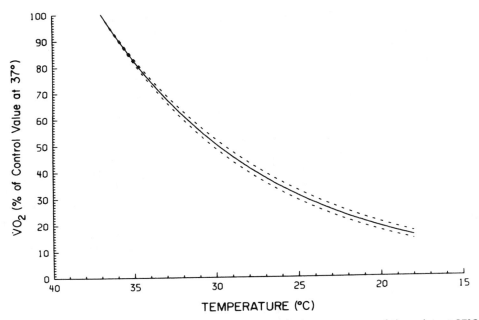

FIG. 27.4. Relationship between oxygen consumption ($\dot{V}O_2$), as a percent of the value at 37°C, and body temperature. The *dotted lines* show the 70% confidence limits. (From Kirklin JW, Barratt-Boyes BG. *Cardiac surgery*, 2nd ed. Vol. 1. New York: Churchill Livingstone, 1993:64, with permission.)

fully discussed in Chapter 12. In the present context it is important to remember that the relation is nonlinear and $\dot{V}O_2$ approaches a minimum of 10% to 15% of the normothermic value at approximately 15°C (Fig. 27.4). Importantly however, this decline in $\dot{V}O_2$ with decreasing temperature may not be the same in all organs. For example, the duration of "safe" circulatory arrest time at 18°C is 45 to 60 minutes regarding neurologic outcome, yet for renal function at 18°C the safe limit is significantly longer. The transplantation literature would suggest even longer "circulatory arrest'" times for transplanted organs (4 to 5 hours for the heart, 24 or more hours for the kidney and the liver), recognizing of course that graft organs are stored at more profound levels of hypothermia (less than 4°C) than are clinically applied in CPB. However, factors other than decreased $\dot{V}O_2$—for example, variable, tissue-specific tolerance for hypoxia—may also contribute to the variability of safe arrest time in different organs maintained at the same temperature.

Effective Flow

During CPB, effective blood flow is blood flow from the oxygenator that actually results in tissue perfusion. It must be understood that arterial blood aspirated from the surgical field represents a loss of effective flow from total CPB flow. In this context, all physiologic and anatomic shunting of arterialized blood around capillary beds to the venous circulation also detracts from effective perfusion. For example,

bronchial blood flow, which is normally the major component of "physiologic" right-to-left shunting of blood (2% to 4% of cardiac output), may be significantly increased in certain congenital lesions associated with decreased pulmonary arterial blood flow and correspondingly increased pulmonary collateral blood flow. In adults with significant chronic obstructive lung disease, bronchial blood flow may also be significantly increased. At a total flow rate of 4 to 5 L/min during CPB, this physiologic shunting may normally be 250 to 500 mL/min that is lost from effective systemic perfusion and pathologic increases in bronchial or pulmonary collateral flow may substantially increase that amount of lost effective blood flow.

Left atrial, left ventricular, or aortic root vents are another common source of loss of effective flow. Blood returned to the oxygenator from these vent lines is lost from effective systemic perfusion. Parenthetically, the requirement for such vents is largely created by the existence of physiologic and anatomic shunts. Finally, if the microcirculation is inhomogenously perfused, for example because of an increased interstitial fluid compartment either locally or systemically, then the net result is an increased effective diffusion distance for oxygen from the capillaries to the cells that results in a loss of effective perfusion. Thus, determination of effective blood flow is not altogether straightforward, and it may be at times significantly less than total CPB systemic output.

Organ Autoregulation

Autoregulation of blood flow to various organ vascular beds during CPB obviously pertains to any discussion of blood flow rate and perfusion pressure requirements during CPB. Physiologically, autoregulation of blood flow refers to the ability of organ vasculature, through neural, chemical, and direct smooth muscle effects, to regulate local resistance to maintain relatively constant flow despite significant changes in perfusion pressure (59). This capability is preserved in some organ vascular beds during CPB despite the superimposition of a nonpulsatile flow pattern, hemodilution, and hypothermia. For example, Govier et al. (60), Prough et al. (61), and Murkin et al. (62) independently examined cerebral blood flow responsiveness to changed perfusion pressure and carbon dioxide tension during CPB. The conclusion from these studies is that CO_2 responsiveness of the cerebral vasculature is maintained during CPB even at 20°C. Also, autoregulation of cerebral blood flow to changes in perfusion pressure is preserved during CPB and the response curve may even be shifted to the left, indicating a decrease of the autoregulatory pressure threshold from the normal of about 50 mm Hg to approximately 30 mm Hg. As discussed by Thomson (63), this lowering of the pressure threshold for autoregulation is linked to the decreased cerebral metabolic rate for oxygen produced by hypothermia. The cerebral perfusion pressure intercept with the maximal vasodilation blood flow line would be expected to be lower as temperature decreases if blood flow and metabolic rate remain coupled during hypothermia, as has been shown by Murkin et al. (62) for alpha-stat pH management (Fig. 27.5). Others have shown in animal studies that cerebral blood flow during moderate hypothermia is primarily regu-lated by arterial blood pressure and not CPB systemic flow rate (64).

The effect of CPB on autoregulation in other organs is clinically less well documented. Likewise, the effect of CPB on distribution of blood flow to (and within) specific organs requires further study in humans despite nearly 50 years of clinical experience and many millions of cases with CPB, as well as a substantial experimental data base. Experimentally, with systemic blood flow in the range of 2.0 to 2.5 $L/min/m^2$, systemic blood flow distribution remains essentially normal (65). Experimentally, hypothermia during CPB is associated with altered local $\dot{V}O_2$, and the associated change in vascular resistance tends to promote regional blood flow distribution in proportion to the local $\dot{V}O_2$ produced by hypothermia.

Monitoring Perfusion Adequacy

Systemic measurements that may indicate the adequacy of total blood flow relative to total $\dot{V}O_2$ during CPB include $S_{\bar{v}}O_2$, pH, and lactate concentration. The latter two are closely linked because accumulation of lactic acid in blood leads to hydrogen ion accumulation through dissociation ($CH_3CHOHCOOH \leftrightarrow CH_3CHOHCOO^- + H^+$). However, there are other sources of hydrogen ion production during oxygen (blood flow) deprivation such as ongoing glycolysis (anaerobic glucose metabolism) and continued adenosine triphosphate hydrolysis, both of which produce a net accumulation of hydrogen ion.

Measurement of hemoglobin oxygen saturation in the venous blood (or venous oxygen partial pressure) during CPB has the same significance as the corresponding PA (mixed venous) measurement during normal circulation.

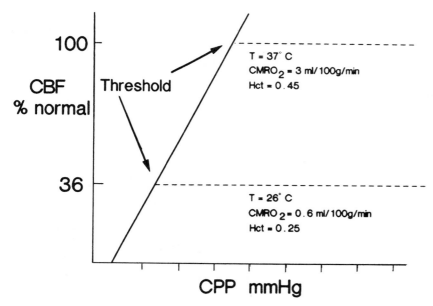

FIG. 27.5. Theoretic effect of hypothermic bypass on the autoregulatory threshold. The *solid line* is the pressure flow relation for the maximally vasodilated state. The autoregulatory threshold is the point where the autoregulatory plateau (represented by the *dashed lines*) intersects the maximal vasodilation pressure flow relation. Given maintained coupling between cerebral metabolic rate and blood flow, a decreased metabolic rate such as that produced by hypothermia will effectively produce a leftward shift of the autoregulatory threshold (*lower dashed line, solid line intersection*). *CBF*, cerebral blood flow; *CPP*, cerebral perfusion pressure. (From Murkin JM, Farrar JK, Tweed A, et al. Cerebral autoregulation and flow/metabolism coupling during cardiopulmonary bypass: the influence of carbon dioxide. *Anesth Analg* 1987;61:825, with permission.)

Given steady-state conditions of hemoglobin concentration, P_{50} (primarily a function of 2,3-diphosphoglyceric acid concentration, temperature, and pH) and arterial oxygenation and then $S_{\bar{v}}O_2$ will change in direct proportion to systemic blood flow at constant $\dot{V}O_2$. Unfortunately, the inverse relationship between $S_{\bar{v}}O_2$ and $\dot{V}O_2$ (predictable from the Fick equation) confounds the simple interpretation of $S_{\bar{v}}O_2$ data. For example, if blood flow and arterial oxygen content are held constant, then $S_{\bar{v}}O_2$ will increase as $\dot{V}O_2$ decreases (66). In the case of a capillary bed that is hypoperfused relative to the local level of $\dot{V}O_2$, the contribution to the systemic $S_{\bar{v}}O_2$ (or pH or lactic acid concentration, for that matter) is a function of the ratio between systemic blood flow volume and the local area blood flow volume. Importantly, an intense hypoxic insult in a focal area of considerable clinical importance (e.g., brain, heart, kidney) may well not produce a major change in $S_{\bar{v}}O_2$. Accordingly, although monitoring $S_{\bar{v}}O_2$ during CPB is a common practice, a normal or increased $S_{\bar{v}}O_2$ value during CPB does not ensure that the CPB systemic blood flow is necessarily meeting regional oxygen delivery (DO_2) requirements. However, a low $S_{\bar{v}}O_2$ during CPB does indicate a problem with systemic DO_2 that may be due to insufficient blood flow, hemoglobin function or concentration, arterial oxygenation, or excessive oxygen consumption due to inadequate anesthesia or hyperthermia.

Relationship Between Perfusion and O_2 Consumption

One method for individualizing blood flow volume relative to $\dot{V}O_2$ during CPB was termed oxygen consumption plateauing by its original describers, Mandl and Motley (67). Using this method, $\dot{V}O_2$ is calculated during CPB and the perfusion is increased until there is no further increase in $\dot{V}O_2$, the $\dot{V}O_2$ plateau. Perfusion is then maintained at this level until an intervention occurs that would be expected to alter $\dot{V}O_2$, for example rewarming, at which point the plateau must be reestablished. One theoretic advantage to this technique is that it calls attention to variables other than flow that have an effect on $\dot{V}O_2$. For example, pharmacologic manipulation of perfusion pressure, if excessive vasoconstriction or vasodilation exist, may improve $\dot{V}O_2$, presumably by improving perfusion to previously under perfused areas. The concept then becomes one of $\dot{V}O_2$ optimization.

The chief difficulty of the technique is the lack of a gold standard against which to compare any given clinical $\dot{V}O_2$ calculation during CPB. The steady-state awake or anesthetized pre-bypass value may be calculated and used as the baseline for CPB, when corrected for the expected temperature effect, but using the uncorrected awake $\dot{V}O_2$ as the baseline would yield excess perfusion during CPB. The anesthetized, paralyzed, mechanically ventilated patient has a substantially lower $\dot{V}O_2$ than the awake patient. Another difficulty is that clinically there is not as clear a plateau to $\dot{V}O_2$ as would be theoretically predicted. Parolari et al. (68)

have further studied $\dot{V}O_2$ and the influence of hemodynamics during CPB in 101 patients managed with conventional systemic flow indices (2.4 L/min/m² during cooling and rewarming and 2.0 L/min/m² when hypothermic at 28 to 30°C). There was a direct relationship between DO_2 and $\dot{V}O_2$ during the three phases of bypass. During cooling, there was no relationship between $\dot{V}O_2$ and either mean arterial pressure or peripheral vascular resistance, but during warming these parameters were inversely related; hence, lower mean arterial pressure and peripheral vascular resistance values were associated with higher $\dot{V}O_2$. This may be attributable to the natural tendency for patients to vasodilate as they rewarm. They could not demonstrate a plateau effect in any patient but acknowledged that only a narrow range of CPB flows and deliveries was used. They recommended higher CPB systemic flows during all phases of CPB but particularly during rewarming to achieve an optimal whole body oxygen metabolism. Optimization of $\dot{V}O_2$ during CPB may provide the best means of assessing adequacy of perfusion during CPB; however, this represents an untested hypothesis, at least as measured against the standard of clinical outcome.

Flow Recommendations

What then are reasonable flow recommendations for CPB? In adults at normothermia, progressive acidosis and increased lactate production are seen with total flows less than 1.6 L/min/m² or 50 mL/kg/min (69,70). Clinical and experimental data support a total flow of 1.8 L/min/m² as predictive of the $\dot{V}O_2$ plateau in normothermic adults (71,72). Kirklin and Barratt-Boyes (73) recommended a flow of 2.2 L/min/m² in adults 28°C or warmer. In patients greater than 2.0 m², a systemic flow of 1.8 to 2.0 L/min/m² is recommended to avoid excessively high flows through the CPB circuit that can increase blood damage and lessen the perfusionist's reaction time. During hypothermia, various nomograms have been proposed (Fig. 27.6) that predominantly rely on the plateauing of $\dot{V}O_2$ to indicate overall adequacy of perfusion for any given temperature. The recommended flow in infants and children is higher at 2.5 L/min/m². Kern et al. (74) delineated minimum flow rates of 30 mL/kg/min at 18°C and 30 to 35 mL/kg/min at 27 to 28°C in pediatric patients for maintenance of adequate cerebral blood flow and unaltered cerebral oxygen consumption using xenon-133 clearance methods.

Perfusion Pressure and Vascular Resistance

Perfusion (arterial) pressure during CPB, like blood flow, remains a topic of some controversy in the management of CPB. In general, blood flow probably outweighs perfusion pressure as a guide to adequacy of perfusion during CPB, especially with hemodilution, but solid data supporting this contention are lacking. In a prospective randomized study investigating outcomes, Gold et al. (75) reported that maintenance of higher perfusion pressures in the range 80 to

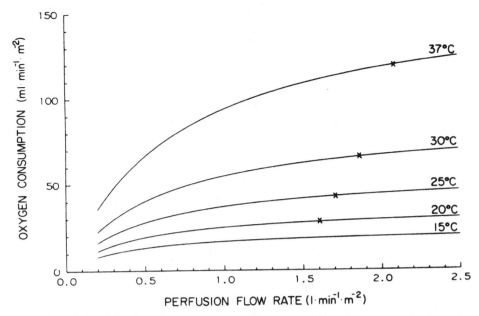

FIG. 27.6. Relationship of oxygen consumption ($\dot{V}o_2$) to perfusion flow rate and temperature. The small *X*s represent commonly clinically used flow rates at the various temperatures. (From Kirklin JW, Barratt-Boyes BG. *Cardiac surgery*, 2nd ed. Vol. 1. New York: Churchill Livingstone, 1993:91, with permission.)

100 mm Hg (actually achieving a mean perfusion pressure of 70 mm Hg) using flow indices of 1.9 to 2.3 L/min/m² and vasoactive drugs was associated with a reduced combined incidence of cardiac and neurologic complications when compared with patients whose pressures were maintained at 50 to 60 mm Hg. Perfusion pressure is determined by the interaction of blood flow and overall arterial impedance. Impedance, in this case, is primarily related to actual friction resistance because the steady-state nonpulsatile nature of most CPB largely negates the elastance, inertial, and reflection components that influence aortic input impedance during pulsatile flow. Friction resistance is primarily a function of the vasomotor tone (cross-sectional area of the arterial system) and blood viscosity. Viscosity, in turn, is a function of temperature (see Chapter 12) and the degree of hemodilution (see Chapter 11). The interaction of temperature and hematocrit with regard to viscosity is depicted graphically in Figure 27.7.

For any given level of hematocrit, viscosity (and therefore resistance to blood flow) increases substantially as temperature decreases. Normal viscosity at 37°C and a hematocrit of 40% approximates that seen at 25°C with hematocrit of 25%. This relationship indicates the importance of hemodilution in CPB, especially with hypothermia. With the onset of CPB, using an asanguineous prime solution there is an immediate fall in systemic vascular resistance that is not seen with a blood prime (Fig. 27.8). This drop in resistance with the onset of CPB is primarily due to the acute decrease in viscosity produced by the hemodilution from the prime

solution (76). Fortunately, this usually transient hypotension appears to have little clinical effect.

A more complex phenomenon pertaining to perfusion pressure during CPB is the increasing vascular resistance seen over time. Because of the third space equilibration of crystalloid prime solutions and the hemoconcentrating effect of the diuresis commonly seen during CPB, the initial drop in viscosity is corrected as the excess crystalloid is removed from the vasculature. Add to this the physical increase in viscosity produced by even moderate hypothermia (Fig. 27.7) and it would seem attractive to accept that viscosity change accounts for both the precipitous drop in vascular resistance with the onset of CPB and the steady increase of resistance over time during CPB. However, even if temperature and blood composition (viscosity) are held constant during CPB, calculated vascular resistance still increases with time (76).

The increase in circulating catecholamines that occurs during CPB is well documented and is to some extent modifiable by the type and depth of the anesthetic, but there remains in most clinical circumstances a significant increase in plasma catecholamines during CPB (77,78). This catecholamine release is but one manifestation of a major stress response elicited by CPB (see Chapters 15 and 17). It is likely that the additive vasomotor effects of circulating catecholamines and other vasoactive mediators of the stress response are responsible for the increased vascular resistance found during and after CPB. Indirect evidence that reflex sympathetic neural activation may also play a role in this

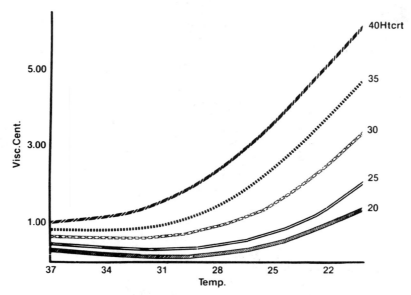

FIG. 27.7. Changes in viscosity of human blood measured *in vitro* with varying temperatures and hematocrit (*Htcrt*). (From Robicsek F, Masters TN, Niesluchowski W, et al. Vasomotor activity during cardiopulmonary bypass. In: Utley JR, ed. *Pathophysiology and techniques of cardiopulmonary bypass*. Baltimore: Williams & Wilkins, 1983:6, with permission.)

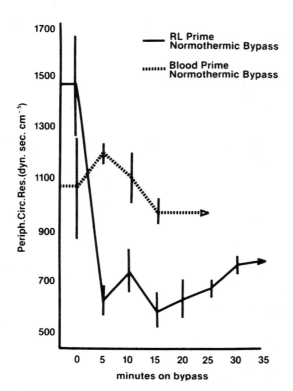

FIG. 27.8. Changes in circulatory resistance comparing data from 15 patients undergoing normothermic bypass with a crystalloid prime (*solid line*) to 8 patients undergoing normothermic bypass with a blood prime. *RL*, Ranger's lactate solution. (From Robiscek F, Masters TN, Niesluchowski W, et al. Vasomotor activity during cardiopulmonary bypass. In: Utley JR, ed. *Pathophysiology and techniques of cardiopulmonary bypass*. Baltimore: Williams & Wilkins, 1983:4, with permission.)

response is provided by the observation that unilateral stellate ganglion blockade ameliorates the hypertensive response after CPB (79).

Arterial Pressure Measurement Artifacts

Another practical point regarding perfusion pressure during and immediately after CPB is the relatively common occurrence of significant measurement artifacts. Especially when hypothermia has been used during CPB, a significant underestimation of central aortic pressure is seen in measured radial artery pressures, sometimes by as much as 30% to 40%. This is counter to the normal state where actual radial artery systolic pressure exceeds central aortic pressure by 10% to 15% or more, largely due to the amplification of effects of pressure waves reflected from the periphery (80).

This artifact is associated with rewarming at the end of CPB and often continues for 30 minutes or more into the post-CPB interval. The physiologic cause of the artifact is not completely understood. In the past, persistent vasoconstriction was often stated to be the cause. However, sufficient proximal conductance vessel constriction to dampen the radial pressure is unlikely, and the effect of distal constriction should be an enhancement of the normal gradient. A more likely explanation is that rewarming initiates uneven vasodilation and intense skeletal muscle vasodilation in the forearm and hand may have the effect of a large arteriovenous shunt, thereby decreasing the pressure measured at the radial artery (81). The final solution to this interesting puzzle remains. But the important clinical message is that apparent hypotension, as measured at the radial artery, at the conclusion of CPB should be confirmed, preferably by a central aortic or femoral arterial pressure measurement, before instituting inotropic or vasoconstrictor therapy. This is easily accomplished using an 18- or 20-gauge needle with pressure tubing connected to a transducer. As an alternative, use of a Doppler probe placed over the brachial artery in conjunction with an ordinary blood pressure cuff and manometer may provide more accurate measurement of arterial pressure than an indwelling radial artery catheter in this situation.

Other common causes of low pressure artifact from the radial artery measurement include surgical retraction and patient size. Significantly obese patients positioned with their arms tucked to the sides will frequently have enough tissue compression of the axillary artery to cause dampening of the radial artery waveform. Even with nonobese patients, this positioning coupled with aggressive use of a sternal retractor for internal mammary artery dissection can lead to axillary artery compression and radial artery waveform dampening. For completeness, the potential disaster of aortic dissection must be mentioned (see Chapter 28 for further discussion). A sudden precipitous drop of radial artery pressure (either left or right, but more classically left) coincident with the onset of CPB should at least raise the question of aortic dissection caused by aortic cannula malposition at the onset of perfusion. Fortunately, the associated findings of a tensely distended aorta with obvious intramural hematoma formation are sufficiently pronounced to make the diagnosis of the problem relatively straightforward. Unfortunately, the treatment of the problem is substantially more complex (see Chapter 34).

Less common, but of equal or greater importance, is the artifact of radial artery pressure measurement during CPB caused by inappropriate aortic perfusion cannula placement so that the flow of blood out of the cannula is directed preferentially into one of the great vessels of the aortic arch. The artifact produced is a high and very pulsatile radial arterial pressure when the radial catheter is ipsilateral to the inadvertent cannulation in the case of either the innominate or left subclavian artery (Fig. 27.9). Another clinical sign of this same complication is lateralized blanching of the face with the onset of CPB in the case of the left carotid artery perfusion (82). The clinical problem presented is one of gross hyperperfusion of the cerebral arterial system leading to cerebral edema or frank neurologic injury and also the probability of significant systemic hypoperfusion. Awareness of the potential problem by perfusionists, surgeons, and anesthesiologists coupled with vigilance for these signs is the key to preventing this potential disaster.

Pulmonary Artery and Left Atrial Pressure Monitoring

Both PA and LA pressure monitoring have a major role in clinical care decisions in cardiac surgical patients. The most important components of this role are found in the pre-

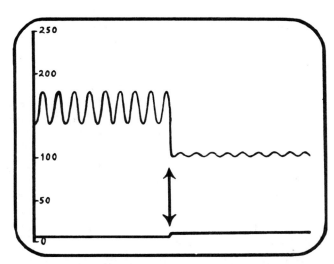

FIG. 27.9. Left radial artery pressure waveform during cardiopulmonary bypass. The high pulsatile pressure is due to the arterial cannula inadvertently directed into the left subclavian system. At the *arrow*, the cannula was redirected into the aortic lumen. (From McCleskey CH, Cheney FW. A correctable complication of cardiopulmonary bypass. *Anesthesiology* 1982;36:214–216, with permission.)

and post-CPB intervals, and both measurements feature prominently in decisions regarding weaning from CPB (see Chapter 29). However, both monitors can be useful during CPB. The LA pressure and, less directly, PA pressure give the same information regarding left ventricular filling during CPB as off CPB. But rather than the usual clinical context of using the measured LA or PA pressure to guide the adjustment of ventricular filling to appropriate physiologic levels, during CPB the expectation is that both PA and LA pressures should be near zero and the monitoring is used to prevent overdistension of the left ventricle. For example, a patient with markedly increased bronchial blood flow due to chronic lung disease or cyanotic congenital heart disease can markedly overdistend the left ventricle if venting is not adequate. Another example is the patient with aortic valve insufficiency. As left ventricular emptying decreases (on CPB and cooling) or stops (on CPB with fibrillation), massive overdistension can rapidly result from blood flow through the incompetent aortic valve. During ventricular fibrillation, surgical manipulation of the heart can result in significant incompetence of even an anatomically normal aortic valve. In most cases, this type of abnormal filling of the left ventricle during CPB can be detected by monitoring either the LA or PA pressure. Importantly, however, because of compliance variation among patients, there is no quantitative predictability of left ventricular volume based on LA or PA pressure. Therefore, one should expect near zero pressures and be wary of any increase during CPB.

As with radial artery catheter pressure measurement, one must be aware of measurement artifacts during CPB in LA and PA pressures. Both LA and PA catheters can be inadvertently kinked or obstructed; LA catheters are more vulnerable to inadvertent dislodgment than are PA catheters, but both are vulnerable. There is a tendency during CPB for a PA catheter that has been properly positioned in the pre-bypass period to migrate distally into the PA by 3 to 5 cm or more as blood volume is taken from the right ventricle into the venous reservoir and the heart empties with initiation of CPB. This can produce a "permanent wedge" phenomenon that has been implicated in PA rupture or pulmonary infarction. Often this malposition is indicated by a distinct increase in the PA pressure reading or $S_{\bar{v}}O_2$ in the case of an oximeter PA catheter. This malposition is sufficiently predictable that it may be clinically prudent to arbitrarily withdraw the PA catheter by 3 to 5 cm at the commencement of CPB. The routine use of a catheter introducer and a sterile protective sheath allows sterile repositioning of the PA catheter at the end of CPB. Some experienced clinicians recommend withdrawal of the PA catheter further, into the superior vena cava (SVC), during CPB. However, refloating the PA catheter at the end of CPB is not always easily accomplished, and difficulty is most likely in the low output management problems where the PA catheter is most useful. Despite the seemingly sound arguments for withdrawing the PA catheter during CPB, it has not been conclusively shown that this practice decreases the already small incidence of PA catheter-induced PA rupture.

CVP measurement is also helpful in guiding clinical decisions during CPB. As with LA and PA pressures, the expectation is that pressure in the vena cava [both SVC and inferior vena cava (IVC)] should be at or near zero or even slightly negative during CPB. In contrast to LA and PA pressure increase, an increased SVC or IVC pressure is not usually associated with cardiac distension. Rather, the increased CVP indicates impaired venous drainage to the venous reservoir due to either venous cannulas of insufficient size, malpositioned venous cannulas, venous cannulas or drainage line obstruction, or insufficient height differential between the heart and the venous reservoir to promote an adequate siphon effect.

The major adverse physiologic effect of elevated venous pressure during CPB is a reduction in effective perfusion pressure for critical organs such as brain, kidneys, and abdominal viscera and an enhanced tendency for edema production. For example, if the mean arterial pressure is 60 mm Hg during CPB and if SVC and IVC pressures are near zero, then the brain, the kidneys, and the splanchnic arterial bed have an effective perfusion pressure of 60 mm Hg. However, if SVC or IVC pressure is elevated to 20 mm Hg, for example, then the net perfusion pressure in these same areas is only 40 mm Hg and the increased back pressure will promote accumulation of edema. From this perspective, the liver is theoretically particularly vulnerable because approximately 75% of hepatic blood flow occurs at

venous pressure via the portal vein. An elevated venous outflow pressure (i.e., IVC pressure) could theoretically have a major adverse effect on hepatic blood flow during bypass.

It is important to recognize that SVC and IVC pressures are not necessarily equal during CPB even with a single two-stage venous drainage cannula. Moreover, there is little visible evidence of IVC engorgement with a median sternotomy incision. Especially with cardiac retraction and a single two-stage venous cannula, it is common to have venous drainage impairment and an increased measured CVP. Venous pressure measurement is also subject to significant artifact during bypass. For example, during total CPB (bicaval cannulation with tourniquets around the cavae), the venous catheter may be entrapped in the tourniquet. If the venous catheter is occluded, the constant flush infusion device on the transducer will rapidly overpressurize the transducer. On the other hand, if the catheter remains patent and passes beyond the tourniquet, then, with the heart open, an artifactually low venous pressure will be measured. In this situation, SVC and IVC pressure can each vary independently. A further CVP measurement artifact, not specific for CPB, is produced when the pressure port of a PA catheter remains within the lumen of the introducer sheath, then an infusion into the sheath via the sidearm can produce a pressure in excess of SVC pressure that is measured at the right atrial port of the PA catheter (Fig. 27.10) (83).

The mixed $S_{\bar{v}}O_2$, as measured from a PA catheter, loses most of its clinical utility during CPB because of the diversion of venous return into the venous reservoir. However, as previously mentioned, a very high PA catheter $S_{\bar{v}}O_2$ can be an indicator of a catheter in "wedged" position during CPB. The value of $S_{\bar{v}}O_2$ measurement of venous blood drained into the venous reservoir is considerable, having much the same significance as the corresponding PA catheter measurement off bypass. As described above in the section on blood flow and perfusion pressure requirements during CPB, if one is aware of the major determinants of the $S_{\bar{v}}O_2$ value (hemoglobin concentration, blood flow, hemoglobin P_{50}, arterial oxygenation, and systemic oxygen consumption), then the $S_{\bar{v}}O_2$ can be used as a guide to adequacy of oxygen delivery during CPB.

Other Cardiovascular Monitors

Another increasingly commonly used clinical cardiovascular monitor is transesophageal echocardiography. Unfortunately, a substantial portion of transesophageal echocardiography utility is lost during CPB with cardioplegia. Blood loss from the cardiac chambers obscures the ultrasound definition of the chambers; there is little or no cavity and therefore little or no ultrasound contrast to define cardiac structures. Likewise, during CPB there is little or no intracardiac blood flow, so that Doppler information on blood flow

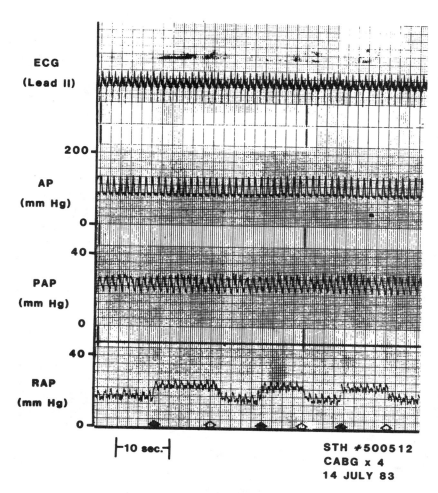

FIG. 27.10. Right atrial pressure (*RAP*) is increased at the onset of the venous infusion port infusion (*solid arrow*) and returns to the preinfusion level when the infusion stops. *AP*, arterial pressure; *PAP*, pulmonary artery pressure; *CABG*, coronary artery bypass graft. (From Davis RF. Yet another CVP artifact. *Anesthesiology* 1984;60:262, with permission.)

velocity and direction and on valvular function is largely irrelevant. However, as the heart is filled near the conclusion of CPB, transesophageal echocardiography regains its ability to visually display intracardiac structures, wall motion, and blood flow direction and velocity and can also be a useful guide to effective air evacuation from the cardiac chambers.

Electrocardiographic monitoring must be continued during CPB. During periods of cardioplegic arrest, it is important to verify that the ECG is isoelectric. After surgical repair, the ECG should return to the baseline state before weaning from CPB (see Chapter 29). Abrupt changes of the ST segment deviation from isoelectric should raise the immediate question of intracoronary embolization of air (particularly to the right coronary artery as typically reflected in leads II, III, and aVF) or particulates. Persistent ST segment deviation should raise the question of ongoing ischemia that should be investigated and corrected before terminating CPB. One should not overlook the value of direct observation of the heart as an adjunct to ECG diagnosis, especially in patients with dysrhythmias.

Neurologic Monitoring

Neurologic monitoring during CPB is directed primarily toward the myoneural junction to confirm adequacy of muscle paralysis and toward the central nervous system (CNS) to detect functional abnormalities developing during CPB. The former is straightforward and needs little attention here except to say that unnecessary oxygen consumption and CO_2 production during moderate hypothermic CPB are decreased when a complete level of skeletal muscle paralysis is maintained. This, coupled with the decreased effective concentration of neuromuscular blocking agents produced by the blood volume expansion from the CPB priming volume (see Chapter 11), explain the common clinical recommendation to redose relaxants with approximately one-half of an expected "intubating dose" at the time of initiating CPB. In this regard there is perhaps some theoretic advantage to the use of *d*-tubocurarine because its ganglionic blocking side effects may help control the increase in vascular resistance during hypothermia and CPB.

CNS monitoring has traditionally relied on electrophysiologic measurement of neurologic activity measured from the body surface and exemplified by the EEG. An enhancement of this passive measurement is the evoked potential. Typically, an evoked potential is measured as the surface electrophysiologic manifestation of the transmission of a stimulus along a given neural pathway. Other nonelectrophysiologic CNS monitoring includes transcranial Doppler and reflectance spectrometry. Transcranial Doppler ultrasound measures blood flow velocity in major arterial segments in the brain and can detect transient artifacts in the velocity signal attributable to particulate or gas emboli. Reflectance spectrometry developments now allow measurement of the signal produced by the mean venous oxygen hemoglobin saturation at discrete loci in the brain. Although the CNS monitoring capabilities applicable to patients undergoing CPB are significant, their clinical use is relatively small compared with the total scope of CPB monitoring. Also, the ability of more intensive CNS monitoring to decrease the frequency of adverse neurologic outcome after CPB remains largely untested.

Recording of a full standard EEG electrode montage on a strip chart with an experienced EEG analyst observing the signals is the ideal method for EEG monitoring. The value of this approach intraoperatively is debated for certain procedures such as carotid endarterectomy; however, application of such technique to CPB is rarely seen outside of specific focused clinical investigation. The processed EEG, either compressed spectral array or density modulated spectral array, provides a smaller volume of data than the raw EEG. However, the data are presented in a user-friendlier format, which allows clinicians to detect lateralized (or global) change in both the dominant frequency and the power of the EEG, even with intermittent observation of the record. Excellent comprehensive reviews of this subject are readily available (84–86).

The process of CPB presents many physiologic changes that markedly complicate the interpretation of the EEG. The primary changes in the EEG indicating hypoperfusion or hypoxia are slowing of the dominant frequency and loss of power in the signal, and similar changes can be produced in the EEG by hemodilution, hypothermia, anesthetics, CPB systemic flow changes, and pulsatility changes, in addition to any imputed hypoxic CNS insult (84). For example, anesthetics have well-known EEG effects, including the ability to produce burst suppression or an isoelectric pattern with barbiturates and with the volatile anesthetic isoflurane. Mild hypothermia itself produces slowing of the EEG, which proceeds through burst suppression to an isoelectric pattern as temperature is further decreased. However, comparing temperature-related EEG changes to hypoxia, there are differences that may become clinically useful (87). Significant hypoxia is marked by a rapid decrease in high-frequency EEG activity. Also, although the burst suppression pattern of hypothermia tends to be regular, that seen with hypoxia is more irregular. Perhaps the situation is analogous to ST segment depression in the ECG. Here, the

unproven but hopeful hypothesis is discrete EEG patterns exist, detectable during CPB and distinguishable from other effects, which reliably indicate CNS hypoxia at a treatable point before frank cytologic injury.

Currently, the use of evoked potentials during CPB is largely limited to surgery involving the descending thoracic aorta, generally repair of aortic coarctation, aortic dissection, and aortic aneurysm repair. Because of the anatomy of the major blood supply to the spinal cord (the anterior spinal artery and the communicating artery of Adamkewicz) (Fig. 27.11), the spinal cord is at risk of ischemic injury when the descending thoracic aorta is clamped to permit surgical repair. By monitoring the progress of an evoked signal at several sites from the periphery to the cerebral cortex, one can monitor the function of each component of the transmission sequence from peripheral nerve through the spinal cord to the cerebral cortex. Theoretically, observation of increased latency or decreased amplitude of the evoked potential signal at any site along the path would allow intervention before neurologic injury. In aortic coarctation, for example, observation of an abnormal evoked potential after application of the aortic clamp could then trigger removal and replacement of the clamp or some other (pharmacologic) maneuver to increase perfusion pressure or cardiac output in an attempt to improve spinal cord blood flow before the repair is undertaken. Unfortunately, the caveats

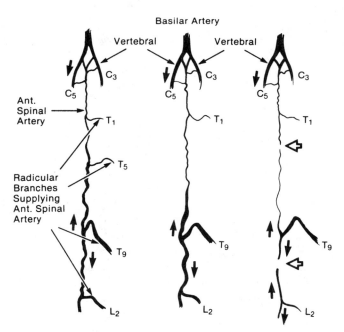

FIG. 27.11. Variation in blood supply to the spinal cord. The variation diagrammed on the right presents a higher risk for spinal cord ischemia with descending aortic surgery. (From Dembitsky WP. Central nervous system injury during surgery of the descending aorta. In: Utley JR, ed. *Pathophysiology and techniques of cardiopulmonary bypass.* Vol. 1. Baltimore: Williams & Wilkins, 1982:80, with permission.)

regarding the interaction of CPB, hypothermia, anesthesia, hemodilution, and the EEG also apply to evoked potentials. Also, the predominant type of evoked potential used clinically is currently the sensory evoked potential. In the case of the somatosensory evoked potential, the motor component of the spinal cord is relatively silent. Cases exist of dense motor paraplegia after thoracic aortic surgery despite persistently normal somatosensory evoked potentials throughout the aortic cross-clamp interval (88).

Temperature Monitoring

Because of the integral relationship between temperature control (manipulation) and CPB, temperature measurement is a core physiologic monitor during CPB. A major difficulty, however, is the simple definition of "core" temperature. The technology available for temperature measurement during CPB is nothing less than abundant. The problem is not how to measure; the technologic capability exceeds the clinical need for accuracy or adaptability. Measurement of nasopharyngeal, esophageal, tracheal, mixed ve-

nous blood, arterial blood, bladder urine, rectal, tympanic membrane, and even great toe temperature are readily available for clinical use. In many cardiac surgical units, measurement of two or more of these is common practice. But what is core temperature? The concept of a single core body temperature is just that—a concept rather than a reality. Figure 27.12 is instructive in this regard. The expectation is that especially during cooling or rewarming, temperature is site-specific and the variability from site to site is significant.

Temperatures are measured during cooling to ensure that the organs believed most vulnerable to potential hypoperfusion actually receive the benefit of the desired degree of hypothermia. In this regard the brain is usually the target, and nasopharyngeal (not airway), tympanic membrane, or esophageal (below tracheal bifurcation) are the usually accepted best estimates of brain temperature. Tympanic membrane temperature monitoring is less popular because of the occurrence of probe-related tympanic membrane injury. Mixed venous temperature in the extracorporeal circuit is a reasonable indicator of average body temperature directly analogous to an $S_{\bar{v}}O_2$ measurement.

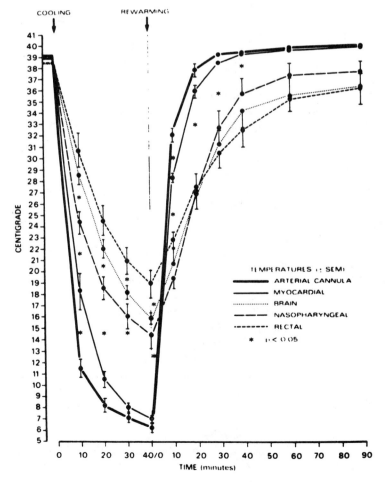

FIG. 27.12. Relationships of temperatures measured at various sites over time during cooling and rewarming from cardiopulmonary bypass. (From Stefaniszyn HJ, Novick RJ, Keith FM, et al. Is the brain adequately cooled during deep hypothermic cardiopulmonary bypass? *Curr Surg* 1983;40: 294–297, with permission.)

During rewarming, the target, obviously, is a normothermic patient at the end of CPB. Success is both time and temperature dependent. For example, the total caloric loss in a series of adult patients cooled to 30°C for 130 minutes on CPB was calculated at 238 kcal (89). The net return during rewarming was approximately 160 kcal, leaving a heat debt of 78 kcal or approximately the equivalent of 1.5 hours of the basal metabolic heat output. This deficit is likely the explanation for the common clinical observation of rebound hypothermia, sometimes termed afterdrop, after termination of CPB. In this regard, the use of vasodilators, nitroprusside or nitroglycerin, to force a vasodilation during CPB theoretically promotes a more uniform rewarming and has been clinically shown to decrease the incidence and severity of rebound hypothermia after CPB (90).

Important considerations for temperature measurement during rewarming are prevention of liberation of free gas bubbles and blood damage. Because of the inverse relationship between gas solubility in blood (or any liquid) and temperature, dissolved gases tend to come out of solution as a fluid is warmed. If this happens clinically, the consequences of gaseous embolization (even microemboli) can be significant. In general, maintenance of a temperature gradient from the heat exchanger to the venous blood of not more than approximately 10°C will prevent significant microbubble formation. Although heat exchangers are highly efficient, there is a temperature gradient produced within the heat exchanger. A boundary layer forms immediately adjacent to the heat exchanger in which blood temperature will equal heat exchanger water temperature, whereas blood farther away from the exchange surface will not fully equilibrate with water temperature. Because blood damage (both cellular elements and protein denaturation) increases with temperature greater than 42°C, this temperature forms the practical upper limit to water temperature within the heat exchanger (91). But as previously mentioned, the minimum exchanger water temperature, approximately 4°C, appears not to damage blood.

Urinary Volume and Renal Function

A detailed discussion of the effect of CPB on renal function is found in Chapter 19. Most cardiac surgical teams closely follow the urine flow of patients during CPB as an indicator of normal renal function. Although a brisk flow of urine during CPB may be comforting and may, in fact, facilitate fluid management during CPB, existing clinical data do not support a close relationship between urine flow while on bypass and postoperative renal function. In the mid-1970s, Abel et al. (92) examined a large number of patients for factors predictive of postoperative renal failure. Two major factors emerged as significant correlates of postoperative renal failure: time on bypass and preexisting renal failure. Other factors, including urine volume on bypass, were not significantly related to postoperative renal failure.

What is the place of diuretic medications, either osmotic (i.e., mannitol) or loop (i.e., furosemide and congeners), in the management of the oliguric patient during CPB? Several considerations are pertinent. The first is to ensure catheter patency. This may seem simplistic, but clinical experience indicates that the bladder is remarkably compliant and that pharmacologic diuresis will rarely fill it to a pressure sufficient to overcome an obstructed catheter. In general, a physiologic urine volume of 0.5 to 1.0 mL/kg/hr requires no treatment. Oliguric or anuric patients may or may not benefit from diuretic therapy. Again, available clinical data do not relate urine volume during CPB to postoperative renal dysfunction. However, oliguria or even normal urine flow in the face of hyperkalemia, hemoglobinemia (presumed hemolysis), or suspected volume overload (excessive hemodilution) are indications for diuresis. Theoretically, in the case of hyperkalemia, loop diuretics would provide the greatest potassium loss. In the case of hemoglobinuria, a large volume of alkaline urine is desired, so either loop or osmotic diuretics (or both) may be useful.

Coagulation Status

Coagulation monitoring is an obviously major area of patient monitoring during CPB. Chapters 22 through 25 provide a detailed review of all relevant aspects of coagulation and CPB.

Laboratory Data

The frequency and type of laboratory data monitored during CPB are relatively institution specific, but laboratory support should minimally include blood gas and pH measurement and rapid access to electrolytes, especially potassium and calcium, and glucose and perhaps lactate. Whether these data are available from a satellite laboratory in close proximity to the operating room, from in-line or in-room monitors, or from the main hospital laboratory is less important than the rapid availability of data. The rapidity and magnitude of intraoperative changes in these parameters in cardiac surgical patients makes their rapid (5- to 10-minute) availability a virtual requirement for safe cardiac surgery.

A common area of controversy in blood gas data interpretation during CPB is the management of P_aCO_2 and pH during hypothermia. The discussion of alpha-stat versus pH-stat management schemes is well presented in Chapters 4 and 12 and does not need to be recapitulated here. The use of potassium-based cardioplegic solutions mandates the capability for rapid and accurate assessment of serum potassium concentration. The metabolic consequences of CPB, especially those involving glucose utilization (see Chapter 17), create the requirement for frequent glucose (and optimally lactate) measurement during and after CPB.

Technologies for in-line, on-line, or local laboratory measurements include cartridge-based electrode systems and intravascular, usually fluorochrome, catheter-based technology. The latter generally couples intensity of fluorescence of the fluorochrome when stimulated by light at a specific wavelength to fiberoptic technology for transmission of the emitted fluorescent light to an analytic instrument. The intensity of fluorescence is proportional to the concentration of the parameter being measured (P_aO_2, P_aCO_2, or pH). Current capabilities in this area include systems that will pass through a 20-gauge catheter, are capable of giving near-continuous P_aO_2, P_aCO_2, and pH data at ambient patient temperature, and still permit pressure measurement via the same catheter. Depending on institutional practices regarding frequency of blood gas analysis and cost of the testing, this new approach may prove to be cost effective, but the clinical value (despite widespread use) of continuous measurement of blood gas data as opposed to intermittent sampling remains to be established.

The cartridge electrode systems are more conventional in that electrochemical reactions form the basis for measurement. The advantage is that the cartridge is a self-contained unit with electrodes and calibration solutions capable of making a defined number of measurements over a defined timespan. For institutions capable of using the full capacity of the cartridge within its lifespan, the result is also often cost effective. Cartridge-based systems are often small enough to be physically attached to the CPB circuit and may be equipped with automatic sampling capability. Although this is not actually a continuous measurement, the sampling frequency is programmable and limited only by the time required for the actual electrode measurement. These instruments also may provide quality management functions such as documentation of quality control testing and control over instrument use by uncertified or untrained individuals, in addition to providing needed laboratory data.

EQUIPMENT MONITORING DURING CARDIOPULMONARY BYPASS

Oxygenator Function

Arguably, the single most important item of equipment in the CPB setup is the oxygenator. Oxygenators in current use are manufactured as single-use disposable items subject to stringent quality control. Problems do occur nevertheless, although rarely. The immediate life-sustaining function of the oxygenator is oxygenation of the blood; ventilation follows. Therefore, the single best monitor of oxygenator function is oxygenation. As just discussed, a variety of instrumentation is available for blood gas (P_aO_2, in this case) analysis ranging from laboratory benchmark instruments to in-line CPB sensors or catheter-based systems. The point is that the adequacy of oxygenation must be reliably determined both early and throughout the CPB course. The emphasis on laboratory determination does not discount

clinical observation. For example, a cyanotic surgical field should be noticed quickly. Having established adequate initial oxygenator function, it is prudent to reassess blood gases at regular intervals throughout CPB or whenever changes are made in oxygenator gas flow or composition or CPB systemic blood flow. Also, recalling the earlier discussion of the value of $S_{\bar{v}}O_2$ measurement to guide perfusion adequacy, CPB venous blood oximetry is a useful monitor used by most perfusionists today.

What then is an appropriate level for arterial blood gas PO_2 during CPB? Two recent studies would suggest hyperoxemia (defined as arterial PO_2 greater than 185 mm Hg) might be deleterious during normothermic and hypothermic CPB (93,94). With the current availability, accuracy and reliability of in-line blood gas sensors, it is relatively easy to maintain the P_aO_2 in the 140- to 180-mm Hg range. Although it is acknowledged that these values are not normoxemic, maintaining blood gas values in this range with in-line sensors displaying contemporary data will provide a margin of safety during CPB, particularly when the aortic cross-clamp is removed and during reversal of hypothermia when the patient's oxygen needs increase.

Cardioplegia Delivery

When cardioplegic solution is delivered by the perfusionist, the flow, pressure, and temperature should be monitored. Depending on the pressure drop through the delivery system and cannula, the aortic root pressure can be monitored and regulated to appropriate levels by adjusting the flow rate. It is particularly important to monitor pressures when cardioplegic solution is delivered directly into coronary ostia or retrograde into the coronary sinus to avoid tissue damage from excessively high pressures and to ensure proper cannula placement. Some cardioplegia cannulas provide for direct measurement of infusion pressure through a second pressure monitoring line or lumen (95). If aortic infusion pressure is not measured directly, the aortic root pressure can be estimated by subtracting the pressure drop of the delivery system from the cardioplegia line pressure. Monitoring the temperatures of both the cardioplegic solution and myocardium can reasonably ensure adequate cardioplegia and guide intervals for reinfusion.

Fluid Management

Fluid administration during CPB in response to decreased circulating volume usually consists of crystalloid solution added directly into the circuit. Extravascular loss of blood at the operative field, fluid shifts within the patient's tissues and organs, and urine output can contribute to the need for supplemental fluid administration. Depending on the patient's recent hematocrit, packed red blood cells may be added per protocol or surgeon or anesthesiologist order. The choice of type of fluid administration (crystalloid or blood products) may be governed by stage of the operation, patient condition, or protocol. For example, if the patient has good diuresis and patient weaning from CPB is expected shortly, blood products may be withheld to avoid donor blood exposure. In other cases such as the elderly, children, or those patients with reduced cardiac function, the threshold for administration of bank blood may be lower. All blood administered should be double checked against the patient name and identification number before administration, with the time of administration recorded on the perfusion record.

When a hemoconcentrator is used during bypass, the volume of plasma water removed should be monitored to avoid excessive fluid removal with concomitant decreases in circulating volume (96). In some settings, a cell-salvage device is used in conjunction with CPB to wash suctioned blood. The time and volume required for such blood processing must be taken into account during CPB because blood being processed may not be immediately available for administration. With hemoconcentration, plasma proteins and platelets are preserved, and use of this device is technically simpler and more cost effective than routine cell salvage during CPB (97,98).

Circuit Alarms

Most CPB circuits have alarms to warn of potentially dangerous conditions such as low reservoir volume or high systemic line pressure. An air bubble detector placed on the arterial line will automatically alarm and shut off the systemic roller pump in the event a bolus of air inadvertently enters the line proximal to the sensor. The location of the air bubble detector within the circuit can vary (99), but for most prompt air detection, the sensor should be placed between the CPB reservoir and systemic pump. Manufacturer recommendations and some practitioners place the sensor after all devices on the arterial flow line, including the arterial line filter. This configuration has the advantage of detecting bubbles that may inadvertently enter this line after all CPB components but the disadvantage of having to remove all air from the arterial line filter before restarting CPB, which can be difficult. Low-level reservoir alarms have a long history of use, and they can be used to warn of low reservoir volume conditions or shut off the systemic blood flow pump if the CPB reservoir volume is too low. However, the use of the alarm is not a substitute for an alert perfusionist monitoring the reservoir level.

Perfusion Record

Record keeping provides permanent documentation of the patient's hemodynamics and metabolic parameters during the period of CPB support. The perfusion record should contain information regarding personnel, patient diagnosis and operation performed, equipment used, and time of ad-

ministration of drugs, fluids, and blood products. The perfusion record also may provide information for other health care personnel responsible for care of the patient after surgery. As such, the perfusion record contains information that may become part of a larger database or serve as documentation for further medical study. The perfusion record also is an important document if legal proceedings arise (100). A complete and legible record can be used in defense if the hospital or perfusionist is named in a lawsuit or the perfusionist is called as a witness. Perhaps one of the most important functions of the perfusion record is to prompt the perfusionist to make observations and in some cases document patient physiologic variables and circuit performance. In this sense, the perfusion record can be viewed as an ongoing checklist during CPB.

The format of the perfusion record varies and may be of the commonly used random time and entry or chart type where data regarding systemic blood flow, patient arterial blood pressure(s), temperature(s), oxygenator ventilating gas flow and composition, and results of laboratory tests such as hemoglobin, arterial and venous blood gases, and electrolytes are recorded.

A second less frequently used perfusion record is the combination flow with time and entry type, which is similar to an anesthesia record. This record also contains information on patient physiologic parameters, but because notations are made at fixed intervals on a grid, it is conceptually easier to determine trends and view in its entirety what occurred during the period of bypass. In practice, the timing of entries should occur every 15 minutes or less in a random entry or a timed entry record.

During CPB, an entry also should be made every time a change is made by the perfusionist in any of the perfusion controls or parameters or any time one of the monitored values change. Use of 24-hour time entries ("military time") is recommended and can clarify the time of day or night for the various entries. Blood gas and other laboratory values should be recorded on the perfusion record at the time they were drawn and not when the results were received. Blood gas samples should be drawn shortly after making a change in systemic blood flow or if there is a major change in patient temperature. Likewise, tests for electrolyte levels should be done after administration of solutions or drugs that can affect such values such as potassium chloride, glucose, or insulin. The use of in-line monitors for arterial and venous blood gas and/or chemistry values may decrease the need for more frequent sampling and documentation. However, the in-line monitor should be calibrated according to the manufacturer's instruction and against a sample using standard laboratory measurements to verify its accuracy.

All fluids added to the CPB circuit should be recorded at the time they are added. These notations, when combined with estimated blood loss and urinary output on bypass, will allow calculation of an estimated fluid balance at the conclusion of bypass and may guide patient management decisions after CPB. Medications added by the perfusionist, whether by protocol or on direction from the surgeon or other physician, should be noted along with who ordered it or whether it was given according to protocol.

COMMUNICATION

It should be apparent from the preceding sections that any medical procedure as invasive, life-sustaining, and complex in execution as CPB depends on close coordination of activities by all team members. Essential and effective communication provides a means to facilitate such coordination. Instructions or announcements from the surgeon to the perfusionist or anesthesia personnel are necessary during conduct of the operation because CPB is being used to facilitate a surgical procedure. Instructions from the anesthesiologist to the perfusionist also often occur during the period of CPB. All instructions or announcements should be followed by an acknowledgment from the person to whom it was directed. In this manner, errors of omission will be minimized and the surgical procedure can proceed expediently. If acknowledgment does not occur, the communication should be repeated until a response is heard, most often by the intended recipient repeating the instruction to avoid possible errors in interpretation.

The perfusionist should communicate to the surgeon activities that are performed according to protocol or according to surgeon preference. Likewise, the anesthesiologist should communicate activities to the perfusionist that also can affect the conduct of CPB and vice versa. An example would be administration of a vasodilator that can alter the circulating volume of blood and CPB reservoir level. Fluid additions to the CPB circuit should be communicated from the perfusionist to the anesthesiologist because of implications for fluid management after CPB.

Both perfusionist and anesthesiologist are obligated to communicate to the surgeon any significant abnormal conditions they observe. Much of the surgeon's attention may be focused on the surgical procedure, and the perfusionist and anesthesiologist are better able to monitor the key parameters outlined earlier.

Some conditions can occur unexpectedly that may potentially jeopardize patient well-being, including: increased CPB arterial line pressure; sustained decreased venous drainage; nonfunctioning vent or sucker; sustained elevated or low patient arterial blood pressure; elevated CVP, LA, or PA pressures; elevated delivery pressure and/or lower than expected flow during cardioplegia administration; and any potentially life-threatening equipment malfunction or failure. In such instances, immediate communication is required.

Often abnormal situations can occur that are less acute but potentially damaging, including: elevated serum potassium; lower than expected hemoglobin or hematocrit (with or without the expected need for blood transfusion that should be ordered by a physician); higher than expected fluid volume requirements; higher than expected use of vasopressors or need for increased systemic blood flow for decreased systemic vascular resistance; lower than expected mixed S_vO_2; resumption of cardiac electrical or mechanical activity during cardioplegic arrest; and air entrainment in the venous line.

If deep hypothermia and low flow or elective circulatory arrest are required, the surgeon should be notified of the duration of cooling, patient temperature(s), and elapsed times of low flow or circulatory arrest. The frequency for such notification should be communicated to the perfusionist before the procedure or at the time of initiation of low flow or circulatory arrest.

Surgical manipulations of the heart or major vessels may affect CPB. For example, retraction of the heart for surgical exposure may restrict venous drainage or allow air to enter the venous line at the venous cannulation site(s) or through side holes in the cannula exposed to atmosphere if the cannula becomes displaced. Such retraction also may distort the aortic valve, causing aortic incompetence with possible left ventricular distention from flow exiting the arterial cannula. Retraction of the heart may increase or decrease vent return. These conditions should be communicated to the surgeon when they occur, and surgeons should alert the perfusionist when they are displacing the unarrested heart such as when a circumflex coronary artery graft anastamoses is checked for bleeding. Collateral blood flow may partially obstruct the surgical field, necessitating a decrease in CPB systemic flow. Application of the aortic cross-clamp usually is preceded by instruction from the surgeon to the perfusionist to momentarily decrease the systemic blood flow to lower pressure in the aorta. The perfusionist should communicate all changes in systemic blood flow, whether in response to direct instruction or by protocol.

POST-CARDIOPULMONARY BYPASS ACTIVITIES

The perfusionist should be prepared to transfuse residual perfusate through the arterial cannula as required and instructed by the surgeon or anesthesiologist. It is important that before any such transfusion occur, the surgeon should check the arterial cannula for any residual air bubbles that may have been liberated from cardiac chambers or vessels since stopping bypass (Fig. 27.13). Often the arterial cannulation site is in the uppermost position the aorta and will become the site of lodgment of residual air due to buoyancy effects.

It is important that the pump sucker(s) or vent(s) not be used if fibrin glue or coagulation-inducing drugs are being used in the operative field (101,102). Aspiration of blood containing this material, even if in a liquid state,

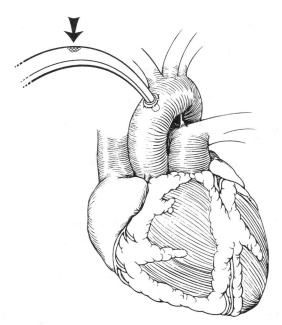

FIG. 27.13. Common site of air lodgment in arterial cannula immediately after cardiopulmonary bypass (*arrow*). The venous cannula(s), which are still in place in the right atrium and/or vena cavae, are not shown for illustrative purposes.

can cause coagulation in the cardiotomy reservoir, venous reservoir, or oxygenator with stasis, thus compromising use of the circuit in the event CPB must be restarted. Similarly, the pump sucker(s) should be turned off after protamine administration is observed to be effective to avoid similar problems. A guideline is for the anesthesiologist to announce when one-fourth to one-half the anticipated protamine dose has been administered as a signal to discontinue use of the pump suckers.

After the arterial cannula has been removed, residual perfusate in the CPB circuit can be salvaged by transfer into a completely de-aired sterile intravenous bag for possible transfusion by anesthesia personnel. Bags containing residual perfusate should be labeled with the patient's name, hospital identification number, and time and date of collection. In practice, residual perfusate is most often administered in the immediate post-bypass period. Alternatively, a cell-salvage device may be used to process blood whereby it is washed before transfusion. A hemoconcentrator can also be used to process residual perfusate before collection. It is important that supplemental protamine sulfate is given after any such transfusion of unwashed residual perfusate to counteract heparin contained in the salvaged perfusate.

The time of administration of protamine sulfate has been temporally related to hemodynamic deterioration in some patients (see Chapter 23). The perfusionist should continue to observe patient hemodynamics at this time and maintain the CPB circuit in a functionally usable state if it is necessary

to urgently restart bypass. If the patient must be placed back on CPB, then the protamine must be stopped and a full loading dose of heparin (300 to 400 units/kg) should be given before restarting bypass to adequately anticoagulate the patient. Sometimes the readministration of heparin will neutralize the heparin–protamine complex and the previously observed hemodynamic deterioration will resolve (103,104). Circuit disassembly and recovery or processing of residual perfusate should not be undertaken until it is reasonably certain that the patient will maintain adequate hemodynamics.

PERFUSION PROTOCOLS, GUIDELINES, AND STANDARDS

Protocols, guidelines, and standards are no substitute for common sense and experience. However, they have been useful in promoting safe conduct of CPB. Perhaps in its simplest form, an institutional protocol outlines the selection of circuit components and required priming volumes (with constituents) according to patient size or diagnosis. These protocols are often determined after review of manufacturer product data and then further developed and updated after a period of use. Such protocols provide some consistency on a case by case basis regardless of perfusion personnel involved. Basic institutional protocols may be customized to a specific surgeon or for specific procedures or patient conditions.

A second type of protocol, which is particularly applicable for pediatric cases or specialty situations, outlines recommended or preferred cannula size and type. Flow charts can be created by performing benchtop measurements or can be provided by manufacturers, showing pressure drops at different flows for arterial cannulas. Similarly, venous cannulas most often are classified by a range of flows with height differentials typically used for gravity siphon drainage.

More detailed protocols may be used to describe various aspects of conduct of CPB and ancillary or more rarely performed procedures such as performing hemodialysis during bypass. Such protocols are usually unique to the institution and sometimes contain specific protocols according to surgeon preference. An example might be desired range of arterial blood pressure while on bypass or treatment regimens for abnormal laboratory results.

Detailed protocols also may list in outline form specific steps for circuit assembly, priming, and management during certain less frequently performed procedures such as cardiac transplantation, left heart bypass for repair of the descending thoracic aorta, or retrograde cerebral perfusion. Protocols should be developed with input from all team members and should be periodically reviewed and updated so that they remain contemporary with current clinical practice. Protocols are especially useful when orienting new personnel who may bring preconceived methods of CPB conduct learned during training or previous job experience. Although it is generally agreed that CPB can be conducted in many ways with acceptable patient outcome, safe conduct on a case by case basis can be facilitated by use of mutually agreed on protocols that clarify personnel roles and expectations and specific patient management issues.

The first national standard of perfusion practice formulated by a professional society appeared in 1978 (105) and contained basic items that were considered important for inclusion on a perfusion record such as names of the surgeon, perfusionist, and anesthesiologist. Also to be recorded were timed entries for specific parameters such as CPB systemic blood flow, patient temperatures and pressures, and blood gas results.

In 1987, a second standard of practice document was published by the American Academy of Cardiovascular Perfusion (106). It acknowledged that although the primary responsibility for care of the patient undergoing CPB rested with the surgeon or physician in charge, it was the responsibility of the perfusionist to assist the surgeon in any way possible in care of the patient and particularly within the defined area of expertise of the perfusionist. It further emphasized the necessity for a written perfusion record, choice of equipment including cost containment and use of available safety devices, personnel (two qualified perfusionists or a qualified assistant for the primary perfusionist per case was deemed preferable), mandatory use of a pre-bypass checklist, and conduct of perfusion.

The standard addressed issues such as maintenance of a safe volume at all times in the CPB reservoir, the volume of which would allow 15 seconds for reaction time in the event of interrupted venous drainage. It specified that systemic blood flow rates should be maintained at such a level that inadequate tissue perfusion not develop, examples of which were development of increasing metabolic acidosis, mixed venous oxygen desaturation, or EEG changes. Specific pressure ranges were not defined in the standard, but the standard did state that the systemic blood pressure "must be maintained at an adequate level so that organ preservation and function are not compromised or impaired function detected." Anticoagulation assessment should be performed on a routine basis and should be adequate to prevent clotting in the extracorporeal circuit and consumption of blood clotting factors. This document was updated in 1994 (107).

AmSECT then developed essentials for perfusion practice that was endorsed by their membership in 1992 (108). In the preamble, the standard reiterated a statement that appeared in an earlier scope of practice (109): "Extracorporeal circulation shall be conducted according to established procedures and protocols in accordance with hospital policy and upon prescription by a physician." Tenets of the standard included: an accurate perfusion record must be maintained; the perfusionist should use a checklist(s); extracorpo-

real circulation should be conducted by a knowledgeable and competent perfusionist; anticoagulation should be monitored; appropriate gas exchange, blood flow, pressures, and volumes should be maintained; appropriate safety and monitoring devices should be used; the perfusionist should make a reasonable effort to contain costs; and the perfusionist must ensure proper maintenance of equipment. Those essential statements dealing with actual conduct of perfusion were qualified by the phrase "according to the established protocol" to permit variations in individual team practice. The intent of these standards was to provide guidance for safe perfusion practice rather than mandating specific practice.

In 1995, AmSECT published guidelines for perfusion practice (110) to augment the earlier essentials document (108). The basis for this document was a national survey on perfusion practice conducted by the organization in 1993 (111). The guidelines are quite specific to each essential. As guidelines, most of the recommendations are phrased in statements using the words "should" or "may," indicating, once again, institutional or surgeon variability in the conduct of perfusion.

CONCLUSIONS

CPB, as noted by Kirklin and Barratt-Boyes (112), is conceptually simple and equipment is now available to accomplish it with ease. In the 1960s, when CPB was just beginning to be practiced routinely in major medical centers, Galletti and Brecher (3) made a plea that it be kept simple, particularly considering the multitude of parameters that could be monitored. Although CPB was not ideal in 1962, nor is it at the current time, it is an established procedure that is well tolerated in most patients who make uneventful recoveries after their cardiac surgery. Until an alternative method is developed to provide the surgeon a motionless blood-free operative field and safely protect vital organs, CPB will likely continue to be used at current levels of a million procedures annually worldwide.

As stated previously, the actual conduct of perfusion practice may vary according to surgeon/perfusionist preference and institutional or even regional practice. However, national consensus on what constitutes adequate and safe conduct of CPB has been delineated and promulgated by professional organizations in the last two decades. Such guidelines and protocols are important to consider in the context of individual practice, but they must be used in perspective. Guidelines and protocols cannot anticipate every contingency or emergency that might arise during CPB. Guidelines and protocols cannot govern all activities of all team members. All personnel involved in the conduct of CPB must rely on experience and deductive reasoning to solve problems or avoid a perfusion crisis. Guidelines and protocols are derived from experience. Experience includes mistakes, accidents, and failures. Guidelines and protocols are meant to eliminate these life-threatening events but should not be totally relied on without constant awareness of the individual patient being supported by CPB and constant vigilance to detect early any abnormal behavior on bypass that could compromise patient safety.

ACKNOWLEDGMENT

The authors acknowledge the artwork of Lee Rose and Steve Schuenke. Terry Crane, Aaron Hill, and John Toomasian critiqued the manuscript in draft form.

KEY POINTS

- The patient's chart should be reviewed before CPB to obtain information regarding the proposed surgical procedure and patient history.
- Assembly of the CPB circuit should be performed in a consistent manner on a day-to-day basis.
- Roller pump occlusion on all pumps should be set before use for each case.
- Centrifugal pump flow probes must be calibrated and zeroed before use for accurate CPB systemic flow measurement.
- Completion of a pre-bypass checklist will greatly ensure the odds of proper CPB assembly and function.
- Minimizing circuit prime volume will result in a higher mixed patient/circuit hematocrit and possibly reduce the need for homologous blood transfusion.
- CPB should be established by activating the systemic pump first (before release of the venous line clamp) to avoid exsanguination in the event of a malfunction of the CPB systemic pump.
- Vents should be tested before use to verify proper suctioning effect.
- The CPB reservoir volume should be continuously monitored so that appropriate changes in systemic blood flow can be made in the event of decreased venous drainage.
- Cooling and warming rates should not exceed an approximate 10°C gradient (arterial blood and patient temperature when cooling; venous blood and heat exchanger water source when rewarming).
- Measuring $S_{\bar{v}}O_2$ does not ensure that CPB systemic flow is meeting regional DO_2 requirements; however, a low $S_{\bar{v}}O_2$ does indicate a problem with systemic DO_2.
- A CPB systemic flow index of 2.2 L/min/m² is recommended when normothermic for adequate perfusion; in children, the flow index should be 2.5 L/min/m².
- Hypothermia allows proportionate reductions in CPB systemic flow guided by nomograms that rely on plateauing of $\dot{V}O_2$.

- Viscosity (and resistance to blood flow) increases substantially with hypothermia, indicating the importance of hemodilution with CPB.
- Pressure measurement artifacts are frequently seen during CPB and result from effects of hypothermia, uneven vasodilation with rewarming, mechanical tissue/vessel compression, or aortic cannula tip malposition.
- Central venous, PA, and LA pressures should be at or near zero during CPB; an increase in any one is a matter for concern requiring assessment of venous cannula(s) position and confirmation of an unrestricted venous drainage line.
- An elevated CVP will reduce the effective perfusion pressure to organs (e.g., brain, kidney, liver) and tissue beds (e.g., gut).
- Changes in the EEG may be induced by hemodilution, hypothermia, anesthetics, CPB systemic flow changes and pulsatility changes, and hypoxia, making interpretation and diagnosis of CNS insult difficult.
- "Core temperature" is conceptually simple, but in reality brain temperature during CPB is best approximated by measuring the nasopharyngeal, tympanic, or esophageal temperature.
- Use of continuous reading in-line blood gas sensors allows precise management of P_aO_2 and P_aCO_2 in the perfusate and provides a margin of safety during CPB.
- The flow, pressure, and temperature of cardioplegic solution and temperature of the myocardium should be monitored to reasonably ensure adequate cardioplegia.
- Use of circuit alarms (e.g., level sensor, air bubble detector) can decrease the risk of air embolism during CPB.

REFERENCES

1. Galletti PM, Brecher GA. *Heart-lung bypass, principles and techniques of extracorporeal circulation.* New York: Grune & Stratton, 1962:194.
2. Commission on Accreditation of Allied Health Education Programs. Standards and guidelines for an accredited educational program for the perfusionist. Adopted 1980; revised 1989, 1994.
3. Galletti PM, Brecher GA. *Heart-lung bypass, principles and techniques of extracorporeal circulation.* New York: Grune & Stratton, 1962:251.
4. Reed CC, Kurusz M, Lawrence AE Jr. *Safety and techniques in perfusion.* Stafford, TX: Quali-Med, 1988:23.
5. Davis RF, Dobbs JL, Casson H. Conduct and monitoring of cardiopulmonary bypass. In: Gravlee GP, Davis RF, Utley JR, eds. *Cardiopulmonary bypass, principles and practice.* Baltimore: Williams & Wilkins, 1993:579.
6. Emergency Care Research Institute. Inspection & preventive maintenance of cardiopulmonary perfusion equipment and an overview of problems. *Health Dev* 1980;9:70–80.
7. Kurusz M, Crane TN, Speer D. Preventive maintenance of

heart-lung machines. *Proc Am Acad Cardiovasc Perfus* 1985;6: 34–37.

8. Young WV, Heemsoth CH, Georgiafandis G, et al. Extracorporeal circuit sterility after 168 hours. *J Extra-Corp Technol* 1997; 29:181–184.

9. Wellons HA, Nolan SP. Prevention of air embolism due to trapped air in filters used in extracorporeal circuits. *J Thorac Cardiovasc Surg* 1973;65:476–478.

10. Hargrove M, McCarthy AP, Fitzpatrick GJ. Carbon dioxide flushing prior to priming the bypass circuit, an experimental derivation of the optimal flow rate and duration of the flushing process. *Perfusion* 1987;2:177–180.

11. Altman PL, Dittmer DS, eds. Respiration and circulation. In: *Biological handbooks*. Bethesda, MD: Federation of American Societies for Experimental Biology, 1971:16–18.

12. Reed CC, Romagnoli A, Taylor DE, et al. Particulate matter in bubble oxygenators. *J Thorac Cardiovasc Surg* 1974;68: 971–974.

13. Reed CC, Stafford TB. *Cardiopulmonary bypass*, 2nd ed. Houston: Texas Medical Press, 1985:376.

14. Rath T, Sutton R, Ploessel. A comparison of static occlusion setting methods: fluid drop rate and pressure drop. *J Extra-Corp Technol* 1996;28:21–26.

15. Lee-Sensiba K, Azzaretto N, Carolina C, et al. New roller pump disposable provides safety and simplifies occlusion setting. *J Extra-Corp Technol* 1997;29:19–24.

16. Mills NL, Ochsner JL. Massive air embolism during cardiopulmonary bypass; causes, prevention and management. *J Thorac Cardiovasc Surg* 1980;80:707–717.

17. Crane TN, Keen WR Jr, Spiller CE, et al. A prebypass checklist-why aren't you using one? *Proc Am Acad Cardiovasc Perfus* 1986; 7:98–100.

18. Kurusz M, Harshaw RC. The contribution of checklists to perfusion safety: lessons from aviation. In: Steenbrink J, Wijers-Hille MJ, deJong DS, eds. *Fourth European Congress on Extracorpeal Circulation Technology*, 12–15 June 1991, Utrecht: Foundation European Congress on Extracorporeal Circulation, 1995: 177–185.

19. American Society of Extra-Corporeal Technology. Suggested pre-bypass perfusion checklist. *Perfus Life* 1990;7:76–77.

20. Rosengart TR, DeBois WJ, O'Hara M, et al. Retrograde autologous priming for cardiopulmonary bypass: a safe and effective means of decreasing hemodilution and transfusion requirements. *J Thorac Cardiovasc Surg* 1998;115:426–439.

21. Darling E, Kaemer D, Lawson S, et al. Experimental use of an ultra-low prime neonatal cardiopulmonary bypass circuit utilizing vacuum-assisted venous drainage. *J Extra-Corp Technol* 1998;30:184–189.

22. Petry AF, Jost T, Sievers H. Reduction of homologous blood requirements by blood-pooling at the onset of cardiopulmonary bypass. *J Thorac Cardiovasc Surg* 1994;107:1210–1214.

23. Jansen PGM, te Velthuis H, Bulder ER, et al. Reduction in prime volume attenuates the hyperdynamic response after cardiopulmonary bypass. *Ann Thorac Surg* 1995;60:544–550.

24. Kolff J, McClurken JB, Alpern JB. Beware centrifugal pumps; not a one-way street, but a potentially dangerous "syphon" [Letter]. *Ann Thorac Surg* 1990;50:512.

25. Fox LS, Blackstone EH, Kirklin JW, et al. Relationship of whole body oxygen consumption to perfusion flow rate during hypothermic cardiopulmonary bypass. *J Thorac Cardiovasc Surg* 1982;83:239–248.

26. Lee-Sensiba K, Azzaretto N, Carolina C, et al. Errors in flow and pressure related to the arterial filter purge line. *J Extra-Corp Technol* 1998;30:77–82.

27. Jones L, Knight PG, Alley R, et al. Adverse effects of Forane,

Ethrane, and Halothane of the William Harvey H-1700 bubble oxygenator. *Proc Am Acad Cardiovasc Perfus* 1987;8:178–181.

28. Maltry DE, Eggers GWN Jr. Isoflurane-induced failure of the Bentley-10 oxygenator [Correspondence]. *Anesthesiology* 1987; 66:100–101.

29. Walls JT, Curtis JJ, McClatchey BJ, et al. Adverse effects of anesthetic agents on polycarbonate plastic oxygenators [Letter]. *J Thorac Cardiovasc Surg* 1988;96:667–668.

30. Gravlee GP, Wong AB, Charles DJ. Hypoxemia during cardiopulmonary bypass from leaks in the gas supply system [Letter]. *Anesth Analg* 1985;64:649–650.

31. Centers for Disease Control. Recommendations for prevention of HIV transmission in health care settings. *MMWR Morb Mortal Wkly Rep* 1989;36:1S–18S.

32. Courington KR, Patterson SL, Howard RJ. Universal precautions are not universally followed. *Arch Surg* 1991;126:93–96.

33. Shelley GA, Howard RJ. A national survey of surgeons' attitudes about patients with human immunodeficiency virus infections and acquired immunodeficiency syndrome. *Arch Surg* 1992; 127:206–212.

34. Gershon RRM, Vlahov D, Felknor SA, et al. Compliance with universal precautions among health care workers at three regional hospitals. *Am J Infect Control* 1995;23:225–236.

35. Megan J, Patterson M, Novak CB, et al. Surgeons' concern and practices of protection against bloodborne pathogens. *Ann Surg* 1998;228:266–272.

36. Akduman D, Kim LE, Parks RL, et al. Use of personal protective equipment and operating room behaviors in four surgical subspecialties: personal protective equipment and behaviors in surgery. *Infect Control Hosp Epidemiol* 1999;20:110–114.

37. Pietrabissa A, Merigliano S, Montorsi M, et al. Reducing the occupational risk of infections for the surgeon: multicentric national survey on more than 15,000 surgical procedures. *World J Surg* 1997;21:573–578.

38. Flum DR, Wallack MK. The surgeon's database for AIDS: a collective review. *J Am Coll Surg* 1997;184:403–412.

39. Lawrence VA, Gafni A, Kroenke K. Preoperative HIV testing: is it less expensive than universal precautions? *J Clin Epidemiol* 1993;46:1219–1227.

40. Klatt EC. Surgery and human immunodeficiency virus infection: indications, pathologic findings, risks, and risk prevention. *Int Surg* 1994;79:1–5.

41. Kirklin JW, Barratt-Boyes BG. *Cardiac surgery*, 2nd ed. New York: Churchill Livingstone, 1993:75.

42. Reed CC, Kurusz M, Lawrence AE Jr. *Safety and techniques in perfusion*. Stafford, TX: Quali-Med, 1988:129.

43. Reed CC, Stafford TB. *Cardiopulmonary Bypass*, 2nd ed. Houston: Texas Medical Press, 1985:407.

44. Collins RL. *Air crashes, what went wrong, why, and what can be done about it.* New York: Macmillan Publishing, 1986:17.

45. Jerabek CF, Walton HG, Doerfler S. The effect of gas scavenging on hollow fiber membrane oxygenator performance. *Proceedings of the 27th International Conference American Society of Extra-Corpeal Technology*, 10–14 March 1989, pp. 24–29.

46. Kurusz M, Andrews JJ, Arens JF, et al. Monitoring oxygen concentration prevents potential adverse patient outcome caused by a scavenging malfunction: case report. *Proc Am Acad Cardiovasc Perfus* 1991;12:162–165.

47. Emergency Care Research Institute. Hazard, scavenging gas from membrane oxygenators. *Health Dev* 1987;16:343–344.

48. Blomback M, Kronlund P, Aberg B, et al. Pathologic fibrin formation and cold-induced clotting of membrane oxygenators during cardiopulmonary bypass. *J Cardiothorac Vasc Anesth* 1995;9:34–43.

49. Donald DE, Fellows JL. Physical factors relating to gas embolism in blood. *J Thorac Cardiovasc Surg* 1961;42:110–118.

50. Stone JG, Young WL, Smith CR, et al. Do standard monitoring sites reflect true brain temperature when profound hypothermia is rapidly induced and reversed? *Anesthesiology* 1995;82: 344–351.

51. Cook DJ, Orszulak TA, Daly RC, et al. Cerebral hyperthermia during cardiopulmonary bypass. *J Thorac Cardiovasc Surg* 1996; 111:268–269.

52. Buss MI, McLean RF, Wong BI, et al. Cardiopulmonary bypass, rewarming, and central nervous system dysfunction. *Ann Thorac Surg* 1996:61:1423–1427.

53. Leigh JM. Oxygen therapy at ambient pressure. In: Scurr C, Feldman S, eds. *Scientific foundations of anaesthesia*, 2nd ed. Chicago: Medical Yearbook, 1974:254.

54. Guyton AC. *Textbook of medical physiology*, 7th ed. Philadelphia: W.B. Saunders, 1986:497.

55. Gregory IC. The oxygen and carbon monoxide capacities of fetal and adult blood. *J Physiol* 1974;236:625–634.

56. Brandfonbrenner M, Landowne M, Shock NW. Changes in cardiac output with age. *Circulation* 1955;12:557–566.

57. Gerstenblith G, Renlund DG, Lakatta EG. Cardiovascular response to exercise in younger and older men. *Federation Proc* 1987;46:1834–1839.

58. Rodenheffer RJ, Gerstenblith G, Becker LC, et al. Exercise cardiac output is maintained with advancing age in healthy human subjects: cardiac dilatation and increased stroke volume compensate for a diminished heart rate. *Circulation* 1984;69: 203–213.

59. Guyton AC. *Textbook of medical physiology,* 7th ed. Philadelphia: W.B. Saunders, 1986:234.

60. Govier AV, Reves JG, McKay RD, et al. Factors and their influence on regional cerebral blood flow during nonpulsatile cardiopulmonary bypass. *Ann Thorac Surg* 1984;38:592–600.

61. Prough DS, Stump DA, Roy RC, et al. Response of cerebral blood flow to changes in carbon dioxide tension during hypothermic cardiopulmonary bypass. *Anesthesiology* 1986;64: 576–581.

62. Murkin JM, Farrar JK, Tweed A, et al. Cerebral autoregulation and flow/metabolism coupling during cardiopulmonary bypass: the influence of carbon dioxide. *Anesth Analg* 1987;66: 825–832.

63. Thomson IR. The influence of cardiopulmonary bypass on cerebral physiology and function. In: Tinker JH, ed. *Cardiopulmonary bypass, current concepts and controversies*. Philadelphia: W.B. Saunders, 1989:21–40.

64. Schwartz AE, Sandhu AA, Kaplon RJ, et al. Cerebral blood flow is determined by arterial pressure and not cardiopulmonary bypass flow rate. *Ann Thorac Surg* 1995;60:165–170.

65. Rudy LW, Heymann MA, Edmunds H. Distribution of systemic blood flow during cardiopulmonary bypass. *J Appl Physiol* 1973;34:194–200.

66. Harris EA, Seelye ER, Barratt-Boyes BG. On the availability of oxygen to the body during cardiopulmonary bypass in man. *Br J Anaesth* 1974;46:425–431.

67. Mandl JP, Motley JR. Oxygen consumption plateauing: a better method of achieving optimum perfusion. *J Extra-Corp Technol* 1979;11:69–77.

68. Parolari A, Alamanni F, Gherli T, et al. Cardiopulmonary bypass and oxygen consumption: oxygen delivery and hemodynamics. *Ann Thorac Surg* 1999;67:1320–1327.

69. Clowes GHA, Neville WE, Sabga G, et al. The relationship of oxygen consumption, perfusion rate, and temperature to acidosis associated with cardiopulmonary bypass. *Surgery* 1958;44: 220–225.

70. Diesh G, Flynn PJ, Marable SA, et al. Comparison of low (azygous) flow and high flow principles of extracorporeal circulation employing a bubble oxygenator. *Surgery* 1957;42:67–72.

71. Moffitt EA, Kirklin JW. Physiologic studies during whole-body perfusion in tetralogy of Fallot. *J Thorac Cardiovasc Surg* 1962; 44:180–188.

72. Levin MB, Theye RA, Fowler WS, et al. Performance of the stationary vertical-screen oxygenator (Mayo-Gibbon). *J Thorac Cardiovasc Surg* 1960;39:417–426.

73. Kirklin JW, Barratt-Boyes BG. *Cardiac Surgery,* 2nd ed. New York: Churchill Livingstone, 1993:80.

74. Kern FH, Ungerleider RM, Reves JG, et al. Effect of altering pump flow rate on cerebral blood flow and metabolism in infants and children. *Ann Thorac Surg* 1993;56:1366–1372.

75. Gold JP, Charlson ME, Williams-Russo P, et al. Improvement of outcomes after coronary artery bypass; a randomized trial comparing intraoperative high versus low mean arterial pressure. *J Thorac Cardiovasc Surg* 1995;110:1302–1314.

76. Robicsek F, Masters TN, Niesluchowski W, et al. Vasomotor activity during cardiopulmonary bypass. In: Utley JR, ed. *Pathophysiology and techniques of cardiopulmonary bypass*. Vol II. Baltimore: Williams & Wilkins, 1983:1–12.

77. Hine IP, Wood WG, Mainwaring-Buton RW, et al. The adrenergic response to surgery involving cardiopulmonary bypass, as measured by plasma and catecholamine concentrations. *Br J Anaesth* 1976;48:355–363.

78. Wallach R, Karp RB, Reves JG, et al. Pathogenesis of paroxysmal hypertension developing during and after coronary artery bypass surgery: a study of hemodynamic and humoral factors. *Am J Cardiol* 1980;46:559–565.

79. Fouad FM, Estafanous FG, Bravo EL. Possible role of cardioaortic reflexes in post-coronary bypass hypertension. *Am J Cardiol* 1979;44:866–872.

80. Murgo JP, Westerhof N. Arterial reflections and pressure waveforms in humans. In: Yin FCP, ed. *Ventricular vascular coupling*. Berlin: Springer-Verlag, 1987:144–146.

81. Stern DH, Gerson JI, Allen FB, et al. Can we trust the radial artery pressure immediately after cardiopulmonary bypass? *Anesthesiology* 1985;62:557–561.

82. Chapin JW, Nance P. Facial paleness. *Anesth Analg* 1982;61: 475.

83. Davis RF. Yet another CVP artifact. *Anesthesiology* 1984;60: 262.

84. Levy WJ. Intraoperative EEG patterns: implications for EEG monitoring. *Anesthesiology* 1984;60:430–434.

85. Levy WJ. Automated EEG processing for intraoperative monitoring. *Anesthesiology* 1980;53:223–236.

86. Levy WJ. Central nervous system monitoring. In: Kaplan JA, Reich DL, Konstadt SN, eds. *Cardiac anesthesia*, 4th ed. New York: W.B. Saunders, 1999:485–505.

87. Levy WJ. Quantitative analysis of EEG changes during hypothermia. *Anesthesiology* 1984;60:291–297.

88. Ginsburg HH, Shetler AG, Raudzeus PA. Postoperative paraplegia with preserved intraoperative somatosensory evoked potentials. *J Neurosurg* 1985;63:296–300.

89. Davis FM, Parimelazhagan KN, Harris EA. Thermal balance during cardiopulmonary bypass with hypothermia in man. *Br J Anaesth* 1977;49:1127–1132.

90. Noback CR, Tinker JH. Hypothermia after cardiopulmonary bypass in man. *Anesthesiology* 1980;53:277–280.

91. Kirklin JW, Barratt-Boyes BG. *Cardiac Surgery,* 2nd ed. New York: Churchill Livingstone, 1993:83.

92. Abel RM, Buckley MJ, Austen WG, et al. Etiology, incidence and prognosis of renal failure following cardiac operations. Results of a prospective analysis of 500 consecutive patients. *J Thorac Cardiovasc Surg* 1976;71:323–333.

93. Joachimsson P-O, Sjoberg F, Forsman M, Johansson M, et al. Adverse effect of hyperoxemia during cardiopulmonary bypass. *J Thorac Cardiovasc Surg* 1996;112:812–819.

94. Ihnken K, Winkler A, Schlensak C, et al. Normoxic cardiopulmonary bypass reduces oxidative myocardial damage and nitric oxide during cardiac operations in the adult. *J Thorac Cardiovasc Surg* 1998;116:327–334.

95. Sievertsen WA, Hankins TD, Lazar HL, et al. A new technique for measuring aortic root pressure during infusion of cardioplegic solution. *Ann Thorac Surg* 1986;41:675–677.

96. Faulkner SC, Kurusz M, Manning JV Jr, et al. Clinical experience with the Amicon Diafilter during cardiopulmonary bypass. *Proc Am Acad Cardiovasc Perfus* 1987;8:66–69.

97. Nakamura Y, Masuda M, Toshima Y, et al. Comparative study of cell saver and ultrafiltration nontransfusion in cardiac surgery. *Ann Thorac Surg* 1990;49:973–978.

98. Boldt J, Zickmann B, Fedderson B, et al. Six different hemofiltration devices for blood conservation in cardiac surgery. *Ann Thorac Surg* 1990;51:747–753.

99. Sarns/3M Health Care. Four out of five regularly use bubble detectors. *Heart-to-Heart Newsletter* 1993;8:5.

100. Roach WH Jr, Aspen Health Law and Compliance Center. *Medical records and the law*, 3rd ed. Gaithersburg, MD: Aspen Publishers, 1998.

101. Lupinetti FM, Stoney WS, Alford WC Jr, et al. Cryoprecipitate-topical glue, initial experience in patients undergoing cardiac operation. *J Thorac Cardiovasc Surg* 1985;90:502–505.

102. Robicsek F, Duncan GD, Born GVR, et al. Inherent dangers of simultaneous application of microfibrillar collagen hemostat and blood-saving devices. *J Thorac Cardiovasc Surg* 1986;92:766–770.

103. Utley JR, Bhatt MA, Stephens DB, et al. Reversal of protamine reaction with heparin. *Perfusion* 1986;1:63–64.

104. Lock R, Hessel EA II. Probable reversal of protamine reactions by heparin administration. *J Cardiothorac Anesth* 1990;4:604–608.

105. American Society of Extra-Corporeal Technology. Standards of practice: recommended minimum standards, permanent perfusion records. *J Extra-Corp Technol* 1978;10:46.

106. American Academy of Cardiovascular Perfusion. Standards of practice. *Proc Am Acad Cardiovasc Perfus* 1987;8:272–274.

107. American Academy of Cardiovascular Perfusion. Standards of practice, revised January 31, 1994. *AACP Newsletter* 1994, Spring:4.

108. American Society of Extra-Corporeal Technology. Essentials for perfusion practice; clinical function: conduct of extracorporeal circulation. *Perfus Life* 1992;9:37.

109. American Society of Extra-Corporeal Technology. Perfusion scope of practice. *Perfus Life* 1991;8:25.

110. American Society of Extra-Corporeal Technology. Guidelines for perfusion practice. *Perfus Life* 1995;12:20–22.

111. American Society of Extra-Corporeal Technology. Perfusion practice survey, September 1993. *Perfus Life* 1994;11:42–45.

112. Kirklin JW, Barratt-Boyes BG. *Cardiac Surgery*, 2nd ed. New York: Churchill Livingstone, 1993:73.

MANAGEMENT OF UNUSUAL PROBLEMS ENCOUNTERED IN INITIATING AND MAINTAINING CARDIOPULMONARY BYPASS

MARK KURUSZ
NOEL L. MILLS

Some preexisting conditions or problems with the operation or function of the cardiopulmonary bypass (CPB) circuit can jeopardize the patient during CPB. Often the experience of a single team member or even several team members may be inadequate to form a plan of management for these problems. This chapter examines several such conditions or incidents that may be encountered infrequently and suggests management strategies derived from the published literature or the authors' experience.

CONDITIONS IDENTIFIABLE BEFORE CARDIOPULMONARY BYPASS

Atherosclerotic Aorta

The atherosclerotic aorta can present problems during cannulation for CPB, application of clamps, delivery of cardioplegia, construction of proximal anastomoses for coronary artery bypass grafts, or valve replacement or repair. A large multicenter study identified the presence of proximal aortic atherosclerosis as the strongest predictor of stroke (1). This lends support to the theory that atherosclerotic emboli liberated by surgical manipulation of the aorta cause most strokes after CPB. Risk factors for ascending aortic atherosclerosis include: significant carotid, abdominal aortic, and left main coronary artery atherosclerosis; aortic wall irregularity on ascending aortic angiogram; adhesions between the ascending aorta and its adventitia; pale appearance of the ascending aorta; and minimal bleeding of an aortic stab wound (2).

In most cases, the surgeon can palpate the aorta at the time of surgery to select a nondiseased section as the site for insertion of the arterial perfusion cannula or proximal anastomoses. Such palpation may be performed before CPB by briefly clamping the superior and inferior venae cavae with straight Satinsky clamps to effect temporary (10- to 12-second) inflow occlusion that will rapidly decrease cardiac ejection and arterial pressure. With lower pressure in the aorta, gentle palpation can be used to assess the quality of the aortic wall to determine the location of disease-free sites for cannulation and placement of the aortic cross-clamp. Preoperative angiogram should also be performed during cardiac catheterization to assess the smoothness of the aortic lumen and detect wall irregularities (2). Transesophageal echocardiography and/or a sterile epiaortic probe placed directly on the aorta during surgery are used increasingly to visualize the ascending aortic lumen, with the latter approach being more sensitive because of the interposition of the tracheal carina between the esophagus and distal ascending aorta. Culliford et al. (3) suggested routine use of transesophageal echocardiography in all patients over 65 years old to assess the degree of aortic atherosclerosis.

In severely diseased aortas, application of an aortic cross-clamp may not be deemed feasible because of increased risk of dislodgment of atherosclerotic debris or aortic dissection (Fig. 28.1). The so-called no-touch technique has evolved to better manage these patients (2). It relies on the internal mammary artery or gastroepiploic artery as conduits for coronary bypass grafts. In some patients requiring extensive revascularization, saphenous vein grafts can be anastomosed to the internal mammary artery. In no-touch cases, a femoral artery, axillary artery, or the underside of the distal aortic arch is used as the arterial cannulation site (2,4,5). Alternatively, either a long arch cannula can be inserted distal to the left subclavian artery (3) or a diffusion-tipped cannula can be used (6) to better disperse the flow jet at the CPB cannula tip. However, these cannulation techniques still

M. Kurusz: Department of Surgery, Division of Cardiothoracic Surgery, University of Texas Medical Branch, Galveston, Texas 77555-0528.

N. L. Mills: Department of Surgery, Division of Cardiothoracic Surgery, Tulane University School of Medicine, New Orleans, Louisiana 70112.

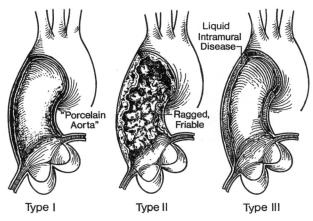

FIG. 28.1. Type 1, type II, and type III ascending aortic atherosclerosis. No clamp is safe on these types of ascending aortic disease. *Type I:* Circumferential ascending aortic calcification, which may be easily diagnosed preoperatively on the angiogram. Palpation of the ascending aorta at operation reveals firm calcification. Embolization or aortic injury that may be difficult to repair may result if the aorta is clamped. *Type II:* This pattern may be diagnosed preoperatively by noting an irregularity of the normally smooth lining of the ascending aorta on the left ventricular angiogram or aortic root injection. Visualization of the ascending aorta is now considered a mandatory part of workup before coronary artery bypass graft. *Type III:* Intraluminal liquid debris is the most elusive of the three patterns to diagnose before clamping the aorta. A pale appearance of the aorta or adherence of the adventitia to the ascending aorta may be the only diagnostic clues. Operative echocardiography wil reveal a thickened ascending aorta that will liberate liquid debris if a cross-clamp or partial occlusion clamp is applied. (From Mills NL, Everson CT. Atherosclerosis of the ascending aorta and coronary artery bypass: pathology, clinical correlates, and operative management. *J Thorac Cardiovasc Surg* 1991;102:546–553, with permission.)

present some risk of stroke hazard from insertion of the cannula in the severely diseased aorta. Cannulating from the left ventricular apex with the cannula advanced through the aortic valve has also been described (7).

We strongly recommend that the anesthesiologist perform simultaneous bilateral proximal (not bifurcation) carotid compression during any surgical manipulation of the severely diseased aorta to minimize atheromatous cerebral embolization. Rather than use conventional approaches to cardioplegia delivery, the surgeon may instead rely on electrical fibrillation or administration of a β-adrenergic blocker such as esmolol to slow the heart during distal anastomoses (4). In these cases, left ventricular venting may be avoided. However, if significant aortic insufficiency is present, conventional venting methods should be used, which then requires needle vent placement in the ascending aorta for de-airing before weaning from CPB and which carries some degree of hazard in the diseased aorta. A case report recommended use of an endoaortic clamp, as designed for minimally invasive cardiac surgery, to isolate the heart from CPB systemic flow (8). A central lumen allows delivery of cardioplegic solution or venting the aortic root. However, the prevailing wisdom is that this approach is unwise in the

presence of severe atherosclerosis because of the risk of dislodging atherosclerotic debris. An aortic filtration system (9) that uses an umbrella screen inserted through a modified 24 French arterial cannula before aortic cross-clamp removal has been shown to capture particulate debris that presumably would have otherwise embolized systemically.

In summary, cannulation of the severely diseased ascending aorta may be associated with significant morbidity after CPB. Modification of conventional CPB cannulation, cardioplegia, and venting techniques can reduce the incidence of stroke in this challenging patient population. Newer diagnostic measurements such as release of S-100 β, a marker of cerebral ischemia (10), and novel perfusion cannulation techniques under development may lead to further reductions in neurologic injury in the patient with diffuse atherosclerosis needing cardiac surgery.

Hematologic Problems

Cryoproteins

Cold agglutinins are serum antibodies that become active at decreased blood temperature and produce agglutination or hemolysis of red blood cells. These antibodies are classically directed against antigens on the red blood cells but can also be nonspecific. The most clinically relevant characteristic of cold agglutinins is thermal amplitude, the temperature below which the antibodies become activated. As temperature drops below this threshold, antibody activity increases exponentially. In general, this activity reverses as rewarming occurs (11). Higher cold agglutinin titers (concentrations) are more clinically significant than low titers. There is no widely accepted definition for high versus low titer; however, Lee et al. (12) suggested titers less than 1:32 as being low and those greater than 1:128 as being high.

Rewarming activates the complement system to induce hemolysis in patients with cold agglutinins. For hemolysis to occur, the cold agglutinin and complement activities must overlap. That is, the temperature must be low enough for the cold agglutinins to activate but warm enough for a complement fixation to occur.

Aside from during hypothermic bypass, cold agglutinins seldom produce symptoms because activation most often occurs at temperatures well below the usual range of body temperature. With cold exposure, clinical signs may include acrocyanosis of digits, tip of the nose, or ears from agglutination-induced ischemia. Most commonly, immediate warming of the affected areas reverses the agglutination and thus the ischemia. A patient with prolonged hypothermic CPB would be at risk for multiorgan damage from prolonged vascular occlusion (13). This is an uncommon but potentially catastrophic consequence of failure to recognize and treat the presence of cold agglutinins.

When patients undergo screening for cold agglutinins, a diagnosis can be easily made based on laboratory test results. If screening at 4°C is negative, no further screening is needed. If the screen is positive at 4°C, the thermal amplitude should be determined and the titer determined for each temperature at which the screen was positive. This will give more precise information for dealing with the cold agglutinin antibodies.

In patients who are not initially screened for cold agglutinins, a diagnosis may be made by astute observation. During hypothermic CPB, agglutination within the vessels may be noted, particularly if the surgeon is wearing magnifying loops. Hemolysis manifested by hemoglobinuria is most often recognized by pink or red-tinged urine. The latter occurrence, however, is relatively common even in the absence of cryoagglutination. If blood cardioplegia is used, the perfusionist may note agglutination in the cardioplegia delivery system as the blood is cooled (14–16). In addition, immediate agglutination of blood in a syringe during phlebotomy may indicate the presence of cold agglutinins. Agglutination also can be confirmed visually by immersing a test tube of blood into an ice slush solution and observing cell clumping on the side of the test tube that often disappears when the tube is warmed. Many cold agglutinins will present during a routine crossmatch done at room temperature. Any of the above findings suggest the presence of clinically significant cold agglutinins, and steps should be taken to prevent adverse reactions during CPB (14,17,18).

Both monoclonal and polyclonal cold agglutinins exist. The monoclonal types usually associated with lymphoreticular neoplasms are generally irreversible. The polyclonal antibodies are often associated with acute infectious diseases such as mycoplasma, infectious mononucleosis, or cytomegalovirus (13). Production of polyclonal cold agglutinins is typically transient and may remit spontaneously in weeks, but when present it may be associated with acute life-threatening intravascular hemolysis (13). Leach et al. (17) developed a comparison of clinically significant and insignificant cold agglutinins (Table 28.1). An important point in assessing the need to screen for cold agglutinins is that a failure to screen may lead to an adverse outcome, such as myocardial infarction, stroke, or acute renal failure. Without knowledge

of the presence of cold agglutinins, these adverse outcomes may be attributed to another cause. For example, hemolysis may be attributed to mechanical trauma to blood from CPB (19). One report suggests that mechanical trauma to blood may be more important than cold-reacting autoantibodies when the thermal amplitude is less than 22°C (20).

Treatment of cold agglutinin disease during CPB essentially consists of prevention of complement activation and ultimately of agglutination or hemolysis. Treatment is based on the etiology and the severity of the problem. In a mild case of cold agglutinins (i.e., a case in which there is a very low thermal amplitude, such as 4°C) and/or a low titer of antibodies, minor or no changes in surgical or CPB techniques and, in some cases, treatment with corticosteroids to avoid hemolysis have been advised (21). For patients with low-titer nonspecific antibodies (and only these patients), Moore et al. (11) concluded that hypothermic CPB can be performed on these patients without increased risks of hemolytic or agglutination crises; further, minor degrees of hemolysis occur in all patients during hypothermic bypass, especially during the rewarming phase, whether or not cold agglutinins are present.

In a case with clinically significant cold agglutinins (i.e., high thermal amplitude, high titer, or clinical symptoms), a number of changes in surgical technique have resulted in successful surgery using CPB. In the case of cold agglutinins caused by acute infection (e.g., a recent viral illness), elective cardiac surgery should be postponed for several weeks, by which time the antibody may have disappeared (19). If the urgency of surgery precludes that approach, the most sensible approach is to use either normothermia or mild hypothermia using blood temperatures continuously maintained above the thermal amplitude to avoid the active temperature range of agglutination (19,22–28). Hence, the presence of cryoagglutinins with high titer or high thermal amplitude may represent a reasonable indication for the use of warm cardioplegia myocardial protection techniques while maintaining normothermic systemic temperatures.

When selecting cold cardioplegia, blood should be ini-

TABLE 28.1. CHARACTERISTICS OF COLD AGGLUTININS[a]

Clinically Significant[b]	Clinically Insignificant[c]
1. Lytic (cause hemolysis)	1. Nonlytic (causes reversible red blood cell agglutination only)
2. Active in saline at 20°C	2. Peak activity 0–4°C
3. Almost always IgM antibodies	3. Seldom IgM antibodies (IgG, IgA, or nonimmunoglobulin)
4. Wide thermal range (4–32°C)	4. Low thermal range 0–6°C
5. Bind complement	5. Seldom bind complement
6. Agglutination irreversible	6. Agglutination reversible
7. Enhance agglutination when incubated at 30°C in albumin	7. Agglutination is not enhanced when incubated at 30°C in albumin.

[a] Adapted from Leach AB, Van Hasset GL, Edwards JC. Cold agglutinins and deep hypothermia. *Anaesthesia* 1983;38:140–143.
[b] These are commonly associated with chronic cold hemagglutinin disease, neoplasm of lymphoid origin, and mycoplasma pneumonia.
[c] These are commonly associated with viral infections (e.g., cytomegalovirus infections and mononucleosis).

tially flushed out of the coronary circulation with warm crystalloid cardioplegic solution followed by cold cardioplegic solution. Just before removal of the aortic cross-clamp, warm cardioplegic solution should be used to prevent agglutination from blood exposed to a cold heart. Refinements of this latter technique consist of bicaval cannulation with tightening of caval tapes to avoid cooling large amounts of blood in the heart. A sump catheter may be placed in the right atrium to retrieve cardioplegic solution until the coronary sinus effluent is clear. In addition, lower than normal CPB systemic flows may be used to decrease the noncoronary collateral flow and subsequent cooling of this blood.

If it is uncertain whether this noncoronary collateral flow will cause problems, the heart may be maintained at a temperature above the thermal amplitude (29). Venting the left ventricle will avoid cooling and stagnation of blood in the left ventricular cavity. Crystalloid cardioplegia has been used rather than blood cardioplegia to avoid agglutination of the cells in the solution when delivered at low temperature (30). Adjuncts may include a myocardial insulation pad to prevent cooling of blood in structures adjacent to the heart. Using a septal temperature probe in the myocardium to keep the temperature greater than the thermal amplitude may prevent significant activation of cold agglutinins. However, once the red blood cells are flushed out of the coronary circulation, the heart can be cooled to provide myocardial protection provided the above adjuncts are used.

In addition, all fluids, blood, plasma, inspired gases, and bolus injections should be warmed (19) in the periods before and after bypass, especially if the cryoagglutinin has a high thermal amplitude. Antibody dilution by the extracorporeal circuit priming solution probably may reduce the tendency for activation of high titer cold agglutinins (W. Rock, personal communication, 1992). It seems reasonable to assume that hemodilution during CPB will reduce the concentration of the cryoagglutinin 30% to 50%; thus, little protection would appear likely unless the cold agglutinin titer is very low (1:2 or less).

The literature contains descriptions of successful cardiac surgery after plasmapheresis (28,31) or total exchange transfusions in patients with high titer high thermal amplitude cold agglutinins. There is some evidence that the patient's own red cells may be protected from hemolysis, and if transfusions are required, autologous packed red cells may be advantageous (19). In the case of unexpected agglutination encountered at the time of surgery, several techniques may be useful: verification by the blood bank that cold agglutination is present rather than an unrecognized alloantibody; the use of crystalloid cardioplegic solution to dilute the antibody in the coronary circulation; use of noncardioplegic techniques (e.g., electrical fibrillation); and maintenance of systemic temperatures greater than 28 to 30°C at which significant amounts of agglutination are unlikely to occur. In addition, the CPB circuit and blood cardioplegia delivery

system should be monitored carefully throughout bypass for presence of cell aggregates, and CPB arterial line filters should be used in all cases.

Several cases of fibrin formation and clotting of membrane oxygenators during hypothermic CPB have been recently reported (32). Although cold agglutination was initially suspected, none of these patients exhibited agglutinin formation either during preoperative screening or postoperative hematologic workup. No abnormalities in blood coagulation factors VII and VIII or von Willebrand factor were demonstrated in blood samples tested postoperatively, nor were there significant differences between the affected patients' blood samples and control patients' blood. However, rapid CPB cooling in conjunction with use of efficient oxygenator heat exchangers having small blood pathways was associated with excessive premembrane CPB line pressure buildup that usually resolved with more moderate cooling strategies or by warming the perfusate.

In summary, all patients undergoing hypothermic CPB should be screened preoperatively for cold agglutinins (22–25,28,33). If an initial screen is positive, the cold agglutinins should be characterized as to thermal amplitude and titer. Clinical symptoms should also be sought. A patient with low titer, low thermal amplitude, and clinically asymptomatic can tolerate CPB with moderate hypothermia at very low risk with little or no alteration in technique. For clinically significant cold agglutinins with high thermal amplitude and/or titer, if due to a transient viral illness, elective surgery may be postponed several weeks in the hope that this will decrease cold agglutinins to insignificant levels. However, in severe cases in which the high titer high thermal amplitude cold agglutinins are not transient, precautions should be taken as outlined above to prevent an agglutination or hemolytic crisis (Fig. 28.2).

Hemoglobinopathy and Erythrocyte Disorders

Sickle Cell Trait and Disease

In the normal adult, hemoglobin A comprises 96% to 97% of all hemoglobin. Hemoglobin A consists of two α and two β chains. Sickle cell hemoglobinopathy is a single-gene recessive abnormality that may be present in a heterozygous recessive form, which is termed sickle cell trait, or in a homozygous recessive form, which is expressed as sickle cell disease. The percentage of hemoglobin S and hemoglobin A varies with the individual, but sickle cell disease patients have predominantly hemoglobin S. This homozygous state found in 0.15% of African-Americans is associated with severe hemolytic anemia and vaso-occlusive phenomena, resulting from the increased blood viscosity that occurs when red cells aggregate and individually typically assume a sickle shape (34). Sickled cells have a very limited capacity to load and unload oxygen.

In contrast, patients with the sickle cell trait have a lower percentage of hemoglobin S, accounting for 20% to 45%

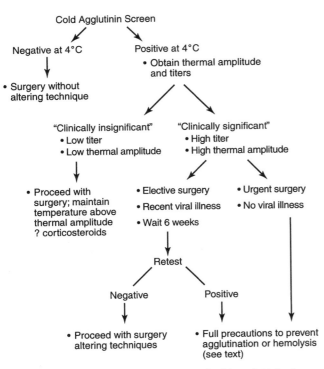

Cold Agglutinin Screen

Negative at 4°C → • Surgery without altering technique

Positive at 4°C
• Obtain thermal amplitude and titers

"Clinically insignificant"
• Low titer
• Low thermal amplitude

• Proceed with surgery; maintain temperature above thermal amplitude ? corticosteroids

"Clinically significant"
• High titer
• High thermal amplitude

• Elective surgery
• Recent viral illness
• Wait 6 weeks

• Urgent surgery
• No viral illness

Retest

Negative

Positive

• Proceed with surgery altering techniques

• Full precautions to prevent agglutination or hemolysis (see text)

FIG. 28.2. Algorithm for management of cold agglutinins in cardiopulmonary bypass.

of their total hemoglobin. Approximately 8% of African-Americans carry the heterozygous recessive trait. These individuals have few clinical problems, and except for severe or provoked conditions, they rarely experience sickle cell crises. Red blood cell sickling results from deoxyhemoglobin formation. The tendency toward sickling increases with hypoxemia, acidosis, increased concentrations of 2,3-diphosphoglyceric acid, infection, hypothermia, and capillary stagnation. A hypertonic environment that may lead to crenation of normal red blood cells also will lead to sickling. Hemoglobin S demonstrates increased osmotic and mechanical fragility, making hemolysis more likely. A hypotonic environment will lyse red blood cells with increased osmotic fragility.

In patients with sickle cell disease, some sickling begins to appear at 85% hemoglobin oxygen saturation, and sickling of red blood cells is complete at 38% hemoglobin oxygen saturation. In patients with sickle cell trait, sickling begins at hemoglobin oxygen saturations of approximately 40%. Sickling is reversible to a degree, but if it is repeated, the sickled cells become permanently damaged, resulting in markedly increased fragility and a shortened cell lifespan. In addition to increased blood viscosity potentially causing vascular occlusion, sickling can cause endothelial cell injury in the microvasculature. This may activate the intrinsic clotting system and exacerbate the vaso-occlusive phenomenon (34–37).

The operative strategy in sickle cell patients is to prevent sickling and thereby prevent hemolysis or vaso-occlusive phenomena intraoperatively and postoperatively. Because sickling results from decreased hemoglobin oxygen saturation, maintaining adequate arterial oxygen tension assumes paramount importance. Adequate capillary perfusion with short capillary transit times and avoidance of low output states (to prevent low mixed venous hemoglobin oxygen saturations) are also important (38–40). Continuous measurement of arterial and mixed venous hemoglobin oxygen saturations help to maintain adequate oxygen saturations. Because sickle crises are frequent when high concentrations of hemoglobin S are present (i.e., homozygous patients), marked reduction of sickling can be achieved by relative dilution of hemoglobin S with respect to hemoglobin A. This can be accomplished by using preoperative or intraoperative exchange transfusions.

Preoperative exchange transfusions, particularly applicable in patients who are already anemic, not only increase the prevalence of hemoglobin A relative to hemoglobin S but also suppress the production of hemoglobin S. This therapy improves the oxygen-carrying capacity of the blood by correcting the anemia and deficiency of hemoglobin A. In nonanemic patients, exchange transfusion may be accomplished intraoperatively. This type of transfusion is usually performed by sequestering the initial CPB venous drainage from the patient after priming the extracorporeal circuit with whole blood containing hemoglobin A (34,40). The goal of exchange transfusion is to achieve a hemoglobin A fraction of 60% to 70%, which is also the level sought when treating a major sickle cell crisis (39).

Acidosis shifts the oxyhemoglobin dissociation curve to the right, which increases the tendency toward sickling. This holds true particularly in venous blood, where sickling is most often initiated. Arterial and mixed venous blood gases should be measured frequently and any developing acidosis aggressively treated with sodium bicarbonate (39,40). Hypoperfusion may result from hypothermia, administration of cardioplegia, diminished intravascular volume, poor patient positioning, tourniquets, low CPB systemic flows, or low cardiac output states. It is important to avoid hypoperfusion because of the tendency of blood to desaturate during the capillary and venous phase of circulation, resulting in low hemoglobin oxygen saturation and red blood cell sickling. Hypoperfusion can usually be prevented by maintaining adequate systemic CPB flows and avoiding low cardiac output states both before and after bypass.

Localized sickling may occur in the heart during aortic cross-clamping because of the absence of coronary blood flow. This phenomenon may be avoided by flushing hemoglobin S out of the coronary arteries using either crystalloid cardioplegia or blood cardioplegia with a high fraction of hemoglobin A. Because mechanical prosthetic valves may predispose the patient to increased hemolysis, such valves are not recommended in these patients (40). Other means of avoiding mechanical blood trauma include minimizing the use of cardiotomy suction and venting. In patients with sickle cell disease, it appears advisable to minimize or avoid hypothermia during CPB. Despite the risks involved, numerous patients with homozygous sickle cell disease have successfully undergone CPB using the techniques described above (41–51). Successful cases have been described even using deep hypothermia with circulatory arrest (52).

Hereditary Spherocytosis

Hereditary spherocytosis, an autosomal dominant defect in red blood cell membranes, results in spherically shaped red blood cells that have increased osmotic and mechanical fragility. The usual treatment for hereditary spherocytosis resulting in hemolysis is splenectomy, which corrects the hemolysis and increases the shortened lifespan of the red blood cells to normal, although the cells retain their abnormal properties. Information describing CPB in these patients is limited. One case report describes a nonsplenectomized patient undergoing bypass with no apparent increase in blood destruction or in osmotic fragility over the baseline level (53). In addition, in a patient who had previously undergone splenectomy, no increase in hemolysis was noted during or after CPB, despite triple valve replacement using Bjork-Shiley mechanical valves (54). Other patients have had porcine valves inserted to minimize mechanically induced hemolysis. One study reported uneventful closure of an atrial septal defect in a 31-year old with hereditary spherocytosis and suggested that a short CPB time was important in avoiding complications (55). Hereditary elliptocytosis is a condition thought to be similar to hereditary spherocytosis; there is infrequent hemolysis and anemia, and no specific precautions are recommended in these patients (34,56).

Miscellaneous

Clinical CPB experience with other hemoglobinopathies is sparse. Another potential problem is that the hospital laboratory may neglect to notify the cardiac surgical team of rare but significant hematologic abnormalities before the patient's surgery.

Thalassemia minor patients exhibit no increase in red blood cell fragility, and therefore one would expect no hemolysis. Anemia in these patients is treated with transfusions. Hemolysis has been induced by a number of drugs in patients with glucose-6-phosphate dehydrogenase deficiency (56). This gender-linked inherited deficiency is present in 10% to 15% of African-American males. Susceptible individuals may develop explosive hemolysis when they receive drugs such as antimalarials, quinidine, phenacetin, or sulfonamides. These drugs should be avoided in susceptible patients undergoing surgery, including those undergoing CPB.

Acute methemoglobinemia may result from increased production of methemoglobin to levels far exceeding the usual amount, which is less than 1% of total circulating hemoglobin (57). Secondary or acquired methemoglobinemia is almost always caused by poisoning with chemicals or drugs classified either as direct oxidants such as nitrites or indirect oxidants such as benzocaine. Other such medications include high-dose methylene blue (58), nitroglycerin (59–61), nitroprusside, prilocaine, silver nitrate, sodium nitrate, flutamide (62), and sulfonamides.

The diagnosis of methemoglobinemia is made when cyanosis or oxygen desaturation occurs in the presence of an adequate arterial oxygen tension and is supported by a chocolate-brown color of blood rather than the usual dark blue of cyanosis (63). The diagnosis can be confirmed by spectrophotometry (64).

Treatment at times may need to precede definitive diagnosis. First, all probable offending drugs should be withdrawn. Next, maximal oxygen concentrations should be delivered to the oxygenator. If cyanosis or oxygen desaturation persists in the presence of high oxygen tension, pharmacologic treatment should begin. The drug of choice is methylene blue, 1 to 3 mg/kg administered in a 1% solution, which converts methemoglobin to active hemoglobin. The response to methylene blue is usually immediate and excellent, and because the treatment is relatively innocuous, its use should not be delayed. However, methylene blue may cause methemoglobinemia when a dose greater than 7 mg/kg is administered (65). If the patient fails to respond to methylene blue, the next line of treatment consists of high-dose vitamin C and, if necessary, exchange transfusion (59).

Polycythemia is defined as increased red cell mass. It occurs with cyanotic congenital cardiac defects as compensation for reduced oxygen delivery to tissues. The preoperative hematocrit in severe cases may exceed 70%, at which level blood viscosity is sufficiently high to compromise blood flow. Hemostatic abnormalities consistent with consumptive coagulopathy can occur (increased prothrombin and activated partial thromboplastin times, increased fibrin degradation products, thrombocytopenia, factor deficiencies, etc.) (66,67). Hemodilution beyond that normally used to prime the CPB circuit may better preserve the patient's coagulation status, so this may be an ideal situation for withdrawal of autologous blood before CPB. The degree of hemodilution needed to achieve a desired patient/pump hematocrit can be calculated using a formula shown in Figure 28.3 (66). Polycythemia vera is a hematologic disease that carries an increased risk of myocardial infarction.

Other Hematologic Problems

Antithrombin III deficiency and heparin-induced thrombocytopenia are discussed thoroughly in Chapters 24 and 25. Other hypocoagulable disorders such as hemophilia A (factor VIII deficiency), hemophilia B (factor IX deficiency), or von Willebrand's disease generally require administration of fresh frozen plasma, cryoprecipitate, or factor VIII con-

Calculation of the volume of crystalloid solution (prime volume) necessary for hemodiluting to a desired hematocrit

I. Determine the patient's EBV according to his/her body weight:

$$EBV\ (ml) = patient's\ weight\ (kg) \times factor^*\ (ml/kg)$$

II. Calculate the total hemodiluted blood volume for the desired hematocrit during CPB

$$Total\ hemodiluted\ blood\ volume\ (ml) = \frac{preperfusion\ hematocrit\ (\%)}{desired\ hematocrit\ (\%)\ during\ CPB} \times EBV\ (ml)$$

III. Determine the prime volume:

$$Prime\ volume\ (ml) = total\ volume\ (ml) - EBV\ (ml)$$

Example: For a 52 kg adult with a hematocrit value of 60%, dilute to 28%:

1. $EBV = 52\ kg \times 70\ ml/kg = 3,640\ ml$
2. $Total\ volume = \frac{0.60}{0.28} \times 3,640\ ml = 7,800\ ml$
3. $Prime\ volume = 7,800\ ml - 3,640\ ml = 4,160\ ml$

Legend: EBV, Estimated blood volume. CPB, Cardiopulmonary bypass.
*Factor (EBV/kg) is assumed to be: 80 ml/kg for <10 kg of body weight; 75 ml/kg for 10-20 kg of body weight; 70 ml/kg for >20 kg of body weight.

FIG. 28.3. Calculation of volume of crystalloid solution (cardiopulmonary bypass prime volume) necessary for hemodiluting to a desired hematocrit. *EBV*, estimated blood volume; *CPB*, cardiopulmonary bypass. *Factor (EBV/kg) is assumed to be 80 mL/kg for less than 10 kg body weight; 75 mL/kg for 10 to 20 kg of body weight; 70 mL/kg for more than 20 kg of body weight. The example addresses the polycythemic adult, but this condition is more prevalent in cyanotic pediatric patients with smaller required CPB circuit prime volumes. (From Milam JD, Austin SF, Nihill MR, et al. Use of sufficient hemodilution to prevent coagulopathies following surgical correction of cyanotic heart disease. *J Thorac Cardiovasc Surg* 1985;89:623–629, with permission.)

centrates to counteract excessive bleeding tendencies after CPB (68,69). Despite the possible temptation to use less heparin for anticoagulation in these situations, standard full-heparin anticoagulation regimes should be used during CPB.

With the increased application of interventional cardiac procedures by cardiologists, patients may present for surgery with antiplatelet or thrombolytic therapy (e.g., aspirin, urokinase, streptokinase, tissue plasminogen activator, IIb/IIIc platelet receptor antagonists) that can cause alterations in results of conventional anticoagulation tests after heparin administration and severe bleeding after CPB. Standard treatment has been to administer platelet concentrates or fresh frozen plasma after CPB subsequent to protamine administration. Abciximab may be removed by hemoconcentration during CPB (70). These patients will still likely require platelet transfusion, but the effect of the transfused platelets will be to provide hemostasis rather than act as receptors for circulating antibodies contained in abciximab.

Patients with a history of thrombophlebitis or other re-

current venous or arterial thromboembolism may be predisposed to hypercoagulability. These patients may require larger than expected and more frequent doses of heparin to maintain adequate anticoagulation during CPB. Cases of fatal thrombosis after CPB in patients with protein C deficiency have been reported (71). Lawson et al. (72) reported a successful CPB case in a patient with heterozygous protein C deficiency and outlined management recommendations that included continuous heparin anticoagulation therapy preoperatively (activated partial thromboplastin time 1.5 to 2.0 times baseline), normal heparin dosing (400 units/kg) just before bypass along with administration of fresh frozen plasma, reinstitution of heparin therapy after control of bleeding in the postoperative period, and discharge on oral warfarin.

Coagulation problems in pediatric patients undergoing CPB are usually more complex than those seen in the adult population (73). Neonates, in particular, have underdeveloped hemostatic systems when compared with older children and adults (74). This, coupled with the massive hemodilution and usual requirement for blood products in the CPB prime, may further obscure the hematologic picture with these patients (75). Use of the freshest bank blood obtainable (preferably less than 48 hours old) and fresh frozen plasma in the CPB circuit prime can minimize bleeding problems postoperatively. Administration of platelet concentrate or cryoprecipitate should improve coagulation parameters postoperatively; fresh frozen plasma administered after platelet transfusion may exacerbate bleeding (76).

In summary, patient history and preoperative testing can diagnose most hematologic disorders. In particular, patients with hepatic dysfunction may have serious bleeding postoperatively. In both elective cases and those presenting for CPB surgery emergently, consultation with an experienced hematologist is advised for safe management during the perioperative period. Dyke and Sobel (68) reviewed coagulation disorders and surgical management issues in greater detail.

Religious Objections to Blood Transfusion

Avoidance of homologous blood transfusion is a desirable goal whenever CPB is used; with patients of the Jehovah's Witness faith it is mandatory because of their strict interpretation of the bible (77). Nearly 40 years ago, Cooley et al. (78) first reported the feasibility of open heart surgery in this patient population. In 1977, Ott and Cooley (79) reported additional results in a large series of Jehovah's Witness patients in whom no blood was transfused. However, there was a 10.7% mortality in those undergoing CPB ($n = 39$), with preoperative or postoperative anemia a contributing factor in 12 deaths.

Using current low prime membrane oxygenator circuits, intraoperative cell salvage, and reinfusion of shed mediastinal blood, CPB can be performed relatively safely, even in pediatric patients (77,80,81), reoperations, or those with

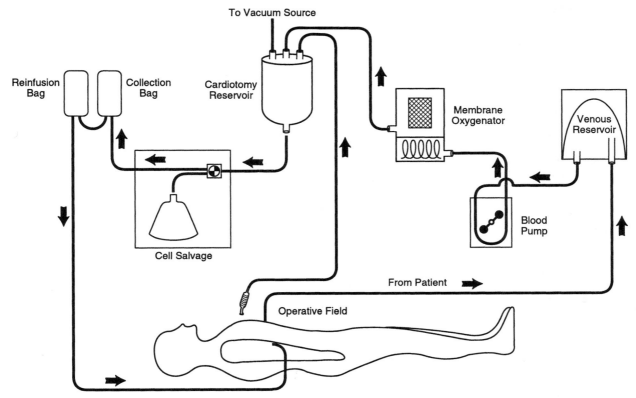

FIG. 28.4. Schematic drawing of cardiopulmonary bypass (CPB) circuit for collection, processing, and reinfusion of blood after bypass while maintaining continuity with the patient's circulation. The reinfusion bag (*top left*) should initially be back-filled with patient's blood from an intravenous site to establish continuity with cell salvaged blood (from collection bag) before CPB. Cardiotomy suction can be used after bypass until protamine is administered with collected blood processed in the cell salvage system. Residual perfusate in the CPB circuit should be transferred to the cardiotomy reservoir and also processed by the cell-salvage system to minimize blood loss. A second cardiotomy reservoir (not shown) is used during CPB for conventional collection of suctioned and vent blood, which is drained into the venous reservoir. (Modified from Milan TP Jr, Whitmore J, Maddi R. Reoperative cardiac surgery in a Jehovah's Witness: role of continuous cell salvage and in-line reinfusion. *J Cardiothorac Anesth* 1989;3:211–214, with permission.)

complex anatomy (82). The lowest safe hematocrit on CPB is not known, but values of approximately 15% have been used successfully provided CPB systemic flows are maintained at levels to prevent development of metabolic acidosis.

To honor the patient's religious beliefs, it is necessary to maintain continuity between removed blood and the patient's vascular system when cell salvage is used (83). Figure 28.4 shows how this can be accomplished pre- and post-bypass. Some authors have further advocated use of heparin-bonded CPB circuits and lower levels of heparinization [activated clotting time (ACT) >280 seconds] with favorable results (84). Use of erythropoietin preoperatively to promote red cell growth and antifibrinolytics perioperatively also have been advocated (85,86). Von Son et al. (81) enumerated management strategies to minimize blood loss in these patients (Table 28.2). Lee and Martin (87) wrote an excellent review of CPB management in this patient population.

Reoperative Surgery

Patients undergoing repeat cardiac surgery often present problems because of adhesions that make a second sternotomy and vascular access for CPB cannulation technically difficult. There is also an increased risk of encountering major bleeding during dissection because cardiac structures or vessels may be adherent to the chest wall, particularly if the pericardium has not been closed during the initial operation (88). Normal anatomic landmarks are often obliterated, prolonging adequate surgical exposure and CPB times. Because of adhesions necessitating sharp dissection, these patients tend to bleed more and have higher transfusion rates than first time cases (89). The surgeon should dissect as little as possible during reoperative surgery to minimize large disrupted tissue surface areas that will bleed. Use of an argon beam coagulator in these cases may also minimize bleeding problems associated with extensive dissection.

TABLE 28.2. PERIOPERATIVE MEASURES TO MINIMIZE BLOOD LOSS IN THE JEHOVAH'S WITNESS PATIENT

1. Pretreat patient with synthetic erythropoeitin if hematocrit <38%.
2. Avoid cardiac catheterization, if possible.
3. Administer antifibrinolytics perioperatively.
4. Use low-energy electrocautery in chest wall, pericardial, and great vessel dissections.
5. Use cell salvage system.
6. Minimize pre-CPB fluid administration.
7. Reduce CPB circuit priming volume.
8. Use moderate CPB systemic flow rates and gentle cardiotomy suction.
9. Use hemoconcentration to remove excess plasma water.
10. Avoid deep levels of hypothermia if possible.
11. Delay heparin neutralization until all bleeding sites have been secured (this will allow continued use of cardiotomy suction).
12. Gradually return entire volume of residual perfusate to patient (after processing by cell salvage system).
13. Administer postoperative iron supplements in patients with depleted red cell mass.

CPB, Cardiopulmonary bypass. (Derived from Von Son Jam, Hovaguimian H, Rao IM, et al. Strategies for repair of congenital heart defects in infants without the use of blood. *Ann Thorac Surg* 1995;59:384–388.

In some cases, groin cannulation of the femoral or iliac artery and femoral vein must be used to establish CPB. Placing an adequately sized femoral arterial cannula can usually be accomplished easily, but placement of an adequately sized venous cannula may be more difficult. New long, thin-walled, kink-resistant femoral venous cannulas are now commercially available to permit positioning the cannula tip near the cavoatrial junction (90). However, because of their length, standard gravity siphonage may be inadequate to permit full CPB systemic flow. If maximizing the height differential between the patient's heart and the CPB venous reservoir or repositioning the cannula does not improve venous drainage, flow may be augmented with a centrifugal pump placed in the venous line (91,92). Activation of the centrifugal pump will exert additional negative pressure beyond that obtainable by height differential alone with a concomitant modest increase in venous line flow. Alternatively, a hard-shell venous reservoir may have regulated vacuum applied to its interior to effect additional venous line flow using the same principles (93).

Both methods of augmented venous drainage require careful monitoring of venous line pressure so that excessive levels of vacuum are not created (94). Excessive vacuum can collapse vascular walls into the venous cannula openings, thus impeding or stopping venous line flow (95). Excessive vacuum may be manifested by intermittent or staccato flow; in severe situations, the venous line may rhythmically jerk and relax as flow stops and is then reestablished with systemic venous return in the patient's cavae or right atrium.

Levels of hemolysis will also quickly rise if excessive vacuum is exerted in the venous line (96).

Establishing CPB via the groin vessels will afford the surgeon more control if massive bleeding in the chest is encountered. Alternatively, if the arterial cannula has been placed, CPB may be established using the pump suckers and a vent as a source of venous return (so-called sucker bypass). This will allow surgical control of bleeding and provide adequate decompression of the heart and preserve patient hemodynamics until the surgeon can place a conventional venous cannula in the right atrium or right atrium/inferior vena cava. The perfusionist should be prepared with additional cannulas, connectors, and tubing if CPB must be established emergently during reoperations (97). It must be recognized that the risk of aortic dissection is much greater when femoral arterial cannulation is used, which is discussed later in this chapter.

In summary, the number of patients presenting for reoperation is increasing. Increased surgical experience, use of antifibrinolytic drugs, and newer CPB technology can reduce the risk of morbidity and mortality associated with these procedures to levels approaching primary cardiac operation (98,99). Augmented venous drainage techniques have also been applied during minimally invasive cardiac surgery (100) and are discussed in greater detail in Chapter 35.

Cardiopulmonary Bypass after Pneumonectomy

CPB techniques for patients who have undergone prior pneumonectomy have only recently been addressed in the literature (101,102). The technical aspects of conducting CPB in such patients are not significantly different from those in patients who have had lobectomy or no pulmonary resection.

Hemodilution for CPB has been associated with a decrease in postoperative pulmonary problems theoretically from dilution of noxious blood elements or from avoidance of noxious elements (e.g., microaggregates present in homologous blood). However, excessive hemodilution may predispose to pulmonary edema, which might be addressed by limiting hemodilution to a hematocrit fraction of more than 20% in postpneumonectomy patients.

Blood transfusions should be avoided not only because of potential infections or transfusion reactions but also because of possible pulmonary damage from such elements as platelets and white blood cells. Washed packed red blood cells appear more appropriate when transfusion is indicated; return of shed blood should be avoided. When platelet transfusion is indicated, steroids and diphenhydramine should be used as pretreatment and leukocyte-depleted platelet concentrate should be used. Leukocyte reduction of all transfused residual perfusate will lessen the potential for pulmonary injury (103).

Technically, the position of the heart may be distorted because of contracted fibrothorax and/or hyperinflation of the remaining lung. This may lead to technical difficulty in gaining exposure, especially after left pneumonectomy. Remote cannulation from the femoral vessels has been helpful in some patients. Monitoring of pulmonary artery or left atrial pressure, with possible left ventricular venting, is important because strict control of the level of pulmonary capillary hydrostatic pressure is critical both intraoperatively and postoperatively to prevent pulmonary edema. Air emboli in the pulmonary circuit would seemingly be less well tolerated, and this is addressed by standard de-airing techniques. CPB time directly correlates with postoperative lung water; therefore, at times, a less complete coronary revascularization may be preferable to incurring a long CPB time. For coronary bypass surgery, the proximal anastomoses may be performed off pump or with low-flow partial CPB.

Minimally Invasive Surgery

This topic is reviewed in detail in Chapter 35.

INITIATION OF CARDIOPULMONARY BYPASS

The initiation of bypass is discussed in detail in Chapter 27. To briefly recapitulate a key issue, patency and continuity between the patient's vascular system (venous and arterial) and the CPB circuit must be assured for uncomplicated initiation of CPB. Cannula malposition, kinks in the CPB tubing, or clamps inadvertently left in place on cannulas or CPB tubing (venous or arterial) can prevent a smooth transition to full CPB flow. The absence of air bubbles in the CPB systemic line or arterial cannula must be visually verified to avoid systemic air embolism when CPB is started. Presence of abnormal anatomy (e.g., persistent left superior vena cava) or patient pathophysiology (e.g., aortic valve insufficiency) may compromise decompression of the heart during CPB. Presence of anatomic shunts may further obscure the surgical site, requiring placement of vents. Problems related to CPB cannulation and venting are discussed thoroughly in Chapters 5 and 6.

Acute dissection of the aorta is a serious often devastating problem that can occur with initiation of CPB. It is associated with a high mortality rate and, when recognized, inevitably leads to modification of the original surgical procedure. Fortunately, the incidence of acute dissection with ascending aortic cannulation is much less than when the femoral artery is used for the CPB systemic flow connection (104). Dissection may be delayed and not recognized until the postoperative period. This most often occurs in patients undergoing coronary artery bypass surgery who have a history of hypertension and severe atherosclerosis (105).

A triad of observations may aid recognition of acute aortic dissection. First and foremost is an unexpectedly increased CPB arterial line pressure as the systemic pump is activated. This often coincides with profoundly decreased systemic pressure measured by the indwelling arterial cathe-

ter. Third, the perfusionist may experience decreased venous drainage to the CPB circuit. At the surgical field, a hematoma may develop near the arterial cannulation site or there may be bleeding around the purse-string sutures.

If aortic dissection is suspected, the perfusionist should immediately stop CPB and notify the surgeon. The perfusionist and surgeon must confirm there are no kinks or clamps on the arterial line responsible for the increased CPB line pressure and/or decreased systemic pressure. The surgeon should palpate the aorta; if it is flaccid, this often indicates a major problem and acute dissection should be strongly suspected. It is important to clamp the venous line in this emergency situation to avoid exsanguinating the patient into the CPB reservoir. If dissection is confirmed, the arterial cannula is removed and reinserted in a different location so that CPB can be resumed. The dissection must be surgically repaired, which may involve replacement of the ascending aorta, quite possibly with deep hypothermia and circulatory arrest.

The risk of acute aortic dissection may be decreased by the surgeon observing a brisk backflow of blood at the time of insertion of the arterial cannula into the aorta. Once the CPB systemic flow line and cannula are joined, the perfusionist should observe and manually palpate pulsation in the CPB line that corresponds with the patient's pulse before starting bypass. Direct continuous measurement of arterial line pressure by aneroid gauge or electronic transducer allows observation of the CPB systemic line pressure during initiation and throughout the course of bypass.

Massive air embolism may occur during aortotomy for cannulation if an intraaortic balloon is in place (106,107). Briefly turning off the balloon pump whenever the aorta is opened, for instance, when placing cannulas (arterial or cardioplegia) or vents, will prevent aspirating room air into the aorta with intraaortic balloon deflation (108).

MAINTENANCE OF CARDIOPULMONARY BYPASS

CPB depends on two basic requirements: adequate blood volume to maintain appropriate blood flow and adequate gas flow (in the correct composition) to maintain appropriate gas exchange. Because of the invasive nature of cardiac surgery and CPB, a third requirement is avoidance of air embolism at all stages of the procedure. Myriad threats exist in accomplishing these objectives. Miscellaneous problems that may jeopardize patient well-being include errors in drug administration, contamination of the circuit or patient, and transfusion reactions or administration of mismatched blood products. Because of the patient's dependence on the CPB circuit and ancillary monitoring devices, equipment malfunction or failure is always a potential concern. Fortunately, the incidence of perfusion accidents is low and the incidence of adverse patient outcome (defined as injury re-

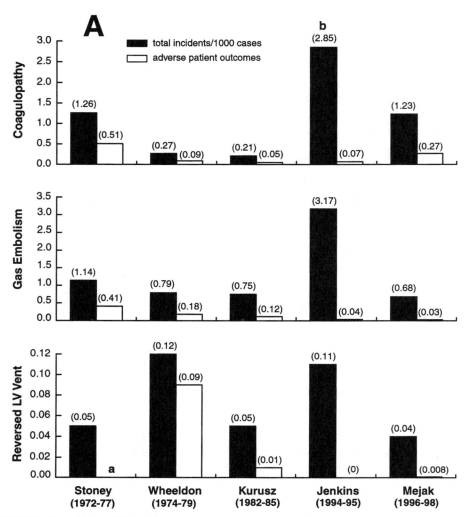

FIG. 28.5. A and B: Specific incidents are compared from the major cardiopulmonary bypass (CPB) perfusion accident surveys in the last three decades. The total caseload experience represented in each survey was as follows: Stoney, 373,819; Wheeldon, ~33,000; Kurusz, 573,785; Jenkins, 27,048; Mejak, 653,621. Total numbers of incidents per 1,000 cases are plotted in *solid bars* with reported adverse patient outcomes (defined as permanent injury, significantly complicated patient recovery, prolonged hospital stay, or death) to the right in *open bars*; incident rates are shown numerically for all categories. [a]Patient outcome for reversed left ventricular vent incidents not reported on Stoney survey.

quiring prolonged hospitalization, permanent injury, or death) is rare.

Publication of case reports and national surveys examining CPB experience has further heightened practitioner awareness of errors and malfunctions associated with CPB. Surveys by Stoney et al. (109), Kurusz et al. (110), and Mejak et al. (111) have elucidated incidence rates in the United States for a variety of perfusion mishaps occurring in the 1970s, 1980s, and 1990s, respectively. Other broad-based surveys by Wheeldon (112) and Jenkins et al. (113) have reported experiences in the United Kingdom and Australasia. The following discussion addresses the more common perfusion incidents based on these survey reports and

the authors' experience (114,115). Although direct comparison of results among different respondents during different survey time frames may be challenged, some sense of trends in the major reported CPB incidents may be discerned in Figure 28.5, A and B.

Inadequate Blood Flow

Acute aortic dissection can be a cause for inadequate blood flow during CPB and was discussed in the previous section because it most often is manifested at the time of initiation of CPB. Other causes of inadequate blood flow include low circulating volume that may result from a variety of causes.

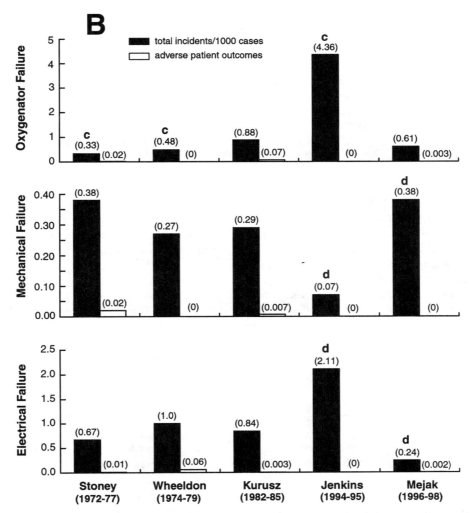

FIG. 28.5. *(continued)* [b]Jenkins reported "coagulation problems" and Mejak reported "coagulation problems following bypass" instead of the more specific "disseminated intravascular coagulopathy" or "consumption coagulopathy" as was used by Stoney, Wheeldon, and Kurusz; these differences in survey question wording could have accounted for the higher incident rates reported by Jenkins and Mejak. [c]Stoney asked about "failure of delivery of oxygen to pump," whereas Kurusz asked about "oxygenator failure"; Jenkins asked about several specific types of "oxygenator failures" and "gas supply failures," the most common being membrane leak; there were 35 cases reported in his survey, for which the oxygenator required replacement before or during CPB. [d]Jenkins and Mejak reported 13 and 140 additional "electrical or mechanical failures," respectively, that were not distinguished.

With the emphasis on reduced priming volumes for the CPB circuit and limited pre-CPB fluid administration by anesthesia personnel, there may be insufficient volume in the reservoir to maintain appropriate CPB systemic flow. Administration of vasodilators can drastically reduce CPB reservoir levels. Undetected blood leaks either from the CPB circuit or, more commonly, in the operative field or under surgical drapes will also reduce circulating blood volume. A particularly insidious blood leak may occur from Swan-Ganz catheter-induced pulmonary artery perforation, which carries a high risk of mortality (116,117). Hypothermia causes the catheter tip to stiffen and may predispose it to perforate the pulmonary artery (118). Deflating the balloon and withdrawing the catheter approximately 3 to 5 cm before or at the onset of CPB should lessen the risk of this complication (116), and a useful rule is to never inflate the balloon after systemic heparinization.

Inappropriate cannula size can reduce venous drainage, as will partial occlusion on the venous line. The venous or arterial cannulas may become malpositioned within the vasculature or inadvertently kinked or clamped, leading to reduced CPB blood flow (119–123). Rarely, the venous cannula may have a manufacturing defect that compromises the available cross-sectional area of its lumen, thus preventing normal venous drainage. Therefore, all cannulas should be inspected before use not only for proper size selection but also to confirm the absence of structural defects. A partially obstructed arterial cannula or oxygenator is manifested by elevated CPB systemic flow line pressures and lower than expected patient arterial pressures (124) or, if a centrifugal pump is being used, higher than expected revolutions per minute to maintain the desired flow (32). Another problem with centrifugal pumps is inaccurate flowmeter readings, which can arise when the flow probe is miscalibrated. With roller pumps, false displays of CPB pump output will result if the flow rate indicator on the CPB console is not set to match the tubing size (124).

Small quantities of entrained venous line air are rarely problematical in leading to a decrease in CPB systemic blood flow. However, if the entire venous line becomes filled with air, the gravity siphon effect will be lost (commonly referred to as air lock). This usually requires slowing or momentarily stopping CPB by clamping the venous line at the pump to allow personnel at the surgical field to refill the venous line with fluid and then "walking" any remaining air down the venous line into the venous reservoir to reestablish effective siphon drainage.

The CPB pump may fail, causing inadequate blood flow. Centrifugal pumps may decouple, meaning that the magnetic force to effectively rotate the pump has been lost between the pump console and base of the disposable pump head. This incident is often manifested by a high-pitched whining sound as the centrifugal pump motor accelerates to very high revolutions per minute; the in-line blood flowmeter also will show decreased flow that can progress to zero forward flow (and even retrograde flow) if not promptly corrected. An in-line valve in the CPB systemic flow line may prevent retrograde flow from the patient's aorta under these conditions (125). Underocclusion of a roller pump may lead to inadequate blood flow; this condition may be more difficult to detect than a centrifugal pump malfunction because in-line flowmeters are rarely used with roller pumps. Manifestations might include lower than expected CPB line or patient arterial pressures and decreased mixed venous hemoglobin oxygen saturation or P_vO_2 with developing acidosis.

Inadequate Gas Exchange

Although there are fundamental physiologic issues related to whole body oxygen consumption and delivery during CPB (discussed in Chapter 27), mechanical problems related to inadequate gas exchange by the oxygenator include oxygenator failure and gas delivery system failures. Oxygenator failure is diagnosed by observing dark-colored blood exiting the oxygenator that cannot be corrected by increasing the concentration of oxygen in the ventilating gas. Blood gas analysis or in-line blood gas sensors can confirm visual assessment of inadequate oxygenation. Causes may include loss of gas supply to the CPB oxygen/air blender or flowmeter or, more rarely, failure of the blender. Leaks or obstructions in the gas delivery system have been reported (126–128). Use of an in-line oxygen analyzer, which is considered standard on anesthesia machines, should be incorporated into the oxygenator gas delivery line to monitor delivery of appropriate concentrations and warn of abnormally low oxygen flow. The optimal position of the sensor is to place it nearest the oxygenator (129). Kirson and Goldman (130) reviewed oxygenator gas delivery problems in detail and proposed a system consisting of an aspirating oxygen sensor and pneumotachography for more accurate detection of such problems. Problems with gas scavenging systems causing inadequate gas transfer in the oxygenator have been reported (131). The patient who is either too lightly anesthetized or is hypothermic with inadequate muscle relaxation may have higher oxygen consumption that can lead to decreased mixed venous hemoglobin oxygen saturation and decreased arterial P_{O_2} if left uncorrected.

Inadequate anticoagulation leading to clotting in the oxygenator can cause inadequate gas transfer. The use of propofol anesthetic administered directly into the membrane oxygenator can potentially affect gas transfer, presumably by blocking pores or otherwise interfering with the membrane surface in the blood-contacting compartment of a microporous membrane. Therefore, propofol should be administered peripherally to permit deemulsification before it reaches the membrane oxygenator (132,133).

Fisher (134) recently provided data from the United Kingdom on the incidence of oxygenator failures requiring change-out. Two time periods were surveyed (1990 to 1992 and 1994 to 1996) during which the incidence was approximately 0.25 per thousand CPB procedures (1:4,000). Major causes for the change-outs differed between the two time periods. In the earlier survey, clotting in the oxygenator, particularly when aprotinin was being used, was the most frequently cited reason. In the latter survey, development of a high transoxygenator pressure gradient or a blood leak in the oxygenator was the major reason for change-out. Table 28.3 outlines steps for oxygenator change-out during CPB. Hart et al. (135) also described a technique for membrane oxygenator change-out that does not require stopping CPB. Earlier techniques with bubble oxygenator change-out required short periods (~2 to 3 minutes) of circulatory arrest (136,137).

Electrical Problems

Minor and major electrical problems are relatively common during CPB but only rarely cause adverse patient outcome. The entire CPB console or individual components can fail to operate as a result of wall power or electrical cord failures. Most hospitals have backup emergency generators to supply

TABLE 28.3. EMERGENCY REPLACEMENT OF MEMBRANE OXYGENATOR

1. Notify surgeon and anesthesiologist of problem; seek qualified assistance (second perfusionist preferable).
2. Turn off water flow to heat exchanger; clamp and disconnect water lines.
3. Turn off gas flow and remove oxygen delivery line.
4. Clamp venous line, turn off stopcock venting arterial line filter, and stop systemic blood flow pump.
5. Remove monitoring/sample line from oxygenator outlet.
6. Double clamp recirculation line (leaving 3″ between clamps while squeezing tubing between clamps to decrease pressure), oxygenator inlet and outlet lines; cut midway between clamps, leaving adequate lengths of tubing for reconnection.
7. Detach oxygenator from bracket; detach oxygenator from hard-shell venous reservoir (if attached).
8. Attach replacement oxygenator to hard-shell venous reservoir (if present) and mount in bracket.
9. Reconnect oxygenator inlet, outlet, and recirculation lines (trace connections to verify proper direction of flow) and band all new connections.
10. Connect water lines to heat exchanger, turn on water source, and inspect for leaks.
11. Connect oxygen line and set blender to deliver 100% oxygen.
12. Remove clamps from recirculation and oxygenator inlet tubing lines (DO NOT UNCLAMP ARTERIAL OUTLET LINE OR VENOUS DRAINAGE LINE)
13. After verifying sufficient volume in venous reservoir, turn on systemic flow pump *slowly* to fill the oxygenator.
14. Recirculate at 4 to 5 L/min to debubble oxygenator.
15. Stop recirculation and clamp recirculation line.
16. Visually inspect entire system to ensure system is free of leaks and gas bubbles.
17. Notify surgeon CPB is ready to be restarted.
18. Remove all clamps from arterial and venous lines, open arterial purge line stopcock, turn on gas flow, and restart CPB.

CPB, Cardiopulmonary bypass.

the operating room with electricity in the event of power outage. Sometimes these backup generators can fail to come on in a timely manner, making it prudent to have alternative electrical backup such as a uninterruptible power supply in the operating room and in-line with the CPB console for dealing with power failures. Some newer CPB consoles have battery power built in to provide continuous function in the event of electrical failure. All CPB systemic pumps should have provision for manual hand cranking readily available in the event backup electrical sources fail. The CPB console can be sabotaged, either by inappropriate conduct by untrained personnel or by malicious actions by those with more sinister intentions. In either situation, performance of a thorough pre-bypass checklist by the primary perfusionist at the time of setup should uncover potential malfunctions before placing the patient on bypass.

Electronic components within the console can fail, leading to erratic operation or cessation of function of individual components. Runaway pumps have been reported (138,139), as have electrical fires that can lead to loss of function of CPB components (140). Power surges or brownouts can lead to inaccurate readings on the CPB console or physiologic monitors. Piezo-electric or static charges created by roller pump rotation can interfere with the electrocardiogram (ECG) (141). This may be prevented by grounding the CPB console to a metal-jacketed temperature port in the oxygenator (142). ECG electrodes, lead wires, and cables should be intact to also avoid ECG "noise" when the patient is on CPB (143). Transducers may "drift" over the course of several hours, leading to inaccurate readings. It is therefore prudent to re-zero transducers before weaning from bypass to ensure accuracy of measured parameters that can influence management decisions (144). Temperature probes may become disconnected or malpositioned, leading to improper displays. It is therefore advisable to place at least two patient temperature probes for redundancy. In-line blood gas monitors or oximeters may display erroneous values unless calibrated against standard laboratory samples. The electrocautery can interfere with monitor displays; use of a shielded ECG cable will minimize such interference.

There are a variety of alarms used on anesthesia, perfusion, and ancillary equipment in the cardiac surgical operating room. Often, similar sounding high-pitched signals can make rapid identification of the source of the alarm difficult. Cases of misinterpreted alarms (e.g., intraaortic balloon and low-level alarm on CPB reservoir) have distracted the perfusionist with serious patient consequences (145). Alarms may be obtrusive, and there may be a tendency among some practitioners to disable alarms that are designed to give early warning or automatically respond if user-set thresholds are exceeded when potentially hazardous patient conditions are met (146,147).

Perfusionists, anesthesiologists, and nurses must know how to troubleshoot equipment used during CPB. Performing team drills for the unexpected perfusion crisis such as oxygenator change-out, hand cranking for electrical failure, or dealing with massive air embolism can be life saving during these rare events. Cooper et al. (148) cited lack of familiarity with equipment as one major factor in operating room mishaps, and Gaba (149) provided an excellent review of human error during conduct of anesthesia that has applicability to performance of CPB.

Air Embolism

Concern over air embolism during CPB has been a constant focus of all involved in the perioperative care of the cardiac surgical patient. Air embolism (venous or arterial) may occur not only from CPB (pump air) but during a variety of surgical procedures (surgical air) or at the head of the table from actions or inaction by anesthesia personnel (anesthetic air) (150). The pathophysiology of air embolism has been extensively studied in laboratory experiments, many of which predated the clinical use of CPB. Case reports detailing mechanisms of air embolism have appeared periodically in the literature. The next sections review the more common etiologies, followed by a discussion of treatment strategies for this complication.

Surgical (Operative) Air

In 1914, the danger of air embolism during cardiac surgery was reported by Carrel (151), who wrote, "The opening of the ventricles or of the pulmonary artery and the aorta is always followed by entrance of air into the heart." Support for his statement was the observation of ventricular fibrillation and death in animals after coronary artery air embolism.

Air embolism on the left side of the heart was well known to thoracic surgeons before the advent of open heart surgery. Reyer and Kohl (152) reported 10 cases of venous or arterial air embolism, 5 of which resulted in the patients' deaths, during a variety of surgical or diagnostic procedures. Kent and Blades (153) further warned that the two major hazards of thoracic surgery were infection and embolic phenomena. In their animal experiments, air embolism was found to be well tolerated on the venous side, in the absence of a patent foramen ovale, but fatal with small injections of air into the pulmonary veins.

Geoghegan and Lam (154) reported that the mechanism of death due to air embolism in dogs (0.25 to 2.0 mL/kg) was either coronary (immediate death) or cerebral (severe brain damage). Benjamin et al. (155) further sought to define the mechanisms of air embolism by injecting varying amounts of air (0.5 to 8.0 mL/kg) into the left atrium, left ventricle, aortic root, common carotid, or descending aorta of dogs. Left atrial air embolism was fatal 100% of the time, whereas the same volumes of air injected into the left ventricle caused death in 83% of the animals. Aortic root and carotid air embolism were better tolerated, and large volumes of air (up to 10 mL/kg) were required to cause death when given into the descending aorta. They, like other investigators (156–164), noted the dangers of left heart air but concluded that small amounts of air in the systemic circulation were generally well tolerated during surgical procedures if appropriate resuscitative maneuvers were undertaken when required.

Many retrospective reviews of early clinical experience with CPB have been published. Callaghan et al. (165) analyzed 60 deaths in 250 CPB patients operated on between 1956 and 1961. A variety of causes described included seven cases of cerebral damage, four of which were from air embolism. Ehrenhaft et al. (166) reported 19 of 244 (7.7%) patients undergoing open heart surgery suffered cerebral damage. Systemic air embolism was the suspected etiology because many operations involved closure of septal defects. Like Carrel nearly 50 years earlier, they warned of air entrance to the left side of the heart or aorta with subsequent embolization when the normal circulation was restored. Allen (167) reported cerebral damage in 18 of 500 (3.6%)

patients undergoing repair of valvular or congenital cardiac defects and warned of the propensity of air to collect in the left atrium near the right superior pulmonary vein. Sloan et al. (168) reported 78 of 600 (13%) patients died after CPB; air trapped in the left ventricle was identified as the source of the air and was believed responsible for 49 deaths. Nicks (169) reported systemic air embolism in 40 of 340 (11.7%) patients undergoing congenital or valvular procedures; 10 patients died. Fishman et al. (170) later confirmed the left atrium and pulmonary veins as locations of trapped air whenever the left heart was opened. Anderson et al. (171) and Lin (172) also warned of the risks of pulmonary hypertension due to right-sided air embolism.

The preference of cannulation of the ascending aorta for CPB, although much safer than the femoral artery site, increased the risk of cerebral air embolism. Gomes et al. (173) found that air embolism via the femoral artery was five times less likely to involve the cerebral vessels if the air originated from the CPB arterial line. Beckman et al. (174) determined the optimum method of placement of the ascending aortic cannula to lessen the risk of air entry. Direct insertion of the cannula without use of a side-biting clamp, which tended to trap a small amount of air, was found to be safest.

In the article by Mills and Ochsner (114) on mechanisms of air embolism, two additional surgical sources were described: unexpected resumption of the heart beat and inadequate steps to remove air after cardiotomy. Coronary air embolism with cardioplegia techniques was reported in 1981 (175) and 1986 (110). Although air embolism was generally thought not to occur during coronary bypass operations, Hughes (176) reported the possibility of intraventricular air with right superior pulmonary vein venting that could draw air in via coronary arteriotomy, especially when the left anterior descending coronary artery was opened. Robicsek and Duncan (177) and Lee (178) subsequently confirmed this mechanism. Air also can be drawn retrograde through an opened coronary artery if an aortic root vent is used and placed under significant negative pressure.

Cardiopulmonary Bypass (Pump) Air

Air embolism originating from the CPB circuit may enter the patient's vascular system either from the arterial line or by other mechanisms, many of which are discussed in other chapters. Reed et al. (179) reviewed the many mechanisms for air embolism from the CPB circuit, some of which have been reported in the literature and others learned through direct or anecdotal experience.

Arterial line air embolism due to emptying of the CPB reservoir, as occurred during Dennis' early case (180), has been a common cause. The current popular use of membrane oxygenators in which the blood is drawn from a venous reservoir and then pumped through the oxygenator may have decreased the incidence of arterial line air embolism that was much more prevalent when bubble oxygenators were widely used (110). However, inattention to the reservoir level can still cause air to be transmitted to the CPB systemic flow line, regardless of oxygenator type. The importance of maintaining an adequate volume in the CPB reservoir was reported in 1958 (181) and has been one of the fundamental safety principles taught in perfusion training programs since their inception.

High pump flows in conjunction with vertical CPB reservoir outlets may cause vortexing of air into the systemic flow line. Newer model reservoirs with angled or horizontal outlets are less prone to this condition.

The arterial roller pump head tubing may rupture, causing arterial air embolism. Cases of electrical malfunction of the arterial pump (roller and centrifugal) were previously mentioned (138,139); in some circumstances the malfunctioning pump can spontaneously accelerate to a high speed, drawing air into the CPB systemic flow line. Less dramatic, but just as dangerous, the arterial roller pump may rotate slowly before or after CPB and may be unnoticed by the perfusionist, leading to emptying of the reservoir and subsequent air embolism. If the arterial pump is not operating, a second roller pump for blood cardioplegia can draw air into both the cardioplegia delivery circuit and the arterial line.

Accidental disconnects, punctures, cuts, or openings, such as stopcocks left open to atmosphere, in the arterial line can cause air embolism depending on flow conditions. Generally, such disruptions will cause blood loss from the circuit, but under low CPB systemic flow conditions air may enter the arterial line (182,183). Centrifugal pumps, when connected directly to the patient's venous system, can draw air into the CPB circuit if intravenous lines are open to atmosphere. Breaks in the integrity of the CPB arterial line are especially favorable for air entry if they occur on the negative (inlet) side of the pump. Strictures in the arterial line on the positive side from kinks, application of clamps, or excessive flows through small-diameter connectors or cannulas can produce air embolism from cavitation effects (184).

The oxygenator or venous or cardiotomy reservoir may become pressurized and transmit air into blood lines connected to the patient if ports designed to vent them to atmosphere become occluded (185,186). The current popularity of vacuum-assisted venous return has the potential for pressurizing the cardiotomy reservoir if vacuum is not maintained and the pump suction or vent pumps continue to operate. Vacuum-assisted venous drainage also has the potential to deprime the arterial line filter or oxygenator if vacuum is applied before establishing CPB. A pressurized cardiotomy reservoir may transmit air retrograde to the patient's heart via the vent line (114) or to the arterial filter if the purge line is connected to the reservoir and a one-way valve is not incorporated into the purge line. Retrograde venous air embolism from bubble oxygenators due to block-

age of the gas scavenging line was described by Wells and Stiles (187) and confirmed by others (188,189). Alternatively, if the gas phase of either a silicone rubber or microporous membrane oxygenator becomes pressurized above blood phase pressure, ventilating gas can enter the arterial line through the membrane material.

Anesthetic Air

The risk of air embolism in the course of anesthetic management of patients undergoing open heart surgery most commonly occurs with intravenous or monitoring lines. Despite controversy regarding the risk of small quantities of venous air, cases of fatal air embolism during neurosurgical procedures with patients in the sitting position were reported as early as 1902 (190). During animal experiments, Goodridge sought to dispel the earlier report by Hare (191) that venous air embolism was innocuous. He concluded (190) ". . .I would say that I believe the statement, 'that large quantities of air may be introduced into the veins without unfavorable results' to be pernicious teaching and not supported by fact."

Inappropriate ventilation of the patient during insertion of CPB cannulas or a left atrial monitoring line can cause air embolism. Expanding the lungs fully to displace pulmonary venous air is an important adjunct to surgical de-airing maneuvers; if not performed properly, air may be retained and later embolize to the arterial circulation.

The risk of greater than 50% nitrous oxide ventilation in promoting bubble growth has been reported by several authors (192–195) and was reviewed by Munson (196). Wells et al. (197) found increased cerebrospinal fluid markers indicative of cerebral ischemia when nitrous oxide anesthesia was used in conjunction with bubble oxygenation. Conventional wisdom is that nitrous oxide should be avoided from the time of cannulation for CPB until emergence from CPB. Many would also advise its avoidance after CPB, because the likelihood of some intravascular air is relatively high, especially in procedures where the heart has been opened.

Treatment of Air Embolism

Peirce (198) wrote that treatment of iatrogenic air embolism has not kept pace with other medical knowledge, perhaps because it is a rare and frequently unrecognized complication. Intraoperative treatment for air embolism in open heart surgical patients is unique when compared with other medical procedures where air embolism may occur. If coronary air embolism results in myocardial dysfunction, the circulatory needs of the patient can be met by the CPB circuit. Systemic heparinization, a requisite for CPB, has been shown to be of benefit in reducing interactions of bubbles with blood but may be deleterious if brain infarction has occurred (199). Hemodilution to levels commonly used during CPB will reduce blood viscosity and improve tissue perfusion when air embolism occurs. With the chest open, the surgeon is able to aspirate air directly from the heart chambers or vessels. Venting, induction of hypothermia (200,201), retrograde coronary sinus (202,203) or cerebral perfusion (114), or direct cardiac massage are all available if air embolism occurs during the open heart operation. If right coronary artery air embolism is suspected (isolated acute ST segment elevation in the inferior ECG leads is highly suggestive), the surgeon can transiently raise the pressure in the proximal aorta by gently pinching the aorta distal to the arterial cannula with the left hand while using the index finger of the other hand to assess proximal aortic pressure. The transiently increased aortic pressure will push intracoronary air bubbles through the coronary circulation, which often can be seen if significant right coronary air embolism has occurred. This maneuver should be tried in all patients before implementing intraaortic balloon counterpulsation when there is difficulty encountered in weaning from CPB.

Drug or fluid therapy by the anesthesiologist also may be instituted immediately via the CPB circuit. Packing the patient's head in ice will decrease cerebral metabolism and may be beneficial (204). Ventilating the patient with 100% oxygen favors bubble resolution and can limit cerebral ischemia (205). If air embolism occurs before or after CPB, conventional means of treatment can immediately be used such as positioning the patient head-down and turning the patient into the left lateral recumbent position (206,207) or instituting cardiopulmonary resuscitation (208).

The source of air must be determined and promptly interrupted to prevent further transmission of air into the patient. If the source of air is the CPB systemic flow line, then CPB should be stopped immediately (114,209). The arterial and venous lines should be clamped to prevent additional embolization or exsanguination. After confirming sufficient volume in the CPB reservoir, air in the arterial line should be purged out by aspirating with a large syringe or refilling the line using the systemic pump. If a pressurized reservoir or CPB component is the source, the pressure should be relieved before releasing clamps on lines directly connected to the patient.

If air has filled the aorta, the arterial line can be disconnected from the arterial cannula. After clamping the venous cannula(s) and disconnecting the venous line, the arterial line and venous line are joined so perfusate can be quickly recirculated back to the CPB reservoir to remove the air. Once cleared of air, the lines are reconnected to the appropriate cannulas and CPB may be resumed. If air has not reached the arterial line filter, it can be vented out the purge line by slowly advancing flow with the systemic pump. Air can be removed from a centrifugal pump by detaching it from the console and positioning the pump head outlet uppermost to take advantage of buoyancy effects; with the pump head de-aired, recirculation or resumption of CPB

can then be accomplished. Air may be removed from the membrane oxygenator by recirculating at high flow via the membrane recirculation line. Tapping and inverting components, as is performed during initial priming, may be required to effectively remove CPB air. If the arterial filter has been filled with air, it may be necessary to clamp the filter out of the circuit and use an arterial filter bypass line to quickly reestablish CPB blood flow. Alarms to detect air embolism often must be turned off to reestablish CPB systemic flow but then should be reengaged after the patient is safely back on bypass.

Placing the patient in the Trendelenburg position after air embolism is common practice but may not aid in bubble removal from cerebral vessels deep within the brain. Butler et al. (210) studied the distribution of carotid artery injections of air (0.5 to 1.0 mL) in dogs placed in 0 to 30-degree Trendelenburg position. They concluded that regardless of the position, if the heart was ejecting blood, bubbles would not be retarded in their distribution into the brain. In additional *in vitro* studies in the same report using a simulated carotid artery, the authors verified that the buoyant properties of the bubbles were not sufficient to prevent the blood from carrying bubbles in the direction of flow. They did suggest, however, that in conditions of circulatory arrest or extremely low flow, bubbles would have a propensity to rise in stagnated blood.

More recently, Mehlhorn et al. (211) studied the effects of body repositioning on the hemodynamic response to large infusions of venous air (2.5 mL/kg at a rate of 5 mL/sec) in dogs. Testing the supine, left lateral recumbent (Durant's maneuver), left lateral recumbent with 10-degree head-down, or right lateral recumbent positions, they found no significant differences among the various body positions in terms of heart rate, blood pressure, pulmonary artery, central venous, or left ventricular end-diastolic pressures, or cardiac output. There also were no significant differences in recovery times regardless of body position.

If large quantities of air are suspected of having entered the cerebral vessels, retrograde cerebral perfusion, as first described by Mills and Ochsner (114), may be used with remarkable results. There are a number of case reports now in the literature (212–220) confirming the benefit of this technique, as well as anecdotal information from survey respondents (110). The fact that retrograde cerebral perfusion is being used electively more frequently during aortic arch surgery may facilitate implementation of this method under emergency condition. Table 28.4 outlines steps to perform retrograde cerebral perfusion for massive air embolism.

Drug therapy for arterial air embolism is aimed first at raising the arterial blood pressure to force bubbles through tissue vasculature to the venous side of the circulation (221). Corticosteroids, diuretics, antiplatelet agents, anticonvulsants, and barbiturates have been advocated to decrease cerebral manifestations of ischemic injury due to air embolism.

TABLE 28.4. STEPS TO PERFORM RETROGRADE CEREBRAL PERFUSION FOR TREATMENT OF MASSIVE AIR EMBOLISM

1. Perfusionist: Stop CPB.
2. Anesthesiologist: Place patient in steep head-down position.
3. Surgeon: Remove aortic cannula from ascending aorta.
4. After purging air and refilling CPB systemic flow line, insert arterial cannula in the SVC above a point where a vascular clamp can be placed; if bicaval cannulation has been used, the arterial cannula may be connected to the snared SVC cannula.
5. Begin retrograde perfusion with hypothermia (20°C) at a flow of 1–2 L/min for 1–3 min or until no more air or froth is seen exiting the opened aorta.
6. Anesthesiologist: Temporarily compress the carotids during the later phase to purge air retrograde through the vertebral system.

CPB, Cardiopulmonary bypass; SVC, superior vena cava.

Lidocaine pretreatment has been shown to be beneficial in an experimental setting (222). Surface tension-reducing agents have been proposed (223–225). More recently, the use of perfluorocarbons to enhance oxygen delivery has been suggested for treatment of air embolism (226); however, it apparently has not been used clinically for treatment of air embolism (227). Such agents may also reduce the surface tension at the bubble–blood interface and would aid in absorption and dissolution of the bubbles (228,229). Speiss et al. (230,231) studied the protective effects of prophylactically administered perfluorocarbon solutions in experimental coronary and cerebral air embolism in the laboratory. Treated animals had significantly fewer dysrhythmias and less decrease in myocardial function when pretreated.

The patient with known or suspected air embolism should be ventilated with 100% oxygen (232). Ventilation with nitrous oxide, if it is being used, should be discontinued to decrease the possibility for bubble expansion (233,234). Hlastala and Van Liew (235) showed that a 2-mm bubble will disappear in approximately 1 hour if the patient is breathing oxygen; if the patient is not being ventilated and is breathing room air, the same size bubble will persist for 9 hours.

Regardless of when air embolism occurs during the intraoperative period, most authors have recommended that the surgical procedure should be completed (114,209). An air embolism incident in the course of an open heart surgical procedure can create confusion on the part of various team members. Having a predetermined treatment plan (209,236) for dealing with this event can be life saving. Tovar et al. (237) recently published an excellent review of management of air embolism. A proposed algorithm from their article is shown in Figure 28.6.

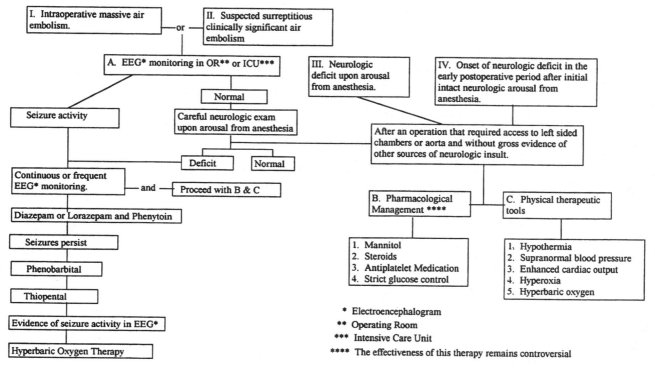

FIG. 28.6. Algorithm for postoperative management of air embolism. (From Tovar EA, DelCampo C, Borsari A, et al. Postoperative management of cerebral air embolism: gas physiology for surgeons. *Ann Thorac Surg* 1995;60:1138–1142, with permission.)

The most effective postoperative treatment for air embolism is compression in a hyperbaric chamber and ventilation with 100% oxygen (238–248). Although the logistics of moving a critically ill patient on a ventilator and with invasive monitoring and multiple intravenous lines can be daunting, treatment in such a facility has been credited for many complete recoveries. Recoveries have been reported even if such treatment is delayed (249,250). However, it must be recognized that access to a multiplace hyperbaric chamber may be limited. There are only approximately 100 such facilities in the United States, most of which are located on the coastlines or near large bodies of water and therefore are at great distances from many hospitals performing open heart surgery. The patient with suspected air embolism should not be transported by air because reduced air pressure during flight will cause intravascular bubbles to expand. Brenner (209) suggested that treatment regimens for air embolism should be continued unless the patient expires or is diagnosed as brain dead. Table 28.5 outlines management strategies for treatment of air embolism.

Miscellaneous Problems

The CPB circuit or its components may become contaminated by inattention to detail during setup or operation. The obvious risk of bacterial contamination via the patient's bloodstream necessitates observing sterile technique at all stages of use of CPB. Infection after cardiac surgery is an uncommon but serious complication leading to prolonged duration of mechanical ventilation and intensive care unit stay. One third of these patients may die of causes related to infection (251).

The practice of dry preassembly of the CPB circuit is not without risk. The Centers for Disease Control and Prevention recently reported an investigation into an outbreak of gram-negative bacteremia in nine cardiac surgery patients at one hospital (252). The source of the infections was found to be caused by housekeeping personnel inadvertently contaminating uncovered preassembled disposable pressure transducers on the CPB console with sprayed cleaning water. This complication can be prevented by ensuring all blood-contacting surfaces and devices on the CPB circuit are kept covered until time of use. Alternatively, the entire CPB circuit can be set up just before use to minimize risk of contamination. Hospital-prepared cardioplegic solution may be the source of contamination by *Enterobacter cloacae* (253,254) due to defective equipment used by manufacturing pharmacy personnel. Thus, meticulous attention to quality control, including batch sterility testing of the cardioplegic solution, will minimize this risk. Alternatively, commercially prepared cardioplegic solutions are usually subject to more stringent quality controls.

Drug errors by any cardiac surgical team member are relatively common and can lead to adverse outcomes. The most commonly cited drug-related problem in one survey (110) was overdosage of either a vasodilator or vasoconstric-

TABLE 28.5. INTRAOPERATIVE AND POSTOPERATIVE MANAGEMENT STRATEGIES FOR TREATMENT OF AIR EMBOLISM

1. Perfusionist: Stop CPB immediately, clamp arterial and venous lines, and notify surgeon and anesthesiologist.
2. Locate and confirm source of air; if due to pressurized CPB component, isolate component from patient before relieving pressure.
3. Perfusionist: Purge air from CPB systemic flow line and refill with fluid.
4. Surgeon: Aspirate air (if present) from arterial cannula; if possible, initiate cardiac massage until CPB restarted.
5. Anesthesiologist: Place patient in steep head-down position; be prepared to temporarily occlude carotid arteries.
6. Confirm sufficient volume in CPB reservoir and resume CPB with active aortic root venting.
7. Administer vasopressors to raise perfusion pressure.
8. If suspected cerebral air embolism, cool patient on CPB and consider instituting retrograde cerebral perfusion; consider packing patient's head in ice.
9. Anesthesiologist: Ventilate lungs vigorously with 100% oxygen; administer corticosteroids (2–4 g methylprednisolone and/or 20 mg dexamethasone, and continue for 72–96 hr postoperatively).
10. Administer 25 g mannitol and maintain for 48 hr postoperatively.
11. Aim for early patient arousal and assess for return of normal mentation.
12. Consult a neurologist if central nervous system damage is suspected.
13. Consider computed tomography or magnetic resonance imaging if patient fails to awaken or develops delayed mental deterioration.
14. Consider hyperbaric oxygen treatment (6 ATA using recommended U.S. Navy dive tables) and make necessary ground transportation arrangements; repeat hyperbaric therapy as necessary.
15. Do not give up resuscitative efforts unless patient expires or is diagnosed brain dead.

CPB, Cardiopulmonary bypass; ATA, atmospheres of absolute pressure.

tor. Although these types of errors may be short-lived and of no clinical consequence, drug errors related to anticoagulation can be fatal. Protamine administration during CPB can effectively render the oxygenator, reservoir, and arterial line filter unusable due to development of gross clot. A case of inadvertent protamine administration instead of heparin has been reported (255). The patient survived, but a massive clot was found in the oxygenator, a smaller clot in the arterial filter, and fibrin strands in the cardiotomy suction tubing. No activated coagulation time or heparin assay testing was performed. The hospital has now changed their policy to no longer store protamine in the operating room; it is now reportedly not drawn up until the surgeon requests that protamine be administered.

Another serious complication is transfusion of ABO-incompatible bank blood. The manifestation is an acute hemolytic reaction that can damage the kidneys. Prevention lies in adherence to strict double checking of blood units against the patient's identification wristband. Maintenance of urine output with diuretics, intravenous fluid support, and administering corticosteroids and cardiotonic drugs has been used with success (256).

PATIENT PATHOPHYSIOLOGY

Pregnancy

Although the rate of cardiovascular disease in pregnancy has steadily declined over the past several decades, it remains a topic of interest because of the high rate of fetal mortality when an operation requiring CPB is needed. The incidence of all maternal cardiovascular disease during pregnancy is currently about 1.5% (257). The most frequently performed procedures include closed mitral commissurotomy, open mitral commissurotomy, mitral valve replacement, and aortic valve replacement. Credit for the first case using CPB in a pregnant patient has been attributed to Leyse et al. (258) in 1958, with three more cases reported subsequently (259,260). Other cardiac problems associated with pregnancy in which operation may be necessary are atrial septal defect, patent ductus arteriosus, ventricular septal defect, and idiopathic hypertrophic subaortic stenosis (261). Because of intravenous drug abuse, infectious endocarditis assumes an increasing role among cardiovascular diseases in pregnancy.

A number of fundamentals in the physiology of pregnancy affect the timing and use of CPB in the pregnant patient. The first trimester is the trimester of organogenesis. Therefore, any injury to the embryo during this period may result in teratogenesis. This is particularly true of drugs. An important example is warfarin, a well-known teratogen. Because of the small size of the warfarin molecule, it can cross the placenta. The neonatal morbidity and mortality for patients taking warfarin throughout their pregnancy may be 40% or greater. For this reason, patients undergoing warfarin therapy are often changed to heparin when pregnancy is confirmed. The large heparin molecule cannot cross the uteroplacental barrier (262). However, the rate of spontaneous abortion increases with heparin.

Other factors associated with CPB that may lead to teratogenesis include hypoxemia and decreased perfusion. During the second trimester of pregnancy, the period of organogenesis is finished; therefore, teratogenesis is not seen. The risk of premature labor is much less than in the third trimester, when the risk rises significantly. The hypervolemia and anemia of pregnancy also are less in the second trimester than in the third trimester, as are the hemodynamic demands because of the smaller size of the fetus and lesser uterine blood flow.

Numerous physiologic changes occur during pregnancy. Because there is no autoregulation of uterine blood flow, nonpulsatile flow during CPB may compromise fetal blood supply. After the 28th to 32nd week of gestation, the patient's blood volume has increased by 30% to 50%. Heart rate increases 10% to 15% and stroke volume increases 30% to 35% with an associated 15% decrease in systemic vascular resistance. During pregnancy, uterine blood flow represents 10% to 15% of the cardiac output, as compared with only 1% in a nonpregnant female (261).

The lowest risk for CPB surgery is believed to occur during the second trimester, with reported maternal mortality risk during this time varying from 1.5% to 5% (263–266). In particular, a survey (257) regarding bypass surgery on pregnant women revealed only 1 maternal death in 68 cases. In general, the maternal risk is probably not increased over that in a nonpregnant patient. Fetal risk, however, is quite high, ranging from 10% to 50% (261,264–272). The previously cited survey (257) revealed a 20% fetal mortality in the same 68 CPB cases.

A closer examination of the causes of fetal risk reveals multiple factors. There are numerous possible causes for fetal hypoxia. Low CPB systemic flows or hypotension during bypass can result in fetal hypoxia because of the lack of autoregulation of the uterine blood flow. Low hemoglobin oxygen saturation and possibly the lack of pulsatile flow, uterine arteriovenous shunts, or uterine arterial spasm may contribute to fetal hypoxia. Hypoxia may result from particulate or bubble embolization to the uteroplacental bed (273). Uterine blood flow also may be compromised by venous obstruction of the inferior vena cava resulting from improper cannula placement (274).

Hypoxia is best diagnosed by noting fetal heart rate (FHR) decelerations. The normal FHR is between 120 and 160 beats/min. The FHR may decrease to 80 to 100 beats/min with hypothermia, but an FHR less than 60 beats/min suggests a high probability of life-threatening fetal distress. Acidosis may contribute to fetal bradycardia. Fetal bradycardia, defined as FHR less than 120 beats/min at normothermia and FHR less than 80 beats/min at hypothermia, may be treated by increasing the CPB systemic flow rate, which usually increases the heart rate toward normal (270,275,276). However, one problem that may occur is a temporary increase in the heart rate followed by a heart rate reduction that does not respond to increased flow. For this reason, time on CPB is a significant factor and should be minimized (265).

The initiation of uterine contractions most frequently causes fetal death (264,265). The dilution of progesterone during CPB secondary to hemodilution may predispose to the onset of uterine contractions (270), which can be detected by a tachodynamometer. When the FHR is monitored simultaneously, the FHR pattern may show late decelerations with each uterine contraction, indicating hypoxia. This usually indicates that blood flow across the myometrium stops as uterine contraction pressure increases to exceed the uteroplacental arteriolar pressure. Most uterine contractions resolve after the termination of CPB. Risk of initiation of uterine contractions does not end, however, with termination of CPB; therefore, it is recommended that uterus be monitored for contractions for 72 hours postoperatively (269). The rewarming cycle during bypass is associated with the onset of uterine contractions (269). Uterine contractions are treated with tocolytic agents (see below). Progesterone may also be useful.

Perfusion problems constitute a potential source of fetal complications. These include nonpulsatile perfusion, inadequate perfusion pressure, inadequate systemic blood flow, embolic phenomena to uteroplacental circulation, or alterations in placental blood flow secondary to cannulation. Meffert and Stansel (262) noted an increase in fetal mortality when mitral valve replacement was performed, as compared with that resulting from mitral commissurotomy. Those authors believed that this difference resulted from the longer CPB times required for mitral valve replacement. Fetal mortality rate has been noted to increase with an increase in CPB time in some reviews (265), yet Weiss et al. (266) could find no correlation between time on CPB and neonatal outcome in their recent survey of the literature.

A number of strategies have evolved to avoid complications, and techniques have been devised to reduce the rate of fetal complications. Because of the marked increase in cardiac output during pregnancy, normal cardiac output during the third trimester of pregnancy may be 6 L/min; therefore, a perfusion flow of 4 L/min represents only two thirds that of the normal flow and could result in fetal hypoperfusion. Using a membrane oxygenator and an arterial line filter in the CPB circuit minimizes particulate and gaseous emboli. FHR can be adequately maintained by perfusion at either normothermia or mild hypothermia. In pregnant patients, most authors recommend systemic pressures ranging from 60 to 75 mm Hg, preferably accomplished with high perfusion flows rather than with α-adrenergic agonists. FHR monitoring should be used to detect the decreases in heart rate associated with poor fetal perfusion. Because FHR is correlated with CPB systemic flow, fetal bradycardia should be treated with an increase in CPB flow rate. Both FHR and uterine activity monitoring should be maintained for 48 to 72 hours postoperatively. Table 28.6 outlines management strategies for the pregnant patient.

In the third trimester of pregnancy, particularly because of the increased rate of premature labor, expectant management of the patient allowing the fetus to stay *in utero* as long as possible plays an increasing role. Options may include expectant management of the mother with delivery or cesarean section followed by maternal cardiac surgery, maternal surgery with the fetus remaining *in utero*, or simultaneous cesarean section and maternal cardiac surgery. The approach selected should balance the maturity of the fetus with the severity of maternal cardiac disease and the risk of labor and delivery with uncorrected cardiac disease. If uteroplacental insufficiency is present (suggested by fetal bradycardia), delivery of the fetus before CPB should be considered. Al-

TABLE 28.6. MANAGEMENT STRATEGIES FOR THE PREGNANT PATIENT

1. If possible, postpone surgery until patient is postpartum.
2. Position patient in left uterine displacement position if gestational age of fetus >20 wk.
3. Monitor fetal heart rate (FHR).
4. Monitor uterine contractile activity.
5. Prime CPB circuit with bank blood if expected mixed patient/circuit hematocrit is <22–25%.
6. Use CPB systemic flow index of 2.5–3.0 L/min/m² and be prepared to increase flow if FHR decreases.
7. Maintain minimum mean arterial pressure 60 mm Hg.
8. Use normothermia or mild hypothermia (32°C); use deep hypothermia and circulatory arrest *only* if surgical conditions necessitate.
9. Do not use potassium-based cardioplegia.
10. Be prepared to administer progesterone, β-agonist, or intravenous alcohol if uterine contractions occur.
11. Minimize CPB time consistent with surgical objective.
12. Have an obstetrician and neonatologist on standby in case cesarean section is required (gestational age >28 wk).

CPB, cardiopulmonary bypass.

though the exact role is not known, avoidance of CPB altogether by using a closed procedure such as closed mitral commissurotomy or balloon valvuloplasty may be an option in patients at particularly high risk for undergoing CPB.

Fetal complications could also be theoretically attributed to nonpulsatile perfusion, hyperoxygenation, or anticoagulation with heparin. At present, none of these factors has been clearly identified as the cause of fetal problems. Hypothermia also causes FHR decelerations; therefore, normothermia or mild hypothermia (32°C) is generally used. However, Buffolo et al. (277) reported use of deep hypothermia with circulatory arrest for aortic arch surgery with survival of the mother and fetus. Others (271,278) also reported successful cases in which hypothermia with a period of circulatory arrest was required. Most sources believe that a hematocrit exceeding 22% should be maintained as well as a CPB systemic flow index of 3.0 L/min/m². To avert the potential effects of aortocaval compression by the gravid uterus, central cannulation is preferable to femoral arterial or venous cannulation. Late in pregnancy, the right flank should be elevated to prevent aortocaval compression (262).

When necessary, tocolytic agents are used. At term, the uterus is more responsive to tocolytic agents than it is earlier in pregnancy (269). A number of tocolytic agents are available. The agent should be chosen because of its effectiveness and its lack of side effects. A number of tocolytic agents may have cardiovascular side effects, particularly β-adrenergic agonists such as terbutaline (261,270,279). Ritodrine and magnesium sulfate have proven most effective in clinical trials (268). Other approaches include ethanol or a combination of a β-adrenergic agonist and progesterone (270).

Because of limited side effects, magnesium sulfate may be the best tocolytic agent for pregnant patients undergoing CPB associated with diabetes mellitus or hypertension.

If measures to avoid or treat fetal complications fail and fetal distress occurs, measures must be taken to correct this problem. If fetal distress can be prevented, fetal mortality will decline. Metabolic acidosis, when present, is treated with sodium bicarbonate. Glucose is given to replenish decreased fetal glycogen stores, and reduced arterial or venous hemoglobin oxygen saturations are promptly corrected by increasing oxygenator gas flow, CPB systemic flow, or hemoglobin concentration as indicated (275). Inotropic or vasopressor agents should be avoided when other treatments may be substituted. For example, if the patient has lost blood and needs volume replacement, transfusion would be preferred over vasopressor agents. Epinephrine has been recommended because of its rapid onset, brief duration, and minimal unwanted side effects at moderate doses. At high doses, epinephrine predominantly manifests α-adrenergic effects. Because blood flow to the gravid uterus is primarily under α-adrenergic control, α-adrenergic agonists will decrease uterine blood flow in normotensive pregnant patients. Drugs that exhibit a combination of α- and β-adrenergic activity are most useful because they increase maternal blood pressure without reducing uterine blood flow (273,280). Examples of such drugs are ephedrine and moderate-dose epinephrine. A reduction in uterine blood flow has been seen in animal studies in which hypotension was treated with dopamine or hypertension was treated with nitroprusside. In addition, nitroprusside crosses the placenta in animals and may liberate free cyanide ions and cause metabolic acidosis. Large doses of nitroprusside in gravid ewes uniformly result in maternal and fetal death (263,281).

In summary, CPB during pregnancy is associated with a low rate of maternal complications but a high risk to the fetus. If possible, bypass surgery should be avoided during pregnancy. If the disease process dictates that surgery is necessary, the first and third trimester are best avoided to minimize teratogenesis or premature initiation of uterine contractions and labor, respectively. It appears likely that fetal distress and complications can be avoided by maintaining a high mean arterial pressure, high CPB systemic flows, normothermia or mild hypothermia, by the use of fetal monitoring, and by early treatment of FHR decelerations and uterine contractions. If fetal distress does become apparent, corrective measures must be taken.

Renal Failure

The effects of CPB on renal function is discussed fully in Chapter 19. However, in patients with preexisting renal disease, cardiac surgery and CPB present difficulties primarily related to their inability to excrete potassium and tendency to become fluid overloaded during the perioperative period. Secondary problems involve anemia, acidosis, plate-

let dysfunction, and hypofibrinogenemia, all of which may be exacerbated by conventional CPB. The patient on chronic hemodialysis may also present with sepsis, bleeding tendencies, malnutrition, and glucose intolerance.

Hemodialysis can be performed concurrently with CPB and offers benefits over either scavenging hyperkalemic cardioplegic solution (282) or using conventional hemoconcentration, which is not as effective in removing potassium. The first case of hemodialysis during CPB has been attributed to Soffer et al. (283) in 1979. The patient was a 55 year old in congestive heart failure from aortic insufficiency secondary to infective endocarditis. The patient had been on maintenance hemodialysis for 10 months before admission for aortic valve replacement. The CPB circuit was primed with two units of packed red blood cells, fresh frozen plasma (900 mL), and balanced electrolyte solution (300 mL), which resulted in an initial hematocrit of 30% on CPB. A conventional hemodialysis machine was connected to the CPB circuit, drawing blood from the venous line and returning it to the cardiotomy reservoir (flow rate 180 mL/min); the dialysate flow rate was 500 mL/min. Serum potassium values ranged from 3.2 to 4.3 mEq/L, and the patient did not require hemodialysis again until postoperative day 3.

In 1984, Geronemus and Schneider (284) reported continuous arteriovenous hemodialysis using a hollow-fiber hemoconcentrator to treat acute renal failure in 10 critically ill patients. Peritoneal dialysis fluid was slowly pumped (15 to 20 mL/min) countercurrent to blood flow that relied on the patient's arterial blood pressure as the driving force. Because of these low flow rates, the duration of continuous arteriovenous hemodialysis was maintained for between 23 and 108 hours. They found that advantages included simplicity of the extracorporeal circuit, hemodynamic stability during treatment, and excellent urea and creatinine clearance. The technique was less effective in treatment of volume overload with fluid removal rates between 25 and 100 mL/hr.

In 1985, Hakim et al. (285) reported a series of 26 patients undergoing cardiac surgery, including cardiac transplantation, who had impaired or absent renal function preoperatively. In five cases a conventional hemodialysis machine was used in the operating room by accessing the patient's circulation via the CPB circuit. The other 21 had hemodialysis performed using continuous arteriovenous hemodialysis via a shunt in parallel with the CPB circuit (blood flow 200 to 300 mL/min). Benefits described were no fluid retention after CPB, no increase in the serum potassium (average 4.5 mEq/L) or blood urea nitrogen, unlimited ability to use potassium cardioplegia, and no need for increased heparin dosages to maintain anticoagulation. Murkin et al. (286) also reported intraoperative hemodialysis in 12 patients with renal failure. All patients underwent conventional hemodialysis the evening before surgery and had a portable dialysis machine connected to the CPB cir-

TABLE 28.7. SIEVING COEFFICIENTS FOR SELECTED DRUGS AND IONS

	PB (%)	PC	S
Ions			
Ca^{2+}	45	5.0 mEq/L	0.55
K$^+$	0	4.4 mEq/L	1.0
Mg^{2+}	0	2.0 mEq/L	1.0
Drugs			
Aprotinin	0	250 KIU/ml	1.0
Bretylium	6	0.63 mg/L	0.94
Digoxin	25	0.0005 mg/L	0.75
Diltiazem	83	0.215 mg/L	0.17
Dobutamine	0	0.025 mg/L	1.0
Fentanyl	71	0.016 mg/L	0.28
Furosemide	95	6.14 mg/L	0.05
Heparin	80	4,821.25 U/L	0.20
Lidocaine	63	1.63 mg/L	0.37
Midazolam	95	0.18 mg/L	0.06
Pancuronium	87	0.20 mg/L	0.13
Vecuronium	70	0.38 mg/L	0.30
Verapamil	90	0.19 mg/L	0.10

The higher the sieving coefficient (S), the more readily ions or drugs will diffuse across the hemoconcentrator or dialyzer membrane. For an S value of 1.0, solute will freely diffuse across the membrane. Other factors affecting sieving coefficients include the percent of the ion or drug that is protein bound, drug membrane interaction, drug charge, molecular size, patient protein concentration, membrane material, membrane design, and blood flow. PB, protein bound; PC, plasma concentration; Ca^{++}, calcium; K$^+$, potassium; Mg^{++}, magnesium. [From Sutton RG. *Intl Anesthesiol Clin* 1996;34:165–176, (as modified from Clar A, Larson DF. *J Extra-Corpor Technol* 1995;27:158–163) with permission.]

cuit. Blood flow was between 150 and 300 mL/min and dialysate flow was 500 mL/min to maintain the serum potassium at 4.0 mEq/L. Benefits included simplicity and intraoperative control of metabolic changes when other methods would have been ineffective.

Wheeldon and Bethune (287) published an excellent review of the principles of hemofiltration (hemoconcentration) and hemodialysis during CPB, including available equipment and suggested circuitry. Besides providing safe intraoperative management of patients in renal failure, they concluded that hemodialysis or hemoconcentration was a simple, efficient, and inexpensive method for control of patient blood volume and blood conservation during CPB. Sutton (288) also recently reviewed CPB management for patients with renal failure and provided a useful table listing sieving coefficients of drugs and ions (Table 28.7).

Other authors (289–292) reported the benefits of intraoperative hemodialysis when compared with routine hemodialysis before and after CPB (usually postoperative day 1) to control serum potassium and reverse fluid overload. A primary benefit appears to be delay of reinstitution of conventional hemodialysis with systemic heparinization until postoperative day 2 or 3. Hamilton et al. (290) described use of a hollow-fiber hemoconcentrator to perform hemodialysis during CPB. They relied on regulated gravity flow of

peritoneal dialysis fluid matched to blood flow (300 to 500 mL/min) through the hemoconcentrator. For increased removal of solutes, the dialysate flow can be increased. However, if the serum potassium is low, dialysate flow can be stopped while maintaining hemoconcentration. If the serum glucose becomes elevated, they recommended using normal saline as the dialysate. They also noted the importance of careful monitoring of the blood pH and HCO$_3$ values, with sodium bicarbonate administration as necessary. A diagram of hemodialysis using two roller pumps to control dialysate flow in and out of the hemoconcentrator is shown in Figure 28.7.

In summary, the leading cause of death in patients undergoing chronic renal dialysis is cardiovascular disease (291), and there are in excess of 180,000 patients currently on hemodialysis for end-stage renal disease in the United States (293). The risk of morbidity or mortality after coronary artery bypass surgery is only slightly increased in this patient population (294), and it is likely that more patients with renal failure will require open heart surgery in the future. Hemodialysis concurrent with CPB can be performed safely using equipment and techniques familiar to perfusionists. Attention to maintenance of adequate hematocrit, electrolyte and fluid balance, and control of hemodynamics during hemodialysis on CPB are important for successful patient outcome.

Acquired Immunodeficiency Syndrome

The AIDS epidemic is unlike previously known epidemics in that the disease may lie clinically silent for 10 years or more after the organism is introduced. In June 1979, a 32-year-old man in New York City, infected with HIV, appeared at first to be a medical curiosity, but the syndrome was rapidly recognized, and by June 1983, over 1,600 cases had been reported in the United States. Health care workers have always lived with the risks associated with contracting potentially fatal diseases; however, rarely in the course of history has a disease provoked such an emotional response, intense debate, and such a plethora of research efforts. The apparently uniform fatal outcome of clinical AIDS mandates introspection and close scrutiny of any invasive procedures performed by health care workers. This section briefly discusses the management of patients harboring an HIV infection who undergo cardiac surgery.

Homologous blood might best be considered a toxic substance. For cardiac surgical team members, exposure to blood is a daily risk. Gerberding et al. (295) studied the risks of exposure in 1,307 consecutive surgical procedures and reported that accidental exposure to blood occurred in 84 instances. The incidence of exposure increased when procedures lasted more than 3 hours and when blood loss exceeded 300 mL. Their data supported the practice of double gloving and the use of waterproof garments and face shields. Blood contact events were reported in 28% of 684 operations in a university medical center setting (296). The

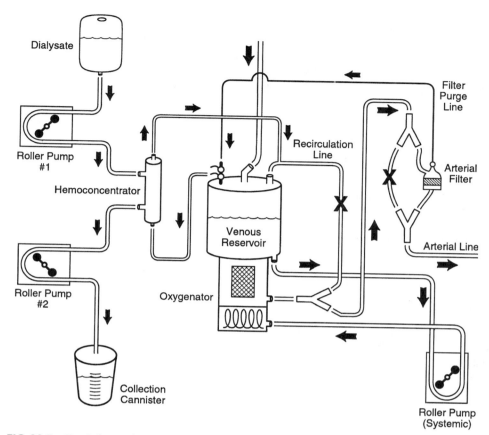

FIG. 28.7. Circuit for performing hemodialysis with a hollow-fiber hemoconcentrator during cardiopulmonary bypass. Blood and fluid flow is in direction of *arrows*, and *bold Xs* represent placement of tubing clamps. The arterial filter purge line (*top right*) is used as a source of blood (estimated flow 150 to 300 mL/min) through the hemoconcentrator and is returned to the venous reservoir. Dialysate fluid is drawn from large bag by roller pump #1 and pumped through the outer chamber of the hemoconcentrator while simultaneously being drawn (roller pump #2) from the hemoconcentrator effluent port where it is discarded into a collection cannister (*lower left*). The speed of pump #1 must always be less than the speed of pump #2 to prevent dialysate from crossing hollow fibers in the hemoconcentrator and entering the bloodstream. For most effective solute removal, blood flow and dialysate flow should be countercurrent. Increasing the flow of dialysate will increase the rate of removal of solutes. Frequent laboratory measurements of serum electrolytes, acid-base status, and whole blood activated clotting time should be performed when using intraoperative hemodialysis. If hemodialysis is not required, hemoconcentration alone can be accomplished by stopping pump #1 and using pump #2 to exert a slight negative pressure in the hemoconcentrator. The volume of fluid collected in excess of that removed by pump #1 from the dialysate bag represents plasma water removed from the patient's circulation. The volume of removed fluid or collected dialysate should be monitored continuously when using this technique. If both hemodialysis and hemoconcentration are not required, both pumps are turned off and blood is simply allowed to shunt through the hemoconcentrator to avoid stasis.

authors concluded that most contacts were preventable and reflected indifference to universal precautions that were part of their standard operating room policy.

The so-called universal precautions advised by the Centers for Disease Control and Prevention did not address the unique problems that occur in the operating room (297). Cardiothoracic cases (298) revealed a 58% contact ($p < 0.001$) with blood by personnel and multiple contacts in 12 cases. Although no case of operating room transmission of HIV had yet been documented, the authors concluded

it had no doubt occurred and would certainly be documented in the future.

AIDS has clearly become a national obsession. The National Commission on AIDS concluded that mass screening programs would interfere with doctor–patient relationships and would encourage a false sense of security. This is because a 6- to 12-week window period normally occurs between infection with the HIV virus and seropositivity with traditional HIV screening tests. The medicolegal ramifications of testing patients present a significant problem, although, in part, this may be obviated by complying with local statutes for informed consent. No solution has been developed for the emergency patient who must rapidly undergo CPB when there is not sufficient time to obtain test results; thus implementation of universal precautions necessitate that all patients be treated as potentially infected.

The extent to which blood should be considered a toxic substance is realized when one studies the history of a nurse health care worker infected in Iowa. The worker was infected during a resuscitative effort on an HIV-positive patient when blood seeped from an intravenous line onto her ungloved left index finger, which had been previously cut during gardening. She became HIV-positive 3 months later. If a patient develops clinical AIDS after open heart surgery, he or she will likely blame the surgery or its personnel, when in fact a positive HIV test may have predated the patient's surgery.

The ELISA screening test, which may be completed in a few hours, has few false-negative results but a significant number of false positives. The confirmatory test is the Western blot, which has a low false-positive rate. Patients confirmed positive with this test should have adequate counseling, which is available in most hospital settings at this time.

The American Medical Association and the American College of Physicians have endorsed statements that doctors may not ethically refuse to treat a patient solely because the patient has AIDS or is seropositive for HIV infection. The subcommittee on AIDS of The American College of Surgeons Governors Committee does not currently recommend discontinuation of practice for HIV-positive surgeons (299). Patient-to-health care worker transmission has been reported and appears to be much more frequent than the reverse.

The Society of Thoracic Surgeons Committee on AIDS has made the following recommendations to thoracic surgeons. First, before elective surgery, make every attempt to identify patients who are positive for infection with the HIV by voluntary testing. In doing so, be careful to comply with any applicable confidentiality statutes and informed consent statutes. Second, use universal precautions against exposure to blood and other body fluids in the operating room and throughout the hospital, regardless of whether the status of the HIV serology is known. Third, take a leadership role to encourage easing the current restrictions on HIV testing so that we may learn about the risk of transmission of HIV, the role that positive HIV status may play in affecting the results of treatment of other disease processes, and the possibility that surgery and bypass may accelerate the development of AIDS in the HIV-positive patient. Finally, encourage hospital laboratories to develop the capability of providing rapid screening of patients for HIV.

In 1989 Condit and Frater (300) surveyed cardiothoracic surgeons' attitudes regarding whether AIDS patients should be operated on. Two thirds of respondents indicated they would operate on this patient population, but the decision would be based on medical indications. However, there was

a concern expressed that CPB might accelerate the progression of the disease. With current treatment regimens, HIV patients are living much longer than they did more than a decade ago at the time of the survey. No association between CPB and progression to AIDS in the HIV-positive patient have been established (301–303), and HIV patients are now operated on with less concern than was expressed in the previous decade.

In summary, the AIDS epidemic has positively and negatively affected the use of CPB. Health care workers have become much more cautious since the identification of its etiology. The modes of HIV transmission have been established with a high degree of certainty, and in infected patients, viral presence has been established in virtually all body fluids (semen, vaginal secretions, blood, urine, saliva, cerebrospinal fluid, mother's milk, and almost certainly feces). All hospitals should have the drug azidothymidine immediately available for health care workers who experience an injury from an HIV-positive patient. There is laboratory evidence that azidothymidine given within 15 minutes of such injury can prevent HIV viral migration into the injured worker's cells (304).

A practical technique to minimize accidental needle punctures or cuts during cardiac surgery is to establish a policy whereby no surgical intruments or needles are handed off or passed directly between the scrub nurse and surgeon. Instead, a white towel on the sterile field can be used to delineate a space for placing and retrieving instruments by only one surgical team member at a time. Full-blown AIDS is still 100% fatal despite intense research efforts and newer drug regimens to control the disease. Health care professionals working in cardiac surgery have an obviously increased risk of exposure, and universal precautions to provide barriers cannot be overemphasized.

Malignant Hyperthermia

Malignant hyperthermia is a syndrome of acute hyperthermia (core temperatures may exceed 42°C) and/or myotonic reactions initiated by a hypermetabolic state of skeletal muscle. This syndrome can be triggered by administration of potent inhalation anesthetics (e.g., halothane, sevoflurane, and isoflurane) and succinylcholine. The syndrome was originally described in 1962 (305). The incidence is approximately 1 in 15,000 children and 1 in 50,000 adults. Early on, management of patients with malignant hyperthermia consisted of copious amounts of chilled intravenous Ringer's lactate solution, lavage of stomach and bladder with iced solutions, and large doses of procainamide or procaine (306). Currently, dantrolene sodium from 1 to 10 mg/kg is the treatment of choice, along with some of the active cooling measures listed above. Unlike previous pharmacologic measures (e.g., procainamide), dantrolene specifically addresses the causative mechanism, which is impaired reuptake of ionized calcium from the cytosol into storage sites located in the sarcoplasmic reticulum of skeletal muscle myocytes. Before the introduction of dantrolene, mortality was greater than 60% (307). Before dantrolene was available, CPB had been used unsuccessfully and later successfully as a method of controlled cooling in the treatment of malignant hyperthermia (308).

Byrick et al. (309) described the anesthetic management of a patient with biopsy-proven malignant hyperthermia who underwent coronary artery bypass grafting. Measures included pretreatment with dantrolene, removal of the halothane vaporizer from the oxygenation-inspired gas pathway, and the use of high-dose fentanyl for anesthesia and pancuronium for muscle relaxation. Cold potassium (10 mEq/L) cardioplegia was used; inotropic agents and calcium (possible trigger agent) were avoided. The patient continued to receive dantrolene every 6 hours for 24 hours after the operation. No evidence of malignant hyperthermia was encountered. Other authors (310) used similar management strategies with success, the common theme of which is avoidance of trigger agents. Pretreatment with dantrolene is no longer recommended.

The diagnosis of malignant hyperthermia may be complicated or delayed by the coincidental use of CPB and may require an increased index of suspicion. Cases in which malignant hyperthermia occurred while on CPB have been reported (311,312). Both patients were successfully treated with a single dose of dantrolene (1 mg/kg). Early recognition and treatment of malignant hyperthermia is important because the marked hypermetabolism may exceed the oxygen delivery capacity of the oxygenator, especially at normothermia. During CPB, unexpected hyperthermia or temperature rises and unexplained metabolic and respiratory acidosis would provide the most likely clues to the diagnosis. When suspected, it appears sensible to induce or maintain CPB hypothermia while awaiting dantrolene-induced resolution of the clinical syndrome. Repeated doses of dantrolene may be required. Dantrolene is known to cause skeletal muscle weakness and causes myocardial depression in animals; caution is advised in its use in cardiac patients (309,310). Schwartz and Hensley (313) presented two cases and reviewed the physiologic basis and clinical diagnosis of this rare complication.

Miscellaneous Pathophysiology

There is no specific contraindication for CPB in the elderly patient, and several reports demonstrated successful outcomes for coronary artery bypass surgery in octogenarians (314–316). Coronary bypass surgery has even been performed in a 100-year-old patient for unstable angina with favorable outcome for 3 years after surgery (C.D. Williams, personal communication, 1999). Others reported a low incidence of cardiac-related mortality in patients after coronary bypass or valve replacement surgery (317). However, the risk of morbidity or mortality is increased in the elderly patient population (318).

Rady et al. (319) statistically determined perioperative predictors of morbidity and mortality in elderly patients (defined as age older than 75 years) having surgery with CPB. They reviewed the records of 1,157 patients who had cardiac surgery within a 30-month period at one hospital (14% of total caseload during the same time frame) and found that predictors of postoperative morbidity were: preoperative intraaortic balloon; preoperative serum bilirubin of more than 1.0 mg/dL; blood transfusion with more than 10 units of packed red blood cells; CPB time more than 120 minutes (aortic cross-clamp time greater than 80 minutes); return to operating room for surgical exploration; heart rate more than 120 beats/min; use of inotropes or vasopressors after CPB and upon admission to the intensive care unit; and anemia beyond postoperative day 2. Predictors of mortality ($n = 90/1,157$ or 8%) were similar and included: preoperative cardiogenic shock; serum albumin less than 4.0 g/dL; systemic oxygen delivery less than 320 mL/min/m² before surgery; blood transfusion more than 10 units; CPB time more than 140 minutes (aortic cross-clamp time more than 120 minutes; return to operating room for surgical exploration; mean arterial pressure less than 60 mm Hg; heart rate more than 120 beats/min; central venous pressure more than 15 mm Hg; stroke volume index less than 30 mL/min/m²; requirement for inotropes; arterial bicarbonate less than 20 mmol/L; plasma glucose more than 300 mg/dL after surgery; and anemia beyond postoperative day 2.

The decision to operate on the elderly patient should consider these findings. Maintenance of higher than normal CPB perfusion pressure (e.g., minimum 70 mm Hg), having a lower target threshold for administration of blood products, and minimizing CPB time may address several of the risk factors outlined above. In addition, the carotid arteries of all patients over 75 years of age should be checked preoperatively by noninvasive examination. For the cachectic patient, an immunologist can perform an anergy skin test battery (tetanus toxoid, diphtheria toxoid, steptococcus, old tuberculin, candida, trichophyton, and proteus), which can be used to screen those patients who would benefit from nutritional therapy before their surgery (320). Those patients determined to be anergic will have a high incidence of morbidity and mortality associated with open heart surgery.

The obese patient may be at a slightly increased risk of superficial wound complications or atrial dysrhythmias, but obesity per se is not a risk factor for adverse outcome after cardiac surgery (321). The standard criteria for CPB systemic flow indices based on body surface area may be safely lowered to 1.8 to 2.0 L/min/m² to avoid very high CPB flows (322), provided acceptable metabolic parameters are maintained. Occasionally, there may be difficulties in achieving adequate venous drainage in the obese patient (323); these problems can be overcome by use of assisted venous drainage methods (see Chapter 27). In the occasional morbidly obese patient, perhaps especially one who is also quite tall, the gas exchange capacity of the oxygenator may prove marginal at normothermia. If this problem develops, possible approaches include deepening anesthesia, cooling the patient, and using two oxygenators in parallel.

Klemperer et al. (324) showed that patients with noncardiac liver cirrhosis (Child class A) tolerate CPB and cardiac surgery with only minor morbidity. However, with moderate to advanced cirrhosis, morbidity and mortality are markedly high (80% mortality). All patients in their series (*n* = 13) had chest tube drainage and requirement for blood transfusion at a rate three times higher than patients without liver disease. Because the liver produces most coagulation factors but also clears activated factors and fibrinolytic components from the circulation (325), bleeding after CPB is the major concern in this patient population. Patients with liver disease also frequently have reduced platelet numbers and function (326) and increased fibrinolysis secondary to low-grade disseminated intravascular coagulopathy (327), which may be aggravated by the hematologic derangement inherent with CPB. Because of the high risk of morbidity in the patient presenting for cardiac surgery with chronic active hepatitis, a liver biopsy should be performed. If white cells are found, elective surgery should be postponed until the infection is controlled.

Patients with gastrointestinal disease may require excessive volume on CPB due to an increased tendency to third-space fluids. Buzzelli and Trittipoe (328) reported a case in which a patient with end-stage renal disease and an acutely perforated Meckel's diverticulum required over 4 L of fluid and blood administration plus 1,500 mL of crystalloid cardioplegic solution during 96 minutes of CPB. After bypass, the patient's abdomen was markedly distended, which required laparotomy and closure of the perforated bowel.

CONCLUSIONS

An unanticipated perfusion mishap or the unusual or unappreciated patient condition can turn a routine CPB case into a challenge that will tax even the most experienced practitioners. Although statistically the current risk of patient serious injury or death directly related to CPB has been reduced to levels of a fraction of 1% and are certainly less than the risk of untreated heart disease in most cases, perfusion safety should continue to be a guiding principle whenever CPB is used (329). For the team that experiences an adverse patient outcome, reexamination of practices can yield rewards for future patients. A systematic approach to how CPB is performed may eliminate inherent potential errors that will occur no matter how diligent the team.

Newer CPB technology will undoubtedly continue to evolve. If device or equipment failure or fluids administered to the patient on CPB are suspected as contributory to an adverse patient outcome, they should be sequestered in a secure area for later examination. Like other endeavors that rely on complex tightly coupled technologies (330), CPB accidents more often result from operator error than from device failure. This chapter was written in the hope that awareness and communication of past failures will educate dedicated clinicians in avoiding their repetition.

KEY POINTS

- To reduce the incidence of stroke after CPB in the patients with severe atherosclerosis of the ascending aorta, transesophageal echocardiographic visualization of the aortic lumen, alternative cannulation sites and techniques, bilateral proximal carotid compression during surgical manipulation of the aorta, electrical fibrillation or β-adrenergic blockers for myocardial protection, and no-touch techniques should be considered.
- All patients undergoing hypothermic CPB should be screened for cold agglutinins.
- Patients found to exhibit low titer (e.g., less than 1: 32) low thermal amplitude for cold agglutinins and who are clinically asymptomatic can tolerate CPB with moderate hypothermia.
- Patients with high thermal amplitude and/or titer (e.g., more than 1:128) with clinical symptoms of cold agglutinins require that the temperature be maintained above the thermal amplitude; additionally, warm crystalloid cardioplegia (followed by cold with insulation of the heart from adjacent structures) may prevent activation of cold agglutinins.
- Sickle cell disease is a homozygous gene recessive abnormality characterized by a predominance of hemoglobin S; sickled cells have a limited capacity to load and unload oxygen, exhibit increased osmotic and mechanical fragility, increase blood viscosity, and can cause vascular occlusion.
- Sickle cell trait is a heterozygous recessive abnormality in which hemoglobin S comprises 20% to 40% of the total hemoglobin.
- Tendency for sickling occurs with hypoperfusion, hypoxemia, acidosis, increased concentrations of 2,3-diphosphoglyceric acid, infection, hypothermia, and capillary stagnation.
- Exchange transfusion before or with the initiation of CPB should raise the hemoglobin A fraction more than 60% to decrease the risk of sickling, which will minimize hemolysis and prevent vaso-occlusive phenomenon.
- Acute methemoglobinemia is most often induced by chemicals or drugs and is diagnosed when cyanosis or oxygen desaturation (chocolate-brown–colored blood) occurs despite an adequate arterial oxygen tension.
- The most effective treatment of methemoglobinemia consists of methylene blue administration (1 to 2.5 mg/kg); additionally, the oxygenator should be venti-

lated with 100% oxygen and high CPB systemic flows should be used.

- Patients with polycythemia may be hemodiluted to normal CPB levels by either removal of blood before bypass or using larger volumes of crystalloid solution in the CPB prime.
- Jehovah's Witness patients may safely undergo CPB by minimizing circuit prime and fluid administration, use of cell salvage and hemoconcentration, and return of residual perfusate after bypass while maintaining continuity between removed blood and the patient to accommodate the patient's religious beliefs.
- Reoperative patients may require alternative cannulation sites and augmented venous drainage techniques to adequately establish CPB.
- Acute aortic dissection should be suspected if the CPB arterial line pressure unexpectedly increases and there is a simultaneous decrease in systemic pressure and/or venous drainage.
- Venous or arterial air embolism may occur from improper operation of CPB, surgical technique, or through intravenous lines.
- Systemic air embolism carries a greater risk than venous air embolism because of the potential for cerebral involvement.
- Air embolism originating from CPB may enter the patient's systemic circulation from the arterial line or by other mechanisms such as improperly operated vents, cardioplegia delivery, or vacuum-assisted venous drainage or from pressurized CPB components.
- Improperly de-aired intravenous lines or inappropriate ventilation of the patient during insertion of cannulas or vents or during surgical de-airing maneuvers can result in air embolism.
- If massive air embolism from the CPB circuit occurs, bypass should be stopped immediately, the source of air determined, and efforts made to remove the air from the circuit and patient's vasculature.
- Retrograde cerebral perfusion may be an effective treatment if significant air is suspected to have entered the patient's cerebral circulation.
- The sterility of preassembled CPB circuits must be maintained by ensuring all blood-contacting surfaces and components are kept secure and covered until time of use.
- CPB in the pregnant patient is associated with a low risk of maternal complications but a high risk to the fetus, particularly during the first and third trimesters when teratogenesis or premature initiation of uterine contractions may occur.
- Maintenance of mean arterial pressures more than 60 mm Hg, CPB flow indices of 2.5 to 3.0 L/min/m², normothermia or mild hypothermia, avoidance of potassium-based cardioplegia, use of FHR monitoring, and prompt treatment of uterine contractions with tocolytic agents can minimize complications in the mother and fetus.

- Hemodialysis during CPB for patients in renal failure can be performed using a hemoconcentrator to lower elevated serum potassium, remove excess fluid, and delay reinstitution of maintenance hemodialysis until postoperative day 2 or 3.
- CPB can be performed safely on HIV-positive patients by using universal precautions and modifying the way surgical instruments are exchanged to prevent blood exposure and accidental needlesticks.
- Malignant hyperthermia may be suspected during CPB in the patient who exhibits unexpected temperature rises and unexplained metabolic and respiratory acidosis; it is treated with dantrolene (1 to 2.5 mg/kg).

REFERENCES

1. Roach GW, Kanchuger M, Mangano CM, et al. Adverse cerebral outcomes after coronary bypass surgery. *N Engl J Med* 1996; 335:1857–1863.
2. Mills NL, Everson CT. Atherosclerosis of the ascending aorta and coronary artery bypass: pathology, clinical correlates, and operative management. *J Thorac Cardiovasc Surg* 1991;102: 546–553.
3. Culliford AT, Colvin SB, Rohrer K, et al. The atherosclerotic ascending aorta and transverse arch: a new technique to prevent cerebral injury during bypass: experience with 13 patients. Updated in 1994. *Ann Thorac Surg* 1994;57:1051–1052.
4. Olearchyk AS. Case report: calcified ascending aorta and coronary artery disease. *Ann Thorac Surg* 1994;59:1013–1015.
5. Sabik JF, Lytle BW, McCarthy PM, et al. Axillary artery: an alternative site of arterial cannulation for patients with extensive aortic and peripheral vascular disease. *J Thorac Cardiovasc Surg* 1995;109:885–891.
6. Groom RC, Hill AG, Kuban B, et al. Aortic cannula velocimetry. *Perfusion* 1995;10:183–188.
7. Tanaka T, Kawamura T, Ohara K, et al. Transapical aortic perfusion with a double-barreled cannula. *Ann Thorac Surg* 1978;25:209–214.
8. Liddicoat JR, Doty JR, Stuart RS. Case report: management of the atherosclerotic ascending aorta with endoaortic occlusion. *Ann Thorac Surg* 1998;65:1133–1135.
9. Reichenspurner HH, Navia J, Berry G, et al. Particulate embolic capture by an intra-aortic filter device during cardiac surgery. *J Thorac Cardiovasc Surg* 2000;119:233–241.
10. Kumar P, Dhital K, Hossein-Nia M, et al. S-100 protein release in a range of cardiothoracic surgical procedures. *J Thorac Cardiovasc Surg* 1997;113:953–954.
11. Moore RA, Geller EA, Mathews ES, et al. The effect of hypothermic cardiopulmonary bypass on patients with low-titer, nonspecific cold agglutinins. *Ann Thorac Surg* 1984;37:233–238.
12. Lee M-C, Chang C-H, Hsieh M-J. Use of a total wash-out method in an open-heart operation. *Ann Thorac Surg* 1989;47: 57–58.
13. Pruzanski W, Shumak KH. Biologic activity of cold-reacting autoantibodies. Part 2. *N Engl J Med* 1977;297:583–589.
14. Dake SB, Johnston MFM, Brueggeman P, et al. Detection of cold hemagglutination in a blood cardioplegia unit before systemic cooling of a patient with unsuspected cold agglutinin disease. *Ann Thorac Surg* 1989;47:314–315.

15. Bracken CA, Gurkowski MA, Naples JJ, et al. Case Conference: Case 6-1993, Cardiopulmonary bypass in two patients with previously undetected cold agglutinins. *J Cardiothorac Vasc Anesth* 1993;7:743–749.

16. Fischer GD, Claypoole V, Collard CD. Increased line pressures in the retrograde blood cardioplegia line: an unusual presentation of cold agglutinins during cardiopulmonary bypass. *Anesth Analg* 1997;84:454–456.

17. Leach AB, Van Hasselt GL, Edwards JC. Cold agglutinins and deep hypothermia. *Anaesthesia* 1983;38:140–143.

18. Pruzanski W, Shumak KH. Biologic activity of cold-reacting autoantibodies. Part 1. *N Engl J Med* 1977;297:538–542.

19. Shahian DM, Wallach SR, Bern MM. Open-heart surgery in patients with cold-reactive proteins. *Surg Clin North Am* 1985; 65:315–322.

20. AuBuchon JP, Stofan BA, Davey RJ. Hemolysis during extracorporeal circulation: significance of cold-reactive auto-antibodies and mechanical trauma [Abstract]. *Blood* 1983;62 [Suppl 1]: 42a.

21. Schreiber AD, Herskovitz BS, Goldwein M. Low-titer cold-hemagglutinin disease: mechanism of hemolysis and response to corticosteroids. *N Engl J Med* 1977;296:1490–1494.

22. Berreklouw E, Moulijin AC, Pegels JG, et al. Myocardial protection with cold cardioplegia in a patient with cold autoagglutinins and hemolysins. *Ann Thorac Surg* 1982;33:521–522.

23. Klein HG, Faltz LL, McIntosh CL, et al. Surgical hypothermia in a patient with a cold agglutinin. *Transfusion* 1980;20: 354–357.

24. Wertlake PT, McGinniss MH, Schmidt PJ. Cold antibody and persistent intravascular hemolysis after surgery under hypothermia. *Transfusion* 1969;9:70–73.

25. Williams AC. Cold agglutinins: cause for concern? *Anaesthesia* 1980;35:887–889.

26. Diaz JH, Cooper ES, Ochsner JL. Cardiac surgery in patients with cold autoimmune diseases. *Anesth Analg* 1984;63: 349–352.

27. Blumberg N, Hicks G, Woll J, et al. Successful cardiac bypass surgery in the presence of a potent cold agglutinin without plasma exchange [Letter]. *Transfusion* 1983;23:363–364.

28. Agarwal SK, Ghosh PK, Gupta D. Collective review: cardiac surgery and cold-reactive proteins. *Ann Thorac Surg* 1995;60: 1143–1150.

29. Landymore R, Isom W, Barlam B. Management of patients with cold agglutinins who require open-heart surgery. *Can J Surg* 1983;26:79–80.

30. Holman WL, Smith SH, Edwards R, et al. Agglutination of blood cardioplegia by cold-reacting autoantibodies. *Ann Thorac Surg* 1991;51:833–836.

31. Paccagnella A, Simini G, Nieri A, et al. Cardiopulmonary bypass and cold agglutinin [Letter]. *J Thorac Cardiovasc Surg* 1988;95: 543.

32. Blomback M, Kronlund P, Aberg B, et al. Pathologic fibrin formation and cold-induced clotting of membrane oxygenators during cardiopulmonary bypass. *J Cardiothorac Vasc Anesth* 1995;9:34–43.

33. Dove SK, Raskin SA, Lawson DS. Cold agglutinins and hypothermic cardiopulmonary bypass. *Perfusion* 1992;7:3–6.

34. Szentpetery S, Robertson L, Lower RR. Complete repair of tetralogy associated with sickle cell anemia and G-6-PD deficiency. *J Thorac Cardiovasc Surg* 1976;72:276–279.

35. Hebbel RP. Beyond hemoglobin polymerization: the red blood cell membrane and sickle disease pathophysiology [Review]. *Blood* 1991;77:214–237.

36. Ballas SK, Mahandas N. Pathophysiology of vaso-occlusion. *Hematol Oncol Clin North Am* 1996;10:1221–1239.

37. Setty BNY, Stuart MJ. Vascular cell adhesion molecule-1 is involved in mediating hypoxia-induced sickle red blood cell adherence to endothelium: potential role in sickle cell disease. *Blood* 1996;88:2311–2320.

38. Chun PKC, Flannery EP, Bowen TE. Open-heart surgery in patients with hematologic disorders. *Am Heart J* 1983;105: 835–842.

39. Fox MA, Abbott TR. Hypothermic cardiopulmonary bypass in a patient with sickle-cell trait. *Anaesthesia* 1984;39:1121–1123.

40. Ingram CT, Floyd JB, Santora AH. Aortic and mitral valve replacement after sickle cell crisis [Letter]. *Anesth Analg* 1982; 61:802–803.

41. Harris LC, Haggard ME, Travis LB. The coexistence of sickle cell disease and congenital heart disease: a report of three cases with repair under cardiopulmonary by-pass in two patients. *Pediatrics* 1964;33:562–570.

42. Yacoub MH, Baron J, Et-Etr A, et al. Aortic homograft replacement of the mitral valve in sickle cell trait. *J Thorac Cardiovasc Surg* 1970;59:568–573.

43. Craenen J, Kilman J, Hosier DM, et al. Mitral valve replacement in a child with sickle cell anemia. *J Thorac Cardiovasc Surg* 1972; 63:797–799.

44. Heiner M, Teasdale SJ, David T, et al. Aortocoronary bypass in a patient with sickle cell trait. *Can Anaesth Soc J* 1979;26: 428–434.

45. Riethmuller R, Grundy EM, Radley-Smith R. Open heart surgery in a patient with homozygous sickle cell disease. *Anaesthesia* 1982;37:324–327.

46. Baxter MRN, Bevan JC, Esseltine DW, et al. The management of two pediatric patients with sickle cell trait and sickle cell disease during cardiopulmonary bypass. *J Cardiothorac Anesth* 1989;3:477–480.

47. Balasundaram MS, Duran CG, Al-Halees Z, et al. Cardiopulmonary bypass in sickle cell anaemia: report of five cases. *J Cardiovasc Surg* 1991;32:271–274.

48. Pagani FD, Polito RJ, Bolling SF. Case report: mitral valve reconstruction in sickle cell disease. *Ann Thorac Surg* 1996;61: 1841–1843.

49. Kingsley CP, Chronister T, Cohen DJ, et al. Case conference. Case 2-1996, anesthetic management of a patient with hemoglobin SS disease and mitral insufficiency for mitral valve repair. *J Cardiothorac Vasc Anesth* 1996;10:419–424.

50. Shulman G, McQuitty C, Vertrees RA, et al. Case report: acute normovolemic red cell exchange for cardiopulmonary bypass in sickle cell disease. *Ann Thorac Surg* 1998;65:1444–1446.

51. Yung GL, Channick RN, Fedullo PF, et al. Successful pulmonary thromboendarterectomy in two patients with sickle cell disease. *Am J Respir Crit Care Med* 1998;157:1690–1693.

52. Longenecker VW, Hartley MB, Dingmann M, et al. Cardiopulmonary bypass in the sickle cell anemia patient using profound hypothermia and circulatory arrest: a case report. *J Extracorp Technol* 1998;30:135–139.

53. Moyes DG, Holloway AM, Hutton WS. Correction of Fallot's tetralogy in a patient suffering from hereditary spherocytosis. *S Afr Med J* 1974;48:1535–1536.

54. Gayyed NL, Bouboulis N, Holden MP. Open heart operation in patients suffering from hereditary spherocytocis. *Ann Thorac Surg* 1993;55:1497–1500.

55. Dal A, Kumar RS. Open heart surgery in presence of hereditary spherocytosis. *J Cardiovasc Surg* 1995;36:447–448.

56. deLeval MR, Taswell HF, Bowie EJW, et al. Open heart surgery in patients with inherited hemoglobinopathies, red cell dyscrasias and coagulopathies. *Arch Surg* 1974;109:618–622.

57. Mansouri A. Methemoglobinemia [Review]. *Am J Med Sci* 1985;289:200–209.

58. Hedlund KD, Sanford DM, Coyne DP. Methemoglobinemia

during cardiopulmonary bypass? A case report and review. *Proc Am Acad Cardiovasc Perfus* 1987;8:232–235.

59. Robicsek F. Acute methemoglobinemia during cardiopulmonary bypass caused by intravenous nitroglycerin infusion. *J Thorac Cardiovasc Surg* 1985;90:931–933.

60. Bojar RM, Rastegar H, Payne DD, et al. Methemoglobinemia from intravenous nitroglycerin: a word of caution. *Ann Thorac Surg* 1987;43:332–334.

61. Zurick AM, Wagner RH, Starr NJ, et al. Intravenous nitroglycerin, methemoglobinemia, and respiratory distress in a postoperative cardiac surgical patient. *Anesthesiology* 1984;61:464–466.

62. Jackson SH, Barker SJ. Case reports: methemoglobinemia in a patient receiving flutamide. *Anesthesiology* 1995;82:1065–1067.

63. Cooper JR, Keats AS. Methemoglobinemia diagnosed as a consequence of cardiopulmonary bypass. *Tex Heart Inst J* 1985;12:103–106.

64. Armstrong D, Schmalfuss V, Reed CC, et al. A case study: methemoglobinemia during cardiopulmonary bypass. *Proc Am Acad Cardiovasc Perfus* 1985;6:179–181.

65. Kastrup EK. Antidotes. In: Kastrup EK, ed. *Drug facts and comparisons.* St. Louis: J.B. Lippincott, 1986:2012–2013.

66. Milam JD, Austin SF, Nihill MR, et al. Use of sufficient hemodilution to prevent coagulopathies following surgical correction of cyanotic heart disease. *J Thorac Cardiovasc Surg* 1985;89:623–629.

67. Ware JA, Reaves WH, Horak JK, et al. Defective platelet aggregation in patients undergoing surgical repair of cyanotic congenital heart disease. *Ann Thorac Surg* 1983;36:289–294.

68. Dyke C, Sobel M. The management of coagulation problems in the surgical patient. *Adv Surg* 1991;24:229–257.

69. Manley NJ, Williams DR, Pierce WS. Double valve replacement in a hemophiliac. *AmSECT Proc* 1976;4:46–50.

70. Poullis M, Manning R, Haskard D, et al. Brief communication: Reopro removal during cardiopulmonary bypass using a hemoconcentrator. *J Thorac Cardiovasc Surg* 1999;117:1032–1034.

71. Ridley PD, Ledingham SJM, Lennox SC, et al. Case report: protein C deficiency associated with massive cerebral thrombosis following open heart surgery. *J Cardiovasc Surg* 1990;31:249–251.

72. Lawson DS, Darling EM, Ware RE, et al. Case report: management considerations for a heterozygous protein C deficient patient undergoing open heart surgery with cardiopulmonary bypass. *J Extra-Corp Technol* 1995;27:172–176.

73. Petaja J, Peltola K, Sairanen H, et al. Fibrinolysis, antithrombin III, and protein C in neonates during cardiac operations. *J Thorac Cardiovasc Surg* 1996;112:665–671.

74. Andrew M, Paes B, Johnston M. Development of the hemostatic system in the neonate and young infant. *Am J Pediatr Hematol Oncol* 1990;12:95–104.

75. Kern FH, Morana NJ, Sears JJ, et al. Coagulation defects in neonates during cardiopulmonary bypass. *Ann Thorac Surg* 1992;54:541–546.

76. Miller BE, Mochizuki T, Levy JH, et al. Predicting and treating coagulopathies after cardiopulmonary bypass in children. *Anesth Analg* 1997;85:1196–1202.

77. Stein JI, Gombotz H, Rigler B, et al. Open heart surgery in children of Jehovah's Witness: extreme hemodilution on cardiopulmonary bypass. *Pediatr Cardiol* 1991;12:170–174.

78. Cooley DA, Crawford ES, Howell JF, et al. Open heart surgery in Jehovah's Witnesses. *Am J Cardiol* 1964;13:779–781.

79. Ott DA, Cooley DA. Cardiovascular surgery in Jehovah's Witnesses: report of 542 operations without blood transfusion. *JAMA* 1977;238:1256–1258.

80. Tsang VT, Mullaly RJ, Ragg PG, et al. Bloodless open-heart surgery in infants and children. *Perfusion* 1994;9:257–263.

81. Van Son JAM, Hovaguimian H, Rao IM, et al. Strategies for repair of congenital heart defects in infants without the use of blood. *Ann Thorac Surg* 1995;59:384–388.

82. St. Rammos K, Bakas AJ, Panagopoulos FG. Mitral valve replacement in a Jehovah's Witness with dextrocardia and situs solitus. *J Heart Valve Dis* 1996;5:673–674.

83. Malan TP Jr, Whitmore J, Maddi R. Reoperative cardiac surgery in a Jehovah's Witness: role of continuous cell salvage and in-line reinfusion. *J Cardiothorac Anesth* 1989;3:211–214.

84. Aldea GS, Shapira OM, Treanor PR, et al. Effective use of heparin-bonded circuits and lower anticoagulation for coronary artery bypass grafting in Jehovah's Witnesses. *J Card Surg* 1996;11:12–17.

85. Rosengart TK, Helm RE, Klemperer J, et al. Combined aprotinin and erythropoietin use for blood conservation: results with Jehovah's Witnesses. *Ann Thorac Surg* 1994;58:1397–1403.

86. Chikada M, Furuse A, Kotsuka Y, et al. Open-heart surgery in Jehovah's Witness patients. *Cardiovasc Surg* 1996;4:311–314.

87. Lee RB, Martin TD. Religious objections to blood transfusion. In: Mora CT, ed. *Cardiopulmonary bypass, principles and techniques of extracorporeal circulation.* New York: Springer-Verlag, 1995:473–480.

88. Dobell ARC, Jain AK. Catastrophic hemorrhage during redo sternotomy. *Ann Thorac Surg* 1984;37:273–278.

89. Bracey AW, Radovancevic R, Radovancevic B, et al. Blood use in patients undergoing repeat coronary artery bypass graft procedures: multivariate analysis. *Transfusion* 1995;35:850–854.

90. Jones RE, Fitzgeral D, Cohn LH. Reoperative cardiac surgery using a new femoral venous right atrial cannula. *J Card Surg* 1990;5:170–173.

91. Praeger PI, Pooley RW, Moggio RA, et al. Simplified method for reoperation on the mitral valve. *Ann Thorac Surg* 1989;48:835–837.

92. Solomon L, Sutter FP, Goldman SM, et al. Augmented femoral venous return. *Ann Thorac Surg* 1993;55:1262–1263.

93. Darling E, Kaemer D, Lawson S, et al. Experimental use of an ultra-low prime neonatal cardiopulmonary bypass circuit utilizing vacuum-assisted venous drainage. *J Extra-Corp Technol* 1998;30:184–189.

94. Toomasian JM, McCarthy JP. Total extrathoracic cardiopulmonary support with kinetic assisted venous drainage: experience in 50 patients. *Perfusion* 1998;13:137–143.

95. Kurusz M, Deyo DJ, Sholar AD, et al. Laboratory testing of femoral venous cannulae: effect of size, position and negative pressure on flow. *Perfusion* 1999;14:379–387.

96. Pedersen TH, Videm V, Svennevig JL, et al. Extracorporeal membrane oxygenation using a centrifugal pump and a servo regulator to prevent negative inlet pressure. *Ann Thorac Surg* 1997;63:1333–1339.

97. Reed CC, Kurusz M, Lawrence AE Jr. Effects of surgical technique on cardiopulmonary bypass. *Safety and techniques in perfusion.* Stafford, TX: Quali-Med, 1988:187–189.

98. Antunes MJ. Techniques of valvular reoperation. *Eur J Cardiothorac Surg* 1992;6[Suppl I]:S54–S58.

99. Watanabe G, Haverich A, Speier R. Third-time coronary artery revascularization. *Thorac Cardiovasc Surg* 1993;41:163–166.

100. Toomasian JM Peters WS, Siegal LC. Extracorporeal circulation for port-access cardiac surgery. *Perfusion* 1997;12:83–91.

101. Berrizbeitia LD, Anderson WA, Laub GW, et al. Case report: coronary artery bypass grafting after pneumonectomy. *Ann Thorac Surg* 1994;58:1538–1540.

102. Soltanian H, Sanders JH Jr, Robb JC, et al. Case report: hybrid myocardial revascularization after previous left pneumonectomy. *Ann Thorac Surg* 1998;65:259–260.

103. Gu YJ, Obster R, Haan J, et al. Biocompatibility of leukocyte

removal filters during leukocyte filtration of cardiopulmonary bypass perfusate. *Artif Organ* 1993;17:660–665.

104. Soorae AS, Cleland J, O'Kane H. Delayed non-mycotic false aneurysm of ascending aortic cannulation site. *Thorax* 1977;32: 743–748.

105. Murphy DA, Craver JM, Jones EL, et al. Recognition and management of ascending aortic dissection complicating cardiac surgical operations. *J Thorac Cardiovasc Surg* 1983;85:247–256.

106. Mills NL, Morris JM. Air embolism associated with cardiopulmonary bypass. In: Waldhausen JA, Orringer MB, eds. *Complications in cardiothoracic surgery*. St. Louis: Mosby, 1991:60–67.

107. Coughlan DWS, Diehl JT, Rice TW, et al. Ascending aortic insertion of the intra-aortic balloon catheter: the potential for air embolism. *Proc Am Acad Cardiovasc Perfus* 1986;7:161–162.

108. Kurusz M, Lick SD, Conti VR. Air embolism with intraaortic balloon counterpulsation during cardiopulmonary bypass [Letter]. *J Thorac Cardiovasc Surg* 1998;115:1393.

109. Stoney WS, Alford WC Jr, Burrus GR, et al. Air embolism and other accidents using pump oxygenators. *Ann Thorac Surg* 1980; 29:336–340.

110. Kurusz M, Conti VR, Arens JF, et al. Perfusion accident survey. *Proc Am Acad Cardiovasc Perfus* 1986;7:57–65.

111. Mejak BL, Stammers A, Rauch E, et al. A retrospective study on perfusion accidents and safety devices. *Perfusion* 2000;15: 51–61.

112. Wheeldon DR. Can cardiopulmonary bypass be a safe procedure? In: Longmore DB, ed. *Towards safer cardiac surgery*. Lancaster, UK: MTP, 1981:427–446.

113. Jenkins OF, Morris R, Simpson JM. Australasian perfusion incident survey. *Perfusion* 1997;12:279–288.

114. Mills NL, Ochsner JL. Massive air embolism during cardiopulmonary bypass-causes, prevention, and management. *J Thorac Cardiovasc Surg* 1980;80:708–717.

115. Kurusz M, Wheeldon DR. Risk containment during cardiopulmonary bypass. *Semin Thorac Cardiovasc Surg* 1990;2:400–409.

116. Fleisher AG, Tyers GFO, Manning GT, et al. Management of massive hemoptysis secondary to catheter-induced perforation of the pulmonary artery during cardiopulmonary bypass. *Chest* 1989;95:1340–1341.

117. Thrush DN, Jeffries D. Pulmonary hemorrhage during cardiac surgery. *J Cardiothorac Vasc Anesth* 1991;5:377–378.

118. Cohen JA, Blackshear RH, Gravenstein N, et al. Increased pulmonary artery perforating potential of pulmonary artery catheters during hypothermia. *J Cardiothorac Vasc Anesth* 1991;5: 234–236.

119. Kulkarni MG. A complication of aortic cannulation. *J Cardiovasc Surg* 1968;9:207–208.

120. Krous HF, Mansfield PB, Sauvage LR. Carotid artery hyperperfusion during open-heart surgery. *J Thorac Cardiovasc Surg* 1973;66:118–120.

121. Ross WT, Lake CL, Wellons HA. Cardiopulmonary bypass complicated by inadvertent carotid cannulation. *Anesthesiology* 1981;54:85–86.

122. McLeskey CH, Cheney FW. A correctable complication of cardiopulmonary bypass. *Anesthesiology* 1982;56:214–216.

123. Sudhaman DA. Accidental hyperperfusion of the left carotid artery during CPB [Letter]. *J Cardiothorac Vasc Anesth* 1991;5: 100–101.

124. Tempe D, Khanna SK. Accidental hyperperfusion during cardiopulmonary bypass: suggested safety features [Letter]. *Ann Thorac Surg* 1998;65:306.

125. Springer MA, Korth DC, Guiterrez PJ, et al. An in vitro analysis of a one-way arterial check valve. *J Extra-Corp Technol* 1995; 27:29–33.

126. Gravlee GP, Wong AB, Charles DJ. Hypoxemia during cardiopulmonary bypass from leaks in the gas supply system [Letter]. *Anesth Analg* 1985;64:646–653.

127. Roth JV, Fried DW. Catastrophic cardiopulmonary bypass accident [Letter]. *J Cardiothorac Vasc Anesth* 1993;7:253–254.

128. Robblee JA, Crosby E, Keon WJ. Hypoxemia after intraluminal oxygen line obstruction during cardiopulmonary bypass. *Ann Thorac Surg* 1989;48:575–576.

129. Kurusz M, Andrews JJ, Arens JF, et al. Monitoring oxygen concentration prevents potential adverse patient outcome caused by a scavenging malfunction: case report. *Proc Am Acad Cardiovasc Perfus* 1991;12:162–165.

130. Kirson LE, Goldman JM. A system for monitoring the delivery of ventilating gas to the oxygenator during cardiopulmonary bypass. *J Cardiothorac Vasc Anesth* 1994;8:51–57.

131. Jerabek CF, Walton HG, Doerfler S. The effect of gas scavenging on hollow fiber membrane oxygenator performance. *Proceedings 27th International Conference American Society of Extracorpeal Technology*, 10–14 March 1989:24–29.

132. Nader-Djalal, Khadra WZ, Spaulding W, et al. Correspondence: Does propofol alter the gas exchange in membrane oxygenators? *Ann Thorac Surg* 1998;66:298–299.

133. Tarr TJ, Kent AP. Sequestration of propofol in an extracorporeal circuit. *J Cardiothorac Anesth* 1989;3[Suppl 1]:75.

134. Fisher AR. The incidence and cause of emergency oxygenator changeovers. *Perfusion* 1999;14:207–212.

135. Hart MA, Abshier DA, Pacheco SL, et al. A technique for the change-out of a malfunctioning membrane oxygenator without terminating cardiopulmonary bypass. *Proc Am Acad Cardiovasc Perfus* 1988;9:105–113.

136. McMillan J, Smith BF, Cooper E, et al. Case report: emergency changing of an oxygenator during total cardiopulmonary bypass. *Anaesth Intens Care* 1979;7:271–272.

137. Reed CC, Stafford TB. *Cardiopulmonary bypass*, 2nd ed. Houston: Texas Medical Press, 1985:408.

138. Kurusz M, Shaffer CW, Christman EW, et al. Runaway pump head: new cause of gas embolism during cardiopulmonary bypass. *J Thorac Cardiovasc Surg* 1979;77:792–795.

139. Ballard S, Biggan DE. Runaway pumphead. In: Stafford TB, Toomasian JM, Kurusz M, eds. *Case reports. I. Clinical studies in extracorporeal circulation*. Houston: PREF Press, 1994:94–99.

140. Kurusz M. Fire in the heart-lung machine during mitral valve replacement. In: Stafford TB, Toomasian JM, Kurusz M, eds. *Case reports. I. Clinical studies in extracorporeal circulation*. Houston: PREF Press, 1994:85–93.

141. Khambatta HJ, Stone JG, Wald A, et al. Electrocardiographic artifacts during cardiopulmonary bypass. *Anesth Analg* 1990;71: 88–91.

142. Metz S. ECG artifacts during cardiopulmonary bypass and alternative method [Letter]. *Anesth Analg* 1991;72:715–716.

143. Emergency Care Research Institute. ECG artifact in the OR. *Health Dev* 1991;20:140–141.

144. Hug CC Jr. The anesthesiologist's response to a low-output state after cardiopulmonary bypass: etiologies and remedies. *J Card Surg* 1990;5:259–262.

145. Kurusz M, Faulkner SC. Anecdotes and case reports from the perfusion accident survey. *Proc Am Acad Cardiovasc Perfus* 1987; 8:261–264.

146. Quinn ML. Semipractical alarms: a parable. *J Clin Monit* 1989; 5:196–200.

147. Beneken JEW, van der Aa JJ. Alarms and their limits in monitoring. *J Clin Monit* 1989;5:205–210.

148. Cooper JB, Newbower RS, Kitz RJ. An analysis of major errors and equipment failures in anesthesia practice—considerations for prevention and detection. *Anesthesiology* 1984;60:34–42.

149. Gaba DM. Human error in anesthetic mishaps. *Int Anesthesiol Clin* 1989;27:137–147.

150. Kurusz M, Butler BD, Katz J, Conti VR. Air embolism during cardiopulmonary bypass. *Perfusion* 1995;10:361–391.

151. Carrel A. Experimental operations on the orifices of the heart. *Ann Surg* 1914;60:1–6.

152. Reyer GW, Kohl HW. Air embolism complicating thoracic surgery. *JAMA* 1926;87:1626–1630.

153. Kent EM, Blades B. Experimental observations upon certain intracranial complications of particular interest to the thoracic surgeon. *J Thorac Cardiovasc Surg* 1942;11:434–445.

154. Geoghegan T, Lam CR. The mechanism of death from intracardiac air and its reversibility. *Ann Surg* 1953;139:351–359.

155. Benjamin RB, Turbak CE, Lewis FJ. The effects of air embolism in the systemic circulation and its prevention during open cardiac surgery. *J Thorac Cardiovasc Surg* 1957;34:548–552.

156. Clowes GHA Jr. Experimental procedures for entry into the left heart to expose the mitral valve. *Ann Surg* 1951;134:957–968.

157. Potts WJ, Riker WL, de Bord R, et al. Maintenance of life by homologous lungs and mechanical circulation. *Surgery* 1952; 31:161–166.

158. Helmsworth JA, Clark LC, Kaplan S, et al. Artificial oxygenation and circulation during complete by-pass of the heart. *J Thorac Cardiovasc Surg* 1952;24:117–133.

159. Lewis FJ, Taufic M. Closure of atrial septal defects with the aid of hypothermia. *Surgery* 1953;33:52–59.

160. Miller BJ, Gibbon JH Jr, Greco VF, et al. The production and repair of interatrial septal defects under direct vision with the assistance of an extracorporeal pump-oxygenator circuit. *J Thorac Surg* 1953;26:598–616.

161. Eguchi S, Bosher LH Jr. Myocardial dysfunction resulting from coronary air embolism. *Surgery* 1962;51:103–111.

162. Goldfarb D, Bahnson HT. Early and late effects on the heart of small amounts of air in the coronary circulation. *J Thorac Cardiovasc Surg* 1963;46:368–378.

163. Taber RE, Maraan BM, Tomatis L. Prevention of air embolism during open-heart surgery: a study of the role of trapped air in the left ventricle. *Surgery* 1970;68:685–691.

164. Justice C, Leach J, Edwards WS. The harmful effects and treatment of coronary air embolism during open-heart surgery. *Ann Thorac Surg* 1972;14:47–53.

165. Callaghan JC, Despres JP, Benvenuto R. A study of the causes of 60 deaths following total cardiopulmonary bypass. *J Thorac Cardiovasc Surg* 1961;42:489–496.

166. Ehrenhaft JL, Claman MA, Layton JM, et al. Cerebral complications of open-heart surgery: further observations. *J Thorac Cardiovasc Surg* 1961;42:514–526.

167. Allen P. Central nervous system emboli in open heart surgery. *Can J Surg* 1963;6:332–337.

168. Sloan H, Morris JD, Mackenzie J, et al. Open heart surgery: results in 600 cases. *Thorax* 1962;17:128–138.

169. Nicks R. Arterial air embolism. *Thorax* 1967;22:320–326.

170. Fishman NH, Carlsson E, Roe BB. The importance of the pulmonary veins in systemic air embolism following open-heart surgery. *Surgery* 1969;66:655–662.

171. Anderson RM, Fritz JM, O'Hae JE. Pulmonary air emboli during cardiac surgery. *J Thorac Cardiovasc Surg* 1965;49:440–449.

172. Lin C-Y. Pulmonary air embolism: reappraisal of the importance in open-heart surgery. *Nagoya J Med Sci* 1967;30:365–372.

173. Gomes OM, Pereira SN, Castagna RC, et al. The importance of the different sites of air injection in the tolerance of arterial air embolism. *J Thorac Cardiovasc Surg* 1973;65:563–568.

174. Beckman CR, Hurley F, Mammana R, et al. Risk factors for air embolization during cannulation of the ascending aorta. *J Thorac Cardiovasc Surg* 1980;80:302–307.

175. Sturm J. Air embolism during mitral valve replacement [Letter]. *J Thorac Cardiovasc Surg* 1981;81:804–805.

176. Hughes D. Air embolism during cardiopulmonary bypass [Letter]. *J Thorac Cardiovasc Surg* 1981;82:639.

177. Robicsek F, Duncan GD. Retrograde air embolization in coronary operations. *J Thorac Cardiovasc Surg* 1987;94:110–114.

178. Lee ME. Air embolism in coronary bypass operations [Letter]. *J Thorac Cardiovasc Surg* 1988;95:543.

179. Reed CC, Kurusz M, Lawrence AE Jr. Air embolism. *Safety and techniques in perfusion.* Stafford, TX: Quali-Med, 1988: 239–246.

180. Dennis C. Perspective in review: one group's struggle with development of a pump-oxygenator. *Trans Am Soc Artif Intern Organ* 1985;31:1–11.

181. Milnes RF, vanderWoude R, Morris JD, et al. Problems related to a bubble oxygenator system. *Surgery* 1958;42:986–992.

182. Baird RJ, Miyagishima RT. The danger of air embolism through a pressure-perfusion cannula. *J Thorac Cardiovasc Surg* 1963;46:212–219.

183. Kumar AS, Jayalakshmi TS, Kale SC, et al. Management of massive air embolism during open heart surgery. *Int J Cardiol* 1985;9:413–416.

184. Tanasawa I, Wotton DR, Yang W-J, et al. Experimental study of air bubbles in a simulated cardiopulmonary bypass system with flow constriction. *J Biomech* 1970;3:417–424.

185. Comer TP, Saxena NC, Hamel NC. Full recovery of a patient after oxygenator replacement during open-heart surgery. *Cardiovasc Dis Bull Tex Heart Inst* 1980;7:165–168.

186. Pfefferkorn RO, Rose MW, Pfefferkorn SP. An unreported pathway for the introduction of air embolism from and unvented hardshell cardiotomy reservoir: a case report. *Proceedings First World Congress on Open Heart Technology, Brighton UK 1981.* London: Franklin Scientific Projects, 1982:78–79.

187. Wells WJ, Stiles QR. Massive venous air embolism during cardiopulmonary bypass. *Ann Thorac Surg* 1981;31:86–89.

188. Pickard LR. Venous air embolism [Letter]. *Ann Thorac Surg* 1982;33:102–103.

189. Emergency Care Research Institute. Hazard: scavenging gas from membrane oxygenators. *Health Dev* 1987;16:343–344.

190. Goodridge M. Entrance of air into the veins, and its treatment. *Am J Med Sci* 1902;124:461–476.

191. Hare HA. The effect of the entrance of air into the circulation. *Therap Gazette* 1889;5:606–610.

192. Tisovec L, Hamilton WK. Newer considerations in air embolism during operation. *JAMA* 1967;201:376–377.

193. Munson ES. Transfer of nitrous oxide into body air cavities. *Br J Anaesth* 1974;46:202–209.

194. Garcia C, Albin MS, Bunegin L. Effect of nitrous oxide on air bubble volume in arterial air embolism [Letter]. *Crit Care Med* 1989;17:1236.

195. Losasso TJ, Black S, Muzzi DA, et al. Detection and hemodynamic consequences of venous air embolism. Does nitrous oxide make a difference? *Anesthesiology* 1992;77:148–152.

196. Munson ES. Pathophysiology and treatment of venous air embolism: a review. *Middle East J Anesthesiol* 1988;9:315–325.

197. Wells DG, Podolakin W, Mohr M, et al. Nitrous oxide and cerebrospinal fluid markers of ischemia following cardiopulmonary bypass. *Anaesth Intens Care* 1987;15:431–435.

198. Peirce EC II. Cerebral gas embolism (arterial) with special reference to iatrogenic accidents. *HBO Rev* 1980;1:161–188.

199. Dutka AJ. A review of the pathophysiology and potential application of experimental therapies for cerebral ischemia to the treatment of cerebral arterial gas embolism. *Undersea Biomed Res* 1985;12:403–421.

200. Spampinato N, Stassano P, Gagliardi C, et al. Massive air embolism during cardiopulmonary bypass: successful treatment with immediate hypothermia and circulatory support. *Ann Thorac Surg* 1981;32:602–603.

201. Steward D, Williams WG, Freedom R. Hypothermia in conjunction with hyperbaric oxygenation in the treatment of massive air embolism during cardiopulmonary bypass. *Ann Thorac Surg* 1977;24:591–593.

202. Fundaro P, Santoil C. Massive coronary gas embolism managed by retrograde coronary sinus perfusion. *Tex Heart Inst J* 1984; 11:172–174.

203. Sandhu AA, Spotnitz HM, Dickstein ML, et al. Retrograde cardioplegia preserves myocardial function after induced coronary air embolism. *J Thorac Cardiovasc Surg* 1997;113: 917–922.

204. Bauer RO, Campbell M, Goodman R, et al. Aeroembolism treated by hypothermia: report of a case. *Aerospace Med* 1965; 36:671–675.

205. Fine J, Fischmann J. An experimental study of the treatment of air embolism. *N Engl J Med* 1940;223:1054–1057.

206. Alvaran SB, Toung JK, Graff TE, et al. Venous air embolism: comparative merits of external cardiac massage, intracardiac aspiration, and left lateral decubitus position. *Anesth Analg* 1978; 57:166–170.

207. Musgrove JE, MacQuigg RE. Successful treatment of air embolism. *JAMA* 1952;150:28.

208. Ericsson JA, Gottlieb JD, Sweet RB. Closed-chest cardiac massage in the treatment of venous air embolism. *N Engl J Med* 1964;270:1353–1354.

209. Brenner WI. A battle plan in the event of massive air embolism during open heart surgery. *J Extra-Corp Technol* 1985;17: 133–137.

210. Butler BD, Laine GA, Leiman BC, et al. Effect of Trendelenburg position on the distribution of arterial air emboli in dogs. *Ann Thorac Surg* 1988;45:198–202.

211. Mehlhorn U, Burke EJ, Butler BD, et al. Body position does not affect the hemodynamic response to venous air embolism in dogs. *Anesth Analg* 1994;79:734–739.

212. Watanabe T, Shimasaki T, Kuraoka S, et al. Retrograde cerebral perfusion against massive air embolism during cardiopulmonary bypass [Letter]. *J Thorac Cardiovasc Surg* 1992;104:532–533.

213. Brown JW, Dierdorf SF, Moorthy SS, et al. Venoarterial cerebral perfusion for treatment of massive arterial air embolism. *Anesth Analg* 1987;66:673–674.

214. Diethrich EB, Koopot R, Maze A, et al. Successful reversal of brain damage from iatrogenic air embolism. *Surg Gynecol Obstet* 1982;154:572–575.

215. Ghosh PK, Kaplan O, Barak J, et al. Massive arterial air embolism during cardiopulmonary bypass. *J Cardiovasc Surg* 1985; 26:248–250.

216. Hendricks FFA, Bogers AJJC, de la Riviere AB, et al. The effectiveness of venoarterial perfusion in treatment of arterial air embolism during cardiopulmonary bypass. *Ann Thorac Surg* 1983;36:433–436.

217. Noritake S, Kitayama H, Matsuno S, et al. Massive air embolism during cardiopulmonary bypass: a case report of successful management by temporary retrograde perfusion through the superior vena cava. *Kyobu Geka* 1985;38:274–277.

218. Stark J, Hough J. Air in the aorta: treatment by reversed perfusion. *Ann Thorac Surg* 1986;41:337–338.

219. Toscano M, Chiavarelli R, Ruvolo G, et al. Management of massive air embolism during open-heart surgery with retrograde perfusion of the cerebral vessels and hyperbaric oxygenation. *Thorac Cardiovasc Surg* 1983;31:183–184.

220. Rozanski J, Szufladowicz M. Successful treatment of massive air embolism. *J Card Surg* 1994;9:430–432.

221. Goldstone J, Towan HJ, Ellis RJ. Rationale for use of vasopressors in treatment of coronary air embolism. *Surg Forum* 1978; 29:237–239.

222. Evans DE, Kobrine AI, LeGrys DC, et al. Protective effect of

223. Padula RT, Eisenstat TE, Bronstein MH, et al. Intracardiac air following cardiotomy: location, causative factors, and a method for removal. *J Thorac Cardiovasc Surg* 1971;62:736–742.

224. Eiseman B, Baxter BJ, Prachuabmoh K. Surface tension reducing substances in the management of coronary air embolism. *Ann Surg* 1959;149:374–380.

225. Malette WG, Fitzgerald JB, Eiseman B. Aeroembolus: a protective substance. *Surg Forum* 1960;11:155–156.

226. Menasche P, Pinard E, Desroches A-M, et al. Fluorocarbons: a potential treatment of cerebral air embolism in open-heart surgery. *Ann Thorac Surg* 1985;40:494–497.

227. Menasche P, Fleury J-P, Piwnica A. Update: fluorocarbons: a potential treatment of cerebral air embolism in open-heart surgery. *Ann Thorac Surg* 1992;54:392–393.

228. Butler BD, Kurusz M. Fluorocarbon treatment for cerebral air embolism [Letter]. *Ann Thorac Surg* 1986;42:350–351.

229. Speiss BD, McCarthy RJ, Tuman KJ, et al. Perfluorocarbon emulsions and air embolism [Letter]. *Ann Thorac Surg* 1987; 44:223.

230. Speiss BD, McCarthy RJ, Ivankovich AD. Protection from coronary air embolism by a perfluorocarbon emulsion (FC-43). *J Cardiothorac Anesth* 1987;1:210–215.

231. Speiss BD, Braverman B, Woronowicz AW, et al. Protection from cerebral air emboli with perfluorocarbons in rabbits. *Stroke* 1986;17:1146–1149.

232. Annane D, Troche G, Delisle F, et al. Effects of mechanical ventilation with normobaric oxygen therapy on the rate of air removal from cerebral arteries. *Crit Care Med* 1994;22: 851–857.

233. Presson RG Jr, Kirk KR, Haselby KA, et al. Effect of ventilation with soluble and diffusible gases on the size of air emboli. *J Appl Physiol* 1991;70:1068–1074.

234. Tuman KJ, McCarthy RJ, Speiss BD, et al. Effects of nitrous oxide on coronary perfusion after coronary air embolism. *Anesthesiology* 1987;67:952–959.

235. Hlastala MP, Van Liew HD. Absorption of in vivo inert gas bubbles. *Respir Physiol* 1975;24:147–158.

236. Schabel RK, Berryessa RG, Justison GA, et al. Ten common perfusion problems: prevention and treatment protocols. *J Extra-Corp Technol* 1987;19:392–398.

237. Tovar EA, Del Campo C, Bosari A, et al. Postoperative management of cerebral air embolism: gas physiology for surgeons. *Ann Thorac Surg* 1995;60:1138–1142.

238. Armon C, Deschamps C, Adkinson C, et al. Hyperbaric treatment of cerebral air embolism sustained during an open-heart surgical procedure. *Mayo Clin Proc* 1991;66:565–570.

239. Bove AA, Clark JM, Simon AJ, et al. Successful therapy of cerebral air embolism with hyperbaric oxygen at 2.8 ATA. *Undersea Biomed Res* 1982;9:75–79.

240. Halliday P, Anderson DN, Davidson AI, et al. Management of cerebral air embolism secondary to a disconnected central venous catheter. *Br J Surg* 1994;81:71.

241. Hart GB. Treatment of decompression illness and air embolism with hyperbaric oxygen. *Aerospace Med* 1974;45:1190–1193.

242. Kindwall EP. Massive surgical air embolism treated with brief recompression to six atmospheres followed by hyperbaric oxygen. *Aerospace Med* 1973;44:663–666.

243. Lar LW, Lai LC, Ren LW. Massive arterial air embolism during cardiac operation: successful treatment in hyperbaric chamber under 3 ATA [Letter]. *J Thorac Cardiovasc Surg* 1990;100: 928–930.

244. Meijne NG, Schoemaker G, Bulterijs AB. The treatment of cerebral gas embolism in a high pressure chamber: and experimental study. *J Cardiovasc Surg* 1963;4:757–763.

245. Menkin M, Schwartzman RJ. Cerebral air embolism: report of five cases and review of the literature. *Arch Neurol* 1977;34: 168–170.

246. Murphy BP, Harford FJ, Cramer FS. Cerebral air embolism resulting form invasive medical procedures: treatment with hyperbaric oxygen. *Ann Surg* 1985;201:242–245.

247. Peirce EC II. Specific therapy for arterial air embolism [Editorial]. *Ann Thorac Surg* 1980;29:300–303.

248. Takita H, Olszewski W, Schimert G, et al. Hyperbaric treatment of cerebral air embolism as a result of open-heart surgery: report of a case. *J Thorac Cardiovasc Surg* 1968;55:682–85.

249. Mader JT, Hulet WH. Delayed hyperbaric treatment of cerebral air embolism: report of a case. *Arch Neurol* 1979;36:504–505.

250. Bitterman H, Melamed Y. Delayed hyperbaric treatment of cerebral air embolism. *Israel J Med Sci* 1993;29:22–26.

251. Ryan T, McCarthy JF, Rady MY, et al. Early bloodstream infection after cardiopulmonary bypass: frequency rate, risk factors, and implications. *Crit Care Med* 1997;25:2009–2014.

252. Rudnick JR, Beck-Sague CM, Anderson RL, et al. Gram-negative bacteremia in open-heart-surgery patients traced to probable tap-water contamination of pressure-monitoring equipment. *Infect Control Hosp Epidemiol* 1996;17:281–285.

253. Hughes CF, Grant AF, Leckie BD, et al. Cardioplegic solution: a contamination crisis. *J Thorac Cardiovasc Surg* 1986;91: 296–302.

254. Talbot GH. Contamination of cardioplegic solution [Letter]. *J Thorac Cardiovasc Surg* 1986;92:966.

255. Metz S. Administration of protamine rather than heparin in a patient undergoing normothermic cardiopulmonary bypass. *Anesthesiology* 1994;80:691–694.

256. Ti LK. Survival after large ABO-incompatible blood transfusion. *Can J Anaesth* 1998;45:916.

257. Becker RM. Intracardiac surgery in pregnant women. *Ann Thorac Surg* 1983;36:453–458.

258. Leyse R, Ofstun M, Dillard DH, et al. Congenital aortic stenosis in pregnancy, corrected by extracorporeal circulation: offering a viable male infant at term but with anomalies eventuating in his death at four months of age-report of a case. *JAMA* 1961; 176:1009–1012.

259. Dubourg G, Broustet P, Bricaud H, et al. Correction complete d'une triade de Fallot en circulation extra-corporelle chez une femme enceinte. *Arch Mal Coeur* 1959;52:1389–1391.

260. Kay CF, Smith K. Surgery in the pregnant cardiac patient. *Am J Cardiol* 1963;12:293–295.

261. Werch A, Lambert HM, Cooley D, et al. Fetal monitoring and maternal open heart surgery [Letter]. *South Med J* 1977;70: 1024.

262. Meffert WG, Stansel HC Jr. Open heart surgery during pregnancy. *Am J Obstet Gynecol* 1968;102:1116–1120.

263. Pedersen H, Finster M. Anesthetic risk in the pregnant surgical patient. *Anesthesiology* 1979;51:439–451.

264. Parry AJ, Westaby S. Cardiopulmonary bypass during pregnancy. *Ann Thorac Surg* 1996;61:1865–1869.

265. Pomini F, Mercogliano D, Cavalletti C, et al. Cardiopulmonary bypass in pregnancy. *Ann Thorac Surg* 1996;61:259–268.

266. Weiss BM, von Segesser LK, Seifert B, et al. Outcome of cardiovascular surgery and pregnancy: a systematic review of the period 1984–1996. *Am J Obstet Gynecol* 1998;179:1643–1653.

267. Izquierdo LA, Kushnir O, Knieriem K, et al. Effect of mitral valve prosthetic surgery on the outcome of a growth-retarded fetus. A case report. *Am J Obstet Gynecol* 1990;163:584–586.

268. Caritis SN, Edelstone DI, Mueller-Heubach E. Pharmacologic inhibition of premature labor. *Am J Obstet Gynecol* 1979;133: 557–578.

269. Lamb MP, Ross K, Johnstone AM, et al. Fetal heart rate monitoring during open heart surgery. *Br J Obstet Gynecol* 1983;88: 669–674.

270. Korsten HHM, Van Zundert AAJ, Mooij PNM, et al. Emergency aortic valve replacement in the 24th week of pregnancy. *Acta Anaesth Belg* 1989;40:201–205.

271. Strickland RA, Oliver WC Jr, Chantigian RC, et al. Anesthesia, cardiopulmonary bypass, and the pregnant patient. *Mayo Clin Proc* 1991;66:411–429.

272. Chambers CE, Clark SL. Cardiac surgery during pregnancy. *Clin Obstet Gynecol* 1994;37:316–323.

273. Conroy JM, Bailey MK, Hollon MF, et al. Anesthesia for open heart surgery in the pregnant patient. *South Med J* 1989;82: 492–495.

274. Harrison EC, Roschke EJ. Pregnancy in patients with cardiac valve prostheses. *Clin Obstet Gynecol* 1975;18:107–123.

275. Koh KS, Friesen RM, Livingstone RA, et al. Fetal monitoring during maternal cardiac surgery with cardiopulmonary bypass. *Can Med Assoc J* 1975;112:1102–1104.

276. Reisner LS. Cardiac dysfunction: special considerations during pregnancy. In: Utley JR, ed. *Pathophysiology and techniques of cardiopulmonary bypass.* Vol. III. Baltimore: Williams & Wilkins, 1985:15–29.

277. Buffolo E, Palma JH, Gomes WJ, et al. Case report: successful use of deep hypothermic circulatory arrest in pregnancy. *Ann Thorac Surg* 1994;58:1532–1534.

278. Daley R, Harrison GK, McMillan IKR. Direct-vision pulmonary valvotomy during pregnancy. *Lancet* 1957;273:875–876.

279. Ravindran R, Viegas OJ, Padilla LM, et al. Anesthetic considerations in pregnant patients receiving terbutylline treatment. *Anesth Analg* 1980;59:391–392.

280. Rolbin SH, Levinson G, Shnider SM, et al. Dopamine treatment of spinal hypotension decreases uterine blood flow in the pregnant ewe. *Anesthesiology* 1979;51:37–40.

281. Naulty JS, Cefalo RC, Lewis P. Fetal toxicity of nitroprusside in the pregnant ewe. *Am J Obstet Gynecol* 1980;139:708–711.

282. Kopman EA. Scavenging of potassium cardioplegic solution to prevent hyperkalemia in hemodialysis-dependent patients. *Anesth Analg* 1983;62:780–782.

283. Soffer O, MacDonell C Jr, Finlayson DC, et al. Intraoperative hemodialysis during cardiopulmonary bypass in chronic renal failure. *J Thorac Cardiovasc Surg* 1979;77:789–791.

284. Geronemus R, Schneider N. Continuous arteriovenous hemodialysis: a new modality for treatment of acute renal failure. *Trans Am Soc Artif Intern Organs* 1984;30:610–613.

285. Hakim M, Wheeldon D, Bethune DW, et al. Haemodialysis and haemofiltration on cardiopulmonary bypass. *Thorax* 1985; 40:101–106.

286. Murkin JM, Murphy DA, Finlayson DC, et al. Hemodialysis during cardiopulmonary bypass: report of twelve cases. *Anesth Analg* 1987;66:899–901.

287. Wheeldon D, Bethune D. Haemofiltration during cardiopulmonary bypass. *Perfusion* 1990;5[Suppl]:39–51.

288. Sutton RG. Renal considerations, dialysis, and ultrafiltration during cardiopulmonary bypass. *Int Anesthesiol Clin* 1996;34: 165–176.

289. Ilson BE, Bland PS, Jorkasky DK, et al. Intraoperative versus routine hemodialysis in end-stage renal disease patients undergoing open-heart surgery. *Nephron* 1992;61:170–175.

290. Hamilton CC, Harwood SJ, Deemar KA, et al. Haemodialysis during cardiopulmonary bypass using a haemofilter. *Perfusion* 1994;9:135–139.

291. Koyanagi T, Nishida, Endo M, et al. Coronary artery bypass grafting in chronic renal dialysis patients: intensive perioperative dialysis and extensive usage of arterial grafts. *Eur J Cardiothorac Surg* 1994;8:505–507.

292. Garrido P, Bobadilla JF, Albertos J, et al. Cardiac surgery in

patients under chronic hemodialysis. *Eur J Cardiothorac Surg* 1995;9:36–39.

293. United States Health Care Financing Administration. *End stage renal disease program highlights [Fact sheet]*. August 1997.

294. Marshall WG Jr, Rossi NP, Meng RL, et al. Coronary artery bypass grafting in dialysis patients. *Ann Thorac Surg* 1986; 42[Suppl]:S12–S15.

295. Gerberding JL, Littell C, Tarkington A, et al. Risks of exposure of surgical personnel to patient's blood during surgery at San Francisco General Hospital. *N Engl J Med* 1990;322: 1788–1793.

296. Popejoy SL, Fry DE. Blood contact and exposure in the operating room. *Surg Gynecol Obstet* 1991;172:480–483.

297. Centers for Disease Control. Recommendation for preventing transmission of infection with human T-lymphotropic virus type III/lymphadenopathy-associated virus in the workplace. *MMWR Morb Mortal Wkly Rep* 1985;35:681–686, 691–695.

298. Centers for Disease Control. Recommendation for preventing transmission of infection with human T-lymphotropic virus Type III/lymphadenopath-associated virus in the workplace. *MMWR Morb Mortal Wkly Rep* 1986;35:21–23.

299. Subcommittee on AIDS of The American College of Surgeons Governors Committee. 1991 Clinical Congress highlights: statement on the surgeon and HIV infection. *ACS Bull* 1991; 76:28–31.

300. Condit D, Frater RWM. Human immunodeficiency virus and the cardiac surgeon: a survey of attitudes. *Ann Thorac Surg* 1989; 47:182–186.

301. Lemma M, Vanelli P, Beretta L, et al. Cardiac surgery in HIV-positive intravenous drug addicts: influence of cardiopulmonary bypass on the progression to AIDS. *Thorac Cardiovasc Surg* 1992;40:279–282.

302. Aris A, Pomar JL, Saura E. Cardiopulmonary bypass in HIV-positive patients. *Ann Thorac Surg* 1993;55:1104–1108.

303. Uva MS, Jebara VA, Fabiani JN, et al. Cardiac surgery in patients with human immunodeficiency virus infection: indications and results. *J Card Surg* 1992;7:240–244.

304. Robicsek F, Duncan GD, Masters TN, et al. Can AIDS be prevented after injury with contaminated instruments? *Ann Thorac Surg* 1990;49:984–986.

305. Denborough MA, Foster VFA, Lovell RRH, et al. Anaesthetic deaths in a family. *Br J Anaesth* 1962;34:395–396.

306. Ryan JF, Kerr WS Jr. Malignant hyperthermia: a catastrophic complication. *J Urol* 1973;109:879–883.

307. Britt BA, Kalow W. Malignant hyperthermia, a statistical review. *Can Anaesth Soc J* 1970;17:293–301.

308. Ryan JF, Donlon JV, Malt RA, et al. Cardiopulmonary bypass in the treatment of malignant hyperthermia. *N Engl J Med* 1974;290:1121–1122.

309. Byrick RJ, Rose DK, Ranganathan N. Management of a malignant hyperthermia patient during cardiopulmonary bypass. *Can Anaesth Soc J* 1982;29:50–54.

310. Bahret PM, Larach DR, Williams DR, et al. Malignant hyper-

thermia: a case report. *Proc Am Acad Cardiovasc Perfus* 1986; 7:177–180.

311. MacGillivray RG, Jann H, Vanker E, et al. Development of malignant hyperthermia obscured by cardiopulmonary bypass. *Can Anaesth Soc J* 1986;33:509–514.

312. Quinn RD, Pae WE Jr, McGary SA, et al. Development of malignant hyperthermia during mitral valve replacement. *Ann Thorac Surg* 1992;53:1114–1116.

313. Schwartz AJ, Hensley FA Jr. Case conference 3, 1990. *J Cardiothorac Anesth* 1990;4:385–399.

314. Utley JR, Leyland SA. Coronary artery bypass grafting in the octogenarian. *J Thorac Cardiovasc Surg* 1991;101:866–870.

315. Tsai T-P, Nessim S, Kass RM, et al. Morbidity and mortality after coronary artery bypass in octogenarians. *Ann Thorac Surg* 1991;51:983–986.

316. Ko W, Kreiger KH, Lazenby D, et al. Isolated coronary artery bypass grafting in one hundred consecutive octogenarian patients. *J Thorac Cardiovasc Surg* 1991;102:532–538.

317. Ranger WR, Glover JL, Shannon FL, et al. Coronary artery bypass and valve replacement in octogenarians. *Am Surg* 1996; 62:941–946.

318. Cane ME, Chen C, Bailery BM, et al. CABG in octogenarians: early and late events and actuarial survival in comparison with a matched population. *Ann Thorac Surg* 1995;60:1033–1037.

319. Rady MY, Ryan T, Starr NJ. Perioperative determinants of morbidity and mortality in elderly patients undergoing cardiac surgery. *Crit Care Med* 1998;26:225–235.

320. Johnson WC, Lurich F, Meguid MM, et al. Role of delayed hypersensitivity in predicting postoperative morbidity and mortality. *Am J Surg* 1979;137:536–542.

321. Moulton MJ, Creswell LL, Mackey ME, et al. Obesity is not a risk factor for significant adverse outcome after cardiac surgery. *Circulation* 1996;94[Suppl II]:II-87–II-92.

322. Kirklin JW, Barratt-Boyes BG. *Cardiac surgery*, 2nd ed. New York: Churchill Livingstone, 1993:80.

323. Babka RM, Caviness ML, Howell J, et al. The effects of obesity on cardiopulmonary bypass using the Bentley BOS-10 oxygenator. *Proc Am Acad Cardiovasc Perfus* 1982;3:60–63.

324. Klemperer JD, Ko W, Kreiger K, et al. Cardiac operations in patients with cirrhosis. *Ann Thorac Surg* 1998;65:85–87.

325. Humphries JE. Transfusion therapy in acquired coagulopathies. *Hematol Oncol Clin North Am* 1994;8:1181–1201.

326. Joist JH. Hemostatic abnormalities in liver disease. In: Colman RW, Hirsh J, Marder VJ, eds. *Hemostasis and thrombosis: basic principles and clinical practice*. Philadelphia: J.B. Lippincott, 1994:906.

327. Rastogi P, Gupta SC, Bisht D. Coagulation studies in patients with cirrhosis of liver: bleeders vs. non-bleeders. *Indian J Pathol Microbiol* 1990;33:323–327.

328. Buzzelli TJ, Trittipoe RE. Massive volume loss during cardiopulmonary bypass and its association with Meckel's diverticulum. *J Extra-Corp Technol* 1997;29:45–48.

329. Kurusz M, Wheeldon DR. Perfusion safety. *Perfusion* 1988;3: 97–112.

330. Perrow C. *Normal accidents, living with high-risk technologies*. New York: Basic Books, 1984.

TERMINATION OF CARDIOPULMONARY BYPASS

STEPHEN J. THOMAS
RICHARD F. DAVIS

Cardiopulmonary bypass (CPB) produces several major physiologic perturbations, including cardiac arrest (diastolic arrest with cardioplegia or ventricular fibrillation), hypothermia, hemodilution, anticoagulation, electrolyte shifts, neuroendocrine stress, and activation of the inflammatory cascade, among others. Restoration of the normal cardiopulmonary circulation after CPB, whether the surgical procedure is myocardial revascularization, valve replacement or repair, repair of congenital heart defects, or other types of surgery, is a period of significant cardiovascular stress. The success of this critical step in cardiac surgery depends on thorough planning and preparation. The cardiothoracic anesthesiologist facilitates this transition by assessing cardiac function and providing appropriate pharmacologic support when intrinsic cardiac function is inadequate to ensure safe termination of CPB. The termination of bypass must be a team effort: communication between surgeon, perfusionist, and anesthesiologist is of paramount importance to its success.

PREPARING FOR SEPARATION

Preparation for separation from CPB must be based on a clear understanding of the patient's preoperative condition and the events of the operative course. Certain routines are common to all cardiac surgical cases, whereas other specific situations demand specific preparations (e.g., anticipation of the need for inotropic therapy for predicted postoperative ventricular dysfunction).

Rewarming

Before termination of CPB, the patient must be rewarmed if hypothermia was used. Moderate hypothermia (25 to

30°C) is often used to slow myocardial rewarming after cold cardioplegia and perhaps reduce central nervous system complications. Deep hypothermia (16 to 25°C) with circulatory arrest is occasionally needed for repairs of certain congenital defects or for aortic arch reconstruction. This process is facilitated by the heat exchanger in the bypass circuit. Temperature measurement must include the arterial and venous blood (because it is customary to keep the arteriovenous gradient less than 10°C) and one or more patient sites such as nasopharyngeal, esophageal, rectal, bladder, or great toe. Rewarming is initiated so that its completion coincides as much as possible with completion of the surgical procedure. Criteria for a degree of rewarming vary between institutions but usually require a nasopharyngeal or esophageal temperature of 37°C, bladder or rectal temperature of 35°C, or great toe temperature of 30°C. Palpation of the patient's head and shoulders can be helpful in assessing the degree of peripheral perfusion and rewarming. However, the high blood flow to tissue mass ratio of the head and neck region will result in more rapid rewarming of these areas, and this clinical assessment can therefore underestimate the adequacy of rewarming in other areas.

Rebound hypothermia results when the heat calories removed from the body during the hypothermic interval exceed the heat calories returned during rewarming. This net negative thermal balance is almost always the case in clinical practice. This heat deficit is often compounded by further convective heat loss from the patient into the cool operating room environment. Inadequate rewarming while on CPB can result in a considerable (2 to 3°C) drop in patient temperature from the end of CPB until arrival in the intensive care unit. This fall in temperature can result in shivering, with increased oxygen consumption, cardiac rhythm disturbances, and increased peripheral vascular resistance. Nitroprusside-induced vasodilation during CPB may facilitate rewarming and decrease the post-bypass fall in temperature (1). However, routine or injudicious use of this technique may lead to a requirement for significant intravascular volume expansion to maintain adequate perfusion pressure.

S. J. Thomas: Department of Anesthesiology, Weill Medical College of Cornell University, New York, New York 10021.

R. F. Davis: Portland VA Medical Center and Department of Anesthesiology, Oregon Health Sciences University, Portland, Oregon 97207.

Also, nitroprusside and other vasodilators can lead to increased pulmonary venous admixture. Together these side effects of vasodilation can complicate early extubation protocols. Shivering should be anticipated when a systemic temperature is less than 35°C. It should be aggressively treated with active rewarming measures. The use of muscle relaxants to prevent active shivering may be appropriate until ventilator weaning is undertaken.

LAMPS

After rewarming, the major factors that must be considered before the termination of CPB should be attended to using some routine procedure or checklist to ensure that important steps are not inadvertently omitted. The mnemonic *LAMPS* for *l*aboratory data, *a*nesthesia machine, *m*onitors, *p*atient (pump), and *s*upport is one useful approach (Table 29.1).

Laboratory Data

CPB results in numerous metabolic abnormalities, which should be normalized before termination of bypass when possible. Arterial blood gases and pH should be measured and significant abnormalities corrected, if necessary. Particular attention should be paid to arterial pH, especially in prolonged cases where metabolic acidosis with a considerable base deficit is likely to occur. Acidemia, from respiratory and/or metabolic acidosis, should be corrected because of its depressant effects on myocardial function, its interference with the action of inotropic drugs (i.e., especially the natural and synthetic catecholamines), and its ability to increase pulmonary vascular tone (2–4). Serum sodium, potassium, and ionized calcium should be measured. Hemodilution and repeated dosing of hyperkalemic cardioplegia solution frequently result in significant electrolyte abnormalities, especially in patients who have poor renal function. Potassium has pronounced deleterious effects on cardiac conduction, and atrioventricular conduction block is common in the presence of hyperkalemia (5). Hyperkalemia can be treated with insulin (10 to 20 units i.v.) with glucose if necessary. It is usually unnecessary to treat mild hyperkalemia (i.e., less than 6.0 mEq/L) in the presence of normal renal function, because serum potassium usually falls after CPB, and overly aggressive treatment of mild hyperkalemia may result in significant by hypokalemia.

Hypokalemia should be avoided after bypass and should be treated promptly because ventricular and atrial dysrhythmias are more common in the presence of acute hypokalemia, particularly in the patient receiving digoxin. Ideally, serum ionized calcium and glucose should also be determined. Hypocalcemia resulting from hemodilution and transfusion of albumin or citrate-containing blood products

TABLE 29.1. MNEMONIC FOR PREPARATIONS BEFORE TERMINATION OF CPB

Laboratory data
pH, Pco_2 of arterial blood
So_2 of venous blood
Serum NA^+, K^+, Ca^{2+}, glucose
Hematocrit
Activated clotting time, heparin concentration, thromboelastogram

Anesthesia/machine
Analgesia–supplemental opioid
Amnesia–benzodiazepine
Muscle relaxation–if needed
Airway and functional oxygen delivery system
   Anesthesia machine on
   Adequate oxygen supply
   Breathing circuit intact
   Endotracheal tube connected, unkinked
   Ventilator functional
   Ability to ventilate both lungs confirmed
   Vaporizers off

Monitors
Invasive blood pressure monitors–zeroed and calibrated
   Arterial catheter–radial, femoral or aortic
   Pulmonary artery catheter
   Central venous (right atrial) catheter
   Left atrial catheter
Electrocardiogram
   Rate—pacing capability
   Rhythm
   Conduction
   Ischemia—review all available leads
Bladder catheter—urine output
Pulse oximeter
Capnometer/mass spectrometer
Safety monitors–oxygen analyzer, circuit pressure alarm, spirometer
Transesophageal echocardiogram
Temperature (37°C nasopharangeal, 35°C rectal or bladder)

Patient/pump
The heart
   Cardiac function—contractility, size
   Rhythm
   Ventricular filling
   Air removed
   Vent removed
The lungs
   Inflation/deflation
   Compliance
The field
   Bleeding
   Oxygenation–blood color
   Movement–a sign of inadequate anesthesia

Support
Pharmacologic
   Inotropes
   Vasodilators
   Vasoconstrictors
   Antidysrhythmics
Electrical
   Atrial and/or ventricular pacing
Mechanical
   Intraaortic balloon counterpulsation
   Left and/or right ventricular assist device

should be corrected with a calcium solution (usually $CaCl_2$ in the dosage range of 3 to 5 mg/kg) to improve myocardial contractility (in the presence of hypocalcemia) and peripheral vascular tone. Hyperglycemia, which is common after CPB, usually returns to normal shortly after termination of CPB but should be treated with insulin, especially in diabetic patients. Even moderate hyperglycemia (more than 200 mg/dL) has significant adverse effects in terms of increasing the risk of postoperative infection and should be aggressively treated (6). More severe hyperglycemia increases serum osmolarity and can cause osmotic diuresis and central nervous system dysfunction and may increase the susceptibility of the brain to hypoxic damage. Treatment should include small incremental intravenous doses or continuous infusion of regular insulin, with close monitoring of blood glucose and potassium levels, to avoid the possibility of hypoglycemia and/or hypokalemia as a result of insulin therapy.

Hemodilution is induced during hypothermic CPB to reduce blood viscosity and improve systemic circulation. The optimal hemoglobin concentration during CPB is usually accepted as being 6 to 8 g/dL, although there is no proven minimum safe level. Healthy adult patients rarely need homologous blood transfusion with appropriate blood conservation measures, although the chronically ill patient may require red cell transfusion. Heparin-induced anticoagulation should be monitored during rewarming and additional heparin given if necessary because of the increased metabolism of heparin at higher body temperatures and the potential consequences of inadequate anticoagulation.

Marked abnormalities in coagulation and platelet function occur during and after CPB (7). Platelet transfusions are occasionally required, especially in patients who have thrombocytopenia or chronic renal failure, who are receiving aspirin therapy, or who require reoperation or a lengthy procedure. Fresh frozen plasma and cryoprecipitate should be available for treating factor deficiencies or coagulopathies but are rarely required. Postoperative bleeding is usually due to one of three factors: inadequate surgical hemostasis, inadequate heparin reversal, or platelet dysfunction.

Anesthesia

The requirements for anesthetics and muscle relaxants are greatly reduced during CPB because of the anesthetic effects of hypothermia and decreased metabolism of most drugs (8). However, rewarming reverses these effects, and care must be taken to ensure adequate anesthetic depth and muscle relaxation to prevent patient awareness and shivering. It is prudent to administer supplementary anesthetic agents (usually a benzodiazepine and opioid) and muscle relaxant empirically when rewarming is initiated, although volatile agents can easily be administered during CPB. Volatile anesthetic agents may also be used to induce vasodilation and facilitate rewarming. However, volatile anesthetic agents

should be discontinued approximately 10 minutes before termination of CPB to eliminate their circulatory depressant effects and avoid myocardial depression during emergence from bypass (9,10). The vaporizers on the anesthesia machine itself should be turned off at the onset of CPB.

The anesthesia machine should also be checked; oxygen should be flowing through the machine and the airway circuit should be properly connected. Failure to wean from CPB has occurred because of the inadvertent administration of a cardiodepressant volatile anesthetic during the weaning process. The lungs should be inflated manually to evaluate compliance and eliminate macroatelectasis. Inspection of the lungs may suggest poor deflation, unilateral inflation, pneumothorax, or pleural fluid accumulation, which should be corrected. When poor or slow deflation of the lungs is observed clinically and potential mechanical causes have been excluded, the prophylactic use of bronchodilators, such as β-adrenergic agonists (e.g., Albuterol or epinephrine) should be seriously considered. Rarely, endotracheal suction will be required to clear the endotracheal tube; this should be done carefully in the anticoagulated patient to avoid mucosal trauma and bleeding. Mechanical ventilation with 100% oxygen and a sufficient minute ventilatory volume to produce an arterial P_{CO_2} of 30 to 35 mm Hg should be initiated before beginning the weaning process.

Monitors

It is important to quickly survey all routine monitors including the pulse oximeter, capnometer, the apnea alarm, and the oxygen monitor and return to operation any that may have been turned off during CPB. Pulse oximeter probes placed on the extremities frequently do not function immediately after CPB because of peripheral hypoperfusion; a probe placed on the ear lobe or lip may perform better. There is usually a larger gradient between the arterial P_{CO_2} and end-tidal P_{CO_2} after CPB than before CPB. Adequate ventilation should be maintained during termination of CPB to prevent hypercapnia and respiratory acidosis with resultant pulmonary hypertension (11,12). Clinically, mild hyperventilation (P_aCO_2 approximately 30 mm Hg) is a useful adjunct in the treatment of increased pulmonary vascular resistance.

Pressure transducers should be zeroed and calibrated with the operating table in its neutral position. Frequently, the radial arterial pressure does not reflect the central aortic pressure after CPB (13–15). If there appears to be a discrepancy between the transduced radial arterial pressure and the aortic pressure estimated by palpation or the pressure cuff, the aortic pressure can be transduced from a needle in the aorta. This central aortic pressure can then be used during termination of CPB to avoid the unnecessary administration of vasoactive drugs. Alternatively, a femoral arterial catheter, which will normally more closely reflect the central aortic pressure, can be placed. Central and peripheral arterial pressures usually equilibrate shortly after CPB is discontinued. The use of potent inotropic and/or vasoconstrictor support must be predicated on an accurate central arterial pressure assessment. If a difficult separation from CPB is anticipated, preparations should be made to measure left ventricular filling pressures (PA catheter, direct left atrial catheter) or LV volume (transesophageal echocardiography) from CPB. Pulmonary artery catheters frequently migrate distally during manipulation of the heart during cardiac surgery. If the pulmonary artery pressure waveform reflects pulmonary artery occlusion pressure, the catheter should be pulled back until the phasic pulmonary artery pressure waveform appears. The left atrial catheter is a useful monitor of left ventricular filling pressure; however, ventricular pressure and intracavity volume are poorly correlated. The left atrial catheter can be used as a route for administration of inotropic drugs, especially those with significant α-adrenergic agonist properties in the context of excessive pulmonary vasoconstriction (see below). The central venous pressure should be measured, especially in those patients with pulmonary hypertension or right ventricular failure. The appropriate right/left ventricular function balance is an important variable in successful weaning.

The electrocardiogram (ECG) should be carefully assessed for rate, rhythm, conduction changes, and evidence of ischemia. Sinus rhythm with a rate of 70 to 90 beats/min appears to be ideal for termination of CPB in the adult. Higher heart rates are desirable in the case of children having repair of congenital lesions or in other cases when stroke volume is fixed, such as after left ventricular aneurysm repair, when left ventricular chamber size and compliance are reduced.

After hyperkalemic diastolic arrest, slow heart rates are commonly observed due to sinus bradycardia, atrial fibrillation with a slow ventricular response, or atrioventricular conduction block. These abnormalities are usually transient. Sinus bradycardia is easily treated with atrial pacing, which can be discontinued when an adequate rate or otherwise normal conduction returns after CPB. Atrial pacing can be used for sinus or junctional bradycardia with normal A-V conduction. Sequential atrioventricular pacing is indicated for atrioventricular conduction block or significant first-degree heart block. This preserves the atrial contribution to ventricular filling, which is a significant advantage in the presence of a noncompliant hypertrophied ventricle (hypertension, aortic stenosis) or enlarged ventricle (aortic or mitral regurgitation). The availability of temporary multifunctional dual chamber pacemakers has significantly increased the pacing capabilities after CPB. Ventricular pacing should only be used when the ventricular rate is too slow and atrial or atrioventricular pacing is not feasible (e.g., atrial fibrillation or flutter with a very slow ventricular response).

Tachycardia (i.e., heart rate more than 120 beats/min in the adult) before termination of CPB is more difficult to manage. In the patient with good ventricular function, sinus tachycardia often slows with ventricular filling and increased arterial pressure; in such a case, termination of CPB may solve the problem. Patients with poorly functioning ventricles often have persistently rapid rates. It is important to consider and treat other common causes of tachycardia, including hypoxemia, hypercapnia, anemia, inadequate anesthesia, and effects of medications. Once these causes are eliminated and if myocardial function is determined to be adequate, the abnormal rate can be reduced with appropriate doses of β-adrenergic receptor or calcium channel blocking drugs. Supraventricular tachycardias are best treated intraoperatively with cardioversion; however, therapy with propranolol, edrophonium, verapamil (in divided doses of 2.5 mg i.v.), or adenosine (6 to 12 mg i.v. bolus centrally) may be effective when cardioversion fails.

Ventricular fibrillation is common during reperfusion and usually responds to direct current defibrillation. Sustained or recurrent ventricular fibrillation during CPB may result in ventricular distension, which can produce irreversible myocardial damage. Potential causes, including hypothermia, hypoxemia, acidosis, hypocalcemia, hypomagnesemia, hypotension, or myocardial ischemia, should be addressed and corrected. Recurrent ventricular fibrillation should be treated with class I and/or III antidysrhythmics (lidocaine, procainamide, or amiodarone) and repeat defibrillation. β-Adrenergic blockers (propranolol 1 mg or esmolol 20 mg by intraaortic injection) are remarkably effective for facilitating defibrillation in resistant cases. Premature ventricular contractions are common after CPB. Correcting hypokalemia, overdrive pacing to a higher heart rate, or antidysrhythmic agents can often treat this condition.

All available ECG leads should be examined and compared with a preoperative tracing before terminating CPB to detect evidence of ventricular damage or ischemia. Ventricular pacemakers, if present, should be momentarily discontinued to make the evaluation. Transient ST segment elevation is common during emergence from CPB but usually resolves over a short time interval (16). Persistent ST segment elevation suggests myocardial ischemia, which may require surgical treatment (i.e., revision of a graft or placement of an additional graft). Another possible cause is intracoronary artery air embolism, which occurs with open heart procedures, usually involves the right coronary artery, and frequently improves after a period of increased perfusion pressure. Coronary artery or internal mammary artery spasm also produces a similar clinical picture and often responds favorably to treatment with intravenous nitroglycerin, phosphodiesterase (PDE) inhibitors, or calcium channel blockers or to elevation of the perfusion pressure. Residual cardioplegia-induced ECG changes may improve with additional reperfusion on CPB.

Urine output is routinely monitored during CPB, but low urinary volume during CPB is not independently predictive of postoperative renal dysfunction (17). Nevertheless, patients with preoperative renal dysfunction or low urine output during or after CPB are often treated with low-dose dopamine infusion (1 to 3 μg/kg/min) for its natriuretic and renal vasodilatory effects (18,19). Although dopamine has been shown to be a more effective diuretic and natriuretic than dobutamine in adults after CPB, dopamine does not appear to be more effective than dobutamine in protecting renal function in children after CPB (19,20). It is not known whether prophylactic use of dopamine preserves renal function. After termination of CPB and the resumption of pulsatile blood flow, many patients exhibit a marked diuresis, particularly if mannitol has been added to the pump prime. In such cases, serum potassium should be monitored frequently and replenished as needed to maintain levels greater than 4.0 mEq/L, especially in patients who have received digoxin or who have dysrhythmias.

Most CPB consoles include an in-line monitor of venous blood hemoglobin oxygen saturation. Changes in this parameter may reflect the adequacy of systemic perfusion and oxygen delivery or increases in oxygen consumption (e.g., shivering) while on CPB. Before terminating CPB, the venous saturation and pump flow should be checked. A low saturation may indicate the need for additional muscle relaxant, red cell transfusion, or vasodilator therapy before weaning from bypass.

Transesophageal echocardiography (TEE) provides information that can be very useful when terminating CPB. Early in the weaning process, TEE provides an excellent assessment of residual air in the heart after open procedures. Later, as the ventricular volume increases and ejection begins, ventricular and vascular function can be assessed. The left ventricular, short-axis, cross-section view provides a useful indicator of left ventricular size and filling. Regional wall motion abnormalities may provide an important indicator of myocardial ischemia, including the failure of a specific coronary artery bypass graft (CABG), although regional wall motion abnormalities may also be due to residual effects of cardioplegia, inhomogeneous myocardial temperature, or preexisting abnormalities. One of the most useful applications of TEE prior to and after the termination of CPB is in evaluating valvular function after valve replacement or repair (21). Epicardial echocardiography and TEE have proven to be useful in evaluating the repair of complex congenital heart defects (22,23). Also, in contrast to routine intravascular (or even intraventricular) pressure measurements, which do not accurately reflect cardiac chamber volumes, TEE provides the capability to accurately assess biventricular filling volumes (24,25).

Patient/Pump

With all of the attention placed on the ECG, invasive pressure monitors, and TEE it is easy for the novice to overlook one of the most important indicators of cardiac function,

direct observation of the heart itself. Inspection of the heart will provide valuable information concerning contractility, rhythm, and ventricular filling. Contractility can be assessed by observing the speed of contraction and the size of the heart compared with that present before CPB. A poorly contracting heart will visibly dilate as diastolic volume is increased to increase stroke volume during weaning from CPB. The presence of sinus rhythm can frequently be verified by observing sequential atrial and ventricular contractions, even if P waves are not evident on the ECG. Right ventricular filling and ejection can be easily observed because the right ventricle is on the anterior surface of the heart; this parameter is a useful monitor for guiding volume infusions from the pump when terminating CPB. It is also important to continually monitor the lungs for bilateral inflation and deflation. An indication of ongoing blood loss can also be obtained by observing the surgical field and the pump suction before protamine administration. This blood can be replaced by infusions from the pump while the arterial cannula is still in place.

Once CPB has been discontinued, direct observation of the heart remains as an important monitor of ventricular function until the chest is closed and is invaluable in guiding volume infusions and the titration of inotropic agents. Observation of blood color is also important but is obviously a late monitor of hypoxemia. The effectiveness of heparin reversal by protamine can also be determined by observing clot formation in the surgical field. Bronchospasm, secondary to reactive airway disease or rarely to protamine administration, may be evident as lung hyperinflation. The importance of direct observation of the patient and the surgical field in the conduct of cardiac anesthesia cannot be overemphasized.

Support

The need for pharmacologic support after CPB is usually assessed by reviewing the ECG and all available hemodynamic data. However, other information available before and during bypass relating to ventricular function is of value in preparing for separation. Such data consist of the primary cardiac diagnosis, including the extent of myocardial dysfunction and the patient's status relative to the natural history of the disease, the effectiveness of intraoperative myocardial protection, and the adequacy of surgical repair.

Relatively few studies have been conducted to help predict which patients will require hemodynamic support during and immediately after CPB. Most published studies have used intraoperative myocardial infarction or postoperative mortality as endpoints. In an Australian study of 12,003 patients undergoing CABG surgery, duration of bypass (especially more than 100 minutes), preoperative unstable angina, and poor left ventricular function predicted a greater frequency of intraoperative myocardial infarction and postoperative mortality (26). Older age and female gender nega-

TABLE 29.2. CHRISTAKIS STUDY: PREDICTORS OF MORTALITY FOLLOWING CORONARY BYPASS SURGERY

- □ 12,471 patients: 9445 with ejection fraction (EF) >40%; 2539 with EF20-4 %;487 with EF <20%
- □ Normal EF mortality predictors: emergency surgery, female gender, left main coronary artery disease; reoperation; age
- □ EF 20–40% predictors: emergency surgery; female gender; age; reoperation; myocardial protection (crystalloid Vs blood)
- □ EF <20% predictors: emergency surgery only

Adapted form Christakis GT, Weisel RD, Frerres SE, et al. Coronary artery bypass grafting in patients with poor ventricular function. *J Thorac Cardiovasc Surg* 1992;103(6): 1083–1092, with permission.

tively influenced mortality-older patients. Coronary Artery Surgery Study (CASS) data also recognized older age, female gender, and heart failure as predictors of operative mortality (27).

In a Canadian study of 12,471 patients undergoing CABG surgery, preoperative left ventricular function was a relevant factor in predicting outcome. In patients with an ejection fraction of more than 40%, the predictors of postoperative mortality were emergency surgery, female gender, reoperation, type of myocardial protection (blood-based cardioplegia appeared to offer greater protection than crystalloid cardioplegia), and age. The presence of left main coronary artery disease was a predictor of death in patients with an ejection fraction greater than 40%. The type of myocardial protection used remained correlated with mortality in patients with ejection fraction between 20% and 40% (28). In patients with an ejection fraction less than 20%, emergency surgery was the only predictor of death (Table 29.2).

These findings are consistent with those of Mangano (29), who evaluated patterns of left ventricular function recovery after cardiac surgery. Two groups of patients emerged. One group experienced early biventricular dysfunction but recovered completely within 4 to 6 hours. The second group of patients had persistent biventricular dysfunction and showed little or no recovery as late as 24 hours postoperatively. Patients with low preoperative ejection fractions and ventricular dyssynergy tended to fall into the second group with prolonged dysfunction, whereas those with normal ejection fractions preoperatively fell into the first group, had less dysfunction, and recovered faster.

Clinically, the need for hemodynamic support may be thought of as a surrogate endpoint to predict postoperative myocardial infarction and mortality. In a retrospective analysis of patients who underwent CABG surgery, predictors of the need for inotropic support were essentially the same as those identified for major morbidity and mortality in the previously discussed studies (30). Preexisting low ejection fraction, a dilated left ventricle, an elevated left ventricular end-diastolic pressure (LVEDP), longer duration of aortic cross-clamp (or total bypass) time, age, and female gender

were positive predictors of the need for postoperative inotropic support. In another study, left ventricular dysfunction, defined by an ejection fraction less than 40%, LVEDP more than 15 mm Hg, and abnormal systolic and diastolic left ventricular volumes, correlated with the need for postoperative hemodynamic support, either pharmacologic or with an intraaortic balloon pump (IABP) (31).

Several factors, including microemboli, reperfusion injury, chest closure, incomplete rewarming, and hemodilution, have been suggested to explain the observed decline in cardiac function postoperatively. In an analysis of data from several previous studies, Royster (32) presented an interesting composite figure that showed a decline in ventricular function immediately after CPB as compared with preoperative values with a consistent early (after CPB) improvement in systolic myocardial performance, reaching the preoperative level 1 to 2 hours after CPB. A decline in function follows, which reaches a nadir 4 to 6 hours after CPB with a subsequent improvement over the next 12 to 18 hours (Fig. 29.1). Interestingly, in patients with normal preoperative ejection fractions (at least 55%), the presence of wall motion abnormalities and an LVEDP at least 10 mm Hg indicated a higher risk for requiring inotropic support. Thus, the intuitive predictors of a requirement support after CPB are supported by clinical data, and preoperative left ventricular dysfunction appears to be a strong predictor of a requirement for postoperative supportive management. Furthermore, the multiple risk factors appear to be additive and/or synergistic in their effects during postoperative recovery.

The specific underlying cause of the preoperative ventricular dysfunction has significant influence on the predicted postoperative ventricular function. Ventricular function is almost always impaired to some extent by aortic cross-clamping. The ischemia imposed by aortic cross-clamping

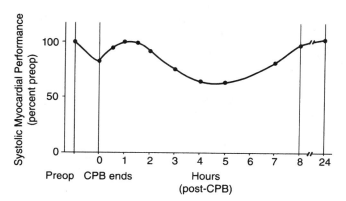

FIG. 29.1. Conceptualized time course of ventricular function change that occurs after cardiopulmonary bypass. (From Royster RL. Myocardial dysfunction after cardiopulmonary bypass: recovery patterns, predictors of inotropic need, theoretical concepts of inotropic administration. *J Cardiothorac Vasc Anesth* 1993; 7[Suppl 2]:19–25, with permission.)

can result in considerable myocardial stunning, which is a condition of prolonged reversible postischemic ventricular dysfunction of viable myocardium that follows reperfusion and which may exacerbate preexisting irreversible ventricular dysfunction (33). In the case of acute myocardial ischemia, successful myocardial revascularization may improve ventricular function by restoring perfusion. However, improvements in ventricular function can be delayed for hours to days because of myocardial stunning or for weeks in the case of prolonged ischemia, resulting in "hibernating" myocardium (34). Improved ventricular function is usually obtained after valve replacement and relief of the pressure overload in aortic stenosis, a condition in which the compensatory response to chronic pressure overload is a concentric hypertrophy of the ventricular wall that tends to normalize wall stress and avoid an overall decrement in contractility (35). In contrast, irreversible myocardial dysfunction is frequently present in the patient with mitral regurgitation. Here, the acute afterload mismatch produced by replacing the mitral valve and removing the low pressure relief effect frequently results in postoperative ventricular dysfunction (35,36). The degree of postoperative dysfunction is less predictable in patients with mitral stenosis or aortic regurgitation, but myocardial depression may exist because of the cardiomyopathy of rheumatic heart disease or eccentric ventricular hypertrophy, respectively. Previous myocardial infarction is an obvious cause for irreversible myocardial dysfunction. Ventricular dysfunction can also result from cardiomyopathy, which may be ischemic (congenital or acquired), viral, hypertrophic (secondary to pressure or volume overload or idiopathic), or drug induced (e.g., adriamycin). Evidence of preoperative myocardial dysfunction is provided by a history of poor exercise tolerance, congestive heart failure, or recent myocardial infarction and/or by evidence of ongoing myocardial ischemia, increased ventricular filling pressures, cardiomyopathy, or a decreased ejection fraction (29).

The adequacy of the surgical repair will also have an impact on postoperative ventricular function. For coronary artery bypass grafting, the number of lesions bypassed, the quality of the distal anastomoses, and the presence of small distal vessels or distal coronary artery disease (as in diabetes mellitus) are important factors. For valvular surgery or surgery to repair congenital defects, the specific valvular or anatomic defect, the adequacy of the valvular or anatomic repair, competency of valve replacements, and resultant changes in intracardiac pressures and flows are important. Procedures requiring a ventriculotomy may have a profound impact on postoperative ventricular function because of transection of important coronary artery branches or resection of viable myocardium or reduced ventricular compliance produced by closure of the ventriculotomy.

The surgeon is an important source for information regarding the adequacy of the surgical procedure. Objective evidence of the adequacy of the surgical repair can be ob-

tained before the termination of CPB by several methods. Among these are flowmeter determination of CABG flows, by epicardial echocardiographic (or TEE) assessment of intracardiac structures, by color-flow Doppler assessment of transvalvular flows and/or intracardiac shunts and by measurement of intracardiac chamber pressures to determine the gradient across a repaired valve or outflow tract.

Evaluation of the factors discussed above before the termination of CPB will give some idea of the need for circulatory support after CPB. If right or left ventricular failure is anticipated, plans should be made for the institution of pharmacologic and/or mechanical support, including inotropic drugs, vasodilators, and/or ventricular assist devices. If the need for support is obvious, then pharmacologic therapy should be initiated in advance of discontinuation of CPB to allow the drug to take effect before the mechanical circulatory support from CPB is removed. The capacity to pace the heart using atrial and/or ventricular pacing electrodes with a sequential atrioventricular pacemaker should be immediately available. A period of partial bypass may benefit cases of severe ventricular dysfunction by allowing the gradual recovery of cardiac function from the effects of ischemia and cardioplegia and the titration of vasoactive drugs. When preoperative findings indicate severe abnormalities of left ventricular function, it is wise to apply a second set of ECG leads before draping the patient at the start of the procedure to facilitate rapid deployment of intraaortic balloon counterpulsation if it is subsequently required. If cardiac function is inadequate and unresponsive to therapy after terminating CPB, it is prudent to reinstitute bypass to prevent ventricular distension and possible ischemic damage. This allows extra time for the heart to recover and for a reassessment of the situation and formulation of a revised plan.

SEPARATION FROM CARDIOPULMONARY BYPASS: TECHNIQUE

Termination of Cardiopulmonary Bypass

Physiologically, separation from bypass converts a circulation in series (venae cavae → oxygenator → aorta) to one in parallel (venae cavae → both → oxygenator and right ventricle/lungs/left ventricle → common return to aorta), and finally to one in series (venae cavae → heart/lungs → aorta). The duration of the transitional period of parallel circulation (partial bypass) is determined by ventricular function. The better the ability of the left ventricular (or, less commonly, the right) to sustain the entire cardiac output, the more rapidly bypass can be terminated. Conversely, poor left ventricular function mandates a period of partial bypass while ventricular loading conditions are carefully adjusted by manipulations of venous return and vascular resistance, and contractility is improved by judicious selection of positive inotropic drug therapy. During separation, ven-

1. Adjust rate & rhythm - pacing if needed
2. Partially occlude venous line - fill the heart
3. Decrease arterial flow from the pump (partial bypass); ejection begins

4. MEASURE ARTERIAL BLOOD PRESSURE

BP	↑	↓

5. Completely occlude venous line
6. Stop arterial pump after ventricle seems
    appropriately full

5. Maintain partial bypass
6. Carefully adjust ventricular volume
7. Begin appropriate vasoactive drugs: inotropes,
    vasoconstrictors (use algorithm)
8. Reduce flow - readjust volume & drugs
9. Stop arterial pump

ESTIMATE OR MEASURE PRELOAD & STROKE VOLUME (CONTRACTILITY)

FIG. 29.2. General approach to the termination of cardiopulmonary bypass. (From Amado WJ, Thomas SJ. Cardiac surgery: intraoperative management. In: Thomas SJ, ed. *Manual of cardiac anesthesia*, 2nd ed. New York: Churchill Livingstone, 1993, with permission.)

tricular distension should be avoided and coronary perfusion pressure must be maintained.

A general approach to the termination of CPB is shown in Figure 29.2. Separation is accomplished by gradual occlusion of the venous line, which decreases flow to the pump and leaves more blood in the patient. Arterial flow rate from the pump is then gradually reduced (e.g., to 2 L/min). Hemodynamics are assessed and appropriate drugs administered, if necessary. Flow can then be reduced further and hemodynamics reassessed. This process is then cycled until separation from CPB is complete. During this period, it is also essential to observe that the lungs are being adequately

ventilated with appropriate peak inspiratory pressures. Hemodynamic management for every patient focuses on regulating four primary determinants of cardiac function: rate and rhythm, arterial pressure, preload or ventricular volume (ventricular filling pressure), and contractility (stroke volume). An algorithm for the diagnosis and treatment of hemodynamic abnormalities at the termination of CPB is shown in Figure 29.3.

Rate and rhythm are controlled as much as possible before separation. Atrial, ventricular, or atrioventricular sequential pacing should be instituted when needed. Blood pressure is then assessed, and preload and contractility are

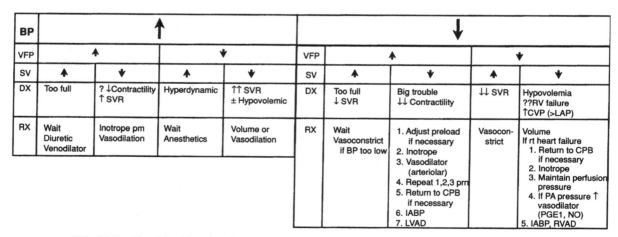

BP	↑				BP	↓			
VFP	↑		↓		**VFP**	↑		↓	
SV	↑	↓	↑	↓	**SV**	↑	↓	↑	↓
DX	Too full	? ↓Contractility ↑ SVR	Hyperdynamic	↑↑ SVR ± Hypovolemic	**DX**	Too full ↓ SVR	Big trouble ↓↓ Contractility	↓↓ SVR	Hypovolemia ??RV failure ↑CVP (>LAP)
RX	Wait Diuretic Venodilator	Inotrope pm Vasodilation	Wait Anesthetics	Volume or Vasodilation	**RX**	Wait Vasoconstrict if BP too low	1. Adjust preload if necessary 2. Inotrope 3. Vasodilator (arteriolar) 4. Repeat 1,2,3 prn 5. Return to CPB if necessary 6. IABP 7. LVAD	Vasoconstrict	Volume If rt heart failure 1. Return to CPB if necessary 2. Inotrope 3. Maintain perfusion pressure 4. If PA pressure ↑ vasodilator (PGE1, NO) 5. IABP, RVAD

FIG. 29.3. Algorithm for the diagnosis and treatment of hemodynamic abnormalities at the termination of CPB. *BP*, systemic blood pressure; *VFP*, ventricular filling pressure; *SV*, stroke volume; *Dx*, diagnosis; *Rx*, treatment; *SVR*, systemic vascular resistance; *CVP*, central venous pressure; *LAP*, left atrial pressure; *IABP*, intraaortic balloon pump; *LVAD*, left ventricular assist device; *RVAD*, right ventricular assist device; *PA*, pulmonary artery; *PGE₁*, prostaglandin E₁; *NO*, nitric oxide; *RV*, right ventricle. (From Amado WJ, Thomas SJ. Cardiac surgery: intraoperative management. In: Thomas SJ, ed. *Manual of cardiac anesthesia*, 2nd ed. New York: Churchill Livingstone, 1993, with permission.)

altered as appropriate. If both ventricular volume and inotropic state are adequate, use of vasoconstrictors or vasodilators for arterial pressure control is warranted. If blood pressure is too low, a search for the etiology of the post-bypass ventricular dysfunction is mandatory before beginning vasoactive drugs. Filling of the heart is assessed by direct inspection of the right ventricle, hemodynamic measurement, or (perhaps more appropriately and accurately) using TEE. It is important to recognize that right ventricular filling and central venous pressure do not accurately indicate left ventricular volume. The pulmonary artery occlusion or diastolic pressure is frequently used to guide volume infusion at the conclusion of CPB. However, the pulmonary artery occlusion pressure correlates poorly with left ventricular end-diastolic volume after coronary artery bypass surgery, possibly because of acute changes in left ventricular compliance (24). With poor left or right ventricular function, a direct measure of left ventricular filling pressure is helpful to better guide volume infusion. Ideal left atrial pressure will vary; however, a value of 10 to 15 mm Hg is almost always adequate in patients after isolated coronary artery bypass surgery. Higher pressures may be required in patients with valvular disease. TEE clearly provides the best available clinical intraoperative estimate of ventricular volumes (25).

After termination of CPB, volume can be infused directly from the pump through the aortic cannula as long as it is in place. The need for additional volume infusion can be judged by evaluating the stroke volume response to volume infused from the pump. Although repeated cardiac output measurement and stroke volume calculation are the best way to judge this Frank-Starling effect of volume expansion, for practical purposes the arterial pressure effect is also useful. This is true because over a short time frame (1 to 2 minutes) after the infusion, one can assume an unchanged vascular resistance so that a pressure increment produced by the volume infusion relates directly to a flow (stroke volume) increment.

After CPB, the clinical management goal is to have an arterial pressure of 90 to 100 mm Hg (somewhat higher in patients with renal, cerebrovascular, or hypertensive disease) and a cardiac output (3.0 L/min) with a left atrial pressure of 10 to 15 mm Hg (15 to 20 mm Hg in patients with chronic preoperative volume or pressure overload). Earlier clinical work by Kirklin and colleagues (37) demonstrated an increased mortality in patients after mitral valve replacement when the cardiac index was less than 2 L/min/m^2. However, adherence to a requirement for a cardiac index more than 2 L/min/m^2 immediately after CPB has not been shown to be beneficial. Assessment of the global context of the patient's cardiopulmonary function is the key to success.

Not infrequently the arterial pressure is observed to be low, whereas the measured filling pressures are moderately high shortly after terminating CPB. If there is no prospective reason to suspect severe ventricular dysfunction, this situation usually responds to limited (bolus) inotropic therapy such as epinephrine (4 to 8 μg i.v.), ephedrine (5 to 10 mg i.v.), or a short-term infusion of an inotrope (e.g., epinephrine 0.02 to 0.04 μg/kg/min i.v.). The absence of preexisting significant risk factors for more severe dysfunction and the rapid response to therapy are key features of this scenario. Hypotension may also be due to vasodilation and/or hypovolemia, particularly if the patient has been rewarmed for a long period. This condition is identified by low arterial pressure and filling pressures with an adequate cardiac output and is effectively treated with an α-adrenergic agonist (e.g., phenylephrine 50 to 100 μg i.v. or an infusion at 10 to 50 μg/min). If the situation does not improve rapidly and cardiac function is worse than anticipated, additional support may be required; if additional inotropes and vasodilators are not already prepared or if the patient's condition continues to deteriorate, partial bypass should be reinstituted while therapy is optimized. Additional time on partial CPB will allow more time for the postischemic recovery of ventricular function (38).

Left Ventricular Failure

Ventricular failure or dysfunction can be defined as inadequate cardiac pump performance, despite appropriate adjustments of preload and afterload, due to a decrease in myocardial contractility that can be either acute (as in ischemia) or chronic (as in cardiomyopathy). A subacute form of ventricular dysfunction, known as "stunning," may also develop after episodes of ischemia and may progress to postischemic ventricular dysfunction (33). Stunned myocardium exhibits recovery of contractile function that is delayed after restoration of coronary blood flow. This phenomenon has been observed after coronary artery bypass grafting and may improve with inotropic therapy (38,39).

Inotropic Therapy

Initial therapy of left ventricular dysfunction is usually achieved with a positive inotropic drug, of which there are several clinically useful categories. A comparison of mild ventricular dysfunction after separation from CPB and the result of inotropic treatment, as analyzed by pressure-volume loops, is shown in Figure 29.4. Calcium chloride or calcium gluconate (Tables 29.3 and 29.4) have a positive inotropic effect in the presence of hyperkalemia or hypocalcemia but are ineffective in the presence of normal ionized calcium concentrations and may actually be harmful because of the detrimental effects of elevated intracellular Ca^{2+} in ischemic cells after reperfusion (40).

β-Adrenergic receptor agonists are the most potent and widely used inotropes. In the myocardium activation of the β_1 receptor by these drugs leads to a process linked to trough the G protein system to the activation of the enzyme adenyl cyclase. This enzyme leads to the formation of cyclic 3',5'-

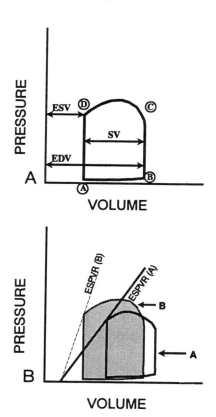

FIG. 29.4. A: Idealized pressure-volume loop with corresponding events of the cardiac cycle under normal conditions. *A,* mitral valve opens and ventricular filling begins; *B,* mitral valve closes: end-diastolic volume (*EDV*) and pressure (*EDP*); *C,* aortic valve opens after isovolumic contraction; *D,* aortic valve closes, end-systolic volume (*ESV*) and pressure (*ESP*). The stroke volume (*SV*) is EDV-ESV. **B:** Pressure-volume loop demonstrating mild ventricular dysfunction after separation from cardiopulmonary bypass. *Loop A* shows an increase in end-diastolic volume, a reduced end-systolic pressure-volume relationship (*ESPVR*) and reduced stroke volume. Inotropic therapy will usually increase contractility as illustrated by the shift from ESPVR (*A*) to ESPVR (*B*). Stroke volume increases, end-systolic and end-diastolic volumes decrease. (From Amado WJ, Thomas SJ. Cardiac surgery: intraoperative management. In: Thomas SJ, ed. *Manual of cardiac anesthesia,* 2nd ed. New York: Churchill Livingstone, 1993, with permission.)

adenosine monophosphate (cyclic AMP) from AMP, which is one of the principal degradation products from adenosine triphosphate. Increased intracellular concentrations of cyclic AMP in the myocardium in turn lead to increased availability of Ca^{2+} to the contractile apparatus in the sarcomere, which increases the speed and force of contraction (Fig. 29.5). In addition to increasing the force of contraction (a positive inotropic effect), β-adrenergic receptor activation leads to an increase in the slope of diastolic depolarization, and in heart rate (positive chronotropic effect), in the speed of conduction of the electrical impulse throughout the myocardium (a positive dromotropic effect), and in the speed of relaxation of the myocardium during diastole (a positive lusitropic effect). Because of these widespread cardiac ef-

fects, β-adrenergic agonists have been at the core of the "therapeutic armamentarium" for treating acute ventricular dysfunction after CPB. A number of different β-adrenergic agonists are available, including the natural catecholamines epinephrine, norepinephrine, and dopamine and the synthetic catecholamines dobutamine and isoproterenol (Table 29.3). These drugs have varying actions at β_1, β_2, and α-adrenergic receptors. Typically, a specific drug is best selected based on the specific hemodynamic abnormality being treated and the drug's relative actions at each receptor type.

Adrenergic therapy of severe ventricular failure usually requires the maximal potency of epinephrine or norepinephrine, frequently in combination with vasodilator therapy (see below). Epinephrine and norepinephrine are also useful when ventricular dysfunction is accompanied by peripheral vasodilation, because they are also potent α-receptor agonists. The vasopressor effect of norepinephrine is greater than that of epinephrine because of the greater potency of epinephrine at the β-2 receptors, which produce considerable vasodilation in skeletal muscle and other major vascular beds. Dobutamine and dopamine are useful when moderate inotropic support is desired, although the wisdom of selecting a drug with less adrenergic agonist potency (i.e., dopamine or dobutamine) as opposed to careful titration of a more potent drug (i.e., epinephrine) has been and is still very debatable. Dobutamine is a β_1 receptor agonist with only minimal α receptor activity and may therefore be useful when further vasoconstriction is undesirable. Dopamine is unique in that it stimulates renal dopamine receptors and causes an increase in both renal blood flow and sodium excretion. It may be especially useful in patients with renal dysfunction (18,19). Use of dopamine as an inotrope at higher doses (more than 8 to 10 μg/kg/min) is complicated by its increasing activity at α-adrenergic receptors, which may produce undesirable increases in systemic and pulmonary vascular resistance. At higher doses both dobutamine and dopamine tend to induce tachycardia and atrial arrhythmias (41,42). At equally effective inotropic doses, dobutamine and dopamine both appear to have stronger dysrhythmogenic potency than does epinephrine (41). The partial dependence of the inotropic effects of dopamine on endogenous catecholamines may also limit its efficacy in patients with chronic ventricular dysfunction and after CPB.

Isoproterenol is a nonselective β receptor agonist that is a potent inotrope (β_1 effect) and peripheral vasodilator (β_2 effect). The potent chronotropic effect of isoproterenol (β_1 and β_2 effect) is not compensated for by the baroreceptor-mediated reflex bradycardia that occurs with β receptor agonists that also possess intrinsic α receptor activity such as epinephrine and norepinephrine. Either isoproterenol or dobutamine may be useful in patients with severe pulmonary hypertension and right ventricular failure, because α receptor stimulation is a potent mechanism producing pul-

TABLE 29.3. INOTROPES USED IN THE TERMINATION OF CPB

Drug	Dose	Mechanism	Actions	Indications	Contraindications	Adverse Effects
Calcium chloride or calcium gluconate	2–10 mg/kg i.v. bolus effects last 10–20 min	↑ Ca$_i^{2+}$	Inotrope if hypocalcemic Vasopressor if normocalcemic	Hypocalcemia (from CPB, albumin, citrate) Hyperkalemia Hypotension (e.g., secondary to protamine) Myocardial depression (e.g., secondary to residual cardioplegia or hypocalcemia) Calcium channel blocker overdose	Hypercalcemia Pancreatitis Digitalis toxicity	Coronary artery spasm (?) Pancreatitis
Epinephrine	Low-dose infusion 1–2 μg/min, primarily β Moderate dose infusion 2–10 μg/min, mixed α and β High-dose infusion 10–20 μg/min, primarily α; potent vasoconstriction 2–8 μg i.v. bolus	α$_1$-Receptor (↑ Ca$_i^{2+}$) β$_1$-Receptor (↑ cAMP) β$_2$-Receptor (↑ cAMP)	Inotrope—β$_1$-effect Vasopressor—α$_1$-effect at higher doses Vasodilator—β$_2$-effect primarily in muscle Chronotrope—β$_1$-effect Bronchodilation—β$_2$-effect	Ventricular dysfunction Vasodilation Anaphylaxis Bronchoconstriction	Idiopathic hypertrophic subaortic stenosis (relative) Tetralogy of Fallot (with RV outflow tract obstruction, relative)	Vasoconstriction (splanchnic, renal) Dysrhythmias
Norepinephrine	4–16 μg/min	β$_1$-Receptor (↑ cAMP) α$_1$-Receptor (↑ Ca$_i^{2+}$)	Inotrope—β$_1$-effect Vasopressor—α$_1$-effect Chronotrope—β$_1$-effect	Ventricular dysfunction Vasodilation Anaphylaxis Shock	See epinephrine	Vasoconstriction (splanchnic, renal) Dysrhythmias
Dopamine	0.5–2 μg/kg/min (activation of DA$_1$ receptors) >2 μg/kg/min (activation of β$_1$ receptors) >5 μg/kg/min (activation of α$_1$ receptors)	α$_1$-Receptor (↑ Ca$_i^{2+}$) β$_1$-Receptor (↑ cAMP) DA$_1$-Receptor (↑ cAMP)	Inotrope—β$_1$-effect Vasopressor—α$_1$-effect Renal vasodilator and natriuretic—DA$_1$ effect Chronotrope—β$_1$-effect	Ventricular dysfunction Vasodilation Renal dysfunction/oliguria	See epinephrine	Tachycardia Peripheral vasoconstriction Dysrhythmias
Dobutamine	2–20 μg/kg/min	β$_1$-Receptor (↑ cAMP) α$_1$-Receptor (↑ Ca$_i^{2+}$)	Inotrope—β$_1$-effect Vasodilator—β$_2$—effect Chronotrope—β$_1$-effect	Vasoconstriction	See epinephrine	Tachycardia
Isoproterenol	1–5 μg/min	β$_1$-Receptor (↑ cAMP) β$_2$-Receptor (↑ cAMP)	Inotrope—β$_1$-effect Vasodilator—β$_2$-effect Bronchodilation—β$_2$-effect Chronotrope—β$_1$-effect	Ventricular dysfunction, especially RV Bronchoconstriction Bradycardia—profound β-blockade, AV block, cardiac transplant Pulmonary hypertension—primary, secondary	See epinephrine	Tachycardia Vasodilation ↑ MVo$_2$
Amrinone	0.5–1.5 mg/kg i.v. bolus (slow) 5–30 μg/kg/min infusion	PDE III inhibition (↑ cAMP) (↑ Ca$_i^{2+}$)	Inotrope—due to ↑ cAMP Vasodilator—due to ↑ cAMP	Ventricular dysfunction Vasoconstriction	Thrombocytopenia	Vasodilation
Ephedrine	5–10 mg i.v. bolus	α$_1$-Effect (↑ Ca$_i^{2+}$) β$_1$-Effect (↑ cAMP)	Vasopressor—α$_1$-effect Inotrope—β$_1$-effect ↓ Venous capacitance	Ventricular dysfunction Vasodilation	See epinephrine	Tachycardia

cAMP, cyclic adenosine monophosphate; RV, right ventricular; DA, dopamine; MVo$_2$, myocardial; O$_2$, consumption; AV, atrioventricular; Ca$_i^{2+}$, intracellular ionized calcium; PDE, phosphodiesterase.

TABLE 29.4. COMPARATIVE EFFECTS OF SUPPORTIVE THERAPIES USED TO FACILITATE TERMINATION OF CPB

Therapy	Preload	SVR	PVR	Contractility	Conduction	Rate	Rhythm	MVO$_2$
Calcium salts	↑ LVEDP	↑	—	↑ dP/dt ↑ SV	↓ AV conduction	↓	Dysrhythmogenic	↑
Epinephrine	↑ PAOP	↑	↑	↑ dP/dt ↑ CO	Enhanced	↑	Dysrhythmogenic	↑
Norepinephrine	↑ PAOP	↑	↑	↑ dP/dt ↑↓ CO	Enhanced	Reflex ↓	Dysrhythmogenic	↑
Dopamine	↑ PAOP	↑ At high doses	↑	↑ dP/dt ↑ CO	±	↑	Dysrhythmogenic	↑
Dobutamine	↓ PAOP, ↓ LVEDP	↓	↓	↑ dP/dt ↑ CO	Enhanced	↑	↑ Automaticity	± or ↓
Isoproterenol	↓ PAOP	↓	↓	↑ dP/dt ↑ CO	Enhanced	↑↑	↑ Automaticity Dysrhythmogenic	↑
Amrinone/milrinone	↓ PAOP	↓	↓	↑ dP/dt ↑ CO	Enhanced	±	±	± or ↓
Ephedrine	↑ CVP	↑	↑	↑ dP/dt ↑ CO	Enhanced	↑	±	↑
Sodium nitroprusside	↓ PAOP, ↓ CVP	↓	↓	± dP/dt ↑ CO	±	Reflex ↑	±	↓
Nitroglycerin	↓ LVEDP, ↓ PAOP ↓ CVP	↓	↓	± dP/dt ↑↓ CO	±	Variable	±	↓
Phenylephrine	↑ PAOP, ↑ CVP	↑	↑	± dP/dt ↑↓ CO	±	Reflex ↓	±	± or ↑
Intraaortic balloon counterpulsation	↓ PAOP, ↓ CVP ↓ LAP	↓ LV afterload	—	↑ CO	±	±	±	↓

SVR, systemic vascular resistance; PVR, pulmonary vascular resistance; MVo$_2$, myocardial; O$_2$ consumption; LVEDP, left ventricular end-diastolic pressure; SV, stroke volume; AV, atrioventricular; PAOP, pulmonary artery occlusion pressure; CO, cardiac output; CVP, central venous pressure; LAP, left atrial pressure; LV, left ventricular; dP/dt, first time derivative of ventricular pressure.

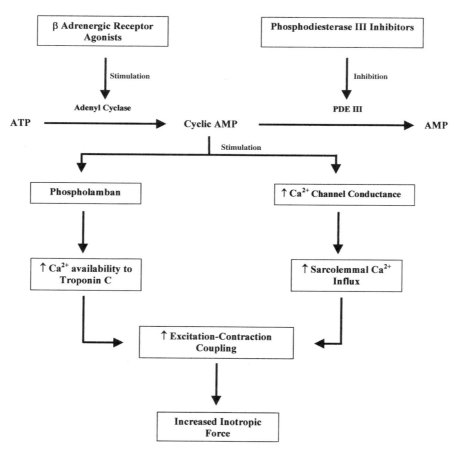

FIG. 29.5. Cyclic AMP-mediated intracellular pathways for inotropic stimulation. Cascade of cyclic AMP effects leading to increased inotropy. ATP, adenosine triphosphate; AMP, adenosine monophosphate.

monary vasoconstriction. Isoproterenol is also useful for the treatment of slow ventricular rates or atrioventricular conduction disturbances when other methods have failed because of the positive chronotropic and dromotropic effects of β-adrenergic stimulation. These effects are also clinically useful in cardiac transplantation dealing with the acutely denervated transplanted heart.

In general, epinephrine appears to be the most useful adrenergic drug for inotropic stimulation for adult cardiac surgical patients after CPB, perhaps because of its combined β_1, β_2, and α-adrenergic actions. Dopamine and isoproterenol are often favored in the pediatric population because of advantages of a higher heart rate in this group. However, patterns of inotrope use show significant institutional variation, and the literature describing comparative effects of the drugs in patients requiring inotropic support, especially larger scale well-designed clinical trials, is somewhat sparse. One well-designed trial documented the increased efficacy of epinephrine as compared with calcium chloride for increasing cardiac performance after CPB (43). In this study, epinephrine had superior hemodynamic effects as compared with calcium. And calcium, when given to normocalcemic patients, had no predictable effect on cardiac output or arterial pressure. In critically ill adults with severe ventricular dysfunction and low urine output, infusion of a low-dose dopamine infusion (1 to 3 μg/kg/min) may help to improve renal perfusion and urine production. When combined with a second inotrope (e.g., epinephrine), this treatment can increase contractility without increasing ventricular filling pressure, as can be seen with higher doses of dopamine (44,45). The use of dopamine or epinephrine as an inotrope in severe left ventricular dysfunction is limited by dose-dependent increases in afterload and preload. These undesirable side effects are the basis for the frequent clinical use of combined inotropic stimulation and afterload reduction with direct acting vasodilators such as nitroprusside or nitroglycerin (46).

Another class of positive inotropic drugs has, over the last 10 to 12 years, significantly improved the menu of available therapies for myocardial failure after CPB. Although these drugs have a shared property with the β-adrenergic agonists, namely the function by increasing the intracellular concentration of cyclic AMP, they produce this effect by an entirely separate mechanism. This class of drugs is the group of inhibitors of the enzyme responsible for the metabolic breakdown of intracellular cyclic AMP, cyclic nucleotide PDE. Several classes of drugs have the property of PDE inhibition (Table 29.5). Benzylisoquinolines (e.g., papavarine) and methylxanthines (e.g., aminophylline) are examples of nonspecific inhibitors of PDE. The PDE enzymes have several isoforms in the body, of which type III predominates in the myocardium and in vascular smooth muscle. The selective type III PDE inhibitors available clinically include the bipyridine derivatives amrinone and milrinone and the imidazolone derivative enoximone. Milrinone and amrinone are available for clinical use in the United States. Both

TABLE 29.5. PHOSPHODIESTERASE INHIBITORS

Nonspecific
 Benzylisoquinolines (e.g., papaverine)
 Methylxanthines (e.g., aminophylline)
Fraction III specific
 Bipyridines (e.g., milrinone, amrinone)
 Imidazolones (e.g., enoximone)

drugs are highly selective PDE III inhibitors and differ primarily in terms of potency and side-effect profile. Milrinone is approximately 20 times more potent as a PDE III inhibitor than amrinone. It has a half-life of about one third of that for amrinone, which may make it a more titratable medication for continuous infusion. The principal side-effect difference is that amrinone has a significant platelet inhibitory effect that is much less pronounced with milrinone.

PDE III inhibitors increase the intracellular concentration of cyclic AMP in myocardium and vascular smooth muscle. In the myocardium, this effect leads to an increased Ca^{2+} concentration similar to that seen with the β-adrenergic receptor agonists, but this effect is independent of β receptor activation. The increased Ca^{2+} concentration leads to increased force of contraction and increased speed of relaxation (positive inotropic and lusitropic effects) (Fig. 29.5). In vascular smooth muscle, this same chain of biochemical events leads to increased concentrations of cyclic AMP and GMP, which produces significant vasorelaxation. Clinically, these drugs produce mild to moderate improvement in cardiac contraction that is often overshadowed by the more marked improvement in cardiac pump performance produced by the combined inotropic, lusitropic, and peripheral vasodilation (afterload reduction) effects. The inotropic activity of the PDE III inhibitors is synergistic with that of β-adrenergic agents and may not be associated with increased myocardial oxygen consumption; these properties have made this agent particularly useful in patients with severe left ventricular dysfunction (47,48).

Advantage can be taken of the inotropic activity of PDE III inhibitors without overt hypotension by combining their use with an α-adrenergic vasoconstrictor, usually phenylephrine or norepinephrine (49,50). Another important methodology for the use of PDE III inhibitors for facilitating termination of CPB is to load the drug before weaning is attempted so that the flow from the pump can be used to counteract the vasodilation which occurs during loading. The recommended dose of milrinone is 50 μg/kg given into the pump during the last 10 minutes of CPB, followed by infusion of 0.5 μg/kg/min. This dosage has been shown to produce effective plasma concentrations of the drug and to help avoid significant hypotension resulting from its vasodilating property (51). However, these drugs can cause hypotension (due to vasodilation) that may be difficult to treat.

Because of this, some clinicians advocate use of these drugs only after weaning from CPB, so that vascular resistance can be assessed before their use.

Another important advantage of the PDE III inhibitors has to do with the significant downregulation of the β-adrenergic receptors that is associated with left ventricular failure. This downregulation is well accepted in the context of chronic congestive heart failure but may also occur in the more acute immediate perioperative context. The desensitization of β-adrenergic receptors that occurs in congestive heart failure significantly limits the efficacy of β-adrenergic agonists. Combined therapy with PDE III inhibitors enhances the inotropic effect of β-adrenergic receptor agonists by potentiating the rise in intracellular cyclic AMP. Such combined therapy may also permit use of a lower dose of the β-adrenergic agonist, thereby avoiding possible adverse side effects such as arrhythmias. PDE III also have a positive lusitropic, or myocardial relaxation, effect (52). This positive lusitropic effect enhances diastolic myocardial relaxation, improves ventricular compliance, facilitates ventricular filling, and decreases ventricular filling pressure and perhaps end-diastolic wall tension at any given filling volume. Thus, myocardial oxygen minute consumption may be decreased while stroke volume is increased.

Vasodilators

Although positive inotropes are useful in improving the contractile state of the failing ventricle, vasodilators can improve ventricular function by optimizing its loading conditions. Indeed, severe heart failure is characterized by both poor left ventricular function (decreased cardiac output with elevated filling pressure) and elevated systemic vascular resistance, and added therapeutic benefit may be obtained by treating both abnormalities (53). Thus, the effects of inotropes and vasodilators are additive in augmenting cardiac output and decreasing filling pressures in the treatment of severe left ventricular failure.

Sodium nitroprusside and nitroglycerin are among the clinically most useful vasodilators in cardiac anesthesia because of their potency, rapid onset, and short duration of action. These properties make them ideal for rapid titration of arterial pressure. Other vasodilators, which are occasionally used but which have slower onset and/or longer duration of action, include hydralazine and phentolamine (an α_1-adrenergic receptor antagonist). Other classes of vasodilating drugs, such as calcium channel blockers (e.g., nicardipine), dopaminergic agonists (e.g., fenoldepam), and natriuretic peptides (e.g., nesritide), have been developed and may be useful in this context (54–56).

Sodium nitroprusside is a potent arterial vasodilator and venodilator, whereas nitroglycerin is a potent venodilator but is less potent as an arterial vasodilator. This differential effect of the two drugs is due to the requirement for metabolic degradation of nitroglycerin by vascular endothelial cells to release the active component, nitric oxide. Nitro-

prusside, in contrast, releases nitric oxide directly. In many vascular beds, especially in the distal arterial and arteriolar circulation, there is relatively little of the enzyme needed for nitroglycerin breakdown; hence, there is relatively less arterial and arteriolar dilation produced by nitroglycerin as compared with nitroprusside. This is clinically evident in the greater efficacy of sodium nitroprusside in reducing arterial pressure in normovolemic patients, whereas both agents are effective in reducing ventricular filling pressures. Nitroglycerin, and to a lesser extent sodium nitroprusside, are also effective pulmonary vasodilators and inhibitors of hypoxic pulmonary vasoconstriction (hence the increased pulmonary shunt frequently observed with their use). Other pulmonary vasodilators useful for the acute control of right ventricular afterload include prostaglandin E_1, prostacyclin, and inhaled nitric oxide (see below). Nitroglycerin also exhibits potent effects on coronary blood flow and is useful in treating myocardial ischemia.

In the perioperative period, sodium nitroprusside (0.5 to 10 μg/kg/min) and nitroglycerin (0.5 to 4 μg/kg/min) are useful in treating ventricular dysfunction with elevated filling pressures, pulmonary hypertension, and systemic hypertension. Sodium nitroprusside appears to be particularly effective in producing systemic vasodilation during rewarming on CPB, treating postoperative hypertension in patients with hyperdynamic circulation, and in reducing afterload and preload in patients with poor ventricular function and acceptable arterial blood pressure. Concurrent volume infusion may be required to maintain adequate filling pressures and achieve increased stroke volume (Fig. 29.6). Both so-

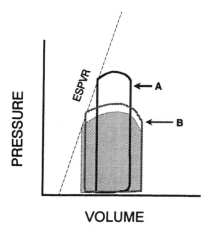

FIG. 29.6. Systemic vasoconstriction and hypertension with concomitant hypovolemia after cardiopulmonary bypass (*loop A*) results in decreased stroke volume. Administration of additional intravascular volume and of a vasodilator results in *loop B*, in which end-diastolic volume and stroke volume have returned toward normal (*shaded loop*) as the blood pressure is reduced. The end-systolic pressure volume relationship (*ESPVR*) is unchanged. (From Amado WJ, Thomas SJ. Cardiac surgery: intraoperative management. In: Thomas SJ, ed. *Manual of cardiac anesthesia*, 2nd ed. New York: Churchill Livingstone, 1993, with permission.)

dium nitroprusside and nitroglycerin have also been used to offset the vasoconstriction produced by inotropes with intrinsic α-adrenergic activity. The use of sodium nitroprusside is complicated by the potential for cyanide toxicity at higher doses (e.g., doses more than 8 to 10 $\mu g/kg/min$), whereas nitroglycerin has the advantage of being relatively nontoxic. All nitrovasodilators have the potential to produce clinically significant tachyphylaxis. This is rarely a problem in the acute perioperative setting but can complicate long-term therapy.

Vasoconstrictors

Vasoconstrictors work by increasing systemic vascular resistance (afterload) and decreasing venous capacitance (increasing preload) due to their action at α-adrenergic receptors (Fig. 29.7). Both phenylephrine and methoxamine are pure α_1 agonists and are useful in the treatment of hypotension secondary to vasodilation, whereas ephedrine and metaraminol act to release endogenous catecholamines and thereby activate both α and β receptors. In general, the use of pure α agonists to increase arterial blood pressure in patients with poor ventricular function or pulmonary hypertension is best avoided because increased afterload without a compensatory increase in contractility results in a decreased stroke volume. If significant arterial vasodilation is combined with poor left ventricular function, norepinephrine, which possesses less β_2-adrenergic activity than epinephrine,

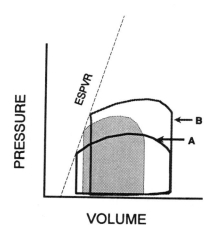

FIG. 29.7. Hypotension due to systemic vasodilation despite hypervolemia results in increased stroke volume and decreased end-systolic volume. **A:** Administration of an arterial vasoconstrictor increases blood pressure and end-systolic volume. **B:** Stroke volume is reduced while the end-systolic pressure-volume relationship (*ESPVR*) is unchanged. Vasoconstriction is indicated only when systemic blood pressure is unacceptably low. *Shaded loop* represents normal hemodynamics. (From Amado WJ, Thomas SJ. Cardiac surgery: intraoperative management. In: Thomas SJ, ed. *Manual of cardiac anesthesia*, 2nd ed. New York: Churchill Livingstone, 1993, with permission.)

may be appropriate to counteract the vasodilation while providing some degree of inotropic increase to meet the increased afterload. Pure α receptor agonists are useful in the treatment of hypotension in patients with good ventricular function; the beneficial increase in coronary perfusion pressure usually outweighs the negative effects of decreased cardiac output and increased filling pressures in the patient with coronary artery disease or ventricular hypertrophy. Short-term use of a vasopressor is frequently required when terminating CPB in the vasodilated patient; this is easily accomplished with small intravenous boluses of phenylephrine (e.g., 50 to 100 μg).

Mechanical Support

If ventricular function remains inadequate despite appropriate inotropic and vasodilator therapy, the addition of mechanical support may be required to allow termination of CPB (57). IABP, in addition to inotropic and vasodilator therapy, should be considered early in the patient with poor preoperative ventricular function and postoperative low cardiac output syndrome; a need for this device can be anticipated in the patient with severe preoperative left ventricular dysfunction (58). If difficulty or failure is encountered when terminating CPB despite maximal pharmacologic therapy, the IABP should be inserted while still on bypass to prevent ventricular distension

Right Ventricular Failure

This condition may occur as a result of right coronary artery damage, occlusion or embolism, inadequate intraoperative right ventricular protection, or in patients with pulmonary hypertension (e.g., secondary to chronic mitral stenosis, left-to-right shunts, massive pulmonary embolism, or a reaction to protamine administration). Increased pulmonary artery and central venous pressures, decreased arterial pressure and cardiac output, and a bulging right ventricle characterize right ventricular failure. Pulmonary artery occlusion pressure (or left atrial) pressure and left ventricular volume assessed by TEE will be low or normal if right ventricular failure is associated with normal left ventricular function. However, these measurements will be abnormal if right ventricular and left ventricular dysfunction coexist. The therapeutic goals in treating right ventricular dysfunction are similar to those in treating left ventricular dysfunction: increase right ventricular contractility and decrease afterload (pulmonary artery pressure) while maintaining adequate preload (central venous pressure) and coronary perfusion pressure. It is more difficult to achieve these objectives, however, given the pulmonary vasoconstriction induced by most adrenergic positive inotropes with α receptor agonist effects when they are administered into the venous circulation. It is critical to maintain adequate systemic arterial pressure in the presence of right ventricular failure to provide adequate coronary perfusion pressure to the distended right ventricle, which has an elevated end-diastolic pressure. Because of the relatively thin wall of the right ventricle, intramyocardial wall tension is higher for any given level of intracavitary pressure than is the case for the left ventricle, as predicted by the La Place relationship. This increases oxygen consumption and compromises coronary blood flow.

The goal in right ventricular failure is maintenance of a normal systemic arterial (coronary perfusion) pressure, an increased ventricular contractility, and a decreased right ventricular afterload. These effects may be best achieved by inhalation of nitric oxide combined with inotropic drugs. Inhaled nitric oxide has been used experimentally as a selective pulmonary vasodilator with encouraging results (60). Unlike other vasodilators, inhaled nitric oxide is very selective for the pulmonary circulation because it is largely taken up by hemoglobin before reaching the systemic circulation. Thus, it can decrease pulmonary artery pressure without producing significant systemic vasodilation. If nitric oxide is unavailable, selective infusion of pulmonary vasodilators into the right atrium and vasopressors into the left atrium is another method to achieve the desired goals. This has been demonstrated by infusing prostaglandin E_1 (30 to 50 ng/kg/min) into the right atrium and norepinephrine into the left atrium in patients with refractory right heart failure after mitral valve replacement (59). Alternatively, nitroglycerin can be infused into the right atrium as the pulmonary vasodilator.

If a left atrial catheter is not available, isoproterenol or dobutamine can be infused into the right atrium. Isoproterenol may be useful for increasing right ventricular contractility without significantly increasing pulmonary artery pressure (afterload), although problems with tachycardia and dysrhythmias may occur. Use of dobutamine may avoid these problems. The PDE III inhibitors are extremely useful in treating right ventricular dysfunction and pulmonary hypertension after CPB because of their ability to increase right ventricular contractility and reduce pulmonary vascular resistance (61). Other manipulations to decrease pulmonary vascular resistance include hyperventilation to induce hypocapnia, a reduction in tidal volume and inspiratory time, and avoidance of hypoxemia and acidemia. If these measures fail, mechanical support may be required either in the form of an IABP or a right ventricular assist device.

SEPARATION FROM CARDIOPULMONARY BYPASS: PROBLEM SITUATIONS

Vasodilation and Hypotension

Systemic vascular resistance progressively decreases with rewarming and continues to decrease during the period after CPB. In some but not all cases, pronounced vasodilation at the termination of CPB appears to be related to the dura-

tion of rewarming; the systemic vascular resistance can be quite low and the cardiac output high if this period is protracted. This condition is effectively treated with a vasopressor such as phenylephrine to restore arterial blood pressure and maintain coronary perfusion pressure.

Vasoconstriction and Hypertension

In the patient with good ventricular function, this condition can occur with inadequate rewarming or in the immediate post-bypass period as the core body temperature drops with thermal equilibration. The cardiac output is usually reduced and the ventricular filling pressure may be low, normal, or high. Treatment is with vasodilator therapy, usually sodium nitroprusside at low doses (0.25 to 0.5 μg/kg/min i.v.) with volume replacement as necessary to maintain preload. Hydralazine (in 2.5- to 5-mg i.v. increments) may also be used in the stable patient.

Hypoxemia

Hypoxemia can be a serious problem in the immediate post-bypass period if not quickly recognized and treated. A frequent etiology is atelectasis, which can be largely corrected by vigorous lung expansion although the addition of positive end-expiratory pressure is occasionally required. Bronchospasm may be due to preexisting pulmonary disease or secondary to protamine administration. It is often recognized by high peak inspiratory pressures, poor lung deflation, and a shallow slope on the expiratory phase of the capnogram. Clinically significant bronchospasm is best treated with aerosolized β_2-adrenergic agonists, volatile anesthetic agents if ventricular function is satisfactory, methylxanthines, or intravenous epinephrine or isoproterenol. Right-to-left intracardiac shunt, which may occur with congenital heart disease or in otherwise normal patients with a patent foramen ovale and elevated right atrial pressure, may require mechanical correction. Early intraoperative diagnosis is made possible by TEE. Low cardiac output is associated with hypoxemia, especially when accompanied by right-to-left shunting, high oxygen consumption, and/or low oxygen delivery (anemia). Vasodilator therapy (especially nitroprusside) increases intrapulmonary shunting due to inhibition of hypoxic pulmonary vasoconstriction. Noncardiogenic pulmonary edema is usually secondary to allergic reactions to drugs or blood products. Pneumothorax, hemothorax, or hydrothorax are usually evident as distended pleurae visible in the surgical field. Many other causes of significant hypoxemia after CPB are not specific to cardiac surgery including inadequate ventilator settings, circuit disconnect, endobronchial intubation, kinking, or obstruction of the endotracheal tube. An arterial blood gas should be checked soon after the termination of CPB to assess the adequacy of ventilation and oxygenation.

Acute Hemodynamic Deterioration

This critical situation can result from a number of causes, including cardiac dysrhythmias, graft or valve malfunction, reactions to medications (often to protamine), or to the adverse hemodynamic effects of closure of the pericardium or the sternum. The latter can result in compression of the heart producing a tamponade effect, which may improve with volume infusion or inotropic support as the heart adjusts to the altered loading conditions. The pericardium may need to be reopened. And in severe cases, sternum may have to be left open for closure at a later date. Another cause of sudden hemodynamic deterioration is ischemia produced by kinking, clotting, or embolization of a vascular graft. This may require surgical revision and is usually associated with acute changes in the ECG, often ST segment elevation and occasionally followed by dysrhythmias. Coronary (or mammary graft) vasospasm is another cause of acute ischemia after CPB. Treatment of spasm includes nitroglycerin or calcium channel blockers. Other causes of acute hemodynamic deterioration include dysrhythmias, which may be secondary to new myocardial ischemia; other metabolic or electrolyte abnormalities; to atrial decannulation; and surgical manipulation of the heart, which should be obvious. In this situation TEE can provide vital diagnostic information regarding new regional wall motion abnormalities, valve function, and ventricular filling to help determine the most appropriate therapy.

Progressive Hemodynamic Deterioration

The hemodynamic status of most patients gradually improves after the termination of CPB as the residual effects of myocardial ischemia and cardioplegia abate, even in patients requiring aggressive inotropic therapy. If this is not the case or if requirements for vasoactive drugs actually increase, correctable causes such as myocardial ischemia or valvular dysfunction should be sought. Early institution of intraaortic balloon counterpulsation may be advantageous to improve myocardial perfusion and salvage ischemic myocardium; otherwise, a return to partial CPB may be necessary to allow further recovery of cardiac function and optimization of pharmacological therapy.

Controversial Issues in the Termination of Cardiopulmonary Bypass

Calcium Administration

Routine administration of calcium salts at the end of CPB is not beneficial and may be harmful. Exceptions include patients with evidence of hyperkalemia or hypocalcemia. The incidence of hypocalcemia during CPB is relatively high, but ionized Ca^{2+} usually approaches normal values immediately before termination of bypass (62). Moreover, considerable evidence suggests that elevated intracellular Ca^{2+} is correlated with increased cell death and injury during ischemia and reperfusion, as occurs frequently during cardiac surgery (40). A recent study suggests that calcium chloride administration, during emergence from CPB in patients with good ventricular function, has no significant effect on cardiac index (43). Use of calcium salts at the conclusion of bypass should be guided by determination of ionized Ca^{2+} levels; significant increases in ventricular function are produced experimentally by Ca^{2+} administration in the presence of hypocalcemia (63). Calcium salts should not be routinely administered to patients with good ventricular function in the absence of hypocalcemia or hyperkalemia because of the potential detrimental effects of iatrogenic hypercalcemia; whether this is true in cases of impaired ventricular function remains to be determined.

Use of Inotropes

Concern exists that inotropic stimulation of the myocardium may have deleterious effects because of increased energy consumption (64). This may be particularly relevant after cardiac surgery with ischemic cardiac arrest, especially in the presence of residual myocardial ischemia caused by disproportionate increases in myocardial oxygen consumption relative to supply (65). Animal data suggest that catecholamines should be avoided in the reperfusion period immediately after release of the aortic cross-clamp to facilitate metabolic recovery of the myocardium (66). Exogenous positive inotropic agents may also potentiate damage because of the already high endogenous catecholamine levels during cardiac surgery (67). Inotropic agents are clearly useful in discontinuing CPB and may even expedite the recovery of stunned myocardium (39). Given their potential to increase myocardial damage, however, their use should probably be delayed until the heart has had a chance to recover from the ischemia immediately after aortic cross-clamp release. Animal data suggest that in the presence of ventricular dysfunction, the potentially deleterious effects of inotropic stimulation on oxygen consumption may be reduced by afterload-reducing agents (68).

KEY POINTS

- Systematic preparation for separation from CPB is critical.
  - LAMPS: Laboratory Data, Anesthesia, Monitors/Machine, Patient, Support.
- Large-scale studies includes: age, emergency surgery, female gender, preoperative ventricular function, left main coronary disease, and reoperation.
  - There is a biphasic postoperative course for ventricular function: early (1 to 2 hours) improvement relative to the end of CPB, nadir of ventricular func-

tion 4 to 6 hours after CPB, and improvement over next 12 to 18 hours.

- Support for ventricular function after CPB includes: optimizing patient physiologic status; preparing before initiating weaning process; anticipation of requirements; pharmacologic support with: positive inotropic drugs (e.g., catecholamines, PDE III inhibitors, calcium, cardiac glycosides); vasoconstrictors (e.g., phenylephrine, norepinephrine); vasodilators (e.g., nitroprusside, nitroglycerin, PDE III inhibitors, prostaglandin E_1, nitric oxide); and mechanical support with IABP or VAD.
- Causes for right ventricular failure include right coronary insufficiency, poor right ventricular (RV) protection, and pulmonary hypertension.
  - Principle findings regarding right ventricular failure include elevated pulmonary artery pressure (PAP), high central venous pressure (CVP), decreased arterial pressure, decreased cardiac output, RV distension, and high RV wall tension.
- Treatment for right ventricular failure include elevation of perfusion pressure [left atrial (LA) infusion of vasoconstrictors] and pulmonary artery vasodilation (nitric oxide, prostaglandin E_1, nitrovasodilators, PDE III inhibitors).
- Problem situations during weaning include: vasodilation and hypotension (e.g., increased with long duration of rewarming and treatment with α-adrenergic agonists); vasoconstriction and hypertension (e.g., inadequate rewarming, decreased cardiac output, treatment with vasodilators); acute hemodynamic deterioration (e.g., utility of TEE); and hypoxemia (e.g., nitroprusside, intracardiac shunt, atelectasis, bronchospasms, which may be produced by protamine and treated with β-2 agonists [inhaled or i.v.], inhaled anesthetic agents [if ventricular function is good], and methylxanthines).
- Controversies include early inotrope use (appropriate if guided by relevant hemodynamic data) and calcium use (left ventricular dysfunction: no data, normal left ventricular function, normocalcemia: no benefit and potential harm, hypocalcemia: useful to normalize ionized calcium level).

REFERENCES

1. Novack CR, Tinker JH. Hypothermia after cardiopulmonary bypass in man. *Anesthesiology* 1980;53:277–280.
2. Cingolani HE, Faulkner SL, Mattiazzi AR, et al. Depression of human myocardial contractility with "respiratory" and "metabolic" acidosis. *Surgery* 1975;77:427–432.
3. Houle DB, Weil MH, Brown EB, et al. Influence of respiratory acidosis on ECG and pressor responses to epinephrine, norepinephrine and metaraminol. *Proc Soc Exp Biol Med* 1957;94:561–564.
4. Rudolph AM, Yuan S. Response of the pulmonary vasculature to hypoxia and H+ ion concentration changes. *J Clin Invest* 1966;45:399–441.
5. Ettinger PO, Regan TJ, Oldewurtel HA. Hyperkalemia, cardiac conduction, and the electrocardiogram: a review. *Am Heart J* 1974;88:360–371.
6. Zerr KJ, Furnary AP, Grunkemeier GL, et al. Glucose control lowers the risk of wound infection in diabetes after open heart operations. *Ann Thorac Surg* 1997;63:356–361.
7. Harker LA, Malpass TW, Branson HE, et al. Mechanism of abnormal bleeding in patients undergoing cardiopulmonary bypass: acquired transient platelet dysfunction associated with selective alpha-granule release. *Blood* 1980;56:824–834.
8. Buylaert WA, Herrengods LL, Mortier EP, et al. Cardiopulmonary bypass and the pharmacokinetics of drugs: an update. *Clin Pharmacokinet* 1989;7:234–251.
9. Price SL, Brown DL, Carpenter RL. Isoflurane elimination via a bubble oxygenator during extracorporeal circulation. *J Cardiothorac Anesth* 1988;2:41–44.
10. Nussmeier NA, Lambert ML, Moskowitz GJ, et al. Wash-in and wash-out of isoflurane administered via bubble oxygenators during hypothermic cardiopulmonary bypass. *Anesthesiology* 1989;71:519–525.
11. Bermudez J, Lichtiger M. Increases in arterial to end-tidal CO_2 tension differences after cardiopulmonary bypass. *Anesth Analg* 1987;66:690–692.
12. Salmenpera M, Heinonen J. Pulmonary vascular responses to moderate changes in PaCO2 after cardiopulmonary bypass. *Anesthesiology* 1986;64:311–315.
13. Stern DH, Gerson JI, Allen FB, et al. Can we trust the direct radial artery pressure immediately after cardiopulmonary bypass? *Anesthesiology* 1985;62:557–571.
14. Mohr R, Lavee J, Goor DA. Inaccuracy of radial artery pressure measurement after cardiac operations. *J Thorac Cardiovasc Surg* 1987;94:286–290.
15. Gallagher JD, Moore RA, McNicholas KW, et al. Comparison of radial and femoral arterial blood pressure in children after cardiopulmonary bypass. *J Clin Monit* 1985;1:168–171.
16. Thomson IR, Rosenbloom M, Cannon JE, et al. Electrocardiographic ST-segment elevation after myocardial reperfusion during coronary artery surgery. *Anesth Analg* 1987;66:1183–1186.
17. Abel RM, Buckley MJ, Austen WG, et al. Etiology, incidence and prognosis of renal failure after cardiac operations: results of a prospective analysis of 500 consecutive patients. *J Thorac Cardiovasc Surg* 1976;71:323–333.
18. Davis RF, Lappas DG, Kirklin JK, et al. Acute oliguria after cardiopulmonary bypass: renal functional improvement with low dose dopamine infusion. *Crit Care Med* 1982;10:852–856.
19. Hilberman M, Moseda J, Stinson EB, et al. The diuretic properties of dopamine in patients after open-heart operation. *Anesthesiology* 1984;61:489–494.
20. Weinstone R, Campbell JM, Booker PD, et al. Renal function after cardiopulmonary bypass in children: comparison of dopamine with dobutamine. *Br J Anaesth* 1991;67:591–594.
21. Cahalan MK, Litt L, Botvinick EH, et al. Advances in noninvasive cardiovascular imaging: implications for the anesthesiologist. *Anesthesiology* 1987;66:356–372.
22. Ungerleider RM, Greeley WJ, Sheikh KH, et al. Routine use of intraoperative epicardial echocardiography and Doppler color flow imaging to guide and evaluate repair of congenital heart lesions. A prospective study. *J Thorac Cardiovasc Surg* 1990;100:297–309.
23. Greeley WJ, Ungerleider RM. Echocardiography during surgery for congenital heart disease. In: DeBruijn NP, Clements FM, eds. *Intraoperative use of echocardiography*. Philadelphia: J.B. Lippincott, 1991:129–175.

24. Hansen RM, Viguerat CE, Matthay MA, et al. Poor correlation between pulmonary arterial wedge pressure and left ventricular end-diastolic volume after coronary artery bypass graft surgery. *Anesthesiology* 1986;64:764–770.

25. Cheung AT, Savino JS, Weiss SJ, et al. Echocardiographic and hemodynamic indexes of left ventricular preload in patients with normal and abnormal ventricular function. *Anesthesiology* 1994; 81:376–387.

26. Iyer VS, Russell WJ, Leppard P, et al. Mortality and myocardial infarction after coronary artery surgery: a review of 12,003 patients. *Med J Aust* 1993;59:166–170.

27. Berger RL, Davis KB, Kaiser GC, et al. Preservation of the myocardium during coronary artery bypass grafting. *Circulation* 1981; 64[Suppl 2]:61–66.

28. Christakis GT, Weisel RD, Fremes SE, et al. Coronary artery bypass grafting in patients with poor ventricular function. *J Thorac Cardiovasc Surg* 1992;103:1083–1092.

29. Mangano DT. Biventricular function after myocardial revascularization in humans: deterioration and recovery patterns in the first 24 hours. *Anesthesiology* 1985;62:571–577.

30. Royster RL, Butterworth JF, Prough DS, et al. Preoperative and intraoperative predictors of inotropic support and long-term outcome in patients having coronary artery bypass grafting. *Anesth Analg* 1991;72:729–736.

31. Goenen M, Jacquemart JL, Galvez, et al. Preoperative left ventricular dysfunction and operative risks in coronary bypass surgery. *Chest* 1987;92:804–806.

32. Royster RL. Myocardial dysfunction after cardiopulmonary bypass: recovery patterns, predictors of inotropic need, theoretical concepts of inotropic administration. *J Cardiothorac Vasc Anesth* 1993;7[Suppl 2]:19–25.

33. Braunwald E, Kloner RA. The stunned myocardium: prolonged, post-ischemic ventricular dysfunction. *Circulation* 1982;66: 1146–1149.

34. Rahimtoola SH. The hibernating myocardium. *Am Heart J* 1989; 117:211–221.

35. Ross J Jr. Afterload mismatch in aortic and mitral valve disease: implications for surgical therapy. *J Am Coll Cardiol* 1985;5: 811–826.

36. Ross J Jr. Left ventricular function and the timing of surgical treatment in valvular heart disease. *Ann Intern Med* 1981;94: 498–504.

37. Appelbaum A, Kouchoukos N, Blackstone EH, et al. Early risks of open heart surgery for mitral valve disease. *Am J Cardiol* 1976; 37:201–209.

38. Takeishi Y, Tono-Oka I, Kubota I, et al. Functional recovery of hibernating myocardium after coronary bypass surgery: does it coincide with improvement in perfusion? *Am Heart J* 1991;122: 665–670.

39. Ellis SG, Wynne J, Braunwald E, et al. Response of reperfusion-salvaged, shinned myocardium to inotropic stimulation. *Am Heart J* 1984;107:13–19.

40. Elz JS, Panagiotopoulos S, Nayler WG. Reperfusion-induced calcium gain after ischemia. *Am J Cardiol* 1989;63:7E–13E.

41. Steen PA, Tinker JH, Pluth JR, et al. Efficacy of dopamine, dobutamine, and epinephrine during emergence from cardiopulmonary bypass in man. *Circulation* 1978;57:378–384.

42. Salomon NW, Plachetka JR, Copeland JG. Comparison of dopamine and dobutamine after coronary artery bypass grafting. *Ann Thorac Surg* 1982;33:48–54.

43. Royster RL, Butterworth JF, Prielipp RC, et al. A randomized, blinded, placebo-controlled evaluation of calcium chloride and epinephrine for inotropic support after emergence from cardiopulmonary bypass. *Anesth Analg* 1992;74:3–13.

44. Richard C, Ricome JL, Rimailho A, et al. Combined hemody-

namic effects of dopamine and dobutamine in cardiogenic shock. *Circulation* 1983;67:620–626.

45. Loeb HS, Bredakis J, Gunnar RM. Superiority of dobutamine over dopamine for augmentation of cardiac output in patients with chronic low output cardiac failure. *Circulation* 1977;55: 375–381.

46. Hess W, Klein W, Muller-Busch C, et al. Haemodynamic effects of dopamine and dopamine combined with nitroglycerin in patients subjected to coronary bypass surgery. *Br J Anesth* 1979;51: 1063–1068.

47. Gage J, Rutman H, Lucido D, et al. Additive effects of dobutamine and amrinone on myocardial contractility and ventricular performance in patients with severe heart failure. *Circulation* 1986;74:367–373.

48. Benotti JR, Grossman W, Braunwald E, et al. Effects of amrinone on myocardial energy metabolism and hemodynamics in patients with severe congestive heart failure due to coronary artery disease. *Circulation* 1980;62:28–34.

49. Robinson RJS, Tchervenkow C. Treatment of low cardiac output after aortocoronary bypass surgery using a combination of norepinephrine and amrinone. *J Cardiothorac Anesth* 1987;1:229–233.

50. Lathi KG, Shulman MS, Diehl JT, et al. The use of amrinone and norepinephrine for inotropic support during emergence from cardiopulmonary bypass. *J Cardiothorac Anesth* 1991;5:250–254.

51. Bailey JM, Levy JH, Kikura M, et al. Pharmacokinetics of milrinone in patients undergoing cardiac surgery. *Anesthesiology* 1994; 81:616–622.

52. Wynands JE. Amrinone: is it the inotrope of choice? *J Cardiothorac Anesth* 1989;3[Suppl 2]:45–52.

53. LeJemtel TH, Sonnenblick EH. Should the failing heart be stimulated? *N Engl J Med* 1984;310:1384–1385.

54. David D, DuBois C, Loria Y. Comparison of nicardipine and sodium nitroprusside in the treatment of paroxysmal hypertension after aortocoronary bypass surgery. *J Cardiothorac Vasc Anesth* 1991;5:357–361.

55. Goldberg ME, Cantillo J, Nemiroff, et al. Fenoldepam infusion for the treatment of postoperative hypertension. *J Clin Anesth* 1993;5:386–391.

56. Mills RM, LeJemtel TH, Horton D, et al. Sustained hemodynamic effects of an infusion of nesritide (human b-type natriuretic peptide) in heart failure: a randomized, double-blind, placebo-controlled clinical trial. *J Am Coll Cardiol* 1999;34:155–162.

57. Sturm JT, Fuhrman TM, Sterling R, et al. Combined use of dopamine and nitroprusside therapy in conjunction with intra-aortic balloon pumping for the treatment of postcardiotomy low-output syndrome. *J Thorac Cardiovasc Surg* 1981;82:13–17.

58. Feola M, Weiner L, Walinsky P, et al. Improved survival after coronary artery bypass surgery in patients with poor left ventricular function: role of intraaortic balloon counterpulsation. *Am J Cardiol* 1977;39:1021–1026.

59. D'Ambra MN, LaRaia PJ, Philbin DM, et al. Prostaglandin E$_1$: a new therapy for refractory right heart failure and pulmonary hypertension after mitral valve replacement. *J Thorac Cardiovasc Surg* 1985;89:567–572.

60. Frostell C, Fratacci MD, Wain JC, et al. Inhaled nitric oxide: a selective pulmonary vasodilator reversing hypoxic vasoconstriction. *Circulation* 1991;83:2038–2047.

61. Hess W, Arnold B, Veit S. The haemodynamic effects of amrinone in patients with mitral stenosis and pulmonary hypertension. *Eur Heart J* 1986;7:800–807.

62. Robertie PG, Butterworth JF, Royster RL, et al. Normal parathyroid hormone responses to hypocalcemia during cardiopulmonary bypass. *Anesthesiology* 1991;75:43–48.

63. Drop LJ, Geffin GA, O'Keefe DD, et al. Relation between ionized calcium concentration and ventricular pump performance

in the dog under hemodynamically controlled conditions. *Am J Cardiol* 1981;47:1041–1051.

64. Katz AM. Potential deleterious effects of inotropic agents in the therapy of chronic heart failure. *Circulation* 1986;73[Suppl 3]: 184–190.

65. Lazar HL, Buckberg GD, Foglia RP, et al. Detrimental effects of premature use of inotropic drugs to discontinue cardiopulmonary bypass. *J Thorac Cardiovasc Surg* 1981;82:18–25.

66. Ward HB, Einzig S, Wang T, et al. Comparison of catecholamine effects on canine myocardial metabolism and regional blood flow during and after cardiopulmonary bypass. *J Thorac Cardiovasc Surg* 1987;87:452–465.

67. Reves JG, Buttner E, Karp RB, et al. Elevated catecholamines during cardiac surgery: consequences of reperfusion of the post-arrested heart. *Am J Cardiol* 1984;53:722–728.

68. Dyke CM, Lee KF, Parmor J, et al. Inotropic stimulation and oxygen consumption in a canine model of dilated cardiomyopathy. *Ann Thorac Surg* 1991;52:750–758.

CARDIOPULMONARY BYPASS IN INFANTS AND CHILDREN

JAMES JAGGERS
IAN R. SHEARER
ROSS M. UNGERLEIDER

HISTORICAL ASPECTS

Cardiac surgery today has grown to enormous proportions. Coronary bypass grafting has become routinely safe throughout the world. Advances in valve repair and replacement have improved outcomes for thousands of patients each year who are afflicted with valvular heart disease. Congenital heart defects can be repaired in tiny infants, even those weighing less than 2 kg, with generally excellent outcomes. Yet less than 50 years ago (within the lifetime of many of today's prominent practitioners), elective cardiac surgery as an option offered to patients was virtually nonexistent. Procedures were limited to those that could be performed without any reliable means of circulatory support (such as extracardiac procedures on the aorta), or to those performed emergently to save patients who had sustained traumatic injury to the heart (often limited to cardiac suture repair and evacuation of pericardial tamponade).

Early pioneers in cardiac surgery were motivated by the predicament of older children with "crippling" congenital heart defects, in addition to the results of good scientific investigation and the belief that application of these results to such children was practical and possible. These practitioners launched a sequence of clinical undertakings that would be rightfully considered as intrepid by any relevant standards.

In the late 1940s and early 1950s, it did not seem that coupling extracorporeal circulation with oxygenation would be achievable. Despite dedicated work by numerous experts, the prospects for success seemed grim. Not to be stopped, surgeons began developing ingenious methods of repairing cardiac defects without the use of extracorporeal circulation. One method that became popular for selected patients was the use of caval occlusion with moderate hypothermia. Bigelow et al. (1) first demonstrated the application of hypothermia to cardiac surgery in 1950. They showed that dogs cooled to 20°C could survive a 15-minute period of total circulatory arrest. In 1952, Lewis and Taufic (2,3) were the first to apply hypothermia and inflow occlusion in the repair of an atrial septal defect in humans.

The idea of coupling extracorporeal circulation and oxygenation and surgical repair of the heart originated with Dr. John Gibbon, Jr. Inspired by the tragic death of a pregnant woman with a pulmonary embolus, he was the first to establish the feasibility of artificially supported circulation during temporary occlusion of the pulmonary artery. In 1953, he successfully used extracorporeal circulation in a young woman, Cecelia Bavolek, to facilitate open cardiac surgery, an atrial septal defect closure (4). After an initial success, however, Dr. Gibbon lost his next 4 patients and "retired" from pursuing open heart surgery. In fact, aside from Dr. Gibbon's initial procedure, early experience with the clinical use of cardiopulmonary bypass (CPB) was uniformly dismal (Table 30.1), and most surgical groups continued to seek alternative methods to correct heart defects. In 1954, Lillehei and associates (5,6) began using the technique of controlled cross-circulation, with a compatible adult as the pump–oxygenator, to repair congenital heart defects. Within a period of 16 months, 45 patients were operated on and 28 survived. This really began the remarkable era of heart surgery, which we now look at without appropriate "marvel." For the first time, surgeons were able to repair intracardiac defects with the "luxury of time" as the patient's body was provided with nutrient perfusion by an "exogenous" (albeit human) pump–oxygenator. Nevertheless, the use of other humans as pump–oxygenators carried impractical risks, and as further investigation led to the development of safer extracorporeal circuits, the field of cardiac surgery was provided with an essential tool for growth and surgeons acquired, as Dr. Denton Cooley put it (6), "the can opener for the biggest picnic they had ever known!"

J. Jaggers, I. R. Shearer, and R. M. Ungerleider: Department of Pediatric Cardiac Surgery, Duke University Medical Center, Durham, North Carolina 27710.

TABLE 30.1. OPEN HEART SURGERY WITH TOTAL CARDIOPULMONARY BYPASS: RESULTS OF ALL REPORTED CASES 1951–1954 (BEFORE CROSS-CIRCULATION, 3/26/54)

Surgeon	No. Patients	Oxygenator Type	Year	No. Survivals	No. Deaths
Dennis	2	Film	1951	0	2
Helmsworth	1	Bubble	1952	0	1
Gibbon	6	Film	1953	1 (ASD repair)	5
Dodrill	1	Autogenous	1953	0	1
Mustard	5	Monkey lungs	1951–1953	0	5
Clowes	3	Bubble	1953	0	3
Total	18			1 (5.5%)	17 (94.5%)

ASD, atrial septal defect.

The addition of heat exchangers allowed core cooling and rewarming of internal organs in a way that surface cooling could not, and this facilitated decreased pump flow rates and prolonged the period of safe operation. Although the basic mechanism of the propulsion of blood with the roller pump has not changed, the mechanisms of oxygenation have undergone an evolution. Gibbon's first oxygenator was a rotating film oxygenator. Kirklin's group adopted the stationary film oxygenator that was developed with technical support from IBM (7). Bubble oxygenators were developed in the late 1950s and were mass-produced in the 1960s. This revolutionized the field of cardiac surgery. Membrane oxygenators utilizing thin sheets of permeable Teflon were developed and had some advantages over bubble oxygenators. However, the rapid expansion of cardiac surgery in the 1960s required a preassembled, sterile, and disposable oxygenator, and the membrane oxygenator was far from ready, so the initial growth of cardiac surgery in the 1960s, with the advent of coronary and valvular surgery, emphasized the use of bubble oxygenators. By the 1970s, many centers were switching to membrane oxygenators because of increased safety and fewer complications with longer exposure time. With the advancement of gas-permeable, extraluminal-flow oxygenator fibers, the production of bubble oxygenators has all but disappeared in the United States.

Because of advances in the techniques of surgery and perioperative care, the numbers of patients being exposed to CPB at both ends of the age spectrum has increased. Miniaturization of some of the elements of the CPB circuit has made neonatal heart surgery safer and more efficient. The next great advances will be in the modulation of the systemic inflammatory response and injury resulting from CPB. In this chapter, we review the basic physiology of CPB, the associated systemic inflammatory effects, strategies employed in the application of CPB, including deep hypothermic circulatory arrest (DHCA), and our current recommendations for how best to manage CPB in infants and children.

DIFFERENCES BETWEEN INFANTS AND ADULTS

Numerous differences between infants and adults (8,9) (Table 30.2) affect the response to CPB, and these must be accounted for in CPB management strategies. Procedures performed in infants and children may require extremes of temperature, hemodilution, and perfusion flow rates. Certain anatomic features, such as the presence of large aortopulmonary collateral vessels or an interrupted aortic arch, require an alteration of bypass strategies and cannulation techniques. Circuit capacity can not currently be reduced in proportion to patient size. Therefore, significant hemodilution in neonates and small infants is unavoidable. In addition to the decrease in hematocrit associated with hemodilution, significant dilution of clotting factors and plasma proteins also occurs, resulting in dilutional coagulopathy. Other organ systems in neonates and infants are not mature. For example, the production of vitamin K-dependent clotting factors by the liver is diminished. Neonates and infants require much higher flow rates per body surface area to meet metabolic demands. Neonates are often perfused at flow rates up to 200 mL/kg per minute. As the temperature is reduced, flow rates can be decreased. This has the benefit of producing less blood in a small and complicated surgical field. Thermoregulation in small children is also impaired, so that close attention to temperature monitoring is re-

TABLE 30.2. DIFFERENCE BETWEEN INFANTS AND ADULTS

Smaller circulating blood volume
Higher oxygen consumption rate
Reactive pulmonary vascular bed
Presence of intracardiac and extra cardiac shunting
Immature organ systems
Altered thermoregulation
Poor tolerance to microemboli

quired. Furthermore, in some instances, patients are cooled to profoundly hypothermic temperatures (e.g., 15° to 18°C) and the pump is then turned off (DHCA). This provides the surgeon with the opportunity to remove the cannulas from the patient and perform a precise repair in an operative field unencumbered by blood, cannulas, or other apparatus related to CPB. When CPB is resumed, patients are rewarmed to their normal temperature.

The period of time from 6 months' gestation to 6 months after birth is critical in the development of the cortical connections of the brain, which are involved in perceptual and cognitive functions (10). Also, neonates and young infants are endowed with "plasticity," which is the potential for remodeling in response to environmental stimuli (11). In general, the immature brain tolerates O_2 deprivation better than the mature brain. This supports the clinical observations that infants tolerate longer periods of DHCA better than do older children or adult patients. The lungs are also immature at birth, and lung development proceeds up to about 8 years of age (12). At birth, the number of alveoli present is approximately one-tenth of what it is in the adult. The lungs of the neonate are quite fragile and are at increased risk for pulmonary edema and hypertension (13). The kidneys of neonates and infants have a high vascular resistance with preferential blood flow away from the outer cortex. Sodium reabsorption and excretion, concentrating and diluting mechanisms, and acid–base balance capacity are limited. These characteristics must be taken into account in the management of CPB in infants. Finally, the immune system of the neonate is immature. Complement generation is low and neonatal mononuclear cells are dysfunctional (14). These differences and many more make CPB in the infant and neonate a specialized endeavor that requires great attention to detail and the ability to adapt to unexpected situations.

PHYSIOLOGY OF CARDIOPULMONARY BYPASS

Improvements in technology have reduced the morbidity associated with CPB. The safe conduct of CPB in the neonate and infant requires a comprehensive understanding of the physiologic alterations associated with CPB, in addition to the implications of circuit design, hemodilution, choice of cannulas, degree of hypothermia, acid–base strategies, and selected flow rates.

Hypothermia

The use of hypothermia in conjunction with CPB provides several advantages. Hypothermia facilitates surgical exposure by allowing decreases in flow rate, which results in less blood returning through the collateral vessels. Systemic hypothermia also decreases the rate of myocardial rewarm-

ing between applications of cardioplegia. Hypothermia is mandatory for brain protection when periods of DHCA are utilized. Hypothermia also affords some protection to other organs during periods of CPB and low-flow states. At deep hypothermia, cellular metabolism is so low and membrane fluidity is reduced to such a large extent that cellular basal metabolic needs can be met and cellular membrane integrity can be maintained for a relatively prolonged period of time. The principal clinical effect of hypothermia is the reduction in metabolic rate and molecular movement. As the temperature is lowered, both basal and functional cellular metabolism is reduced and the rate of adenosine triphosphate (ATP) consumption is decreased. Whole body O_2 consumption decreases directly with body temperature (Fig. 30.1). According to Arrhenius's equation, the logarithmic rate of chemical reactions is inversely proportional to the reciprocal of the absolute temperature. The multiple by which the reaction rate decreases for every 10°C is the Q^{10}. Repeated analysis of published data suggests a Q^{10} of 3.65 for infants, compared with approximately 2.6 for adults (15). This higher Q^{10} in infants suggests a greater metabolic suppression related to hypothermia, which might enable them to tolerate longer periods of "imperfect" perfusion or ischemia. During CPB, as the temperature of the patient decreases, O_2 consumption becomes independent of the flow rate. This is the basis for predicting the minimal pump flow rate (MPFR)—the minimal flow necessary to meet metabolic demands (16). Table 30.3 shows that as the temperature decreases, the cerebral metabolic rate of O_2 extraction ($CMRo_2$) decreases and the predicted MPFR decreases proportionally. Although hypothermia attentuates the hypoxia-induced depression of cellular ATP content and membrane injury, there is evidence to suggest that hypothermia and hypoxia result in a significant increase in intracellular calcium and sodium during subsequent reperfusion (17). This has important implications for the management of oxygenation during the resumption of CPB after hypothermic circulatory arrest. In the heart, the contribution of hypothermia to lowering the basal metabolic rate is relatively small compared with the effects of stopping electromechanical work. There also appears to be a marked increase in the resting tension of the myocardium in response to a sudden decrease in perfusion temperature. This is referred to as a *rapid cooling contracture* (18), which may be the consequence of a sudden release of intracellular calcium stores within the sarcoplasmic reticulum. This cold-induced increase in resting myocardial tone may lead to impaired recovery of systolic and diastolic function after reperfusion, which has led some groups to avoid cold perfusion of the heart before the aortic cross-clamp is applied and to use warm induction cardioplegia when possible (19,20). However, ventricular function may not be impaired by rapid cooling in an appropriate metabolic environment. Lowering the serum ionized calcium levels with citrate may ameliorate some of the adverse effects of hypothermic cardiac perfusion

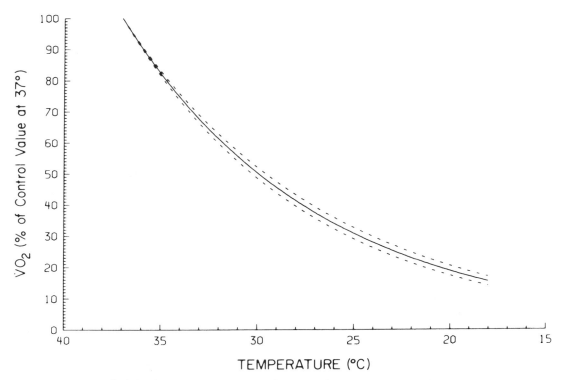

FIG. 30.1. Whole body O_2 consumption as a function of body temperature. (Adapted by Blackstone and Kirklin from data reported by Bigelow WG, Callaghan JC, Hopps JA. General hypothermia for experimental intra-cardiac surgery: the use of electrophrenic respirations, an artificial pacemaker for cardiac standstill and radio frequency re-warming in general hypothermia. *Ann Surg* 1950;132:531–539, with permission.)

(21). With the "hypocalcemic" primes commonly used in neonatal heart surgery today, rapid cooling and cold induction of ischemia does not seem to be deleterious (22).

The adverse effects of rapid cooling have also been demonstrated experimentally in the kidneys, liver, and lungs. However, many variables are involved clinically, and there does not appear to be any readily apparent injury to the patient resulting from rapid cooling on CPB. It does appear

TABLE 30.3. PREDICTED MINIMAL PUMP FLOW RATES

Temperature (°C)	CMR_{O_2} (mL/100 g/min)	Predicted MPFR (mL/kg/min)
37	1.48	100
32	0.823	56
30	0.654	44
28	0.513	34
25	0.362	24
20	0.201	14
18	0.159	11
15	0.112	8

CMR_{O_2}, cerebral metabolic rate of oxygen; MPFR, minimal pump flow rate.

that neonates are able to tolerate the "stresses" of profound hypothermia without difficulty. This has previously been attributed to a greater glycolytic activity and higher glycogen reserves in neonates. However, they may also have differential ionic channel density or different membrane function in comparison with older subjects. These theories remain speculative. The degree of hypothermia selected depends on the needs for reduced flow to enhance surgical repair. Three distinct degrees of hypothermia are (a) mild (30° to 34°C, (b) moderate (25° to 30°C), and (c) deep (15° to 22°C). Deep hypothermia is often used when periods of low flow or DHCA are desired. The technique selected is based on (a) required surgical conditions, (b) patient size, (c) type and expected duration of the operation, and (d) potential physiologic impact on the patient. Mild and moderate hypothermic CPB is principally employed in older children and adolescents. In these patients, venous cannulas are less obtrusive and the heart can easily accommodate cannulation of the superior and inferior venae cavae. Bicaval cannulation reduces right atrial blood return and improves the surgeon's ability to visualize intracardiac anatomy. Mild hypothermia may also be chosen for less demanding cardiac procedures in infants, such as repair of an atrial septal defect, ventricular septal defect, or uncomplicated atrioventricular septal de-

TABLE 30.4. RECOMMENDED PUMP FLOW RATES

Patient Weight (kg)	Pump Flow Rate (mL/kg/min)
<3	150–200
3–10	125–175
10–15	120–150
15–30	100–120
30–50	75–100
>50	50–75

fect. More complex procedures, such as a pulmonary autograft aortic valve replacement, might lead to selection of moderate hypothermia to help maintain adequate cardiac protection during a longer aortic cross-clamp period. Recommendations for optimal pump flow rates for children are based on body surface area and on the maintenance of efficient organ perfusion as determined by arterial blood gases, acid–base balance, and whole body O_2 consumption during CPB. Table 30.4 lists recommended normothermic flow rates for children based on body weight. At hypothermic temperatures, metabolism is reduced and therefore pump flow rates may be further reduced accordingly. Decisions on flow rates determine the size of cannulas chosen.

Deep hypothermic CPB is generally reserved for neonates and infants requiring complex cardiac repairs. However, certain older children with complex cardiac disease or aortic arch anomalies may benefit from a short period of circulatory arrest. For the most part, deep hypothermia is selected to allow the surgeon to operate under conditions of low flow (e.g., in repairing the pulmonary arteries of patients with substantial aortopulmonary collateral flow) or DHCA (e.g., in repairing the aortic arch). Low pump flows improve the operating conditions for the surgeon by providing a nearly bloodless field and better visualization of critical portions of the repair at selected times during the procedure. When the strategy is to use DHCA for the intracardiac portion of the repair, venous return can be accomplished with a single atrial cannula. This has the advantage of providing optimal venous return, concomitant venting of the heart, and generally uncomplicated venous return.

During DHCA, the surgeon can remove the atrial or aortic cannula. With this technique, surgical repair is more precise because of the bloodless and cannula-free operative field. Arresting the circulation, even at deeply hypothermic temperatures, introduces the question of how well deep hypothermia preserves organ function, with the brain being of greatest concern. This is discussed in more detail in a later section (see Hypothermic Injury to the Brain). Hypothermia preserves organ function by maintaining cellular ATP stores despite reduced O_2 delivery, reducing excitatory neurotransmitter release, and preventing calcium entry into the cell. In summary, some degree of hypothermia is necessary and beneficial during CPB in neonates and infants.

Hypothermia helps to preserve organ function during ischemia, aids in the operative exposure, and increases the safety of CPB.

Pulsatile versus Nonpulsatile Flow

The desirability of pulsatile perfusion has been contemplated and studied since the introduction of extracorporeal circulation in the 1950s. Hundreds of experiments have been performed to try to prove that pulsatile perfusion is preferable to the more commonly employed nonpulsatile or laminar-flow perfusion. The inability to reproduce normal physiologic pulsatile blood flow, in addition to the additional complexity of these systems, led to the adoption of laminar flow systems. In some studies, the use of pulsatile perfusion results in a decrease in systemic vascular resistance following CPB and an increase in the cardiac index in adult patients (23). Others have found that production of the potent vasodilator nitric oxide from cultured endothelial cells is increased during pulsatile flow in comparison with laminar flow (24). This may be important at the microcirculatory level, affecting vascular endothelial function, thrombogenicity, and overall vascular tone. Many have reported beneficial hemodynamic effects of pulsatile perfusion, with reduction of the need for inotropes and intraaortic balloon pump therapy (25). It appears that the major benefit of pulsatile perfusion is a reduction in post-CPB vasoconstriction and resultant improvement in cardiac index (23). There is also evidence that pulsatile perfusion allows for better splanchnic perfusion in comparison with nonpulsatile perfusion (26,27). In our own experience with a neonatal porcine model of CPB and circulatory arrest, we found no difference in cerebral blood flow either before or after the arrest period. Before arrest, renal blood flow was improved, and myocardial blood flow was better both before and after arrest (27–29). The availability of effective pulsatile pumps is limited, and the clinical superiority of this technique is yet to be proved.

Strategies for Carbon Dioxide Management: Alpha-Stat and pH-Stat

The role of CO_2 management in CPB has been studied extensively in animals and adult patients. Based on the effect of CO_2 on arterial and intracellular pH at hypothermic temperatures, two divergent blood gas management strategies have been championed: alpha-stat (temperature uncorrected) and pH-stat (temperature corrected) (17,18,30–35). Alpha-stat strategy maintains a pH of 7.40, measured without mathematical correction for the effects of temperature, whereas pH-stat uses a mathematical correction for the effects of temperature on pH. With temperature-corrected measurements, blood pH becomes increasingly alkaline as the blood cools. To correct for this alkalotic pH, CO_2 is added to maintain a temperature-corrected pH of 7.40 (pH-stat). The addition of CO_2, however, lowers the intracellular pH (pH$_i$), which results in an imbalance between H$^+$ and OH$^-$ ions (i.e., the loss of electrochemical neutrality). Intracellular enzymatic function depends on the maintenance of a normal pH$_i$, and therefore cellular enzyme function is impaired when pH-stat is used. An acidotic pH$_i$ is problematic because at hypothermic temperatures the normal buffering systems (NH$_3^-$, HCO$_3^-$) become ineffective. At hypothermia, buffering capacity is limited to negative charges of the amino acids composing intracellular proteins. The amino acid histidine is the most important buffer at hypothermia because it contains an α-imidazole ring with many negatively charged moieties, which can buffer H$^+$ ions. The "alpha" in the term alpha-stat, which denotes uncorrected blood gas measurement, refers to the α-imidazole ring of histidine. The principal advantage of alpha-stat strategy therefore is the preservation of intracellular electrochemical neutrality, in which an appropriate pH$_i$ and the efficiency of intracellular enzymatic function are maintained (36). During moderate hypothermia, selecting one blood gas management strategy over the other appears less critical because intracellular pH differences in the brain are small (37,38). During deep hypothermia with or without DHCA, the addition of CO_2 during active brain cooling could potentially improve the distribution of the cold perfusate to deep brain structures. Recent evidence suggests that pH-stat management enhances the distribution of extracorporeal perfusate to the brain and may help cool the brain more thoroughly and rapidly (32,39). Although improved cooling was demonstrated in these studies, metabolic recovery after circulatory arrest was shown to be impaired, suggesting that the acid load induced by pH-stat has a negative effect on enzymatic function after cerebral rewarming. In an effort to retain the benefits of pH-stat on cooling and eliminate its negative effects on enzymatic function, our group has suggested a combined strategy for blood gas management in which pH-stat and alpha-stat are used in succession. In a group of neonatal pigs that underwent initial cooling with pH-stat followed by a switch to alpha-stat before DHCA, metabolic suppression was improved over that achieved with alpha-stat alone; in addition, a significant enhancement in metabolic recovery after rewarming was noted. This suggests that initial cooling with pH-stat, followed by a switch to alpha-stat to normalize the pH in the brain before ischemic arrest, may be an alternative and effective approach. Other factors that may result in maldistribution of pump flow away from the cerebral circulation and contribute to inefficient cerebral cooling include anatomic variants (large aortopulmonary collateral vessels) (40–42) and technical problems (aortic and venous cannula misplacement) (43). Cyanotic patients with known aortopulmonary collateral vessels may benefit from the cerebral vasodilation of pH-stat during early cooling (44). Once they are cool, however, if DHCA or deep hypothermia with low flow is planned, converting to an alpha-stat strategy may help preserve intra-

cellular brain pH and improve neurologic outcome following the procedure.

Myocardial Protection

Neonatal repair is the preferred approach to most congenital heart defects. As the complexity of the repair and the time required for surgery increase, the need for outstanding myocardial protection also increases. Some laboratory evidence suggests that the immature myocardium has structural and functional characteristics different from those of the adult myocardium (45). The immature heart is less compliant and has less preload reserve, which results in a very limited range on the Starling curve. The normal neonatal heart operates at maximal saturation of adrenergic stimulation and shows an exaggerated negative inotropic response to anesthetic agents; therefore, when inotropic agents are required, larger doses are needed (46). The immature myocardium relies on glucose as its major substrate and also is more dependent on extracellular calcium for calcium-mediated excitation–contraction coupling (47,48). It is widely accepted that the immature heart has a greater tolerance to ischemia than the adult or mature heart. However, most of these laboratory data have been obtained from normal hearts. It is unclear what the ischemic tolerance is when preexisting conditions such as cyanosis, hypertrophy, or acidosis are present. Many of these conditions are present in neonates and infants who require surgical correction of a heart defect and can compromise myocardial protection. Infants and children with chronic cyanosis as a result of inadequate pulmonary blood flow often have an increased bronchial collateral flow. This increased blood return to the left side of the heart can result in insufficient myocardial protection as the heart is warmed and cardioplegia is washed out (49). Hypertrophic ventricles may also have inadequate myocardial protection and subendocardial ischemia during prolonged periods of arrest. Hypothermia remains the most important factor for successful myocardial protection in infants (50). Electromechanical arrest, ventricular decompression (by venting), and hypothermia all work together to decrease myocardial O_2 consumption. Topically applied iced saline solution may be helpful; however, it often interferes with the operative procedure and can result in phrenic nerve palsy. Therefore, many groups use topical cooling intermittently.

Typically, cardioplegia is delivered through a catheter or needle in the aortic root after the cross-clamp has been applied. In the presence of an interrupted aortic arch or hypoplastic left heart syndrome, the aorta may be quite small, and a small butterfly needle can be useful to deliver the cardioplegia in an atraumatic manner. Retrograde delivery of cardioplegia has received significant attention in the adult population; however, its applicability is limited in neonates except for those with severe aortic insufficiency or severe ventricular hypertrophy. Blood cardioplegia may be superior to crystalloid cardioplegia, especially with longer (>1 hour) periods of myocardial ischemia (50).

In general, the calcium concentration of cardioplegia solutions should be below the serum concentration (51). Despite the potential for excessive calcium influx secondary to hyperkalemia-induced membrane depolarization, potassium remains the most widely used cardiac arresting agent in all of cardiac surgery. Magnesium helps to maintain the negative resting membrane potential and also inhibits sarcolemmal calcium influx (52). The addition of magnesium to blood cardioplegia results in significantly improved functional recovery (53). Typically, an initiating dose of 30 mL of cardioplegia solution per kilogram is delivered at 4°C. Although there is no conclusive evidence to support or refute the practice, many surgeons use multiple doses of cardioplegia at approximately 20- to 30-minute intervals during the ischemic period. This can be helpful when a significant number of bronchial collateral vessels are present, or when operations are performed with mild or moderate hypothermia; in both these cases, the heart may be rewarmed prematurely.

In certain operations on the right side of a heart in which the septa are intact (i.e., tricuspid valve repair or pulmonary valve repair or replacement), a technique referred to as "empty beating" may be employed, in which myocardial ischemia is limited and a cross-clamp is not applied. This is a reasonable technique so long as there is no significant communication between the right and left sides of the heart. Also, mild hypothermia with fibrillator arrest can be used in operations on the right side of the heart, especially when a significant intracardiac communication exists, such as an atrial septal defect.

Intramyocardial air has also been suggested as a contributing factor for right ventricular dysfunction after pediatric cardiac surgery (54,55). In 4% of 350 consecutive pediatric patients undergoing repair of congenital cardiac defects, intramyocardial air was detected in the immediate post-bypass period by means of echocardiography with Doppler imaging (55). Echo-Doppler demonstrated increased echogenic areas localized to the right ventricular free wall and along the inferior portion of the intraventricular septum. Hemodynamic instability was a significant finding in many of these patients. The distribution of air was localized to the area supplied by the right coronary artery. The right coronary artery is a likely source for embolization of retained left ventricular air because of the location of the ostium of the right coronary artery on the anterior aspect of the aorta. Therefore, residual left ventricular air is more likely to enter the right coronary artery and result in right ventricular ischemia and dysfunction. For this reason, we now rarely place our patients in the Trendelenburg position while deairing the heart. We leave the aortic cross-clamp in place and use the cardioplegia needle site to vent air from the left ventricle. Placing the patient in the Trendelenburg position increases the likelihood that air will enter the right coronary

rather than exit the cardioplegia needle vent site. After deairing, the cross-clamp is removed with little concern for cerebral injury. This has greatly reduced the incidence of intramyocardial air in our experience.

Therapy for air embolism is directed at increasing the perfusion pressure to propel air through the arterioles and capillary bed. Dramatic hemodynamic and echocardiographic improvements have been demonstrated in patients with intramyocardial air after the administration of phenylephrine or reperfusion of the heart with high pump flow rates and perfusion pressures on CPB (55).

Another important mechanism of cardiac dysfunction that can occur in neonates and infants relates to the "inflammatory response" to CPB and the tendency for the microvasculature to "leak," thereby increasing the water content of important end-organs such as the heart and lungs. When the heart becomes edematous, it also becomes stiffer (less compliant), and higher filling pressures are required for an adequate preload. This problem is especially prominent in infants and may be related to the hemodilution that occurs once they are placed on CPB (56) (Fig. 30.2). Decreases in ventricular compliance can be measured by using echocardiographic indices of filling. Normally, flow into the left ventricle from the left atrium proceeds throughout most of diastole. In patients with altered (decreased) compliance, filling of the left ventricle from the left atrium may stop midway through diastole, and there may actually be a mid-diastolic reversal of flow. In an interesting clinical report published recently (57), it was noted that in those infants undergoing repair of transposition of the great arteries or interrupted aortic arch, which is a population believed to be at risk for excess fluid accumulation during CPB, all cases of operative mortality in the series were in infants

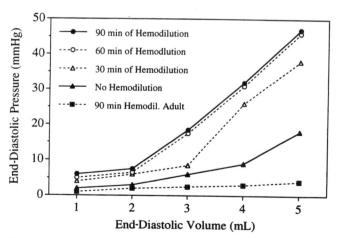

FIG. 30.2. Duration of hemodilution related to left ventricular end-diastolic volume and end-diastolic pressure in neonates: comparison with effects in adults. (From Mavroudis C, Ebert PA. Hemodilution causes decreased compliance in puppies. *Circulation* 1978;58:155–159, with permission.)

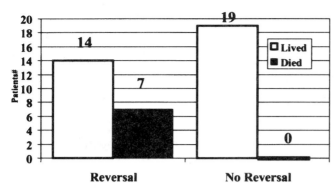

FIG. 30.3. The effects on hospital mortality of middiastolic flow reversal seen on transesophageal echocardiography immediately after cardiopulmonary bypass. (Data compiled from Li JS, Bengur AR, Ungerleider RM, et al. Abnormal left ventricular filling after neonatal repair of congenital heart disease: association with increased mortality and morbidity. *Am Heart J* 1998;136: 1075–1080, with permission.)

with middiastolic flow reversal noted by transesophageal echocardiography on the post-CPB echocardiogram (Fig. 30.3). Therefore, techniques of myocardial protection during CPB need to include some method to limit the development of myocardial edema.

Endocrine Response

Cardiopulmonary bypass is associated with tremendous increases in native catecholamines, particularly epinephrine and norepinephrine. This is partly a consequence of surgical stress, but also of peripheral vasoconstriction with relative ischemia, lack of pulsatile blood flow, and acidosis (27,58). The elevation of catecholamines extends into the postoperative period (59). It seems that the initially increased catecholamine levels fall considerably during reperfusion of the lungs. This is probably related to the uptake and metabolism of the catecholamines in the lungs. When the lungs are excluded from the circulation (total CPB), a significant accumulation of norepinephrine is noted. Hypothermia also has the effect of raising the serum catecholamine levels, not only by increasing production, but also by downregulating catecholamine receptors and decreasing the metabolic rate. Circulatory arrest also results in increases of catecholamines, but it is likely the rewarming, reperfusion phase of circulatory arrest is most associated with catecholamine surge (60,61). Catecholamine levels tend to fall rapidly once normothermia is achieved and bypass is discontinued. It is clear that the level of anesthesia has a great influence on the surge of catecholamines associated with CPB and surgery. The anesthetic management of neonates has been shaped largely according to the findings of Anand and Hickey (62). High-dose narcotic induction and maintenance can result in reduction of catecholamine and reduce postoperative complications. There is a rise in serum cortisol following induction

of anesthesia and surgery. Following the onset of CPB, the cortisol levels fall secondary to hemodilution. After CPB, the level again begins to rise, and this continues for 24 hours, after which it gradually falls to normal. The effect of ultrafiltration on the levels of glucocorticoids is not known.

It appears that hypothermia and CPB result in a decrease in the level of insulin and also in a decreased peripheral response to the insulin. The net result is an increase in the serum glucose level. The level of insulin increases after reperfusion and rewarming (63). Glucagon and human growth hormone are released as part of the general stress response. Growth hormone is an anabolic hormone that tends to rise in both adults and children during and following CPB. A few studies show an increase in glucagon during the CPB period, and there is a clear gradual rise in glucagon levels after surgery that peaks at about 6 hours (14).

Thyroid hormones decrease during the CPB period and into the first several days following surgery (64,65). The reasons for this include hemodilution, decreased thyroid-binding globulin, and increased glucocorticoid levels. The lowest levels seem to be associated with a poor outcome. For this reason, the administration of triiodothyronine intravenously after CPB has been proposed to augment cardiac contractility. However, a controlled trial in adults failed to demonstrate a beneficial effect (66).

Renal Response

Renal dysfunction is an important cause of morbidity and mortality following CPB. The general stress of surgery results in a decrease in renal blood flow and the glomerular filtration rate secondary to central nervous system influences. Additionally, an increase in vasopressin release results in fluid accumulation. Cortical blood flow within the kidney is decreased in favor of medullary blood flow. The elevation of vasopressin may last for 48 to 72 hours after surgery (67). There is also an activation of the renin–angiotensin system with increased aldosterone production and fractional excretion of potassium. Hypothermia has been shown to decrease renal perfusion (27,31). A longer duration of CPB is a risk factor for injury, as is preoperative renal dysfunction and heart failure. It is not uncommon for temporary oliguric renal dysfunction to occur after neonatal heart surgery and generally improve by 24 to 48 hours after surgery. Placement of peritoneal dialysis catheters routinely at the time of cardiac surgery has been recommended by some in high-risk infants. However, once peritoneal dialysis is instituted after cardiac surgery, it has been our experience that native urinary output diminishes, related in part to decreases in the glomerular filtration rate as a result of reduced cardiac output, and we worry that this may further impair or delay the recovery of renal function. Because renal function generally returns to normal as cardiac function and systemic perfusion improve in the first 24 to 48 hours after bypass, the use of peritoneal dialysis following neonatal heart surgery should be reserved for those infants with severely impaired renal function.

Pulmonary Dysfunction

Pulmonary injury can be manifested in several ways, as the lungs have both a parenchymal and a vascular component. Parenchymal effects of CPB are reflected by alterations in pulmonary compliance, most commonly related to an increase in lung water. The impact of this on the patient is a requirement for increased ventilatory support and a diminished ability of the lungs to perform their function in gas exchange. Vascular effects are manifested by changes in pulmonary vascular resistance, which in turn affect the function of the right ventricle. The lungs are in a unique position in the circulation and may be vulnerable to different mechanisms of injury.

The multiple specialized cells within the lung include many cells of inflammation. The lung is an important source and target of the inflammatory response to CPB. Part of the pulmonary derangement that occurs is related to the inflammatory response to CPB (see below). This is manifested as decreased functional residual capacity, compliance, and gas exchange and increased pulmonary vascular resistance and pulmonary artery pressure.

However, inflammation is not the only factor causing impaired pulmonary function related to CPB. When patients are placed on bypass, the lungs undergo a sudden and significant decrease in perfusion via the pulmonary artery. During "total" bypass, the lungs receive only "nutrient" flow from their bronchial supply. This "ischemic" effect of CPB is added to its inflammatory effect to produce clinical pulmonary dysfunction (68). It seems that low-flow CPB produces worse pulmonary injury than does circulatory arrest (69,70), which suggests that the interaction between the inflammatory and ischemic components is complex. Both the inflammatory and ischemic factors damage the pulmonary endothelium (68,71–73). This leads to increases in post-CPB pulmonary vascular resistance and pulmonary artery pressure, both of which can have significant implications in neonates and small infants, especially following certain types of procedures, such as a Norwood procedure for hypoplastic left heart syndrome.

A number of ways to limit pulmonary dysfunction have been suggested. Some studies of liquid lung ventilation, in which a fluorocarbon solution was infused into the lungs before bypass, have shown that the antiinflammatory and O_2-carrying capabilities of this compound can have a dramatic effect on post-bypass pulmonary parenchymal and vascular function (74,75). The use of steroids at least 8 hours before exposure to CPB reduces the accumulation of lung water, improves post-CPB pulmonary compliance, and limits post-CPB pulmonary hypertension (76).

The pulmonary function of patients who undergo modified ultrafiltration following CPB seems to be greatly improved immediately in comparison with that of patients who do not undergo ultrafiltration (77–85). All this suggests that some significant advances can be made with respect to the pulmonary response to CPB.

Neurologic Injury

The very real incidence of neurologic injury (10% to 25% of patients in some series) (14,86–88) following infant cardiac repair has stimulated intensive investigation into the effects of CPB on the brain. Clearly, the neonate or infant with congenital heart disease is a patient at risk for neurologic impairment. This risk seems to be comprised of three elements: (a) *preexisting risk* associated with various congenital heart lesions, (b) injury induced by CPB and the various *CPB strategies* employed by the surgical team, and (c) injury sustained during the *"vulnerable"* period following exposure to CPB. When neurologic injury is manifested following CPB, it is often difficult to ascertain which of these elements has played the most prominent role, and indeed, it is often a combination of all three in some part that relates to clinically apparent neurologic injury.

The associated risk for abnormal neurologic development, even without exposure to CPB or without repair of the lesion, ranges from 2% to 10% for a variety of congenital heart lesions. This may relate to abnormal cerebral perfusion patterns or to actual associated structural anomalies within the brain. The cardiac defects of certain syndromes (e.g., complete atrioventricular septal defect in Down syndrome) are associated with an even higher incidence of abnormal brain development, irrespective of whether the patient is exposed to CPB. The natural history of neurologic development without cardiac surgery is not known and is impossible to obtain because several serious and life-threatening cardiac lesions (e.g., hypoplastic left heart syndrome) present in infancy, and surgery is required for survival. Nevertheless, available data suggest that cerebral flow patterns are extremely abnormal in these infants before they are placed on CPB. Finally, the condition of infants at the time they present with congenital heart disease can greatly affect their neurologic outcome (89). From all of this, it can be easily appreciated that patients with congenital heart disease comprise a group with a high inherent risk for neurologic abnormality following cardiac surgery (90).

The physiology of CPB produces many "alterations" that may be related to neurologic injury. During CPB, microembolic events occur commonly and can contribute significantly to end-organ injury (30,91). Air and particulate emboli have been demonstrated by middle cerebral artery transcranial Doppler, retinal angiography, and echocardiography. Direct evidence of air embolism is visualization of air in the coronary vessels, electrocardiographic changes of ST-segment elevation, and blanching of the skin of the head (55,92,93). Neurologic events have been correlated with the presence of focal dilatations of the microvasculature or very small aneurysms in terminal arterioles and capillaries within the cerebral circulation. The use of membrane oxygenators, arterial filters, and adequate heparinization (activated clotting time >400 s) during CPB decreases the number of microemboli and may reduce the incidence of embolic events (94–96). Yet despite these methods, air embolism remains an important factor in postoperative neurologic dysfunction. During pediatric CPB, the frequency with which the left side of the circulation is exposed to air increases the likelihood of systemic air embolization. In a recent report of perioperative neurologic effects in neonates undergoing the arterial switch operation for transposition of the great arteries, the presence of a ventricular septal defect was associated with an increased incidence of postoperative seizure activity (97). Although this may be related to longer periods of DHCA, the data also suggest a higher incidence of air embolism as a cause of neurologic dysfunction. When it occurs, cerebral air embolism can be treated by reducing gas bubble size, either by reestablishing hypothermic CPB or by using hyperbaric O_2 therapy in the early postoperative period (98). Major cerebral air embolism has also been treated with retrograde cerebral perfusion in adult patients, although experience with this modality in children is limited. Both hypothermia and hyperbaric therapy reduce the size of gaseous microbubbles and allow them to pass through the arterial and capillary beds, so that tissue damage is reduced.

Hypothermic Injury to the Brain

Early experience with deep hypothermia suggested that the use of extremely low temperatures (esophageal temperatures <10°C) caused a dramatic increase in neurologic and pulmonary injury. Neurologic sequelae, especially choreoathetosis, were commonly reported (99–101). Neuropathologic examination of the brain of animals undergoing profound levels of hypothermia revealed microvascular lesions compatible with the no-reflow phenomenon (102,103). Similar histologic brain lesions were observed in children who died after cardiac surgery in which circulatory arrest was used (104). These early reports diminished the enthusiasm for profound levels of hypothermia, and most institutions limited hypothermic temperatures to 18° to 20°C.

More recent, and probably more accurate, information suggests that some of these early fears were unfounded. Profound hypothermia does not seem to create cerebral injury (105), and in fact it may correlate with improved cerebral protection during periods of DHCA. However, the risk for injury can be affected by the type of blood gas management strategy used during DHCA (pH-stat vs. alpha-stat), the duration of the period of cooling, the duration of the period of DHCA, and the number of significant aortopulmonary collaterals (32,33,40–42,44,102,106–111). The lower limit at which hypothermia causes significant end-organ damage is not known. Current clinical practice suggests,

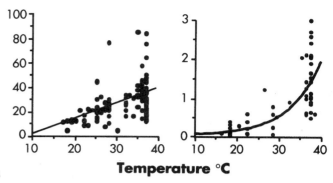

FIG. 30.4. A: Data obtained from patients based on xenon clearance methodology showing that cerebral blood flow (*CBF*) decreases in a linear fashion with decreasing temperature. (From Greeley WJ, Ungerleider RM, Kern FH, et al. Effects of cardiopulmonary bypass on cerebral blood flow in neonates, infants, and children. *Circulation* 1989;80:1209–1215, with permission.) **B:** The cerebral metabolic rate of O_2 (*CMRo$_2$*) decreases exponentially with temperature reduction such that cerebral metabolism is extremely low, but still present, at 18°C. (From Kern FH, Greeley WJ, Ungerleider RM. The effects of bypass on the developing brain. *Perfusion* 1993;8:49–54, with permission.)

however, that temperatures of 15°C and below are probably no worse than temperatures of 18° to 20°C, so long as appropriate hemodilution is used.

It is now well recognized that the relationship between decreases in cerebral blood flow and decreases in temperature is *linear*, whereas cerebral *metabolism* is reduced exponentially as temperature is decreased (Fig. 30.4). This accounts for most of the cerebral protection afforded the brain by cooling, as cerebral metabolic needs for O_2 are significantly lowered and cerebral blood flow becomes "luxurious." Nevertheless, cerebral metabolism persists, even at very low temperatures, and the brain is therefore susceptible to ischemic injury despite hypothermia if cerebral blood flow is eliminated (e.g., in DHCA).

During the past decade, much has been learned about the effects of DHCA on the brain. Although it was felt for years that DHCA was potentially detrimental to the neurologic outcome, the advantages of DHCA made it a very attractive CPB strategy, especially for complex repairs or almost any intracardiac repair in infants. In general, it was believed that the likelihood of DHCA resulting in neurologic impairment was "small" if the DHCA period could be kept under 45 minutes at 18°C (14) (Fig. 30.5). The perception that the potential for injury from DHCA was related to the duration of the DHCA appears to be accurate (99,112,113). However, the type of information displayed in Fig. 30.6 creates a misperception that the neurologic risk of DHCA occurs primarily when the duration of the arrest period extends beyond some minimal time period. In a series of clinical studies performed between 1988 and 1991 (15,114–116), Greeley and colleagues described an interesting pattern of blood flow and metabolic recovery observed

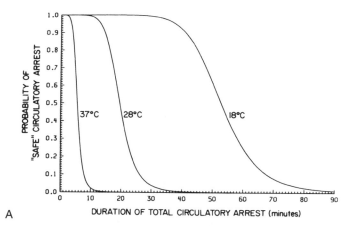

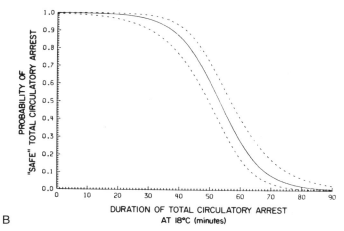

A

B

FIG. 30.5. A: The probability of "safe" circulatory arrest is related to the duration of arrest and to the temperature at which it occurs. **B:** At 18°C, the likelihood of neurologic injury becomes exponentially greater beyond 45 minutes. (From Kirklin JW, Barratt-Boyes BG. *Cardiac surgery*, 2nd ed. New York: Churchill Livingston, 1993, with permission.)

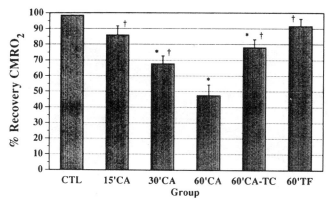

FIG. 30.6. Impairment of the recovery of the cerebral metabolic rate of O$_2$ (*CMR*o$_2$) after deep hypothermic circulatory arrest (*DHCA*) is greater [in comparison with control (*CTL*) animals exposed to hypothermic cardiopulmonary bypass without arrest] with longer times of DHCA. This metabolic impairment can be ameliorated by packing the head in ice (*60′ CA-TC*) or by using continuous trickle flow (*60′ TF*) for a 60-minute period of DHCA. *p <0.05 vs. CTL; †p <0.05 vs. 60′ CA. (From Mault JR, Ohtake S, Klingensmith ME, et al. Cerebral metabolism and circulatory arrest: effects of duration and strategies for protection. *Ann Thorac Surg* 1993;55:57–63, with permission.)

in the brains of patients exposed to varying periods of DHCA in comparison with the brains of "control" patients exposed to deep hypothermia without circulatory arrest. They observed that cerebral blood flow and cerebral metabolism (CMRo$_2$) failed to return to normal, pre-bypass levels in patients exposed to DHCA, whereas in those patients not exposed to DHCA, cerebral blood flow and CMRo$_2$ recovered to normal levels. Impairment of CMRo$_2$ appeared to be an excellent "marker" for cerebral injury from DHCA. In a complementary series of laboratory experiments, the same group described the relationship of duration of DHCA and degree of impairment to CMRo$_2$ recovery, and the relationship appeared to be linear (106) (Fig. 30.7). These data suggest that DHCA produces a "dose-dependent" injury. Current investigation is helpful in identifying practical strategies that the surgical team can employ to lessen the effects of prolonged DHCA, but duration of DHCA remains the factor with the most influence on out-

come. Simply packing the head in ice (topical cooling, or TC) or providing some small amount of continuous flow (trickle flow, or TF), for example, can greatly diminish the impact of duration on the metabolic recovery of the brain (106) (Fig. 30.6). It is possible to predict the amount of

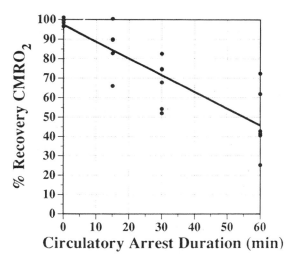

FIG. 30.7. At 18°C, the metabolic impairment seen following a period of deep hypothermic circulatory arrest (*DHCA*) is related in a linear fashion to the *duration* of DHCA (r^2 = 0.73):

Percentage Recovery CMRo$_2$ = (-0.86 × CA Duration) + 97

(From Mault JR, Ohtake S, Klingensmith ME, et al. Cerebral metabolism and circulatory arrest: effects of duration and strategies for protection. *Ann Thorac Surg* 1993;55:57–63, with permission.)

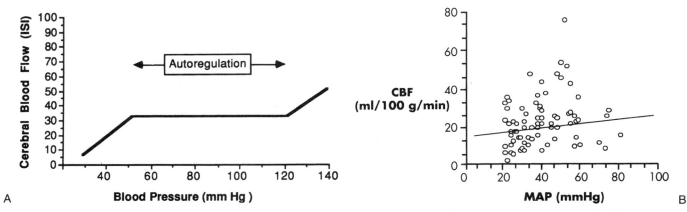

FIG. 30.8. A: Cerebral blood flow is "autoregulated" throughout a wide range of pressures in the normal adult patient. (From Venn GE. Cerebral vascular autoregulation during cardiopulmonary bypass. *Perfusion* 1989;4:105, with permission.) **B:** Data from human infants based on xenon clearance methodology demonstrate that "autoregulation" of cerebral blood flow also exists in pediatric patients at moderate hypothermia (temperatures >25°C). CBF, cerebral blood flow; MAP, mean arterial pressure. (From Kern FH, Greeley WJ, Ungerleider RM. Cardiopulmonary bypass. In: Nichols DG, Cameron DE, Greeley WJ, et al., eds. *Critical heart disease in infants and children.* St. Louis: Mosby, 1995:497–530, with permission.)

blood flow required to support cerebral metabolic needs at decreasing temperatures, and this is the rationale behind continuous low-perfusion CPB (5,16,38) (Table 30.3).

Cerebral blood flow is regulated by several controllable parameters. Although cerebral blood flow seems to be "autoregulated" at normothermic and moderately hypothermic temperatures (8,9,117,118) (Fig. 30.8), autoregulation is lost at temperatures below 22°C (15,114–116) (Fig. 30.9), and cerebral flow is more dependent on mean arterial pressure. Fortunately, at these cold temperatures, the brain needs very little blood flow (16). The acid–base strategy employed during cooling also affects cerebral blood flow and metabolism. Alpha-stat is more commonly used throughout the country, but enthusiasm has recently been expressed by some centers for more routine use of pH-stat strategies (34,35). CO_2 added to the CPB circuit during cooling (pH-stat) is a potent cerebral vasodilator. Its addition to the circuit significantly increases blood flow to the brain (32,119). Although this might promote more homogeneous cerebral cooling, the addition of CO_2, especially at temperatures below 15°C, creates significant acidosis (pH <6.9) in the circulating blood. This acidosis at the time of circulatory arrest may be the reason for substantial impairment in cerebral metabolic recovery in animals subjected to these conditions experimentally (32). However, if pH-stat methodology is used during cooling and then the added CO_2 is removed from the circuit (i.e., the patient is returned to alpha-stat, or temperature-"uncorrected" blood gas management) before DHCA is established, the acidotic effects of pH-stat with respect to cerebral metabolic recovery appear to be alleviated (33).

One group of patients that seems to be at increased risk for neurologic injury, especially choreoathetosis, is the

group with significant aortopulmonary collateral vessels (e.g., older, cyanotic patients) (42,120). This has been demonstrated in an elegant experimental model by Kirshbom et al. (40,41), which also demonstrated how utilization of pH-stat cooling protected the brains of these particular animals (44). It is important to note, however, that neither alpha-stat nor pH-stat protects the brain from significant structural or metabolic derangement following prolonged periods of DHCA. The types of damage induced with either strategy are indistinguishable (107).

It seems that the surgical team can do several practical things to limit injury from DHCA. Intravenous methylprednisolone (10 mg/kg) given at least 8 hours before CPB exposure significantly improves cerebral metabolic response to DHCA (Langley et al., unpublished data from our laboratory, submitted for presentation). There is also evidence that aprotinin (121), thromboxane A_2 receptor blockade (122), platelet-activating factor inhibitors, and free radical scavengers may improve cerebral recovery following DHCA, but none of the above, except for aprotinin, is currently clinically useful, and aprotinin has potential side effects that limit its use. The recognition of high-risk groups (patients with severe cyanosis, substantial aortopulmonary collateral vessels) might prompt the utilization of pH-stat cooling, although we recommend a switch to alpha-stat before DHCA is induced. It is important to cool for at least 20 minutes to promote adequate cerebral metabolic suppression. Patients cooled for less time are more likely to sustain brain injury (15,108–111,123,124). If measurement of jugular venous hemoglobin O_2 saturations is available, then this value can be used to guide the duration of DHCA. It is probably unwise to use prolonged periods of DHCA if the jugular venous hemoglobin O_2 saturation re-

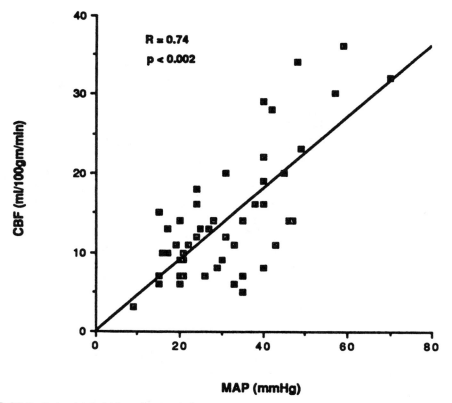

FIG. 30.9. Data obtained from human infants demonstrate that cerebral "autoregulation" is lost at deep hypothermia (temperature <22°C), with cerebral blood flow (*CBF*) related in a linear manner to mean arterial pressure (*MAP*). (From Greeley WJ, Kern FH, Ungerleider RM, et al. The effect of hypothermic cardiopulmonary bypass and total circulatory arrest on cerebral metabolism in neonates, infants, and children. *J Thorac Cardiovasc Surg* 1991;101:783–794, with permission.)

mains below 95% (15,111). If continuous low-flow CPB can be used, this might afford better cerebral protection, although the effects of continuous low-flow perfusion on the lung and the microvasculature might be deleterious in comparison with DHCA (69,70). DHCA should be used only for the period of time necessary for the patient to benefit from its advantages, as brain injury does seem to be related to the duration of the arrest period (106,112,113,125,126). Perhaps the most exciting and practical information for the surgical team was recently provided by Langley et al. (107) and Mault et al. (127), who demonstrated that periods of DHCA of up to 60 minutes can be associated with absolutely normal recovery of cerebral metabolism and preservation of neural microarchitecture if the brain is simply perfused from the pump for 1 minute (50 mL/kg per minute) every 15 to 20 minutes. This means that sequential periods of DHCA can be utilized by the surgical team so long as they are not prolonged beyond 15 to 20 minutes. If the brain is perfused between periods of DHCA, the durations of the DHCA periods are not additive (128). Similar findings have been alluded to by Miura et al. (129) and Robbins et al. (130). During the period of DHCA, the head should be packed in ice (106). Although

little can be done during reperfusion to improve cerebral recovery (123), the use of modified ultrafiltration following weaning from CPB does seem to improve recovery of cerebral metabolism (85,131). Of equal importance following DHCA, cardiac output and cerebral O_2 delivery should be maintained, as this is the period when the brain is most "vulnerable" to injury (132–134). Recent information suggests that the brain might be better protected following DHCA if the patient is removed from CPB at rectal temperatures of 34°C, as opposed to 36°C or warmer (135). There is also a suggestion by some that cerebral protection is improved with the use of higher hematocrits (30% vs. 20%) during hypothermic bypass.

Systemic Inflammatory Response

The systemic inflammatory response to CPB is indeed multifaceted. It involves a complex interaction of many systems and cellular elements in the body, all of which are, teleologically, normal responses to noxious stimuli. It is important to consider the biochemical events and pathways not individually but as a complex interaction with regulatory and counterregulatory effects. With the exposure of the blood to foreign surfaces of the circuit and oxygenator, the initiating event appears to be contact activation of the blood elements. Other factors, including tissue ischemia and reperfusion, hypotension with nonpulsatile perfusion, relative anemia, and administration of blood products, heparin, and protamine, may also play a role in the inflammatory response to CPB. One of the initial responses is complement activation (136). The complement system is composed of more than 30 different proteins. It appears that the alternate pathway of activation is the most important in CPB. This results in the formation of C3a and C5a (14), which are important anaphylatoxins, chemotactic agents for neutrophils, and inflammatory mediators, followed in turn by the production of other cytokines and the activation of cellular elements, such as macrophages and platelets. Complement also has intrinsic lytic properties (137–140). The next major step in the process is neutrophil activation and the neutrophil–endothelial cell interaction, which can cause direct tissue injury and the elaboration of many toxic substances, including other cytokines. Neutrophils probably play a major role in the ischemia–reperfusion injury associated with pulmonary and neurologic injury. Complement activation also results in the elaboration of many different cytokines from monocytes, macrophages, and endothelial cells. These cytokines mediate many of the inflammatory reactions, some regulatory (tumor necrosis factor, interleukin-1, IL-6, IL-8, and LPS) (141) and some counterregulatory (IL-4 and IL-10). The cytokines have been associated with CPB, and levels have been shown to increase with the duration of bypass (142). CPB is also a very procoagulant stimulus. Heparin inhibits the formation of clot; however, it does not prevent the expression of tissue factor on endothelial cells. Tissue factor results in the production of thrombin, which by itself has significant inflammatory and thrombotic properties (143). It appears that initially following CPB, a relative thrombolytic state exists. However, shortly thereafter, a hypercoagulable state prevails, which predisposes patients to some of the major venous (or shunt) thromboses occasionally seen following neonatal operations. Arachidonic acid pathway activation also occurs in cells that are irritated or ischemic, especially in the lung. This results in production of thromboxanes, leukotrienes, and prostaglandins. Endothelial injury results in altered microcirculatory function, which is responsible for elevations in pulmonary, cerebral, and systemic vascular resistance—a common finding after hypothermic CPB. Endothelial injury impairs the release of important vasodilators, such as nitric oxide and prostacyclin, and promotes the release of vasoconstrictors such as thromboxane A_2 and endothelin (also known to have inotropic effects in the myocardium) (144–146). The endothelial surface (pulmonary endothelium in particular) is also responsible for the metabolism of vasoconstrictors such as angiotensin, catecholamines, and eicosanoids (147). Injured endothelium, by virtue of reduced production of nitric oxide and impaired metabolism of mediators of vaso-

dilation, promotes vasoconstriction (68,71,73,147). Endothelial cells also play an important regulatory role in water and solute transport. Abnormalities in endothelial function promote increased capillary permeability and increases in interstitial edema (148).

The worst responses are at the extremes of age, the very young and the very old. In infants and neonates, the response is characterized by post-bypass acute respiratory distress syndrome, pulmonary hypertension, total body edema, coagulation abnormalities, myocardial dysfunction, and hemodynamic instability. These adverse sequelae translate into prolonged ventilation, prolonged inotropic support, renal dysfunction, bleeding and later thrombosis, inability to close the chest in the operating room, and potentially the need for mechanical support after cardiotomy. In particular, the pulmonary injury seems to be quite profound and is a major source of morbidity. Injury to the lungs results in increased pulmonary vascular resistance and loss of endothelium-dependent pulmonary vasorelaxation. This is likely a neutrophil-mediated injury produced by ischemia–reperfusion.

Potential areas of therapeutic intervention include: heparin-bonded circuits to prevent contact activation; circuit miniaturization to reduce priming volumes and oxygenator exposure; DHCA, which seems to limit the duration of CPB exposure and is associated with less post-bypass edema (69,70); anticytokine or anti-adhesion molecule therapy; simple leukocyte depletion; serine protease inhibition; modified ultrafiltration; and antiinflammatory agents.

Corticosteroids have been used for many years with CPB. Steroids affect the inflammatory process at many levels. They may reduce complement activation and decrease complement-mediated neutrophil adhesion and degranulation. They may act to inhibit the release of some cytokines and to promote the release of others. They decrease the production of acute-phase reactants and decrease the production of antibody. The more powerful effects of steroids occur through inhibition of the signal transduction pathways within cells. This results in the decreased production of messenger RNA for the protein synthesis of inflammatory mediators and cellular products of inflammation. Because some of these processes take time, it is not surprising that the administration of high doses of steroids several hours before the patient is exposed to CPB effects a more significant reduction in the inflammatory response than does administration in the pump prime (immediately on exposure to CPB) or no administration at all (76) (Fig. 30.10).

In the not-so-distant past, mortality rates in pediatric cardiac surgery depended mostly on the technical ability of surgeons. With improved bypass techniques and pediatric critical care and cardiology in addition to surgical technical advances, the mortality rates have decreased markedly during the last 10 years. There still remain, however, the adverse inflammatory effects of CPB and the occasional severe inflammatory responses that add significantly to perioperative

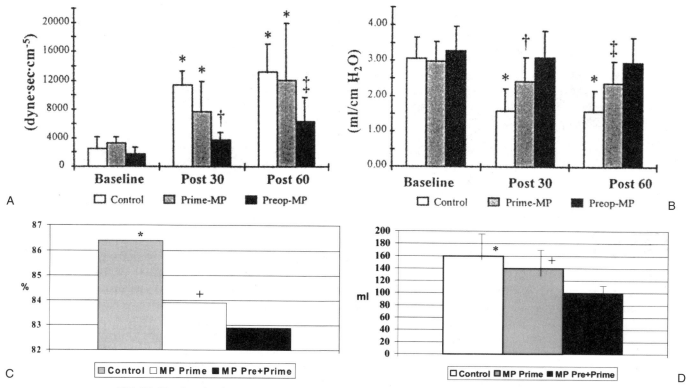

FIG. 30.10. Graphs demonstrating the effect of high-dose steroids administered at least 8 hours before exposure to cardiopulmonary bypass (*CPB*) versus steroids in the pump prime only or no steroids at all on pulmonary vascular resistance **(A)**, pulmonary compliance **(B)**, total lung water accumulation (lung water in a normal piglet not exposed to CPB is 82%) (*p = 0.001 vs. preop-mp; †p = 0.026 vs. preop-mp) **(C)**, and total body water accumulation (*p = 0.003 vs. preop-mp; †p = 0.01 vs. preop-mp) **(D)**. [From Lodge AJ, Chai PJ, Daggett CW, et al. The use of corticosteroids to reduce post-CPB inflammatory syndrome in neonates: impact of dose timing. *J Thorac Cardiovasc Surg* (*in press*), with permission.]

morbidity and mortality. Because of explosions in knowledge by so many investigators in this area, the entire process of the whole body inflammatory response seems considerably more complex than it did several years ago. Once the molecular mechanisms of inflammation have been unraveled, improved outcomes after repair of the most complex of congenital cardiac defects will be realized.

THE PEDIATRIC EXTRACORPOREAL CIRCUIT

Prime

The trend in modern pediatric bypass equipment is to reduce the size of the extracorporeal circuit to reduce the prime volume. The priming volume may actually exceed the blood volume of a neonate by as much as 200% to 300%, whereas in an adult patient, the priming volume accounts for only 25% to 33% of the blood volume. Recently, with the development of smaller tubing and oxygenators, it has been possible to reduce the priming volume significantly.

High priming volume can produce a low (<15%) hematocrit on CPB in small infants. This mandates the use of donor blood in the prime. What constitutes the lowest acceptable hematocrit is debated, but it is generally considered to be between 15% and 20%. The use of donor blood has several disadvantages, including transmission of viral particles; complement activation; induction of a transfusion reaction; lactate, potassium, and glucose infusion; and CPD (citrate–phosphate–dextrose) infusion (149,150). Hemodilution during CPB results in reductions in plasma proteins and clotting factors, decreases in colloid osmotic pressure (resulting in increased interstitial edema), electrolyte imbalance, and an exaggerated release of stress hormones, with activation of complement, white blood cells, and platelets. For these reasons, priming volumes should be kept to a minimum and transfusions avoided as much as possible. Blood viscosity increases as temperature is lowered. Hematocrits of 40% coupled with hypothermia and the nonpulsatile flow of CPB impairs blood flow through the microcirculation (31). The optimal level of hemodilution during pediatric CPB is based on providing adequate O_2 delivery at hypothermic temperatures and during rewarming. Hematocrits as low as 10% appear to provide adequate O_2 delivery during hypothermic CPB. During rewarming, however, when the O_2 demand rises, such low hematocrits may be insufficient to meet the body's recovering metabolic needs (151–153). Cerebral O_2 delivery is an especially important consideration because cerebral autoregulation is impaired at deep hypothermic temperatures in infants (15) and after DHCA. In neonates undergoing deep hypothermic CPB (15° to 20°C), a hematocrit of 20% ± 2% is generally targeted; however, hematocrits as low as 15% are sometimes considered acceptable. The following formula estimates the amount of red blood cells that must be added to achieve a target hematocrit of 20%:

$$RBC_{added} (cm^3) =$$
$$(BV_{pt} + TPV) (Hct_{desired}) - (BV_{pt}) (Hct_{pt})$$

where RBC_{added} is the packed red blood cells in cubic centimeters added to the prime volume, BV_{pt} is the patient's blood volume (80% to 85% of body weight in infants), TPV is the total priming volume, $Hct_{desired}$ is the desired hematocrit on CPB, and Hct_{pt} is the starting hematocrit of the patient.

Most institutions use packed red blood cells in their priming solutions. However, some institutions substitute whole blood. The advantage of adding whole blood to the priming solution is that it maintains colloid oncotic pressure and increases the level of circulating clotting factors. The disadvantage of a whole blood prime is a much higher glucose content in the priming solution. Hyperglycemia is a risk factor for neurologic injury in the presence of cerebral ischemia. Whole blood may also be used following CPB when priming with blood is avoided. This preserves much of the clotting factor and platelet functions of the donor blood and also increases the hematocrit. Fresh whole blood has the added advantage of being beneficial for hemostasis.

The addition of colloid to the prime increases the protein content and therefore the oncotic pressure of the perfusate. This may prevent some capillary leak of fluid and result in improved organ function following CPB. Alternatively, whole blood may be used as part of the priming solution. Reduction in the plasma protein concentration has been shown experimentally to impair lymphatic flow and alter pulmonary function by increasing capillary leak. Although studies in adults have not demonstrated any advantage to adding albumin to pump prime, one study has suggested that maintaining normal colloid osmotic pressure may improve survival in infants undergoing CPB (154,155).

Pediatric priming solutions contain variable levels of electrolytes, buffer [sodium bicarbonate or tromethamine (THAM)], calcium, glucose, and lactate. Electrolytes, glucose, and lactate levels may be quite high if the prime includes large amounts of stored blood, or quite low if a minimal amount of bank blood is added. Calcium levels are generally very low in priming solutions, and this may ac-

count for the rapid slowing of the heart with the initiation of bypass. Primes low in calcium are generally preferred because of the potentially deleterious effects of ionized calcium during periods of ischemic arrest (20). Buffer is added to maintain a physiologic pH. Controversial supplementary additives included in pediatric priming solutions include mannitol and steroids. Mannitol is added to promote an osmotic diuresis and to scavenge oxygen free radicals from the circulation. Steroids are added to reduce ion shifts during periods of ischemia, reduce the inflammatory response and capillary leak, and decrease secondary injury after a period of ischemia.

Oxygenators

In the pediatric population, oxygenators must provide efficient gas exchange over a wide range of temperatures (10° to 40°C), pump flow rates (0 to 200 mL/kg per minute), hematocrits (15% to 30%), line pressures, and gas flow rates. Both bubble and membrane oxygenators can achieve effective gas exchange under these diverse conditions. Bubble oxygenators allow fresh gas, in the form of microbubbles, to mix directly with circulating blood in an oxygenating column. The direct interface of blood and gas is traumatic to blood cellular elements, causing an increase in red blood cell hemolysis, platelet microaggregation, complement activation, and release of mediators of the inflammatory response (156–159). These undesirable effects are minimized with the use of membrane oxygenators.

The membrane oxygenator acts as a synthetic alveolar–capillary membrane; a direct interface between blood and fresh gas is minimized or absent. Most membrane oxygenators used for CPB are composed of microporous hollow fibers. A microporous membrane contains pores 3 to 5 μm in size, which allows for minimal contact between blood and gas. The advantage of micropores is improved gas exchange with a smaller total membrane surface area. The disadvantage is that if negative pressure develops on the blood side of the membrane, gas emboli can be entrained into the blood, resulting in gas embolization in the arterial blood of the patient.

Examples of microporous hollow fiber membrane oxygenators used for pediatric CPB include the COBE VPCML, Dideco Miniflow, Dideco Lilliput 1 and 2, Medtronic Minimax, Terumo Capiox II, and the newer COBE Micro (Table 30.5). These oxygenators attempt to minimize priming volume and provide effective gas exchange for the pediatric patient. The COBE VPCML, Dideco Miniflow, Terumo Capiox, and Medtronic Minimax allow for lower priming volumes (50 to 140 mL).

Newer devices such as the COBE Micro and Dideco Lilliput 1 have been designed to be an exclusive neonatal oxygenator. The heat exchanger–oxygenator module requires a priming volume of just 60 mL, and the device includes a volume control reservoir system with a maximum

TABLE 30.5. COMPARISON OF PEDIATRIC OXYGENATORS

Membrane Oxygenators	Prime Volume (mL)	Maximum Flow Rate (mL/min)
Dideco Miniflow	140	4,500
Dideco Lilliput 1	60	800
Medtronic Minimax	140	1,500
Terumo Capiox II	80	1,000
COBE Micro	52	800

TABLE 30.6. CARDIOPULMONARY BYPASS CIRCUIT RECOMMENDATIONS

Weight Range (kg)	Boot Size (ID)	Arterial Line (ID)	Venous Line (ID)
0–3	3/16	3/16	3/16
3–5	3/16	3/16	1/4
6–10	1/4	1/4	1/4
11–15	1/4	1/4	3/8
16–30	3/8	1/4	3/8
31–50	3/8	3/8	3/8
>50	3/8	3/8	1/2

kg, kilograms; ID, internal diameter (in inches).

priming volume of 90 mL. Despite the low oxygenator priming volumes, recommended flow rates of 800 mL/min are achievable. This would allow perfusion flow rates of 150 mL/kg in neonates and young infants up to 5.3 kg. In conjunction with reduced tubing length and more thoughtful system designs, the COBE and Lilliput devices may allow total prime volumes of 250 mL to be achieved (159).

A third type of membrane oxygenator is composed of nonporous silicone rubber and is arranged in folded sheets. Silicone rubber membrane oxygenators are more expensive and require a larger surface area for gas exchange than do microporous membrane oxygenators. Oxygenators with silicone membranes provide no clear advantage for short-term perfusion, but they are the only membrane oxygenators recommended for long-term perfusion, such as extracorporeal membrane oxygenator (ECMO) support. (See Chapter 31).

Pumps

Two types of pumps are currently used for CPB: roller pumps and centrifugal pumps. Roller pumps, the most widely used type in pediatric perfusion, consist of two rollers oriented 180 degrees from each other. They provide continuous blood flow by partially occluding the tubing between the roller and the pump casing. Blood is displaced in a forward direction by the roller, resulting in continuous, nonpulsatile flow. The second roller acts as a valve to minimize backward flow. The rollers are never totally occlusive because that would promote hemolysis. Ideally, the occlusion for each roller should be set independently of the other. This is especially true in neonatal and infant perfusion, in which maladjustment of occlusion can result in a higher percentage of error in estimating pump flow rate and an increase in red cell hemolysis.

Centrifugal pumps are newer devices that have gained increasing acceptance because of the experience gained during ECMO and ventricular assist cases. Flow is maintained by the entrainment of blood against spinning impellers (curved blades) or by the creation of a vortex with a centrifugal cone. The advantages of centrifugal pumps include a reduced priming volume, less damage to formed blood elements, and the concept that vortex design may assist in air removal (160). These pumps are also capable of producing pulsatile blood flow, which may improve flow in the microcirculation. An example of this type is the Biomedicus pump. (See Chapter 3).

Tubing

Tubing sizes should be kept as small as possible to reduce prime volume, but they must be large enough to achieve effective flow rates and low line pressure. Both the length and the diameter of the tubing contribute to prime volume. In neonates, 3/16-in internal diameter (ID) tubing is used for the arterial and 1/4-in tubing for the venous limbs of the circuit. Tube length is kept as short as possible by positioning the pump close to the surgical field. The 1/4-in ID tubing requires approximately 30 mL of volume per meter of tube length. A 3.5-kg newborn, for example, has a blood volume of approximately 300 mL. Each meter of tubing therefore requires an increase in prime volume equal to 10% of the newborn's circulating blood volume. Moving the pump heads closer to the patient, and the use of vacuum-controlled rather than gravity-siphon venous drainage, can significantly reduce tubing length and priming volume. Table 30.6 represents current recommendations regarding patient weight versus tubing diameter. Overall, prime volume increases as the diameter and length of tubing increases. Tubing diameter for the circuit should be chosen to provide the maximal flow with a minimum of prime volume (Tables 30.7 and 30.8).

TABLE 30.7. APPROXIMATE PRIME VOLUME PER LENGTH OF TUBING

Tubing (ID)	Volume per Length (mL/ft)	Estimated Total for 6 ft (mL)
3/16	5	30
1/4	9.65	57.9
3/8	21.7	130.4
1/2	38.6	232

ID, internal diameter (in inches).

TABLE 30.8. MAXIMAL FLOW RATES

Tubing Size (ID)	Maximum Arterial Flow Rate (mL/min)	Maximum Venous Return Rate (mL/min)
3/16	<1,300	500–650
1/4	<3,000	1,200–1,600
3/8	>5,000	4,000–4,500
1/2	>5,000	>5,000

ID, internal diameter (in inches).

Cardiotomy Circuit

The cardiotomy circuit is used to suction blood from the field and return it to the patient's circulation. It requires its own reservoir, roller pump, and filters. Suction tubing from the cardiotomy circuit can be attached to suckers, which are used in the operative field, or to aortic, atrial, or ventricular vents. Once collected, the blood is drained into a venous reservoir, which can then be added to the venous inflow of the oxygenator. The size of the venous reservoir and the efficiency of its filtering system also contribute to prime volume.

Cannulas

Cannulas must be flexible and durable enough to maintain their shape and flow characteristics despite rapid changes in temperature and pressure and the operative manipulation required during hypothermic CPB. In neonates and infants, the aortic cannula tip needs to be small to facilitate insertion into a tiny aorta and not impede the normal flow of aortic blood around the cannula. Maintaining flow around the cannula is particularly important before initiation of CPB and after weaning from CPB, when it can significantly impede aortic outflow in small infants. Adequate perfusion flow rates must be attainable at relatively low perfusion pressures. Excessive pressure in the cannula tip may create a powerful jet of blood, which can damage the intima of the aorta and blood cellular elements.

Arterial Cannulation

The arterial cannula is generally placed into the ascending aorta; however, the great vessel anatomy of the patient and the type of surgical procedure may influence arterial cannula placement. For example, in hypoplastic left heart syndrome, the ascending aorta is 1 to 5 mm in size, which is too small to accommodate a cannula capable of providing systemic perfusion. As an alternative, the arterial cannula is placed in the main pulmonary artery. Systemic perfusion is maintained from the pulmonary artery through the ductus arteriosus and down the descending aorta. Coronary perfusion is retrograde through the hypoplastic ascending aorta. The right and left pulmonary arteries are occluded with snares

to prevent excessive perfusion of the pulmonary vascular bed. In newborns with transposition of the great arteries, the arterial cannula is placed in a more distal aspect of the ascending aorta because a large portion of the surgery is performed on the aortic root. Infants with interrupted aortic arch require two aortic cannulas—one in the ascending aorta to perfuse the head vessels and one in the descending aorta to perfuse the body. Cannulation of the femoral artery is not commonly used in neonatal or infant heart surgery because the femoral vessels are too small. In older children requiring reoperation, sternotomy is associated with a high risk of inadvertently entering a conduit or a ventricular chamber. In these patients, femoral or iliac arterial cannulation should be considered. The choice of cannula size depends not only on the lesion but also on the size of the patient.

Problems with aortic cannula placement are possible in neonates and infants. The position of the aortic cannula may promote preferential flow down the aorta or induce a Venturi effect, in which flow is stolen from the cerebral circulation. This problem has been suggested during xenon cerebral blood flow monitoring by the identification of large discrepancies in cerebral blood flow between the right and left hemispheres after initiation of CPB (111). Placement of the aortic cannula in a more distal location, commonly used in procedures in which ascending aorta or proximal aortic arch reconstruction is required (e.g., arterial switch procedure), may play a role in altering brain blood flow. Cooling patterns are substantially different in neonates and infants from those generally observed in adults or older children (43). The surgical team should be notified if the rectal temperature does not fall as quickly as the nasopharyngeal temperature. This might indicate a significant aortic obstruction from the cannula or even a native coarctation. Delayed rectal cooling is also noted in patients who present with low cardiac output resulting from increased peripheral vascular resistance. When this pattern is present, it might be reasonable to avoid prolonged periods of DHCA, as significant abnormalities in the pattern of cooling might indicate regions that would be suboptimally protected. Patients with large left-to-right shunts into the pulmonary bed might have an increase in the amount of shunted blood as cooling proceeds (161). If the nasopharyngeal temperature does not fall as fast as the rectal temperatures, there should be some concern regarding the degree of cerebral cooling, and strategies involving prolonged exposure to DHCA may need to be revised (15,107).

Venous Cannulation

Venous anatomy can be very complex. Bilateral superior venae cavae, inferior venae cavae that drain into an azygos vein or hemiazygous vein, or hepatic veins that drain directly into an atrial chamber are common anatomic variations in the venous systems of patients with congenital cardiac defects. Venous cannulation must account for these variables if the repair is to take place during continuous-flow CPB.

If the repair is going to take place under DHCA, CPB is used as a cooling modality. The repair occurs during the arrest period. Venous cannulation can therefore be simplified. A large single venous cannula is placed in the right atrium to achieve effective venous drainage. Once cooling has occurred, the cannulas are removed and surgery proceeds in a cannula-free field. In contrast, repairs performed during continuous flow must address the complex venous anatomy. This is particularly true in heterotaxic patients with a single ventricle, in whom bilateral superior venae cavae are commonly found.

In the repair of defects associated with anomalies of systemic venous return, three venous cannulas may be required. Venous drainage is more effective and the cannulas are less obtrusive in the surgical field if right-angle venous cannulas are used. The inferior vena cava (IVC) is cannulated with a short right-angle cannula, which is inserted below the pericardial reflection. A short cannula avoids placing the cannula tip beyond the hepatic veins and causing hepatic venous obstruction. A third venous cannula may be required if a large left superior vena cava (SVC) with no bridging innominate vein is present. It is often easiest to place this cannula after the patient is on CPB. The venous tubing circuit can be constructed for these patients in a manner that will accommodate the addition of a third venous cannula.

To meet the surgical requirements, a large assortment of venous cannulas should be available. The type of venous cannula used and the amount of venous return it yields will vary depending on cannula size, patient anatomy, site of insertion, and adequacy of cannula position.

Appropriate placement of venous cannulas is important in achieving effective systemic perfusion. A poorly positioned venous cannula has the potential to cause vena caval obstruction. This may result in cerebral venous or splanchnic congestion. The problems of venous obstruction are magnified during CPB because of low perfusion pressures, particularly in neonates. Large, relatively stiff venous cannulas easily distort the very pliable great veins, and the use of such cannulas should be avoided.

A cannula in the IVC can obstruct venous return from the splanchnic bed, resulting in ascites from increased hydrostatic pressure, or it can directly reduce perfusion pressure across the mesenteric, renal, and hepatic vascular beds. Significant renal, hepatic, and gastrointestinal dysfunction may ensue and should be anticipated in the patient with unexplained ascites after weaning from CPB. Similarly, obstruction of the SVC is possible. This problem can elevate jugular venous pressure, decrease cerebral perfusion pressure, and cause cerebral edema. In the operating room, monitoring the SVC pressures directly via an internal jugular line or looking at the patient's head for signs of increased puffiness or venous distension after initiation of bypass may be ways to detect systemic venous congestion. Discussions

with the perfusionist regarding the adequacy of venous return should alert the anesthesiologist and the surgeon to potential venous cannula problems.

Initiation of Cardiopulmonary Bypass

Once the aortic and venous cannulas are positioned and connected to the arterial and venous limbs of the extracorporeal circuit, bypass is initiated. The technique for initiating bypass varies depending on the size of the patient and the temperature of the perfusate. In older children and adolescents, bypass is initiated slowly. The venous line is unclamped, and blood is siphoned from the right atrium into the oxygenator by gravity drainage. The rate at which venous blood is drained from the patient is determined by the difference in height between the patient and the oxygenator reservoir inlet, and by the diameter of the venous cannula and line tubing. Increasing the difference in height between the oxygenator and the patient can enhance venous drainage. Venous drainage can be reduced either by decreasing the difference in height between the reservoir and the patient or by partially clamping the venous line. Some groups have advocated collecting from the patient 20 mL of whole blood per kilogram immediately after institution of CPB, to be infused after completion of the repair and when the patient has been weaned from CPB. This, in theory, returns functional platelets and clotting factors back to the patient and aids in hemostasis and stability. More recently, a system of assisted venous drainage has been developed in which negative pressure is applied to the venous reservoir and blood is actively evacuated from the atria. This may allow for decreased priming volumes and reduced sizes of venous cannulas. The immediate effects of negative pressure on blood components have not, however, been fully explored.

Once venous blood begins to accumulate in the reservoir, the arterial pump is slowly started. Its speed is gradually increased until full flow is reached. If return is diminished, the arterial line pressure is high, or the mean arterial pressure is excessive, then pump flow rates must be reduced until the difficulty is corrected. High line pressure and inadequate venous return are usually caused by malposition or kinking of the arterial and venous cannulas, respectively.

In neonates and infants, deep hypothermia is commonly used. For this reason, the pump prime is usually cold (18° to 22°C). When the cold perfusate contacts the myocardium, the heart rate immediately slows and contraction is severely impaired. The contribution to total blood flow pumped by the heart rapidly diminishes. Therefore, to sustain adequate systemic perfusion at or near normothermic temperatures, the arterial pump must reach full flows quickly. A major difference between the initiation of bypass in neonates and infants and that in older children is the speed at which full support must be achieved. One method for initiating CPB in infants is to begin the arterial inflow first; once the aortic flow is certain, the venous line is unclamped and blood is siphoned out of the right atrium into the inlet of the oxygenator. Flow before the venous line is unclamped prevents the potential problem of patient exsanguination if aortic dissection, malposition of the aortic cannula, or systemic pump failure have occurred. Pump flow rates are then rapidly increased to sustain systemic perfusion. Because coronary artery disease is not a consideration, the myocardium should cool evenly. When a cold prime is used, caution must be exercised in using the pump to infuse volume before initiating CPB. Infusion of cold perfusate can result in bradycardia and impaired cardiac contractility before the surgeon is prepared to initiate CPB.

Once CPB begins, it is essential to observe the heart. Ineffective venous drainage can rapidly result in ventricular distension. This is especially true in infants and neonates, in whom ventricular compliance is low and the heart is relatively intolerant of excessive preload augmentation because of a flat Starling curve. If distension occurs, pump flow must be reduced and the venous cannula repositioned. Alternatively, the heart may be vented or a pump sucker can be placed into the right atrium.

Management of Anticoagulation and Bleeding

Controlling anticoagulation during CPB is crucial. The activated clotting time (ACT) has been used as the standard because of reproducibility and ease of use. The amount of heparin to be delivered has been determined by the patient's weight in kilograms and a dose–response curve, described by Bull et al. (162). This very simple approach is used by many centers; however, it does not take into account the patient's blood volume and the effects of hypothermia, hemodilution, and previous heparin therapy. Another approach is to measure heparin levels indirectly with the Hepcon heparin management system (Medtronic, Inc., Minneapolis, MN). With this method, a "heparin level" is calculated in a 2-mL sample of blood by means of an automated protamine titration method. Both heparin and protamine doses are calculated based on the patient's blood volume. In infants and neonates, most centers add blood to the circuit prime and consequently add heparin also. Adequate anticoagulation is crucial; otherwise, intravascular coagulation, thrombosis, oxygenator dysfunction, and consumption of clotting factors may occur. Several CPB-related bleeding complications are related to heparin. These include antithrombin III (AT III) deficiency, heparin-induced thrombocytopenia, and inadequate heparin neutralization. The AT III concentration in healthy newborns is only half that of adults. Using a standard dose of heparin may result in inadequate anticoagulation and intravascular coagulation. Administration of fresh-frozen plasma or recombinant AT III easily remedies this problem. Some pediatric patients present with unusual and potentially dangerous hematologic problems, such as protein C deficiency, that can greatly increase their risk during CPB without careful management of anticoagulation (163).

There can be many reasons for abnormal coagulation in the perioperative period, and it is clearly beyond the scope of this chapter to discuss them. However, a few important points should be emphasized. First, coagulation factors are decreased during CPB and into the postoperative period. Hemodilution is responsible for some of this decrease. Also, ongoing activation of the extrinsic clotting system during bypass results in consumption of factors. Secondly, a qualitative and quantitative platelet defect is present. Platelet activation results from initial contact with the artificial surfaces of the circuit and oxygenator. The ongoing production of thrombin also results in significant activation of platelets. Finally, CPB results in an alteration of normal fibrinolytic and antifibrinolytic processes. During and shortly after the cessation of CPB, a fibrinolytic state exists that is characterized by an elevation of tissue plasminogen activator (t-PA). After a few hours, t-PA levels begin to fall, and the natural inhibitor of t-PA, plasminogen activator inhibitor, increases throughout the first 24 hours. There are few studies addressing the use of heparin in infant heart surgery. Much of what we practice is extrapolated from adult literature. Excess anticoagulation can result in excessive bleeding and a risk for intracranial hemorrhage. Too little heparin can result in ongoing intravascular coagulation and malfunction of the circuit and oxygenator. Young children seem to require higher doses of heparin to maintain ACTs of 350 to 450 seconds. It is important to realize that ACTs are highly variable and do not correlate with actual heparin levels. Newer anticoagulants are being examined in adult populations, but few studies in children have been performed.

Weaning

When a patient is weaned from CPB, filling of the heart is accomplished by partially clamping the venous return line and reducing the arterial inflow until adequate blood volume is achieved. It is important that the anesthesiologist resume ventilation of the lungs. Blood volume is assessed by direct visualization of the heart and by measurement of right atrial or left atrial filling pressures. When filling pressures are adequate, the venous cannula is clamped and the arterial inflow is stopped. The arterial cannula is left in place so that a slow infusion of residual perfusate can be used to optimize filling pressures. Myocardial function is assessed by direct cardiac visualization, intracardiac monitoring, and intraoperative echocardiography (55,164–168). In corrected physiology, the pulse oximeter can also be used as a crude measure of cardiac output. Low saturations or the inability of the oximeter probe to register a pulse may be a sign of very low output and high systemic resistance (169). After the repair of complex congenital heart defects, the anesthesiologist and surgeon may have difficulty in weaning patients from CPB. Under these circumstances, a distinction must be made among (a) a poor surgical result with a residual defect requiring repeated repair or a residual defect that cannot be repaired (an "inoperable" lesion), (b) pulmonary artery hypertension, and (c) right or left ventricular dysfunction. Two methods of evaluation are used in the operating room. First, an intraoperative "cardiac catheterization" can be performed to assess isolated pressure measurements from the various chambers of the heart. Catheter measurements in various chambers and at various locations can help uncover residual pressure gradients across valves, repaired sites of stenosis, and conduits. Furthermore, blood samples can be obtained and analyzed for O_2 saturation data to look for residual shunts. Tiny (3F) pressure catheters can be left in various chambers via a transthoracic approach to help in postoperative management (170).

In addition, intraoperative echocardiography with Doppler color flow has been used to provide an intraoperative "picture" of structural or functional abnormalities that might exist. If structural abnormalities are found, the patient can be put back on CPB and residual defects repaired before the patient leaves the operating room. Leaving the operating room with a significant residual structural defect adversely affects survival and increases patient morbidity and cost (164–167). With the introduction of improved probes, transesophageal echocardiography can now be used in babies as small as 2 kg. This has the advantage of being less obtrusive to the surgical team and enables accurate preoperative and postoperative evaluations to be performed without delaying the operation (164). Functional problems can also be identified by echocardiography. Once they have been diagnosed, therapy can be directed to the specific problem (55,171) (Fig. 30.11). Left ventricular dysfunction can be treated by optimizing preload and heart rate, increasing coronary perfusion pressure, correcting ionized calcium lev-

els, and adding inotropic support. Inotropic support is usually begun with calcium supplementation (10 mg/kg) and dopamine (5 to 15 μg/kg per minute). If function remains poor, a second drug is usually added. For left ventricular dysfunction, a more potent inotrope is generally administered, such as epinephrine at a dose of 0.05 to 0.1 μg/kg per minute and titrated to effect. Dobutamine can be used as an alternative second-line drug. However, because of their weak β-agonist effect and the uncoupling of the β-receptor during CPB, it may not be efficacious to use β-specific drugs, such as dobutamine, during weaning from CPB. In addition, dobutamine can produce significant tachycardia in neonates and infants. Amrinone in conjunction with epinephrine has been shown to improve left ventricular contractility and reduce systemic afterload. Milrinone, a newer phosphodiesterase inhibitor, has fewer side effects and is easier to titrate safely. The combination of milrinone and epinephrine is very effective for left ventricular dysfunction because it addresses left ventricular contractility through non–β-receptor-mediated mechanisms (epinephrine, α-receptor; milrinone, phosphodiesterase inhibition), an important approach after pediatric CPB. If very high doses of inotrope are required to wean from CPB, mechanical circulatory support with ECMO or a left ventricular assist device should be considered.

Pulmonary artery hypertension is a common problem after CPB in children. It is best treated with ventilatory manipulations. The goal is to reduce pulmonary vascular resistance by regulating P_aCO_2 (arterial), pH, P_{AO_2} (alveolar), P_aO_2 (arterial), and lung volumes. Arterial pH is a potent mediator of pulmonary vascular resistance, especially

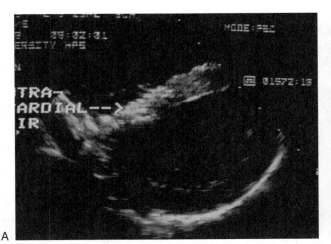
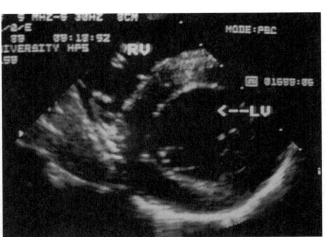

FIG. 30.11. **A:** Intraoperative echo reveals air in the septal portion of the heart after removal of the patient from cardiopulmonary bypass. **B:** The patient was treated by increasing the blood pressure and the air was "removed," thus restoring normal ventricular function. (From Greeley WJ, Ungerleider RM, Kern FH, et al. Intra-myocardial air causes right ventricular dysfunction after repair of congenital heart lesions. *Anesthesiology* 1990;73:1042–1046, with permission, and Ungerleider RM. Epicardial echocardiography during repair of congenital heart defects. In: Karp RS, Laks H, Wechsler AS, eds. *Advances in cardiac surgery.* Chicago: Mosby–Year Book, 1992:285–312, with permission.)

in the newborn (172). Maintaining a pH of 7.50 to 7.60 by manipulating the P_aCO_2 or pH is effective in modulating pulmonary vascular resistance (173,174). Increases in both P_aO_2 and P_AO_2 decrease the peripheral vascular resistance (175). Because increasing the fraction of inspired O_2 (FIO_2) reduces the peripheral vascular resistance in patients with intracardiac shunts, one can infer a direct pulmonary vasodilator effect of the alveolar rather than the arterial PO_2.

Adjusting lung volumes through ventilatory mechanics also plays a major role in controlling pulmonary vascular resistance. After CPB, total lung water is increased, lung compliance is reduced, and closing capacity exceeds functional residual capacity. Airway closure occurs before end-exhalation, producing areas of lung that are perfused but underventilated. These segments of lung become increasingly hypoxemic, and secondary hypoxic vasoconstriction occurs. The result is elevated pulmonary vascular resistance and reduced pulmonary blood flow. A large discrepancy can be noted between set tidal volume (recorded at the ventilator) and delivered tidal volume (measured at the endotracheal tube). Maintaining lung volumes by using large set tidal volumes will maintain lung volumes, restore functional residual capacity, and decrease peripheral vascular resistance. Therefore, not only hyperventilation and alkalosis are important; achieving and maintaining lung volumes are also crucial. Care must be taken to avoid excessive positive end-expiratory pressure or high mean airway pressure, which can result in alveolar overdistension, compression of capillaries in the alveolar wall and interstitium, elevated pulmonary vascular resistance, reduced pulmonary blood flow, and decreased left ventricular filling (176). Therefore, high tidal volume ventilation with inspiratory–expiratory ratios of 1:3 or longer may be necessary to optimize lung volumes and reduce pulmonary vascular resistance during weaning from CPB.

High-frequency jet ventilation provides improved CO_2 removal at lower mean airway pressures. Because high-frequency jet ventilation reduces mean airway pressure and pulmonary vascular resistance, it should be ideally suited for patients with right ventricular dysfunction and for those with pulmonary artery hypertension. For example, in postoperative Fontan patients, the cardiac index is adversely affected by increased pulmonary vascular resistance and mean airway pressure. High-frequency jet ventilation can significantly decrease mean airway pressure, reduce pulmonary vascular resistance, and increase cardiac index in this group of patients (177).

Nitric oxide is an endothelium-derived vasodilator that can be administered as an inhaled gas. Although a nonselective smooth-muscle vasodilator, nitric oxide is rapidly inactivated by hemoglobin, and therefore when it is administered via an inhaled route, the systemic circulation is protected from its vasodilating properties. Reduction in pulmonary vascular resistance has been demonstrated in adult patients with mitral valve stenosis and recently in children

with reactive pulmonary hypertension after congenital heart surgery (178). Experience with nitric oxide in the operating room has been limited, but this drug shows great promise in treating elevations in pulmonary vascular resistance.

If right ventricular dysfunction and pulmonary artery hypertension persist, the cardiac output can be augmented by creating a small atrial septal defect or by leaving a residual persistent foramen ovale to allow blood to shunt at the atrial level. This approach improves left ventricular filling, augments cardiac output, and improves O_2 delivery to tissue. Finally, leaving the chest open allows the right ventricle to obtain a larger end-diastolic dimension, which improves diastolic filling and right ventricular stroke volume. This may occasionally be necessary in neonates and infants with right-sided heart dysfunction after weaning from CPB. It also prevents the effects of decreased chest wall compliance and mediastinal swelling on pulmonary and cardiac mechanics. If these methods fail, mechanical circulatory support should be considered.

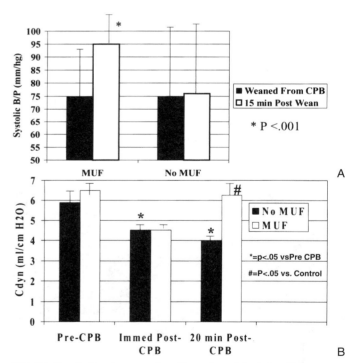

FIG. 30.12. A: Graph shows the effect of modified ultrafiltration (*MUF*) on ventricular function, represented by improvements in systolic blood pressure. (From Naik SK, Knight A, Elliott MJ. A prospective randomized study of a modified technique of ultrafiltration during pediatric open-heart surgery. *Circulation* 1991; 84[Suppl III]:III-422–III-431, with permission, and Naik SK, Elliott MJ. Ultrafiltration and paediatric cardiopulmonary bypass. *Perfusion* 1993;8:101–112, with permission.) **B:** Graph demonstrates how MUF improves the injury to pulmonary compliance observed after cardiopulmonary bypass. (From Meliones JN, Gaynor JW, Wilson BG, et al. Modified ultrafiltration reduces airway pressures and improves lung compliance after congenital heart surgery. *J Am Coll Cardiol* 1995; [Special Issue]:271A, with permission.)

Modified Ultrafiltration

Total body water can accumulate significantly during even routine open cardiac procedures. Edema develops not only in the periphery but also in vital areas such as the brain, heart, gut, and lungs. The increase in total body water can be partially controlled by limiting the excess crystalloid given with the pump prime and also by removing the fluid by various means during or following CPB. Various techniques include peritoneal dialysis, aggressive diuresis, conventional (on-pump) ultrafiltration, and post-CPB (modified) ultrafiltration (80,179,180). The technique of modified ultrafiltration is performed in the immediate postbypass period. Most commonly, blood is removed from the aortic cannula, passed through a hemofilter, and then returned as oxygenated, concentrated, and ultrafiltered blood to the cannula in the right atrium. Modified ultrafiltration has the advantage of filtering only the patient's extracellular blood volume and not the CPB circuit, which results in greater hemoconcentration (85). Both conventional and modified ultrafiltration have been shown to remove inflammatory mediators from the circulation (181). However, modified ultrafiltration may be more effective in concentrating the patient's blood and in improving both pulmonary compliance and ventricular functional recovery (82–84,182) (Fig. 30.12). In a recent survey (183), 50 pediatric open heart surgery programs were contacted, and it was found that 22 centers were using modified ultrafiltration. This report also outlined some of the complications associated with the conduct of modified ultrafiltration. It is notable that most complications are minor and seem to disappear as the team acquires experience with the technique (184). Figure 30.13 displays the schema for the conduct of modified ultrafiltration used by our group. This circuit involves using the cardioplegia "warmer" to prevent infants from cooling down during the period of modified ultrafiltration. Alternative circuit designs are also readily available, including designs for the use of venovenous modified ultrafiltration after modified ultrafiltration (78,183,184).

SUMMARY

Cardiopulmonary bypass and extracorporeal support have evolved from futuristic visions of surgical pioneers to safe and efficient means of support for infants and children undergoing complex cardiac procedures. CPB in infants and neonates poses many challenges and should be undertaken in centers specializing in the care of infants with congenital heart disease. The physiology of CPB and hypothermia has been gradually elucidated, pathophysiologic effects determined, and therapies addressed. Our technical ability to address the most complex of problems surgically has im-

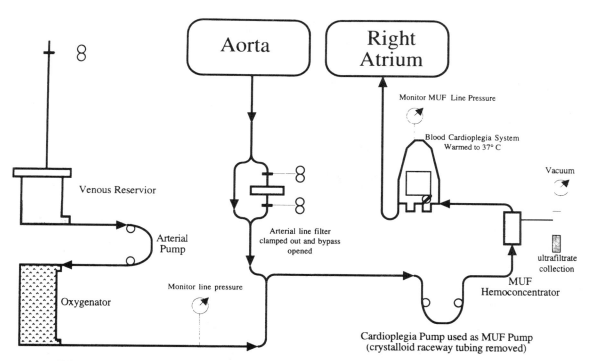

FIG. 30.13. A schematic for modified ultrafiltration (*MUF*) in which the cardioplegia warmer is used to prevent the patient from cooling during the MUF period. (From Darling E, Nanry K, Shearer I, et al. Techniques of paediatric modified ultrafiltration: 1996 survey results. *Perfusion* 1998;13: 93–103, with permission.)

proved during the last decade, with a reduction in mortality rates to less than 5% for most complex lesions. However, CPB is still associated with significant morbidity. Miniaturization of bypass circuitry, modulation of the inflammatory response, advancement of technology, and improvement in techniques of perfusion will maximize the safety of extracorporeal circulation and provide the next major step in producing better outcomes.

KEY POINTS

- Historically, the need to correct serious congenital cardiac abnormalities has been a primary impetus to the advances in the discipline of cardiac surgery.
- The pathophysiology of CPB in neonates and infants generally parallels that in older children and adults but differs in some significant ways.
  - During hypothermia, the "Q_{10}" is greater for infants than for adults, so that a greater degree of metabolic suppression occurs for a given degree of hypothermia.
  - DHCA may be best conducted with two different pH management strategies:
  - pH stat during cooling to augment brain blood flow and therefore improve cooling.
  - Alpha-stat before and during the circulatory arrest period.
  - The significant physiologic and metabolic characteristics of the immature myocardium require protection strategies different from those used in adults.
  - The immature lung may respond to CPB differently than does the adult lung, and in some cases it may benefit from liquid ventilation with fluorocarbon compounds.
  - Neurologic abnormalities following congenital heart surgery are common; however, the pathophysiology is not uniform and the causes are often unclear.
  - Preexisting abnormalities of the central nervous system are a possibility.
  - Hypothermia *per se* does not appear to be responsible for central nervous system damage.
  - Steroid therapy, to be most effective, should be started several hours before the circulatory arrest period.
  - The most severe inflammatory responses to CPB appear to occur in patients at the extremes of age.
- Smaller blood volumes in infants compound the mechanical difficulties of CPB.
  - Prime volumes and their content must be carefully controlled.
  - Nonporous silicone rubber membrane oxygenators may be beneficial for long-term perfusion.

- The need for miniature tubing and cannulas presents a significant technical challenge in small patients.
- Anticoagulation can be more difficult to manage in neonates and infants.
  - The pharmacokinetic and pharmacodynamic properties of heparin and protamine differ between pediatric patients and adults.
  - Intrinsic coagulation abnormalities are present, especially in deeply cyanotic patients.
- Modified ultrafiltration is a very valuable method for controlling body fluid balance during and after CPB in neonates and infants.

REFERENCES

1. Bigelow WG, Callaghan JC, Hopps JA. General hypothermia for experimental intra-cardiac surgery: the use of electrophrenic respirations, an artificial pacemaker for cardiac standstill and radio frequency re-warming in general hypothermia. *Ann Surg* 1950;132:531–539.
2. Lewis FJ, Taufic M. Closure of atrial septal defects with the aid of hypothermia: experimental accomplishments and the report of the one successful case. *Surgery* 1953;33:52–59.
3. Ungerleider RM. Direct-vision aortic valvotomy: predecessor to modern aortic surgery. *Ann Thorac Surg* 1994;57:1351–1353.
4. Gibbon JH. Application of mechanical heart–lung apparatus to cardiac surgery. *Minn Med* 1954;37:171–185.
5. Lillehei CW, Cohen M, Warden HE, et al. Direct vision intracardiac surgery by means of controlled cross-circulation or continuous arterial reservoir perfusion for correction of ventricular septal defects, atrioventricularis communis, isolated infundibular pulmonic stenosis, and tetralogy of Fallot. In: Lam CR, ed. *Proceedings of Henry Ford Hospital Symposium.* Philadelphia: WB Saunders, 1955:371–392.
6. Lillehei CW, Varco RL, Cohen M, et al. The first open-heart repairs of ventricular septal defect, atrioventricular communis, and tetralogy of Fallot using extracorporeal circulation by cross-circulation: a 30-year follow-up. *Ann Thorac Surg* 1986;41:4–21.
7. Kirklin JA, Dushane JW, Wood EH. Intra-cardiac surgery with the aid of a mechanical pump oxygenator system: report of eight cases. *Proc Mayo Clin* 1955;30:201–206.
8. Kern FH, Greeley WJ, Ungerleider RM. Cardiopulmonary bypass. In: Nichols DG, Cameron DE, Greeley WJ, et al., eds. *Critical heart disease in infants and children.* St. Louis: Mosby, 1995:497–530.
9. Gaynor JW, Kern FH, Greeley WJ, et al. Management of cardiopulmonary bypass in infants and children. In: Baue AE, Geha AS, Laks H, et al., eds. *Glenn's thoracic and cardiovascular surgery.* Stamford, CT: Appleton & Lange, 1996.
10. Purpura D. Normal and aberrant neuronal development in the cerebral cortex of the human fetus and young infant. In: Brazier MAB, ed. New York: Raven Press, 1975:33–49.
11. Moore RY. *Normal development of the nervous system. Prenatal and perinatal factors associated with brain disorders.* NIH publication. Washington, DC: US Government Printing Office, 1985:33–51.
12. Thurlbeck WM, Angus GE. Growth and development of the normal human lung. *Chest* 1975;35:67.
13. Kirklin JK, Kirklin JW, Pacifico AD. Deep hypothermia and total circulatory arrest. In: Arcinegas E, ed. *Pediatric cardiac surgery.* Chicago: Year Book, 1985.

14. Kirklin JW, Barratt-Boyes BG, eds. *Cardiac surgery*, 2nd ed. New York: Churchill Livingstone, 1993.

15. Greeley WJ, Kern FH, Ungerleider RM, et al. The effect of hypothermic cardiopulmonary bypass and total circulatory arrest on cerebral metabolism in neonates, infants, and children. *J Thorac Cardiovasc Surg* 1991;101:783–794.

16. Kern FH, Ungerleider RM, Reves JG, et al. The effects of altering pump flow rate on cerebral blood flow and metabolism in neonates, infants and children. *Ann Thorac Surg* 1993;56:1366–1372.

17. Navas JP, Anderson W, Marsh JD. Hypothermia increases calcium content of hypoxic myocytes. *Am J Physiol* 1990;

18. Sakai TH, Kurihara S. Rapid cooling contracture of toad cardiac muscle. *Jpn J Physiol* 1974;365:131–146.

19. Williams W, Rebeyka I, Tibsirani R. Warm induction blood cardioplegia in the infant, a technique to avoid rapid cooling myocardial contracture. *J Thorac Cardiovasc Surg* 1990;100:896–901.

20. Rebeyka IM, Hanan SA, Borges MR, et al. Rapid cooling contracture of the myocardium: the adverse effect of pre-arrest cardiac hypothermia. *J Thorac Cardiovasc Surg* 1991; :240–249.

21. Aoki M, Nomure F, Kawata H, et al. The effect of calcium and pre-ischemic hypothermia on recovery of myocardium after cardioplegic ischemia in neonatal lambs. *J Thorac Cardiovasc Surg* 1993;104:207–213.

22. Heinle JS, Lodge AJ, Mault JR, et al. Myocardial function is normal following rapid cooling of the *in vivo* neonatal heart. *Ann Thorac Surg* 1994;57:326–333.

23. Taylor KM. Cardiopulmonary bypass. In: Taylor KM, ed. *Cardiopulmonary bypass*. London: Chapman & Hall, 1986.

24. Noris M, Morigi M, Donadelli R, et al. Nitric oxide synthesis by cultured endothelial cells is modulated by flow conditions. *Circ Res* 1995;76:536–543.

25. Bregman D, Bowman F, Parodi E. An improved method of myocardial protection with pulsation during cardiopulmonary bypass. *Circulation* 1977;56:156–159.

26. Gaer J, Shaw A, Wild R. Effect of cardiopulmonary bypass on gastrointestinal perfusion and function. *Ann Thorac Surg* 1994;57:371–375.

27. Lodge AJ, Undar A, Daggett CW, et al. Regional blood flow during pulsatile cardiopulmonary bypass and after circulatory arrest in an infant model. *Ann Thorac Surg* 1997;63:1243–1250.

28. Undar A, Lodge AJ, Daggett CW, et al. Error associated with the choice of an aortic cannula in measuring regional cerebral blood flow with microspheres during pulsatile CPB in a neonatal piglet model. *ASAIO J* 1997;43:M482–M486.

29. Undar A, Lodge AJ, Runge TM, et al. Design and performance of a physiologic pulsatile flow neonate–infant cardiopulmonary bypass system. *ASAIO J* 1996;42:M580–M583.

30. Clark RE, Dietz DR, Miller JG. Continuous detection of microemboli during cardiopulmonary bypass in animals and man. *Circulation* 1976;54:74–78.

31. Utley R, Wachtel C, Cain RB, et al. Effects of hypothermia, hemodilution and pump oxygenation on organ water content, blood flow and oxygen delivery and renal function. *Ann Thorac Surg* 1981;31:121–133.

32. Skaryak LA, Chai PJ, Kern FH, et al. Blood gas management and degree of cooling: effects on cerebral metabolism before and after circulatory arrest. *J Thorac Cardiovasc Surg* 1995;110:1649–1657.

33. Kern FH, Greeley WJ. Pro: pH-stat management of blood gases is not preferable to alpha-stat in patients undergoing brain cooling for cardiac surgery. *J Cardiothorac Vasc Anesth* 1995;9:215–218.

34. Jonas RA, Bellinger DC, Rappaport LA, et al. Relation of pH strategy and developmental outcome after hypothermic circulatory arrest. *J Thorac Cardiovasc Surg* 1993;106:362–368.

35. Aoki M, Nomura F, Stromski ME, et al. Effects of pH on brain energetics after hypothermic circulatory arrest. *Ann Thorac Surg* 1993;55:1093–2103.

36. Somero GN, White FN. Enzymatic consequences under alpha-stat regulation. In: Rahn H, Prakash O, eds. *Acid–base regulation and body temperature*. Boston: Nijhoff, 1985:55–80.

37. Bashein G, Townes BD, Nessly BS, et al. A randomized study of carbon dioxide management during hypothermic cardiopulmonary bypass. *Anesthesiology* 1990;72:7–15.

38. Swain JA, McDonald JT, Griffith PK, et al. Low-flow hypothermic cardiopulmonary bypass protects the brain. *J Thorac Cardiovasc Surg* 1990;102:76–84.

39. Watanabe T, Hrita H, Kobayashi M, et al. Brain tissue pH oxygen tension and carbon dioxide tension in profoundly hypothermic cardiopulmonary bypass. *J Thorac Cardiovasc Surg* 1989;97:396–401.

40. Kirshbom PM, Skaryak LA, DiBerardo LR, et al. Effect of aorto-pulmonary collateral vessels on cerebral cooling and metabolic recovery during cardiopulmonary bypass and circulatory arrest. *Circulation* 1995;92[Suppl II]:II-490–II-494.

41. Kirshbom PM, Skaryak LA, DiBernardo et al. Aorto-pulmonary collateral vessels decrease the rate of cerebral cooling and alter regional cerebral perfusion during cardiopulmonary bypass. *Surg Forum* 1994;XLV:258–259.

42. Wong PC, Barlow CF, Hickey PR, et al. Factors associated with choreoathetosis after cardiopulmonary bypass in children with congenital heart disease. *Circulation* 1992;86[Suppl II]:II-118–II-126.

43. Kern FH, Johas RA, Mayer JE. Temperature monitoring during infant CPB: does it predict efficient brain cooling? *Ann Thorac Surg* 1992;54:749–754.

44. Kirshbom PM, Skaryak LA, DiBernardo LR, et al. pH-Stat cooling improves cerebral metabolic recovery after circulatory arrest in a piglet model of aorto-pulmonary collateral vessels. *J Thorac Cardiovasc Surg* 1996;111:147–157.

45. Billingsley A, Laks H, Haas G. Myocardial protection in children. In: Baue A, Geha A, Hammond G, eds. *Glenn's textbook of cardiovascular surgery*. East Norwalk, CT: Appleton & Lange, 1991.

46. Boudreaux J, Schieber R, Cook D. Hemodynamic effects of halothane in the newborn piglet. *Anesth Analg* 1984;63:731–737.

47. Boucek R, Citak M, Braham T, et al. Postnatal development of calcium release from cardiac sarcoplasmic reticulum. *Pediatr Res* 1984;18:948.

48. Rolph T, Jones C. Regulation of glycolytic flux in the heart of the fetal guinea pig. *J Dev Physiol* 1983;5:31–39.

49. Hetzer R, Warnecke H, Wittock H. Extracoronary collateral myocardial blood flow during cardioplegic arrest. *J Thorac Cardiovasc Surg* 1980;28:191–196.

50. Corno AF, Bethencourt DM, Laks H. Myocardial protection in the neonatal heart: a comparision of topical hypothermia and crystalloid and blood cardioplegia solutions. *J Thorac Cardiovasc Surg* 1987;93:163–172.

51. Baker E, Olinger G, Baker J. Calcium content of St. Thomas II cardioplegic solution damages ischemic immature myocardium. *Ann Thorac Surg* 1991;52:993–999.

52. Kraft L, Katholi R, Woods W. Attenuation by magnesium of the electrophysiologic effects of hyperkalemia on human and canine heart cells. *Am J Cardiol* 1980;45:1189–1195.

53. Rebeyka I, Diaz R, Waddell J. Magnesium-based blood cardioplegia in a neonatal heart model. *Circulation* 1992;86[Suppl I]:I-630.

54. Bell C, Rimar S, Barash P. ST-segment changes consistent with

myocardial ischemia in the neonate: a report of three cases. *Anesthesiology* 1989;71:601–604.

55. Greeley WJ, Ungerleider RM, Kern FH, et al. Intra-myocardial air causes right ventricular dysfunction after repair of congenital heart lesions. *Anesthesiology* 1990;73:1042–1046.

56. Mavroudis C, Ebert PA. Hemodilution causes decreased compliance in puppies. *Circulation* 1978;58:155–159.

57. Li JS, Bengur AR, Ungerleider RM, et al. Abnormal left ventricular filling after neonatal repair of congenital heart disease: association with increased mortality and morbidity. *Am Heart J* 1998;136:1075–1080.

58. Malm JR, Manger WM, Sullivan SF. The effects of acidosis on sympatho-adrenal stimulation. *JAMA* 1966;197:121–125.

59. Engleman RM, Haag B, Lemeshow S. Mechanism of plasma catecholamine increases during coronary artery bypass and valve procedures. *J Thorac Cardiovasc Surg* 1983;86:608–615.

60. Turley K, Roizen M, Vlahakes GJ. Catecholamine response to profound hypothermia and circulatory arrest in infants. *Circulation* 1980;62[SupplI]:I-175–I-179.

61. Wood M, Shang DG, Wood AJ. The sympathetic response to profound hypothermia and circulatory arrest in infants. *Can Anaesth Soc J* 1980;27:125.

62. Anand KJS, Hickey PR. Halothane–morphine compared with high-dose sufentanil for anesthesia and post-operative analgesia in neonatal cardiac surgery. *N Engl J Med* 1992; :327.

63. Ratcliffe JM, Wyse FKH, Hunter S. The role of priming fluid in the metabolic response to cardiopulmonary bypass in children less than 15 kg of body weight undergoing open heart surgery. *J Thorac Cardiovasc Surg* 1988;36:65.

64. Mitchell IM, Pollock JCS, Jamieson MPG, et al. The effects of cardiopulmonary bypass on thyroid function in infants weighing less than five kilograms. *J Thorac Cardiovasc Surg* 1992;103:800–805.

65. Chu SH, Huang TS, Hsu RB. Thyroid hormone changes after cardiovascular surgery and the clinical implications. *Ann Thorac Surg* 1991;52:791–796.

66. Bennett-Guerrero E, Jimenez JL, White WD, et al. Cardiovascular effects of intravenous tri-iodothyronine in patients undergoing coronary artery bypass graft surgery. A randomized, double-blind, placebo-controlled trial. Duke T_3 Study Group. *JAMA* 1996;275:687–692.

67. Philbin DM, Levine FH, Emerson CW, et al. Plasma vasopressin levels and urinary flow during cardiopulmonary bypass in patients with valvular heart disease. *J Thorac Cardiovasc Surg* 1979;78:779.

68. Chai PJ, Williamson A, Lodge AJ, et al. Effects of ischemia on pulmonary dysfunction following cardiopulmonary bypass. *Ann Thorac Surg* (in press).

69. Wernovsky G, Wypij D, Jonas RA, et al. Postoperative course and hemodynamic profile after the arterial switch operation in neonates and infants. A comparison of low-flow cardiopulmonary bypass and circulatory arrest. *Circulation* 1995;92:2226–2235.

70. Skaryak LA, Lodge AJ, Kirshbom PM, et al. Low-flow cardiopulmonary bypass produces greater pulmonary dysfunction than circulatory arrest. *Ann Thorac Surg* 1996;62:1284–1288.

71. Kirshbom PM, Tsui SL, DiBernardo LR, et al. Blockade of endothelin-converting enzyme significantly reduces pulmonary hypertension after cardiopulmonary bypass and circulatory arrest. *Surgery* 1995;118:440–445.

72. Kirshbom PM, Jacobs MT, Tsui SSL, et al. Effects of cardiopulmonary bypass and circulatory arrest on endothelium-dependent vasodilation in the lung. *J Thorac Cardiovasc Surg* 1996;111:1248–1256.

73. Kirshbom PM, Page SO, Jacobs MT, et al. Cardiopulmonary bypass and circulatory arrest increase endothelin-1 production and receptor expression in the lung. *J Thorac Cardiovasc Surg* 1997;113:777–783.

74. Cannon ML, Cheifetz IM, Craig DM, et al. Optimizing liquid ventilation as a lung protection strategy for neonatal cardiopulmonary bypass: full-FRC dosing is more effective than half-FRC dosing. *J Crit Care Med* (in press).

75. Cheifetz IM, Cannon ML, Craig DM, et al. Liquid ventilation improves pulmonary function and cardiac output in a neonatal swine model of cardiopulmonary bypass. *J Thorac Cardiovasc Surg* 1998;115:528–535.

76. Lodge AJ, Chai PJ, Daggett CW, et al. The use of corticosteroids to reduce post-CPB inflammatory syndrome in neonates: impact of dose timing. *J Thorac Cardiovasc Surg* (in press).

77. Koutlas TC, Gaynor JW, Nicolson SC, et al. Modified ultrafiltration reduces postoperative morbidity after cavopulmonary connection. *Ann Thorac Surg* 1997;64:37–43.

78. Bando K, Vijay P, Turrentine MW, et al. Dilutional and modified ultrafiltration reduces pulmonary hypertension after operations for congenital heart disease: a prospective randomized study. *J Thorac Cardiovasc Surg* 1998;115:517–527.

79. Wang M-J, Chiu I-S, Hsu C-M, et al. Efficacy of ultrafiltration in removing inflammatory mediators during pediatric cardiac operations. *Ann Thorac Surg* 1996;61:651–656.

80. Elliott MJ. Ultrafiltration and modified ultrafiltration in pediatric open-heart operations. *Ann Thorac Surg* 1993;56:1518–1522.

81. Journois D, Poupard P, Greeley WJ, et al. Hemofiltration during cardiopulmonary bypass in pediatric cardiac surgery. *Anesthesiology* 1994;81:1181–1189.

82. Meliones JN, Gaynor JW, Wilson BG, et al. Modified ultrafiltration reduces airway pressures and improves lung compliance after congenital heart surgery. *J Am Coll Cardiol* 1995; [Special Issue]:271A(abst).

83. Naik SK, Knight A, Elliott MJ. A prospective randomized study of a modified technique of ultrafiltration during pediatric open-heart surgery. *Circulation* 1991;84[Suppl III]:III-422–III-431.

84. Naik SK, Elliott MJ. Ultrafiltration and paediatric cardiopulmonary bypass. *Perfusion* 1993;8:101–112.

85. Ungerleider RM. Effects of cardiopulmonary bypass and use of modified ultrafiltration. *Ann Thorac Surg* 1998;65:S35–S39.

86. Ferry PC. Neurological sequelae of cardiac surgery in children. *Am J Dis Child* 1987;141:309–312.

87. Ferry PC. Neurological sequelae of open-heart surgery in children. An "irritating question." *Am J Dis Child* 1990;144:369–373.

88. Fessatidis IT, Thomas VL, Shore DF, et al. Brain damage after profoundly hypothermic circulatory arrest: correlations between neurophysiologic and neuropathologic findings. An experimental study in vertebrates. *J Thorac Cardiovasc Surg* 1993;106:32–41.

89. Grayck EN, Meliones JN, Kern FH, et al. Elevated serum lactate correlates with intracranial hemorrhage in neonates treated with extracorporeal life support. *Pediatrics* 1995;96:914–917.

90. Tasker RC. Cerebral function and heart disease. In: Nichols DG, Cameron DE, Greeley WJ, et al., eds. *Critical heart disease in infants and children.* St. Louis: Mosby, 1995:157–184.

91. Orenstein JM, Sato N, Aaron B, et al. Microemboli observed in deaths following cardiac surgery. *Hum Pathol* 1982;13:1082–1090.

92. Deverall PB, Padayachee TS, Parson S, et al. Ultrasound detection of microemboli in the middle cerebral artery during cardiopulmonary bypass surgery. *Eur J Cardiothorac Surg* 1988;2:256–260.

93. Blauth CI, Arnold JV, Schulenberg WE, et al. Cerebral microembolism during cardiopulmonary bypass. *J Thorac Cardiovasc Surg* 1988;95:668–676.

94. Young JA, Kisker CT, Doty DB. Adequate anticoagulation during cardiopulmonary bypass determined by activated clotting time and the appearance of fibrin monomer. *Ann Thorac Surg* 1978;26:231–240.

95. Semb BKH, Pedersen T, Hatteland K, et al. Doppler ultrasound estimation of bubble removal by various arterial line filters during extracorporeal circulation. *Scand J Thorac Cardiovasc Surg* 1982;16:55–62.

96. Blauth C, Smith P, Newman S, et al. Retinal microembolism and neuropsychiatric deficit following clinical cardiopulmonary bypass: comparison of a membrane and a bubble oxygenator. *Eur J Cardiothorac Surg* 1989;3:135–139.

97. Newburger JW, Jonas RA, Wernovsky G, et al. A comparison of the perioperative neurological effects of hypothermic circulatory arrest versus low-flow cardiopulmonary bypass in infant heart surgery. *N Engl J Med* 1993;329:1057–1064.

98. Armon C, Deschamps C, Adkinson C, et al. Hyperbaric treatment of cerebral air embolism sustained during an open-heart surgical procedure. *Mayo Clin Proc* 1991;66:565–571.

99. Egerton N, Egerton WS, Kay JH. Neurological changes following profound hypothermia. *Ann Surg* 1962;157:366–373.

100. DeLeon S, Ilbawi M, Arcilla R, et al. Choreoathetosis after deep hypothermia without circulatory arrest. *Ann Thorac Surg* 1990; 50:714–719.

101. Brunberg JE, Doty DB, Reilly EL. Choreoathetosis in infants following cardiac surgery with deep hypothermia and circulatory arrest. *J Pediatr* 1974;84:232–235.

102. Norwood WI, Norwood CR, Castaneda AR. Cerebral anoxia: effect of deep hypothermia and pH. *Surgery* 1986;86:203–210.

103. Treasure T, Naftel DC, Conger KA, et al. The effect of hypothermic circulatory arrest on cerebral function, morphology, and biochemistry. *J Thorac Cardiovasc Surg* 1983;86:761–770.

104. Bjork VO, Hultquist G. Contraindications to profound hypothermia. *J Thorac Cardiovasc Surg* 1962;44:1–9.

105. Gillinov AM, Redmond JM, Zehr KJ, et al. Superior cerebral protection with profound hypothermia during circulatory arrest. *Ann Thorac Surg* 1993;55:1432–1439.

106. Mault JR, Ohtake S, Klingensmith ME, et al. Cerebral metabolism and circulatory arrest: effects of duration and strategies for protection. *Ann Thorac Surg* 1993;55:57–63.

107. Langley S, Mault JR, Chai PJ, et al. Hemodynamic, metabolic and electron microscopic evidence supporting the use of intermittent perfusion during deep hypothermic circulatory arrest. *Ann Thorac Surg* (in press).

108. Bellinger DC, Wernovsky G, Rappaport LA, et al. Rapid cooling of infants on cardiopulmonary bypass adversely affects later cognitive function. *Circulation* 1988;78:A358(abst).

109. Bellinger DC, Jonas RA, Rappaport LA, et al. Developmental and neurological status of children after heart surgery with hypothermic circulatory arrest or low-flow cardiopulmonary bypass. *N Engl J Med* 1995;332:549–555.

110. Greeley WJ, Kern FH, Mault JR, et al. Mechanisms of injury and methods of protection of the brain during cardiac surgery in neonates and infants. *Cardiol Young* 1993;3:317–330.

111. Kern FH, Ungerleider RM, Schulman SR, et al. Comparison of two strategies of cardiopulmonary bypass cooling on jugular venous oxygen saturation in neonates and infants. *Ann Thorac Surg* 1995;60:1198–1202.

112. Fisk GC, Wright JS, Hicks RG, et al. The influence of duration of circulatory arrest at 20°C on cerebral changes. *Anaesth Intensive Care* 1976;4:126–134.

113. Wells FC, Coghill S, Caplan HL, et al. Duration of circulatory arrest does influence the psychological development of children after cardiac operation in early life. *J Thorac Cardiovasc Surg* 1983;86:823–831.

114. Greeley WJ, Ungerleider RM, Smith LR, et al. Cardiopulmonary bypass alters cerebral blood flow in infants and children during and after cardiovascular surgery. *Circulation* 1988; 78[Suppl II]:II-356–II-363.

115. Greeley WJ, Ungerleider RM, Smith LR, et al. The effects of deep hypothermic cardiopulmonary bypass and total circulatory arrest on cerebral blood flow in infants and children. *J Thorac Cardiovasc Surg* 1989;97:737–745.

116. Greeley WJ, Ungerleider RM, Kern FH, et al. Effects of cardiopulmonary bypass on cerebral blood flow in neonates, infants, and children. *Circulation* 1989;80:1209–1215.

117. Croughwell N, Smith LR, Quill T, et al. The effect of temperature on cerebral metabolism and blood flow in adults during cardiopulmonary bypass. *J Thorac Cardiovasc Surg* 1992;103: 549–554.

118. Venn GE. Cerebral vascular autoregulation during cardiopulmonary bypass. *Perfusion* 1989;4:105.

119. Kern FH, Ungerleider RM, Quill TJ, et al. Cerebral blood flow response to changes in arterial carbon dioxide tension during hypothermic cardiopulmonary bypass in children. *J Thorac Cardiovasc Surg* 1991;101:618–622.

120. DuPlessis AJ, Treves ST, Hickey PR, et al. Regional cerebral perfusion abnormalities after cardiac operations. *J Thorac Cardiovasc Surg* 1994;107:1036–1043.

121. Aoki M, Jonas RA, Nomura F, et al. Aprotinin enhances acute recovery of cerebral metabolism after circulatory arrest. *Circulation* 1993;86[Suppl 1]:182.

122. Tsui SSL, Kirshbom PM, Davies MJ, et al. Thromboxane A$_2$-receptor blockade improves cerebral protection for deep hypothermic circulatory arrest. *Eur J Cardiothorac Surg* 1997;12: 228–235.

123. Greeley WJ, Bracey VA, Ungerleider RM, et al. Recovery of cerebral metabolism and mitochrondrial oxidation state are delayed after hypothermic circulatory arrest. *Circulation* 1991; 82[Suppl III]:III-412–III-418.

124. Hindman BJ, Dexter F, Cutkomp J, et al. Brain blood flow and metabolism do not decrease at stable brain temperature during cardiopulmonary bypass in rabbits. *Anesthesiology* 1992; 77:342–351.

125. Fallon P, Roberts I, Kirkham FJ, et al. Cerebral hemodynamics during cardiopulmonary bypass in children using near-infrared spectroscopy. *Ann Thorac Surg* 1993;56:1473–1477.

126. Greeley WJ, Bracey VA, Ungerleider RM, et al. Recovery of cerebral metabolism and mitochrondrial oxidation state is delayed after hypothermic circulatory arrest. *Circulation* 1991; 84[Suppl 3]:400–415.

127. Mault JR, Whitaker EG, Heinle JS, et al. Intermittent perfusion during hypothermic circulatory arrest: a new and effective technique for cerebral protection. *Surg Forum* 1992;XLIII:314–316.

128. Mault JR, Whitaker EG, Heinle JS, et al. Effects of a second period of circulatory arrest on the brain. *Ann Thorac Surg* (in press).

129. Miura T, Laussen PL, Lidov GW, et al. Intermittent whole-body perfusion with "somatoplegia" versus blood perfusate to extend duration of circulatory arrest. *Circulation* 1996;94[Suppl II]:II-56–II-62.

130. Robbins RC, Balaban RS, Swain JA. Intermittent hypothermic asanguineous cerebral perfusion (cerebroplegia) protects the brain during prolonged circulatory arrest. *J Thorac Cardiovasc Surg* 1990;99:878–884.

131. Skaryak LA, Kirshbom PM, DiBernardo LR, et al. Modified ultrafiltration improves cerebral metabolic recovery after circulatory arrest. *J Thorac Cardiovasc Surg* 1995;109:744–752.

132. Mezrow CK, Midulla P, Sadeghi A, et al. A vulnerable interval for cerebral injury: comparison of hypothermic circulatory arrest and low-flow cardiopulmonary bypass. *Cardiol Young* 1993;3: 287–298.

133. Mezrow CK, Sadeghi AM, Gandsas A, et al. Cerebral effects of low-flow cardiopulmonary bypass and hypothermic circulatory arrest. *Ann Thorac Surg* 1994;57:532–539.

134. Mezrow CK, Gandsas A, Sadeghi AM, et al. Metabolic correlates of neurological and behavioral injury after prolonged hypothermic circulatory arrest. *J Thorac Cardiovasc Surg* 1995;109:959–975.

135. Shum-Tim D, Nagashima M, Shinoka T, et al. Postischemic hyperthermia exacerbates neurological injury after deep hypothermic circulatory arrest. *J Thorac Cardiovasc Surg* 1998;116:780–792.

136. Sonntag J, Dahnert I, Stiller B, et al. Complement and contact activation during cardiovascular operations in infants. *Ann Thorac Surg* 1998;65:525–531.

137. Moat NE, Shore DF, Evans TW. Organ dysfunction and cardiopulmonary bypass: the role of complement and regulatory proteins. *Eur J Cardiothorac Surg* 1993;7:563–573.

138. Kirklin JK, Westaby S, Blackstone EH. Complement and the damaging effects of cardiopulmonary bypass. *J Thorac Cardiovasc Surg* 1983;86:845–857.

139. Butler J, Rocker GM, Westaby S. Inflammatory responses to cardiopulmonary bypass. *Ann Thorac Surg* 1993;55:552–559.

140. Seghaye MC, Duchateau J, Grabitz RG, et al. Complement, leukocytes, and leukocyte elastase in full-term neonates undergoing cardiac operations. *J Thorac Cardiovasc Surg* 1994;108:29–36.

141. Finn A, Naik S, Klein N, et al. Interleukin-8 release and neutrophil degranulation after pediatric cardiopulmonary bypass. *J Thorac Cardiovasc Surg* 1993;105:234–241.

142. Steinberg JB, Kapelanski DP, Olson JG, et al. Cytokine and complement levels in patients undergoing cardiopulmonary bypass. *J Thorac Cardiovasc Surg* 1993;106:1008–1016.

143. Boyle EM, Verrier ED, Speiss BD. Endothelial cell injury in cardiovascular surgery: the procoagulant response. *Ann Thorac Surg* 1996;62:1549–1557.

144. Finn A, Dreyer WJ. Neutrophil adhesion and the inflammatory response induced by cardiopulmonary bypass. *Cardiol Young* 1993;3:244–250.

145. Cave AC, Manache A, Derias NW, et al. Thromboxane A₂ mediates pulmonary hypertension after cadiopulmonary bypass in the rabbit. *J Thorac Cardiovasc Surg* 1993;106:959–967.

146. Bui KC, Hammerman C, Hirshl RB, et al. Plasma prostanoids in neonates with pulmonary hypertension treated with conventional therapy and with extracorporeal membrane oxygenation. *J Thorac Cardiovasc Surg* 1991;101:973–983.

147. Watkins L Jr, Lucas SK, Gardner TJ, et al. Angiotensin II levels during cardiopulmonary bypass: a comparison of pulsatile and nonpulsatile flow. *Surg Forum* 1978;29:229–235.

148. Seghave MC, Grabitz RG, Duchateau J, et al. Inflammatory reaction and capillary leak syndrome related to cardiopulmonary bypass in neonates undergoing cardiac operations. *J Thorac Cardiovasc Surg* 1996;112:687–697.

149. Ratcliffe JM, Elliott MJ, Wyse RKH, et al. The metabolic load of stored blood. Implications for major transfusions in infants. *Arch Dis Child* 1986;61:1208–1214.

150. Salama A, Meuller C. Delayed hemolytic transfusion reactions: evidence for complement activation involving allogeneic autologous red cells. *Transfusion* 1984;214:188–193.

151. Kawashima Y, Yamamoto Z, Manabe H. Safe limits of hemodilution in cardiopulmonary bypass. *Surgery* 1974;76:391–397.

152. Henling CE, Carmichael MJ, Keats AS, et al. Cardiac operation for congenital heart disease in children of Jehovah's Witnesses. *J Thorac Cardiovasc Surg* 1985;89:914–920.

153. Leone BJ, Spahn DR, McRae RL, et al. Effects of hemodilution and anesthesia on regional function of compromised myocardium. *Anesthesiology* 1990;73:A596(abst).

154. Marelli D, Paul A, Samson CP. Does the addition of albumin to the prime solution in cardiopulmonary bypass affect the clinical outcome? *J Thorac Cardiovasc Surg* 1989;98:751–756.

155. Haneda K, Sato S, Ischizawa E, et al. The importance of colloid oncotic pressure during open-heart surgery in infants. *Tohou J Exp Med* 1985;147:65–71.

156. VanOerversen W, Kazatchkine MD, Descamp-Latscha, et al. Deleterious effects of cardiopulmonary bypass: a prospective study of bubble versus membrane oxygenators. *J Thorac Cardiovasc Surg* 1985;89:888–899.

157. Sade RM, Bartles DM, Dearing JP, et al. A prospective randomized study of membrane versus bubble oxygenators in children. *Ann Thorac Surg* 1979;29:502–511.

158. Pearson DT, McArdle B, Poslad SJ, et al. A clinical evaluation of the performance characteristics of one membrane and five bubble oxygenators: haemocompatibility studies. *Perfusion* 1986;1:81–98.

159. Menghini A. Oxygenator design: a global approach. *Perfusion* 1993;8:87–92.

160. Horton AM, Wutt W. Pump-induced haemolysis: is the constrained vortex pump better or worse than the roller pump? *Perfusion* 1992;7:103–108.

161. Mavroudis C, Brown GL, Katzmark SL, et al. Blood flow distribution in infant pigs subjected to surface cooling, deep hypothermia, and circulatory arrest. *J Thorac Cardiovasc Surg* 1984;87:665–672.

162. Bull HS, Huse WM, Brauer FS, et al. Heparin therapy during extracorporeal circulation II: use of a dose response curve to individualize heparin and protamine dosage. *J Thorac Cardiovasc Surg* 1975;69:685–689.

163. Lawson DS, Darling EM, Ware RE, et al. Management considerations for a heterozygous protein C-deficient patient undergoing open heart surgery with cardiopulmonary bypass. *J Extra-Corporeal Technol* 1995;27:172–176.

164. Bengur AR, Li JS, Herlong JR, et al. Intraoperative transesophageal echocardiography in congenital heart disease. *Semin Thorac Cardiovasc Surg* 1998;10:255–264.

165. Ungerleider RM, Kisslo JA, Greeley WJ, et al. Intraoperative echocardiography during congenital heart operations: experience from 1,000 cases. *Ann Thorac Surg* 1995;60[6 Suppl]:S539–S542.

166. Ungerleider RM, Greeley WJ, Kanter RJ, et al. The learning curve for intraoperative echocardiography during congenital heart surgery. *Ann Thorac Surg* 1992;54:691–698.

167. Ungerleider RM, Greeley WJ, Sheikh KH, et al. The use of intraoperative echo with Doppler color flow imaging to predict outcome after repair of congenital cardiac defects. *Ann Surg* 1989;210:526–534.

168. Ungerleider RM. Decision making in pediatric cardiac surgery using intraoperative echo. *Int J Card Imaging* 1989;4:33–35.

169. Severinghaus JW, Spellman BA. Pulse oximeter failure thresholds in hypotension and vasoconstriction. *Anesthesiology* 1990;73:532–537.

170. Gold JP, Jonas RA, Lang P, et al. Transthoracic intracardiac monitoring lines in pediatric surgical patients: a ten-year experience. *Ann Thorac Surg* 1986;42:185.

171. Ungerleider RM. Epicardial echocardiography during repair of congenital heart defects. In: Karp RS, Laks H, Wechsler AS, eds. *Advances in cardiac surgery.* Chicago: Mosby–Year Book, 1992:285–312.

172. Drummond WH, Gregory GA, Heyman MA, et al. The independent effects of hyperventilation, tolazoline, and dopamine in infants with persistent pulmonary hypertension. *J Pediatr* 1981;98:603–608.

173. Lyrene RK, Welch KA, Godoy G, et al. Alkalosis attenuates

hypoxic pulmonary vasoconstriction in neonatal lambs. *Pediatr Res* 1985;19:1268.

174. Morray JP, Lynn AM, Mansfield PB. Effects of pH and P_{CO_2} on pulmonary and systemic hemodynamics after surgery in children with congenital heart disease and pulmonary hypertension. *J Pediatr* 1988;113:474.

175. Rudolph AM, Yuan S. Response of the pulmonary vasculature to hypoxia and H^+ ion concentration changes. *J Clin Invest* 1966;45:399.

176. Jenkins J, Lynn A, Edmonds J, et al. Effects of mechanical ventilation on cardiopulmonary function in children after open-heart surgery. *Crit Care Med* 1985;13:77–80.

177. Meliones JN, Bove EL, Dekeon MK, et al. High-frequency jet ventilation improves cardiac function after the Fontan procedure. *Circulation* 1991;84[Suppl III]:III-364–III-368.

178. Roberts JD, Chen TY, Kawai N, et al. Inhaled nitric oxide reverses pulmonary vasoconstriction in the hypoxic and acidotic newborn lamb. *Circ Res* 1993;72:246–254.

179. Giuffe RM, Tam KH, Williams WW, et al. Acute renal failure complicating pediatric cardiac surgery: a comparison of survi-

vors and non-survivors following acute peritoneal bypass. *Pediatr Cardiol* 1992;13:208–213.

180. Paret G, Cohen AJ, Bohn DJ. Continuous arterio-venous hemofiltration after cardiac operation in infants and children. *J Thorac Cardiovasc Surg* 1992; :1225–1230.

181. Millar AB, Armstrong L, van der Linden J. Cytokine production and hemofiltration in children undergoing cardiopulmonary bypass. *Ann Thorac Surg* 1993;56:1499–1502.

182. Daggett CW, Lodge AJ, Scarborough JE, et al. Modified ultrafiltration versus conventional ultrafiltration: a randomized prospective study in neonatal piglets. *J Thorac Cardiovasc Surg* 1998;115:336–342.

183. Darling E, Nanry K, Shearer I, et al. Techniques of paediatric modified ultrafiltration: 1996 survey results. *Perfusion* 1998;13:93–103.

184. Darling EM, Shearer IR, Nanry K, et al. Modified ultrafiltration in pediatric cardiopulmonary bypass. *J Extra-Corporeal Technol* 1994;26:205–209.

185. Kern FH, Greeley WJ, Ungerleider RM. The effects of bypass on the developing brain. *Perfusion* 1993;8:49–54.

31

EXTRACORPOREAL MEMBRANE OXYGENATION FOR RESPIRATORY OR CARDIAC SUPPORT

SCOTT K. ALPARD
JOSEPH B. ZWISCHENBERGER

During the last two decades, two major developments in extracorporeal life support (ECLS) have occurred: (a) technology has progressed to the point where injured lungs can be supported for several days and, if necessary, for several weeks in newborns, children, and adults; and (b) specific patient populations with potentially reversible respiratory failure have been identified (1,2). Extracorporeal membrane oxygenation (ECMO) should be considered in the patient with severe respiratory failure (SRF) unresponsive to optimal management if the patient is a newborn infant past 34 weeks' gestational age, or a child or adult with treatable and reversible pulmonary disease of less than 5 days' duration. However, ECMO *should not* be considered if the patient has extensive pulmonary fibrosis, other incurable disease, or necrotizing pneumonitis, or has been treated with a ventilator with high pressure and a high O_2 concentration for 1 week or longer. ECMO can also be used for cardiac failure in all age groups, but only if there is reason to believe that the patient will recover from the cardiac disease within a week. Severe left ventricular failure may be better managed by left atrial-to-aortic ECLS or a total artificial heart as a bridge to transplantation (see Chap. 8). Venoarterial (VA) ECMO is reserved for patients with right ventricular or biventricular failure, unresponsive to other modes of therapy, in whom heart recovery or replacement is anticipated within 5 to 7 days.

Extracorporeal membrane oxygenation is the term used to describe prolonged extracorporeal cardiopulmonary bypass (CPB) achieved by extrathoracic vascular cannulation. A modified heart–lung machine is used, most often consisting of a distensible venous blood drainage reservoir, a servo-regulated roller pump, a membrane lung to exchange O_2 and CO_2, and a countercurrent heat exchanger to maintain temperature (Figs. 31.1 and 31.2). The patient must be continuously anticoagulated with heparin to prevent thrombosis within the circuit and possible development of thromboemboli. Institutional expertise and need dictate the availability of pediatric ECMO for respiratory or cardiac support, and adult ECMO for respiratory failure. Investigational treatment modalities such as nitric oxide, partial liquid ventilation, and ECMO have shown isolated spectacular outcomes, but their application is limited by cost, complications, their labor-intensive nature, and a lack of validation by prospective randomized trials (Fig. 31.3). Even when randomized trials have been proposed or attempted, the nature of the new treatment modalities precludes blinding of the treatment arms. "Protective" mechanical ventilation, designed to minimize barotrauma and volutrauma, has become the standard supportive treatment for acute respiratory distress syndrome (RDS). The search continues for ventilator management and gas exchange techniques that will provide atraumatic ventilation while allowing the lungs to recover from severe respiratory failure. Treatment alternatives such as nitric oxide, high-frequency ventilation and other investigational ventilation techniques, and surfactant have affected the potential enrollment of patients with SRF into ECMO protocols.

This chapter reviews key events in the history of ECMO for respiratory and cardiac support and describes current ECMO techniques. The chapter emphasizes ECMO for respiratory failure in newborns because ECMO has been established as a standard treatment for this group of patients. However, many of the principles described in that discussion also apply to the use of ECMO for children and adults, and pertinent differences are detailed. The expanding use of ECMO for cardiac failure after surgical repair of congenital heart defects, for perioperative support in pediatric heart transplantation, and for cardiac failure after adult cardiac surgery are also described.

S. K. Alpard and J. B. Zwischenberger: Department of Surgery, Division of Cardiothoracic Surgery, University of Texas Medical Branch, Galveston, Texas 77555-0528.

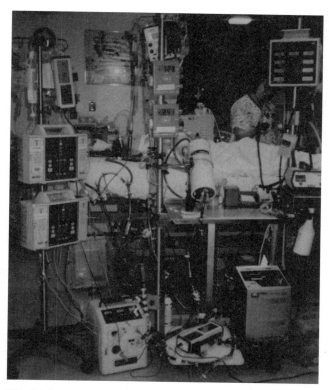

FIG. 31.1. An extracorporeal membrane oxygenation (*ECMO*) circuit in use.

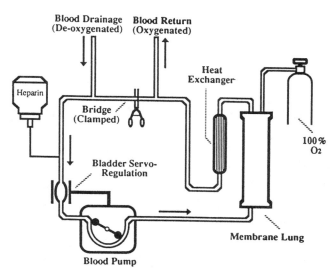

FIG. 31.2. Schematic diagram of an extracorporeal membrane oxygenation (*ECMO*) circuit.

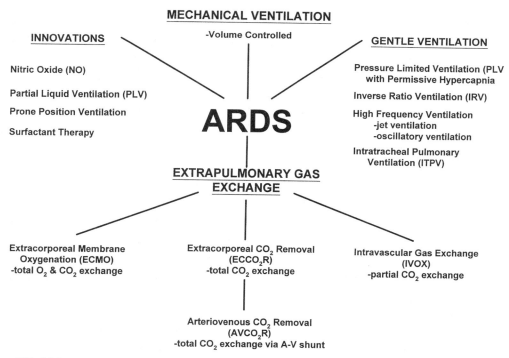

FIG. 31.3. Treatment options for adult respiratory distress syndrome (*ARDS*), which also apply to neonates, infants, and children.

HISTORY

John Gibbon, Jr. (3) and others developed the heart–lung machine in the 1930s and opened the era of cardiac surgery in the early 1950s (see Chapters 1 and 2). The use of an artificial pump and lung, however, was limited to 1 to 2 hours—not because of the pump but because of the oxygenator, which severely altered blood cells and proteins. Early oxygenators exposed blood directly to gas mixtures to provide oxygenation and CO_2 removal; these devices have been called *bubble oxygenators*. Their success resulted in the development of disposable, single-use bubble oxygenators used for cardiac surgery. A time-dependent pathologic response resulting in thrombocytopenia, hemolysis, coagulopathy, generalized edema, and multiple organ failure appeared to result from this direct exposure of blood to gaseous O_2. The first attempts to separate the blood phase from the gas phase (similar to what occurs in the native lung) utilized semipermeable membranes constructed of cellophane or polyethylene. These plastics were found to have low gas permeability and thus required very large surface areas to achieve adequate gas exchange (4,5). The first membrane oxygenator built and used clinically was reported in 1956 (4). With the introduction of silicone rubber as a membrane for gas transfer, the membrane oxygenator became practical for long-term CPB (6,7). In the absence of direct gas expo-

sure to blood, extracorporeal circulation could be carried out for weeks without hemolysis, significant capillary leak, or organ deterioration. Table 31.1 provides a chronology of key events in the history of ECMO.

Partial systemic anticoagulation was an important development in ECLS. Heparin anticoagulation sufficient to achieve an infinite clotting time had been used since the development of the first heart–lung machines. Bartlett et al. (8) demonstrated that lower doses of systemic heparin could be safely used by carefully regulating the activated clotting time (ACT) at the bedside within narrow ranges (e.g., ACT of 240 to 280 seconds). As a result, thrombosis in the extracorporeal circuit could be prevented while the potential for systemic bleeding complications was reduced.

Concurrently with the development of open heart surgery, the concept of intensive care units (ICUs) developed during the 1960s and early 1970s. Many patients with various forms of respiratory failure required mechanical ventilation to maintain adequate oxygenation and ventilation. Native lungs were subjected to whatever pressures and volumes were necessary in an effort to provide adequate gas exchange (9). At this time, a new pathophysiologic process called adult respiratory distress syndrome (ARDS) came to be recognized. Failure of the lungs, either as primary pathology or as a component of multiple organ failure, caused or contributed to more than 50% of all ICU deaths. ECMO was

TABLE 31.1. KEY EVENTS IN THE HISTORY OF EXTRACORPOREAL MEMBRANE OXYGENATION FOR RESPIRATORY FAILURE

Date	Event
1965–1975	Unsuccessful attempts to support infants with both bubble and membrane oxygenators by Rashkind (12), Dorson (210), White (211), Pyle (212).
1972	First successful treatment of adult respiratory distress syndrome with ECMO and partial venoarterial bypass for 3 days by Hill (23).
1975	First neonatal ECMO survivor at University of California, Irvine, by Bartlett (11).
1975–1979	U.S. National Institutes of Health ECMO study of adults with respiratory failure shows 9% survival in both treatment and control groups (26).
1982	Forty-five newborn cases with 23 survivors reported by Bartlett at University of Michigan, Ann Arbor (13).
1985, 1989	Randomized prospective studies of ECMO for neonatal respiratory failure show superiority over conventional therapy (18, 19).
1986	Gattinoni (31) reports 49% survival with extracorporeal CO_2 removal in ARDS.
1988	Treatment of selected adult patients resumes in United States (213).
1988	ECMO registry report: 715 neonatal cases at 18 centers with >80% survival (214).
1989	Extracorporeal Life Support Organization (ELSO) study group formed.
1989	Development (116) and first successful treatment of neonates with single-cannula double-lumen venovenous ECMO (77).
1990	Overall survival rate of 83% in 3,500 newborns with respiratory failure (215).
1992	ELSO Registry on ECMO for cardiac support with 46% survival in 553 cases following cardiac surgery (216).
1993	ELSO Registry on 285 pediatric cases at 52 centers with 49% survival (217).
1994	Double-lumen venovenous ECMO has higher survival and lower complication rate (118) (probably biased by selection; later reports show venovenous equal to venoarterial).
1997	Percutaneous double-lumen venovenous ECMO; Bartlett proposes "best management" algorithm for adult ARF (35).
1999	ELSO Registry report (20): 15,636 neonatal cases with 76% survival 3,372 pediatric cases with 47% survival 742 adult cases with 43% survival 1,642 pediatric cardiac cases with 39% survival

ARDS, Adult respiratory distress syndrome; ARF, adult respiratory failure.

proposed as a possible solution to the problem of life-threatening respiratory failure, just as hemodialysis had been developed to support the failing kidney until organ recovery occurred or transplant was performed.

In 1975, investigators studying prolonged extracorporeal support met near Copenhagen to define goals and produce a benchmark publication (10). In the United States, the National Institutes of Health (NIH) began a multicenter prospective, randomized study of ECMO in life-threatening respiratory failure. During this trial, many patients who were placed on ECMO continued to receive very high-pressure mechanical ventilation, which may have contributed to ongoing lung injury. The study was terminated after 92 patients had been enrolled (less than a third of the projected study size) when survival rates of the ECMO and control groups were both less than 10%. Death was frequently the result of technical complications, and autopsies uniformly revealed extensive pulmonary fibrosis (an irreversible injury). As a result of these findings, ECMO therapy for adults essentially stopped in the United States. Conclusions of the study were the following: (a) application of ECMO to patients with irreversible pulmonary fibrosis is ineffective; (b) application to patients with reversible lung injury may work; (c) technical conduct of ECMO is critically important because complications during ECMO are often life-threatening and must be reduced to a minimum for ECMO to be successful; and (d) lungs will not heal when exposed to extremely high ventilator pressures.

Bartlett et al. (11) persisted with application of the technique to a select population of neonates with life-threatening but potentially reversible respiratory failure characterized by pulmonary hypertension and right-to-left shunting associated with hypoxemia. The technique of neonatal ECMO involved extrathoracic cannulation of the right internal jugular vein and right common carotid artery for partial venoarterial (VA) CPB. Partial systemic anticoagulation with heparin was used to prevent circuit thrombosis and minimize hemorrhagic complications. The most physiologically significant concept to come from this experience was that of "lung rest." Early in the ECMO experience, it became apparent that even profoundly injured lungs could recover if they were allowed to heal without the application of high-pressure mechanical ventilation.

Although ECMO had been used since 1975, aside from the NIH-sponsored study, the systematic collection of data did not begin until 1985. Since 1989, participating ECMO centers have voluntarily registered all patients with the Neonatal, Pediatric, and Adult ECMO Registry of the Extracorporeal Life Support Organization (ELSO). Use of this database has permitted information about patient demographics, pre-ECMO clinical features, ECMO indications, medical and technical complications, and outcome to be collected and updated continuously. Table 31.2 displays the number of cases in the database as of mid-1999 along with the average number of hours of ECMO support stratified by patient population.

TABLE 31.2. CASES IN EXTRACORPOREAL LIFE SUPPORT ORGANIZATION DATABASE AS OF JULY 1999

	Total No. of Cases	Average No. of Hours on ECMO
Neonatal respiratory	14,543	150.18
Neonatal and pediatric cardiac	2,727	140.86
Pediatric respiratory	1,711	276.08
Adult respiratory	483	224.23
Adult cardiac	244	104.63

ECMO, extracorporeal membrane oxygenation.

Neonatal Application

Extracorporeal circulation for respiratory failure was first attempted in newborns in the 1960s (12). Bartlett et al. (11) began clinical trials in 1972 and reported the first successful use of ECMO in newborn respiratory failure in 1976. During the initial experience, neonates undergoing ECMO had an overall survival rate of 75% to 95% (13–15). These results helped to establish the therapeutic effectiveness of ECMO in infants who had met criteria predicting 80% to 100% mortality. In 1986, Bartlett et al. (16) reported the first 100 cases of neonatal respiratory failure managed with ECMO; the overall survival rate was 72%. The collaborative United Kingdom ECMO Trial (17) concluded that ECMO support reduces the risk for death without a concomitant rise in severe disability. In a comparison of ECMO with conventional treatment, 61% of the ECMO group ($n = 92$) were alive at 1 year versus 41% of the conventionally treated group ($n = 93$). ECMO has become the standard treatment for SRF in newborn infants based on successful phase I studies (11), two prospective randomized studies (18,19), and worldwide application in more than 14,543 patients, with an overall 80% survival rate in neonates thought to have a survival rate of 20% without ECMO (20).

Neonatal respiratory failure can be severe, progressive, and rapidly fatal. Although there are a number of causes of respiratory failure in newborns [meconium aspiration, persistent fetal circulation (PFC), persistent pulmonary hypertension (PPHN), congenital diaphragmatic hernia (CDH), sepsis], they all share a common pathophysiologic mechanism—pulmonary artery hypertension with persistent fetal circulation. Hypoxia, hypercarbia, and acidosis cause pulmonary vasoconstriction that results in right-to-left shunting at the atrial, ductal, and intrapulmonary levels. Shunting worsens the hypoxia, which in turn increases pulmonary vascular resistance, creating a downward cycle. Conventional methods for treating pulmonary artery hypertension have included mechanical ventilation with paralysis, induced respiratory alkalosis, and sometimes vasodilators.

Pediatric Application

Concurrently with the adult collaborative study, ECMO was evaluated in children. Bartlett et al. (14) and Kolobow et al. (21) reported an ECMO survival rate of 30% in children and infants with acute respiratory failure (ARF) whose predicted survival rate with conventional therapy was thought to be less than 10%. Familiarity with ECMO use and success in neonates fostered confidence in the technique and an understanding of complications sufficient to initiate use in children and adults. Unlike neonatal ECMO trials, in which the pathology has a rapid onset and tends to be isolated in the lungs, pediatric clinical trials are subjected to many of the same problems experienced in trials of adult populations, notably diverse underlying disease processes and initiation of therapy after the onset of irreversible pulmonary changes. Green et al. (22) reported in the results from the Pediatric Critical Care Study Group multicenter analysis of ECMO for pediatric respiratory failure that ECMO was associated with a significant reduction in mortality versus conventional or high-frequency ventilation (74% survival with ECMO vs. 53% survival in controls). As of July 1998, ECMO had been used in more than 1,710 children with respiratory failure, with an overall survival rate of 55% (20). In children needing cardiac support, ECMO has also been used to yield a survival rate of 39% (20). As currently applied to children and adults, ECMO is indicated in acute, potentially lethal respiratory failure that does not respond to conventional therapy when the underlying condition is potentially reversible.

Adult Application

In 1972, Hill et al. (23) reported the first successful clinical use of ECMO in adults. A number of small patient series soon followed from the United States and Europe (24,25). Initially, the overall survival rates were relatively low, but the successes were individually dramatic. In response to this early enthusiasm, the United States NIH sponsored a multi-institutional prospective, randomized study of conventional mechanical ventilation versus ECMO in an adult population (26). In 90 adults with SRF, the survival rate with ECMO was 9.5%, compared with 8.3% when conventional treatment was used. The national experience at that time was only marginally better, with a reported pool survival rate of 15% (27). ECMO did not change the outcome in a group of patients with SRF for whom therapy was begun after several days of high-pressure mechanical ventilation and high O_2 concentration. The cause of death in patients in the ECMO and control groups was pulmonary fibrosis or necrotizing pneumonitis. ECMO provided safe and stable life support, and it seemed that ECMO would be effective for high-risk patients if begun early, before pulmonary fibrosis or necrosis occurred. With the development of new equipment, a more clinically homogenous study group, ear-

lier intervention, use of a lower fraction of inspired O_2 (F_{IO_2}), and ventilation techniques less traumatic to the lung, the survival rates of adult ECMO patients are improving (28).

The first successful application of VA ECMO for status asthmaticus in an adult was reported in 1981 (29), as severe reactive airway disease is reversible, with most deaths resulting from complications of mechanical ventilation (30). Gattinoni and co-workers (31), using a modified ECMO technique [low-frequency positive-pressure ventilation with extracorporeal CO_2 removal (LFPPV-$ECCO_2R$)] achieved 49% survival in adult patients with ARF. Improved survival rates were also partly attributable to better patient selection, venovenous (VV) perfusion, better regulation of anticoagulation, and ventilator management directed toward "lung rest." With this information at hand, Morris et al. (32) initiated a controlled trial of a three-step therapy for ARDS. Patients were randomly assigned to a control arm of protocol-controlled continuous positive-pressure ventilation or a new treatment arm of pressure-controlled inverse-ratio ventilation; if the patient failed to improve, LFPPV-$ECCO_2R$ was used. The overall survival rate was 39% in the $ECCO_2R$ and conventional therapy groups. Bartlett's experience, initially reported by Anderson et al. (33) in 1993, reported 47% survival in adults with ARF and 40% survival with ECMO for cardiac support. Most recently, in a retrospective review of 100 adult patients with ARF treated by Bartlett's group, Kolla et al. (34) reported a 54% overall survival using ECMO. Pre-ECMO independent predictors of outcome included the number of days of mechanical ventilation, pre-ECMO P_{aO_2}/F_{IO_2} (P/F) ratio, and patient age. Rich et al. (35) also retrospectively evaluated Bartlett's standardized management protocol for ARF by utilizing "lung-protective" mechanical ventilation and ECMO in 141 patients. Forty-one patients showed improvement with the initial protocol of ventilator management (83% survival), whereas 100 did not and required ECMO support (54% survival). Overall, lung recovery occurred in 67% of the ARF patients, with a 62% survival. Detailed protocols for respiratory management to ensure consistent and uniform respiratory care may yield results superior to those of historical or non–protocol-controlled critical care and may decrease the need for ECMO. As of July 1999, 483 adults with SRF treated with ECMO had been entered in the ELSO Registry. The overall survival rate in those patients was 40% (20). Clearly, the results of ECMO support for adult ARF have been much less impressive than those for neonates.

Trauma

Respiratory failure adds significant morbidity, mortality, and cost to the care of patients with multiple trauma. High peak airway pressures, F_{IO_2} values, and respiratory rates are often needed to maintain oxygenation and CO_2 removal, all of which are associated with barotrauma and O_2 toxicity (21). ECMO can provide cardiorespiratory support for the trauma patient, allowing reduction of ventilatory support to less damaging levels (36,37). The primary risk with ECLS in trauma patients is severe bleeding because of the need for systemic heparinization. Among 24 moribund pediatric and adult patients with respiratory failure from trauma, Anderson and associates (36) reported 15 (63%) survivals to discharge with the use of ECMO. Early intervention was found to be a key factor in successful outcome.

PATHOPHYSIOLOGY

The immediate beneficial effects of ECMO relate to decreasing the lung injury associated with mechanical ventilation by using ventilator settings that "rest" the lungs. In general, ECMO provides pulmonary, cardiac, or cardiopulmonary support for a period of days to several weeks to allow resolution of the primary injury.

Neonates

Persistent fetal circulation, also known as PPHN of the newborn, is a major pathophysiologic mechanism of hypoxemia in full-term infants, regardless of whether the primary condition is CDH, meconium aspiration, respiratory distress syndrome, sepsis, or primary PFC (38). In this condition, pulmonary arteriolar spasm increases pulmonary vascular resistance to cause right-to-left shunting through the patent ductus arteriosus and foramen ovale. During ECMO, exposure of the lungs to a low FIO_2, low ventilator rate, and low airway pressures allows reversal of PFC and promotes recovery by minimizing the harmful effects of high-pressure mechanical ventilation.

Children and Adults

In adults and children, the challenge is to identify the causes of ARF that may be reversible within the safe time limits (2 to 3 weeks) of ECMO. Conditions treated successfully by ECMO include bacterial and viral pneumonias, fat and thrombotic pulmonary embolism, thoracic or extrathoracic trauma, shock, sepsis, and near-drowning. As in neonates, lung rest from the harmful effects of positive-pressure ventilation may be the primary benefit of ECMO (39).

Physiology of Other Organs during Extracorporeal Membrane Oxygenation

Whereas red blood cell destruction occurs after several hours of bypass when a bubble oxygenator is used, red cell loss is minimal across modern membrane lungs. Potential sources of red blood cell damage during long-term ECMO include mechanical injury from the roller pump and negative pres-

sures within the circuit. Homologous blood transfusions may be needed to replace blood lost through wounds, blood sampling, and the small amount of red cell destruction that occurs. Platelets adhere to the prosthetic surface, where fibrinogen is deposited within minutes of exposure. Released adenosine diphosphate and serotonin attract additional platelets, causing platelet aggregates to form. These "clumps" of platelets, including some white cells (and red cells in stagnant areas of the circuit), are released into the circulating blood and infused into the patient, where they eventually separate and are removed by the reticuloendothelial system (40,41). Platelets are continuously consumed during ECMO. If platelet consumption is balanced by increased platelet production, platelet counts stabilize in the range of 30,000 to 60,000/μL (1). In newborns and children, platelet production does not match destruction, and platelet transfusion is virtually always required. The functional effects of ECMO on white blood cells is less well known, but total and differential white blood cell counts remain nearly normal at 5,000 to 15,000/mm³ (42,43).

Fluid and electrolytes are managed as they would be in any patient. Capillary permeability is usually increased to some degree because of the patient's underlying disease in addition to complement activation when ECMO is initiated (44). Both loop diuretics and osmotic agents can be used to treat fluid overload or edema. Preexisting renal failure can be treated by dialysis with a hemofilter placed within the circuit. Although rarely a problem, significant amounts of free water are lost from the membrane lung. Cool, dry sweep gas exits the lung warmed and saturated with vapor. An infant can lose more than 150 mL of free water per day in this fashion. Serum ionized calcium levels may fall when ECMO is started (45), which is especially significant when VV ECMO is initiated, and can result in hypotension from low cardiac output. It remains unclear whether this derives from the citrate present in banked blood or from dilution.

Direct hyperbilirubinemia, likely from hemolysis, is common and may be severe, but it typically resolves without sequelae. One group reported biliary calculi in 2 of 121 patients with post-ECMO follow-up (46). The hemolysis, total parenteral nutrition, diuretics, and prolonged fasting associated with ECMO may predispose neonates to early calculous disease. Although gastrointestinal function may be normal, it has not been customary to use enteral nutrition during ECMO; however, recent emphasis on its beneficial effects to the integrity of the intestinal mucosa is changing this practice. Piena et al. (47) prospectively evaluated changes in small intestinal integrity in neonatal ECMO patients. Although intestinal integrity is typically compromised in neonates on ECMO, introducing enteral nutrition did not result in further deterioration. Pettignano et al. (48) compared enteral and parenteral nutrition in neonates on ECMO. Although the differences did not reach statistical significance, these authors reported 100% survival in their enterally fed group and 79% in the parenterally fed group.

They concluded that enteral nutritional support can be safely administered to pediatric patients undergoing VA or VV ECMO.

Central nervous system function appears to be unaffected by ECMO. Infants may be awake and alert, and adults may be communicative during ECMO. The effects of microembolization from the extracorporeal circuit, although potentially harmful, seem to be of little practical significance. Organ function usually remains normal during prolonged ECMO. Tissue infarcts are rarely seen at autopsy, which suggests that microembolization during ECMO is not functionally significant. VV ECMO has a theoretical advantage over VA ECMO because of the reduced potential for systemic embolization (assuming the absence of anatomic right-to-left shunting). Neurologic and audiologic sequelae have been reported in 10% to 20% of VA ECMO survivors (49–57). Another 20% to 30% who had no evidence of severe handicap at 1 to 3 years of age manifested cognitive and visual–motor deficiencies at early school age (51,58). Graziani et al. (59) followed 271 infants treated with ECMO between 1985 and 1996 and concluded that (a) hypotension before or during ECMO and the need for cardiopulmonary resuscitation before ECMO contribute to cerebral palsy; (b) profound hypocarbia before ECMO and delayed ECMO intervention are associated with a significantly increased risk for hearing loss; and (c) the type and severity of neurologic and cognitive sequelae depend, in part, on the primary cause of the neonatal cardiorespiratory failure.

Physiology of the Native Lung during Extracorporeal Membrane Oxygenation

During VA ECMO, left ventricular outflow falls in proportion to the extracorporeal blood flow, which results in a decreased pulse pressure. During VA ECMO, a significant portion of the pulmonary blood flow is diverted through the extracorporeal circuit. There appear to be no major deleterious effects of reduced pulmonary blood flow unless normal ventilation is maintained. With normal ventilation of the native lungs during ECMO, pulmonary capillary pH can be as high as 8.0. Hemolysis and pulmonary hemorrhage can result, even without marked systemic hypocarbia (60,61). When ECMO is initiated, ventilatory settings are rapidly decreased to prevent further damage from overdistension and to prevent local tissue alkalosis. A low respiratory rate and normal inspiratory pressure or continuous positive airway pressure can be used during ECMO. A few sustained inflations above the alveolar opening pressure are provided periodically to prevent total lung collapse.

During VV ECMO, right ventricular output is normal and probably higher than before ECMO because cardiac output increases after severe hypoxia is corrected. This exposes the pulmonary arterioles to blood with a relatively high P_{O_2}, which may reduce pulmonary hypertension.

Oxygen Delivery

Management with ECMO requires a thorough understanding of O_2 delivery and the physiology of O_2 consumption. O_2 consumption ($\dot{V}_{O_2}$) reflects the aerobic metabolic activity of tissues. Newborns use 5 to 8 mL of O_2 per kilogram per minute, children 4 to 6 mL, and adults 3 to 5 mL. O_2 consumption is decreased by hypothermia, sedation, and muscle paralysis induced by neuromuscular blocking drugs, and it is increased by exercise, shivering, catecholamines, hyperthermia, and infection. Under normal steady-state conditions, the amount of O_2 taken up across the lungs into the pulmonary circulation equals the amount of O_2 consumed by the tissues. This concept, the Fick principle, is summarized by the following equation:

$$\dot{V}_{O_2} = CO\,(Ca_{O_2} - Cv_{O_2})$$

where CO is cardiac output, Ca_{O_2} is arterial O_2 content, and Cv_{O_2} is mixed venous O_2 content. The amount of O_2 delivered to the tissues (D_{O_2}) is the product of CO and Ca_{O_2}. Under most circumstances, O_2 consumption is independent of O_2 delivery, and D_{O_2} exceeds $\dot{V}_{O_2}$ by a factor of 4 to 1. When D_{O_2} is substantially reduced, $\dot{V}_{O_2}$ can become supply-limited and fall below tissue demands for O_2, which results in lactic acidosis and circulatory failure (i.e., shock) (62).

During ECMO, extracorporeal flow is set at the minimum amount that allows an acceptable $P_{a_{O_2}}$ and mixed venous O_2 saturation ($S\bar{v}_{O_2}$). Pump flow may be decreased as $P_{a_{O_2}}$ rises when $S_v{O_2}$ is normal, indicating lung recovery. Air–O_2 sweep gas mixtures can be used to reduce the P_{O_2} of the perfusate if significant arterial hyperoxia is present. ECMO is most often applied to treat low D_{O_2} in the face of arterial hypoxia (hypoxic shock). During VA ECMO, total D_{O_2} is expressed as follows:

$$\begin{aligned} \text{Total } D_{O_2} \\ = (\text{Extracorporeal Flow})\,(Ca_{O_2}\ \text{Postmembrane Lung}) \\ + (CO)\,(Ca_{O_2}\ \text{Left Ventricle}) \end{aligned}$$

This concept must be appreciated to interpret arterial blood gases sampled from the patient on VA ECMO.

Blood oxygenation in the membrane lung is a function of the thickness of the blood film, membrane material and thickness, $F_{I_{O_2}}$, residence time of red cells in the gas exchange area, hemoglobin concentration, and inlet saturation. All these factors are included in a single descriptor of membrane lung function called *rated flow* (63), which is the amount of normal venous blood that can be raised from 75% to 95% oxyhemoglobin saturation in a given period. We use this information to plan which membrane lung to use and to evaluate membrane lung performances during perfusion. In planning the size of the circuit and extracorporeal flow rate, one assumes that there will be no gas exchange across the native lung.

As long as extracorporeal blood flow is less than the rated

flow of the membrane lung (and the device is functioning normally), the blood leaving the lung will be fully saturated. If the hemoglobin concentration is low or the venous blood saturation is high, the amount of O_2 that can be taken up by the membrane lung decreases, which can be compensated for by increasing blood flow. Conversely, a given DO_2 can be achieved at a lower blood flow by maintaining a higher hemoglobin concentration.

During VV bypass, P_aO_2 will be identical to the mixed right atrial PO_2, assuming there is no contribution from native lung gas exchange. Because some unsaturated blood is not captured by the venous drainage catheter, right atrial saturation is rarely greater than 90% and often resides closer to 80%. The resulting P_aO_2 may be as low as 40 mm Hg. The patient will therefore be relatively hypoxic and even cyanotic, but if the cardiac output is normal and the hemoglobin concentration is adequate, O_2 delivery will be adequate and recovery can occur. Recovery is indicated by an increase in P_aO_2 as the native lung begins to contribute O_2 to pulmonary blood flow.

In VA bypass, the perfusate blood is typically 100% saturated, with a PO_2 of 500 mm Hg. During VA bypass, an increase in systemic PO_2 may signify improving lung function at constant flows, decreasing native cardiac output at constant extracorporeal flow, or increasing extracorporeal flow at constant native output. An interesting physiologic property of the lung has been recognized with application of ECMO. Even the most severely injured lungs are capable of O_2 transfer if they are not required to provide any ventilatory function. This is the rationale behind $ECCO_2R$ and "apneic oxygenation," as developed by Gattinoni et al. (31). The lungs are inflated to moderate pressures (15 to 20 cm H_2O) and O_2 concentration is reduced while CO_2 is removed by low-flow partial VV bypass.

Carbon Dioxide Removal

Metabolic production of CO_2 approximates $\dot{V}O_2$ (respiratory quotient = 1). Excretion of CO_2 across normal native lungs is exquisitely sensitive to alveolar ventilation, with the rate and depth of breathing controlled to maintain P_aCO_2 at or below 40 mm Hg. The amount of CO_2 eliminated in the extracorporeal circulation is a function of membrane lung geometry, material, surface area, blood PCO_2, blood flow, and membrane lung ventilating gas flow. Usually, the ventilating gas contains no CO_2, so the gradient for CO_2 transfer is the difference between the blood PCO_2 and zero (when the gas flow rate is high). As the PCO_2 drops during the passage of blood through the membrane lung, the gradient decreases, so CO_2 excretion is less at the blood outlet than at the inlet. Consequently, the amount of CO_2 transfer is relatively independent of blood flow and only moderately dependent on inlet PCO_2, with the major determinants being total surface area and flow rate of sweep gas (analogous to minute ventilation in normal lungs). The capacity for

CO_2 removal is considerably greater than the capacity for O_2 uptake at the rated flow. For any silicone rubber or microporous membrane oxygenator, CO_2 clearance will always be more efficient than oxygenation when the oxygenator is well ventilated and functioning properly. Because of the efficiency of $ECCO_2R$, the systemic PCO_2 can be "set" at any level by matching the membrane lung surface area and gas flow with the systemic production of CO_2.

During VV bypass, oxygenated venous blood is returned to the venous circulation and mixed with systemic venous blood, which raises its O_2 content. The final O_2 content depends on native lung function, O_2 saturation of blood from the ECMO circuit, and the amount of recirculation through the circuit. Some of the mixed blood returns (recirculates) to the extracorporeal circuit, and some enters the right ventricle and traverses the pulmonary vasculature on its way to the systemic arterial circulation. VV ECMO is limited by the amount of systemic venous return in the extracorporeal circuit. If systemic venous return is insufficient, adequate support may not be achieved. VV ECMO depends solely on native cardiac output to provide flow and is most useful in pure respiratory failure or in respiratory failure accompanied by cardiac failure solely attributable to hypoxia or to excessive intrathoracic pressures generated by mechanical ventilation.

PATIENT SELECTION

Patients selected for ECMO must have a potentially reversible underlying pathologic process. Indications include acute reversible respiratory or cardiac failure that is unresponsive to optimal ventilator and pharmacologic management but from which recovery can be expected within a reasonable period (10 to 20 days) of extracorporeal support. The requirement for systemic heparinization limits ECMO support to patients without a bleeding diathesis, so that premature infants (younger than 35 weeks' gestation) (64) and patients with active bleeding are relatively excluded. Other contraindications include conditions incompatible with normal life after lung recovery (such as major brain injury), congenital or acquired immunodeficiency state, and mechanical ventilation for more than 5 to 10 days (an indication of irreversible ventilator-induced lung injury).

Neonates

Extracorporeal membrane oxygenation has been applied to infants with a mortality risk of 80% or greater by retrospective analysis of local patient populations. Included are neonates who, despite optimum medical management, have demonstrated acute deterioration (P_aO_2 <40 mm Hg or pH <7.15 for 2 hours), failure to improve (P_aO_2 <55 mm Hg and hypotension requiring inotropic support), uncontrolled air leak, pneumomediastinum, or deterioration after

CDH repair. Excessive alveolar-to-arterial O_2 gradients [$P(A-a)O_2$] have been proposed as a qualification for ECMO. In a retrospective review by Krummel and associates (65), a $P(A-a)O_2$ above 620 mm Hg for 12 consecutive hours correlated with a mortality rate above 90%. Many programs currently use the oxygenation index: mean airway pressure times F_{IO_2} times 100 divided by postductal P_aO_2. Based on data generated before ECMO availability, an oxygenation index consistently above 25 after optimal conventional therapy implies a 50% mortality rate, and an index above 40 defines an 80% mortality rate.

Contraindications to neonatal ECMO include any evidence of intracerebral hemorrhage, other brain damage, multiple congenital anomalies, and irreversible lung damage. In CDH, PFC cannot be distinguished from pulmonary hypoplasia; in most centers, therefore, all patients with diaphragmatic hernias are treated who otherwise meet local ECMO criteria (66). In some centers, a P_aO_2 value above 70 mm Hg or a P_aCO_2 below 80 mm Hg is required at some time in the neonate's life as evidence of sufficient functional pulmonary parenchyma to avoid the use of ECMO in infants with fatal pulmonary hypoplasia. Potential ECMO candidates are evaluated with cranial ultrasonography to rule out intraventricular hemorrhage and with cardiac ultrasonography to rule out congenital cardiac anomalies. Entry criteria should be evaluated at each hospital before ECMO therapy is begun because of regional differences in patient populations and treatment protocols.

Children and Adults

Despite advances in ventilatory support, antibiotic therapy, and critical care, mortality from ARDS remains at 50% to 80% (67–69). The disappointing outcomes with the conventional management of ARDS have resulted in an increased urgency for developing alternative strategies that provide sufficient oxygenation, CO_2 removal, and "lung rest," with the recognition that the primary goal of respiratory support is to accomplish CO_2 removal and O_2 exchange while avoiding high tidal volumes and airway pressures (70).

Reversible ARF in adults is difficult to define; therefore, adult criteria for ECMO are controversial (26,28,71). Table 31.3 lists selection criteria based on a predicted 90% mortality risk without ECMO. Most investigators use the entry criteria from the NIH ECMO study (26). Many use a P/F ratio of less than 100. Care must be taken to avoid therapy in patients with established pulmonary fibrosis, for which lung biopsy may be necessary.

TECHNIQUES AND MANAGEMENT

Extracorporeal membrane oxygenation has evolved into several formats, each with advantages and disadvantages depending on the physiology to be corrected and the expertise of the ECMO team. A comparison of different extracorporeal treatment modalities appears in Table 31.4.

Neonates

After the decision to begin ECMO is made, parental consent is obtained while the circuit is prepared and primed with heparinized blood. Because the blood volume in the circuit is as much as twice that of the neonate, the appropriate hematocrit, pH, and electrolyte concentrations must be obtained in the circuit before CPB is instituted. Patients are cannulated with VA access if cardiac support is required for acute hemodynamic compromise (cardiac arrest) or for transport on ECMO (Fig. 31.4). VV access is the method of choice for patients with isolated respiratory failure (Fig. 31.5).

Dissection and cannulation are performed under local anesthesia in the ICU. An oblique incision in the right side of the neck anterior to the sternocleidomastoid muscle exposes the internal jugular vein and common carotid artery (if VA ECMO is to be used). The infant is given a heparin bolus of 100 U/kg as a loading dose. The vessels are ligated cephalad, and cannulas are inserted toward the heart from the ligation site. The venous cannula is threaded through the right internal jugular vein into the right atrium, and the arterial cannula is inserted into the common carotid artery so that its tip rests at the entrance to the aortic arch (Fig. 31.6). The right common carotid artery in a neonate can be successfully ligated with a relatively low complication rate, presumably because of abundant collateral flow (72).

TABLE 31.3. EXTRACORPOREAL MEMBRANE OXYGENATION SELECTION CRITERIA FOR ADULTS WITH 90% MORTALITY RISK OR GREATER

Indications	Contraindications
Failure of optimal conventional therapy	Age >60 yr
Transpulmonary shunt >30%	Mechanical ventilation >5–7 days
Static lung compliance <0.5 mL/cm H_2O/kg	Incurable condition
Diffuse abnormal chest radiographic findings (four quadrants)	Potential for severe bleeding
Cardiac failure or cardiac arrest	

TABLE 31.4. COMPARISON OF EXTRACORPOREAL MEMBRANE OXYGENATION (ECMO), CARDIOPULMONARY BYPASS (CPB), EXTRACORPOREAL CARBON DIOXIDE REMOVAL (ECCO₂R), ARTERIOVENOUS CARBON DIOXIDE REMOVAL (AVCO₂R), AND TOTAL ARTIFICIAL LUNG

	ECMO	CPB	ECCO$_2$R	AVCO$_2$R	Total Artificial Lung
Setting	Respiratory and/or cardiac failure	Cardiac surgery	Respiratory failure	Respiratory failure (investigational)	Respiratory failure (experimental)
Location	Extrathoracic	Intrathoracic	Extrathoracic	Extrathoracic	Extrathoracic
Type of support	VA (cardiac) VV (respiratory)	VA (total bypass)	VV (respiratory) (CO_2)	AV (respiratory) (CO_2)	PA→PA or PA→LA
Cannulation	VA: neck VV: neck and groin 2 cannulas (surgical or percutaneous) 1 cannula (VVDL)	Direct cardiac 2 cannulas (surgical)	Neck and groin 2 cannulas (surgical or percutaneous) 1 cannula (VVDL)	Groin 2 cannulas (percutaneous)	Transthoracic to major vessels
Blood flow	High (70–80% CO)	Total (100% CO)	Medium (30% CO)	Low (10–15% CO)	Total (100%)
Ventilatory support	Pressure-controlled ± high PEEP 10–12 breaths/min	None (anesthesia)	High PEEP 2–4 breaths/min High F$_{IO_2}$	Volume controlled (algorithm driven)	None necessary
Blood reservoir	Small (50 mL)	Yes (>1 L)	Small (50 mL)	No	No
Arterial filter	No	Yes	No	No	No
Blood pump	Roller or centrifugal	Roller or centrifugal	Roller or centrifugal	None	None
Heparinization	ACT 200–260 s	ACT >400 s	ACT 200–260 s	ACT 200–260 s	ACT 200–260 s
Average length of extracorporeal support	Days to weeks	Hours	Days to weeks	Days to weeks	Days
Complications	Bleeding Organ failure	Intraoperative	Bleeding	Bleeding	Bleeding
Causes of death	Support terminated: PAP >75% systemic Irreversible lung disease Cardiac dysrhythmias	Intraoperative air embolism	Multiple organ failure Septic shock Hemorrhage	Respiratory failure	Right-sided heart failure

VA, venoarterial; VV, venovenous; AV, arteriovenous; PA, pulmonary artery; LA, left atrium; CO, cardiac output; PEEP, positive end-expiratory pressure; F$_{IO_2}$, fraction of inspired oxygen; ACT, activated clotting time; VVDL, venovenous double-lumen; PAP, pulmonary artery pressure.

The largest catheters [8 French (F) to 14F] that fit "comfortably" inside the artery and vein are used. Catheter positions are confirmed by chest radiography or ultrasonography. Positioning and flow resistance of the venous drainage catheter determine the maximum blood flow; the catheter should be capable of delivering total cardiac support of 120 mL/kg per minute.

After cannulation is accomplished and bypass initiated, blood drains by gravity through the venous catheter to a servo-regulated roller pump. The pump then perfuses the blood through a 0.6-, 0.8-, 2.5-, 3.5-, or 4.5-m² membrane lung (Avecor Cardiovascular, Inc., Minneapolis, MN) matched to the size of the patient. Gas exchange takes place in the membrane lung as O_2 is added to the blood, while water vapor and CO_2 are removed. Because CO_2 removal is much more efficient than O_2 transfer, exogenous CO_2

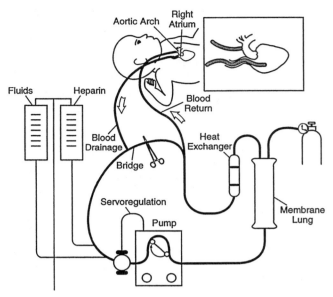

FIG. 31.4. Venoarterial extracorporeal membrane oxygenation (*VA ECMO*) circuit. Inset shows optimal locations for venous (right atrium) and arterial (near junction of aorta and innominate artery) cannula tips.

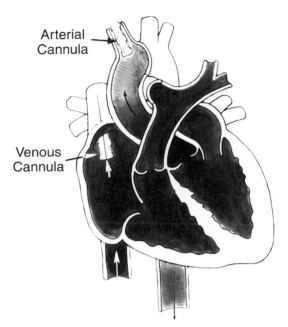

FIG. 31.6. The arterial catheter is positioned to reinfuse blood via the ascending aorta. The venous catheter aspirates blood from the atrium beyond the superior cavoatrial junction.

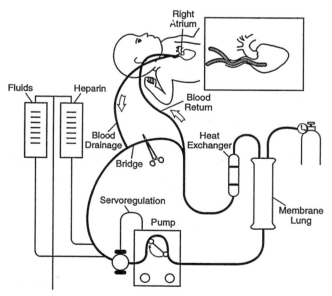

FIG. 31.5. Venovenous extracorporeal membrane oxygenation (*VV ECMO*) circuit with a double-lumen catheter. Inset depicts cannulation of the right atrium by way of the right internal jugular vein. Side holes on the return lumen of the catheter direct oxygenated blood toward the tricuspid valve.

often must be added to the O_2 inflow to avoid hypocapnic alkalosis. The blood then passes through a heat exchanger and returns to the patient. Blood flow is gradually increased during the initial 15 to 20 minutes of bypass until approximately 80% of the infant's cardiac output flows through the circuit. Figure 31.7 plots a typical sequence in an adult, which would differ from that in a neonate only in the magnitude of flows. Oxygenated blood from the circuit mixes in the aortic arch with poorly oxygenated blood from the left ventricle and ductus arteriosus to yield a mixed arterial O_2 content adequate for the infant's metabolic requirements (73).

Once ECMO is established and appropriate pH, P_aO_2, and P_aCO_2 values are obtained, ventilator settings are reduced to minimize barotrauma and O_2 toxicity (peak inspiratory pressure, 20 cm H_2O; rate, 10 breaths per minute; FIO_2, 0.3). The optimum peak end-expiratory pressure (PEEP) is uncertain, but many programs use high PEEP (12 to 15 cm H_2O) with mean airway pressures of 13 to 16 cm H_2O, based on experimental studies in a neonatal lamb model of meconium aspiration (74) showing that this approach decreases the time of ECMO without increasing barotrauma. A prospective, randomized study in neonates concluded that higher PEEP safely prevents deterioration of pulmonary function during ECMO and results in more rapid lung recovery (75).

The ECMO flow is maintained to achieve full respiratory support until lung improvement occurs. Pulmonary function is assessed by monitoring the saturation of venous drainage blood and arterial blood (with a pulse oximeter).

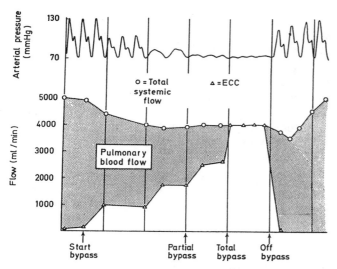

FIG. 31.7. Hemodynamic changes during venoarterial bypass. Total flow and arterial blood pressure are shown during various levels of bypass. As blood is diverted from the right atrium to the extracorporeal circuit, pulmonary blood flow (and left ventricular flow) gradually decrease to nil, so that total bypass is achieved. Pulse amplitude decreases, reaching nearly a nonpulsatile state during total bypass.

The usual flow for full support is 80 to 120 mL/kg per minute (average, 300 to 400 mL/min), and the target arterial P_aO_2 range is 70 to 90 mm Hg. Adequate support is defined as that level of extracorporeal flow that results in normal arterial and mixed venous oxygenation, mean arterial pressure, and organ function. During ECMO, chest physiotherapy continues, and suctioning is accomplished through the endotracheal tube. Neuromuscular blocking and vasoactive drugs are discontinued, and patients are maintained alert and awake. Standard treatment for severe lung dysfunction is continued during ECMO, including bronchoscopy when necessary, prone positioning, and diuresis to achieve the appropriate calculated "dry" patient weight. Although not necessary for management, we monitor native lung $\dot{V}O_2$ and $\dot{V}CO_2$ and membrane lung $\dot{V}O_2$ and $\dot{V}CO_2$ daily. We determine the total $\dot{V}O_2$ (calculate the respiratory quotient) and use that number to calculate calorimetry indirectly for purposes of nutritional planning (76). We calculate the percentage of total $\dot{V}O_2$ achieved through the native lung. If that percentage is less than 25% of total $\dot{V}O_2$ after the first week on support, the prognosis for lung recovery is poor.

Anticoagulation must be maintained during the entire course of treatment. Heparin is administered into the circuit with a loading dose of 100 U/kg, followed by a constant infusion of approximately 30 U/kg per hour (20 to 70 U/kg per hour). The whole blood ACT is measured each hour and maintained at two to three times normal values (220 to 260 seconds). Platelets, which may be destroyed by the membrane lung, are administered when thrombocytopenia

of 100,000/μL or less (or 150,000/μL—the exact number is controversial) is observed. The hematocrit is maintained between 35% and 45% with packed red blood cell transfusions. Maintenance intravenous (IV) fluids are delivered directly into the bypass circuit, as is total parenteral nutrition, which is begun on the second or third day of life. Antibiotics (ampicillin and gentamicin) are administered until ECMO is completed. A chest radiograph and cranial ultrasonographic study are obtained daily.

When the lungs begin to recover, extracorporeal blood flow is reduced in a stepwise fashion until 10% to 20% of the infant's cardiac output (usually 40 to 50 mL/min) is diverted through the circuit while arterial PO_2 is again maintained between 70 and 90 mm Hg. After an idling period of 8 to 12 hours to ensure continued lung function, the circuit is disconnected, cannulas are removed, and the vessels are ligated. The vessels can be repaired, but this procedure is unnecessary and may be harmful if thrombi form and embolize. After decannulation, the infant is maintained with mechanical ventilation but is usually weaned to an O_2 hood within 48 to 72 hours. During the first 3 to 4 days off ECMO, the platelet count must be monitored closely for a precipitous drop while damaged platelets are removed from the circulation.

The ductus arteriosus usually closes spontaneously during the course of ECMO. If it does not, surgical closure is indicated while the patient remains on bypass. Termination of ECMO is indicated when the lungs have recovered or when signs of irreversible brain damage, uncontrollable bleeding, or irreversible lung damage (patient dependent on ECMO for >20 days) are present. ECMO may be continued longer than 20 days if progressive improvement is seen or if open lung biopsy demonstrates a reversible condition. In recent years, VV ECMO, with a single cannula placed in the internal jugular vein, has been used to provide ECLS with excellent results in newborns (77).

Children and Adults

For VA bypass, the same vessels used for neonatal ECMO (common carotid artery and internal jugular vein) are cannulated to deliver the oxygenated blood into the aortic arch. For VV access, we prefer the right internal jugular vein for drainage and the right femoral vein for reinfusion (Fig. 31.8). Rich et al. (78) recently compared atriofemoral and femoroatrial flow in adult VV ECMO. Femoroatrial bypass provided higher maximal extracorporeal flow and higher pulmonary arterial mixed venous O_2 saturation, and it required less flow to maintain equivalent mixed venous O_2 saturation than did atriofemoral bypass. In adults, 80 to 100 mL/kg per minute is an adequate blood flow rate. As in the neonate, the extracorporeal flow is increased until satisfactory gas exchange is achieved with low ventilator settings. Large membrane lungs (up to 4.5 m²) are used, and if necessary, two lungs may be placed in parallel for increased

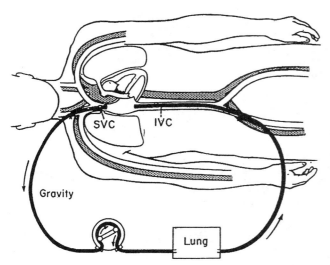

FIG. 31.8. Venovenous bypass in which the superior vena cava (*SVC*) (via jugular vein) is used as the venous outflow tract and the inferior vena cava (*IVC*) (via femoral vein) is used as the arterial inflow tract.

gas exchange. Management and weaning of adults is similar to that for neonates, but survivors require a longer time on ECMO. When pulmonary or cardiac function has recovered sufficiently to sustain reasonable hemodynamic and metabolic parameters off ECMO, the patient is decannulated. Complications are primarily related to bleeding and circuit component failure.

Because the patient is on extracorporeal support and does not have to breathe, aspects of airway management unique to ECMO can be undertaken. If a large bronchopleural fistula is present, we manage it by selectively ventilating the opposite lung for a period of time, selectively occluding the offending bronchus with a balloon catheter for 1 or 2 days, or stopping ventilation altogether while the air leak seals. Once the air leak has been sealed for 48 hours, we re-recruit the atelectatic lung by continuous static airway pressure in the range of 20 to 30 cm H_2O. If the primary problems include excessive exudate or occlusion of the airways, the patient undergoes bronchoscopy, with lengthy periods devoted to airway cleaning and lavage. The use of perfluorocarbon liquid ventilation in these patients to lavage the airways and improve alveolar recruitment and oxygenation shows promise (79). Some centers favor early tracheostomy in patients with respiratory failure, in general because of the decreased incidence of nosocomial pneumonia caused by pharyngeal bacteria, easier airway access, and easier ventilator weaning (80,81). If a tracheostomy has not been placed before ECMO, some undertake that procedure by percutaneous access on the first or second day of bypass (82). However, this involves some risk for bleeding at the tracheal stoma, so if the patient will be weaned off bypass within a few days, we delay tracheostomy until the patient is off bypass.

Rarely, we have used ECMO to manage patients with severe airway obstruction in status asthmaticus or with airway occlusion by blood clots or other foreign material (83). In these circumstances, oxygenation is usually adequate, and the problem is CO_2 retention, high intrathoracic pressures, cardiovascular collapse, or barotrauma; relatively low-flow ECMO is used to remove CO_2 (ECCO$_2$R) and permit nondamaging ventilator settings.

Hemodynamics and cardiac status are monitored by pulse contour, pulmonary capillary wedge pressure, systemic blood pressure, and signs of systemic perfusion. Mixed venous O_2 saturation is distorted in the VV access patient because of recirculation. If there is any question about ventricular dysfunction, valvular dysfunction, clots in the heart, or pericardial tamponade, we evaluate the heart by echocardiography. Usually, it is possible to wean the patient from inotropic drugs completely within a day or two of starting ECMO. If severe myocardial dysfunction is present that is unresponsive to small doses of inotropes, we convert to VA access, usually by direct cutdown to the right common carotid artery. If we begin VA bypass for reasons of transporting the patient or because of severe hemodynamic instability, we convert to VV access as soon as adequate myocardial function is demonstrated.

A progressive increase in pulmonary vascular resistance toward systemic levels is an ominous sign and usually represents progressive and irreversible fibrosis in the lung parenchyma. When the mean pulmonary artery pressure is consistently greater than two-thirds of the systemic pressure, the risk for right ventricular failure is high, and arrhythmias leading to ventricular tachycardia and fibrillation may occur. It is possible to support the circulation by converting to VA access at this point, but this situation has been uniformly fatal because of progressive lung injury, so we consider right ventricular failure after days or weeks of VV support to be a sign of irreversibility and do not attempt cardiac resuscitation if it occurs. Conversely, if we have been managing ECMO for 3 or 4 weeks with no sign of lung improvement, but pulmonary artery pressure is less than half the systemic pressure, we continue ECMO with the expectation of recovery.

Patients who are started on ECMO have usually been heavily sedated and perhaps intentionally paralyzed with neuromuscular blockers to facilitate ventilator management. As soon as stable ECMO is achieved, we stop (or actively reverse) all sedative and paralytic drugs until we can document the status of brain function. Most of these patients have had prolonged periods of hypoxia, usually associated with low blood flow, and they may not return to normal consciousness during the initial testing. However, we expect to see the patient moving all extremities and the eyes and tongue, and to be able to respond to simple commands. After verifying that level of neurologic function, we provide minimal sedation with morphine or midazolam titrated to apparent patient comfort. After sufficient sedation has been achieved (including the use of an amnestic agent such as midazolam), we frequently paralyze patients, particularly when the ventilator is managed with a very long inspiratory phase and short expiratory phase. In addition, paralysis is sometimes necessary when patient agitation and activity increase the $\dot{V}O_2$ beyond what our delivery system can match. Our preference, however, is to keep patients awake and alert during prolonged support. If the patient is paralyzed and heavily sedated, we reverse the agents every 1 to 2 days to evaluate brain function. In the course of testing, if it is apparent that the patient has sustained a significant decrease in brain function, we then perform computed tomography of the head to look for diffuse cerebral edema resulting from preexisting hypoxic ischemic encephalopathy, localized intracranial bleeding, or infarction. When severe brain damage becomes apparent, the entire procedure is discontinued if the situation does not improve within 24 hours. On occasion, the diagnosis of cortical brain death can be made by physical examination after reversal of pharmacologic agents (lack of spontaneous movement, pupillary reflexes, and response to cold caloric stimulation of the ears). In such a case, we do not find computed tomography of the head or electroencephalography necessary to confirm the diagnosis, although these studies may be reassuring to team members or family members before ECMO support is discontinued.

When we are managing the patient at low ACT and high platelet count, either for operations or to control bleeding, thrombosis may occur in the circuit. We monitor the circuit carefully by examining it directly for clots and by noting pressure drops across the membrane lungs. The first sign of circuit clotting is an increased pressure drop across the membrane lung and loss of gas exchange function, in which case the entire circuit is exchanged for a fresh one.

Occasionally, it becomes necessary to conduct a surgical operation while a patient is receiving ECMO therapy. Usually, this is an elective tracheostomy or related to active bleeding in the chest or abdomen. However, we have undertaken such operations as diaphragmatic hernia repair, liver transplantation, lung transplantation, heart transplantation, and evacuation of intracranial hematoma in patients on ECMO. Table 31.5 lists some of the operative procedures that have been performed on ECMO. When undertaking elective or emergent operations (other than cardiac procedures requiring complete CPB) while a patient is on ECMO, we decrease the heparin dose until the whole blood ACT is 140 seconds, give platelets until the count is above $100,000/\mu L$, and prepare to use autotransfusion if necessary.

Congenital Diaphragmatic Hernia

In 1981, the first cases of infants with CDH treated with ECMO were reported (84). The rationale for using ECMO in infants with CDH is to rest the lungs as pulmonary hypertension resolves to avoid subjecting them to unneces-

TABLE 31.5. SURGICAL PROCEDURES PERFORMED DURING EXTRACORPOREAL MEMBRANE OXYGENATION FOR CARDIOPULMONARY SUPPORT

Thoracotomy for intrathoracic bleeding
Transthoracic repair of congenital diaphragmatic hernia
Ligation of patent ductus arteriosus
Open lung biopsy
Lung lobectomy for bronchopleural fistula
Lung lobectomy for arteriovenous malformation
Lung lobectomy for cystic adenomatoid malformation
Pericardial window to release tamponade
Repair of aortic puncture wound
Tracheal reconstruction
Laparotomy for gastrointestinal perforation
Gastrectomy for bleeding
Transabdominal repair of congenital diaphragmatic hernia
Splenectomy for bleeding
Exploratory laparotomy for hemoperitoneum

Extracorporeal Life Support Organization Registry Report, July 1999.

sary barotrauma. Since the introduction of ECMO as a treatment strategy for respiratory failure associated with CDH, improved survival rates have been reported (85–94). The impact on mortality, however, has been institution-dependent, with survival rates varying from 34% to 87% (90). CDH has the lowest survival rate of all neonatal ECMO diagnostic categories. Current multicenter ELSO Registry data show that CDH infants treated with ECMO have a survival rate of 58% (20). Despite no reliable predictors to govern ECMO utilization, ECMO remains the mainstay of CDH treatment.

Although the role of ECMO as a treatment for CDH has been widely accepted, the timing of the surgical repair of the defect in relation to ECMO therapy remains controversial. It has been suggested that there is a survival advantage to performing CDH repair after ECMO decannulation (95–99). With this operative strategy, survival rates have been variable and as high as 80% (95,97,100). CDH patients have a higher risk for complications than do other ECMO patients. They have longer ECMO runs and are generally kept less anticoagulated, which leads to more mechanical complications. Because they undergo a major operation (CDH repair) either just before or during ECMO, CDH patients experience more hemorrhagic complications. In a review of 483 cases of CDH, the overall incidence of hemorrhage was 43%, with fatal hemorrhage occurring in 4.8% of cases (101). Locations of bleeding in descending order were surgical site (24%), intracranial (11%), cannulation site (7.5%), gastrointestinal (5%), pleural cavity (3.5%), abdominal (2.8%), and pulmonary (1.9%).

The criteria for determining ECMO use in infants with CDH have been based on factors predicting a mortality of 80% or higher for all cases of neonatal respiratory failure treated with conventional mechanical ventilation, although such criteria are variable and institution-specific. In neonates with CDH, ECMO is indicated in the presence of inadequate O_2 delivery despite adequate volume resuscitation, pharmacologic support, and ventilation. If emergent repair is required, infants are placed on ECMO postoperatively. As delayed repair has become more common, the perioperative use of ECMO (including during hernia repair) has also increased. Favorable results have also been reported when repair is delayed until the child is off ECMO (102,103).

Although the overall survival rate for neonates with CDH is unknown, the outcome from various institutions is shown in Table 31.6. Past studies have suggested that the mortality rate has remained approximately 50%, even with the increased utilization of ECMO support (90,104–107). Variation in published survival rates is quite high and represents institutional differences in management strategies and perhaps patient accrual. The continued evolution of mechanical ventilation techniques, extracorporeal support, surfactant use, nitric oxide use, and timing of surgical intervention complicates the interpretation of all studies.

Clinically, chronic lung disease has been reported in CDH survivors requiring ECMO (108,109). Whether this is related to the pathophysiology of the disease or is induced iatrogenically remains unclear. Studies have identified a number of nonpulmonary morbidities in CDH survivors, particularly in those infants requiring aggressive management of SRF. Neurologic abnormalities have been the most common problems found in a number of series. Abnormalities in both motor and cognitive skills have been identified (96,108) in addition to visual disturbances, hearing loss, seizures, abnormal cranial computed tomographic and magnetic resonance imaging findings, and abnormal electroencephalogram studies (108,109).

VENOVENOUS EXTRACORPOREAL MEMBRANE OXYGENATION

Development and Clinical Experience

The most widely used strategy for long-term perfusion support has been VA ECMO. Of the 13,708 neonatal ECMO cases reported to the ELSO Registry, 10,051 were supported with VA perfusion and only 220 with VV ECMO. However, the VV approach is not new; its use in animals was first described in 1969 (110). In 1973, Hanson and colleagues (111) showed that VV perfusion could be used to support adequate gas exchange in lambs breathing nitrogen. Lamy and colleagues (112) investigated the effects of various cannulation routes, including VV support, on the pulmonary circulation, and in 1979, Delaney and co-workers (113) studied the effects of VV in comparison with VA flow on lung transvascular fluid dynamics. The technique of VV ECMO, as performed by Gattinoni et al. (31) and Kolobow (28), is different from VA ECMO (114) (Table 31.7). This

TABLE 31.6. CONGENITAL DIAPHRAGMATIC HERNIA PATIENT OUTCOME WITH EXTRACORPOREAL MEMBRANE OXYGENATION

ECMO Before Repair		
Authors	**Year**	**Survival**
Bailey et al. (94)	1989	2/3 (67%)
Breaux et al. (218)	1991	5/11 (45%)
West et al. (100)	1992	7/9 (78%)
Wilson et al. (98)	1992	24/64 (38%)
Coughlin et al. (219)	1993	4/7 (57%)
Walker (220)	1993	50/114 (44%)
Vazquez and Cheu (101)	1994	181/258 (70%)
Lessin et al. (90)	1995	11/22 (50%)
Rais-Bahrami et al. (221)	1995	16/27 (59%)
Sigalet et al. (103)	1995	13/20 (65%)
Reickert et al. (222)	1996	5/10 (50%)
Azarow et al. (223)	1997	32/61 (52%)
Wilson et al. (224)	1997	23/52 (44%)
Nagaya et al. (225)	1998	7/17 (41%)
ECMO During Repair		
Authors	**Year**	**Survival**
Lally et al. (99)	1992	18/42 (43%)
Steimle et al. (226)	1994	6/17 (35%)
Vazquez and Cheu (101)	1994	88/173 (51%)
Wilson et al. (97)	1994	13/31 (42%)
Azarow et al. (223)	1997	37/61 (61%)
Ssemakula et al. (227)	1997	15/31 (48%)
Wilson et al. (224)	1997	51/74 (69%)
Weber et al. (228)	1998	16/27 (59%)
ECMO After Repair		
Author	**Year**	**Survival**
Langham et al. (229)	1987	5/7 (71%)
Langham et al. (230)	1987	52/93 (56%)
Redmond et al. (92)	1987	7/12 (58%)
Johnston et al. (231)	1988	11/11 (100%)
Stolar et al. (232)	1988	12/14 (86%)
Bailey et al. (94)	1989	10/20 (50%)
Heiss et al. (86)	1989	13/15 (87%)
Newman et al. (233)	1990	15/25 (60%)
Van Meurs et al. (91)	1990	10/17 (59%)
Atkinson et al. (89)	1991	9/13 (69%)
O'Rourke et al. (234)	1991	9/26 (35%)
West et al. (100)	1992	8/11 (73%)
Coughlin et al. (219)	1993	6/13 (46%)
Van Meurs et al. (235)	1993	18/34 (53%)
Steimle et al. (226)	1994	21/29 (72%)
Vazquez and Cheu (101)	1994	35/52 (67%)
Lessin et al. (90)	1995	12/23 (52%)
Azarow et al. (223)	1997	28/54 (52%)
Keshen et al. (236)	1997	6/14 (43%)
McGahren et al. (237)	1997	9/34 (26%)
Ssemakula et al. (227)	1997	21/29 (72%)
Wilson et al. (224)	1997	21/50 (43%)
Nagaya et al. (225)	1998	11/15 (73%)
Weber et al. (228)	1998	20/32 (62%)
Overall Survival (unspecified or mixed categories)		
Author	**Year**	**ECMO Patients**
D'Agostino et al. (108)	1995	16/20 (80%)
Heiss and Clark (238)	1995	679/1089 (62%)
Heiss and Clark (239)	1995	9/14 (64%)
Clark et al. (240)	1998	141/261 (54%)
Reickert et al. (241)	1998	104/189 (55%)
Thibeault et al. (242)	1998	22/36 (61%)

TABLE 31.7. COMPARISON OF VENOARTERIAL AND VENOVENOUS EXTRACORPOREAL MEMBRANE OXYGENATION (NEONATES)

	Venoarterial	Venovenous
Cannulation sites	Internal jugular vein, right atrium, or femoral vein plus right common carotid, axillary, or femoral artery or aorta (directly)	Internal jugular vein alone (double-lumen or single-lumen tidal flow) Jugular-femoral Femorofemoral Saphenosaphenous Right atrium (directly)
Organ support	Gas exchange and cardiac output	Gas exchange only
Systemic perfusion	Circuit flow and cardiac output	Cardiac output only
Pulse contour	Reduced pulsatility	Normal pulsatility
CVP	Unreliable	Accurate guide to volume status
PA pressure	Unreliable	Reliable
Effect of R → L shunt	Mixed venous into perfusate blood	None
Effect of L → R shunt (PDA)	Pulmonary hyperperfusion	No effect on flow
Blood flow for full gas exchange	80–100 mL/kg/hr	100–120 mL/kg/hr
Circuit Svo_2	Reliable	Unreliable
Circuit recirculation	None	15–30%
Arterial PO_2	60–150 mm Hg	45–80 mm Hg
Arterial oxygen saturation	≥95%	80–95%
Indicators of O_2 insufficiency	Mixed venous saturation or Po_2 Calculated oxygen consumption	Cerebral venous saturation Da-vo$_2$ across the membrane Patient Pao_2 Premembrane saturation trend Combinations of all of the above
Carbon dioxide removal	Sweep gas flow and membrane lung size-dependent	Sweep gas flow and membrane lung size-dependent
Oxygenator (m²)	0.4 or 0.6	0.6 or 0.8
Ventilator settings	Minimal	Minimal-moderate (dependent on patient size)
Decrease initial vent settings	Rapidly	Slowly

CVP, central venous pressure; PA, pulmonary artery; PDA, patent ductus arteriosus.

technique prevents damage to diseased lungs by reducing their motion (pulmonary rest), although three to five "sighs" with low-frequency positive-pressure ventilation (LFPPV) are provided each minute to preserve the functional residual capacity. With this method, O_2 uptake and CO_2 removal are dissociated; oxygenation is accomplished primarily through the lungs, whereas CO_2 is cleared through extracorporeal removal ($ECCO_2R$). LFPPV-$ECCO_2R$ is performed at an extracorporeal blood flow that is 20% to 30% of cardiac output. Vascular access can be jugulofemoral, femorofemoral, or saphenosaphenous. VV access, emphasizing CO_2 removal, is promising, although most infants and children go through a phase of diminished lung function requiring oxygenation support. It is possible to supply all O_2 requirements during VV bypass by increasing the flow to 100% to 120% of cardiac output. Oxygenator O_2 transfer efficiency is decreased because of the elevated saturation of the venous blood (recirculation). This can be offset by increasing blood flow. In a recent retrospective review of 94 patients, Bartlett's group (115) concluded that percutaneous cannulation can be utilized for VV ECMO in adults.

Advantages

Venovenous ECMO has the advantage of maintaining normal pulmonary blood flow and avoiding arterial cannulation with its risk of systemic microemboli. Total support of gas exchange with VV perfusion, with return of the perfusate blood into the venous circulation through the femoral vein or a modified jugular venous drainage catheter, also has the advantage of avoiding carotid artery ligation (116).

Bartlett's group (77,117) had developed a polyurethane double-lumen catheter for single-site cannulation of the internal jugular vein. A tidal flow VV system with a single-lumen catheter (116) has also been developed to aid venous gas exchange. Efficient wire-wound cannulas, which are capable of sufficient flow for total gas exchange, can be inserted in large children (>15 kg) and adults by percutaneous insertion (Seldinger technique). Although jugulofemoral VV bypass is feasible in neonates, the advantages do not outweigh the disadvantages (longer operative time for separate cannulation sites, problems with groin wound, and potential for leg swelling) (114).

Outcome

Since the 14F VV double-lumen catheter became commercially available in 1989, more than 2,120 neonates have been treated, with a 90% overall survival (20). A multicenter retrospective comparison of VA access versus VV double-lumen catheter access for newborns with respiratory failure undergoing ECMO was undertaken (117). Overall survival in patients undergoing VA bypass was 87%, whereas survival in the patients undergoing VV double-lumen catheter bypass was 95%. Eleven patients required conversion from VV double-lumen catheter to VA bypass because of insufficient support, with 10 survivors. Average bypass time for newborns on VA bypass was 132 ± 7.4 hours, in comparison with 100 ± 5.1 hours for those on VV double-lumen catheter bypass, and neurologic complications were more common in VA bypass. Hemorrhagic, cardiopulmonary, and mechanical complications, other than kinking of the VV double-lumen catheter, occurred with equal frequency in each group.

When the entire ELSO Registry experience of VA versus VV double-lumen bypass was analyzed, the survival for VA bypass (1990 to 1992, $n = 3146$) was 81%, whereas that for VV double-lumen catheter bypass (1990 to 1992, $n = 576$) was 91% (118). The average duration of VA ECMO was 141 ± 89 hours, and the duration of VV double-lumen catheter ECMO was 120 ± 64 hours. A comparison of specific mechanical complications demonstrated that the VV double-lumen catheter technique was associated with a significantly higher prevalence of restrictive sutures and kinking in the cannulas. When the specific patient complication rates for the two techniques were compared, the patients undergoing VV double-lumen catheter bypass had a much lower rate of major neurologic complications. The prevalence of seizures and cerebral infarction was significantly lower with VV double-lumen catheter ECMO, which seemed to have a substantial impact on overall survival. Therefore, during the initial experience, VV double-lumen catheter ECMO was associated with a higher survival rate and a lower rate of major neurologic complications (118). As of July 1998, VA survival is 79% and VV double-lumen catheter survival is 79% to 89% (20).

Although VV double-lumen catheter cases may have been more carefully selected and "more stable" than VA ECMO cases, early success may lead to an important conceptual change in the use of ECMO technology. The current practice of waiting until the natural lungs become severely dysfunctional and then having to support cardiopulmonary function almost completely, as with VA ECMO, may give way to the concept of early lung assistance. Single-site cannulation may soon become the method of choice for most newborn patients. Likewise, continued catheter development will allow percutaneous access for VV double-lumen catheter ECMO. A single-cannula tidal flow VV ECMO system has been developed that allows percutaneous access (119,120).

MANAGEMENT OF COMPLICATIONS

The success of a course of therapy including ECMO depends completely on prompt recognition and management of related complications as they emerge. Complications during ECMO are the rule, not the exception (118,121). Unfortunately, the nature of long-term heart–lung bypass is that potentially catastrophic complications arise unexpectedly and progress rapidly. An understanding of the physiology relevant to ECMO, familiarity with the ECMO circuit, and the attainment of a certain level of confidence in managing patients on ECMO prepare one to handle most of the routinely encountered problems. The complications can be classified as mechanical or patient-related. Any mechanical component of the ECMO apparatus may fail, and constant system checks and monitoring prevent most complications from becoming management disasters. Although patient complications span the entire field of critical care, they are often related to systemic heparinization and include intracranial hemorrhage, gastrointestinal hemorrhage, and bleeding at the cannula site.

Mechanical Complications

The collective experience of complications during ECMO from the ELSO Registry has been reviewed (20). In 18,371 ECMO cases, 12,310 mechanical complications were reported, or an average of 0.67 mechanical complications per case. Mechanical complications, in descending order of frequency, are listed in Table 31.8. Revealingly, the most common mechanical complication listed in the ELSO Registry for the pediatric, cardiac, and adult groups is that of "other." This reflects the fact that in addition to the identifiable components listed above, the entire circuit is subject to failure, including the bladder box, connectors, electrical components, power sources, plugs, O_2 sources, carbogen tanks, blenders, and circuit-monitoring equipment.

Clots in the circuit are the single most common mechanical complication, representing approximately a third (32.8%) of the mechanical complications reported (20). Major clots can lead to oxygenator failure or a consumption coagulopathy in addition to the potential for pulmonary or systemic emboli. The extracorporeal circuit presents a large foreign surface for the activation of neutrophils, lymphocytes, and platelets, which release inflammatory mediators and promote free radical activity (122–126). Recently, heparin-coated ECMO systems have been used, which may help decrease bleeding during major surgery on ECMO (127–129).

Cannulas are inserted with great care to avoid vascular damage; loss of control of the internal jugular vein can result in massive mediastinal bleeding, and dissection of the carotid artery intima can progress to a lethal aortic dissection. The venous cannula, however, can be advanced too little or too much, which in either case can cause cannula obstruc-

TABLE 31.8. MECHANICAL COMPLICATIONS

Neonatal	Incidence (%)	Pediatric/Cardiac/Adult	Incidence (%)
Clots in circuit	41	Other	46.2
Cannula problems	15	Oxygenator failure	22.3
Other	12.8	Cannula problems	18.2
Air in circuit	8.4	Tubing rupture	7.2
Oxygenator failure	7.8	Pump malfunction	4.6
Cracks in connectors	5.2	Heat exchanger	1.6
Pump malfunction	2.3		
Cannula kinking	2.2		
Heat exchanger	1.5		
Hemofilter malfunction	1.3		
Other tubing rupture	1.2		
Restrictive sutures	0.6		
Raceway rupture	0.5		

Extracorporeal Life Support Organization Registry Report, July 1999.

tion. Likewise, the venous catheter can enter the subclavian vein or cross the foramen ovale. Anatomic variations of the right atrium (aneurysmal atrial septum or redundant eustachian valve) can also interfere with venous return. The use of echocardiography to confirm cannula position has been recommended because routine chest radiography can fail to demonstrate cannula malposition (130,131). Problems with arterial cannulation include insertion too far into the ascending aorta, insertion too far down the descending aorta, or misdirection into the subclavian artery. Insertion too far into the ascending aorta can obstruct left ventricular outflow, which can contribute to left ventricular failure. In addition, the cannula can cross the aortic valve, causing aortic insufficiency. Insertion too far down the descending aorta can compromise coronary and cerebral oxygenated blood flow and cause "streaming" of hyperoxygenated blood from the ECMO circuit without adequate mixing. The distance from the orifice of the innominate artery to the takeoff of the right subclavian artery can be a remarkably short 1.0 to 1.5 cm. If the arterial cannula is pulled out to the point at which the arterial infusion selectively enters the right subclavian artery, the right upper extremity can be infused with the entire post-oxygenator blood flow while the rest of the body is hypoxic and cyanotic. Cannula-induced vertebral steal during VA ECMO is characterized by decreased blood flow to the right arm and retrograde flow in the right vertebral artery, although arm ischemia is rare (132).

Oxygenator failure has decreased in frequency to 10.7%. Any failing membrane should be changed immediately on recognition to prevent an air–blood leak. A double-diamond tubing arrangement with dual connectors, both pre- and post-oxygenator, allows in-line replacement of the oxygenator without interruption of ECMO flow. Air in the circuit (6.7%) can be a few small bubbles seen in the bladder or a complete venous air lock. Venous air lock usually results from dislodgment of the venous cannula so that one or

more of the side holes are outside the vessel (133). Massive air lock requires the patient to come off ECMO support so that either the air can be removed or the entire ECMO circuit can be reprimed. Small amounts of air in the venous line can be "walked" into the venous reservoir for evacuation.

The ECMO circuit is designed to pump blood safely and efficiently, but a large bolus of air can develop and circulate rapidly. This complication, although rare, is commonly fatal. There are several potential sources for such an embolus. When the P_{O_2} in the blood is very high, as seen post-oxygenator, O_2 can easily be forced out of solution. Bumping into the membrane or operating the circuit in an environment of low ambient pressure (such as during flight in a nonpressurized cabin) can produce foam in the top of the oxygenator. Operating the pump with a clamp on the venous side of the circuit, with the bladder in the "prime" mode or with the outlet arm of the bladder kinked, can generate a markedly negative pressure in the blood path and pull large amounts of gas out of solution, which results in cavitation. The bladder box system is designed to avoid this latter problem.

Probably the most dramatic air embolus occurs when a small tear develops in the membrane, allowing blood to leak into the gas path of the oxygenator. The blood gradually moves down to the gas exhalation port, where it may either be blown out in small drops onto the floor or accumulate and form a clot. If this clot obstructs the egress of gas, back pressure will develop inside the gas path of the oxygenator. When the gas pressure exceeds that of the blood, a large bolus of gas crosses the membrane and appears in the blood path. As it surges out of the membrane to the heat exchanger (and the arterial line filter, if one is used), the gas-trapping capacity of these two devices (on the order of 45 mL for each) may rapidly be exceeded, and the embolus will push into the arterial line toward the aorta.

The solution to these problems rests on prevention and

a rapid response when air embolism is recognized. Keeping the PO_2 in the membrane blood at 600 mm Hg or less, carefully monitoring the bladder box, strictly prohibiting the placement of extraneous clamps on the circuit, and adherence to precautions such as "walking the raceway" will eliminate most problems. Lightly touching the gas exhalation port of the membrane with a finger as a part of the hourly circuit check will alert the practitioner when blood is being expelled. However, occluding the gas exhalation port even briefly can cause a precipitous rise in the gas phase pressure across the membrane, which creates the risk for a membrane rupture, air embolus, or both.

If air is headed toward the arterial cannula, a clamp is immediately placed on the arterial tubing close to the patient. The pump is immediately turned off, the main bridge is unclamped, and the venous line is clamped. The patient should be hand-ventilated, or the ventilator should be returned to its pre-ECMO settings and the problem in the circuit identified and corrected. Once the patient is "off bypass," the patient's head should be lowered relative to his or her body as much as possible to move any air pockets away from the cerebral circulation. With a sterile catheter-tipped syringe, aspirate any accessible air back out of the arterial cannula. If a hyperbaric chamber is available and the patient is stable, its immediate use should also be considered.

Tubing rupture has become much less frequent with the introduction of Super Tygon (S65HL) (Norton Performances Plastics, Inc., Akron, OH) raceway tubing (134). Previously, polyvinyl chloride tubing required advancing the raceway every 24 hours to prevent tube fatigue and rupture. With prolonged ECMO, the raceway should be advanced approximately every 36 hours for neonates with 1/4-in Super Tygon tubing and every 96 to 120 hours in older patients with 3/8-in Super Tygon tubing. Pump failure, likewise, has become more rare as direct and belt drive pumps have been manufactured specifically with long-term extracorporeal support in mind. Occasionally, the pump "cuts out" and quits pumping blood. This is a manifestation of inadequate venous return, which may simply be a response to hypovolemia that can be corrected easily with intravascular volume expansion. Although heat exchanger malfunction occurs in only 1% of cases, it may cause severe hypothermia or hemodilution in an infant. Also, defective heat exchangers have been responsible for aluminum particle emboli (135); however, redesign has eliminated this problem.

Patient Complications

Management of the patient on ECMO, including patient-related complications, spans the entire field of critical care. In our recent review of complications during neonatal ECMO in the ELSO Registry (20), there were 40,826 patient complications, or an average of 2.2 complications per case. Of the registered ECMO patients, 32% had no medical complications, and these patients had a 94% survival rate. The incidence of patient-related complications is three times that of the mechanical circuit-related events. Bleeding is one of the most devastating and difficult problems encountered. Patient complications in descending order of frequency are listed in Table 31.9.

Moderate bleeding (>10 mL/hr in neonates) is frequently seen at the neck cannulation site. This problem is minimized by liberal use of electrocautery at the time of surgical exposure, systemic anticoagulation, and cannulation, and liberal use of a topical hemostatic agent, such as Gelfoam thrombin. At many centers, neck wounds are packed with a topical hemostatic agent before closure, which decreases the incidence of bleeding for the duration of the ECMO course and is easily removed at decannulation.

TABLE 31.9. PATIENT COMPLICATIONS[a]

Complication	Incidence (%)
Hemofiltration/dialysis	8.4
Intracerebral hemorrhage	6.2
Abnormal creatinine	5.8
Seizures	5.3
Inotropes on ECMO	5.2
Hypertensive	4.9
Surgical site bleeding	4.9
Hemolysis	4.8
Other hemorrhage	3.9
Sepsis (culture +)	3.9
Abnormal potassium	3.9
Other cardiovascular	3.5
Acid–base abnormalities	3.4
Hyperbilirubinemia	3.2[a]
Arrhythmias	3.2
Abnormal glucose	2.9
Pneumothorax	2.8
Other pulmonary	2.6
Abnormal sodium	2.3
Myocardial stun	2.2
Other neurologic	1.9
Cannula site bleeding	1.8
Abnormal calcium	1.4
CPR required	1.4
Symptomatic PDA	1.3[a]
Other metabolic	1.3
Pulmonary hemorrhage	1.2[a]
Brain death	1.1
WBC count abnormal	1.1
Other renal	1.1
Other infections	1.0
GI hemorrhage	1.0
Abnormal hemoglobin	1.0
Intracerebral infarct	0.2
Complications	0.1

[a] Extracorporeal Life Support Organization Registry Report, July 1999.
ECMO, extracorporeal membrane oxygenation; CPR, cardiopulmonary resuscitation; PDA, patent ductus arteriosus; WBC, white blood cell; GI, gastrointestinal.

If bleeding from the neck incision is observed, local pressure, topical placement of hemostatic agents (Gelfoam thrombin, Oxycel, topical thrombin), and injection of cryoprecipitate topical glue into the wound have all been successful. If topical treatment methods are unsuccessful, consider decreasing the heparin infusion rate to keep the ACT between 180 and 220 seconds and the platelet count above $100,000/\mu L$. Anytime the neck incision bleeds more than 10 mL/hr for 2 hours despite the treatment strategies outlined above, the wound should be explored. Once hemostasis is achieved with electrocautery, the wound should be packed with a topical hemostatic agent and reclosed.

Bleeding into the site of a previous invasive procedure is a frequent complication. Intracranial, gastrointestinal, intrathoracic, abdominal, and retroperitoneal bleeding have all been observed in neonates on ECMO. A decreasing hematocrit, rising heart rate, fall in blood pressure, or progressive rise in the P_aO_2 on VA ECMO disproportionate to observed improvements in a patient's pulmonary status all suggest bleeding, which should be pursued aggressively.

Minor surgical procedures may be required during ECMO and should not be taken lightly. Bleeding complications have occurred after seemingly trivial procedures. Arterial cutdown may be needed if appropriate access cannot be obtained before the initiation of ECMO or if access is lost. Tube thoracostomy may be required to drain hemothorax or pneumothorax. Cannulation sites may bleed, in which case reexploration is required. Skin incisions can be made with the cutting mode of an electrocautery instrument. Muscles should be cauterized and not torn. Fibrin glue (cryoprecipitate, calcium, and thrombin solution) applied to wounds will help decrease bleeding complications. Although bleeding may be a significant problem, liberal use of cautery, application of fibrin glue, and a low threshold for reexploration permit nearly any procedure to be performed.

The development of safe and reliable heparin-bonded, nonthrombogenic surfaces may usher in an entirely new era in ECMO (136–138) by allowing the safer application of ECMO to patients with conditions currently considered as contraindications. Presently, a randomized, prospective trial of a heparin-bonded circuit with neonates is in progress. The use of heparin-bonded circuits also appears to decrease platelet, leukocyte, complement, and kinin system activation (139).

Aminocaproic acid and aprotinin have been recommended as drugs to decrease bleeding and complications of intracranial hemorrhage during ECMO (97,140–147). Wilson and colleagues (97,141) reported that aminocaproic acid, an inhibitor of fibrinolysis, administered just before or after cannulation (bolus of 100 mg/kg, then 30 mg/kg per hour as an infusion) significantly decreased bleeding in high-risk neonates. The incidence of intracranial hemorrhage was also reduced. Presently, a randomized, prospective study is ongoing. Brunet and colleagues (140) reported that infusion of aprotinin (loading dose of 2×10^6 kallikrein-inhibitory units (KIU), then 5×10^5 KIU/hr) added to heparin stopped life-threatening bleeding in two adult patients during prolonged $ECCO_2R$. Further clinical trials will be required to determine its safety and efficiency during prolonged ECMO.

The subject of intracranial hemorrhage in neonates has been reviewed extensively (148). As a rule, the appearance of a new intracranial hemorrhage or the enlargement of a preexisting bleed are indications to discontinue ECMO support if possible. Factors that increase the pressure gradient between the blood vessel lumen and the surrounding brain tissue increase the likelihood of small-vessel rupture and hemorrhage. Factors contributing to intracranial hemorrhage in critically ill neonates include hypoxia, hypercapnia, acidosis, ischemia, hypotension, sepsis, coagulopathy, thrombocytopenia, venous hypertension, seizures, birth trauma, and rapid infusions of colloid or hypertonic solution. Mechanical ventilation has also been associated with an increased rate of intracranial hemorrhage in premature infants with respiratory distress syndrome. Before ECMO treatment, cranial ultrasonography is mandatory in all patients to identify those neonates in whom significant intracranial hemorrhage is already present (149,150).

Patients in whom VA ECMO is used commonly have a ligation of the right common carotid artery and internal jugular vein. Potentially decreased cerebral blood flow and increased cerebral venous hypertension have been considered as a source of intracranial hemorrhage (132,151–153). Schumacher et al. (154) reported right-sided central nervous system lesions in 8 of 69 ECMO patients, although these patients were also profoundly hypoxic and hypotensive at initiation of ECMO. Others have shown no evidence of a higher incidence of right-sided central nervous system lesions (72). Blood flow to the right cerebral hemisphere is preserved after right carotid artery ligation by collateral circulation via the external carotid artery and the anterior communicating artery of the circle of Willis. Noninvasive vascular studies have demonstrated that cerebral blood flow is adequate during ECMO, early after decannulation (155,156), and in late follow-up (55,157). Ten infants also underwent digital IV angiography; in each case, there was prompt bilateral filling of both middle cerebral arteries (156). No consistently lateralized electroencephalographic abnormalities were observed during or after ECMO in comparison with tracings obtained before cannulation of the right common carotid artery (158). These studies suggest that in neonates, when the common carotid artery is ligated, collateral circulation is readily established. Because of continued concerns about long-term common carotid artery ligation, a few centers reconstruct the artery at decannulation (159–161). Carotid reconstruction, however, introduces the potential for carotid dissection, thrombosis, emboli, or late stenosis.

Instability of previously well-controlled coagulation parameters (ACT, platelet count, fibrinogen) can be an early predictor of an intracranial event (162,163). Hemolysis may also often be related to the ECMO membrane or circuit (164). Thrombocytopenia is expected during the use of ECMO, as platelets are altered and platelet aggregates form in the extracorporeal circuit and are preferentially sequestered in the lung, liver, and spleen (124,125,165). Thrombocytopenia in the neonate is significant in that existing bleeding may be exacerbated or bleeding may occur spontaneously. A platelet count of less than $100,000/\mu L$ is considered abnormal. Thrombocytopenia must be avoided by using platelet transfusion as often as necessary to maintain adequate platelet counts during ECMO (165).

Ultrasonography of the kidneys to exclude major anatomic anomalies is mandatory in the presence of elevated creatinine or a persistently poor response to furosemide (1 to 2 mg/kg). Oliguria during ECMO is common, especially during the first 24 to 48 hours. Sell et al. (166) reported the use of continuous hemofiltration for renal failure during ECMO. Continuous hemofiltration removes plasma water and dissolved solutes while proteins and cellular components of the intravascular space are retained. The classic indications for dialysis hold true with continuous hemofiltration on ECMO: hypervolemia, hyperkalemia, and azotemia. Hyperkalemia and hypervolemia are easily managed with continuous hemofiltration, but azotemia is more difficult to manage because of chronic hemolysis and occult gastrointestinal bleeding. The continuous hemofiltration apparatus is easily added in-line to the ECMO circuit and allows removal of up to 10 mL/kg per hour.

Systolic hypertension is a dangerous side effect of ECMO. Sell et al. (167) reported that systolic blood pressures above 90 mm Hg developed in 38 of 41 newborns treated with ECMO. Detectable intracranial hemorrhage developed in 44%, and clinically significant intracranial hemorrhage in 27%. With the development of a medical management protocol including the use of hydralazine, nitroglycerine, and captopril, the incidence of clinically significant intracranial hemorrhage has decreased. We currently use 0.1 mg of hydralazine per kilogram intravenously for systolic hypertension above 90 mm Hg.

Ionized hypocalcemia is a frequent occurrence after initiation of ECMO and can contribute to hypotension on ECMO (45). "Stunned myocardium" after ECMO is defined as a left ventricular shortening fraction decreasing by 25% or more with initiation of ECMO and returning to normal after 48 hours on ECMO (168–170). This syndrome occurs despite relief of hypoxia. Underlying congenital heart disease can be "masked" by respiratory failure in 2% of cases requiring ECMO (171). VA ECMO is preferred over VV support in these cases.

If cardiac arrest, dysrhythmia, or a drop in cardiac output secondary to severe myocardial dysfunction occurs, the initial treatment of choice during VA ECMO is simply to turn up the pump flow. This may require the addition of blood volume to the circuit. Continued ECMO with circulatory support is likely to be one of the most effective therapeutic

measures. Treatment may include the administration of standard "arrest" medications, some adjustments of the electrolyte levels, addition of antiarrhythmic agents, treatment with sympathomimetics or inotropes, or even countershock. If pump flow cannot be increased sufficiently to compensate for the fall in intrinsic cardiac output, or if the patient is on VV ECMO, the episode must be handled in much the same way as a cardiac arrest in any other patient. Do not forget that the most common cause of cardiac dysfunction in ventilated neonates is hypoxia resulting from respiratory (not cardiac) failure. Assess the infant for inadvertent extubation or the development of a tension pneumothorax. The reason why one cannot achieve the desired ECMO flows may be that venous return to the heart is being impeded by the accumulation of blood or air in the chest or pericardium (66). The triad of increased $P_{a}O_{2}$ and decreased peripheral perfusion (evidenced by decreased pulse pressure and decreased $S_{\overline{v}}O_{2}$) followed by decreased ECMO flow with progressive hemodynamic deterioration is consistently associated with tension pneumothorax (66). An echocardiogram will demonstrate a pericardial effusion and may also localize a hemothorax.

For emergency treatment of both tension hemothorax and pneumothorax and pericardial tamponade, we recommend placement of a percutaneous drainage catheter to reverse the developing pathophysiology (172,173). For pericardial tamponade, placement of an angiocatheter into the pericardium under ultrasonographic guidance seems most safe and reliable. Once partial drainage through the angiocatheter has relieved the tamponade, a guidewire may be passed via a modified Seldinger technique to place a multiholed drainage tube. We have successfully used a No. 5F pediatric feeding tube for this purpose. For tension hemothorax and pneumothorax, a needle, angiocatheter, and chest tube are all options for emergent decompression (172, 173).

Sepsis is both an indication for and a complication of ECMO. However, according to the ELSO Registry, positive blood cultures develop in only 5% of all patients requiring ECMO. This is a remarkably low incidence given the duration of cannulation, the large surface area involved, and the frequency of access to the circuit.

The pathophysiology of PFC is a right-to-left shunt and a patent ductus arteriosus during severe respiratory failure in the newborn. Therefore, when ECMO is initiated, a patent ductus arteriosus is always present. When pulmonary vasospasm relaxes, flow through the ductus reverses (becomes left-to-right shunting). A persistent left-to-right shunt across the ductus arteriosus may lead to pulmonary edema. Decreased systemic oxygenation may result both from pulmonary edema and from decreased systemic blood flow. Both of these effects will require the operator to increase the ECMO flow to maintain adequate gas exchange and perfusion. Likewise, if renal failure occurs and a previous hypoxic or ischemic insult cannot be identified, then the possibility of decreased renal perfusion during ECMO as a result of a patent ductus arteriosus must be considered. Therefore, a patent ductus arteriosus on ECMO may present with (a) a decreased P_aCO_2, (b) decreased peripheral perfusion, (c) decreased urine output, (d) acidosis, and (e) rising ECMO flow and volume requirements. The clinical diagnosis can be confirmed as in other neonatal patients with Doppler echocardiography or angiography. Some centers have tried using intravenous indomethacin to treat patent ductus arteriosus in patients on ECMO. However, many practitioners strongly discourage this approach because of its effects on platelet function, which increase the risks for bleeding in patients on ECMO. Once the diagnosis is established, most programs will "run the patient relatively dry" while maintaining supportive ECMO flow until the patent ductus arteriosus closes. Although this often means a few additional days on ECMO, surgical ligation is rarely necessary.

Occasionally, after 2 to 3 weeks of ECMO, a patient is unable to be weaned. Ventilator support is increased to the maximal acceptable pressures and levels of inspired O_2. An echocardiogram is repeated to ensure that a patent ductus arteriosus with predominant left-to-right shunt is not present and once again to rule out total anomalous venous return. We then attempt a trial off ECMO with increased ventilator settings. If the trial off ECMO is unsuccessful, then cardiac catheterization or open lung biopsy must be considered to rule out potentially correctable problems or irreversible diseases such as congenital pulmonary lymphangiectasis. If no correctable lesions are found, a decision must be made to discontinue ECMO support or to continue indefinitely if there are objective signs of improvement without any complications.

CARDIAC SUPPORT

The pioneering use of ECMO in patients with severe cardiac failure was first reported in the 1950s, but ECMO was not commonly used until the 1980s (174). Although prior experience had shown success in infants with SRF, early results in postoperative cardiac failure were disappointing. Later experience demonstrated the effectiveness of ECMO in some postcardiotomy patients. The goal of ECMO support in patients after cardiac surgery is to maintain adequate tissue perfusion while providing complete or nearly complete cardiac bypass. Considerations for ECMO include the complexity of the heart defects, the need for continued heparinization to prevent clotting in the circuit, and the incidence of infection related to the surgical implantation of the system (26,175–178).

The use of ECMO has been extended to cardiac and pulmonary support after cardiac surgery in children and infants (179,180). The first successful application of ECMO in postcardiotomy failure was reported by Soeter et al. in 1973 (181). Advantages include support of both

the right and left ventricles, improvement of systemic oxygenation, and ease of placement. ECMO support in postcardiotomy patients can be provided with either VA or VV cannulation. VA cannulation provides the optimal cardiac support when ventricular dysfunction dominates the clinical picture. However, one group used VV bypass to provide cardiac recovery and support for a Blalock-Taussig procedure (182).

Cannulation

Venoarterious ECMO can be performed by extrathoracic cannulation (carotid artery and jugular vein, or femoral artery and femoral vein), or more commonly by transthoracic cannulation through the median sternotomy incision (aorta and right atrium). Carotid–jugular cannulation may best be used in patients who are weaned from CPB in the operating room and in whom myocardial dysfunction with cardiogenic shock develops after operation. Advantages of this approach are a separate incision site remote from the median sternotomy wound and a lower incidence of bleeding from the mediastinal wound. Both of these factors may contribute to a decreased risk for mediastinal infection (183).

In patients with a cavopulmonary connection (Glenn or Fontan circulation), direct access from the jugular vein to the right atrium is not feasible. A transthoracic approach is therefore needed in these cases. Femoral arteriovenous cannulation can be used in certain older children, with placement of intravascular catheters into the inferior vena cava or right atrium through the femoral vein and into the common femoral or iliac artery for arterial return. The venous return with this type of cannulation may be restrictive unless a centrifugal type pump is used that provides active venous drainage. The advantage of this peripheral technique includes the noninvasive surgical approach and a more secure cannula fixation.

Transthoracic cannulation is preferable in patients who cannot be weaned from CPB in the operating room or who had their chest opened for the purpose of resuscitation in the postoperative period. The major disadvantages of the transthoracic approach include the potential risks for mediastinal hemorrhage, infection, and cannula dislodgement during repositioning or transport. Anticoagulation with ACTs of approximately 200 seconds is maintained by means of a continuous intravenous heparin infusion. If bleeding persists, the ACT can be lowered to 180 seconds. The platelet count should be maintained above 100,000/μL, with platelet transfusions given as needed. The development of heparin-bonded circuits may help reduce the need for significant anticoagulation and its attendant risks (184), and some centers have adopted this approach to ECMO-based cardiac support following cardiac surgery. Heparin-bonded circuits have been used for ECMO in patients with major coagulopathies who are bleeding significantly at the time ECMO is instituted. This advance makes it possible to use ECMO for patients who cannot come off conventional CPB in the operating room, those with major trauma and active bleeding, and those who have undergone major operations such as thoracotomy for lung transplantation. The standard cannulas for bypass can be converted to the ECMO circuit and brought out through or below the median sternotomy incision. Whenever possible, the sternum should be closed unless this is prevented by edema of the myocardium.

Flows are titrated to levels needed to reduce right and left atrial pressures while providing adequate systemic perfusion; as much as 150 mL/kg may be required in neonates, but generally 50 to 75 mL/kg is sufficient in adults. When left atrial pressures remain elevated despite optimal flow, a scenario frequently found in patients with multiple aortopulmonary collaterals, the left atrium should be vented to the venous drainage system. High flows are most often maintained for 48 to 72 hours before weaning from ECMO is attempted.

The preoperative use of ECMO in infants with congenital heart disease is controversial. In patients with unoperated cyanotic heart disease and cardiopulmonary collapse associated with hypercyanotic spells, pulmonary hypertension, or sepsis, indications for ECMO included an arterial O_2 saturation of less than 60% on maximal medical therapy with hypotension and metabolic acidosis despite maximal support including hyperventilation with 100% O_2 and inotropes, vasodilators, or both (183). Duration of ECMO support ranged from 1 to 38 days. Seven of eight patients underwent corrective or palliative surgery while on ECMO or within 48 hours after decannulation. The survival rate was 62%, and survivors had normal growth and development. Other groups have described the successful use of ECMO as a bridge to transplant in pediatric patients (185) and a lifesaving therapy after lung transplantation (186). ECMO has also been used for circulatory support in adults and children who could not be weaned from CPB despite maximal pharmacologic (and possibly intraaortic balloon) support after cardiac surgical procedures.

The diagnoses most often associated with the development of postoperative low cardiac output in children requiring ECMO support are listed in Table 31.10. This list could be extended to include any cardiac surgical procedure in

adults, although the need would most often occur in higher-risk patients (e.g., advanced age, poor left ventricular function, emergency procedure, complex or combined procedures). These patients usually present with decreased urine output (<1 mL/kg per hour), poor peripheral perfusion, low systemic venous saturation (wide S_aO_2 - S_vO_2), and elevated filling pressures despite maximal inotropic and diuretic support. Myocardial injury in these patients is usually less than in those who cannot be weaned from CPB. The interval between surgery and initiation of ECMO may provide sufficient time for recovery of normal coagulation, an important factor that can positively affect the outcome of these patients (177).

Weaning

A decreased need for inotropic support and an improvement in renal function and diuresis of retained fluid are initial indicators of myocardial recovery. After a period of time in which myocardial contractility is permitted to improve, an attempt is made to wean from ECMO. With reasonable inotropic support, ECMO flow is gradually reduced. If myocardial contractility remains satisfactory and the filling pressures are low, decannulation can be accomplished.

Complications

As previously discussed, mechanical support with ECMO results in several possible complications. The major complication of postcardiotomy ECMO is hemorrhage. To minimize the magnitude of bleeding, the ACT is maintained at approximately 200 seconds and the platelet count is kept above 100,000/μL, or a heparin-coated circuit without systemic heparinization is used (187). The primary determinant of significant hemorrhage is the duration of ECMO (188). Keeping the chest open is sometimes necessary to facilitate reexploration and to prevent periods of cardiac tamponade.

Clinical Results

The results of ECMO for pediatric cardiac support have been summarized (Table 31.11). Early survival was 40% to 44%, with somewhat better survival (43% to 54%) when the lesion was tetralogy of Fallot, truncus arteriosus, atrioventricular canal, or total anomalous pulmonary venous return. Lower survival rates (14%) have been reported for single ventricle, hypoplastic left heart syndrome, and other malformations requiring a Fontan procedure. Differences in survival rates suggest that improved survival is associated with a complete biventricular operative repair, whereas operations with shunt-dependent pulmonary blood flow are associated with lower recovery rates. A decreased survival rate, of 0 to 27%, is found when patients cannot be weaned

TABLE 31.10. DIAGNOSES AFTER PEDIATRIC CARDIAC SURGERY REQUIRING ECMO USE

Atrioventricular septal defect
Truncus arteriosus
Total anomalous pulmonary venous return
Tetralogy of Fallot
Anomalous coronary artery
Ebstein's malformation of the tricuspid valve
Heart and/or lung transplantation
Fontan procedure

ECMO, extracorporeal membrane oxygenation.

TABLE 31.11. EXTRACORPOREAL MEMBRANE OXYGENATION FOR CARDIAC SUPPORT

Author	Year	No. Patients	Survival
Bartlett et al. (174)[a]	1977	4	25%
Pennington et al. (243)	1984	4	75%
Redmond et al. (244)	1987	9	55.6%
Kanter et al. (179)[b]	1987	13	26%
Rogers et al. (245)	1989	10	70%
Weinhaus et al. (246)	1989	14	35.7%
Klein et al. (178)	1990	36	61%
Delius et al. (247)[c]	1990	6	33.3%
Galantowicz and Stolar (248)	1991	20	20%
Ziomek et al. (249)[b]	1992	24	54%
Raithel et al. (250)[a]	1992	65	35%
Hunkeler et al. (251)[b]	1992	8	62.5%
del Nido et al. (252)[d]	1992	11	64%
del Nido et al. (253)[c]	1994	14	50%
Walters et al. (254)[b]	1995	73	57.5%
Black et al. (255)[a]	1995	31	45%
del Nido (256)[a,c,f]	1996	68	38%
		(14 bridge to transplant)[c]	(50%)
		(resuscitation after arrest)[f]	(53%)
Wang et al. (257)[g]	1996	18	33.3%
Kulik et al. (258)[b]	1996	64	33%
Ishino et al. (259)[c]	1996	6	33.3%
Doski et al. (260)[d]	1997	839	60.8%
Peek et al. (261)[a]	1997		43–61%
Ko et al. (262)[c]	1997	3	100%
Saker et al. (263)[e]	1997	1	100%
Goldman et al. (264)[a]	1997	12	66%
Trittenwein et al. (265)[b]	1997	3	100%
Langley et al. (266)[b]	1998	9	22%
Duncan et al. (267)[f]	1998	11	64%
Delius (268)[c]	1998	22	50%

[a] Cardiac failure.
[b] Congenital heart disease (preoperative, postoperative, cardiac failure).
[c] Heart transplant (bridge, post-transplant).
[d] During cardiopulmonary resuscitation.
[e] After myocardial infarction.
[f] Resuscitation after arrest.
[g] Cardiogenic shock.
(No symbol signifies unspecified group.)

from CPB, which suggests a greater degree of myocardial damage in these patients.

FUTURE

The future of extracorporeal support depends on the development of techniques and devices to make the technique less invasive, safer, and simpler in management. It is hoped that the availability of heparin-coated circuits will allow a reduction in bleeding, the main cause of complications of extracorporeal support.

The future of ECMO also includes: laminar-flow oxygenators; safe, simple automatic pumps; nonthrombogenic surfaces to eliminate bleeding complications; advances in respiratory and cardiac care; and new approaches to clinical trials. A system for long-term ECMO with reduced heparin-ization and minimal plasma leakage has been reported (189). Although initial trials with the intra-venacaval gas exchange device (IVOX) identified problems of inadequate gas exchange and technical placement difficulties, they also showed that nonthrombogenic coating and a totally implantable prosthetic lung is possible. In the future, temporary or permanent implantable devices may play a major role in mechanical support for respiratory failure. The servo-regulated roller pump will be replaced by simpler, safer pumps, including electronically servo-regulated centrifugal pumps, mechanically servo-regulated peristaltic pumps, or mechanically servo-regulated ventricle pumps.

Heparin-bonded oxygenators, pump chambers, and extracorporeal circuits may allow ECMO to continue for days without bleeding or clotting, and the requirement for heparin may be decreased or eliminated. Most often, low-level systemic heparinization (ACT of 170 to 200 seconds) is still administered because if ECMO must be interrupted, blood in the circuit will clot very quickly, although this hazard also exists with uncoated circuits at the ACT levels most often used. Unfortunately, the thrombocytopenia and platelet dysfunction that accompany ECMO have not been eliminated by the availability of heparin-bonded circuits.

In the future, combinations of surface coatings including heparin and modifications to minimize platelet adherence with low-level anticoagulation will further extend the use of ECMO. Various groups have tested heparin-coated circuits and reported reduced thrombogenicity and reductions in required systemic heparinization for prolonged support (190–193). Recently, the use of nitric oxide in the sweep gas to decrease platelet adhesion has been proposed (194).

If technique improves and ECMO is simplified, the indications may be expanded. With improved circuit safety, single-vein access, and minimal anticoagulation, ECMO may be indicated not only for moribund patients but also for those with moderate respiratory and cardiac failure. ECMO may become an adjunct to conventional ventilation and pharmacologic management rather than something to be tried when standard ventilation and pharmacology are failing. At the same time, simpler methods of treatment of acute pulmonary and cardiac failure may significantly decrease the need for ECMO. We believe that ECMO will continue to gain wider application as a means of temporary mechanical support of the circulation in children and adults with cardiac failure. Heparin-bonded nonthrombogenic circuits will provide a major advance in cardiac operations and other procedures during which extracorporeal circulation with circulatory arrest or control of local blood flow is desirable.

Various techniques (nitric oxide, pressure-controlled inverse-ratio ventilation and permissive hypercapnia, intravenous oxygenation, arteriovenous CO_2 removal, and liquid ventilation) highlight the fact that the tools used to sustain gas exchange in the patient with respiratory failure in the near future may be very different from those employed now. The availability of ECMO has made it possible to study these innovative and numerous methods of lung management.

Arteriovenous Carbon Dioxide Removal

Arteriovenous CO_2 removal (AVCO$_2$R) has been developed as a less labor-intensive, less complex technique of extracorporeal gas exchange to minimize blood–surface interactions while providing an exchange membrane of sufficient surface area for nearly total CO_2 removal. The use of a simple AV shunt eliminates a substantial portion of tubing and ECMO-related components, which in turn reduces the foreign surface area, priming fluid, and blood transfusion volume. In addition, the amount of CO_2 exchange is not limited by surface area (as with intravascular devices such as the IVOX), and moderate hypercapnia can be used to advantage. AVCO$_2$R can be utilized to supplement mechanical ventilatory support for ARDS patients, which allows

positive-pressure ventilation to be reduced and therefore decreases hemodynamic compromise and barotrauma. Prior studies have reported adequate support of gas exchange with use of an AV shunt with apneic oxygenation in both acute and chronic settings. However, tubing and oxygenator resistance proved to be the limiting factor in effective gas exchange (195).

Our group (196) has developed a technique of simplified extracorporeal AVCO$_2$R with a low-resistance membrane gas exchanger to provide lung rest in the setting of severe respiratory failure. The extremely low resistance of the AVCO$_2$R gas exchange device (pressure difference <10 mm Hg) allows blood flows of as much as 25% of the animal's cardiac output (>1,300 mL/min). Surgical cannulation for vascular access in AVCO$_2$R is identical to the setup performed in conventional ECMO; however, the prime volume is as low as 200 mL. During initial trials, AVCO$_2$R proved capable of removing as much as 96% of the animal's total CO_2 production with a reduction of ventilator support to 16% of baseline minute ventilation. At shunt flows of less than 500 mL/min, moderate hypercapnia (40 to 70 mm Hg) occurred, but it was well tolerated without adverse hemodynamic effects.

Blood flow during AVCO$_2$R depends on three variables: (a) device resistance, (b) the pressure gradient between the arterial and venous systems, and (c) cannula resistance. The effect of venous resistance is minimized by using venous cannulas 4F larger in size than their paired arterial cannulas. Percutaneous arterial cannulas 12F or larger allow sufficient flow for maintaining normocapnia with reserve capacity (197).

The decrease in volume- and pressure-controlled ventilation facilitated by AVCO$_2$R significantly reduces the influence of excessive positive-pressure ventilation on hemodynamic variables (198). AVCO$_2$R, however, does not provide substantial O_2 transfer when the arterial P_aO_2 level is adequate because inflow to the device is already saturated (>90%), with an O_2-carrying capacity close to maximum.

In our clinically relevant large-animal model of severe respiratory failure (199), we evaluated percutaneous AVCO$_2$R and its effect on ventilator-dependent days and survival. The P_aO_2/FIO_2 ratio improved from 151.5 ± 40.0 at the introduction of AVCO$_2$R to more than 200 within 36 hours, with further improvement to more than 300 by 72 hours (200). AVCO$_2$R also allowed animals to be weaned from mechanical ventilation almost three times earlier than algorithm-directed, mechanical ventilator managed survivors. Percutaneous AVCO$_2$R allowed reductions in airway pressures and ventilator-dependent days and improvement in survival in a prospective, randomized outcomes study of percutaneous AVCO$_2$R in adult sheep with severe respiratory failure.

For our initial patient experience with AVCO$_2$R (201), five patients with unresponsive, severe ARDS and CO_2 retention despite maximum medical management with "permissive hypercapnia" were treated at the University of Texas

Medical Branch and the Louisiana State University Medical Center. The feasibility and safety of AVCO$_2$R by percutaneous femoral cannulation (10F to 12F arterial and 12F to 15F venous) were evaluated in a 72-hour trial. All five patients were successfully cannulated for AVCO$_2$R at the bedside and completed the 72-hour trial. Three of five were discharged from the hospital. This initial study demonstrated that percutaneous AVCO$_2$R can achieve approximately 70% CO$_2$ removal in adults with SRF and CO$_2$ retention to allow decreased barotrauma and volutrauma without hemodynamic compromise or instability.

The safety and efficacy of AVCO$_2$R have been demonstrated in a preliminary adult human trial, which could be extended to infants and children with the use of smaller devices and priming volumes. Controlled clinical trials of AVCO$_2$R in patients with ARDS, CO$_2$ retention syndromes, and smoke inhalation/cutaneous burn injuries are needed to define the merits and limitations of this treatment to provide optimal gas exchange, limit ventilator-induced barotrauma, and ultimately improve survival in patients with severe respiratory failure.

Artificial Lung

Intended for temporary implantation as a bridge to lung transplantation in chronic pulmonary insufficiency or to allow a natural healing process in advanced respiratory failure, implantable artificial lungs have been developed (202,203). These devices are designed to be implanted into the thoracic cavity and therefore are not as limited by the venacaval vascular space as is IVOX and other intra-venacaval devices. As a result, the surface area can be as large as that of a conventional membrane oxygenator (1.95 to 2.20 m^2), which results in total gas exchange support.

At implantation, the inflow and outflow anastomoses are attached to the pulmonary artery and left atrium, or to the proximal and distal pulmonary artery. Blood flow is perpendicular to the fiber bundle, and inlet and outlet gas lines exit through the chest wall. With a large frontal plane, the pressure drop in such devices is minimal. *In vitro* and *in vivo* studies showed O$_2$ and CO$_2$ transfer rates above 200 mL/min with normal physiologic values of blood flow, hemoglobin concentration, and gas pressure gradient. These results are significantly better than those achieved with IVOX and appear to result from the larger surface area. In an acute animal study, Lynch et al. (204) reported minimal hemodynamic effects and significant O$_2$ transfer with a low-resistance artificial lung attached to the proximal and distal pulmonary artery; the right ventricle was used as a pulsatile pump. Our group has completed a series of four animals in which a pulmonary artery–pulmonary artery configuration was used, with survivals up to 1 week. Animals tolerated occlusion of the pulmonary artery with no significant hemodynamic changes or complications. Although the implantation of such devices does not seem to affect hemodynamic

stability, open chest surgery and vascular anastomoses would certainly limit their clinical applicability, and chronic animal models and clinical trials are needed to evaluate safety, long-term efficacy, and management of such devices.

Intra-venacaval Gas Exchange Device

The intra-venacaval gas exchange device should not be used as a substitute for ECMO or to provide total support for patients with acute respiratory failure. Our experience with IVOX in animal and human studies demonstrated an average CO$_2$ and O$_2$ exchange of 40 mL/min, about 25% to 30% of the metabolic demand of the patients in whom the device was implanted (205,206). An international multicenter clinical trial of IVOX was conducted for a phase I and phase II Food and Drug Administration study in major critical care centers in the United States and Europe. From February 1990 to May 1993, a total of 164 IVOX devices were utilized in 160 patients as a means of temporary augmentation of gas exchange in patients who had severe but potentially reversible ARF (207). Basic entry criteria in the United States and Europe were similar: (a) mechanical ventilation for more than 24 hours; (b) P$_{aO_2}$ of 60 mm Hg or less on F$_{IO_2}$ of 0.5 or greater and PEEP of 10 cm H$_2$O or greater, P$_{aCO_2}$ greater than 40 mm Hg with minute ventilation of 150 mL/min per kilogram or greater. All patients were adults with ARF of various causes, including lung infection, trauma, sepsis, and ARDS. In a majority of patients, the use of IVOX was associated with immediate blood gas improvement sufficient to allow a reduction in ventilator settings: F$_{IO_2}$, PEEP, mean or peak airway pressure, and minute ventilation were decreased by more than 10% in more than 60% of patients, and by more than 25% in more than 40% of patients. Although the overall survival of patients receiving IVOX is 30%, survival is directly related to the severity of lung injury and patient selection; patients with increasingly severe lung injury or pulmonary malfunction, as indicated by the Murray score, oxygenation index, or intrapulmonary shunt, have a decreasing rate of survival. Unfortunately, there was no control arm to this study to evaluate the improvement in survival with IVOX. Complications or adverse events associated with use of IVOX included mechanical and performance problems (29%) and patient complications such as bleeding, thrombosis, infection, venous occlusion, and dysrhythmia, in addition to user errors, which reflected the learning curve with a new device. Based on the experience with IVOX worldwide to date, IVOX demonstrates feasibility as a "booster" lung in patients with ARF. Measurable gas exchange (usually 30% of the metabolic demand of the patients implanted with the device) can be achieved to allow a measurable reduction in ventilator settings. Improvements in gas exchange efficiency and ease of insertion will be necessary for IVOX to have greater clinical applicability.

Despite the religious zeal with which many such strategies are defended, few prospective clinical trials can confirm the effectiveness in terms of improving survival. "Cousins" of ECMO, intravascular gas exchange devices (IVOX), and $AVCO_2R$ are designed to supply supplemental gas exchange with the potential for percutaneous access and "routine" ICU management. Despite spectacular results in reported individuals, the results of multicenter trials of IVOX, nitric oxide, and partial liquid ventilation have all been disappointing. As we explore the appropriate application and continued development of these newer modalities, one can only hope that industry support will prevail as the Food and Drug Administration approval process and research and development costs continue to run headlong into cost-containment policies by hospitals and health maintenance organizations.

Clinical experiments comparing ECMO with other treatments are difficult because blinding is impossible, "standard therapy" is not standardized and changes frequently, an extensive learning curve is required for many of the newer techniques before definitive study is undertaken, and randomization may be refused. The best way to evaluate new methods in life support technology will continue to be the approach used by Green et al. (208,209) in the pediatric respiratory failure evaluation. Data for patients undergoing ECMO and conventional ventilator management were prospectively pooled into a common database and evaluated by multivariate analysis to determine which factors were associated with death or survival. Data were then further analyzed by a matched-pairs analysis. This prospective approach to the evaluation of life support techniques has significant pragmatic advantages over randomized studies and offers great promise for the future.

KEY POINTS

- ECMO as a means of support for life-threatening respiratory failure has been used sparingly since the 1970s, but recent investigations and technologic advances have made this approach more attractive, especially in neonates.
- Although still experimental to some degree and available in a limited but growing number of medical centers, ECMO is indicated primarily in patients with ARF unresponsive to optimal ventilator management from which recovery can be expected within a reasonable period (10 to 20 days) of extracorporeal support. Examples include PFC with PPHN in the newborn resulting from such entities as CDH, meconium aspiration, respiratory distress syndrome, and sepsis.
- ECMO reduces the chance of further pulmonary injury and may facilitate pulmonary recovery by permitting reductions in FIO_2, ventilator rate, and airway pressures. As with short-term CPB for cardiac surgery,

the goal is to provide physiologic O_2 delivery and CO_2 elimination.

- Vascular access can be provided through VA or VV approaches, typically via the internal jugular vein (VV and VA) and common carotid artery (VA). Moderate systemic heparinization is used (ACT of 200 to 260 seconds). When possible, patients are kept awake or lightly sedated to facilitate neurologic assessment.
- In regard to the use of ECMO to support patients with CDH, controversy exists about whether to perform surgical repair before, during, or after a period of ECMO support.
- The VV approach to ECMO emphasizes extracorporeal CO_2 removal and leaves some of the O_2 loading to the native lung. In recent studies, this approach has been associated with enhanced survival (approximately 90% vs. approximately 80%), reduced ECMO support times, and reduced neurologic complications in comparison with the VA approach. To work best, this approach may need to be implemented earlier in the course of the pulmonary disease process than has traditionally been the case for VA ECMO.
- Complications are typically classified as mechanical (clot in the circuit, cannula problems, air in the circuit, and oxygenator failure are most common) or as patient complications (bleeding, hemofiltration/dialysis, intracerebral hemorrhage, seizures, and hemolysis are most common). Heparin-bonded circuits may potentially reduce some of these complications while permitting lesser degrees of systemic anticoagulation.
- ECMO has been used successfully for postoperative cardiac support in children and adults undergoing cardiac surgical procedures. Typically, this would be most appropriate in the presence of severe ventricular dysfunction that is thought to be reversible. Because the predominant problem is cardiac failure, the VA approach is most often used, generally via transthoracic cannulation of the right atrium and aorta. Depending on the clinical setting, survival rates of 35% to 61% have been reported in larger series.
- Investigational technologies offering promise for the future include $AVCO_2R$, intrathoracic artificial lungs, and intravenous oxygenators.

REFERENCES

1. Bartlett RH, Gazzaniga AB. Extracorporeal circulation for cardiopulmonary failure. *Curr Probl Surg* 1978;15:1–96.
2. Bartlett RH. Extracorporeal life support for cardiopulmonary failure. *Curr Probl Surg* 1990;27:621–705.
3. Gibbon JH Jr. Artificial maintenance of circulation during experimental occlusion of pulmonary artery. *Arch Surg* 1937;34:1105.
4. Clowes JJ, Hopkins AL, Nevill WE. An artificial lung dependent upon diffusion of oxygen and carbon dioxide through plastic membranes. *J Thorac Cardiovasc Surg* 1956;32:630.

5. Kolff WJ, Effler DB. Disposable membrane oxygenator (heart–lung machine) and its use in experimental and clinical surgery while the heart is arrested with potassium citrate according to the Melrose technique. *ASAIO Trans* 1956;2:13–21.

6. Kammemeyer K. Silicone rubber as a selective barrier. *Indian Eng Chem* 1957;49:1685.

7. Kolobow T, Bowman RL. Construction and evaluation of an alveolar membrane artificial heart lung. *ASAIO Trans* 1963;9:238–243.

8. Bartlett RH, Drinker PA, Burns NE, et al. The toroidal membrane oxygenator: design, performance, and prolonged bypass testing of a clinical model. *ASAIO Trans* 1972;18:369–374.

9. Kolobow T. Extracorporeal respiratory gas exchange: a look into the future. *ASAIO Trans* 1991;37:2–3.

10. Zapol WM, Qvist J. *Artificial lungs for acute respiratory failure.* New York: Academic Press, 1976.

11. Bartlett RH, Gazzaniga AB, Jefferies MR, et al. Extracorporeal membrane oxygenation (ECMO) cardiopulmonary support in infancy. *ASAIO Trans* 1976;22:80–93.

12. Rashkind WJK, Freeman A, Klein D. Evaluation of a disposable plastic, low-volume, pumpless oxygenator as a lung substitute. *J Pediatr* 1965;66:94–102.

13. Bartlett RH, Andrews AF, Toomasian JM, et al. Extracorporeal membrane oxygenation for newborn respiratory failure: forty-five cases. *Surgery* 1982;92:425–433.

14. Bartlett RH, Gazzaniga AB, Wetmore NE, et al. Extracorporeal membrane oxygenation (ECMO) in the treatment of cardiac and respiratory failure in children. *ASAIO Trans* 1980;26:578–581.

15. Kirkpatrick BV, Krummel TM, Mueller DG, et al. Use of extracorporeal membrane oxygenation for respiratory failure in term infants. *Pediatrics* 1983;72:872–876.

16. Bartlett RH, Gazzaniga AB, Toomasian J, et al. Extracorporeal membrane oxygenation (ECMO) in neonatal respiratory failure. 100 cases. *Ann Surg* 1986;204:236–245.

17. Anonymous. The Collaborative UK ECMO (Extracorporeal Membrane Oxygenation) Trial: follow-up to 1 year of age. *Pediatrics* 1998;101:E1.

18. O'Rourke PP, Crone RK, Vacanti JP, et al. Extracorporeal membrane oxygenation and conventional medical therapy in neonates with persistent pulmonary hypertension of the newborn: a prospective randomized study. *Pediatrics* 1989;84:957–963.

19. Bartlett RH, Roloff DW, Cornell RG, et al. Extracorporeal circulation in neonatal respiratory failure: a prospective randomized study. *Pediatrics* 1985;76:479–487.

20. Anonymous. *Extracorporeal Life Support Organization ECMO Registry Report.* Ann Arbor, MI: Extracorporeal Life Support Organization, 1998.

21. Kolobow T, Stool EW, Sacks KL. Acute respiratory failure, survival following ten days' support with a membrane lung. *J Thorac Cardiovasc Surg* 1975;69:947–953.

22. Green TP, Timmons OD, Fackler JC, et al. The impact of extracorporeal membrane oxygenation on survival in pediatric patients with acute respiratory failure. Pediatric Critical Care Study Group. *Crit Care Med* 1996;24:323–329.

23. Hill JD, O'Brien TG, Murray JJ, et al. Prolonged extracorporeal oxygenation for acute post-traumatic respiratory failure (shock-lung syndrome). Use of the Bramson membrane lung. *N Engl J Med* 1972;286:629–634.

24. Gille JP, Bagniewski AM. Ten years of use of extracorporeal membrane oxygenation (ECMO) in the treatment of acute respiratory insufficiency (ARI). *ASAIO Trans* 1976;22:102–109.

25. Gille JP. World census on long-term perfusion for respiratory support. In: Zapol WM, Qvist J, eds. *First International Conference on Membrane Technology.* Copenhagen, 1975.

26. Zapol WM, Snider MT, Hill JD, et al. Extracorporeal membrane oxygenation in severe acute respiratory failure. A randomized prospective study. *JAMA* 1979;242:2193–2196.

27. Peirce EC 2d. Is extracorporeal membrane oxygenation a viable technique? *Ann Thorac Surg* 1981;31:102–104.

28. Kolobow T. An update on adult extracorporeal membrane oxygenation–extracorporeal CO_2 removal. *ASAIO Trans* 1988;34:1004–1005.

29. MacDonnell KF, Moon HS, Sekar TS, et al. Extracorporeal membrane oxygenator support in a case of severe status asthmaticus. *Ann Thorac Surg* 1981;31:171–175.

30. Conrad SA. Selection criteria for use of ECMO in adults. In: Zwischenberger JB, Bartlett RH, eds. *ECMO. Extracorporeal cardiopulmonary support in critical care.* Ann Arbor, MI: Extracorporeal Life Support Organization, 1995:385–400.

31. Gattinoni L, Pesenti A, Mascheroni D, et al. Low-frequency positive-pressure ventilation with extracorporeal CO_2 removal in severe acute respiratory failure. *JAMA* 1986;256:881–886.

32. Morris AH, Menlove RL, Rollins RJ. A controlled clinical trial of a new 3-step therapy that includes extracorporeal CO_2 removal for ARDS. *ASAIO Trans* 1988;34:48–53.

33. Anderson H III, Steimle C, Shapiro M, et al. Extracorporeal life support for adult cardiorespiratory failure. *Surgery* 1993;114:161–173.

34. Kolla S, Awad SS, Rich PB, et al. Extracorporeal life support for 100 adult patients with severe respiratory failure. *Ann Surg* 1997;226:544–566.

35. Rich PB, Awad SS, Kolla S, et al. An approach to the treatment of severe adult respiratory failure. *J Crit Care* 1998;13:26–36.

36. Anderson HL, Shapiro MB, Delius RE. Extracorporeal life support for respiratory failure after multiple trauma. *J Trauma* 1994;37:266–272.

37. Anderson HL, Coran AG, Schmeling DJ. Extracorporeal life support (ECLS) for pediatric trauma: experience with five cases. *J Pediatr Surg* 1990;5:302.

38. Bartlett RH. Respiratory support with extracorporeal membrane oxygenation in newborn respiratory failure. In: Welch K, Randolph J, Ravitch M, eds. *Pediatric surgery*, 4th ed. Chicago: Year Book Medical Publishers, 1986:74–77.

39. Kolobow T. Acute respiratory failure. On how to injure healthy lungs (and prevent sick lungs from recovering). *ASAIO Trans* 1988;34:31–34.

40. Hicks RE, Dutton RC, Ries CA, et al. Production and fate of platelet aggregate emboli during venovenous perfusion. *Surg Forum* 1973;24:250–252.

41. Dutton RC, Edmunds LH Jr, Hutchinson JC, et al. Platelet aggregate emboli produced in patients during cardiopulmonary bypass with membrane and bubble oxygenators and blood filters. *J Thorac Cardiovasc Surg* 1974;67:258–265.

42. Hocker JR, Wellhausen SR, Ward RA, et al. Effect of extracorporeal membrane oxygenation on leukocyte function in neonates. *Artif Organs* 1991;15:23–28.

43. DePalma L, Short BL, Van Meurs K, et al. A flow cytometric analysis of lymphocyte subpopulations in neonates undergoing extracorporeal membrane oxygenation. *J Pediatr* 1991;118:117–120.

44. Westfall SH, Stephens C, Kesler K, et al. Complement activation during prolonged extracorporeal membrane oxygenation. *Surgery* 1991;110:887–891.

45. Meliones JN, Moler FW, Custer JR, et al. Hemodynamic instability after the initiation of extracorporeal membrane oxygenation: role of ionized calcium. *Crit Care Med* 1991;19:1247–1251.

46. Almond PS, Adolph VR, Steiner R, et al. Calculous disease of the biliary tract in infants after neonatal extracorporeal membrane oxygenation. *J Perinatol* 1992;12:18–20.

47. Piena M, Albers MJ, Van Haard PM, et al. Introduction of enteral feeding in neonates on extracorporeal membrane oxygenation after evaluation of intestinal permeability changes. *J Pediatr Surg* 1998;33:30–34.

48. Pettignano R, Heard M, Davis R, et al. Total enteral nutrition versus total parenteral nutrition during pediatric extracorporeal membrane oxygenation. *Crit Care Med* 1998;26:358–363.

49. Glass P. Patient neurodevelopmental outcomes after neonatal ECMO. In: Arensman RM, Cornish JD, eds. *Extracorporeal life support.* Boston: Blackwell Science, 1993:241–251.

50. Glass P, Miller MK, Short BL. Morbidity for survivors of extracorporeal membrane oxygenation: neurodevelopmental outcome at 1 year of age. *Pediatrics* 1989;83:72–78.

51. Glass P, Wagner AE, Papero PH. Neurodevelopmental status at age five years of neonates treated with extracorporeal membrane oxygenation. *J Pediatr* 1995;127:447–457.

52. Gleason CA. ECMO and the brain. In: Arensman RM, Cornish JD, eds. *Extracorporeal life support.* Boston: Blackwell Science, 1993:138–155.

53. Graziani LJ, Baumgart S, Desai S, et al. Clinical antecedents of neurologic and audiologic abnormalities in survivors of neonatal ECMO. *J Child Neurol* 1997;12:415–422.

54. Graziani LJ, Streletz LJ, Baumgart S. The predictive value of neonatal electroencephalograms before and during extracorporeal membrane oxygenation. *J Pediatr* 1994;125:969–975.

55. Towne BH, Lott IT, Hicks DA, et al. Long-term follow-up of infants and children treated with extracorporeal membrane oxygenation (ECMO): a preliminary report. *J Pediatr Surg* 1985;20:410–414.

56. Vaucher YE, Dudell GG, Bejar R. Predictors of early childhood outcome in candidates for extracorporeal membrane oxygenation. *J Pediatr* 1996;128:109–117.

57. Wildin SR, Landry SH, Zwischenberger JB. Prospective, controlled study of developmental outcome in survivors of extracorporeal membrane oxygenation: the first 24 months. *Pediatrics* 1994;93:404–408.

58. Gringlas MB, Stanley C, McKee L. Developmental assessment of survivors of extracorporeal membrane oxygenation at early school age: a longitudinal analysis. *Dev Med Child Neurol* 1995;37:21.

59. Graziani LJ, Gringlas M, Baumgart S. Cerebrovascular complications and neurodevelopmental sequelae of neonatal ECMO. *Clin Perinatol* 1997;24:655–675.

60. Kolobow T, Spragg RG, Pierce JE. Massive pulmonary infarction during total cardiopulmonary bypass in unanesthetized spontaneously breathing lambs. *Int J Artif Organs* 1981;4:76–81.

61. Foster AH, Kolobow T. A potential hazard of ventilation during early separation from total cardiopulmonary bypass. *J Thorac Cardiovasc Surg* 1987;93:150–151.

62. Bartlett RH. Physiology of extracorporeal life support. In: Zwischenberger JB, Bartlett RH, eds. *ECMO. Extracorporeal cardiopulmonary support in critical care.* Ann Arbor, MI: Extracorporeal Life Support Organization, 1995:27–52.

63. Galletti PM, Richardson PD, Snider MT. A standardized method for defining the overall gas transfer performance of artificial lungs. *ASAIO Trans* 1972;18:359–368.

64. Cilley RE, Zwischenberger JB, Andrews AF, et al. Intracranial hemorrhage during extracorporeal membrane oxygenation in neonates. *Pediatrics* 1986;78:699–704.

65. Krummel TM, Greenfield LJ, Kirkpatrick BV. Alveolar–arterial oxygen gradients versus the neonatal pulmonary insufficiency index for prediction of mortality in ECMO candidates. *J Pediatr Surg* 1984;19:380–384.

66. Zwischenberger JB, Bartlett RH. Extracorporeal circulation for respiratory or cardiac failure. *Semin Thorac Cardiovasc Surg* 1990;2:320–331.

67. Cox CS, Zwischenberger JB, Graves D. Mortality from ARDS remains unchanged. *Am Rev Respir Dis* 1992;145:A83.

68. Cunningham AJ. Acute respiratory distress syndrome—two decades later. *Yale J Biol Med* 1991;64:387–402.

69. Dal Nogare AR. Adult respiratory distress syndrome. *Am J Med Sci* 1989;298:413–430.

70. Morris AH, Wallace CJ, Menlove RL, et al. Randomized clinical trial of pressure-controlled inverse ratio ventilation and extracorporeal CO_2 removal for adult respiratory distress syndrome. *Am J Respir Crit Care Med* 1994;149:295–305.

71. Bone RC. Extracorporeal membrane oxygenation for acute respiratory failure. *JAMA* 1986;256:910.

72. Campbell LR, Bunyapen C, Holmes GL, et al. Right common carotid artery ligation in extracorporeal membrane oxygenation. *J Pediatr* 1988;113:110–113.

73. Cilley RE, Wesley JR, Zwischenberger JB. Metabolic rates of newborn infants with severe respiratory failure treated with extracorporeal membrane oxygenation. *Curr Surg* 1987;44:48–51.

74. Kolobow T, Moretti MP, Mascheroni D, et al. Experimental meconium aspiration syndrome in the preterm fetal lamb: successful treatment using the extracorporeal artificial lung. *ASAIO Trans* 1983;29:221–226.

75. Keszler M, Ryckman FC, McDonald JV. A prospective multicenter randomized study of high vs. low positive end-expiratory pressure during extracorporeal membrane oxygenation. *J Pediatr* 1992;120:107–113.

76. Bartlett RH, Dechert RE, Mault J, et al. Measurement of metabolism in multiple organ failure. *Surgery* 1982;92:771–778.

77. Anderson HL 3d, Otsu T, Chapman RA, et al. Venovenous extracorporeal life support in neonates using a double-lumen catheter. *ASAIO Trans* 1989;35:650–653.

78. Rich PB, Awad SS, Crotti S, et al. A prospective comparison of atrio-femoral and femoro-atrial flow in adult venovenous extracorporeal life support. *J Thorac Cardiovasc Surg* 1998;116:628–632.

79. Hirschl RB, Pranikoff T, Gauger P, et al. Liquid ventilation in adults, children, and full-term neonates. *Lancet* 1995;346:1201–1202.

80. Rodriguez JL, Steinberg SM, Luchetti FA. Early tracheostomy for primary airway management in the surgical critical care setting. *Surgery* 1990;108:655–659.

81. Bryant LR, Trinkle JK, Mobin-Uddin K. Bacterial colonization profile with tracheal intubation and mechanical ventilation. *Arch Surg* 1972;104:647–651.

82. Anderson HL, Bartlett RH. Elective tracheostomy for mechanical ventilation by the percutaneous technique. In: Jeffer, ed. *Clinic in chest medicine.* Philadelphia: WB Saunders, 1991:555–560.

83. Shapiro MB, Kleaveland AC, Bartlett RH. Extracorporeal life support for status asthmaticus. *Chest* 1993;103:1651–1654.

84. Hardesty RL, Griffith BP, Debski RF, et al. Extracorporeal membrane oxygenation. Successful treatment of persistent fetal circulation following repair of congenital diaphragmatic hernia. *J Thorac Cardiovasc Surg* 1981;81:556–563.

85. Finer NN, Tierney AJ, Hallgren R, et al. Neonatal congenital diaphragmatic hernia and extracorporeal membrane oxygenation. *Can Med Assoc J* 1992;146:501–508.

86. Heiss K, Manning P, Oldham KT, et al. Reversal of mortality for congenital diaphragmatic hernia with ECMO. *Ann Surg* 1989;209:225–230.

87. vd Staak FH, de Haan AF, Geven WB, et al. Improving survival for patients with high-risk congenital diaphragmatic hernia by

using extracorporeal membrane oxygenation. *J Pediatr Surg* 1995;30:1463–1467.

88. Weber TR, Connors RH, Pennington DG, et al. Neonatal diaphragmatic hernia. An improving outlook with extracorporeal membrane oxygenation. *Arch Surg* 1987;122:615–618.

89. Atkinson JB, Ford EG, Humphries B, et al. The impact of extracorporeal membrane support in the treatment of congenital diaphragmatic hernia. *J Pediatr Surg* 1991;26:791–793.

90. Lessin MS, Thompson IM, Deprez MF, et al. Congenital diaphragmatic hernia with or without extracorporeal membrane oxygenation: are we making progress? *J Am Coll Surg* 1995;181: 65–71.

91. Van Meurs KP, Newman KD, Anderson KD, et al. Effect of extracorporeal membrane oxygenation on survival of infants with congenital diaphragmatic hernia. *J Pediatr* 1990;117: 954–960.

92. Redmond C, Heaton J, Calix J, et al. A correlation of pulmonary hypoplasia, mean airway pressure, and survival in congenital diaphragmatic hernia treated with extracorporeal membrane oxygenation. *J Pediatr Surg* 1987;22:1143–1149.

93. Mallik K, Rodgers BM, McGahren ED. Congenital diaphragmatic hernia: experience in a single institution from 1978 through 1994. *Ann Thorac Surg* 1995;60:1331–1335.

94. Bailey PV, Connors RH, Tracy TF Jr, et al. A critical analysis of extracorporeal membrane oxygenation for congenital diaphragmatic hernia. *Surgery* 1989;106:611–615.

95. Connors RH, Tracy T Jr, Bailey PV, et al. Congenital diaphragmatic hernia repair on ECMO. *J Pediatr Surg* 1990;25: 1043–1046.

96. Stolar CJ, Crisafi CA, Driscoll YT. Neurocognitive outcome for neonates treated with extracorporeal membrane oxygenation: are infants with congenital diaphragmatic hernia different? *J Pediatr Surg* 1995;30:366–371.

97. Wilson JM, Bower LK, Lund DP. Evolution of the technique of congenital diaphragmatic hernia repair on ECMO. *J Pediatr Surg* 1994;29:1109–1112.

98. Wilson JM, Lund DP, Lillehei CW, et al. Delayed repair and preoperaitve ECMO does not improve survival in high-risk congenital diaphragmatic hernia. *J Pediatr Surg* 1992;27:368–372.

99. Lally KP, Paranka MS, Roden J, et al. Congenital diaphragmatic hernia. Stabilization and repair on ECMO. *Ann Surg* 1992;216: 569–573.

100. West KW, Bengtson K, Rescorla FJ, et al. Delayed surgical repair and ECMO improves survival in congenital diaphragmatic hernia. *Ann Surg* 1992;216:454–460.

101. Vazquez WD, Cheu HW. Hemorrhagic complications and repair of congenital diaphragmatic hernias: does timing of the repair make a difference? Data from the Extracorporeal Life Support Organization. *J Pediatr Surg* 1994;29:1002–1005.

102. Adolph V, Flageole H, Perreault T, et al. Repair of congenital diaphragmatic hernia after weaning from extracorporeal membrane oxygenation. *J Pediatr Surg* 1995;30:349–352.

103. Sigalet DL, Tierney A, Adolph V, et al. Timing of repair of congenital diaphragmatic hernia requiring extracorporeal membrane oxygenation support. *J Pediatr Surg* 1995;30:1183–1187.

104. Adzick NS, Harrison MR, Glick PL, et al. Diaphragmatic hernia in the fetus: prenatal diagnosis and outcome in 94 cases. *J Pediatr Surg* 1985;20:357–361.

105. Harrison MR, Adzick NS, Estes JM, et al. A prospective study of the outcome for fetuses with diaphragmatic hernia. *JAMA* 1994;271:382–384.

106. Sharland GK, Lockhart SM, Heward AJ, et al. Prognosis in fetal diaphragmatic hernia. *Am J Obstet Gynecol* 1992;166:9–13.

107. Wilson JM, Lund DP, Lillehei CW, et al. Congenital diaphragmatic hernia: predictors of severity in the ECMO era. *J Pediatr Surg* 1991;26:1028–1033.

108. D'Agostino JA, Bernbaum JC, Gerdes M, et al. Outcome for infants with congenital diaphragmatic hernia requiring extracorporeal membrane oxygenation: the first year. *J Pediatr Surg* 1995;30:10–15.

109. Lund DP, Mitchell J, Kharasch V, et al. Congenital diaphragmatic hernia: the hidden morbidity. *J Pediatr Surg* 1994;29: 258–262.

110. Kolobow T, Zapol W, Pierce J. High survival and minimal blood damage in lambs exposed to long-term (1 week) venovenous pumping with a polyurethane chamber roller pump with and without a membrane blood oxygenator. *ASAIO Trans* 1969; 15:172–177.

111. Hanson EL, Bartlett RH, Burns NE, et al. Prolonged use of a membrane oxygenator in air-breathing and hypoxic lambs. *Surgery* 1973;73:284–298.

112. Lamy M, Eberhart RC, Fallat RJ, et al. Effects of extracorporeal membrane oxygenation (ECMO) on pulmonary hemodynamics, gas exchange and prognosis. *ASAIO Trans* 1975;21: 188–198.

113. Delaney AG, Zapol WM, Erdmann AJ III. Lung transvascular fluid dynamics with extracorporeal membrane oxygenation in unanesthetized lambs. *J Thorac Cardiovasc Surg* 1979;77: 252–258.

114. Klein MD, Andrews AF, Wesley JR, et al. Venovenous perfusion in ECMO for newborn respiratory insufficiency. A clinical comparison with venoarterial perfusion. *Ann Surg* 1985;201: 520–526.

115. Pranikoff T, Hirschl RB, Remenapp R, et al. Venovenous extracorporeal life support via percutaneous cannulation in 94 patients. *Chest* 1999;115:818–822.

116. Zwischenberger JB, Toomasian JM, Drake K, et al. Total respiratory support with single-cannula venovenous ECMO: double-lumen continuous flow vs. single-lumen tidal flow. *ASAIO Trans* 1985;31:610–615.

117. Anderson HL 3d, Snedecor SM, Otsu T, et al. Multicenter comparison of conventional venoarterial access versus venovenous double-lumen catheter access in newborn infants undergoing extracorporeal membrane oxygenation. *J Pediatr Surg* 1993; 28:530–534.

118. Zwischenberger JB, Nguyen TT, Upp JR Jr, et al. Complications of neonatal extracorporeal membrane oxygenation. Collective experience from the Extracorporeal Life Support Organization. *J Thorac Cardiovasc Surg* 1994;107:838–849.

119. Chevalier JY, Couprie C, Larroquet M, et al. Venovenous single-lumen cannula extracorporeal lung support in neonates. A five-year experience. *ASAIO J* 1993;39:M654–M658.

120. Kolla S, Crotti S, Lee WA, et al. Total respiratory support with tidal-flow extracorporeal circulation in adult sheep. *ASAIO J* 1997;43:M811–M816.

121. Upp JR Jr, Bush PE, Zwischenberger JB. Complications of neonatal extracorporeal membrane oxygenation. *Perfusion* 1994; 9:241–256.

122. Cavarocchi NC, England MD, Schaff HV, et al. Oxygen free radical generation during cardiopulmonary bypass: correlation with complement activation. *Circulation* 1986;74:III-130–III-133.

123. Eberhart RC. Interactions of blood and artificial surfaces: in search of "heparin-free" cardiopulmonary bypass. In: Arensman RM, Cornish JD, eds. *Extracorporeal life support*, 1st ed. Boston: Blackwell Science, 1993:105–125.

124. Robinson TM, Kickler TS, Waler LK, et al. Effect of extracorporeal membrane oxygenation on platelets in newborns. *Crit Care Med* 1993;21:1029–1034.

125. De Puydt LE, Schuit KE, Smith SD. Effect of extracorporeal membrane oxygenation on neutrophil function in neonates. *Crit Care Med* 1993;21:1324–1327.

126. Bergman P, Belboul A, Friberg LG, et al. The effect of prolonged perfusion with a membrane oxygenator (PPMO) on white blood cells. *Perfusion* 1994;9:35–40.

127. Toomasian JM, Hsu LC, Hirschl RB, et al. Evaluation of Duraflo II heparin coating in prolonged extracorporeal membrane oxygenation. *ASAIO Trans* 1988;34:410–414.

128. Koul B, Wetterberg T, Ohqvist G, et al. Veno-venous extracorporeal membrane oxygenation with a heparin-coated system in adult respiratory distress syndrome. *Scand J Thorac Cardiovasc Surg* 1991;25:199–206.

129. Rossaint R, Slama K, Lewandowski K, et al. Extracorporeal lung assist with heparin-coated systems. *Int J Artif Organs* 1992;15:29–34.

130. Nagaraj HS, Mitchell KA, Fallat ME, et al. Surgical complications and procedures in neonates on extracorporeal membrane oxygenation. *J Pediatr Surg* 1992;27:1106–1109.

131. Rais-Bahrami K, Martin GR, Schnitzer JJ, et al. Malposition of extracorporeal membrane oxygenation cannulas in patients with congenital diaphragmatic hernia. *J Pediatr* 1993;122:794–797.

132. Alexander AA, Mitchell DG, Merton DA, et al. Cannula-induced vertebral steal in neonates during extracorporeal membrane oxygenation: detection with color Doppler US. *Radiology* 1992;182:527–530.

133. Faulkner SC, Chipman CW, Baker LL. Trouble shooting the extracorporeal membrane oxygenator circuit and patient. *J Extracorporeal Technol* 1993;24:120–129.

134. Toomasian JM, Kerby KA, Chapman RA, et al. Performance of a rupture-resistant polyvinyl chloride tubing. *Proc Am Acad Cardiovasc Perfus* 1987;8:56–59.

135. Vogler C, Sotelo-Avila C, Lagunoff D, et al. Aluminum-containing emboli in infants treated with extracorporeal membrane oxygenation. *N Engl J Med* 1988;319:75–79.

136. Lazzara RR, Magovern JA, Benckart DH, et al. Extracorporeal membrane oxygenation for adult post-cardiotomy cardiogenic shock using a heparin-bonded system. *ASAIO J* 1993;39:M444–M447.

137. Shanley CJ, Hultquist KA, Rosenberg DM, et al. Prolonged extracorporeal circulation without heparin. Evaluation of the Medtronic Minimax oxygenator. *ASAIO J* 1992;38:M311–M316.

138. Tsuno K, Terasaki H, Otsu T, et al. Newborn extracorporeal lung assist using a novel double-lumen catheter and a heparin-bonded membrane lung. *Intensive Care Med* 1993;19:70–72.

139. Plotz FB, van Oeveren W, Bartlett RH, et al. Blood activation during neonatal extracorporeal life support. *J Thorac Cardiovasc Surg* 1993;105:823–832.

140. Brunet F, Mira JP, Belghith M, et al. Effects of aprotinin on hemorrhagic complications in ARDS patients during prolonged extracorporeal CO_2 removal. *Intensive Care Med* 1992;18:364–367.

141. Wilson JM, Bower LK, Fackler JC, et al. Aminocaproic acid decreases the incidence of intracranial hemorrhage and other hemorrhagic complications of ECMO. *J Pediatr Surg* 1993;28:536–540.

142. Feindt P, Volkmer I, Seyfert U, et al. Activated clotting time, anticoagulation, use of heparin, and thrombin activation during extracorporeal circulation: changes under aprotinin therapy. *Thorac Cardiovasc Surg* 1993;41:9–15.

143. Spannagl M, Dietrich W, Beck A, et al. High-dose aprotinin reduces prothrombin and fibrinogen conversion in patients undergoing extracorporeal circulation for myocardial revascularization. *Thromb Haemost* 1994;72:159–160.

144. Wachtfogel YT, Kucich U, Hack CE, et al. Aprotinin inhibits the contact, neutrophil, and platelet activation systems during simulated extracorporeal perfusion. *J Thorac Cardiovasc Surg* 1993;106:1–9.

145. Fraedrich G, Weber C, Bernard C, et al. Reduction of blood transfusion requirement in open heart surgery by administration of high doses of aprotinin—preliminary results. *Thorac Cardiovasc Surg* 1989;37:89–91.

146. Dietrich W, Barankay A, Dilthey G, et al. Reduction of homologous blood requirement in cardiac surgery by intraoperative aprotinin application—clinical experience in 152 cardiac surgical patients. *Thorac Cardiovasc Surg* 1989;37:92–98.

147. van Oeveren W, Jansen NJ, Bidstrup BP, et al. Effects of aprotinin on hemostatic mechanisms during cardiopulmonary bypass. *Ann Thorac Surg* 1987;44:640–645.

148. Tarby TJ, Volpe JJ. Intraventricular hemorrhage in the premature infant. *Pediatr Clin North Am* 1982;29:1077–1104.

149. Lazar EL, Abramson SJ, Weinstein S, et al. Neuroimaging of brain injury in neonates treated with extracorporeal membrane oxygenation: lessons learned from serial examinations. *J Pediatr Surg* 1994;29:186–191.

150. von Allmen D, Babcock D, Matsumoto J, et al. The predictive value of head ultrasound in the ECMO candidate. *J Pediatr Surg* 1992;27:36–39.

151. Gleason LA. ECMO and the brain. In: Arensman RM, Cornish JD, eds. *Extracorporeal life support*, 1st ed. Boston: Blackwell Science, 1993:138–155.

152. Schumacher RE. Risks of neonatal ECMO. In: Arensman RM, Cornish JD, eds. *Extracorporeal life support*, 1st ed. Boston: Blackwell Science, 1993:226–240.

153. Taylor GA, Walker LK. Intracranial venous system in newborns treated with extracorporeal membrane oxygenation: Doppler US evaluation after ligation of the right jugular vein. *Radiology* 1992;183:453–456.

154. Schumacher RE, Barks JD, Johnston MV, et al. Right-sided brain lesions in infants following extracorporeal membrane oxygenation. *Pediatrics* 1988;82:155–161.

155. Raju TN, Kim SY, Meller JL, et al. Circle of Willis blood velocity and flow direction after common carotid artery ligation for neonatal extracorporeal membrane oxygenation. *Pediatrics* 1989;83:343–347.

156. Lohrer RM, Bejar RF, Simko AJ, et al. Internal carotid artery blood flow velocities before, during, and after extracorporeal membrane oxygenation. *Am J Dis Child* 1992;146:201–207.

157. Taylor GA, Short BL, Fitz CR. Imaging of cerebrovascular injury in infants treated with extracorporeal membrane oxygenation [see Comments]. *J Pediatr* 1989;114:635–639.

158. Streletz LJ, Bej MD, Graziani LJ, et al. Utility of serial EEGs in neonates during extracorporeal membrane oxygenation. *Pediatr Neurol* 1992;8:190–196.

159. Spector ML, Wiznitzer M, Walsh-Sukys MC, et al. Carotid reconstruction in the neonate following ECMO. *J Pediatr Surg* 1991;26:357–359.

160. Moulton SL, Lynch FP, Cornish JD, et al. Carotid artery reconstruction following neonatal extracorporeal membrane oxygenation. *J Pediatr Surg* 1991;26:794–799.

161. Baumgart S, Streletz LJ, Needleman L, et al. Right common coartoid artery reconstruction after extracorporeal membrane oxygenation: vascular imaging, cerebral circulation, electroencephalographic, and neurodevelopmental correlates to recovery. *J Pediatr* 1994;125:295–304.

162. Hirthler MA, Blackwell E, Abbe D, et al. Coagulation parameter instability as an early predictor of intracranial hemorrhage during extracorporeal membrane oxygenation. *J Pediatr Surg* 1992;27:40–43.

163. Stallion A, Cofer BR, Rafferty JA, et al. The significant relationship between platelet count and haemorrhagic complications on ECMO. *Perfusion* 1994;9:265–269.

164. Steinhorn RH, Isham-Schopf B, Smith C, et al. Hemolysis during long-term extracorporeal membrane oxygenation. *J Pediatr* 1989;115:625–630.

165. Anderson HL 3d, Cilley RE, Zwischenberger JB, et al. Thrombocytopenia in neonates after extracorporeal membrane oxygenation. *ASAIO Trans* 1986;32:534–537.

166. Sell LL, Cullen ML, Whittlesey GC, et al. Experience with renal failure during extracorporeal membrane oxygenation: treatment with continuous hemofiltration. *J Pediatr Surg* 1987;22: 600–602.

167. Sell LL, Cullen ML, Lerner GR, et al. Hypertension during extracorporeal membrane oxygenation: cause, effect, and management. *Surgery* 1987;102:724–730.

168. Martin GR, Short BL, Abbott C. Cardiac stun in infants undergoing extracorporeal membrane oxygenation. *J Thorac Cardiovasc Surg* 1991;101:607–611.

169. Hirschl RB, Heiss KF, Bartlett RH. Severe myocardial dysfunction during extracorporeal membrane oxygenation. *J Pediatr Surg* 1992;27:48–53.

170. Holley DG, Short BL, Karr SS, et al. Mechanisms of change in cardiac performance in infants undergoing extracorporeal membrane oxygenation. *Crit Care Med* 1994;22:1865–1870.

171. Palmisano JM, Moler FW, Custer JR, et al. Unsuspected congenital heart disease in neonates receiving extracorporeal life support: a review of ninety-five cases from the Extracorporeal Life Support Organization Registry. *J Pediatr* 1992;121: 115–117.

172. Zwischenberger JB, Bowers RM, Pickens GJ. Tension pneumothorax during extracorporeal membrane oxygenation. *Ann Thorac Surg* 1989;47:868–871.

173. Zwischenberger JB, Cilley RE, Hirschl RB, et al. Life-threatening intrathoracic complications during treatment with extracorporeal membrane oxygenation. *J Pediatr Surg* 1988;23: 599–604.

174. Bartlett RH, Gazzaniga AB, Fong SW, et al. Extracorporeal membrane oxygenator support for cardiopulmonary failure. Experience in 28 cases. *J Thorac Cardiovasc Surg* 1977;73: 375–386.

175. Anderson HL, Attorri RJ, Custer JR. Extracorporeal membrane oxygenation for pediatric cardiopulmonary failure. *J Thorac Cardiovasc Surg* 1990;99:1011–1019.

176. Raithel SC, Pennington DG, Boegner E, et al. Extracorporeal membrane oxygenation in children after cardiac surgery. *Circulation* 1992;86:II-305–I-310.

177. Weihaus L, Carter C, Noetzel M. Extracorporeal membrane oxygenation for circulatory support after repair of congenital heart defects. *Ann Thorac Surg* 1989;48:206–212.

178. Klein MD, Shaheen KW, Whittlesey GC, et al. Extracorporeal membrane oxygenation for the circulatory support of children after repair of congenital heart disease. *J Thorac Cardiovasc Surg* 1990;100:498–505.

179. Kanter KR, Pennington G, Weber TR, et al. Extracorporeal membrane oxygenation for postoperative cardiac support in children. *J Thorac Cardiovasc Surg* 1987;93:27–35.

180. Bavaria JE, Ratcliff MB, Gupta KB. Changes in left ventricular systolic wall stress during biventricular circulatory assistance. *Ann Thorac Surg* 1988;45:526–532.

181. Soeter JR, Mamiya RT, Sprague AY. Prolonged extracorporeal oxygenation for cardiorespiratory failure after tetralogy correction. *J Thorac Cardiovasc Surg* 1973;66:214–218.

182. Miyamura H, Sugawara MA, Watanabe H, et al. Blalock-Taussig operation with an assist of venovenous extracorporeal membrane oxygenation. *Ann Thorac Surg* 1996;62:565–566.

183. Karl TR, Lyer KS, Mee RB. Infant ECMO cannulation technique allowing preservation of carotid and jugular vessels. *Ann Thorac Surg* 1990;50:105.

184. Fosse E, Moen O, Johnson E. Reduced complement and granulocyte activation with heparin-coated cardiopulmonary bypass. *Ann Thorac Surg* 1994;58:472–474.

185. Jurmann MJ, Haverich A, Demertzis S. Extracorporeal membrane oxygenation as a bridge to lung transplantation. *Eur J Cardiothorac Surg* 1991;5:94–97.

186. Zenati M, Pham SM, Keenan RJ, et al. Extracorporeal membrane oxygenation for lung transplant recipients with primary severe donor lung dysfunction. *Transpl Int* 1996;9:227–230.

187. Karl TR. Extracorporeal circulatory support in infants and children. *Semin Thorac Cardiovasc Surg* 1994;6:154–160.

188. Sell LL, Cullen ML, Lerner GR. Hemorrhagic complications during extracorporeal membrane oxygenation. Prevention and treatment. *J Pediatr Surg* 1986;21:1087–1091.

189. Kitano Y, Takata M, Miyasaka K, et al. Evaluation of an extracorporeal membrane oxygenation system using a nonporous membrane oxygenator and a new method for heparin coating. *J Pediatr Surg* 1997;32:691–697.

190. Weerwind PW, van der Veen FH, Lindhout T, et al. *Ex vivo* testing of heparin-coated extracorporeal circuits: bovine experiments. *Int J Artif Organs* 1998;21:291–298.

191. Moen O, Fosse E, Braten J, et al. Differences in blood activation related to roller/centrifugal pumps and heparin-coated/uncoated surfaces in a cardiopulmonary bypass model circuit. *Perfusion* 1996;11:113–123.

192. Nojiri C, Hagiwara K, Yokoyama K, et al. Evaluation of a new heparin-bonding process in prolonged extracorporeal membrane oxygenation. *ASAIO J* 1995;41:M561–M567.

193. Palmer K, Ehren H, Benz R, et al. Carmeda surface heparinization in neonatal ECMO systems: long-term experiments in a sheep model. *Perfusion* 1995;10:307–313.

194. Mellgren K, Friberg LG, Mellgren G, et al. Nitric oxide in the oxygenator sweep gas reduces platelet activation during experimental perfusion. *Ann Thorac Surg* 1996;61:1194–1198.

195. Barthelemy R, Galletti PM, Trudell LA, et al. Total extracorporeal CO_2 removal in a pumpless artery-to-vein shunt. *ASAIO Trans* 1982;28:354–358.

196. Brunston RL Jr, Zwischenberger JB, Tao W, et al. Total arteriovenous carbon dioxide removal ($AVCO_2R$): simplifying extracorporeal support for severe respiratory failure. *Ann Thorac Surg* 1997;64:1599–1605.

197. Brunston RL Jr, Tao W, Bidani A, et al. Determination of low blood flow limits for arteriovenous carbon dioxide removal ($AVCO_2R$). *ASAIO J* 1996;M4:845–851.

198. Brunston RL Jr, Tao W, Bidani A, et al. Prolonged hemodynamic stability during arteriovenous carbon dioxide removal ($AVCO_2R$) for severe respiratory failure. *J Thorac Cardiovasc Surg* 1997;114:1107–1114.

199. Alpard SK, Zwischenberger JB, Tao W, et al. Dose-dependant development of severe respiratory failure in an ovine model of smoke inhalation and cutaneous flame burn injury. *Crit Care Med* 1999 (*in press*).

200. Alpard SK, Zwischenberger JB, Tao W, et al. Reduced ventilator pressure and improved P/F ratio during percutaneous arteriovenous carbon dioxide removal ($AVCO_2R$) for severe respiratory failure. *Ann Surg* 1999;230:215–224.

201. Zwischenberger JB, Conrad SA, Alpard SK, et al. Percutaneous extracorporeal arteriovenous carbon dioxide removal ($AVCO_2R$) in adult patients with severe respiratory failure: initial clinical experience. *South Thorac Surg Assoc* 1999;68: 181–187.

202. Vaslef SN, Cook KE, Leonard RJ, et al. Design and evaluation of a new, low pressure loss, implantable artificial lung. *ASAIO J* 1994;40:M522–M526.

203. Fazzalari DL, Montoya JP, Bonnell MR, et al. The development

of an implantable artificial lung. *ASAIO J* 1994;40: M728–M731.

204. Lynch W, Montoya P, Schreiner R, et al. Hemodynamic effects of a low-resistance artificial lung in series with native lungs of sheep: a 24-hour study. *Soc Thorac Surg Program* 1999;166.

205. Cox CS Jr, Zwischenberger JB, Traber LD, et al. Use of an intravascular oxygenator/carbon dioxide removal device in an ovine smoke inhalation injury model. *ASAIO Trans* 1991;37: M411–M413.

206. Zwischenberger JB, Cox CS Jr. A new intravascular membrane oxygenator to augment blood gas transfer in patients with acute respiratory failure. *Tex Med* 1991;87:60–63.

207. Conrad SA, Bagley A, Bagley B, et al. Major findings from the clinical trials of the intravascular oxygenator. *Artif Organs* 1994; 18:846–863.

208. Green TP, Moler FW, Goodman DM. Probability of survival after prolonged extracorporeal membrane oxygenation in pediatric patients with acute respiratory failure. *Crit Care Med* 1995; 23:1132–1139.

209. Philips JB. Treatment of PPHNS. In: Long WA, ed. *Fetal and neonatal cardiology*. Philadelphia: WB Saunders, 1990: 691–701.

210. Dorson W Jr, Meyer B, Baker E, et al. Response of distressed infants to partial bypass lung assist. *ASAIO Trans* 1970;16: 345–351.

211. White JJ, Andrews HG, Risemberg H, et al. Prolonged respiratory support in newborn infants with a membrane oxygenator. *Surgery* 1971;70:288–296.

212. Pyle RB, Helton WC, Johnson FW, et al. Clinical use of the membrane oxygenator. *Arch Surg* 1975;110:966–970.

213. Anderson HL 3d, Delius RE, Sinard JM, et al. Early experience with adult extracorporeal membrane oxygenation in the modern era. *Ann Thorac Surg* 1992;53:553–563.

214. Toomasian JM, Snedecor SM, Cornell RG, et al. National experience with extracorporeal membrane oxygenation for newborn respiratory failure. Data from 715 cases. *ASAIO Trans* 1988; 34:140–147.

215. Stolar CJ, Snedecor SM, Bartlett RH. Extracorporeal membrane oxygenation and neonatal respiratory failure: experience from the extracorporeal life support organization. *J Pediatr Surg* 1991; 26:563–571.

216. Zwischenberger JB, Cox CS Jr. ECMO in the management of cardiac failure. *ASAIO J* 1992;38:751–753.

217. O'Rourke PP, Stolar CJ, Zwischenberger JB, et al. Extracorporeal membrane oxygenation: support for overwhelming pulmonary failure in the pediatric population. Collective experience from the Extracorporeal Life Support Organization. *J Pediatr Surg* 1993;28:523–528.

218. Breaux CW Jr, Rouse TM, Cain WS, et al. Improvement in survival of patients with congenital diaphragmatic hernia utilizing a strategy of delayed repair after medical and/or extracorporeal membrane oxygenation stabilization. *J Pediatr Surg* 1991; 26:333–336.

219. Coughlin JP, Drucker DE, Cullen ML, et al. Delayed repair of congenital diaphragmatic hernia. *Am Surg* 1993;59:90–93.

220. Walker LK. Use of extracorporeal membrane oxygenation for preoperative stabilization of congenital diaphragmatic hernia. *Crit Care Med* 1993;21:S379–S380.

221. Rais-Bahrami K, Robbins ST, Reed VL, et al. Congenital diaphragmatic hernia. Outcome of preoperative extracorporeal membrane oxygenation. *Clin Pediatr* 1995;34:471–474.

222. Reickert CA, Hirschl RB, Schumacher R, et al. Effect of very delayed repair of congenital diaphragmatic hernia on survival and extracorporeal life support use. *Surgery* 1996;120:766–772.

223. Azarow K, Messineo A, Pearl R, et al. Congenital diaphragmatic hernia—a tale of two cities: the Toronto experience. *J Pediatr Surg* 1997;32:395–400.

224. Wilson JM, Lund DP, Lillehei CW, et al. Congenital diaphragmatic hernia—a tale of two cities: the Boston experience. *J Pediatr Surg* 1997;32:401–405.

225. Nagaya M, Kato J, Niimi N, et al. Analysis of patients with congenital diaphragmatic hernia requiring pre-operative extracorporeal membrane oxygenation (ECMO). *Pediatr Surg Int* 1998;14:25–29.

226. Steimle CN, Meric F, Hirschl RB, et al. Effect of extracorporeal life support on survival when applied to all patients with congenital diaphragmatic hernia. *J Pediatr Surg* 1994;29:997–1001.

227. Ssemakula N, Stewart DL, Goldsmith LJ, et al. Survival of patients with congenital diaphragmatic hernia during the ECMO era: an 11-year experience. *J Pediatr Surg* 1997;32: 1683–1689.

228. Weber TR, Kountzman B, Dillon PA, et al. Improved survival in congenital diaphragmatic hernia with evolving therapeutic strategies. *Arch Surg* 1998;133:498–502.

229. Langham MR Jr, Krummel TM, Greenfield LJ, et al. Extracorporeal membrane oxygenation following repair of congenital diaphragmatic hernias. *Ann Thorac Surg* 1987;44:247–252.

230. Langham MR Jr, Krummel TM, Bartlett RH, et al. Mortality with extracorporeal membrane oxygenation following repair of congenital diaphragmatic hernia in 93 infants. *J Pediatr Surg* 1987;22:1150–1154.

231. Johnston PW, Bashner B, Liberman R, et al. Clinical use of extracorporeal membrane oxygenation in the treatment of persistent pulmonary hypertension following surgical repair of congenital diaphragmatic hernia. *J Pediatr Surg* 1988;23:908–912.

232. Stolar C, Dillon P, Reyes C. Selective use of extracorporeal membrane oxygenation in the management of congenital diaphragmatic hernia. *J Pediatr Surg* 1988;23:207–211.

233. Newman KD, Anderson KD, Van Meurs K, et al. Extracorporeal membrane oxygenation and congenital diaphragmatic hernia: should any infant be excluded? *J Pediatr Surg* 1990;25: 1048–1052.

234. O'Rourke PP, Lillehei CW, Crone RK, et al. The effect of extracorporeal membrane oxygenation on the survival of neonates with high-risk congenital diaphragmatic hernia: 45 cases from a single institution. *J Pediatr Surg* 1991;26:147–152.

235. Van Meurs KP, Robbins ST, Reed VL, et al. Congenital diaphragmatic hernia: long-term outcome in neonates treated with extracorporeal membrane oxygenation. *J Pediatr* 1993;122: 893–899.

236. Keshen TH, Gursoy M, Shew SB, et al. Does extracorporeal membrane oxygenation benefit neonates with congenital diaphragmatic hernia? Application of a predictive equation. *J Pediatr Surg* 1997;32:818–822.

237. McGahren ED, Mallik K, Rodgers BM. Neurological outcome is diminished in survivors of congenital diaphragmatic hernia requiring extracorporeal membrane oxygenation. *J Pediatr Surg* 1997;32:1216–1220.

238. Heiss KF, Clark RH. Prediction of mortality in neonates with congenital diaphragmatic hernia treated with extracorporeal membrane oxygenation. *Crit Care Med* 1995;23:1915–1919.

239. Heiss KF, Clark RH, Cornish JD, et al. Preferential use of venovenous extracorporeal membrane oxygenation for congenital diaphragmatic hernia. *J Pediatr Surg* 1995;30:416–419.

240. Clark RH, Hardin WD Jr, Hirschl RB, et al. Current surgical management of congenital diaphragmatic hernia: a report from the Congenital Diaphragmatic Hernia Study Group. *J Pediatr Surg* 1998;33:1004–1009.

241. Reickert CA, Hirschl RB, Atkinson JB, et al. Congenital diaphragmatic hernia survival and use of extracorporeal life support

at selected level III nurseries with multimodality support. *Surgery* 1998;123:305–310.

242. Thibeault DW, Haney B. Lung volume, pulmonary vasculature, and factors affecting survival in congenital diaphragmatic hernia. *Pediatrics* 1998;101:289–295.

243. Pennington DG, Merjavy JP, Codd JE, et al. Extracorporeal membrane oxygenation for patients with cardiogenic shock. *Circulation* 1984;70:I-130–I-137.

244. Redmond CR, Graves ED, Falterman KW, et al. Extracorporeal membrane oxygenation for respiratory and cardiac failure in infants and children. *J Thorac Cardiovasc Surg* 1987;93:199–204.

245. Rogers AJ, Trento A, Siewers RD. Extracorporeal membrane oxygenation for postcardiotomy shock in children. *Ann Thorac Surg* 1989;47:903–906.

246. Weinhaus L, Canter C, Noetzel M, et al. Extracorporeal membrane oxygenation for circulatory support after repair of congenital heart defects. *Ann Thorac Surg* 1989;48:206–212.

247. Delius RE, Zwischenberger JB, Cilley R, et al. Prolonged extracorporeal life support of pediatric and adolescent cardiac transplant patients. *Ann Thorac Surg* 1990;50:791–795.

248. Galantowicz ME, Stolar CJ. Extracorporeal membrane oxygenation for perioperative support in pediatric heart transplantation. *J Thorac Cardiovasc Surg* 1991;102:148–152.

249. Ziomek S, Harrell JE Jr, Fasules JW, et al. Extracorporeal membrane oxygenation for cardiac failure after congenital heart operation. *Ann Thorac Surg* 1992;54:861–878.

250. Raithel SC, Pennington DG, Boegner E, et al. Extracorporeal membrane oxygenation in children after cardiac surgery. *Circulation* 1992;86:II-305–II-310.

251. Hunkeler NM, Canter CE, Donze A, et al. Extracorporeal life support in cyanotic congenital heart disease before cardiovascular operation. *Am J Cardiol* 1992;69:790–793.

252. del Nido PJ, Dalton HJ, Thompson AE, et al. Extracorporeal membrane oxygenator rescue in children during cardiac arrest after cardiac surgery. *Circulation* 1992;86:II-300–II-304.

253. del Nido PJ, Armitage JM, Fricker FJ, et al. Extracorporeal membrane oxygenation support as a bridge to pediatric heart transplantation. *Circulation* 1994;90:II-66–II-69.

254. Walters HL 3rd, Hakimi M, Rice MD, et al. Pediatric cardiac surgical ECMO: multivariate analysis of risk factors for hospital death. *Ann Thorac Surg* 1995;60:329–336.

255. Black MD, Coles JG, Williams WG, et al. Determinants of success in pediatric cardiac patients undergoing extracorporeal membrane oxygenation. *Ann Thorac Surg* 1995;60:133–138.

256. del Nido PJ. Extracorporeal membrane oxygenation for cardiac support in children. *Ann Thorac Surg* 1996;61:336–339.

257. Wang SS, Chen YS, Ko WJ, et al. Extracorporeal membrane oxygenation support for postcardiotomy cardiogenic shock. *Artif Organs* 1996;20:1287–1291.

258. Kulik TJ, Moler FW, Palmisano JM, et al. Outcome-associated factors in pediatric patients treated with extracorporeal membrane oxygenator after cardiac surgery. *Circulation* 1996;94:II-63–II-68.

259. Ishino K, Weng Y, Alexi-Meskishvili V, et al. Extracorporeal membrane oxygenation as a bridge to cardiac transplantation in children. *Artif Organs* 1996;20:728–732.

260. Doski JJ, Butler TJ, Louder DS, et al. Outcome of infants requiring cardiopulmonary resuscitation before extracorporeal membrane oxygenation. *J Pediatr Surg* 1997;32:1318–1321.

261. Peek GJ, Firmin RK. Extracorporeal membrane oxygenation for cardiac support. *Coron Artery Dis* 1997;8:371–388.

262. Ko WJ, Chen YS, Chou NK, et al. Extracorporeal membrane oxygenation in the perioperative period of heart transplantation. *J Formos Med Assoc* 1997;96:83–90.

263. Saker DM, Walsh-Sukys M, Spector M, et al. Cardiac recovery and survival after neonatal myocardial infarction. *Pediatr Cardiol* 1997;18:139–142.

264. Goldman AP, Kerr SJ, Butt W, et al. Extracorporeal support for intractable cardiorespiratory failure due to meningococcal disease. *Lancet* 1997;349:466–469.

265. Trittenwein G, Furst G, Golej J, et al. Preoperative ECMO in congenital cyanotic heart disease using the AREC system. *Ann Thorac Surg* 1997;63:1298–1302.

266. Langley SM, Sheppard SV, Tsang VT, et al. When is extracorporeal life support worthwhile following repair of congenital heart disease in children? *Eur J Cardiothorac Surg* 1998;13:520–525.

267. Duncan BW, Ibrahim AE, Hraska V, et al. Use of rapid-deployment extracorporeal membrane oxygenation for the resuscitation of pediatric patients with heart disease after cardiac arrest. *J Thorac Cardiovasc Surg* 1998;116:305–311.

268. Delius RE. As originally published in 1990: Prolonged extracorporeal life support of pediatric and adolescent cardiac transplant patients. Updated in 1998. *Ann Thorac Surg* 1998;65:877–878.

EXTRACORPOREAL CARDIOPULMONARY SUPPORT FOR RESUSCITATION AND INVASIVE CARDIOLOGY OUTSIDE THE OPERATING SUITE

BENJAMIN C. SUN
WALTER E. PAE, JR.

Extracorporeal cardiopulmonary support (CPS) is not widely employed for resuscitation and procedures outside the operating suite. The logistics of initiating support in a timely fashion are often prohibitive in a truly emergent setting. In addition, survival results have been predictably poor in most adult populations with the use of this modality. Nevertheless, the judicious use of extracorporeal CPS in situations in which inciting events are treatable and reversible can lead to dramatic patient recovery.

HISTORICAL BACKGROUND

It was the lack of a rapid effective treatment for moribund patients with pulmonary embolus that led Dr. John Gibbon, Jr. to begin his pioneering work with extracorporeal CPS. Gibbon himself was never able to treat such a patient, but in 1961, Cooley et al. (1) utilized emergency CPS for a patient with a massive pulmonary embolus. The patient was eventually transported to the operating theater and the embolus was removed with CPS. This patient ultimately survived to be discharged from the hospital. In their case report, Cooley and his co-workers suggested the need for a less cumbersome system specially adapted for use in emergency and resuscitative situations. The early years of CPS saw many other reports on the use of this modality as a resuscitative device (1–3).

Stuckey (2) in 1958 reported a series of three patients treated with CPS for cardiogenic shock following acute myocardial infarction. Despite criteria requiring patients be moribund before inclusion, one patient survived to hospital discharge. This was a time when open chest cardiopulmonary resuscitation (CPR) was limited mostly to the operating room, and closed chest CPR and cardiac resuscitation were just beginning to become accepted practice (4).

In the 1960s, an explosion of new operative techniques was made possible by the new and rapidly improving technology of CPS. Investigators continued to explore the role of CPS as a resuscitative tool (3,5). In 1966, Proctor (6) evaluated the technique, being interested in whether the left side of the heart could be adequately decompressed, an issue that remains unresolved today. He concluded that ". . . there appears to be no insoluble problem in the use of the technique of closed-chest, veno-arterial bypass by peripheral cannulation in acute myocardial infarction with severe shock or cardiac arrest." However, the technique was not immediately grasped and put into widespread use.

May et al. (7) in 1971 suggested that the technology could be utilized in the growing number of community hospitals. They reported 10 patients who required resuscitation and support with CPS during noncardiac emergency operations. These included pulmonary embolectomy and repair of a traumatic rupture of the aorta, aortopulmonary fistula, and aortic arch injury. Nine of the 10 patients were transferred while on CPS, from as far away as 75 miles. However, during the next 20 years, interest in using CPS as a resuscitative measure was only sporadic. Most investigators were discouraged with the overall poor clinical outcome resulting from the long periods of time necessary to institute CPS, the skill required to perform femoral artery cut-downs, and the difficulties encountered during the performance of CPR (8). Furthermore, the equipment necessary was cumbersome and patients often exsanguinated during transport.

The first percutaneous initiation of CPS was described by Phillips et al. (9) in 1983. Using two 30-cm 12 French (F) venous cannulas and a single 15-cm 12F arterial cannula, they were able to achieve flow rates of 2 to 2.5 L/min. This and other more recent developments caused a resurgence of

B. C. Sun and W. E. Pae, Jr.: Department of Surgery, Section of Cardiothoracic Surgery, The Pennsylvania State University College of Medicine, Hershey, Pennsylvania 17033.

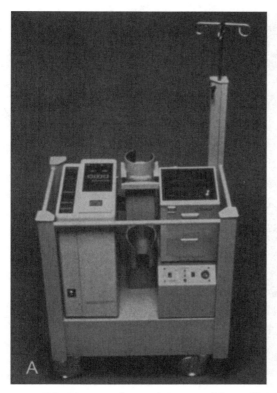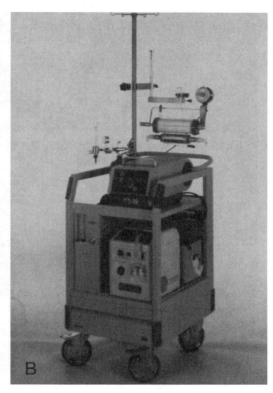

FIG. 32.1. A: The Bard CPS portable cardiopulmonary bypass system. (Photo courtesy of Bard Cardiopulmonary Division, C. R. Bard, Inc., Billerica, MA.) **B:** The Sarns Percart unit. (Photo courtesy of Sarns 3M Health Care, Ann Arbor, MI.)

interest in extracorporeal cardiopulmonary support (ECPS), both as a resuscitative tool outside the operating room environment and as an adjunctive measure in interventional cardiology. Cannulas have been developed that can rapidly be placed percutaneously by the Seldinger technique, and these provide adequate systemic flow and venous drainage to decompress the heart. Commercial compact portable bypass systems have been developed that use vortex pumps without venous reservoirs (Fig. 32.1).

TECHNIQUES

The institution of CPS in the emergency setting by cannulation of the femoral vessels has been accepted since the early days of bypass. Cannulation under direct visualization of the vessels through a groin incision is cumbersome and time-consuming in emergency situations. It also requires the availability of a surgeon capable of performing the procedure in an expeditious manner. This method of access may have excluded many patients from receiving support, or unnecessarily delayed initiation of support. Percutaneous approaches to arterial and venous access for CPS can be created more rapidly in these settings, require less surgical expertise, and are currently the preferred approach.

Insertion Techniques

Percutaneous

The femoral vessels are the vessels most commonly used for cannulation because of their accessibility. The internal jugular vein can also be readily accessed and should not be overlooked, and the carotid artery is also routinely used in children. Typically, the groins are prepared with an antiseptic agent and draped. The femoral artery and vein are then punctured with a thin-walled needle and a guidewire is placed. In the catheterization laboratory, fluoroscopy can be utilized to assist in cannulation. In elective settings, a femoral arteriogram is obtained to define the anatomy and ensure the patency and caliber of the femoral artery. The skin is then incised and the patient is systemically heparinized with 300 U/kg. Activated whole blood clotting times are measured and maintained above 300 seconds with additional doses of heparin as needed. The vessel is successively dilated with 8F, 12F, and 14F dilators passed over a long, stiff guidewire. The cannulas are then exchanged over the guidewire. A 19-cm-long 20F multihole venous cannula and 17F or 18F short arterial cannulas are most commonly utilized. The cannulas are allowed to fill with blood and clamped until connected to the bypass circuit (Fig. 32.2).

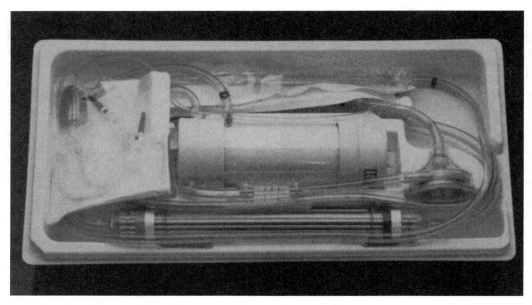

FIG. 32.2. The preassembled tubing pack for the Bard CPS system. (Photo courtesy of Bard Cardiopulmonary Division, Billerica, MA.)

Direct Visualization

Cannulation of the artery and vein under direct vision and removal with repair of the puncture site is preferred to percutaneous cannulation except in emergency situations or when a prolonged support period is anticipated, as in the case of extracorporeal membrane oxygenation. Again, the femoral vessels are most often accessed. The subclavian artery and axillary artery can be used when severe aortoiliac disease is present, and the carotid artery can also be used in children.

For femoral cannulation, standard aseptic conditions and local or general anesthesia are used. A longitudinal incision is made from the inguinal ligament inferiorly for approximately 10 cm, and the femoral artery and vein are exposed. For arterial cannulation, the common femoral, deep femoral, and superficial femoral arteries are isolated with Dacron tapes (proximal and distal arterial control). Following the administration of heparin, the superficial and deep femoral arteries are clamped with noncrushing vascular clamps. A pseudo-Rummel tourniquet is placed around the common femoral artery, and a transverse arteriotomy is performed. A 17F or 19F arterial cannula is then passed and secured with the pseudo-Rummel tourniquet. Venous cannulation with a long 19F or 20F multiholed cannula is performed in a similar fashion. Alternatively, the Seldinger technique can be used, with the vessels in direct vision without isolation. This eliminates the time needed to encircle the vessels and allows for more rapid insertion, although there is less control if the vessel tears.

Bypass Circuit

The early emergency pump oxygenator circuits used for resuscitation were simply scaled-down versions of the pump oxygenator circuit used in the operating room, with a battery pack attached. The development of smaller, more efficient, and less traumatic membrane oxygenators, in addition to the widespread acceptance of centrifugal pumps, has contributed greatly to the resurgence of interest in emergency ECPS. A silicone rubber membrane oxygenator (Avecor Cardiovascular, Inc., Minneapolis, MN) can be used when prolonged CPS is anticipated. However, the most commonly used systems for emergency ECPS consist of a hollow fiber membrane oxygenator and a centrifugal pump head (Fig. 32.3). No venous reservoir bag is utilized in most circumstances. Commercial packs are sold that have an entire circuit connected with the oxygenator and pump head in place (Bard Cardiopulmonary, C. R. Bard, Inc., Billerica, MA; Medtronic, Inc., Grand Rapids, MI). These systems can be rapidly primed within minutes. The absence of a venous reservoir in the circuit allows improved flow rates because venous drainage is by suction rather than by gravity. The centrifugal (vortex) pumps employed also provide a certain margin of safety in comparison with roller head pumps in that they prevent the pumping of massive amounts of air. Because of the aspirating nature of venous return, however, care must be taken that all central venous lines are closed to air, and no central venipunctures should be attempted while the patient is on ECPS.

Devices to monitor mixed venous oxygenation, arterial

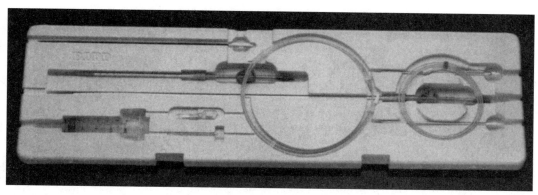

FIG. 32.3. Prepackaged cannulas for percutaneous bypass, available from Bard Cardiopulmonary. (Photo courtesy of Bard Cardiopulmonary Division, Billerica, MA.)

blood gases, and electrolytes as well as hemofiltration circuits can be readily spliced into the system to enhance patient management. The pulmonary artery catheter remains useful to assess pulmonary artery pressures but is rendered useless in measuring cardiac output because of the diversion of blood flow to the bypass circuit.

Initiation of Bypass

Before the initiation of bypass, it is imperative to ascertain that all central catheters are closed to air and to confirm that heparin has been given by measuring the activated clotting time. The venous line is opened first. The arterial line is then opened while pump revolutions per minute (rpm) is increased to prevent retrograde flow. When the clamp is fully opened, pump speed is increased until a corresponding increase in blood flow cannot be seen. Pulmonary ventilation should continue, especially if the left ventricle is ejecting. "Venous chatter" and decreasing pump flows are often the effect of intravascular hypovolemia and can be reduced by the administration of fluid. Although fluid can be rapidly transfused via the circuit priming line, care must be taken not to introduce air when this is done. This route is best reserved for situations in which large volumes are needed immediately to maintain adequate pump flows. Small amounts of air may become trapped in the centrifugal pump or diffuse out through the membrane lung but care should still be exercised to prevent inadvertent introduction of additional air.

Once the patient has been stabilized on CPS, attempts to correct the underlying problems can begin. If the patient has been in intractable ventricular fibrillation, defibrillation should again be attempted. Continued CPR may be of value to decompress the heart further. A pulmonary artery catheter should be used to confirm that the heart is decompressed; however, it cannot be used to assess cardiac output. Kolobow et al. (10) have suggested that a percutaneously placed springlike device, directed into the pulmonary artery, could be used to aid in decompression of the left side of the heart.

Aortic insufficiency is a relative contraindication to closed chest CPS. The failing heart may not be able to eject into the higher CPS pressure, and massive ventricular distension can occur. Additionally, in some patients with ventricular fibrillation, left ventricular decompression will be difficult to achieve with closed chest bypass coupled with the lack of direct ventricular venting. An injured heart that remains distended will not recover. Myocardial wall stress and myocardial oxygen consumption both increase in the unvented heart (11).

Once support is initiated, cardiac catheterization or angioplasty can be performed as indicated. In elective angioplasty situations, central venous catheters should be placed before the initiation of bypass. In emergency situations, extreme care must be taken not to allow air to be aspirated into the system while the cannulas are positioned and flushed. Patients can be transported while on bypass from the nursing unit to the catheterization laboratory, from the catheterization laboratory to the operating room, or from hospital to hospital.

Intrahospital and interhospital transfers of patients supported by CPS can be quite challenging. Before patients are transported, a secure and transportable oxygen source and a reliable battery must be available. It is also mandatory to secure the bypass lines carefully to the patient to prevent dislodgement during transport. Transport demands prior planning to ensure that patient, equipment, and personnel will all fit safely into the vehicles and that the personnel are familiar with the transportation vehicles (12).

Weaning from Bypass and Decannulation

By reduction of the blood pump speed, blood flow through the system is gradually reduced while the patient's hemodynamic status is monitored. The need for inotropic or intraaortic balloon pump support is assessed by the pulmonary capillary wedge pressure, cardiac output, systemic blood pressure, and calculated systemic vascular resistance. Transesophageal echocardiography is critical in assessing myocardial recovery and should be used as CPS is withdrawn and the heart is volume loaded. When flow through the vortex pump reaches 0.5 L/min, the arterial line is clamped. When bypass is discontinued in the operating room, protamine sulfate is always given to reverse the heparin, and the cannulas are removed under direct vision with operative repair.

When the procedure is performed in the catheterization laboratory, the cannulas can be removed in the intensive care unit, after it has been confirmed that the activated clotting time is less than 240 seconds. The cannulas are then removed and a C-clamp device is left in place in the groin for several hours (13). Complications requiring operative intervention have occurred in as many as 10% of patients who have had cannulas placed percutaneously and removed without direct visualization and repair of the vessels (14). We have also found that this practice carries a high risk for complications related to the cannulation site and suggest that removal under direct vision and repair offers the best chance of avoiding these complications (15).

INDICATIONS

The indications for the use of CPS outside the operating room can be grouped into two broad categories, assisted angioplasty and resuscitation. Certainly there is some overlap between these two categories, as patients resuscitated from cardiac arrest have undergone subsequent cardiac catheterization and angioplasty while on extracorporeal support. Also, successful results for survival following resuscitation with bypass have been observed in patients whose arrest occurred in or near the catheterization laboratory, in the intensive care unit, or in the emergency room. Other indications, such as pulmonary emboli, multiple trauma, severe exposure hypothermia, and drug overdoses, have been anecdotally reported.

Assisted Angioplasty

When angioplasty was first introduced in 1977 (14), it was applied to stable patients with preserved left ventricular function and single-vessel coronary artery disease. Since that time, the application of the technique has exploded dramatically to encompass patients with multivessel disease and impaired left ventricular function. Despite advances in techniques, coronary angioplasty still carries a 2% to 8% risk for acute vessel closure (16), which may require emergency CPS and coronary bypass surgery. This emergency surgery has been associated with higher rates of morbidity and mortality (17).

Coronary angioplasty is also performed in patients who are not considered to be candidates for coronary artery bypass. These include patients with severely depressed left ventricular function (ejection fraction <20%), poor bypass conduits or poor target vessels for coronary bypass, and comorbid conditions that prohibit surgical intervention. However, many of these patients also would not be able to tolerate the transient vessel occlusion associated with balloon inflation, or the delay associated with the institution of CPS and surgical revascularization if acute vessel occlusion were to occur. Multiple techniques have been suggested to support this type of patient during coronary angioplasty. These include intraaortic balloon counterpulsation, antegrade coronary perfusion with either a "bail-out" catheter or a perfusion balloon catheter, retrograde perfusion via the coronary sinus, and CPS (18).

Kanter et al. (19) extrapolated the use of CPS as a resuscitative tool into the catheterization laboratory in 1988. They reported six patients resuscitated from cardiac arrest or cardiogenic shock with CPS. Shawl and his group (20,21) have reported a number of patients who have had CPS in both the emergency and elective situations of high-risk angioplasty and valvuloplasty (20). These include 35 patients who had percutaneous CPS instituted before angioplasty (21).

The National Registry for Supported Angioplasty began accumulating data in 1988 on patients undergoing elective supported angioplasty and has been expanded to include patients given standby supported angioplasty. The Registry previously published the initial experience of 13 centers with 105 patients who underwent supported angioplasty in 1988 (22). The entrance criteria included a left ventricular ejection fraction of less than 25%, a target vessel that supplied more than half the myocardium, severe or unstable angina, and the presence of at least one vessel likely to be dilatable. In this group, the angioplasty success rate was 95%. However, 27 patients suffered a complication related to vessel cannulation, and 14 had ischemia or infarction after angioplasty. Although no patients became bypass-dependent, there were eight (7.6%) in-hospital deaths.

The Registry recently published the data on 801 enrolled patients (23). Among these, 728 patients underwent elective supported angioplasty and 73 patients underwent standby-supported angioplasty. The average age was 65 years, and 76% of the patients were male. The overall in-hospital mortality for the Registry improved to 6.8%. There appeared to be no differences in mortality between men and women, between patients considered operable or inoperable, and between patients with left ventricular ejection fractions below 20% or above 20%. Increasing age was a risk factor [12% mortality >70 years vs. 5.9% mortality <70 years (p <0.05)], as was degree of left main stenosis [12% mortality >60% stenosis vs. 5.9% mortality <60% stenosis (p <0.05)]. Overall survival was a very good 82% at 1 year, 80% at 2 years, and 77% at 3 years. With the growth of interventional cardiology, the use of assisted angioplasty is expected to increase.

In elective situations (most supported angioplasties), the patient can be managed awake or lightly sedated. Supplemental oxygen and sedation with benzodiazepines (e.g., midazolam) and opiates (e.g., fentanyl) are commonly provided by an anesthesiologist. Some centers opt for general anesthesia and endotracheal intubation with mechanical ventilation for these procedures. Although perhaps it provides a more controlled situation, clinical experience suggests that intubation is not required.

Patients with acute myocardial infarction and cardiogenic shock are poor candidates for medical (thrombolytic) reperfusion. Percutaneous transluminal coronary angioplasty has been utilized with a 56% survival rate in selected patients (24). Certainly the optimal therapy in these patients is lacking, and as knowledge accumulates regarding reperfusion injury, perhaps more suitable strategies and results will follow. For example, Okamoto et al. (25) have proposed a system to allow for assisted angioplasty and controlled reperfusion with substrate-enriched blood cardioplegia during total vented bypass without thoracotomy. Their proposed system includes institution of bypass early to slow infarction and direct left ventricular venting with a transaortic cannula, followed by angioplasty and direct reperfusion. This constitutes an interesting concept with future promise.

Resuscitation

Since the early 1960s, closed chest massage for CPR has been used routinely (26). Despite the advancement of cardiac life support and the modification of techniques (27), the survival rate after CPR for in-hospital cardiac arrest has remained a disappointingly low 21.9% discharge rate (28). In 1813, LeGallois proposed that organ function could be supported by an external source of oxygenated blood (29). Modern heart–lung machine technology represents an outgrowth of this concept. However, when ECPS has been employed as a resuscitative measure, the results have not been uniformly successful. Among 10 patients with medical cardiac arrest supported in the emergency department at the Henry Ford Hospital in Detroit, there were no survivors (30). However, recent results from the Emergency Supported Angioplasty Registry (a subset of the National Cardiopulmonary Bypass Registry) appear encouraging.

The future development of systems specifically designed for resuscitation may allow for future improvement in these results.

When data were analyzed from 238 patients in the Emergency Supported Angioplasty Registry who were resuscitated from cardiovascular collapse with CPS, it was found that 196 (83%) survived to leave the operating room or angioplasty suite, although only 81 (34%) were discharged improved (31). The authors felt that criteria for implementation included a potentially reversible condition, an arrest time of less than 15 minutes, and presentation where CPS could be instituted rapidly (intensive care unit, catheterization laboratory, emergency department). These results and conclusions have been supported by others (32,33). CPS can also be used for acute resuscitation in patients awaiting cardiac transplantation as a bridge to a long-term ventricular assist device. (See Chapter 8).

Other Indications

Emergency CPS has been utilized as a resuscitative adjunct for several other groups of patients. In 1976, Mattox and Beall (34) expanded on the earlier work of Cooley et al. (35) and reported 39 patients who underwent emergency bypass instituted outside the operating room. Thirteen of 19 patients with massive pulmonary embolus survived operation. Twenty-six of the 39 were able to be weaned from CPS, and 15 were considered to be long-term survivors. In this report, 10 patients were placed on portable bypass because of massive thoracic trauma. Only one patient in this group survived to discharge. The use of CPS in the setting of massive trauma has been reported since this time (36,37), but because of the need for systemic heparinization, results have remained disappointing. Recently, however, Perchinsky et al. (38) reported support with a heparin-bonded circuit of six patients who had had multiple trauma, three of whom survived. The patients were supported until hypothermia, coagulopathy, surgical bleeding, and survivability could be assessed. It is possible that this technology will open CPS to a whole new group of patients.

Cardiopulmonary bypass with active rewarming has been used to salvage patients with severe hypothermia secondary to environmental exposure. Because many of these patients die as a result of ventricular dysrhythmias or circulatory collapse, CPS is an attractive method of rewarming. The introduction of rapid femoral cannulation techniques (39) should lead to a greater utilization and easier application of CPS in these patients.

Future

Attempts are under way at several institutions to decrease the size of support systems and also blood contact and activation by these systems. Many systems are based on the Archimedes water screw (impeller) principle. The Hemopump (Medtronic, Inc., Grand Rapids, MI; Fig. 32.4) is one such device that shows great promise (40,41). An impeller (24F or 14F) is introduced through an artery and across the aortic valve. As the device is actuated, a high-speed rotor aspirates blood from the left ventricle and ejects it into the ascending aorta. This device has the advantage of decompressing the heart while providing support. In addition, an oxygenator or a bypass circuit is not required, as the blood remains within the vessels.

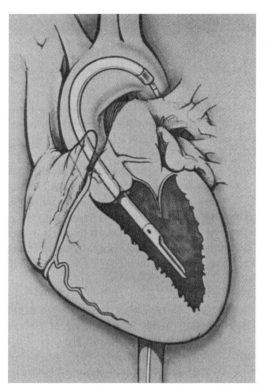

FIG. 32.4. Artist's rendition of the Hemopump cardiac assist system. (Courtesy of Medtronic, Inc., Grand Rapids, MI.)

CONCLUSIONS

The use of emergency CPS systems is expanding rapidly because of the increasing availability of compact commercial systems and femoral catheters with more acceptable flow characteristics. Familiarity with these systems has also been acquired during increasing numbers of assisted angioplasties. The indications for CPS have also expanded. Data from the National Cardiopulmonary Bypass Registry are encouraging, if not spectacular, and suggest that improved results can be achieved.

Emergency CPS systems can provide meaningful survival to a select group of patients previously considered unsalvageable. Still, certain guidelines appear necessary. Patients with unwitnessed cardiac arrest who are not profoundly hypothermic are not candidates. Patients who have correctable underlying pathology, whether anatomic or metabolic, have improved survival. A prolonged period of conventional CPR (>30 minutes) is a relative contraindication to the use of CPS. Presently, patients with multiple trauma or intracranial hemorrhage are poor candidates because of the necessity for anticoagulation. The use of heparin-bonded circuits may further improve survival and increase the usefulness of extracorporeal life support in these groups.

The increasing ease of setup and initiation of bypass, coupled with the greater availability of portable bypass systems, will tempt those not now familiar with CPS to initiate emergency bypass. This may become an acceptable reality in the future as our overall experience grows, but at present it appears that only cardiac surgeons, interventional cardiologists, perfusionists, and a few other highly trained specialists should undertake this endeavor.

KEY POINTS

- Emergency implementation of CPS with extracorporeal circulation is a concept that has roots in the earliest development of cardiopulmonary bypass.
- Femoral arterial and venous cannulation, performed either percutaneously or via surgical exposure of the vessels, is the most common method to secure vascular access.
- Circuitry for emergency CPS is most commonly prepackaged and includes an oxygenator and pump head (centrifugal) to permit rapid setup and priming.
- Broad categories of uses of emergency CPS include assisted interventions in the catheterization laboratory and resuscitation of patients with cardiac arrest, severe hypothermia, pulmonary embolism, or multiple trauma.
- Assisted angioplasty is associated with a 1- to 3-year survival of 75% to 80%, and interventional procedures may be possible in patients who would otherwise not be expected to survive them. Survival following emergency bypass for resuscitation is much less (approximately 30% to 35%).

REFERENCES

1. Cooley DA, Beall AC, Alexander JK. Acute massive pulmonary embolism: successful surgical treatment using temporary cardiopulmonary bypass. *JAMA* 1961;177:283–286.
2. Stuckey JA. The use of the heart lung machine in selected cases of acute myocardial infarction. *Surg Forum* 1958;8:342–344.
3. Joseph WL, Maloney JV Jr. Extracorporeal circulation as an adjunct to resuscitation of the heart. *JAMA* 1965;193:117–118.
4. Kouwenhoven WB, Jude JE, Knickerbocker GG. Closed chest cardiac massage. *JAMA* 1960;173:1064–1067.
5. Kennedy JH. The role of assisted circulation in cardiac resuscitation. *JAMA* 1965;197:97–100.
6. Proctor E. Closed-chest circulatory support by pump–oxygenator in experimental ventricular fibrillation at normal temperature. *Thorax* 1966;21:385–390.
7. May IA, Hardy KL, Samson PC. Emergency bypass for the community. *Am J Surg* 1971;122:256–259.
8. Phillips SJ, Zeff RH, Kongtahworn C. Percutaneous cardiopulmonary bypass: application and indication for use. *Ann Thorac Surg* 1989;47:121–123.
9. Philips SJ, Ballentine B, Slonine D, et al. Percutaneous initiation of cardiopulmonary bypass. *Ann Thorac Surg* 1983;36:223–225.
10. Kolobow T, Rossi F, Borelli M, et al. Long-term closed chest partial and total cardiopulmonary bypass by peripheral cannula-

tion for severe right and/or left ventricular failure, including ventricular fibrillation. *ASAIO Trans* 1988;34:485–489.

11. Scholz K, Schroder T, Hering J, et al. Need for active left-ventricular decompression during percutaneous cardiopulmonary support in cardiac arrest. *Cardiology* 1994;84:222–230.

12. Faulkner S, Chipman, C, Taylor B, et al. Performance of mobile extracorporeal life support. *Proc Am Acad Cardiovasc Perfus* 1993; 14:80–86.

13. Shawl FA, Domanski MJ, Wish MH, et al. Percutaneous cardiopulmonary bypass support in the catheterization laboratory: technique and complications. *Am Heart J* 1990;120:195–203.

14. Gruentzig A. Transluminal dilatation of coronary artery stenosis. *Lancet* 1978;1:263–265.

15. Davis PK, Iams WB, Myers JL. Clinical experience with a new portable rapid access cardiopulmonary support (CPS) system. Unpublished results, presented at the circulatory support topical meeting of the Society of Thoracic Surgeons, St. Louis, MO, 1988.

16. Landau C, Lange RA, Hillis LD. Medical progress: percutaneous transluminal coronary angioplasty. *N Engl J Med* 1994;330: 981–993.

17. Roubin GS, Talley JD, Anderson HV, et al. Morbidity and mortality associated with emergency bypass graft surgery following elective coronary angioplasty. *J Am Coll Cardiol* 1987;9: 124A(abst).

18. Lincoff AM, Popura JJ, Ellis SG, et al. Percutaneous support devices for high-risk or complicated coronary angioplasty. *J Am Coll Cardiol* 1991;17:770–780.

19. Kanter KR, Pennington DG, Vandormael M. Emergency resuscitation with extracorporeal membrane oxygenation for failed angioplasty. *J Am Coll Cardiol* 1988;11:149A(abst).

20. Shawl FA. Percutaneous cardiopulmonary support in high-risk angioplasty. *Cardiol Clin* 1989;7:865–875.

21. Shawl FA, Domanski MS, Punja S, et al. Percutaneous cardiopulmonary bypass to support high-risk elective coronary angioplasty. *J Am Coll Cardiol* 1989;13:160A(abst).

22. Vogel RA, Shawl F, Tommaso C, et al. Initial report of the National Registry of Elective Cardiopulmonary Bypass-Supported Coronary Angioplasty. *J Am Coll Cardiol* 1990;15:23–29.

23. Tommaso C, Vogel R. National Registry for Supported Angioplasty: results and follow-up of three years of supported and standby supported angioplasty in high-risk patients. *Cardiology* 1994;84:238–244.

24. Hibbard MD, Holmes DR, Gersh BJ, et al. Coronary angioplasty for acute myocardial infarction complicated by cardiogenic shock. *Circulation* 1990;82:III-511(abst).

25. Okamoto F, Allen BS, Buckberg GD, et al. Studies of controlled reperfusion after ischemia VII. Regional blood cardioplegic reperfusion during total vented bypass without thoracotomy: a new concept. *J Thorac Cardiovasc Surg* 1986;92:553–563.

26. Kouwenhoven WB, Jude JR, Knickerbocker GG. Closed chest cardiac massage. *JAMA* 1960;173:1064–1067.

27. American Heart Association. Standards and guidelines for cardiopulmonary resuscitation and emergency cardiac care. *JAMA* 1980;244:462–468.

28. Cooper S, Cade J. Predicting survival, in-hospital cardiac arrests: resuscitation survival variables and training effectiveness. *Resuscitation* 1997;35:17–22.

29. Nelson RM. Era of extracorporeal respiration. *Surgery* 1975;78: 685–693.

30. Martin GB, Rivers EP, Paradis NA, et al. Emergency department cardiopulmonary bypass in the treatment of human cardiac arrest. *Chest* 1998;113:743–751.

31. Overlie P, Walter P, Hurd H II, et al. Emergency cardiopulmonary support with circulatory support devices. *Cardiology* 1994; 84:231–237.

32. Mooney MR, Arom KV, Joyce LD, et al. Emergency cardiopulmonary bypass support in patients with cardiac arrest. *J Thorac Cardiovasc Surg* 1991;101:450–454.

33. Kolla S, Lee WA, Hirschl RB, et al. Extracorporeal life support for cardiovascular support in adults. *ASAIO J* 1996;42: M809–M819.

34. Mattox KL, Beall AC Jr. Resuscitation of the moribund patient using portable cardiopulmonary bypass. *Ann Thorac Surg* 1976; 22:436–442.

35. Cooley DA, Beall AC. A technique of pulmonary embolectomy using temporary cardiopulmonary bypass: experimental and clinical considerations. *J Cardiovasc Surg* 1961;2:469–476.

36. Reichman RT, Joyo CI, Dembitsky WP. Improved patient survival after cardiac arrest using a cardiopulmonary support system. *Ann Thorac Surg* 1990;49:101–105.

37. Phillips SJ. Percutaneous cardiopulmonary bypass and innovations in clinical counterpulsation. *Crit Care Clin* 1986;2: 297–318.

38. Perchinsky MJ, Long WB, Hill JG, et al. Extracorporeal cardiopulmonary life support with heparin-bonded circuitry in the resuscitation of massively injured trauma patients. *Am J Surg* 1995; 169:488–491.

39. Lamb GW, Banaszak D, Kupferschmid J. Percutaneous cardiopulmonary bypass for the treatment of hypothermic circulatory collapse. *Ann Thorac Surg* 1989;47:608–611.

40. Wampler RK, Frazier OH, Lansing AM, et al. Treatment of cardiogenic shock with the Hemopump left ventricular assist device. *Ann Thorac Surg* 1991;52:506–513.

41. Casimir-Ahn H, Lonn U, Peterzen B. Clinical use of the hemopump cardiac assist system for circulatory support. *Ann Thorac Surg* 1995;59:S39–S45.

NONCARDIOVASCULAR APPLICATIONS OF CARDIOPULMONARY BYPASS

MICHAEL J. MURRAY
DAVID J. COOK

The development of cardiopulmonary bypass (CPB) for repair of cardiac anomalies during the 1950s stimulated an appraisal of its potential in assisting with the management of other disease processes. Complications associated with this technique tempered the initial enthusiasm for bypass for noncardiac applications. With time, however, a more reasoned approach to the use of CPB for noncardiovascular applications has developed, and many of the early problems and complications have been overcome.

The development of CPB was secondary to many advances, not only in surgery but also in physiology, anesthesiology, cardiology, and bioengineering (1). For example, neurosurgeons and neuroanesthesiologists with expertise in brain protection and monitoring made significant contributions to the management of all patients undergoing bypass.

The current noncardiovascular applications of CPB involve four main areas. First, bypass is used to induce profound hypothermia so that circulatory arrest can be instituted; this provides a bloodless surgical field for the repair of vascular abnormalities such as intracranial aneurysms and the resection of tumors and thromboses of the vena cava and right atrium. Before the availability of CPB, surgeons did use hypothermia, with a safe limit of 28° to 30°C (2), in conjunction with occlusion of cardiac inflow to manage some of these cases. The application of CPB made it possible to achieve cerebral electrical silence via profound hypothermia for circulatory arrest (3).

Second, although CPB is used primarily to facilitate cardiac surgery, the lungs are also bypassed in this technique. In fact, Gibbon developed his pump oxygenator to operate on patients with pulmonary embolism (4). Patients with significant pulmonary disease who require surgery that must be performed within a bloodless pulmonary field constitute the second largest group benefiting from the noncardiovascular application of CPB.

A third group of patients undergoing CPB for noncardiac surgery includes those in whom operations on the inferior vena cava necessitate a bypass procedure to return blood to the heart. Occasionally, venoarterial bypass can be utilized in these patients, but more frequently, venovenous (VV) bypass is instituted. This technique makes use of advances and knowledge gained during the development of CPB.

Finally, patients who have a variety of unusual disease processes may also benefit from the use of bypass techniques to manage their illness.

The experience and techniques gained in the application of CPB to the "traditional" cardiovascular patient are used in managing all these situations.

Anesthetic Considerations

The anesthetic considerations in the noncardiovascular applications of CPB are similar to those in cardiac surgery. It is important to note, though, that bypass can be expected to cause adverse effects in the same organ systems whether it is used for cardiac surgery or noncardiac applications. Thus, depending on the specific application, brain, lung, kidney, and the hemostatic system remain at risk. This level of risk may be further increased when these organ systems are the focus of the operation (5). Therefore, special care must be taken to provide relevant supplemental organ protection when indicated. These considerations are discussed in greater detail below.

Surgical Considerations

Although the preferred technique for the use of CPB in cardiac surgery is a midline sternotomy with cannulation of the right atrium and ascending aorta (6), certain circumstances require the institution of bypass with lower extremity access (7)—typically, femorofemoral bypass (8–10). Access via the upper extremities is not possible because the blood vessels are too small to accommodate sufficiently large cannulas (11). Although the access site depends primarily

M. J. Murray and D. J. Cook: Department of Anesthesiology, Mayo Medical Center, Rochester, Minnesota 55905.

on the surgery being planned, femorofemoral bypass is used more often in CPB for noncardiovascular than for cardiac applications.

The degree of hemodilution (12,13), degree of hypothermia (14–18), pump flows (19), and type of oxygenator (20) are similar to those previously described for the more common uses of CPB, although femorofemoral bypass has the potential to limit flows because of reduced venous return and to decrease cooling efficiency because of its remoteness from the vessels of the head (21).

Complications

Patients undergoing CPB for noncardiovascular applications experience similar complications to those of cardiac surgical patients. Neurologic (22–25), pulmonary (26,27), renal (28,29), gastrointestinal (30), cardiac (31), bleeding (32,33), immunologic (34,35), and infectious (36) complications are probably as prevalent in the noncardiac population as in the "traditional" patient population. Also, the use of femoral arterial cannulation adds the potential for hypoperfusion, dissection of the great arteries, and vascular or neurologic injury to the lower extremity (37). Because patients undergoing noncardiovascular applications of CPB may not have significant cardiac disease, theoretically they should have a lower cardiac risk. Although the incidence of cardiac complications should be lower, if hypothermia and circulatory arrest are used or if the pump time is long, the risk for dysrhythmias and left ventricular dysfunction increases (38). Personnel in the operating room involved in the surgical monitoring and anesthetic management must be well versed and experienced in the implementation and use of CPB (39). Although obvious, this can not be overemphasized because these procedures may take place in "noncardiac" areas where shifting of personnel and material resources require considerable advance planning.

CARDIOPULMONARY BYPASS WITH PROFOUND HYPOTHERMIA AND CIRCULATORY ARREST

Hypothermia

Historical Perspective

In 1958, Sealy and colleagues (40) described open heart surgery in which hypothermia was used as an adjunct to CPB. By the following year, they had used the technique to operate on 95 patients, with an overall survival rate of 83% (41). Also in 1959, Drew and Anderson (18) reported three cases in which they used CPB with profound hypothermia and circulatory arrest. Unique to their technique was the use of the patients' own lungs to provide oxygenation during surgery. Although one child died during the perioperative period of heart block following correction of an atrioventricular canal defect, complications from the hypothermia *per se* were minimal.

During that same year (1959), Woodhall, working with Sealy's group, used hypothermia to repair an intracranial vascular aneurysm (42). Several other techniques had been used to repair these intracranial vascular malformations, but problems occurred with all of them. Before 1959, surface cooling to 28° to 30°C was used (to avoid inducing ventricular fibrillation), but this limited the maximum vascular occlusion time to 8 to 10 minutes (43). Isolated cerebral perfusion techniques with selective brain cooling have also been described (44), but it is difficult to provide uniform cerebral cooling by cannulating just the carotid arteries. Extracorporeal perfusion with profound hypothermia and circulatory arrest became the preferred technique for repairing a number of neurovascular abnormalities.

Initially, there was a great deal of enthusiasm for the induction of hypothermia and circulatory arrest, not only in neurosurgical procedures but also in the repair of intracardiac lesions. As expertise with membrane oxygenation improved, the majority of cardiac cases were repaired with the use of CPB, an oxygenator, and moderate hypothermia to approximately 25° to 30°C. This temperature provided a 50% reduction in metabolic rate and therefore extended the safe ischemic time not only for the brain and heart but for all organ systems. There continue to be surgical cases, however, that can be managed most effectively with profound hypothermia and circulatory arrest.

Management of Hypothermia

When profound hypothermia is used, one cools the patient to 15° to 17°C before circulatory arrest is established. Monitoring core temperature and neurologic function (45) intraoperatively is very important. In patients undergoing a craniotomy, in which electroencephalographic (EEG) documentation of electrical brain silence is technically difficult, it is of primary importance to document core temperature. Because thoracotomy is not always surgically indicated, bypass can be established with use of the femoral artery and vein for access (46,47). Initially, the Q_{10} for humans was thought to be approximately 2 (the metabolic rate doubling for every increase in temperature of 10°C). Michenfelder and Milde (48,49) demonstrated in dogs that the slope of the Q_{10} curve is nonlinear, becoming significantly steeper below 27°C. In that study, the cerebral metabolic rate was found to be approximately 3.9, 1.8, and 0.5 mL/100 g per minute at 37°, 27°, and 18°C, respectively. Virtually identical numbers during CPB have been measured more recently (50). Michenfelder attributed the decrease in the Q_{10} between 37°C and 27°C to a reduction in cerebral O_2 demand without the inhibition of integrated neuronal function. Between 27°C and 18°C, the larger decrease in the cerebral metabolic rate (increase in the Q_{10}) is attributed to the

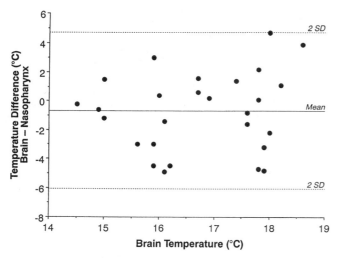

FIG. 33.1. Individual temperature differences between the brain and nasopharynx as a function of brain temperature at circulatory arrest. (From Stone JG, Young WL, Smith CR, et al. Do standard monitoring sites reflect true brain temperature when profound hypothermia is rapidly induced and reversed? *Anesthesiology* 1995;82:344–351, with permission.)

inhibition of integrated neuronal function as reflected in the development of an isoelectric EEG.

The lower the temperature, the lower the cerebral metabolic rate (49). Because electrocerebral silence occurs frequently at 20°C, some authors have cooled patients to 20°C and then instituted circulatory arrest, with satisfactory results (51). However, circulatory arrest is most often instituted, with a core temperature of 17°C or less. We argue that this is prudent because under some bypass conditions the brain may cool more slowly than the body core (52,53) (Fig. 33.1). Additionally, the brain may not cool homogeneously, and warmer areas are presumably at greater risk for ischemic injury (44). The congenital heart literature regarding circulatory arrest has made a strong argument for slow cooling to reduce cerebral temperature gradients before circulatory arrest (54,55). Because of concerns about the long-term sequelae of circulatory arrest (56), profound hypothermia with low flow and intermittent circulatory arrest is being increasingly advocated (57).

The nasopharyngeal temperature during the circulatory arrest period may show modest increases in temperature with time. In the absence of circulation, this probably reflects some minor equilibration of tissue temperatures, but an increase secondary to air temperature may be more significant. External cranial cooling is suggested as an important means for the *maintenance* of hypothermia within the central nervous system during circulatory arrest (58). Although this may offer advantages, surface cooling of the brain alone does not provide adequate cerebral protection during circulatory arrest (59). Therefore, a method that directly cools the blood and decreases the core temperature, in conjunc-

tion with surface cooling of the brain, may provide the best means of establishing and maintaining a low brain temperature and extending the safe circulatory arrest time (60). The majority of reports have indicated that a nasopharyngeal temperature of between 15° and 18°C should be achieved before circulatory arrest is induced, although temperatures of less than 10°C are associated with a higher incidence of complications (61,62).

The longer the circulatory arrest, the greater the incidence of neurologic complications, even with adequate levels of hypothermia (63). Neurologic dysfunction correlates better with the degree of hypoxia that occurs during extended circulatory arrest than it does with the lack of perfusion *per se* (64). The safe ischemic time can be prolonged, therefore, by preliminary hyperbaric oxygenation, but this is not usually practical (65). The safe time limit for circulatory arrest, however, has not been fully delineated (66). Early reports demonstrated a reluctance to use circulatory arrest for more than 30 minutes (67). The majority of more recent reports suggest that a core temperature of 15°C will provide up to 60 minutes of safe ischemic time during circulatory arrest (Table 33.1) (68–80).

Management of Circulatory Arrest

Although hypothermia itself should provide maximum cerebral protection (81), drugs such as a long-acting muscle relaxant (pancuronium) or antibiotics should be considered before circulatory arrest because these agents cannot be administered once the bypass machine is turned off. Experimental evidence suggests that tissue acidosis after circulatory arrest is decreased if hyperventilation and mild hypocapnia are induced before circulatory arrest (82). However, important work from the Boston Children's Hospital indicates that cerebral outcome is improved with a pH-stat CO_2 management strategy (54|83). The elevation of P_aCO_2 increases cerebral blood flow and may facilitate more uniform brain cooling; additionally, the relative acidosis may help shift the oxyhemoglobin dissociation curve rightward, compensating for some of the effect of hypothermia. After the patient is on bypass, during the induction and documentation of hypothermia, a barbiturate should be administered for its neuroprotective effects only if evidence of cerebral electrical activity is present on the EEG (84,85). Barbiturates may be indicated for those patients who do not have EEG monitoring or in whom a central nervous system temperature of 15°C cannot be documented, but this is controversial (86). Rapid cooling and significant temperature gradients or reduced flows during cooling are relative indications for the use of barbiturates. Corticosteroids and mannitol may also be given empirically in an attempt to decrease neurologic complications, but no studies of patients undergoing circulatory arrest have demonstrated a definitive improvement in outcome with these drugs.

TABLE 33.1. USE OF CARDIOPULMONARY BYPASS WITH PROFOUND HYPOTHERMIA AND CIRCULATORY ARREST FOR NEUROSURGICAL PROCEDURES

Author[a]	No. of Patients	Year	Diagnosis	Anesthesia[b]	Access[c]	Hypothermia[d]	Duration of Circulatory Arrest	Complication
Woodhall (42)	1	1959	Subcortical tumor cyst	I		E 11	10 min	
Uihlein (68)*	2	1960	Intracranial aneurysms	I	Open	E 14	25–44 min	Bleeding
Patterson (46)	7	1962	Intracranial aneurysms	I	Closed	E ~4–7 B ~14–17	9–42.5 min	Bleeding
Drake (69)	10	1964	Intracranial aneurysms		8 Open 2-Closed Closed	E 9.6–16.8 B 5–18	5–18 min	Spasm (5/10)
Patterson (70)	8	1965	Intracranial aneurysms		Closed	E 4–14	9–29 min	
Neville (71)	4	1966	Intracranial aneurysms (3), vascular malignancy (1)		Closed	B <15	<40 min	
Uihlein (72)*	67	1966	Intracranial aneurysms		17 Open 49 Closed	E <15		
Sundt (73)	1	1972	Basilar artery aneurysm		Closed	Surface cooling E 13	30 min	
McMurty (74)	12	1974	Basilar artery aneurysms	I	Open	Surface, cooling E 28–29	1–28 min	
Patterson (75)	1	1975	Hemangioblastoma brainstem		Open	E 10	19 min	
Silverberg (76)	1	1980	Giant cerebral aneurysm		Closed	E 20	28 min	
Baumgartner (77)	14	1983	Middle cerebral artery aneurysm (8), internal carotid artery aneurysm (3), basilar artery aneurysm (2), hemangioblastoma (2)	N	Closed	E 16–20	5–51 min	
Gonski (78)	40	1986	Intracranial aneurysms		Open	E <17.5	5–39 min	
Richards (79)	11	1987	Intracranial aneurysms	I				
Williams (80)	10	1991	Intracranial aneurysms (4), glomus tumors (3), arteriovenous malformations (2), hemangioblastoma (1)	N + I	Closed	E 10–12	1–60 min	Edema, swelling

[a] Name of first author only given, to conserve space. * Same institution.
[b] I, inhalational; N, narcotic.
[c] Access refers to whether cannulation was performed through an open chest vs. the groin (closed).
[d] B, brain; E, esophageal; expressed in degrees Centigrade.

Use in Neurosurgery

In the late 1950s, multiple, simultaneous developments took place in the field of CPB. The studies of hypothermia in dogs by Bigelow et al. (87) stimulated other investigators, who used the animal work to serve as a basis for clinical experimentation. In 1960, Woodhall and colleagues (42) at Duke University reported the first use of bypass and profound hypothermia with quinidine administered to protect the myocardium. With a 10-minute period of circulatory arrest, they drained a subcortical tumorlike cyst involving the left parietal lobe. Their case stimulated Uihlein and colleagues (68) at the Mayo Clinic to use extracorporeal circulation with profound hypothermia and circulatory arrest to repair intracranial aneurysms in two patients. Although the basic principles were the same, the reports highlight the anesthetic and surgical differences that can be found between physicians and institutions utilizing these techniques.

Other investigators, notably Patterson and Ray (46), expanded the technique and instituted closed chest extracorporeal circulation. Venous cannulas were advanced into the venae cavae via internal jugular and femoral veins, and an arterial cannula was placed in the femoral artery. This technique solved some of the technical difficulties in performing a simultaneous thoracotomy and craniotomy and was quickly adopted by other groups. The decision to use thoracic or femoral cannulation sites should be made following consultation between the members of the neurosurgical and cardiac teams.

In 5 years, between 1961 and 1966, Uihlein and colleagues (72), using extrathoracic cannulation, had operated on a total of 66 patients with intracranial aneurysms. The mortality rate, although relatively high (14.5%), was thought acceptable given the alternative. Not everyone, however, was enamored of this technique to repair intracranial aneurysms. Using the closed chest technique, Drake and colleagues (69) in London, Ontario, had difficulties in 10 aneurysm patients because of the poor venous return with extrathoracic cannulation. More importantly, from their perspective, cerebral arterial spasm continued to be a problem with ruptured cerebral aneurysms, and 5 of their 10 patients died within 2 to 3 months of the operative procedure. They abandoned this technique and developed other surgical therapies that dramatically changed the way neurosurgeons approached intracranial aneurysms. These techniques, simultaneously developed by Sundt and Nofzinger (88) of the Department of Neurosurgery at the Mayo Clinic, led this group also to abandon the use of profound hypothermia and circulatory arrest for the management of intracranial pathology.

At the same time, Michenfelder (89) was performing pioneering work in the field of neuroanesthesia that would affect the management of these patients. The refinements of the surgical approach to aneurysms, including the operating microscope, withdrawal of cerebrospinal fluid, controlled hypotension, and sophisticated neuroanesthesia, made surgery for most intracranial pathology much safer without the use of extracorporeal circulation. By the beginning of 1965, the majority of neurosurgical centers in the United States and Canada had abandoned the intraoperative use of profound hypothermia and circulatory arrest.

In 1972, however, Sundt et al. (73) reported a case in which an otherwise inoperable giant basilar artery aneurysm was managed successfully with CPB, profound hypothermia, and circulatory arrest. It was the first case in which this technique was used at the Mayo Clinic since 1964. The repair went well, and during the intervening 25 years, several reports have delineated the limited but important role of bypass, hypothermia, and circulatory arrest in managing neurosurgical pathology. In our own practice, we have used profound hypothermia and circulatory arrest 13 times within the past 10 years to manage patients with intracranial aneurysms (Robert Grady, M.D., Mayo Clinic, Rochester, MN, personal communication).

Indications

Since 1972, the majority of cases in which circulatory arrest was employed have involved the surgical treatment of giant basilar and cerebral aneurysms and hemangioblastomas, frequently of the brainstem. In current practice, hypothermia and circulatory arrest allow the only chance for resection in this subgroup of patients. Baumgartner et al. (77) used a modified hypothermic approach in managing all forms of intracranial aneurysms, but this technique has not been utilized elsewhere.

Anesthetic Management

The successful management of these difficult patients mandates frequent, open communication between the neurovascular and cardiovascular surgical and anesthesia teams. Unlike most patients presenting for cardiac surgery, many of these patients are young and without coronary artery disease. The majority, however, do have vascular pathology, frequently a ruptured cerebral aneurysm. Therefore, careful management of the hemodynamics to avoid hypotension and hypertension is as important as it is in the cardiac patient undergoing CPB. Many of these patients, therefore, should receive vasoactive drugs, most frequently β-blockers, to attenuate hemodynamic instability.

Positioning these patients can also be a major problem. Although the literature shows that closed chest techniques were preferred in the past, several cardiac surgeons currently cannulate the great vessels through a midline sternotomy. There are some circumstances in which the cranial pathology can be approached only posteriorly, so that the patient must be in a prone position. Under these circumstances, femoral cannulation is difficult, and a posterolateral thoracotomy, allowing access to the atria for venous cannulation, may be necessary.

Monitoring for these patients may include a pulmonary artery catheter and an intrathecal catheter. A pulmonary artery catheter is placed because myocardial dysfunction can be a problem even in the absence of coronary artery disease when circulatory arrest is prolonged. Furthermore, during circulatory arrest, if the left ventricle or pulmonary vasculature is not vented, left ventricular distension or pulmonary edema can be a serious complication. Left ventricular distension is a primary concern in these operations because an aortic cross-clamp is not placed and cardioplegia is not administered. Therefore, ventricular fibrillation can occur in a "full" heart with serious consequences, and a preoperative echocardiographic examination is essential in these patients to rule out aortic valvular insufficiency. The placement of a pulmonary artery catheter can be an important adjunct in managing these patients as an indicator of left ventricular distension during CPB and hemodynamic management in the post-bypass period.

Occasionally, drainage of cerebrospinal fluid helps the surgeon better visualize the vascular pathology. This benefit must be weighed against the risk for an epidural hematoma in a heparinized, hypothermic patient. Drainage is often achieved with a malleable needle, but in current practice, catheters designed for epidural use can be placed in the intrathecal space by the use of an 18- or 17-gauge Tuohy needle. The catheter is then taped to the patient's back, which allows for the monitoring of cerebrospinal fluid pressure and withdrawal of fluid. The larger the catheter, the better the dynamic response for pressure monitoring and the easier it is to withdraw cerebrospinal fluid. Some catheters have a spiral wire incorporated into the wall that prevents kinking and facilitates pressure monitoring and fluid withdrawal.

The maintenance of stable hemodynamics in the immediate preoperative period is a most important component of the anesthetic protocol. Therefore, a neuroanesthetic technique that employs β-blockers and control of hypotension with nitroprusside is often used. When intracranial hypertension is a problem, controlled hyperventilation and the use of an anesthetic agent such as isoflurane are preferred. As pointed out, the majority of these patients do not have coronary artery disease, and an inhalation anesthetic, as was frequently described in early case reports, can be used. More recent case reports have described the use of a narcotic technique. The choice of an inhalation versus a narcotic technique, or a combination of the two, is at the discretion of the anesthesiologist(s) providing care to the patient.

Neurologic dysfunction is a major postoperative concern, but because these patients are anesthetized, hypothermic, and undergoing craniotomy, there is no effective way to monitor neurologic function intraoperatively. Careful attention to detail in managing the hemodynamic response to the induction of anesthesia and surgery, in addition to controlling P_aCO_2 and core temperature, is the most important adjunct in improving outcome in these patients. To ensure the adequacy of cerebral cooling, a No. 25 needle temperature probe directly applied to the cortex can also be used by the neurosurgical team. Following the surgical procedure, early neurologic assessment of function in the operating room is also important and will sometimes dictate the choice of anesthetic agents. The use of propofol in these cases has not been fully explored, but based on its short half-life, it might be a reasonable agent to achieve these goals as long as hypotension is avoided by titrating the propofol to effect.

Complications

The complications experienced by these patients may be similar to those experienced by patients undergoing CPB for cardiac procedures. Although this neurosurgical population may be at reduced atheroembolic risk relative to the cardiac surgical population, it may be at greater overall risk for bleeding and neurologic injury. In addition to heparinization for CPB, the profound hypothermia required for these procedures increases the risk for bleeding (90). Many case reports underscore the major morbidity that these patients experience secondary to postoperative bleeding (Table 33.1). The anesthesiologist must establish baseline coagulation function on the patient's arrival in the operating room and monitor to identify any coagulation defects as the patient comes off CPB. These defects include transfusion-related thrombocytopenia and decreased coagulation factors that may necessitate the use of transfused platelets, fresh-frozen plasma, or cryoprecipitate. The use of thrombin glue

by the neurosurgical team, although it is associated with identified risks, might be of benefit in managing these patients. Increasingly, an antifibrinolytic agent (e.g., aprotinin or tranexamic acid) is used in this patient population based on experience with CPB and circulatory arrest for other surgical procedures (91).

The incidence of neurocognitive dysfunction following bypass for cardiac surgery can run as high as 70% depending on the sensitivity of the neuropsychiatric test used (23). Neurosurgical patients undergoing CPB may be at risk for bypass-related neurologic injury in addition to brain injury specifically related to the neurosurgery. A temperature probe may be necessary to document that the temperature of the brain is indeed below 15°C, the temperature most frequently cited as allowing maximal cerebral protection.

Finally, cerebral edema may pose major neurologic problems in patients undergoing neurosurgery with CPB. Brain swelling is common during and following intracranial surgery; CPB is also independently associated with cerebral edema (92,93). It is the practice at the Mayo Clinic to use relatively high doses of mannitol in these cases; some cerebral edema is anticipated in all patients. Finally, if an intrathoracic approach is used for venous cannulation, special attention must be paid to the position of the right atrial cannula, as the right atrial cannula can partially obstruct the superior vena cava. This has marked effects in increasing intracranial pressure and decreasing cerebral perfusion pressure.

Use in Urologic Surgery

The use of CPB techniques to facilitate the resection of renal malignancies came about serendipitously. Whereas the benefits of bypass with deep hypothermia and circulatory arrest were quickly appreciated and utilized for the resection of intracranial aneurysms, it was not until 1970, after more than 10 years of CPB use in neurosurgical procedures, that reports began to appear describing the technique of bypass with hypothermia and circulatory arrest for removal of tumor invading the inferior vena cava with right atrial extension. It had been recognized for some time that patients with renal cell carcinomas extending into the inferior vena cava had a poor prognosis (94), but if the tumor could be resected in its entirety, then the prognosis was improved (95). The critical aspect of surgery, therefore, was removal of the tumor with a technique that did not significantly increase morbidity. In 1970, Marshall and colleagues (96) reported several cases of surgical excision of hypernephromas that extended into the inferior vena cava, including one in which they attempted to isolate the inferior vena cava alone, and another in which they attempted to isolate both the inferior vena cava and the kidney. The latter patient sustained a cardiac arrest following caval occlusion. Pulmonary embolism was diagnosed, the patient underwent emergency thoracotomy with cardiac massage, and a pulmonary arteriotomy was made to remove a pulmonary thromboembolus. Based on this experience, in a subsequent case the authors placed two femoral vein cannulas below the obstructing tumor and shunted this blood to the superior vena cava via a cannula in the internal jugular vein. No pump was required in this case because the inferior caval pressure was sufficiently elevated to allow adequate flow from the femoral vein to the superior vena cava. During the procedure, however, the systemic arterial pressure began to fall, so extracorporeal circulation was begun. This was the first time that VV bypass was used in the resection of kidney tumors extending into the right atrium.

The second report in which bypass was utilized in "urologic" surgery was in a patient with a right atrial tumor. The preoperative diagnosis was myxoma; the patient was placed on full CPB and the tumor was resected from the atrium. The pathologic report indicated that the resected mass was in fact a "hypernephroma" (97).

Indications

The main indication for CPB in urologic surgery is for resection of renal tumors, primarily renal cell carcinomas or hypernephromas that extend into the inferior vena cava superiorly past the diaphragm. In children, Wilms' tumors can present in this same way (98). Tumors not extending above the diaphragm or into the right atrium can frequently be resected by surgical techniques without the necessity of a bypass procedure. Depending on the extension of the tumor, VV bypass can occasionally be used to shunt blood from the inferior to the superior vena cava. Many, however, have found that collateral circulation is sufficient, so that this is not usually necessary. The primary use for CPB in the resection of caval tumors is to allow for profound hypothermia, circulatory arrest, and complete exsanguination during the resection of tumors extending into the right atrium. Because complete removal of the tumor is critical to survival, several authors have noted that a quiet, motionless, bloodless right atrium allows the best chance for complete resection (99–101). In addition, given the high incidence of pulmonary artery embolization associated with this surgical procedure, bypass is occasionally instituted in those patients who sustain an intraoperative pulmonary embolus (96,102,103), for whom pulmonary embolectomy offers the only chance for survival.

Management

The successful management of these patients requires full cooperation between the cardiac and urologic teams. The anesthetic management of these cases is infrequently described, but based on the available literature describing anesthetic management, it is obvious that an opioid anesthetic technique is most common (104). This should not necessarily be the case, however. Intravenous induction with thiopental and succinylcholine has also been used, followed by maintenance of anesthesia with inhalation agents, enflurane, and nitrous oxide (103). Standard monitoring of the electrocardiogram, pulse oximeter, esophageal temperature, and systemic arterial pressures was utilized. A pulmonary artery catheter is relatively contraindicated in these patients, depending on the extent and location of the tumor thrombus. Many patients with documented extension of the tumor into the right atrium will have cardiac symptoms and signs present before the surgical procedures (101,105). Several case reports have documented that during positioning of the patient, the tumor can become dislodged or displaced further into the right atrium, causing a precipitous drop in blood pressure. The left lateral decubitus position seems to be the position in which this is most likely to occur (100,103). For most of these cases, transesophageal echocardiographic visualization of the right atrium and tricuspid valve can assist in both surgical assessment and diagnosis in the event of sudden hemodynamic changes. Transesophageal echocardiography should probably be considered as standard monitoring in this patient population.

After the induction of anesthesia, either a thoracoabdominal or a midline abdominal incision extended into a sternotomy is made. The cardiac and urologic surgical teams can begin their procedure simultaneously, but the patient is not heparinized for bypass (to avoid excessive bleeding) until the urologist has the kidney and inferior vena cava dissected free. Once the urologist is ready, the patient is placed on CPB and, when necessary, cooled to 15°C. Some physicians report packing the patient's head in ice to keep the brain at a sufficiently low temperature (106–108), perhaps a worthwhile technique if inefficient cooling is anticipated during femoral arterial cannulation. However, in some centers, circulatory arrest is instituted with only moderate degrees of hypothermia (approximately 25°C) (103). From the literature, it is apparent that the time necessary to resect the caval and right atrial tumor ranges from 10 to 45 minutes (Table 33.2) (109–116). Therefore, profound hypothermia should be instituted when circulatory arrest is anticipated.

During the institution of bypass, a double filter or a filter with a smaller pore size may be placed in the bypass arterial line to prevent the embolization of tumor (117). Because of the concern about malignant emboli, these patients have not been considered candidates for the use of an intraoperative cell saver (103), although the latter recommendation is not based on any reported adverse sequelae. There does not appear to be a clear contraindication to the use autotransfusion because the tumor is already in the bloodstream; furthermore, if cardiotomy suckers are used on bypass, autotransfusion, in effect, is already being used.

Complications

The problems encountered in using this technique are similar to those described for the repair of intracranial aneu-

TABLE 33.2. USE OF CARDIOPULMONARY BYPASS FOR PATIENTS WITH RENAL TUMOR (NON-CASE REPORTS)

Author[a]	No. of Patients	Year	Type	Anesthesia[b]	Access[c]	Technique[d]	Complications[e]	Arrest Time
Marshall (96)	4	1970	—	ND	V-FV, SVC	Standard CPB	Cardiac arrest in 1 patient, no circulatory arrest in 2 patients	
Theman (99)	2	1978	Wilms' adrenal carcinoma	ND	V-SVC A-aorta	CPB	Systolic hypertension	43 min 15 min
Klein (109)	4	1984	Renal cell	ND	V-SVC A-aorta, FA	CPB 25°C	1 patient with filter extrusion, hemorrhage	ND
Montie (110)	13	1988	Renal cell	ND	V-SVC A-aorta	CPB 18–20°C	Bleeding DVT	12–47 min
Hedderich (111)	4	1987	Renal cell	ND	V-SVC, FV A-aorta	1 with CPB with arrest, 3 without CPB		
Marshall (112)	9	1988	Renal cell	ND				
Welch (104)*	20	1989	95% with renal cell	Narcotic technique Thiopental	V-SVC A-aorta	CPB 15.8°C	Bleeding, pulmonary dysfunction	12–44 min
Novick (113)*	43	1990	39 with renal cell					10–44 min
Shahian (114)	10	1990	Renal cell	ND	V-SVC A-aorta	7 with CPB 16–18°C with EEG monitoring	Jaundice, low cardiac output,	10–38 min
Swierzewski (115)	100	1994	Renal cell	ND	V-SVC, FV A-aorta	Shahian technique	54% 5-year survival	NA
Matthews (116)	7	1995	Renal cell	ND	V-R atrium A-aorta	12–15°C	No complications	NA

[a] Name of first author only given, to conserve space. * Same institution.
[b] ND, not described.
[c] V, venous cannula; FV, femoral vein; SVC, superior vena cava; A, arterial cannula; FA, femoral artery.
[d] CPB, cardiopulmonary bypass; EEG, electroencephalogram.
[e] DVT, deep venous thrombosis.

rysms. Neurologic dysfunction is difficult to quantify in this patient population because the majority of reports are of single cases. In only two series were more than 10 patients studied (110,113). Bleeding, especially from retroperitoneal beds, was the major perioperative complication in both of these series. Once the inferior vena cava is resected, postoperative ascites and edema of the lower extremity can develop until adequate collateral flow is established. This is not a problem in most cases, however, because sufficient collateral flow is present preoperatively. In the large series from the Cleveland Clinic, femoral venous cannulation was found to be unnecessary because collateralization around the tumor allowed sufficient venous drainage of the lower half of the body (104). Other complications, including postoperative pulmonary dysfunction and sepsis, are similar to those with standard CPB. Because most of these cases include a nephrectomy, postoperative renal failure is common. The intravenous contrast agents used preoperatively to establish the diagnosis of renal cell carcinoma and inferior vena cava occlusion may contribute to this high incidence of postoperative renal dysfunction. It is important for the anesthesiologist to avoid the administration of any nephrotoxic drugs, to monitor urine output and central venous pressure carefully, and to intervene as appropriate if either decreases below safe levels.

CARDIOPULMONARY BYPASS WITHOUT CIRCULATORY ARREST FOR THORACIC PROCEDURES

In 1959, the same year in which Woodhall and colleagues (42) utilized CPB for excision of an intracranial aneurysm, Woods et al. (118) used CPB for resection of a carinal tumor. The procedure went well but was complicated by postoperative bleeding. An obstructing blood clot was emergently suctioned from the tracheostomy and was attributed to the combination of the operative procedure and the sequelae of bypass. As in other uses of CPB, problems with coagulation remained formidable. Nissen (119) used bypass combined with hypothermia to resect a malignant adenoma of the trachea. In a third case, reported by Adkins and Izawa (120), a cylindroma was resected with use of bypass. In their case report, they emphasized the importance of having the CPB machine primed and ready and the patient's groin prepared. If the patient's airway becomes obstructed during the induction of general anesthesia because of the intratracheal tumor, femoral CPB can be instituted immediately.

In 1965, Neville and colleagues (121) reported using bypass for tracheal resections. Depending on the location of the tumor, they used either a right, left, or anterior thoracotomy. They cannulated the superior vena cava from the right atrium, drained the inferior vena cava via a femoral venous cannula, and returned arterialized blood to their patients via a cannula in the femoral artery. Of the 11 patients studied, CPB was used in eight and partial CPB in three. Of these patients, two died of complications of hemorrhage, four of pulmonary complications, and one of a myocardial infarction. The authors attempted to minimize bleeding by completing the major portion of the operation before instituting bypass. However, it would appear from their outcomes that this was not wholly adequate. In addition, as during CPB for cardiac and vascular procedures, postoperative pulmonary complications were common. Other investigators continued to advocate CPB for pulmonary bypass based on the ease with which sterility could be maintained (no manipulation of tumor or carina around a contaminated endotracheal tube), the unencumbered nature of the surgical incision, and the ease of performance (122).

A technically interesting report was provided in 1996 by Horita et al. (123), who used VV bypass with an oxygenator via a percutaneous femoral venous approach to undertake carinal reconstruction. These authors placed bilateral femoral venous cannulas and interposed a centrifugal pump and oxygenator. Venous blood was drained from a cannula placed in the inferior vena cava, and arterialized blood flowed into the right atrium via the second femoral cannula, which had been advanced into the right atrium (Fig. 33.2). This was accomplished with partial heparinization wherein the activated clotting time was targeted to be greater than

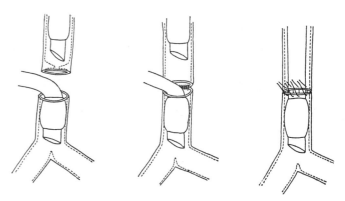

FIG. 33.3. Procedure for resection of a high tracheal lesion. After the trachea is transected below the lesion, the distal tracheal segment is intubated through the operating field. After resection of the lesion, as the trachea is reanastomosed, the distal endotracheal tube is removed and the anastomosis is completed. (Modified from Geffin B, Bland J, Grillo H. Anesthetic management of tracheal resection reconstruction. *Anesth Analg* 1969;48: 884–890, with permission.)

250 seconds. In the two cases described, total flows of approximately 3,000 mL/min were obtained. The reconstructions were performed without ventilation, but the authors did not provide blood gas data obtained during use of this technique (123).

Although CPB continues to be used occasionally for tracheal surgery, primarily in infants and small children in whom adequate ventilation with traditional endotracheal tubes is difficult to maintain (124), current management of tracheal and carinal pathology was pioneered by Grillo and colleagues (125) at the Massachusetts General Hospital. In 1969, they reported the cases of 31 patients who had undergone tracheal resection during a 7-year period in which bypass was not utilized. They emphasized the importance of advances in surgical techniques, anesthetic practice, and management of perioperative complications. For tracheal lesions, anesthesia is induced, an oral endotracheal tube is placed, the chest is opened, and the trachea is transected distally; the distal tracheal segment is later intubated through the operating field (Fig. 33.3). The tracheal lesion can then be resected and the trachea reanastamosed as shown. For more distal lesions, including lesions of the carina, Grillo and colleagues advocated intubating one of the main bronchi through the operative field, with obstruction of the contralateral pulmonary artery to optimize ventilation and perfusion during resection of the carinal lesion (Fig. 33.4). It is currently unusual, then, to use CPB for carinal or tracheal lesions (126). However, because distal airway obstruction can occur following induction of general anesthesia, the use of CPB must be considered as a viable alternative for patients at increased risk for this complication. This management is reported in a case report by Jensen and colleagues (127).

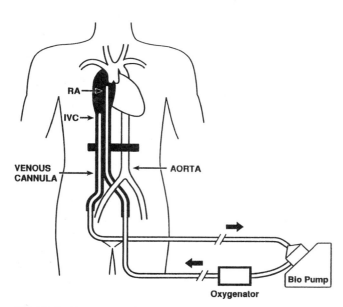

FIG. 33.2. Venovenous bypass system consisting of a centrifugal pump and a hollow-fiber membrane oxygenator. *RA*, right atrium; *IVC*, inferior vena cava. (From Horita K, Itoh T, Furukawa K, et al. Carinal reconstruction under veno-venous bypass using a percutaneous cardiopulmonary bypass system. *Thorac Cardiovasc Surg* 1996;44:46–49, with permission.)

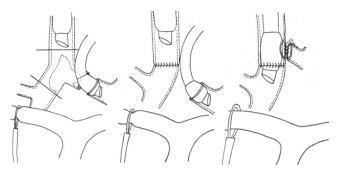

FIG. 33.4. Procedure for resection of a carinal lesion. (Modified from Geffin B, Bland J, Grillo H. Anesthetic management of tracheal resection reconstruction. *Anesth Analg* 1969;48:884–890, with permission.)

Pulmonary Embolectomy

As noted previously, Gibbon initially developed CPB to manage massive pulmonary embolism (4). It was not until 1961, however, that Cooley et al. (128) reported the first successful use of bypass to resect a pulmonary embolus. Previously, pulmonary embolectomy had been occasionally performed with the use of cardiac inflow occlusion under generalized systemic hypothermia without CPB, the same technique that had been used to resect cardiac lesions. It was obvious to those authors that CPB might have important advantages for the resection of large pulmonary emboli, otherwise a uniformly fatal condition. In 1966, Rosenberg and colleagues (129) reviewed the experience with CPB for pulmonary embolectomy and made several recommendations. Based on their review, if pulmonary embolectomy was to be successful, resection had to be attempted within 2 hours of the embolization.

In 1967, Beall and Cooley (130) summarized their experience at the Texas Heart Institute in using CPB for resuscitation and treatment of pulmonary emboli. Their success rate was only 33% for long-term survival, but they believed that the technique was indicated because the mortality rate would otherwise have been 100%, in their estimation.

Sautter (131), at the Marshfield Clinic, also reported similar survival rates (4 of 11) and, based on his experience, recommended that CPB be used only for those patients who were hypotensive and whose lives were immediately threatened. He used hypothermic low-flow hemodilution because no blood was required to prime the bypass machine. Because large cannulas were unnecessary, peripheral cannulization could be used to facilitate the emergent implementation of bypass, which he believed was most important in managing patients and improving survival. In his experience, mortality had more to do with the underlying disease process than with the surgical procedure. He strongly recommended that bypass for pulmonary embolectomy be instituted as rapidly as possible when the patient's cardiopulmonary condition was still reversible, before a series of

events began that would make resuscitation impossible, even after embolus resection.

Garcia and colleagues (132), recognizing the importance of the early use of CPB to resuscitate patients, advocated partial bypass for resuscitation, and employing a combined approach, they used total bypass for resection of the pulmonary embolus. In current practice, transthoracic pulmonary embolectomy without CPB has met with such limited success that the procedure has been all but abandoned. CPB for open pulmonary embolectomy should be utilized for those patients who are hypotensive (systolic pressure <90 mm Hg), have a P_aO_2 of less than 60 mm Hg on 100% oxygen, and have a urinary output of less than 20 mL/hr (133). These guidelines were developed more than 20 years ago, but they are still being used today (134). There are no prospective, controlled studies comparing pulmonary embolectomy with and without bypass, nor are such studies likely to be performed in the future. Pulmonary catheter embolectomy is a new technique that has been advocated for managing these critically ill patients, but its role is still being investigated (135).

In summary, when CPB is indicated, it should be instituted as soon as possible for resuscitation of the patient, frequently via the groin; then, the thromboembolus should be resected with the bypass in effect. Problems with bleeding and postoperative pulmonary complications (e.g., pulmonary edema, atelectasis) must be managed aggressively. Despite the best efforts, a high mortality rate (30 days) is not unusual, but depending on the level of experience, some centers are reporting very good (84%) survival rates (136).

Pulmonary Transplantation

At this time, single-lung transplantation, with the donor lung frequently transplanted into the recipient's right chest, is the most frequently utilized approach. This can be achieved 70% to 80% of the time without using CPB. During resection of the native lung, the contralateral lung is ventilated via an endotracheal tube inserted through the operative field while the donor lung is implanted in the chest and the pulmonary artery anastomosed. In some patients, however, it is impossible to provide adequate gas exchange with one lung because of the underlying disease process in the nonoperative side. Currently, no good preoperative test is available to predict which patients with obstructive lung disease will require CPB.

In our practice, after the patient is anesthetized and intubated, while we wait for the "go ahead" from the procurement team, we attempt one-lung ventilation to get an idea whether CPB will be required, but even this test is not very specific. For patients with restrictive lung disease, it is possible to predict preoperatively, based on exercise tolerance and right ventricular ejection fraction, who will require CPB intraoperatively (137). When CPB is used, insertion of the arterial and venous cannulas is usually through the groin, with the chest kept free of cannulas to improve the surgical field for the transplant surgeon (138); however, many surgeons prefer a standard approach with the cannulas in the cava and aortic root.

In addition to the occasional use of bypass in the management of pulmonary transplantation, CPB has also been used for "domino" procedures, in which the first recipient's heart and lungs are removed *en bloc*; the (normal) heart is then given to a second recipient while the first recipient receives a heart–lung transplant (139). Also, donors are increasingly being placed on bypass for the procurement of combined heart–lung preparations, which allows the rapid induction of hypothermia, viewed as an optimal preservation technique for the procurement of multiple organs (140).

OTHER USES

In a few case reports, CPB has been used for pulmonary lesions that cannot be managed by any other means. Shuman (141) reported a sarcoma of the lung with extension into the left atrium that was successfully managed with bypass, similar to the experience reported for resection of renal cell carcinomas extending into the right atrium (142). In addition to the elective surgical resection of tracheal lesions, CPB has also been used in certain airway emergencies (143,144). Maharaj et al. (145) reported a case in which a patient was placed on bypass for removal of an intratracheal foreign body. Femoral CPB has been used with traumatic tracheal disruptions (146) and in a case of massive sand aspiration that required bronchoscopy and pulmonary lavage (147). Similarly, several case reports have described the use of this technique for bilateral lung lavage in alveolar proteinosis (148,149). In most cases, however, alveolar proteinosis can be effectively managed without the use of CPB (150). Even patients with a single lung and alveolar proteinosis have been managed by more conservative techniques (151).

Anterior Mediastinal Masses

The resection of large anterior mediastinal masses may require the use of CPB. Most commonly, these masses are teratomas, seminomas, or lymphomas (152–154), and their presence in the mediastinum can compromise either oxygenation or cardiac output following the induction of general anesthesia (155). For patients who show respiratory distress in the preoperative period or who are unable to sleep in a supine position, it is prudent to have the groins prepared for femoral cannulation before the induction of anesthesia. For these patients, an awake intubation in a semi-sitting position may be indicated, but placement of an endotracheal tube does not guarantee adequate gas exchange when negative pressure ventilation ceases because airway obstruction may occur distal to the endotracheal tube. Addi-

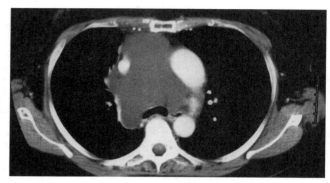

FIG. 33.5. Large anterior mediastinal mass in a 73-year-old woman. Computed tomogram of the chest at the level of the tracheal bifurcation. The mass impacts on the bifurcation, displacing the superior vena cava and pulmonary artery.

tionally, placing the patient in the supine position may cause acute right ventricular failure and cardiac arrest from either pulmonary arterial obstruction or compression of the superior vena cava and insufficient venous return to the right side of the heart. The anesthesiologist and surgical team must specifically review the computed tomogram (Fig. 33.5) and discuss these possibilities, although the anatomy as defined by the computed tomogram alone cannot clearly predict the anatomic changes that may occur during loss of negative pressure ventilation and placement of the patient in the supine position.

Venovenous Bypass

Marshall and colleagues (96) in 1970 used a passive VV bypass to manage a patient with renal cell carcinoma extending into the inferior vena cava and right atrium. The need for a shunt that could drain blood from the lower extremities and portal system was obvious in the 1960s, but the first clinical trials for patients with liver disease that utilized bypass without a pump were unsuccessful. Either clots formed in the bypass circuit so that it did not function, or clots released from the bypass tubing caused lethal pulmonary embolization. When heparinization was used, the addition of anticoagulant therapy to patients with preexisting liver-associated coagulopathy produced unacceptable bleeding and increased morbidity and mortality. It was not until the early 1980s that VV bypass in which heparin-bonded circuits with a centrifugal pump were used instead of systemic heparinization with a roller pump came into practice (155,156).

Definition

Venovenous bypass differs from CPB in many ways: (a) an oxygenator is not used in the circuit; (b) the arterial system is not perfused, so that pressures within the system are lower;

and (c) the circuit, in essence, is serving only as a conduit for blood to flow from one or more regions of the body to the right side of the heart. Therefore, VV bypass frequently utilizes flows less than those seen on CPB, and although occasionally flows as high as 6 L/min can be achieved, flows between 1 and 2 L/min are more common.

Indications

Venovenous bypass can be used for the treatment of respiratory failure (extracorporeal CO_2 removal; see Chapter 31) and in the management of surgical procedures on the liver, most frequently liver transplantation during the anhepatic phase and combined resections of the liver *and* vena cava.

Management

When VV bypass is instituted, depending on the organ bed to be bypassed, the cannula is usually placed in one femoral vein and advanced to the bifurcation of the inferior vena cava. In circumstances in which the portal system must be drained, a second catheter is placed in the portal vein. The drainage from these cannulas is then directed to a centrifugal pump, with return to the patient most frequently via an axillary or internal jugular vein. (The use of centrifugal pumps is discussed in Chap. 3.) For procedures involving the liver, no heparin is used. For extracorporeal CO_2 removal, more aggressive heparinization is mandatory.

As stated previously, because VV bypass in this context is intended only to return blood to the heart, without the requirement for oxygenation, CO_2 removal or systemic perfusion flows much lower than those maintained with CPB are employed. In our own practice, flows are considered adequate as long as they are not less than 1 L/min (157) and cardiac preload is maintained. Flows must be maintained to prevent clot development in the circuit and to provide adequate filling of the right side of the heart, although it is not clear whether any flow can guarantee that no clot will form in the total absence of heparinization. Because there is no reservoir in a VV system, the total flow possible with these systems is a function of blood return to the pump. Additionally, VV bypass systems are "closed," so no volume can be added directly once the circuit is primed. Decreased flows usually indicate a problem with the cannulas or some other obstruction to the venous system, although gradual decreases in flows may be a function of surgically related hypovolemia.

Complications of VV bypass are few. Improvements in material biocompatibility, such as heparin coating of catheters, tubing, and pumps, and the use of centrifugal pumps (158) have decreased the complications of clotting or excessive bleeding that were previously reported. Air embolism can occur in VV bypass (159), just as in CPB, with potentially lethal sequelae. In studies of VV bypass, no clinically significant coagulopathy has been described (155,160).

However, decreases in core temperature, heart rate, and arterial pressure with increases in central venous pressure have been reported (160). The blood volume becomes concentrated, as evidenced by increases in hematocrit, colloid oncotic pressure, serum osmolality, and serum sodium. These data, along with an accumulating base deficit, suggest that VV bypass is associated with some hypoperfusion of the abdominal viscera and lower extremities. Flow-dependent, third-space fluid accumulation (161) may be a primary contributor to decreasing cardiac output and pump flow during the procedure. However, these limitations, although important, do not limit the use of VV bypass for those surgical procedures, in which it has clearly proved to be beneficial.

Liver Transplantation

Fewer than 5% of liver transplantation procedures are carried out with VV bypass. Originally, in the United States, it was thought that a liver transplantation surgical procedure would be improved by the use of a bypass technique that would shunt blood from the lower extremities and mesenteric beds to the right atrium. For many years, the majority of liver transplant centers throughout the United States and Europe utilized VV bypass (162–164). It was this technique that greatly facilitated the development of liver transplantation. The use of VV bypass for up to 4 to 5 hours without obvious harm to the recipient extended the surgeon's time, which allowed for the modification of many aspects of the recipient operation. With the hemodynamic stability afforded by VV bypass, it was possible for the surgeon to perform the resection of the native liver in a more determined and careful manner. Once the liver was isolated and resected, the raw surfaces created during the hepatectomy were closed. This aspect of the surgical procedure, in which the surgeon can utilize the additional time to obtain surgical hemostasis, significantly decreased the bleeding problems associated with liver transplantation.

With the development of liver transplantation, as more experience has been gained, surgeons have been able to use a side-bite clamp on the inferior vena cava and create vascular anastomoses without cross-clamping the entire inferior vena cava. This technique has decreased the need for VV bypass, although, as stated, approximately 5% of patients still require VV bypass because of severe venous congestion and other surgical considerations.

Management

Venovenous bypass has been suggested for venous decompression, improved hemodynamic stability, and decreased intraoperative blood loss during the anhepatic phase of liver transplantation. Because hypothermic coagulopathy is a problem and because VV bypass systems lack a heat exchanger, the maintenance of normothermia during the operative procedure is important. In many centers, patients are positioned on a heating blanket on the operating table. In our own practice, an air-warming device is placed over the lower and upper extremities during surgery. Routine hemodynamic monitoring should include electrocardiography to measure the heart rate and detect the presence of ischemia, use of a core temperature probe, pulse oximetry, placement of an arterial cannula to measure systemic arterial pressure, and placement of a pulmonary artery catheter to determine cardiac filling pressures and cardiac outputs. In addition, metabolic monitoring should include the measurement of arterial blood gases, sodium, potassium, ionized calcium, blood glucose, and coagulation (through the use of a thromboelastogram and, increasingly, a prothrombin and activated partial thromboplastin time). These measurements are obtained at baseline and then repeated at discrete intervals during the operative procedure.

When VV bypass is used for liver transplantation, it is necessary to drain both the systemic and portal systems with cannulas in the femoral and portal veins. In circumstances in which the portal vein cannot be easily cannulated, the placement of catheters in the mesenteric venous system of the abdomen has been described (165). During the recipient hepatectomy, when bypass is ready for implementation, the surgeon ligates the hepatic artery and common duct and mobilizes the liver. The portal vein and femoral cannulas are inserted to allow both the splanchnic and systemic venous drainage to be brought into the VV circuit. Entry into the proximal systemic venous system is usually via the axillary or internal jugular vein. The surgeon then proceeds with mobilization of the liver and divides all structures, including the infrahepatic vena cava.

Following the initiation of bypass, frequently a transient decrease in blood pressure is noted that rarely persists for more than 15 to 30 seconds. One study found a decrease of 4°C in core temperature, a statistically significant decrease in heart rate and systemic arterial pressure, and an increase in the central venous pressure with the initiation of bypass (160). Electrocardiographic changes, attributable to the effects of temperature and alterations in potassium, were also noted. It is important to monitor and prevent hypothermia aggressively during the transplant procedure because in "heparinless" VV bypass, a standard heat exchanger cannot be used because of the large, potentially thrombogenic surface area of these devices.

When bypass is discontinued, any coagulopathies must be corrected. This is accomplished through the infusion of platelets, fresh-frozen plasma, and cryoprecipitate based on the findings of the thromboelastogram and other clotting studies. Calcium, potassium, and glucose abnormalities must be monitored and treated. Hypocalcemia is readily corrected with the intravascular administration of calcium chloride; hyperkalemia is usually transient. Hyperglycemia is infrequently treated intraoperatively because many of these patients become hypoglycemic within 6 to 10 hours of the operative procedure.

Resection of the Vena Cava

Indications

As surgical and anesthetic techniques common to transplantation of the liver improved, these advances were used in procedures on the liver (resections) (165) and vena cava (relief of obstructions) (166), and in combined hepatic and inferior vena caval resections (167). Resection of vena caval leiomyosarcomas (168), surgical correction of the Budd-Chiari syndrome (169), and repair of traumatic vena caval disruption (170) have all been reported with the use of VV bypass, but in most cases, the technique is indicated for combined hepatic and vena caval resections. Frequently, it is impossible to isolate the liver and achieve acceptable cancer-free margins without resecting the inferior vena cava (167).

Management

During a combined liver and vena caval resection, decompression of the portal system is not necessary. The cross-clamp time is usually only 15 to 30 minutes, and it would be unusual for the bowel and mesentery not to tolerate venous outflow obstruction for this brief period. It is necessary, however, to shunt the lower systemic circulation. In these circumstances, the systemic circulation is drained via a catheter in the inferior vena cava, and the venous effluent is returned to the patient through a large-bore cannula in the internal jugular. Most of these patients undergo surgery in a thoracoabdominal position, and unlike the supine position used for liver transplantation, the thoracoabdominal position makes access to the axillary vein more difficult to achieve. During bypass, a flow of more than 1 L/min is the goal. As in liver transplantation, the use of VV bypass permits better surgical exposure, which in turn allows more meticulous dissection, resection of the tumor mass and vena cava, and insertion of a polytetrafluoroethylene graft (Gore-Tex, WL Gore, Inc., Flagstaff, AZ) when indicated.

CARDIOPULMONARY AND VENOVENOUS BYPASS FOR OTHER INDICATIONS

Management of Pharmacologic Problems

Before the clinical use of dantrolene, malignant hyperthermia was treated with support therapies, including hyperventilation and systemic cooling of the patient. In one case in which these maneuvers were unsuccessful, CPB with hypothermia was instituted via a femorofemoral approach (171). The patient was cooled from 41°C to 37°C, with excellent outcome. However, the development of dantrolene made such maneuvers generally unnecessary. Another interesting application of CPB related to drug activity was in flecainide poisoning (172). Flecainide overdose suppresses myocardial function, so in extreme cases drug clearance can be impaired secondary to myocardial failure. This case report describes a patient with flecainide overdose who was placed on CPB for 10 hours. During this period, redistribution and clearance allowed plasma levels to decrease to therapeutic levels, after which cardiac rhythm and blood pressure were reestablished. Although CPB reduced flecainide levels and hemodynamics were reestablished, the patient ultimately died of the neurologic injury sustained during profound hypotension before CPB (172).

Cardiopulmonary Bypass and Accidental Hypothermia

Accidental hypothermia has been a problem for millennia. Only in the 20th century did the realization come that many patients who might otherwise be declared dead could be resuscitated. In 1967, Kugelberg and colleagues (173) described the management of a patient who arrived at their hospital with a core body temperature of 21.7°C. Because of concerns about gradually warming the patient and the risk for cardiac arrest resulting from ventricular fibrillation, the authors rewarmed the patient rapidly with bypass in which a heat exchanger and oxygenator were used. Cannulation was via the left femoral artery and vein. The patient was successfully rewarmed without the development of ventricular fibrillation. The postoperative period was complicated by bronchopneumonia and renal failure, but the patient eventually had a complete recovery. The authors emphasized the use of bypass for the management of accidental hypothermia based on their observations that the patient could be rewarmed more rapidly; the risk for ventricular fibrillation was diminished, and in the event of ventricular fibrillation, circulation and oxygenation could be supported until the heart was defibrillated (frequently once the core temperature was >28°C). In other circumstances, patients have been managed more emergently, usually while profoundly hypothermic, and partial bypass has been instituted during cardiopulmonary resuscitation for ventricular fibrillation.

Several series have examined the use of CPB in accidental hypothermia. Following a tragedy on Mount Hood in Oregon, 11 patients were brought to the hospital emergency department profoundly hypothermic; 10 of the patients were warmed via bypass, and there were two long-term survivors (174). There were no survivors among those patients who presented with a core temperature below 22°C. This would substantiate previous reports in which successes were rarely observed if the core temperature was this low. The two survivors had spontaneous respiratory activity on admission to the hospital.

The issue of age in identifying patients who are candidates is controversial. Based on the Bellevue experience, youth itself is not protective when core temperatures are below 26°C (175). In a series reported from England, Duguid et al. (176) described an 87% mortality rate in 23

elderly patients treated via active external warming and concluded that elderly patients should not be actively rewarmed. A review of the literature since the initial report in 1967 from Kugelberg et al. would indicate a much higher success rate (approximately 50% to 70%), but the success rate is only 50% if isolated case reports are excluded. A recent report from Switzerland (177) described 32 patients in whom CPB was attempted; 15 (47%) were long-term survivors who had minimal sequelae. Most of the patients were young (mean age 25 years), well-conditioned mountain climbers. Based on these results and other work, Lazar (178) advocates CPB as the treatment of choice for any patient with accidental hypothermia, cardiac arrest, and core temperatures of less than 32°C. CPB should also be considered for any patient with a core temperature below 32°C, even if hemodynamics are stable (because of the risk for ventricular fibrillation). CPB is contraindicated in patients with a temperature of 32°C or higher, and in patients with a serum potassium level of 10 mEq/L or higher. Advanced age (>65 years) is a relative contraindication (178).

A review of the previous reports would indicate a dire prognosis if the core temperature is less than 16°C. The duration of the hypothermic insult, independently of core temperature, is another factor in determining the prognosis. Furthermore, the prognosis for patients without some evidence of respiratory activity or with chronic health problems is sufficiently poor that aggressive rewarming with bypass needs to be considered carefully in these particular circumstances. In managing these patients, hemoconcentration, electrolyte abnormalities, hyperkalemia, hypokalemia, and pulmonary and cardiac problems have been reported, and renal failure secondary to myoglobinuria is a major concern.

Whether or not CPB is useful in these profoundly hypothermic patients remains, however, controversial. In a recent study from New York, 16 patients with core temperatures between 25° and 32°C were successfully managed with warmed intravenous fluids, heated aerosol masks, and occasionally warm peritoneal dialysis (179). The decision of whether to use bypass to warm a profoundly hypothermic patient is best made by the physicians managing the patient based on their assessment of the patient's status and the availability of resources.

Several case reports have indicated that patients who are hypothermic following an overdose of barbiturates can also be successfully resuscitated with the use of bypass (180). In contrast to patients who experience accidental hypothermia, the patients with barbiturate-induced comas have higher core temperatures and tend to be older. Outcome is improved if the patient can be rewarmed, and one of the advantages of bypass is that it is possible to include a filter to dialyze barbiturates (181).

Vascular Procedures

Although uncommon, bypass with and without hypothermia has been used for a number of rare and exotic vascular problems. These reports all include the presence of a fistula or aneurysm that would not be amenable to repair without either circulatory arrest or a degree of hypothermia necessitating bypass. There are reports of aortovenous fistulas affecting the aorta and vena cava (182) and the aorta and renal vein (183) repaired with the use of bypass, hypothermia, and circulatory arrest. A variety of aneurysms and fistulas (184,185), hemangiomas (186), and vascular malformations of the face have also been reported (187). Although the surgical repair of renal artery abnormalities is commonly performed *in situ*, occasionally autotransplantation with or without extracorporeal surgery is required. In cases in which extracorporeal surgery is performed, the kidney can be placed in a Euro-Collins slush on a workbench and perfused with cold (4° to 7°C) Euro-Collins solution (188).

Orthopedic Procedures

In the 1950s and 1960s, bypass was used to administer high concentrations of chemotherapeutic agents to discrete regions of the body (189). In this technique, applied most frequently in patients with neoplasms of the lower extremities, the artery and vein supplying the tumor area were isolated and cannulated in a small oxygenator. For the lower extremities, the common femoral artery and vein were most frequently cannulated. The arm could likewise be treated with cannulation of an axillary artery and vein. Complete isolation of the limb was accomplished by applying a tourniquet proximal to the cannulas. Perfusion was usually brief, lasting from 15 to 30 minutes. Although regional perfusion held promise, other treatment modalities have largely supplanted it. However, some centers continue to use this technique experimentally.

Extracorporeal Filtration of Schistosoma

Several reports in the late 1960s described a bypass procedure in which the portal system was drained via a cannula placed in the splenic vein and advanced into the portal vein (190). The blood was filtered to trap schistosomes; a roller pump in the circuit infused blood back into a femoral vein. Heparinization was required for this procedure. Complications were minimal, although the technique was not always successful. Several hundred patients were treated in this way, but newer antiparasitic drugs make the technique unnecessary today.

SUMMARY

Despite enthusiasm in the 1960s for the use of CPB as an adjunct in a variety of surgical cases, its primary use today is to facilitate the surgical correction of cardiac and aortic lesions. However, bypass techniques developed for these procedures have indications in other cases, in which they

are clearly life-saving. Certain neurosurgical and urologic procedures can be undertaken and successfully completed only when CPB, profound hypothermia, and circulatory arrest are used. Furthermore, certain pulmonary procedures are possible only when systemic oxygenation is supplied via CPB. The principles developed for CPB have led to the evolution of effective VV bypass techniques used in hepatic transplantation and other procedures involving the abdominal viscera. In certain other uncommon conditions, CPB and VV bypass can be used to improve patient survival and decrease morbidity.

It is imperative that the surgical and anesthetic teams have adequate experience in the use of these techniques, which is frequently gained in the application of CPB during cardiac procedures. A well-trained, experienced, and knowledgeable team significantly decreases morbidity and improves survival.

KEY POINTS

- The noncardiovascular applications of CPB comprise four major categories:
  - Deep hypothermic circulatory arrest for control of surgical bleeding and for organ (central nervous system) protection.
  - Noncardiac thoracic (pulmonary) applications.
  - Surgical procedures requiring occlusion of the inferior vena cava.
  - Miscellaneous unusual procedural applications.
- The principle application of deep hypothermic circulatory arrest is in neurosurgery, to facilitate the resection of intracranial vascular abnormalities.
- The major use of CPB to occlude the inferior vena cava is in urologic surgery, to allow the resection of renal cell carcinomas extending into the inferior vena cava.
- Noncardiac thoracic surgical applications of CPB include resection of pulmonary thromboembolism, lung transplantation, and carinal resection.
- The principle use of VV bypass is in certain cases of hepatic transplantation, although in current practice it is used only in approximately 5% of liver transplants.
- Miscellaneous uses of CPB include the resuscitation of patients with accidental hypothermia and the application of regional perfusion to facilitate antineoplastic therapy.

REFERENCES

1. Burchell HB. Contributions of the basic sciences to successful clinical application of cardiopulmonary bypass. *Mayo Clin Proc* 1980;55:754–757.
2. Stephen CR, Bourgeois-Gavardin M, Dent S, et al. Anesthetic

management in open-heart surgery: electroencelphalographic and metabolic findings in 81 patients. *Anesth Analg* 1959;38: 198–205.

3. Michenfelder JD. The hypothermic brain. In: Michenfelder JD, ed. *Anesthesia and the brain.* New York: Churchill Livingstone, 1988:23–34.

4. Curtis LE. An early history of extracorporeal circulation. *J Cardiovasc Surg* 1966;7:240–247.

5. Norlander O, Pitzele S, Edling I, et al. Anesthesiological experience from intracardiac surgery with the Craoford-Senning heart–lung machine. *Acta Anaesth Scand* 1958;2:181–210.

6. Serry C, Najafi H, Dye WS, et al. Superiority of aortic over femoral cannulation for cardiopulmonary bypass, with specific attention to lower extremity neuropathy. *J Cardiovasc Surg* 1978;19:277–279.

7. Berger RL, Barsamian EM. Iliac or femoral vein-to-artery total cardiopulmonary bypass. An experimental and clinical study. *Ann Thorac Surg* 1966;2:281–289.

8. Berger RL, Saini VK, Dargan EL. Clinical applications of femoral vein-to-artery cannulation for mechanical cardiopulmonary support and bypass. *Ann Thorac Surg* 1973;15:163–169.

9. Smith CR, Getrajdman GI, Hsu DT. Venous cannulation for high-flow femorofemoral bypass. *Ann Thorac Surg* 1990;49: 674–675.

10. MacDonald JL, Cleland AG, Mayer RL, et al. Extracorporeal circuit design considerations for giant intracranial aneurysm repair. *Perfusion* 1997;12:193–196.

11. Abouna GM. Brachial arteriovenous shunts for hemodialysis and extracorporeal procedures. *Eur Surg Res* 1973;5:390–400.

12. Lilleaasen P, Stokke O. Moderate and extreme hemodilution in open-heart surgery: fluid balance and acid–base studies. *Ann Thorac Surg* 1978;25:127–133.

13. Kawashima Y, Yamamoto Z, Manabe H. Safe limits of hemodilution in cardiopulmonary bypass. *Surgery* 1974;76:391–397.

14. Kabat H, Rosomoff HL, Holaday DA. Recovery of function following arrest of the brain circulation. *Am J Physiol* 1941;132: 737–747.

15. Rosomoff HL, Holaday DA. Cerebral blood flow and cerebral oxygen consumption during hypothermia. *Am J Physiol* 1954; 179:85–88.

16. Swan H, Zeavin I, Holmes JH, et al. Cessation of circulation in general hypothermia. I. Physiologic changes and their control. *Ann Surg* 1953;138:360–376.

17. Parkins WM, Jensen JM, Vars HM. Brain cooling in the prevention of brain damage during periods of circulatory occlusion in dogs. *J Thorac Cardiovasc Surg* 1954;140:284–287.

18. Drew CE, Anderson IM. Profound hypothermia in cardiac surgery. Report of three cases. *Lancet* 1959;1:748–750.

19. Garman JK. Optimal pressures and flows during cardiopulmonary bypass. Pro: a low-flow, low-pressure technique is acceptable. *J Cardiothorac Vasc Anesth* 1991;5:399–401.

20. Silvay G, Ammar T, Reich DL, et al. Cardiopulmonary bypass for adult patients: a survey of equipment and techniques. *J Cardiothorac Vasc Anesth* 1995;9:420–424.

21. Dexter F, Hindman BJ, Cutkomp J, et al. Blood warms as it flows retrograde from a femoral cannulation site to the carotid artery during cardiopulmonary bypass. *Perfusion* 1994;9: 393–397.

22. Silverstein A, Krieger HP. Neurologic complications of cardiac surgery. *Arch Neurol* 1960;3:601–605.

23. Shaw PJ, Bates D, Cartlidge NE, et al. Early neurological complications of coronary artery bypass surgery. *Br Med J Clin Res Ed* 1985;291:1384–1387.

24. Christakis GT, Abel JG, Lichtenstein SV. Neurological outcomes and cardiopulmonary temperature: a clinical review. *J Card Surg* 1995;10:475–480.

25. Roach GW, Kanchuger M, Mangano CM, et al. Adverse cerebral outcomes after coronary bypass surgery. *N Engl J Med* 1996; 335:1857–1863.

26. Redmond JM, Gillinow M, Stuart RS, et al. Heparin-coated bypass circuits reduce pulmonary injury. *Ann Thorac Surg* 1993; 56:474–479.

27. Johnson D, Kelm C, To T, et al. Postoperative physical therapy after coronary artery bypass surgery. *Am J Respir Crit Care Med* 1995;152:953–958.

28. Valentine S, Barrowcliffe M, Peacock J. A comparison of effects of fixed and tailored cardiopulmonary bypass flow rates on renal function. *Anaesth Intensive Care* 1993;21:304–308.

29. Lema G, Meneses G, Urzua J, et al. Effects of extracorporeal circulation on renal function in coronary surgical patients. *Anesth Analg* 1995;81:446–451.

30. Allen KB, Salam AA, Lumsden AB. Acute mesenteric ischemia after cardiopulmonary bypass. *J Vasc Surg* 1992;16:391–396.

31. Hermens WT, Willems GM, van der Vusse GJ. Minimal myocardial injury after uncomplicated coronary bypass surgery. Various sources of overestimation. *Clin Chim Acta* 1988;173: 243–250.

32. Nuttall GA, Oliver WC, Ereth MH, et al. Coagulation tests predict bleeding after cardiopulmonary bypass. *J Cardiothorac Vasc Anesth* 1997;11:815–823.

33. Dacey LJ, Munoz JJ, Baribeau YR, et al. Reexploration for hemorrhage following coronary artery bypass grafting: incidence and risk factors. *Arch Surg* 1998;133:442–447.

34. Kollef MH, Wragge T, Pasque C. Determinants of mortality and multiorgan dysfunction in cardiac surgery patients requiring prolonged mechanical ventilation. *Chest* 1995;107:1395–1401.

35. Oudemans-van Straaten HM, Jansen PGM, Hoek FJ, et al. Intestinal permeability, circulating endotoxin, and postoperative systemic responses in cardiac surgery patients. *J Cardiothorac Vasc Anesth* 1996;10:187–194.

36. Bell DM, Goldmann DA, Hopkins CC, et al. Unreliability of fever and leukocytosis in the diagnosis of infection after cardiac valve surgery. *J Thorac Cardiovasc Surg* 1978;75:87–90.

37. Sekela ME, Noon GP, Holland VA, et al. Differential perfusion: potential complication of femoral–femoral bypass during single lung transplantation. *J Heart Lung Transplant* 1991;10: 322–324.

38. Reed WA, Kittle CF. Survival rate and metabolic acidosis after prolonged extracorporeal circulation with total cardiopulmonary bypass. *J Thorac Cardiovasc Surg* 1958;148:219–225.

39. Tinker JH, ed. *Cardiopulmonary bypass: current concepts and controversies.* Philadelphia: WB Saunders, 1989.

40. Sealy WC, Brown IW Jr, Young WG Jr. A report of the use of both extracorporeal circulation and hypothermia for open heart surgery. *Ann Surg* 1958;147:603–613.

41. Sealy WC, Brown IW Jr, Young WG Jr, et al. Hypothermia and extracorporeal circulation for open heart surgery: its simplification with a heat exchanger for rapid cooling and rewarming. *Ann Surg* 1959;150:627–639.

42. Woodhall B, Sealy WC, Hall KD, et al. Craniotomy under conditions of quinidine-protected cardioplegia and profound hypothermia. *Ann Surg* 1960;152:37–44.

43. Botterell EH, Lougheed WM, Scott JW, et al. Hypothermia and interruption of carotid, or carotid and vertebral circulation, in the surgical management of intracranial aneurysms. *J Neurosurg* 1956;13:1–42.

44. Bachet J, Guilmet D, Goudot B, et al. Cold cerebroplegia. A new technique of cerebral protection during operations on the transverse aortic arch. *J Thorac Cardiovasc Surg* 1991;102: 85–93; discussion 93–84.

45. Coselli JS, Crawford ES, Beall AC Jr, et al. Determination of

brain temperatures for safe circulatory arrest during cardiovascular operation. *Ann Thorac Surg* 1988;45:638–642.

46. Patterson RH, Ray BS. Profound hypothermia for intracranial surgery: laboratory and clinical experiences with extracorporeal circulation by peripheral cannulation. *Ann Surg* 1962;156: 377–393.

47. Michenfelder JD, Kirklin JW, Uihlein A, et al. Clinical experience with a closed-chest method of producing profound hypothermia and total circulatory arrest in neurosurgery. *Ann Surg* 1964;159:125–131.

48. Michenfelder JD, Milde JH. The relationship among canine brain temperature, metabolism, and function during hypothermia. *Anesthesiology* 1991;75:130–136.

49. Michenfelder JD, Milde JH. The effect of profound levels of hypothermia (below 14 degrees C) on canine cerebral metabolism. *J Cereb Blood Flow Metab* 1992;12:877–880.

50. Cook DJ, Orszulak TA, Daly RC: Minimum hematocrit at differing cardiopulmonary bypass temperatures in dogs. *Circulation* 1998;98:II-170–II-175.

51. Rittenhouse EA, Mori H, Dillard DH, et al. Deep hypothermia in cardiovascular surgery. *Ann Thorac Surg* 1974;17:63–98.

52. Olsen RW, Hayes LJ, Wissler EH, et al. Influence of hypothermia and circulatory arrest on cerebral temperature distributions. *J Biomech Eng* 1985;107:354–360.

53. Stone JG, Young WL, Smith CR, et al. Do standard monitoring sites reflect true brain temperature when profound hypothermia is rapidly induced and reversed? *Anesthesiology* 1995;82: 344–351.

54. Jonas RA, Bellinger DC, Rappaport LA, et al. Relation of pH strategy and development outcome after hypothermic circulatory arrest. *J Thorac Cardiovasc Surg* 1993;106:362–368.

55. Kurth CD, O'Rourke MM, O'Hara IB, et al. Brain cooling efficiency with pH-stat and α-stat cardiopulmonary bypass in newborn pigs. *Circulation* 1997;96:II-358–II-363.

56. Bellinger DC, Jonas RA, Rappaport LA, et al. Developmental and neurologic status of children after heart surgery with hypothermic circulatory arrest or low-flow cardiopulmonary bypass. *N Engl J Med* 1995;332:549–555.

57. Newburger JW, Jonas RA, Wernovsky G, et al. A comparison of the perioperative neurologic effects of hypothermic circulatory arrest versus low-flow cardiopulmonary bypass in infant heart surgery. *N Engl J Med* 1993;329:1057–1064.

58. Crittenden MD, Roberts CS, Rosa L, et al. Brain protection during circulatory arrest. *Ann Thorac Surg* 1991;51:942–947.

59. Michenfelder JD, Terry HR Jr, Daw EF, et al. Induced hypothermia: physiologic effects, indications and techniques. *Surg Clin North Am* 1965;45:889–898.

60. Lim RA, Rehder K, Harp RA, et al. Circulatory arrest during profound hypothermia induced by direct bloodstream cooling: an experimental study. *Surgery* 1961;49:367–374.

61. Bjork VO, Hultquist G. Brain damage in children after deep hypothermia for open-heart surgery. *Thorax* 1960;15:284–291.

62. Edmunds LH Jr, Folkman J, Snodgress AB, et al. Prevention of brain damage during profound hypothermia and circulatory arrest. *Ann Surg* 1963;157:637–649.

63. Svensson LG, Crawford ES, Hess KR, et al. Deep hypothermia with circulatory arrest. Determinants of stroke and early mortality in 656 patients. *J Thorac Cardiovasc Surg* 1993;106:19–31.

64. Ausman JI, McCormick PW, Stewart M, et al. Cerebral oxygen metabolism during hypothermic circulatory arrest in humans. *J Neurosurg* 1993;79:810–815.

65. Smith G, Ledingham IM, Norman JN, et al. Prolongation of the time of "safe" circulatory arrest by preliminary hyperbaric oxygenation and body cooling. *Surg Gynecol Obstet* 1963;117: 411–416.

66. Mault JR, Ohtake S, Klingensmith ME, et al. Cerebral metabolism and circulatory arrest: effects of duration and strategies for protection. *Ann Thorac Surg* 1993;55:57–64.

67. Kirklin JW, Dawson B, Devloo RA, et al. Open intracardiac operations: use of circulatory arrest during hypothermia induced by blood cooling. *Ann Surg* 1961;154:769–776.

68. Uihlein A, Theye RA, Dawson B, et al. The use of profound hypothermia, extracorporeal circulation and total circulatory arrest for an intracranial aneurysm. Preliminary report with reports of cases. *Staff Meet Mayo Clin* 1960;35:567–576.

69. Drake CG, Barr HWK, Coles JC, et al. The use of extracorporeal circulation and profound hypothermia in the treatment of ruptured intracranial aneurysm. *J Neurosurg* 1964;21:575–581.

70. Patterson RH Jr, Bronson SR. Profound hypothermia for intracranial surgery using a disposable bubble oxygenator. *J Neurosurg* 1965;23:184–190.

71. Neville WE, Thomason RD, Peacock H, et al. Cardiopulmonary bypass during noncardiac surgery. *Arch Surg* 1966;92: 576–587.

72. Uihlein A, MacCarty CS, Michenfelder JD, et al. Deep hypothermia and surgical treatment of intracranial aneurysms. A five-year survey. *JAMA* 1966;195:639–641.

73. Sundt TM Jr, Pluth JR, Gronert GA. Excision of giant basilar aneurysm under profound hypothermia. Report of case. *Mayo Clin Proc* 1972;47:631–634.

74. McMurtry JG, Housepian EM, Bowman FO Jr, et al. Surgical treatment of basilar artery aneurysms. Elective circulatory arrest with thoracotomy in 12 cases. *J Neurosurg* 1974;40:486–494.

75. Patterson RH Jr, Fraser RAR. Vascular neoplasms of the brainstem: a place for profound hypothermia and circulatory arrest. *Adv Neurosurg* 1975;3:425–428.

76. Silverberg GD, Reitz BA, Ream AK, et al. Operative treatment of a giant cerebral artery aneurysm with hypothermia and circulatory arrest: report of a case. *Neurosurgery* 1980;6:301–305.

77. Baumgartner WA, Silverberg GD, Ream AK, et al. Reappraisal of cardiopulmonary bypass with deep hypothermia and circulatory arrest for complex neurosurgical operations. *Surgery* 1983; 94:242–249.

78. Gonski A, Acedillo AT, Stacey RB. Profound hypothermia in the treatment of intracranial aneurysms. *Aust N Z J Surg* 1986; 56:639–643.

79. Richards PG, Marath A, Edwards JM, et al. Management of difficult intracranial aneurysms by deep hypothermia and elective cardiac arrest using cardiopulmonary bypass. *Br J Neurosurg* 1987;1:261–269.

80. Williams MD, Rainer WG, Fieger HG Jr, et al. Cardiopulmonary bypass, profound hypothermia, and circulatory arrest for neurosurgery. *Ann Thorac Surg* 1991;52:1069–1074; discussion 1074–1075.

81. Hickey PR, Andersen NP. Deep hypothermic circulatory arrest: a review of pathophysiology and clinical experience as a basis for anesthetic management. *J Cardiothorac Anesth* 1987;1: 137–155.

82. Watanabe T, Miura M, Inui K, et al. Blood and brain tissue gaseous strategy for profoundly hypothermic total circulatory arrest. *J Thorac Cardiovasc Surg* 1991;102:497–504.

83. Aoki M, Nomura F, Stromski ME, et al. Effects of pH on brain energetics after hypothermic circulatory arrest. *Ann Thorac Surg* 1993;55:1093–1103.

84. Lafferty JJ, Keykhah MM, Shapiro HM, et al. Cerebral hypometabolism obtained with deep pentobarbital anesthesia and hypothermia (30°C). *Anesthesiology* 1978;49:159–164.

85. Quasha AL, Tinker JH, Sharbrough FW. Hypothermia plus thiopental: prolonged electroencephalographic suppression. *Anesthesiology* 1981;55:636–640.

86. Michenfelder JD. Hypothermia plus barbiturates: apples plus oranges [Editorial]. *Anesthesiology* 1978;49:157–158.

87. Bigelow WG, Mustard WT, Evans JG. Some physiologic concepts of hypothermia and their applications to cardiac surgery. *J Thorac Surg* 1954;28:463–480.

88. Sundt TM Jr, Nofzinger JD. Clip-grafts for aneurysm and small vessel surgery. 1. Repair of segmental defects with clip-grafts; laboratory studies and clinical correlations. 2. Clinical application of clip-grafts to aneurysms; technical considerations. *J Neurosurg* 1967;27:477–489.

89. Tinker JH. ASA Award: John D. Michenfelder. *Anesthesiology* 1990;73:596–598.

90. Valeri CR, Feingold H, Cassidy G, et al. Hypothermia-induced reversible platelet dysfunction. *Ann Surg* 1987;205:175–181.

91. Okita Y, Takamoto S, Ando M, et al. Coagulation and fibrinolysis system in aortic surgery under deep hypothermic circulatory arrest with aprotinin: the importance of adequate heparinization. *Circulation* 1997;96:II-376–II-381.

92. Harris DNF, Bailey SM, Smith PLC, et al. Brain swelling in the first hour after coronary artery bypass surgery. *Lancet* 1993; 342:586–587.

93. Harris DNF, Oatridge A, Dob D, et al. Cerebral swelling after normothermic cardiopulmonary bypass. *Anesthesiology* 1998;88: 340–345.

94. Myers GH Jr, Fehrenbaker LG, Kelalis PP. Prognostic significance of renal vein invasion by hypernephroma. *J Urol* 1968; 100:420–423.

95. Riches EW. Factors in the prognosis of carcinoma of the kidney. *J Urol* 1958;79:190–195.

96. Marshall VF, Middleton RG, Holswade GR, et al. Surgery for renal cell carcinoma in the vena cava. *J Urol* 1970;103:414–420.

97. Ardekani RG, Hunter JA, Thomson A. Hidden hypernephroma simulating right atrial tumor. *Ann Thorac Surg* 1971;11: 371–375.

98. Utley JR, Mobin-Uddin K, Segnitz RH, et al. Acute obstruction of tricuspid valve by Wilms' tumor. *J Thorac Cardiovasc Surg* 1973;66:626–628.

99. Theman T, Williams WG, Simpson JS, et al. Tumor invasion of the upper inferior vena cava: the use of profound hypothermia and circulation arrest as a surgical adjunct. *J Pediatr Surg* 1978; 13:331–334.

100. Choh JH, Gurney R, Shenoy SS, et al. Renal-cell carcinoma: removal of intracardiac extension with aid of cardiopulmonary bypass. *N Y State J Med* 1981;81:929–932.

101. Prager RL, Dean R, Turner B. Surgical approach to intracardiac renal cell carcinoma. *Ann Thorac Surg* 1982;33:74–77.

102. Daughtry JD, Stewart BH, Golding LA, et al. Pulmonary embolus presenting as the initial manifestation of renal cell carcinoma. *Ann Thorac Surg* 1977;24:178–181.

103. Wilkinson CJ, Kimovec MA, Uejima T. Cardiopulmonary bypass in patients with malignant renal neoplasms. *Br J Anaesth* 1986;58:461–465.

104. Welch M, Bazaral MG, Schmidt R, et al. Anesthetic management for surgical removal of renal carcinoma with caval or atrial tumor thrombus using deep hypothermic circulatory arrest. *J Cardiothorac Anesth* 1989;3:580–586.

105. Paul JG, Rhodes MB, Skow JR. Renal cell carcinoma presenting as right atrial tumor with successful removal using cardiopulmonary bypass. *Ann Surg* 1975;181:471–473.

106. Marshall FF, Reitz BA, Diamond DA. A new technique for management of renal cell carcinoma involving the right atrium: hypothermia and cardiac arrest. *J Urol* 1984;131:103–107.

107. Lachance SL, Murray GF. Surgical management of renal cell carcinoma involving the hepatic vena cava (using cardiopulmonary bypass, profound hypothermia, cardiac arrest). *W V Med J* 1987;83:378–380.

108. Appoo JJ, Ralley F, Baslaim G, et al. Anesthesia for deep hypo-
thermic circulatory arrest in adults: experience with the first 50 patients. *J Cardiothorac Vasc Anesth* 1998;12:260–265.

109 Klein FA, Smith MJ, Greenfield LJ. Extracorporeal circulation for renal cell carcinoma with supradiaphragmatic vena caval thrombi. *J Urol* 1984;131:880–883.

110. Montie JE, Jackson CL, Cosgrove DM, et al. Resection of large inferior vena caval thrombi from renal cell carcinoma with the use of circulatory arrest. *J Urol* 1988;139:25–28.

111. Hedderich GS, RJ OC, Reid EC, et al. Caval tumor thrombus complicating renal cell carcinoma: a surgical challenge. *Surgery* 1987;102:614–621.

112. Marshall FF, Dietrick DD, Baumgartner WA, et al. Surgical management of renal cell carcinoma with intracaval neoplastic extension above the hepatic veins. *J Urol* 1988;139:1166–1172.

113. Novick AC, Kaye MC, Cosgrove DM, et al. Experience with cardiopulmonary bypass and deep hypothermic circulatory arrest in the management of retroperitoneal tumors with large vena caval thrombi. *Ann Surg* 1990;212:472–476; discussion 476–477.

114. Shahian DM, Libertino JA, Zinman LN, et al. Resection of cavoatrial renal cell carcinoma employing total circulatory arrest. *Arch Surg* 1990;125:727–732.

115. Swierzewski DJ, Swierzewski MJ, Libertino JA. Radical nephrectomy in patients with renal cell carcinoma with venous, vena caval, and atrial extension. *Am J Surg* 1994;168:205–209.

116. Matthews PN, Evans C, Breckenridge IM. Involvement of the inferior vena cava by renal tumour: surgical excision using hypothermic circulatory arrest. *Br J Urol* 1995;75:441–444.

117. Gleason DM, Reilly RJ, Anderson RM, et al. Removal of hypernephroma and inferior vena cava: right atrial tumor thrombus. *Arch Surg* 1972;105:795–797.

118. Woods FM, Neptune WB, Palatchi A. Resection of the carina and main-stem bronchi with the use of extracorporeal circulation. *N Engl J Med* 1961;264:492–494.

119. Nissen VR. Extrakorporelle zirkulation für langdauernde (30 minuten) Atemunterbrechung zur operation bifurkationsnaher trachealgeschwülste. *Schweiz Med Wochenschr* 1961;91: 957–960.

120. Adkins PC, Izawa EM. Resection of tracheal cylindroma using cardiopulmonary bypass. *Arch Surg* 1964;88:405–409.

121. Neville WE, Langston HT, Correll N, et al. Cardiopulmonary bypass during pulmonary surgery. Preliminary report. *J Thorac Cardiovasc Surg* 1965;50:265–276.

122. Crastnopol P, Platt N, Phillips WR, et al. Resection of solitary tracheal papilloma using cardiopulmonary bypass. *N Y State J Med* 1967;67:1166–1169.

123. Horita K, Itoh T, Furukawa K, et al. Carinal reconstruction under veno-venous bypass using a percutaneous cardiopulmonary bypass system. *Thorac Cardiovasc Surg* 1996;44:46–49.

124. Louhimo I, Leijala M. Cardiopulmonary bypass in tracheal surgery in infants and small children. *Prog Pediatr Surg* 1987;21: 58–63.

125. Geffin B, Bland J, Grillo HC. Anesthetic management of tracheal resection and reconstruction. *Anesth Analg* 1969;48: 884–890.

126. Mathisen DJ, Grillo HC. Carinal resection for bronchogenic carcinoma. *J Thorac Cardiovasc Surg* 1991;102:16–22; discussion 22–23.

127. Jensen V, Milne B, Salerno T. Femoral-femoral cardiopulmonary bypass prior to induction of anaesthesia in the management of upper airway obstruction. *Can Anaesth Soc J* 1983;30: 270–272.

128. Cooley DA, Beall AC Jr, Alexander JK. Acute massive pulmonary embolism. Successful surgical treatment using temporary cardiopulmonary bypass. *JAMA* 1961;177:283–286.

129. Rosenberg DM, Schmidt R, Warren S, et al. Partial circulatory

support in massive pulmonary embolism. *Ann Thorac Surg* 1966;2:217–225.

130. Beall AC Jr, Cooley DA. Use of cardiopulmonary bypass for resuscitation and treatment of acute massive pulmonary embolism. *Pacific Med Surg* 1967;75:67–70.

131. Sautter RD. The technique of pulmonary embolectomy with the use of cardiopulmonary bypass. *J Thorac Cardiovasc Surg* 1967;53:268–274.

132. Garcia JB, Barankay A, Grimshaw VA, et al. Pulmonary embolectomy using heart–lung bypass. Report of successful case. *J Cardiovasc Surg* 1969;10:165–171.

133. Sasahara AA. Clinical studies in pulmonary thromboembolism. In: Sasahara AA, ed. *Pulmonary embolic disease.* New York: Grune & Stratton, 1965.

134. Del Campo C. Pulmonary embolectomy: a review. *Can J Surg* 1985;28:111–113.

135. Greenfield LJ. Catheter pulmonary embolectomy [Editorial; Comment]. *Chest* 1991;100:593–594.

136. Kleny R, Charpentier A, Kleny MT. What is the place of pulmonary embolectomy today? *J Cardiovasc Surg* 1991;32:549–554.

137. de Hoyos A, Demajo W, Snell G, et al. Preoperative prediction for the use of cardiopulmonary bypass in lung transplantation. *J Thorac Cardiovasc Surg* 1993;106:787–796.

138. Lee BS, Sarnquist FH, Starnes VA. Anesthesia for bilateral single-lung transplantation. *J Cardiothorac Vasc Anesth* 1992;6:201–203.

139. Baumgartner WA, Traill TA, Cameron DE, et al. Unique aspects of heart and lung transplantation exhibited in the "domino-donor" operation. *JAMA* 1989;261:3121–3125.

140. Adachi H, Ueda K, Koyama I, et al. Donor core cooling for multiple organ retrieval: new application of portable cardiopulmonary bypass for transplantation. *Transplant Proc* 1989;21:1200–1202.

141. Shuman RL. Primary pulmonary sarcoma with left atrial extension via left superior pulmonary vein. *En bloc* resection and radical pneumonectomy on cardiopulmonary bypass. *J Thorac Cardiovasc Surg* 1984;88:189–192.

142. Murphy JP, Adyanthaya AV, Adams PR, et al. Peripheral pulmonary artery aneurysm in a patient with limited respiratory reserve: controlled resection using cardiopulmonary bypass. *Ann Thorac Surg* 1987;43:323–325.

143. Hall KD, Friedman M. Extracorporeal oxygenation for induction of anesthesia in a patient with an intrathoracic tumor. *Anesthesiology* 1975;42:493–495.

144. Bricker DL, Parker TM, Dalton ML Jr. Cardiopulmonary bypass in anesthetic management of resection. Its use for severe tracheal stenosis. *Arch Surg* 1979;114:847–849.

145. Maharaj RJ, Whitton I, Blyth D. Emergency extracorporeal oxygenation for an intratracheal foreign body. *Anaesthesia* 1983;38:471–474.

146. Yamazaki M, Sasaki R, Masuda A, et al. Anesthetic management of complete tracheal disruption using percutaneous cardiopulmonary support system. *Anesth Analg* 1998;86:998–1000.

147. Mellema JD, Bratton SL, Inglis A Jr, et al. Use of cardiopulmonary bypass during bronchoscopy following sand aspiration. A case report. *Chest* 1995;108:1176–1177.

148. Seard C, Wasserman K, Benfield JR, et al. Simultaneous bilateral lung lavage (alveolar washing) using partial cardiopulmonary bypass. *Am Rev Respir Dis* 1970;101:877–884.

149. Zapol WM, Wilson R, Hales C, et al. Venovenous bypass with a membrane lung to support bilateral lung lavage. *JAMA* 1984;251:3269–3271.

150. Moazam F, Schmidt JH, Chesrown SE, et al. Total lung lavage for pulmonary alveolar proteinosis in an infant without the use of cardiopulmonary bypass. *J Pediatr Surg* 1985;20:398–401.

151. Heymach GJD, Shaw RC, McDonald JA, et al. Fiberoptic bronchopulmonary lavage for alveolar proteinosis in a patient with only one lung. *Chest* 1982;81:508–510.

152. Øvrum E, Birkeland S. Mediastinal tumours and cysts. A review of 91 cases. *Scand J Thorac Cardiovasc Surg* 1979;13:161–168.

153. Simpson I, Campbell PE. Mediastinal masses in childhood: a review from a paediatric pathologist's point of view. *Prog Pediatr Surg* 1991;27:92–126.

154. Morrissey B, Adams H, Gibbs AR, et al. Percutaneous needle biopsy of the mediastinum: review of 94 procedures. *Thorax* 1993;48:632–637.

155. Pullerits J, Holzman R. Anaesthesia for patients with mediastinal masses. *Can J Anaesth* 1989;36:681–688.

156. van der Hulst VP, Henny CP, Moulijn AC, et al. Veno-venous bypass without systemic heparinization using a centrifugal pump: a blind comparison of a heparin-bonded circuit versus a non–heparin-bonded circuit. *J Cardiovasc Surg* 1989;30:118–123.

157. Shaw BW Jr, Martin DJ, Marquez JM, et al. Advantages of venous bypass during orthotopic transplantation of the liver. *Semin Liver Dis* 1985;5:344–348.

158. Memsic L, Quinones-Baldrich W, Kaufman R, et al. A comparison of porcine orthotopic liver transplantation using a venous-venous bypass with and without a nonpulsatile perfusion pump. *J Surg Res* 1986;41:33–40.

159. Prager MC, Gregory GA, Ascher NL, et al. Massive venous air embolism during orthotopic liver transplantation. *Anesthesiology* 1990;72:198–200.

160. Paulsen AW, Whitten CW, Ramsay MA, et al. Considerations for anesthetic management during veno-venous bypass in adult hepatic transplantation. *Anesth Analg* 1989;68:489–496.

161. Demling RH, Hicks RE, Edmunds LH Jr. Changes in extravascular lung water during venovenous perfusion. *J Thorac Cardiovasc Surg* 1976;71:291–294.

162. Wall WJ, Grant DR, Duff JH, et al. Liver transplantation without venous bypass. *Transplantation* 1987;43:56–61.

163. Ringe B, Bornscheuer A, Blumhardt G, et al. Experience with veno-venous bypass in human liver transplantation. *Transplant Proc* 1987;19:2416.

164. Persson NH, Brown M, Goldstein R, et al. Inferior mesenteric vein cannulation for veno-venous bypass during liver transplantation: alternative access in difficult hilar dissection. *Transplant Proc* 1990;22:174.

165. Bismuth H, Castaing D, Garden OJ. Major hepatic resection under total vascular exclusion. *Ann Surg* 1989;210:13–19.

166. Bergan JJ, Yao JS, Flinn WR, et al. Surgical treatment of venous obstruction and insufficiency. *J Vasc Surg* 1986;3:174–181.

167. Miller CM, Schwartz ME, Nishizaki T. Combined hepatic and vena caval resection with autogenous caval graft replacement. *Arch Surg* 1991;126:106–108.

168. Kieffer E, Bahnini A, Koskas F. Nonthrombotic disease of the inferior vena cava: surgical management of 24 patients. In: Bergan JJ, ed. *Venous disorders.* Philadelphia: WB Saunders, 1991:501–516.

169. Murphy JP Jr, Gregoric I, Cooley DA. Budd-Chiari syndrome resulting from a membranous web of the inferior vena cava: operative repair using profound hypothermia and circulatory arrest. *Ann Thorac Surg* 1987;43:212–214.

170. Launois B, de Chateaubriant P, Rosat P, et al. Repair of suprahepatic caval lesions under extracorporeal circulation in major liver trauma. *J Trauma* 1989;29:127–128.

171. Ryan JF, Donlon JV, Malt RA, et al. Cardiopulmonary bypass in the treatment of malignant hyperthermia. *N Engl J Med* 1974;290:1121–1122.

172. Yasui RK, Culclasure TF, Kaufman D, et al. Flecainide overdose: is cardiopulmonary support the treatment? *Ann Emerg Med* 1997;29:680–682.

173. Kugelberg J, Schuller H, Berg B, et al. Treatment of accidental hypothermia. *Scand J Thorac Cardiovasc Surg* 1967;1:142–146.

174. Hauty MG, Esrig BC, Hill JG, et al. Prognostic factors in severe accidental hypothermia: experience from the Mt. Hood tragedy. *J Trauma* 1987;27:1107–1112.

175. White JD. Hypothermia: the Bellevue experience. *Ann Emerg Med* 1982;11:417–424.

176. Duguid H, Simpson RG, Stowers JM. Accidental hypothermia. *Lancet* 1961;2:1213–1219.

177. Walpoth BH, Walpoth-Aslan BN, Mattle HP, et al. Outcome of survivors of accidental deep hypothermia and circulatory arrest treated with extracorporeal blood warming. *N Engl J Med* 1997;337:1500–1505.

178. Lazar HL. The treatment of hypothermia. *N Engl J Med* 1997;337:1545–1547.

179. Shields CP, Sixsmith DM. Treatment of moderate-to-severe hypothermia in an urban setting. *Ann Emerg Med* 1990;19:1093–1097.

180. Kennedy JH, Barnette J, Flasterstein A, et al. Experimental barbiturate intoxication: treatment by partial cardiopulmonary bypass and hemodialysis. *Cardiovasc Res Center Bull* 1976;14:61–68.

181. Fell RH, Gunning AJ, Bardhan KD, et al. Severe hypothermia as a result of barbiturate overdose complicated by cardiac arrest. *Lancet* 1968;1:392–394.

182. Gutierrez-Perry L, Boland JP, Burke A, et al. Under deep hypothermia, circulatory arrest. Repair of traumatic arteriovenous fistula of the aortic arch. *W V Med J* 1987;83:219–221.

183. Griffin LH Jr, Fishback ME, Galloway RF, et al. Traumatic aortorenal vein fistula: repair using total circulatory arrest. *Surgery* 1977;81:480–483.

184. Anagnostopoulos CE, Kabemba JM, Stansel HC Jr. Control of a bleeding intercostal aneurysm with the aid of partial pump–oxygenator bypass. *Ann Thorac Surg* 1969;8:358–360.

185. Fletcher JP, Klineberg PL, Hawker FH, et al. Arteriovenous fistula following lumbar disc surgery—the use of total cardio-pulmonary bypass during repair. *Aust N Z J Surg* 1986;56:631–633.

186. Milligan NS, Edwards JC, Monro JL, et al. Excision of giant haemangioma in the newborn using hypothermia and cardio-pulmonary bypass. *Anaesthesia* 1985;40:875–878.

187. Mulliken JB, Murray JE, Castaneda AR, et al. Management of a vascular malformation of the face using total circulatory arrest. *Surg Gynecol Obstet* 1978;146:168–172.

188. Stormont TJ, Bilhartz DL, Zincke H. Pitfalls of "bench surgery" and autotransplantation for renal cell carcinoma. *Mayo Clin Proc* 1992;67:621–628.

189. Creech O, Krementz ET, Ryan RF, et al. Chemotherapy of cancer: regional perfusion utilizing an extracorporeal circuit. *Ann Surg* 1958;148:616–632.

190. Kessler RE, Amadeo JH, Tice DA, et al. Extracorporeal filtration of schistosomes in unanesthetized man. *Surg Forum* 1970;21:378–380.

34

PERFUSION FOR THORACIC AORTIC SURGERY

JOSEPH S. COSELLI
SCOTT A. LEMAIRE
STEVE A. RASKIN

The three major segments of the thoracic aorta require different perfusion techniques to prevent ischemic complications. The ascending aortic segment begins at the aortic valve annulus and ends just proximal to the origin of the innominate artery. The transverse aortic arch is the segment from which the three brachiocephalic branches arise. Perfusion techniques for these first two segments often overlap—therefore, they are considered together as proximal aortic operations. The thoracoabdominal, or distal, aortic segment extends from just beyond the left subclavian artery to the aortoiliac bifurcation.

PROXIMAL AORTIC OPERATIONS

Selection of Technique

Conventional cardiopulmonary bypass (CPB) is used for nonemergent operations limited to the ascending aortic segment. In the setting of aneurysm rupture or acute dissection, however, hypothermic circulatory arrest (HCA) is routinely used. Although acute proximal aortic dissection can be repaired without circulatory arrest, this technique eliminates the need for distal aortic clamping. The "open" distal anastomosis technique, originally advocated by Cooley and Livesay in 1981 (1), avoids clamp injury of the fragile dissecting membrane, allows identification of tears within the transverse arch, and facilitates assessment of the aortic arch diameter. Circulatory arrest also is used when graft replacement of the transverse aortic arch is performed. To optimize cerebral protection during HCA, retrograde cerebral perfusion is used as an adjunct whenever possible.

Cardiopulmonary Bypass

Oxygenated blood is returned to the patient from the CPB circuit through an arterial cannula placed in either the as-

cending aorta or the femoral artery. The size of the cannula is chosen to minimize the pressure gradient across the cannula at the patient's calculated flow rate, which is based on a standard index of 2.2 to 2.4 L/min per square meter (m^2) body surface for adults at normothermic temperatures. The minimum size of the cannula is then determined by the smallest cannula that will provide the calculated flow rate with a gradient of less than 100 mm Hg (2).

After an aortic cannula is inserted, it is connected to the circuit tubing as the perfusionist slowly advances perfusate through the CPB systemic flow line to facilitate air removal at the connection. Femoral cannulas are initially attached to the tubing and then inserted into the artery with the same technique. After a femoral arterial cannula is placed, reverse flow is briefly allowed to ensure unimpeded return. Poor arterial return into the cannula during this maneuver is an indication of a proximal arterial obstruction and is a situation that requires repositioning of the cannula.

Venous cannulation is accomplished with use of a cavoatrial (dual-stage) cannula, bicaval cannulas, or a combination of femoral venous and superior vena caval (SVC) cannulas. The latter approach is routinely used in hemodynamically unstable patients who require pump support before sternotomy and is particularly useful in patients who are at risk for aortic injury during sternotomy. This includes patients undergoing reoperations and those with large ascending aortic aneurysms abutting the sternum. In these situations, the femoral cannulas are placed before sternotomy and the SVC is cannulated after the chest is opened.

In addition to the arterial and venous cannulas, a left ventricular sump cannula is inserted through a purse-string suture placed at the junction of the right superior pulmonary vein and the left atrium. The sump minimizes preload, prevents ventricular distension, reduces myocardial rewarming, prevents ejection of air, and facilitates exposure of the aortic valve. An in-line pressure relief valve is located between the sump cannula and a roller pump; the pump returns the vented blood to the CPB circuit via the cardiotomy

J. S. Coselli, S. A. LeMaire, and S. A. Raskin: Department of Surgery, Baylor College of Medicine, Houston, Texas 77030.

reservoir. Because inadequate suction will allow ventricular distension and excess suction can cause ventricular collapse and injury, the degree of sump suction must be constantly regulated by the perfusionist (3).

Myocardial protection is achieved by means of systemic hypothermia and a combination of antegrade and retrograde cardioplegia. The use of these complementary techniques optimizes myocardial protection by facilitating adequate delivery of cardioplegic solution to all areas of the heart. We use a one-pass cardioplegia delivery system to administer 4°C blood–crystalloid (4:1) cardioplegia. The retrograde cardioplegia cannula is inserted into the coronary sinus after venous cannulation; this avoids dislodgement of the coronary sinus cannula during positioning of the venous cannula in the inferior vena cava (IVC). Antegrade cardioplegia is delivered either through an aortic cannula placed proximal to the aortic cross-clamp or directly into each of the coronary ostia after the aorta is opened.

Hypothermic Circulatory Arrest with Retrograde Cerebral Perfusion

Since the first successful replacement of an aortic arch in 1957 by DeBakey and associates (4), various methods of cerebral protection have been devised, including direct cannulation of all three brachiocephalic arteries. A major advance in cerebral protection occurred with the popularization of HCA by Griepp and associates in 1975 (5). Soon thereafter, Crawford and Saleh (6) adopted this technique and demonstrated its efficacy in reducing morbidity and mortality. Additionally, HCA provides a bloodless operative field uncluttered by brachiocephalic clamps, cannulas, and tourniquets. However, some investigators have reported that HCA is neither completely safe nor satisfactory in meeting cerebral metabolic demands. Separate canine studies by Nojima et al. (7) and Mezrow et al. (8) indicated that significant cerebral metabolic activity occurs at temperatures used routinely for the initiation of HCA; this activity promotes cerebral ischemia and the accumulation of metabolic waste products (9,10). Clinically, these observations are supported by the findings of Takamoto and associates (11), who reported O_2 extraction of 88.5% and CO_2 production of 71.1% during retrograde cerebral perfusion (RCP) at a rectal temperature of 15°C in 11 subjects. The protective limits of HCA were further defined in 1993 by Svensson et al. (12), who reported Crawford's experience with 656 patients who underwent HCA during surgical repair of proximal aortic disease. The overall incidence of transient or permanent stroke was 7%, and early mortality was 10%. When the HCA time exceeded 40 minutes, however, a high incidence of perioperative neurologic complications resulted; similarly, HCA for longer than 65 minutes was associated with a dramatic increase in mortality.

Retrograde cerebral perfusion was first described in 1980 by Mills and Ochsner (13) as a method for treating massive air embolism during CPB. Two years later, Lemole et al.

(14) described the use of intermittent RCP for the repair of proximal aortic dissection. Continuous RCP during circulatory arrest was introduced by Ueda et al. in 1990 (15,16). The theoretical advantages of RCP over HCA alone include more homogeneous cerebral cooling; washout of air bubbles, embolic debris, and metabolic waste products; prevention of cerebral blood cell microaggregation; and delivery of O_2 and nutritional substrates to brain tissue (17,18). These factors may extend the "safe period" of circulatory arrest.

Although experimental data regarding the efficacy of cerebral protection via RCP are conflicting (19–25), clinical data support its use. RCP has contributed to the improving results of surgery on the ascending and transverse aortic arch. A study of 14 patients by Takamoto and associates (11) demonstrated that RCP affords significant protection from neurologic injury, evidenced by early postoperative awakening, the absence of cerebral infarcts on postoperative computed tomograms, and the absence of abnormalities on postoperative electroencephalograms (EEG) in 11 patients. In addition, Takamoto et al. noted significant levels of cerebral CO_2 production and O_2 consumption even at rectal temperatures of 15°C, which suggests that the oxygenated blood of RCP assists in meeting cerebral metabolic demands. Kitamura et al. (26) recently reported an early survival of 95.8% and a 3-year survival of 91.7% in 24 patients who underwent repair of proximal aortic dissections with HCA and RCP; none of these patients suffered strokes. By retrospective analysis, the Tokyo group demonstrated significant improvements in both early and long-term survival when RCP was used, in comparison with operations performed either without cerebral perfusion techniques or with antegrade cerebral perfusion. Additionally, their report suggested that HCA with RCP facilitates a more complete aortic resection, thereby reducing the risk for subsequent rupture of residual aneurysm distal to the graft. The retrospective analysis of Usui and associates (27) of the Japanese experience with RCP in 228 patients suggests that RCP extends the "safe period" of circulatory arrest up to 60 minutes, after which the risk for stroke rises markedly.

Although cerebral ischemia may be reduced by RCP, prolonged elevated venous pressures associated with the retrograde flow may lead to cerebral edema. Nojima and colleagues (7) demonstrated that during RCP with pressures of 20 mm Hg, 48% of regional cerebral blood flow is maintained at an aerobic level and cerebral water content does not increase significantly over baseline. Usui and associates (17) demonstrated that cerebral blood flow is maximized at RCP pressures of 25 mm Hg. Together, these studies suggest that the optimal RCP pressure is in the range of 20 to 25 mm Hg.

Technique

The closed system CPB circuit includes a soft, collapsible venous reservoir that prevents air from entering the system

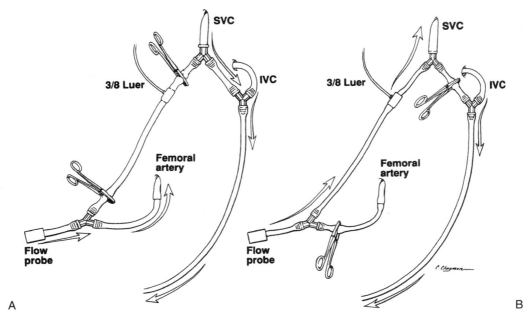

FIG. 34.1. Perfusion setup for hypothermic circulatory arrest with use of femoral artery and bicaval cannulation. During cardiopulmonary bypass and cooling (**A**), venous drainage is achieved via the superior (*SVC*) and inferior (*IVC*) vena caval cannulas. At initiation of circulatory arrest, clamps are repositioned (**B**) to allow flow of oxygenated blood into the SVC in a retrograde direction. (From Ensign RG, Sowel SA, Raskin SA. Marfan syndrome: diagnosis and replacement of the aortic arch utilizing retrograde cerebral perfusion. *Perfusion* 1993;8:377–383, with permission.)

and overflow spillage during exsanguination. The system includes a large cardiotomy reservoir and a cardiotomy return line with a bifurcation spike that allows removal of large amounts of blood from the system during the exsanguination period. The circuit also includes an oxygenator with a high-efficiency-coefficient heat exchanger, a cardiotomy filter, a hemoconcentrator, 1/2-in venous tubing, a 3/8-in bifurcated arterial line, and a high-efficiency cooling/heating unit for temperature control. One limb of the bifurcated arterial line is attached to the SVC cannula via a Y-connector. In addition to the SVC cannula, a second venous cannula drains either the IVC (Fig. 34.1) or the femoral vein (Fig. 34.2). A flow probe located between the arterial filter and the arterial bifurcation allows accurate measurement of blood flow through the arterial line during CPB and through the RCP line during HCA. A centrifugal pump is used to reduce the possibility of generating inadvertently high perfusion pressures during RCP.

The CPB priming fluid consists of approximately 2,100 mL of lactated Ringer's solution (based on the patient's body surface area), 25 of mannitol (100 mL), 5,000 U porcine heparin, 10 g aminocaproic acid, and 2 g of magnesium sulfate. When aprotinin is substituted for aminocaproic acid, it is given by the low Hammersmith method. After a test dose is given to the patient, 1 million kallikrein inhibitory units (KIU) of aprotinin is added to the prime and

an infusion of 500,000 KIU/hr is delivered by anesthesia personnel throughout the case.

Safe performance of HCA requires careful monitoring of several temperatures throughout the procedure. This includes the patient's nasopharyngeal and core (bladder or rectal) temperatures. In the perfusion circuit, the temperatures of the arterial blood at the oxygenator outlet, the venous blood before it enters the venous reservoir, and the water for the heat exchanger unit are all monitored.

In addition to standard hemodynamic parameters, we routinely measure the RCP pressure directly via a pressure line connected to a stopcock in the 3/8-in tubing. A 10-channel EEG is used to monitor brain wave activity. The development of electrocerebral silence on the EEG indicates that adequate cerebral cooling has been achieved and circulatory arrest can be initiated. In the setting of aortic dissection, intraoperative transesophageal echocardiography is extremely useful for assessing aortic valve competency before and after resuspension is performed.

Blood gas analyses are performed before the onset of CPB, before circulatory arrest, 10 to 15 minutes after bypass is resumed, and every 30 minutes thereafter. Acid–base status is managed by the alpha-stat strategy (28,29). The target blood gas values include a P_aO_2 between 300 and 600 mm Hg, a P_aCO_2 between 35 and 45 mm Hg, and a pH between 7.35 and 7.45. During

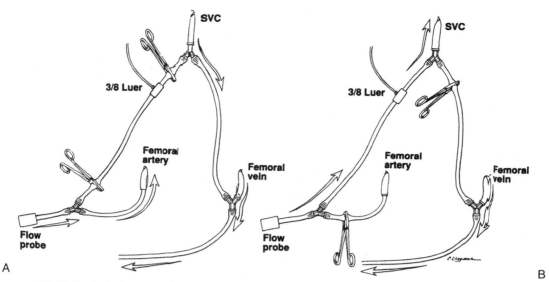

FIG. 34.2. Perfusion setup for hypothermic circulatory arrest with use of femoral–femoral arteriovenous cannulation and subsequent placement of a superior vena caval (*SVC*) cannula. During cardiopulmonary bypass and cooling (**A**), venous drainage is achieved via the SVC and femoral venous cannulas. At initiation of circulatory arrest, clamps are repositioned (**B**) to allow flow of oxygenated blood into the SVC in a retrograde direction. (From Ensign RG, Sowel SA, Raskin SA. Marfan syndrome: diagnosis and replacement of the aortic arch utilizing retrograde cerebral perfusion. *Perfusion* 1993;8:377–383, with permission.)

CPB, the activated clotting time (ACT) is kept above 480 seconds at all times. If aprotinin is to be used, the ACT is kept above 760 seconds by using celite tubes. The hematocrit is deliberately diluted to a range of 18% to 21% to prevent sludging of the blood during HCA and RCP. Coagulation abnormalities associated with HCA generally necessitate administration of fresh-frozen plasma and platelets. Platelet counts of 100,000 to 150,000/mm³ and fibrinogen levels of 150 to 200 mg/dL are targeted in the immediate post-bypass period (30).

Aortic perfusion is provided through a cannula placed either in the femoral artery or in the ascending aorta (Figs. 34.3 and 34.4). The former is well suited for cases of acute dissection or rupture, in which the proximal aorta is too fragile to allow safe cannulation. However, in most cases of elective surgery for chronic dissection or stable aneurysm, direct cannulation of the ascending aorta is a safe and effective alternative. When femoral artery cannulation is used in the setting of aortic dissection, careful attention is required to ensure cannulation of the true lumen. Because the false lumen usually progresses down the left iliac artery, the right femoral artery is preferentially used. Poor backward flow into the arterial cannula during a brief reverse flow test may indicate cannulation of the false lumen; to prevent retrograde malperfusion, the cannula should be repositioned before bypass is initiated. Cannulation of the axillary or subclavian arteries is another option that is particularly useful in patients with contraindications to aortic and femoral cannulation, such as coexisting acute proximal aortic dissection and iliofemoral arterial occlusive disease (31).

Whenever possible, venous blood returning to the right side of the heart is drained by gravity to the CPB reservoir via an SVC cannula in combination with either an IVC cannula (bicaval) or a femoral venous cannula. In the setting of cardiac reoperations, however, a single dual-stage (cavoatrial) venous cannula is often required (2,3). The major disadvantage of the single venous cannula is the inability to use RCP. For this reason, bicaval cannulation is the preferred technique. Total CPB is achieved by placing heavy tapes or caval clamps around each cava and its cannula to divert all venous return to the pump, thereby reducing hemorrhage into the operative field and preventing premature rewarming of the heart (2). A retrograde cardioplegia catheter is often placed into the coronary sinus to assist with providing myocardial protection during the early rewarming phase.

Cardiopulmonary bypass is initiated and a left ventricular sump catheter is placed via the right superior pulmonary vein. This is especially important in patients who are prone to ventricular distension, such as those with aortic valve insufficiency. Ventricular distension can also result from fibrillation caused by systemic hypothermia. To prevent this complication, therefore, the sump is generally placed before systemic cooling is begun. Immediately after the initiation of CPB in patients with a femoral arterial cannula, particularly those with aortic dissection, the possibility of malperfu-

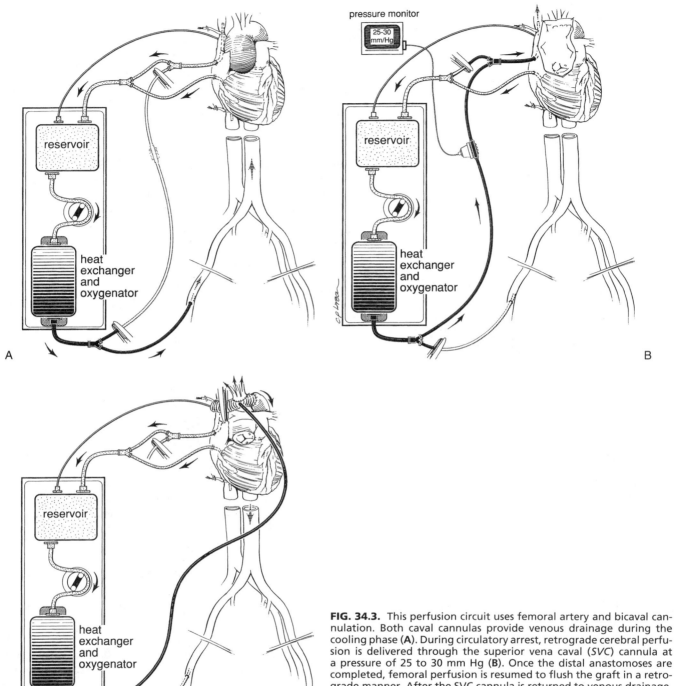

A

B

C

FIG. 34.3. This perfusion circuit uses femoral artery and bicaval cannulation. Both caval cannulas provide venous drainage during the cooling phase (**A**). During circulatory arrest, retrograde cerebral perfusion is delivered through the superior vena caval (*SVC*) cannula at a pressure of 25 to 30 mm Hg (**B**). Once the distal anastomoses are completed, femoral perfusion is resumed to flush the graft in a retrograde manner. After the SVC cannula is returned to venous drainage, the 3/8-in tubing between the arterial line and SVC cannula is cut and used to cannulate the clamped graft, thereby providing antegrade perfusion while the aortic valve and proximal anastomosis are addressed (**C**).

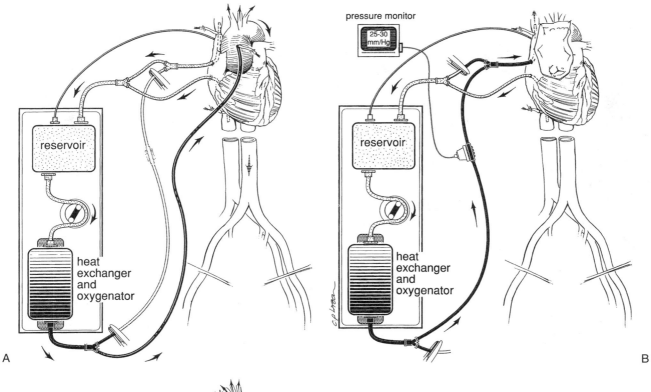

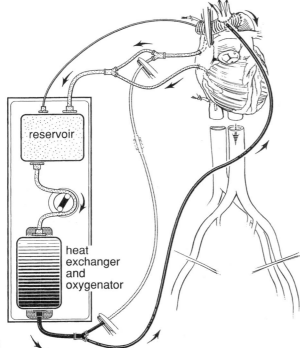

FIG. 34.4. As an alternative to femoral arterial cannulation, the ascending aorta can be directly cannulated for arterial return during the cooling phase (**A**). Once circulatory arrest is initiated, retrograde cerebral perfusion (*RCP*) is provided through the superior vena caval (*SVC*) cannula, the aortic cannula is removed, and the aorta is opened (**B**). After the distal anastomoses are completed, the aortic cannula is placed into the graft and the SVC cannula is returned to venous drainage, which restores antegrade perfusion for the remainder of the procedure (**C**).

sion must be investigated. Any evidence of malperfusion requires cannulation of an axillary or subclavian artery to restore perfusion of the true lumen.

Once systemic cooling has begun, each decrease of 10°C in body temperature reduces the rate of O_2 consumption by about 50%. As the temperature and metabolic rate decrease, pump flows are reduced to 1.6 to 1.8 L/min per square meter. In addition, for every decrease of 10°C in core temperature, there is a 20% to 25% increase in blood viscosity (32,33). In the past, and before the use of hemodilution perfusion, substantial morbidity (e.g., stroke and visceral infarction) and mortality were related to hypothermia-induced hyperviscosity. Currently, patients are routinely hemodiluted to a hematocrit of 20% to 30% until the reconstruction is completed, at which time rewarming and hemoconcentration are initiated. Although hemodilution decreases the O_2-carrying *capacity*, overall O_2 *delivery* is improved because decreased viscosity allows improved microcirculatory flow.

During the initial period of CPB and cooling, the 3/8-in arterial line to the SVC cannula is clamped to provide flow from the bicaval or SVC/femoral vein cannulas to the aorta or femoral artery (Figs. 34.3A and 34.4A). Rapid cooling is continued until the EEG (at an instrument sensitivity of 2 mV/mm) demonstrates the absence of cerebral electrical activity (28,30,34). This state of electrocerebral silence generally takes 20 to 25 minutes to achieve and occurs when brain temperature reaches 18° to 20°C (28,35). When EEG is not available, cooling for at least 25 minutes with a target core temperature of 18° to 20°C is recommended.

After an adequate cooling period, the patient is placed in extreme Trendelenburg position, the CPB systemic flow line is clamped, and the centrifugal pump head is slowed to 800 revolutions per minute (rpm) to prevent a backward flow of blood down the arterial line. The clamp occluding the 3/8-in RCP line to the SVC is then removed slowly, and hypothermic (8°C) retrograde blood flow is initiated through the line (Figs. 34.3B and 34.4B). The number of rpm is increased, and the blood flow is maintained at a rate of 200 to 300 mL/min; flows are not allowed to exceed 500 mL/min. The RCP pressure, measured at the SVC/RCP line connection, is kept at or below 25 to 30 mm Hg. The patient is allowed to exsanguinate into the venous and cardiotomy reservoirs to provide a bloodless field (28). If the ascending aorta had been cannulated, the cannula is removed.

The aorta is opened and blood flowing retrograde from the great vessels into the arch is collected and returned via the pump suctions. Based on the extent of repair needed, the end of the Dacron graft is sewn to the proximal descending thoracic aorta, the transverse arch, or the distal ascending aorta. On completion of the distal anastomoses, RCP is stopped. The RCP line is then clamped, venous drainage via the SVC/IVC or SVC/femoral vein is reestablished, and flow through the arterial line is resumed. After the graft is flushed and checked for anastomotic leaks, a cross-clamp is placed on the graft. If an ascending aortic cannula was used during cooling, the same cannula may now be inserted into an incision in the side of the graft (Fig. 34.4C); the cannula is secured with a purse-string suture. If the femoral artery was the original cannulation site, the RCP line may be clamped and cut. The graft is then cannulated with a 20 French (F) aortic cannula attached to the RCP line with a 3/8 × 3/8-in connector (Fig. 34.3C). This technique eliminates the problem of retrograde malperfusion from the femoral cannula.

The patient is returned to a horizontal position, and rewarming commences for the remainder of the procedure, which is focused on the proximal portion of the aortic reconstruction. The water temperature of the cooler/heater is set at 30°C. During this portion of the procedure, topical myocardial cooling and intermittent retrograde or antegrade cardioplegia protect the heart. Myocardial preservation is achieved by directly infusing cold, dilute, hyperkalemic blood–cardioplegic solution (4:1) into the right and left main coronary arteries. In patients undergoing reoperations or those with extensive coronary disease, retrograde cardioplegia is utilized. When the temperature reaches 28°C, warming is stopped, and this temperature is maintained if the proximal repairs are not yet complete. When the repair is nearly finished, the set cooler/heater water temperature is increased to 40°C and rewarming continues. The patient is warmed to a rectal temperature of 37°C; cardiac function is then reestablished (28). The period of rewarming generally requires 60 to 70 minutes to reach this point. In the setting of valve repair, the bypass flow is reduced, and transesophageal echocardiography is used to determine whether valve leaflet coaptation and function are normal before the separation from bypass is completed. In the event of significant valve dysfunction, the patient is recooled and the appropriate reconstruction performed.

Results

Since January 1987, 767 consecutive patients have undergone surgical repair of ascending aortic or transverse aortic arch pathology by the senior author. HCA was used in 596 of these patients (77.7%). Of the HCA patients, 321 (53.9%) had aneurysms without dissection, 114 (19.1%) had acute dissection, and 161 (27%) had chronic dissection. Thirty-seven patients (6.2%) had Marfan syndrome. RCP—in routine use since May 1991—was applied in 347 cases (58.2%), and HCA was used without RCP in 249 cases (41.8%). The non-RCP group had a higher prevalence of rupture, chronic aortic dissection, and diabetes in comparison with the RCP group. The patients in the RCP group had a higher incidence of aortic valvular insufficiency.

Among the 596 patients who underwent proximal aortic surgery with HCA, there were seven (1.2%) intraoperative deaths; these seven patients were excluded from the analysis regarding neurologic complications. Overall 30-day and in-hospital survival rates were 91.9% and 90.8%, respectively. The 30-day mortality rate was 5.2% (18 of 347) in the RCP group and 12.1% (30 of 249) in the non-RCP group ($p = 0.002$). Postoperative strokes occurred in 27 patients overall (4.6%). Stroke rates were 3.5% (12 of 347) in the RCP group versus 6.2% (15 of 249) in the non-RCP group ($p = 0.122$). Cardiac complications were less common in the RCP group (38 of 347, or 11.0%) than in the non-RCP group (42 of 249, or 16.9%; $p = 0.037$). Subgroup analysis revealed that patients with aortic dissection had the greatest benefit from RCP with respect to early mortality; reductions in stroke rates were present in each RCP subgroup, but no difference reached statistical significance. An additional analysis confirmed a strong association between stroke and early mortality. Long-term survival was also improved in patients who underwent HCA with RCP; actuarial 3-year survival rates were 83.5% for the RCP group and 68.2% for the non-RCP group ($p = 0.0001$).

DISTAL AORTIC OPERATIONS

Selection of Technique

The extent of aortic replacement required during distal thoracic aortic operations ranges from a short graft limited to a few centimeters of the descending thoracic aorta to a graft that spans the entire thoracoabdominal aorta from the left subclavian artery to the aortoiliac bifurcation. The central issue in terms of limiting perioperative morbidity and mortality is the prevention of distal ischemia during aortic cross-clamping. Ischemic injuries involving the spinal cord, kidneys, and other abdominal viscera often have catastrophic consequences. The risk for ischemic morbidity generally increases as the extent of repair increases. The selection of perfusion techniques, therefore, is also based on the extent of aneurysm (Fig. 34.5). Additional factors that increase the

risk for ischemic complications, such as acute dissection and preexisting renal insufficiency, must also be considered carefully as the operative strategy is planned.

It must be emphasized that the prevention of postoperative paraplegia, paraparesis, and renal failure does not rest on perfusion techniques alone. Our strategy includes moderate heparinization, permissive mild hypothermia, sequential aortic clamping, and aggressive reattachment of critical intercostal arteries (T-8 to L-1). For, renal protection, 600 to 800 mL of 4°C lactated Ringer's solution, augmented with 12.5 g of mannitol and 125 mg of methylprednisolone per liter, can be instilled into the renal artery origins via balloon perfusion catheters. When this multimodality strategy is used consistently, ischemic complications following less extensive repairs (i.e., descending thoracic aortic aneurysms and extents III and IV thoracoabdominal aortic aneurysms) are fortunately rare. Therefore, perfusion techniques are not used for less extensive repairs unless other risk factors are present. The surgical treatment of extensive thoracoabdominal aortic aneurysms (extents I and II), however, warrants the use of left-sided heart bypass based on extent alone.

In two specific situations, we use HCA during distal aortic operations: (a) when concomitant graft repair of transverse aortic arch pathology is needed, and (b) when proximal control with a cross-clamp cannot be safely achieved because of rupture or severe atheromatous debris. The largest experience with HCA for spinal cord protection during descending thoracic and thoracoabdominal aortic operations was recently reported by Rokkas and Kouchoukos (36). In their series of 96 consecutive patients, the St. Louis group reported a 30-day mortality rate of 7.3% and a 3.3% incidence of paraplegia or paraparesis. In other contemporary reports, however, early mortality rates range from 14.3% to 33.3% and paraplegia rates range from 7.1% to 14.3% (37–43). Intrapulmonary bleeding, adult respiratory distress syndrome, and other pulmonary complications have remained a major source of morbidity and mortality (37,43,44). Despite the protective effect of profound hypothermia against spinal cord ischemia, the additional risks incurred with CPB and HCA in this setting argue against its routine use.

Left-sided Heart Bypass and Selective Visceral Perfusion

The goal of left-sided heart bypass (LHB) is to provide perfusion to the segment of aorta that is distal to the cross-clamp. This results in shorter ischemic times, which translates into a reduction in ischemic complications. Several reports (45–51) advocate the use of LHB to minimize spinal cord ischemia during thoracoabdominal aortic aneurysm repair. Conclusions regarding its role in this setting, however, have been difficult to substantiate because of several common limitations: failure to report data for descending tho-

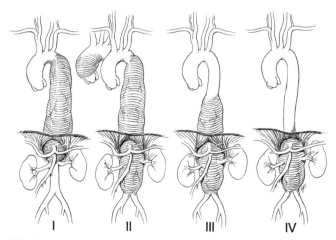

FIG. 34.5. Crawford's classification of thoracoabdominal aortic aneurysm extent.

racic and thoracoabdominal aortic aneurysms separately; lack of comparative data for LHB and non-LHB patients; and limited information regarding thoracoabdominal aortic aneurysm extent and the presence of dissection or rupture, which are critical factors in the evaluation of a study population's risk for paraplegia (52). Two recent retrospective comparative studies, however, do suggest a potential benefit to using LHB during repair of extensive thoracoabdominal aortic aneurysms. The 1995 report by Bavaria et al. (53) demonstrated substantial reduction in postoperative neurologic deficits in 26 patients who survived operations with LHB; statistical significance was not achieved, however, because of the sample size. More recently, Safi et al. (54) demonstrated a similar decrease in paraplegia rates with LHB; this benefit was statistically significant in patients with extent II thoracoabdominal aortic aneurysms. Unfortunately, both studies also used cerebral spinal fluid drainage in the LHB groups; therefore, clear conclusions regarding the individual benefits of either adjunct are difficult to support.

Technique

The bypass circuit is composed of an inflow and an outflow cannula, 3/8-in polyvinylchloride tubing, and a centrifugal pump. No reservoir or heat exchanger is incorporated into the circuit. For selective visceral/renal perfusion, balloon perfusion catheters are connected to the return limb with use of a three-way, large-bore, high-flow stopcock (Fig. 34.6). Although intravenous heparin is not necessary when a centrifugal pump is used for LHB, we routinely administer 100 U of heparin per kilogram to maintain patency of the small intercostal and spinal arteries. Proximal cannulation for LHB can be achieved by directly cannulating the left atrial appendage after the pericardium is opened. Alternatively, the left atrium can be accessed via either of the left pulmonary veins without opening the pericardium; this option is especially useful in patients who have undergone a previous cardiac operation. In either location, a 3-0 polypropylene mattress suture with Teflon felt pledgets and a Rumel tourniquet are used to secure a 26F right-angled aortic cannula. For distal cannulation, standard femoral arterial cannulation (Fig. 34.6) is often used. Cannulation of the distal descending thoracic or abdominal aorta (Fig. 34.7), however, also provides reliable distal perfusion while eliminating the need for a groin incision and femoral arteriotomy. Preoperative imaging studies (i.e., computed tomography and magnetic resonance imaging) are used to select a site without extensive mural thrombus. A 3-0 polypropylene suture with Teflon felt pledgets is placed at the selected location, and a 20F right-angled aortic cannula is inserted into the aorta. During extensive thoracoabdominal aortic aneurysm repairs that may require prolonged visceral and renal ischemic times, selective visceral/renal perfusion is often used. This is achieved by placing 9F balloon perfusion

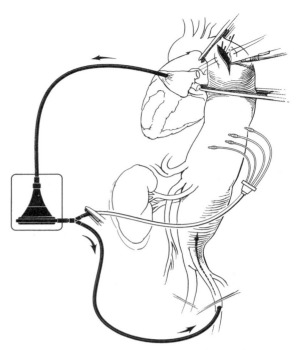

FIG. 34.6. Atriofemoral left-sided heart bypass with use of a centrifugal pump during extensive thoracoabdominal aortic aneurysm repair provides distal aortic perfusion during the proximal anastomosis, thereby reducing spinal and visceral ischemic times. The balloon perfusion cannulas arising from the return line (*right*) allow selective renal and visceral perfusion during the intercostal and visceral arterial reattachment procedure.

catheters into the ostia of the celiac, renal, and superior mesenteric arteries (55). The catheters are attached to the circuit via a stopcock in the arterial limb of the bypass circuit (55) (Fig. 34.6). To prevent retrograde flow on initiation of LHB, the pump is started at 1,000 rpm before the clamp on the perfusion loop is slowly removed. Distal aortic perfusion is conducted at a rate of 1.5 L to 2.5 L/min, with careful attention paid to maintaining a mean proximal aortic pressure near 70 mm Hg and a mean pulmonary artery pressure of 20 mm Hg. The patient's core temperature is allowed to fall 3° to 4°C to achieve mild hypothermia; a heat exchanger is not used to maintain normothermia or rewarm the patient.

After the proximal anastomosis is completed, the distal clamp is either sequentially moved down the aorta or LHB is discontinued entirely and the distal clamp removed. The aneurysm is then opened to its distal extent. For patients with extent II thoracoabdominal aortic aneurysms, selective visceral/renal perfusion is applied during intercostal, visceral, and renal artery reattachment. By clamping the outflow tube, selective visceral/renal bypass via the left atrium is provided. The tips of the four balloon irrigation catheters are inserted into the celiac axis, superior mesenteric artery, and both renal arteries. Although the perfusion rate to each

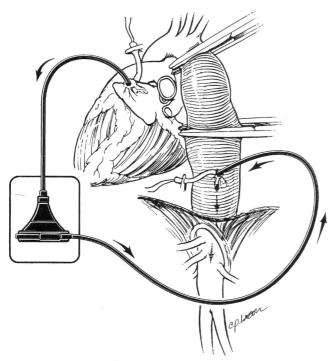

FIG. 34.7. As an alternative to femoral artery cannulation, the distal descending thoracic aorta can be cannulated for left-sided heart bypass during thoracoabdominal aortic aneurysm repair.

vessel is not controlled independently, a total delivery of 400 mL/min to the four branches is effective in preventing critical ischemic damage. This simple method dramatically reduces major organ ischemic time.

Results

Of 710 consecutive patients who underwent repair of extensive thoracoabdominal aortic aneurysms (extents I and II) between January 1986 and March 1998, 49 (6.9%) presented with rupture, 38 (5.4%) had acute dissection, and 205 (28.9%) had chronic dissection. Eleven patients (1.5%) who had preoperative paraplegia or paraparesis were excluded from calculations regarding postoperative neurologic deficits. The overall 30-day and in-hospital survival rates were 94.8% (673 patients) and 91.8% (652 patients), respectively. There were four (0.6%) intraoperative deaths; these patients were excluded when the postoperative morbidity rates were calculated. Paraplegia or paraparesis developed in 42 patients (6.0%), renal failure in 75 patients (10.6%), and bleeding complications in 17 (2.4%).

In 312 (43.9%) cases, LHB was used; 398 (56.1%) operations were performed without this adjunct. In separate analyses for extents I and II repairs, the patients in the LHB and non-LHB groups had similar predicted risks, which supports the validity of the comparison. In patients who underwent extent I repairs, there were no significant differences in outcome between the groups; paraplegia rates were similar (3.7% without LHB vs. 4.9% with LHB). Although LHB did not reduce the paraplegia rate in extent I patients, the incidence did remain stable despite a significantly longer aortic clamp time in the LHB group. Therefore, by reducing intercostal ischemic time, LHB appears to allow the aorta to be clamped safely for longer periods of time. Among the patients with extent II thoracoabdominal aortic aneurysms, the incidence of paraplegia was strikingly lower in the LHB patients (4.8% vs. 13.1%; $p = 0.007$). This marked reduction in paraplegia in extent II patients who underwent repair with LHB was achieved despite significantly longer aortic clamp times. The frequencies of all other complications, including early mortality, were similar between the two groups.

In a comparison of the patients who underwent LHB via femoral arterial cannulation (122 of 312, or 39.1%) with those who had distal aortic cannulation (190 of 312, or 60.9%), both groups were at similar risk for postoperative paraplegia based on aneurysm extent, acute dissection, and rupture. There were no significant differences in early mortality, paraplegia, paraparesis, or stroke. Interestingly, and for unclear reasons, acute renal failure was less common in the distal aortic cannulation group; there were no differences in preoperative risk factors such as age, renal insufficiency, and renal arterial occlusive disease to explain this difference. There were no cases of retrograde dissection in either group and no differences in femoral thromboembolism, limb ischemia, wound infections, or graft infections, all of which were rarely encountered. Of course, the use of distal aortic cannulation eliminated groin wound complications, which occurred in 4.1% of the femoral cannulation group.

SUMMARY

In closing, the use of modified CPB techniques as outlined herein has afforded surgeons more control, protected vital organs, and resulted in improved morbidity and mortality rates in this challenging patient population.

KEY POINTS

- Conventional CPB is used for nonemergent operations limited to repair of the ascending aorta.
- CPB with HCA is used for ruptured aortic aneurysm or acute dissection involving the proximal aorta.
- Depending on patient pathophysiology and surgical objectives, arterial blood is returned from the CPB circuit via a cannula placed in the ascending aorta or femoral artery.
- Unrestricted patency between the CPB systemic flow

line and the patient's arterial system should be ensured by momentarily observing reverse flow after placement of the arterial cannula.

- Venous cannulation for CPB is accomplished by placement of a cavoatrial cannula, bicaval cannulas, or a combination of femoral venous and SVC cannulas.

- A left ventricular sump should be inserted in the left atrium to (a) minimize preload, (b) prevent ventricular distension, (c) reduce myocardial rewarming, (d) prevent cardiac ejection of air, and (e) facilitate aortic valve exposure.

- Antegrade and retrograde blood cardioplegia is routinely used to provide myocardial protection.

- Continuous RCP during HCA was introduced by Ueda in 1990 and has the following potential advantages: (a) more homogeneous cerebral cooling; (b) washout of air bubbles, embolic debris, and metabolic waste products; (c) prevention of cerebral blood cell microaggregation; and (d) delivery of O_2 and nutritive substrates to the brain.

- Cerebral blood flow during RCP is optimized by maintaining a pressure of approximately 25 mm Hg in the SVC.

- RCP is accomplished by incorporation of a Y-connector in the CPB arterial line; one limb is for conventional CPB systemic blood flow, and the other is used for connection to the SVC cannula during HCA.

- During RCP with HCA, temperatures should be monitored in the following: nasopharynx and bladder or rectum, arterial perfusate, venous blood, and heat exchanger water source.

- The development of electrocerebral silence on the EEG (with instrument sensitivity of 2 mV/mm) indicates adequate cerebral cooling for induction of HCA.

- During distal thoracic operations, limiting ischemia of the spinal cord, kidneys, and other abdominal viscera is important to minimize perioperative morbidity and mortality.

- The goal of LHB is to provide perfusion to the segment of aorta that is distal to the cross-clamp.

- The LHB circuit consists of outflow and inflow cannulas (placed in the left atrium and distal aorta or femoral artery, respectively), tubing, and a centrifugal pump; no oxygenator, reservoir, or heat exchanger is required.

- During LHB, the distal aortic perfusion flow is 1.5 to 2.0 L/min; a mean proximal aortic pressure near 70 mm Hg and a mean pulmonary artery pressure of 20 mm Hg are maintained.

- During extensive repair of the thoracoabdominal aorta, selective visceral or renal perfusion is accomplished by placing 9F balloon perfusion catheters into ostia of the celiac axis and renal and superior mesenteric arteries.

REFERENCES

1. Cooley DA, Livesay JJ. Technique of "open" distal anastomosis for ascending and transverse arch resection. *Cardiovasc Dis Bull Tex Heart Inst* 1981;8:421–426.
2. High KM, Williams DR, Kurusz M. Cardiopulmonary bypass circuits and design. In: Hensley FH, Martin DE, eds. *A practical approach to cardiac anesthesia* 2nd ed. Boston: Little, Brown, 1995:466–481.
3. Hessel EA. Cardiopulmonary bypass circuitry and cannulation techniques. In: Gravlee GP, Davis RF, Utley JR, eds. *Cardiopulmonary bypass: principles and practice.* Baltimore: Williams & Wilkins, 1993:55–92.
4. DeBakey ME, Crawford ES, Cooley DA, et al. Successful resection of fusiform aneurysm of aortic arch with replacement by homograft. *Surg Gynecol Obstet* 1957;105:657–664.
5. Griepp RB, Stinson EB, Hollinsworth JF, et al. Prosthetic replacement of the aortic arch. *J Thorac Cardiovasc Surg* 1975;70: 1051–1063.
6. Crawford ES, Saleh SA. Transverse aortic arch aneurysm: improved results of treatment employing new modifications of aortic reconstruction and hypothermic cerebral arrest. *Ann Surg* 1981;194:180–188.
7. Nojima T, Magara T, Nakajima Y, et al. Optimum perfusion pressure for experimental retrograde cerebral perfusion. *J Cardiovasc Surg* 1994;9:548–559.
8. Mezrow CK, Midulla PS, Sadeghi AM, et al. Evaluation of cerebral metabolism and quantitative electroencephalography after hypothermic circulatory arrest and low-flow cardiopulmonary bypass at different temperatures. *J Thorac Cardiovasc Surg* 1994; 107:1006–1019.
9. Joyce JW, Fairbairn JF, Kincaid OW, et al. Aneurysms of the thoracic aorta: a clinical study with special reference to prognosis. *Circulation* 1964;29:176–181.
10. Campbell DE, Raskin SA. Cerebral dysfunction after cardiopulmonary bypass: etiology, manifestations and interventions. *Perfusion* 1990;10:51–57.
11. Takamoto S, Matsuda T, Harada M, et al. Simple hypothermic retrograde cerebral perfusion during aortic arch surgery. *J Cardiovasc Surg* 1992;33:560–567.
12. Svensson LG, Crawford ES, Hess KR, et al. Deep hypothermia with circulatory arrest: determinants of stroke and early mortality in 656 patients. *J Thorac Cardiovasc Surg* 1993;106:19–31.
13. Mills NL, Ochsner JL. Massive air embolism during cardiopulmonary bypass: causes, prevention, and management. *J Thorac Cardiovasc Surg* 1980;80:708–717.
14. Lemole GM, Strong MD, Spagna PM, et al. Improved results for dissecting aneurysms: intraluminal sutureless prosthesis. *J Thorac Cardiovasc Surg* 1982;83:249–255.
15. Ueda Y, Miki S, Kusuhara K, et al. Surgical treatment of aneurysm or dissection involving the ascending aorta and aortic arch using circulatory arrest and retrograde cerebral perfusion. *J Cardiovasc Surg* 1990;31:553–558.
16. Ueda Y, Miki S, Kusuhara K, et al. Deep hypothermic systemic circulatory arrest and continuous retrograde cerebral perfusion for surgery of aortic arch aneurysm. *Eur J Cardiothorac Surg* 1992; 6:36–41.
17. Usui A, Hotta T, Hiroura M, et al. Retrograde cerebral perfusion through a superior vena caval cannula protects the brain. *Ann Thorac Surg* 1992;53:47–53.
18. Ergin MA, Griepp EB, Lansman SL, et al. Hypothermic circulatory arrest and other methods of cerebral protection during operations on the thoracic aorta. *J Card Surg* 1994;9:525–537.
19. Pagano D, Boivin CM, Faroqui MH, et al. Retrograde perfusion through the superior vena cava perfuses the brain in human beings. *J Thorac Cardiovasc Surg* 1996;111:270–272.

20. Safi HJ, Iliopoulos DC, Gopinath SP, et al. Retrograde cerebral perfusion during profound hypothermia and circulatory arrest in pigs. *Ann Thorac Surg* 1995;59:1107–1112.

21. de Brux JL, Subayi JB, Pegis JD, et al. Retrograde cerebral perfusion: anatomic study of the distribution of blood to the brain. *Ann Thorac Surg* 1995;60:1294–1298.

22. Imamaki M, Koyanagi H, Hashimoto A, et al. Retrograde cerebral perfusion with hypothermic blood provides efficient protection of the brain: a neuropathological study. *J Card Surg* 1995; 10:325–333.

23. Boeckxstaens CJ, Flameng WJ. Retrograde cerebral perfusion does not perfuse the brain in nonhuman primates. *Ann Thorac Surg* 1995;60:319–328.

24. Juvonen T, Zhang N, Wolfe D, et al. Retrograde cerebral perfusion enhances cerebral protection during prolonged hypothermic circulatory arrest: a study in a chronic porcine model. *Ann Thorac Surg* 1998;66:38–50.

25. Bavaria JE, Pochettino A. Retrograde cerebral perfusion (RCP) in aortic surgery: efficacy and possible mechanisms of brain protection. *Semin Thorac Cardiovasc Surg* 1997;9:222–232.

26. Kitamura M, Hashimoto A, Akimoto T, et al. Operation for type A dissection: introduction of retrograde cerebral perfusion. *Ann Thorac Surg* 1995;59:1195–1199.

27. Usui A, Abe T, Murase M. Early clinical results of retrograde cerebral perfusion for aortic arch operations in Japan. *Ann Thorac Surg* 1996;62:94–104.

28. Coselli JS, Poli de Figueiredo LF. Surgical techniques for symptomatic aortic arch disease. In: Calligaro KD, ed. *Management of extracranial cerebrovascular disease*. Philadelphia: Lippincott–Raven Publishers, 1997:93–110.

29. Davis RF, Dobbs JL, Casson H. Conduct and monitoring of cardiopulmonary bypass. In: Gravlee GP, Davis RF, Utley JR, eds. *Cardiopulmonary bypass: principles and practice*. Baltimore: Williams & Wilkins, 1993:578–602.

30. Raskin SA, Fuselier VW, Reeves-Viets JL, et al. Deep hypothermic circulatory arrest with and without retrograde cerebral perfusion. In: Stammers AH, ed. Cardiopulmonary bypass: emerging trends and continued practices. *Int Anesthesiol Clin* 1996;34: 177–193.

31. Bichell DP, Balaguer JM, Aranki SF, et al. Axilloaxillary cardiopulmonary bypass: a practical alternative to femorofemoral bypass. *Ann Thorac Surg* 1997;64:702–705.

32. Cooper JR, Slogoff S. Hemodilution and priming solutions for cardiopulmonary bypass. In: Hensley FH, Martin DE, eds. *A practical approach to cardiac anesthesia*, 2nd ed. Boston: Little, Brown, 1995:124–137.

33. Rand PW, Lacombe E, Hunt HE, et al. Viscosity of normal human blood under normothermic and hypothermic conditions. *J Appl Physiol* 1964;19:117–122.

34. Coselli JS, Crawford ES, Beall AC Jr, et al. Determination of brain temperatures for safe circulatory arrest during cardiovascular operation. *Ann Thorac Surg* 1988;45:638–642.

35. Mizrahi EM, Patel VM, Crawford ES, et al. Hypothermic-induced electrocerebral silence, prolonged circulatory arrest, and cerebral protection during cardiovascular surgery. *Electroencephalogr Clin Neurophysiol* 1989;72:81–85.

36. Rokkas CK, Kouchoukos NT. Profound hypothermia for spinal cord protection in operations on the descending thoracic and thoracoabdominal aorta. *Semin Thorac Cardiovasc Surg* 1998;10: 57–60.

37. Szentpetery S, Crisler C, Grinnan GLB. Deep hypothermic arrest and left thoracotomy for repair of difficult thoracic aneurysms. *Ann Thorac Surg* 1993;55:830–833.

38. Kieffer E, Koskas F, Walden R, et al. Hypothermic circulatory arrest for thoracic aneurysmectomy through left-sided thoracotomy. *J Vasc Surg* 1994;19:457–464.

39. Stone CD, Greene PS, Gott VL, et al. Single-stage repair of distal aortic arch and thoracoabdominal dissecting aneurysms using aortic tailoring and circulatory arrest. *Ann Thorac Surg* 1994;57: 580–587.

40. Grabenwoger M, Erlich M, Simon P, et al. Thoracoabdominal aneurysm repair: spinal cord protection using profound hypothermia and circulatory arrest. *J Card Surg* 1994;9:679–684.

41. Ergin MA, Galla JD, Lansman SL, et al. Hypothermic circulatory arrest in operations on the thoracic aorta: determinants of operative mortality and neurologic outcome. *J Thorac Cardiovasc Surg* 1994;107:788–799.

42. Takamoto S, Okita Y, Ando M, et al. Retrograde cerebral circulation for distal aortic arch surgery through a left thoracotomy. *J Card Surg* 1994;9:576–583.

43. Safi HJ, Miller CC III, Subramaniam MH, et al. Thoracic and thoracoabdominal aortic aneurysm repair using cardiopulmonary bypass, profound hypothermia, and circulatory arrest via left side of the chest incision. *J Vasc Surg* 1998;28:591–598.

44. Crawford ES, Coselli JS, Safi HJ. Partial cardiopulmonary bypass, hypothermic circulatory arrest, and posterolateral exposure for thoracic aortic aneurysm operation. *J Thorac Cardiovasc Surg* 1987;94:824–827.

45. Frank SM, Parker SD, Rock P, et al. Moderate hypothermia, with partial bypass and segmental sequential repair for thoracoabdominal aortic aneurysm. *J Vasc Surg* 1994;19:687–697.

46. Schepens MA, Defauw JJ, Hamerlijnck RP, et al. Use of left heart bypass in the surgical repair of thoracoabdominal aortic aneurysms. *Ann Vasc Surg* 1995;9:327–338.

47. Kitamura M, Hashimoto A, Tagusari O, et al. Operation for type B aortic dissection: introduction of left heart bypass. *Ann Thorac Surg* 1995;59:1200–1203.

48. Hessmann M, Dossche K, Wellens F, et al. Surgical treatment of thoracic aneurysm: a 5-year experience. *Cardiovasc Surg* 1995; 3:19–25.

49. Griepp RB, Ergin MA, Galla JD, et al. Looking for the artery of Adamkiewicz: a quest to minimize paraplegia after operations for aneurysms of the descending thoracic and thoracoabdominal aorta. *J Thorac Cardiovasc Surg* 1996;112:1202–1215.

50. Morishita K, Inoue S, Baba T, et al. Our distal aortic perfusion system in descending thoracic and thoracoabdominal aortic aneurysm repairs. *Artif Organs* 1997;21:822–824.

51. Jacobs MJHM, de Mol BAJM, Legemate DA, et al. Retrograde aortic and selective organ perfusion during thoracoabdominal aortic aneurysm repair. *Eur J Vasc Endovasc Surg* 1997;14: 360–366.

52. Acher CW, Wynn MM, Hoch JR, et al. Combined use of cerebral spinal fluid drainage and naloxone reduces the risk of paraplegia in thoracoabdominal aortic aneurysm repair. *J Vasc Surg* 1994; 19:236–248.

53. Bavaria JE, Woo YJ, Hall RA, et al. Retrograde cerebral and distal aortic perfusion during ascending and thoracoabdominal aortic operations. *Ann Thorac Surg* 1995;60:345–353.

54. Safi HJ, Campbell MP, Miller CC III, et al. Cerebral spinal fluid drainage and distal aortic perfusion decrease the incidence of neurological deficit: the results of 343 descending and thoracoabdominal aortic aneurysm repairs. *Eur J Vasc Endovasc Surg* 1997; 14:118–124.

55. Coselli JS, LeMaire SA, Ledesma DF, et al. Initial experience with the Nikkiso centrifugal pump during thoracoabdominal aortic aneurysm repair. *J Vasc Surg* 1998;27:378–383.

CARDIOPULMONARY BYPASS FOR PORT-ACCESS CARDIAC SURGERY

GORDON R. HADDOW
JOHN M. TOOMASIAN
CHRISTINA T. MORA MANGANO

During the past two decades, improvements in endoscopic equipment and operative techniques have permitted the growth of minimally invasive surgical approaches to both general and thoracic procedures. Interest has evolved in applying these advances to cardiovascular surgery. It is hoped that minimally invasive techniques will decrease patient morbidity, reduce pain and scarring, and reduce the duration of short- and long-term recovery. In addition, reductions in intensive care or hospital lengths of stay may provide some cost benefit.

One approach to minimally invasive cardiac surgery is minimally invasive direct coronary artery bypass (MID-CAB). Coronary grafts are placed on the beating heart via a mini-thoracotomy, mini-sternotomy, or full sternotomy without the use of cardiopulmonary bypass (CPB). This technique has been widely described (1–3). Although the technique appears cost-effective, it is technically challenging for both the surgeon and anesthesiologist (4). Stabilization of the heart by mechanical or pharmacologic means is essential to performing a satisfactory anastomosis. Without the assistance of CPB, some coronary arteries are difficult to access, and intracardiac procedures are not possible. Although MIDCAB has been applied to large numbers of patients, the long-term patency of the coronary grafts completed on a "beating heart" remains unknown.

Other approaches to minimally invasive cardiac surgery retain CPB support but permit smaller incisions, such as a mini-sternotomy or mini-thoracotomy. These techniques allow both epicardial and intracardiac procedures to be conducted, either on a fibrillating or protected heart. Port-Access* cardiac surgery (PACS) is a minimally invasive approach that provides cardiopulmonary support while permitting both antegrade and retrograde approaches to the delivery of myocardial protective solutions.

In 1993, Peters (5) first proposed a system of peripheral endovascular CPB in which a multiple-orifice catheter system provided aortic occlusion. Although no working prototype was ever evaluated, this proposal paved the way for the current PACS system. The components of the endovascular catheter system provide three principal functions (6,7): (a) peripheral vascular access for cardiopulmonary support, (b) myocardial protection/arrest with antegrade or retrograde cardioplegia, and (c) ventricular decompression via an aortic root vent or pulmonary artery vent.

Initial testing of the PACS platform in a canine model demonstrated that placing an internal mammary artery-to-coronary artery graft could be accomplished on an arrested protected heart during total CPB (8–11). In canine experiments, investigators replaced the mitral valve and demonstrated similar reductions in myocardial temperature in PACS and conventional treatment groups (12–14).

After it had been demonstrated that the Port-Access platform was feasible, experiments were extended to human cadaver studies and then to a series of patients (11,15–17). Results from these clinical trials were satisfactory, although performing coronary artery bypass grafts with endoscopic equipment proved technically so difficult that this approach was abandoned in favor of a mini-thoracotomy. To date, the PACS platform has been used for a variety of cardiac procedures, including multiple-vessel coronary artery bypass grafting, mitral valve replacements and repairs, closure of atrial septal defects, and combined procedures.

G. R. Haddow and **C. T. Mora Mangano:** Department of Anesthesia, Stanford University Medical Center, Stanford, California 94305.

J. M. Toomasian: Perfusion Services, Stanford University Medical Center, Stanford, California 94305.

* Port-Access is a registered trademark of Heartport, Inc., Redwood City, CA. Port-Access and EndoDirect are trademarks of Heartport, Inc.

TABLE 35.1. FREQUENTLY USED ABBREVIATIONS (IN ALPHABETICAL ORDER)

AVD	Assisted venous drainage
EAC	Endoaortic occlusion clamp
EARC	Endoarterial reinfusion cannula
ECSC	Endocoronary sinus retrograde cardioplegia catheter
EPV	Endopulmonary artery vent
EVD	Endovenous drainage cannula
KAVD	Kinetically-assisted venous drainage
MIDCAB	Minimally invasive direct coronary artery bypass
PACS	Port-access cardiac surgery
PAIR	Port-access international registry
TEE	Transesophageal echocardiography
VAVD	Vacuum-assisted venous drainage

ENDOVASCULAR CATHETER SYSTEM

The endovascular catheter system (EndoCPB system, Heartport, Redwood City, CA) consists of a specialized femoral endoarterial reinfusion cannula (EARC), an endovenous drainage cannula (EVD), an endoaortic occlusion clamp (EAC), an endocoronary sinus retrograde cardioplegia catheter (ECSC), and an endopulmonary artery vent (EPV). These and other frequently used abbreviations in this chapter are listed in Table 35.1.

The EARC is an extremely thin-walled, wire-wound femoral artery cannula [21(F) French or 23F] designed to accommodate both the shaft of the EAC and the arterial blood inflow from the heart–lung machine (Fig. 35.1). The inflow connection to the EARC contains a Y-connector. One side of the connector is attached to the arterial tubing from the heart–lung machine, and the opposite side accepts the EAC through a hemostatic valve. The EndoDirect aortic cannula, a variation of the EARC, permits cannulation of the ascending aorta under direct vision via a small incision in the upper thorax. The dilator incorporates a knife to incise the aorta. Because the latter device is placed directly into the ascending aorta, like a conventional aortic cannula, retrograde embolic phenomena or retrograde aortic dissec-

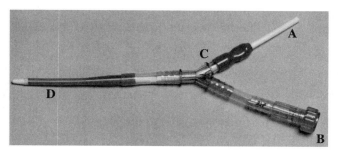

FIG. 35.1. Endoarterial return cannula. **A:** Dilator. **B:** Hemostatic valve for endoaortic clamp. **C:** Arterial return port. **D:** Wire-wound cannula with a soft tip. (Courtesy of Heartport, Inc., Redwood City, CA, with permission.)

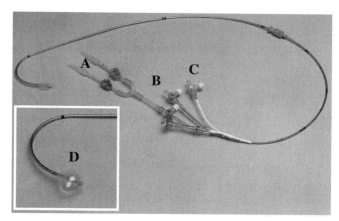

FIG. 35.2. Endoaortic clamp (*EAC*). **A:** Cardioplegia–aortic root vent port. **B:** Balloon inflation port. **C:** Aortic root pressure port. **D:** EAC occlusion balloon; note that it is eccentric in shape to keep the central lumen oriented correctly in the aorta. (Courtesy of Heartport, Inc., Redwood City, CA, with permission.)

tion should not occur. EAC migration is also possibly less likely.

The EVD (28F) is a long, thin-walled venous drainage cannula that couples with the venous tubing of the heart–lung machine. This cannula contains multiple side holes and is advanced into the right atrium via a femoral vein cut-down with fluoroscopic or transesophageal echocardiographic (TEE) guidance.

The EAC (10.5F) is an inflatable, polyurethane aortic occlusion balloon containing individual lumina that allow aortic occlusion, cardioplegia administration or aortic root venting, and aortic root pressure monitoring (Fig. 35.2). The EAC is passed through the lumen of the femoral artery cannula into the aorta and positioned in the ascending aorta by fluoroscopy or TEE.

It is essential that the EARC and the EAC be placed by means of a Seldinger wire technique with fluoroscopic assistance. The anesthesiologist uses TEE to confirm the correct intraluminal position of these wires in the descending aorta before the surgeon advances the cannulas. No resistance should be felt to the EARC or EAC during passage through the arterial system. This method of insertion is recommended to decrease the likelihood of vascular injury or retrograde aortic dissection.

In addition to antegrade delivery through the EAC, retrograde delivery of cardioplegia is possible through the ECSC (Fig. 35.3). The ECSC (9.0F) is inserted through an 11.5F jugular venous sheath and advanced into the coronary sinus with fluoroscopic or TEE guidance. Once positioned, the catheter is connected to cardioplegia delivery tubing. Manual inflation of the ECSC occlusion balloon facilitates the retrograde administration of cardioplegia.

The endopulmonary vent catheter (8.3F) returns blood not drained by the EVD to the CPB circuit (Fig. 35.4) and

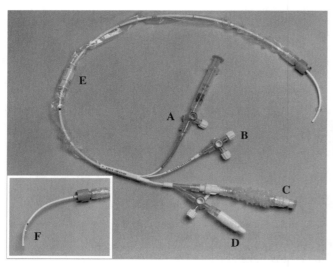

FIG. 35.3. Endocoronary sinus catheter (*ECSC*). **A:** Balloon inflation port. **B:** Coronary sinus pressure port. **C:** Steering stylet. **D:** Cardioplegia infusion port. **E:** Steering attachment. **F:** ECSC showing the inflation balloon and multiple-orifice soft catheter tip. (Courtesy of Heartport, Inc., Redwood City, CA, with permission.)

thus further decompresses the heart during CPB. The EPV, introduced via a second jugular venous sheath, has a 5F flow-directed balloon catheter that acts as a guide to position the catheter into the main pulmonary artery. Figure 35.5 diagrams the final positioning of all catheters.

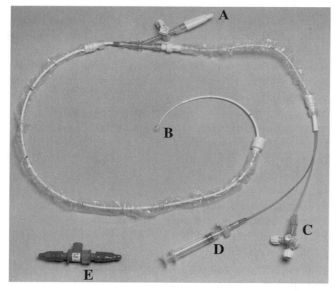

FIG. 35.4. Endopulmonary vent. **A:** Drainage port. **B:** Flotation guide catheter balloon. **C:** Flotation catheter pressure port. **D:** Balloon inflation port. **E:** Negative pressure relief valve. (Courtesy of Heartport, Inc., Redwood City, CA, with permission.)

INTERFACING THE ENDOVASCULAR CATHETERS AND THE CARDIOPULMONARY BYPASS CIRCUIT

Extracorporeal support for PACS adapts a cardiopulmonary circuit used for conventional cardiac procedures to the endovascular catheter system (Fig. 35.6). Individual pumps control arterial blood flow, cardioplegia delivery, pulmonary artery venting, aortic root venting, and cardiotomy suction. An additional pump is needed to augment venous return.

In integrating the endovascular catheter system to the heart–lung machine, the proximal end of the EAC is divided to accommodate the antegrade cardioplegia infusion line and the aortic root vent line (Fig. 35.2). The aortic root vent line contains a negative (-80 mm Hg) pressure relief valve that allows aortic root venting while precluding excessive negative pressure. Cardioplegia delivery and aortic root venting occur through the same lumen. The aortic root can be vented following cardioplegia infusion (if the heart has not been incised directly).

The EPV catheter is connected to 1/4-in internal diameter (ID) tubing containing a second negative (-80 mm Hg) pressure relief valve. The tubing is connected to a standard roller pump that aspirates blood from the pulmonary artery. A blood flowmeter placed between the EPV catheter and pressure relief valve directly measures the EPV blood flow.

In conventional CPB, right atrial drainage occurs through a large-bore cannula via a gravity siphon to an open or closed venous reservoir, after which blood is pumped through an integrated heat exchanger–membrane oxygenator and back into the arterial circulation. In the PACS system, gravity-assisted venous drainage is usually inadequate because the venous cannula is long and has a relatively small diameter.

Extrathoracic vascular cannulation has been widely used in long-term extracorporeal respiratory or cardiac life support (18,19), portable or emergency bypass for supported angioplasty (20), resuscitation from exposure hypothermia (21), surgical clipping of giant cerebral aneurysms (22,23), and cardiovascular rescue (24,25). The jugular vein, carotid artery, or femoral vessels are acceptable vascular access sites for connection to the heart–lung machine. Vascular access cannulas used for extrathoracic circulatory procedures are typically smaller and longer than standard right atrial cannulas, and some can be inserted percutaneously. Although this method of partial support for the circulation can be maintained for a prolonged period of time, total cardiopulmonary support via peripheral cannulas is difficult to achieve for sustained periods (26). Under optimal conditions with these techniques, gravity drains only 75% to 80% of the venous return to the heart. Unless the left ventricle is completely decompressed, the heart continues to eject blood. Thus, extrathoracic gravity-based venous drainage systems cannot reliably provide sufficient support to meet the pa-

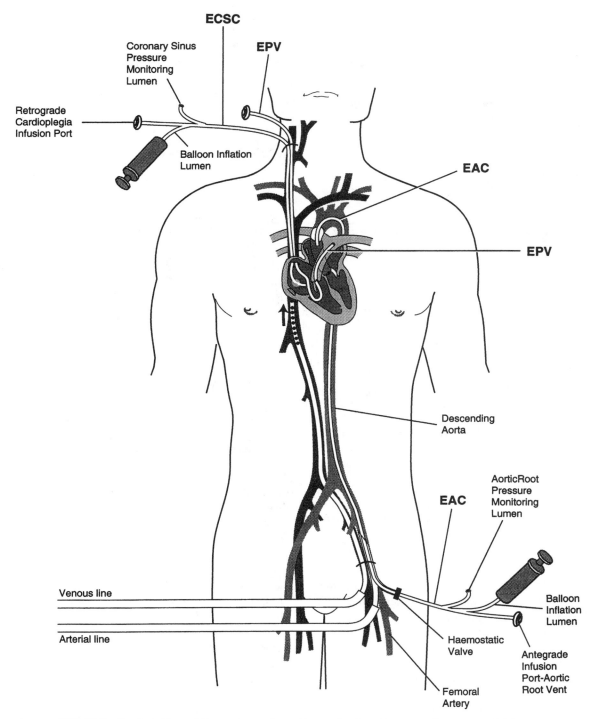

FIG. 35.5. Final position of the endovascular catheters for Port-Access cardiac surgery. EAC, endoaortic occlusion clamp; ECSC, endocoronary sinus retrograde cardioplegia catheter; EPV, endopulmonary artery vent. (From Toomasian JM, Peters WS, Siegel LC, et al. Extracorporeal circulation for Port-Access cardiac surgery. *Perfusion* 1997;12:83–93 with permission)

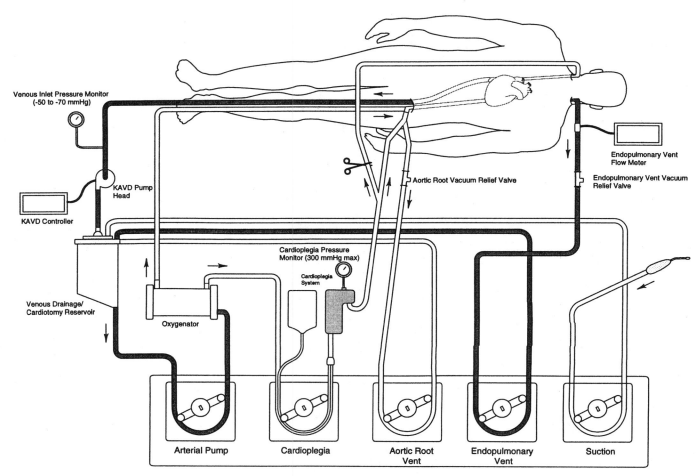

FIG. 35.6. Typical cardiopulmonary bypass circuit for Port-Access cardiac surgery. Note the use of kinetically assisted venous drainage. The bifurcated cardioplegia line allows for antegrade or retrograde cardioplegia delivery and aortic root venting. (Reproduced from the Heartport training manual, revision 1, Fig. 4.3, with permission.)

tient's O_2 requirements. Therefore, some form of augmented venous blood return must be considered to provide complete cardiopulmonary support.

Assisted venous drainage (AVD) enhances the drainage siphon to increase the venous blood flow to the heart–lung machine. A variety of methods are available to implement AVD, but two different techniques are widely used: kinetically-assisted venous drainage (KAVD) and vacuum-assisted venous drainage (VAVD).

Kinetically-assisted venous drainage utilizes a centrifugal or kinetic pump between the venous drainage cannula and the venous reservoir. The kinetic pump generates a siphon, which enhances venous return. This method improves venous drainage by 20% to 40% in comparison with a gravity siphon (27). With KAVD, venous blood is actively pumped into either an open or closed venous reservoir. The inertia of the kinetic pump regulates the siphon. As the pump speed is increased, more suction is generated. Monitoring pressure

in the venous conduit at a point proximal to the kinetic pump inlet assists the perfusionist in regulating the amount of siphon, which can be controlled manually or automatically (28). Excessive negative pressure can cause cavitation, blood trauma, and hemolysis. Excessive negative pressure can also cause the right atrium to collapse around the venous cannula, impeding venous return. KAVD has successfully supplemented venous return in PACS and in other cardiothoracic procedures (27,29).

The other form of assisted venous drainage, VAVD, utilizes a standard vacuum suction source to enhance venous return. Applying vacuum to an open (hard-shell) venous reservoir applies suction to the entire venous drainage system to increase venous return. VAVD requires close regulation of the vacuum source to avoid the negative pressure variations found in most hospital wall suction systems. Excessive VAVD negative pressures can cause blood trauma in addition to venous reservoir cracking or implosion. Step-down vacuum regulators maintain precise vacuum pressures. Positive and negative pressure relief valves must be incorporated into the reservoir to prevent both overpressure and underpressure and to ensure consistent extracorporeal flow rates. VAVD cannot be applied to closed systems utilizing a (soft-shell) venous reservoir bag.

Once venous blood has been collected into the venous reservoir, it is pumped sequentially through the oxygenator, heat exchanger, arterial tubing, and arterial cannula into the systemic arterial circulation by a standard roller pump. Conventional in-line blood gas sensors, monitors, blood filters, and other safety features (e.g., pressure and flow monitors, air detectors) are utilized just as they are in conventional CPB.

PATIENT SELECTION AND CONTRAINDICATIONS

A number of conditions preclude the use of PACS (Table 35.2). These conditions largely relate to the potential for vascular injury with the Port-Access system, difficulties in maintaining the correct catheter position, and the potential for retrograde embolization of particulate matter. Both preoperative screening and intraoperative TEE (and occasionally arteriography) identify patients who are inappropriate candidates for a PACS approach.

Peripheral vascular disease and aortic atheromatous disease predispose to retrograde embolization of atheromatous plaque and retrograde arterial dissection. The increased incidence of aortic dissection in the first group of patients managed with the Port-Access system initiated recommendations for patient screening, EAC and guidewire design changes, and modified insertion techniques. Tortuous femoral and iliac arteries, which make it very difficult to place the endovascular system, increase the risk for vascular injury. Thus, preoperative arterial screening is recommended for all patients with coronary artery disease (or risk factors for ischemic heart disease), age of 55 years or more, or weight of less than 60 kg. An aortoiliac run-off cineangiographic contrast study performed at the time of cardiac catheterization can fulfill this requirement. Alternatively, cross-sectional imaging (spiral computed tomography, magnetic resonance imaging) or angiography can be used. These latter tests, however, raise the cost of the procedure. The cardiologist should inform the surgical team of any problems encountered during catheterization, as this might lead the surgeon to cannulate the contralateral femoral vessels. At the time of operation, the anesthesiologist should examine the thoracic aorta (by TEE) for evidence of atheromatous disease, especially mobile plaque. Grades 3 to 5 atheromatous disease of the aorta is a contraindication to PACS. Because inflation of the EAC results in balloon pressures of 250 to 350 mm Hg, patients with an aortic aneurysm or conditions such as Marfan syndrome should not be considered for the PACS approach.

In the presence of aortic valvular incompetence, an increased stroke volume combined with exaggerated cyclical fluctuations in the proximal aortic blood flow make correct positioning of the EAC difficult. Aortic insufficiency also compromises the delivery of antegrade cardioplegia, which would tend to flow across the aortic valve into the left ventricle rather than into the coronary ostia. Although EAC inflation is possible with mild to moderate aortic incompetence, severe aortic insufficiency contraindicates PACS. Other contraindications to PACS include (a) conditions preventing the placement of a TEE probe (TEE is essential to the management of PACS), and (b) a persistent left superior vena cava draining into the coronary sinus (this may decrease drainage of the right side of the heart and prevent ECSC balloon occlusion of the coronary sinus). Relative contraindications include pleural scarring and obesity, both of which complicate surgical access.

PERFUSION MANAGEMENT DURING PORT-ACCESS CARDIAC SURGERY

Perfusion management during PACS utilizes conventional protocols for the perfusion flow rate, anticoagulation, temperature management, myocardial protection, and acid–base regulation. However, Port-Access CPB requires additional monitoring and instrumentation.

Gravity-dependent venous drainage initiates partial CPB. Once a stable blood flow is achieved, AVD is begun. The magnitude of the venous siphon is increased to a negative pressure of approximately -50 to -80 mm Hg, so a pressure transducer capable of measuring negative pressure is required. Siphon pressures more negative than -100 mm Hg can diminish the extracorporeal flow rate by causing the venous conduits to "chatter" or collapse.

Venous blood not drained by the EVD will be vented from the pulmonary circulation by the EPV, although the flow capacity of this catheter is limited rather substantially by its relatively small caliber and long length. The EPV pressure relief valve allows for a mixture of air and blood

TABLE 35.2. CONTRAINDICATIONS TO PORT-ACCESS CARDIAC SURGERY

Peripheral vascular disease
Aortic atheromatous disease (grades 3–5)
Aortic aneurysm
Conditions predisposing to aortic aneurysm (e.g., Marfan's syndrome)
Severe aortic valvular incompetence
TEE contraindicated, or inability to place TEE probe
Obesity (relative)
Pleural scarring (relative)

TEE, transesophageal echocardiography.

to be vented while preventing excessive negative pressures. A nonpulsatile arterial waveform accompanied by an EPV flow of less than 100 mL/min indicates that complete support has been achieved. In contrast to what occurs in conventional CPB, several minutes usually elapse before a steady state of extracorporeal circulation is established.

To facilitate EAC balloon inflation, the pump flow is reduced while full venous decompression is maintained in an effort to decrease the systemic pressure and keep the heart empty, which prevents left ventricular ejection against the EAC balloon as it is inflated. The EAC occlusion balloon is inflated with a mixture of contrast dye and saline solution (10% to 30%). Fluoroscopy or TEE should demonstrate EAC balloon inflation and occlusion of the ascending aorta. A small amount of contrast dye infused into the aortic root through the distal vent/cardioplegia lumen confirms proper balloon position. Following documentation of correct EAC positioning, the extracorporeal flow rate is gradually increased to normal levels. The EAC balloon pressure is continuously monitored after inflation (ideally 250 to 350 mm Hg). When systemic hypothermia is desired, it is usually initiated after inflation of the EAC to avoid any unintentional cold-induced ventricular fibrillation, although some clinicians prefer the onset of ventricular fibrillation before EAC balloon inflation, as the lack of ejection makes positioning easier.

With EAC inflation, cardioplegia solution can be infused antegrade or retrograde through the EAC cardioplegia–aortic root vent lumen or through the ECSC, respectively. During antegrade delivery, one must verify the pressure and pathway of the cardioplegic solution to avoid inadvertent cardioplegia recirculation down the aortic root vent line. The cardioplegia infusion pressure is measured continuously, and the line pressure should not exceed 350 mm Hg at a maximum cardioplegia flow rate of 250 to 300 mL/min. As the cardioplegia is infused into the EAC, the aortic root pressure may rise and create a pressure gradient of 20 to 40 mm Hg between the aortic root and distal aorta. Failure of the aortic root pressure to rise may indicate leakage across an incompetent aortic valve or a malpositioned EAC. Myocardial temperature can be measured directly by inserting a temperature probe into the myocardium.

Retrograde cardioplegia infusion begins at a low rate (50 mL/min) and is slowly increased to a flow rate of 100 to 250 mL/min. The infusion rate is carefully controlled to avoid excessive flow that can displace the ECSC or overpressurize the coronary sinus. The coronary sinus pressure should not exceed 40 mm Hg, but it will often exceed 30 mm Hg at peak flows during retrograde cardioplegia infusion.

Following cardioplegia infusion, the aortic root can be vented through the EAC aortic root lumen. The aortic root vent flow is initiated by slowly engaging the aortic root roller pump and monitoring the aortic root pressure. If the aortic root pressure is negative, the aortic root vent flow is reduced or discontinued because the potential exists for air to be entrained into the aortic root from a coronary arteriotomy or for the EAC to migrate toward the aortic valve. In most instances, the aortic root vent is not used for any procedure in which the heart is incised because it would principally aspirate air under such circumstances.

To deflate the EAC, the extracorporeal flow rate is decreased and the EAC balloon contents are aspirated into the inflation syringe. The aortic root is usually vented following deflation of the EAC. Following EAC deflation, blood flow to the coronary arteries is reestablished. As the patient warms to 37°C, the left ventricle is permitted to eject, ventilation is reestablished, aortic and pulmonary root venting is discontinued, and the EAC is withdrawn during a brief suspension of pump flow. Weaning from PACS CPB is similar to weaning from conventional CPB procedures. After the administration of protamine, all the Port-Access cannulas [other than the internal jugular introducer(s)] should be removed, including the EPV, which can be replaced with a traditional multilumen pulmonary artery catheter if desired.

Perfusion management is more complex and requires a greater number of monitors and instruments during PACS than during a traditional CPB procedure. In addition to monitoring of the usual perfusion parameters (e.g., arterial and central venous pressures, blood flow, venous reservoir volume, cardioplegia and circuit pressures), careful monitoring of the position and function of the endovascular catheters is required. Venous siphon pressure, endopulmonary and endoaortic root vent flows, EAC balloon pressure, and the relationship of the aortic root pressure and the systemic arterial pressure are all influenced by management of the heart–lung machine. Changes and manipulations to the circuit are often very subtle, and more time and more precise technique are required than in traditional CPB. Surges in systemic or cardioplegia flow can potentially dislodge the endovascular catheters, which require repositioning to prevent patient injury. Constant vigilance is therefore necessary to maintain proper function of the PACS system. Table 35.3 lists normal pressures and flows during Port-Access CPB.

MONITORING AND TROUBLESHOOTING

To ensure the safety and adequacy of perfusion during PACS, the surgical team (surgeon, anesthesiologist, and perfusionist) must monitor venous drainage, arterial inflow, cardioplegia, cardiac venting rates, aortic balloon occlusion, and cerebral perfusion. In addition, TEE and fluoroscopy are used to assess the unique aspects of Port-Access CPB (30,31). The nearly constant attendance of an anesthesiologist skilled in TEE is crucial to PACS management. In many centers, fluoroscopy is used primarily to aid placement of

TABLE 35.3. NORMAL FLOWS AND PRESSURE AND VOLUME MEASUREMENTS DURING PORT-ACCESS CARDIAC SURGERY

Aortic root pressure during	
Delivery of antegrade cardioplegia	60–80 mm Hg
Delivery of retrograde cardioplegia	0–20 mm Hg
Venting	0–10 mm Hg
Cardioplegia line pressure	<350 mm Hg
Coronary sinus pressure	20–40 mm Hg
Endocoronary sinus balloon inflation volume	0.5–2.0 mL
Endoaortic clamp balloon pressure	250–350 mm Hg
Endoaortic balloon clamp volume	20–35 mL
Endoaortic perfusion cannula line pressure	<350 mm Hg
Endopulmonary vent flow	
Initial phase	up to 250 mL/min
Maintenance phase (may increase during cardioplegia delivery)	<40 mL/min
Mean arterial pressure	40–70 mm Hg
Venous line inlet pressure	−40 to −80 mm Hg

From the *Heartport Training Manual,* Heartport, Inc., Redwood City, CA, with permission.

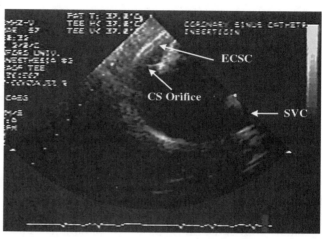

FIG. 35.7. Bicaval transesophageal echocardiography image of the endocoronary sinus catheter (*ECSC*) in position in the coronary sinus (*CS*) orifice. The image approximates a "bicaval" view, which is usually accomplished in an imaging plane of 90 to 110 degrees with use of a multiplane echocardiography probe. In this imaging plane, the inferior vena cava (not seen in this image) is often seen below and to the left of the CS orifice. The chamber separating the CS orifice and the superior vena cava (*SVC*) is the right atrium.

the ECSC and then held on "standby" for potential difficulties with the ECSC or EARC. Monitoring considerations unique to the Port-Access CPB system can be divided into two phases: (a) pre-bypass placement of the Port-Access CPB system, and (b) monitoring during bypass.

Monitoring Considerations for Catheter Insertion

The ECSC is usually the first catheter placed to avoid confusion with other catheters placed in the right atrium. TEE, either alone or combined with fluoroscopy, is utilized (32). A bicaval TEE view with the probe rotated slightly to the left at a viewing angle of 90 to 110 degrees will often bring the coronary sinus, both venae cavae, and the tricuspid valve into a plane, allowing the ECSC to be advanced into position (Fig. 35.7). Some anesthesiologists may prefer a standard horizontal view of the coronary sinus for placing the catheter. Fluoroscopy can also be used to orient the ECSC tip (Fig. 35.8). The injection of contrast dye through the ECSC confirms correct positioning of the catheter in the coronary sinus. Occlusive inflation of the ECSC balloon yields a characteristic pressure waveform that resembles a somewhat dampened right ventricular tracing. Experience appears to improve the success rate for ECSC placement. One group has reported a success rate exceeding 95% with a mean catheter placement time of 5.2 ± 3.5 minutes (33). However, some reports suggest a steep learning curve for this skill (34,35).

Although pressure monitoring is usually sufficient to

guide the EPV into the pulmonary artery, TEE, fluoroscopy, or both can be used in difficult cases. Successful placement of the EPV in the proximal pulmonary artery is more difficult than placement of a traditional, flow-directed, multilumen pulmonary artery catheter. Some practitioners be-

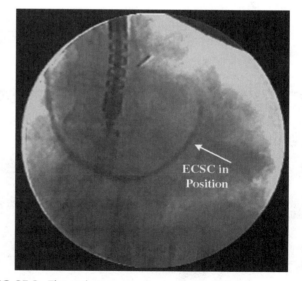

FIG. 35.8. The endocoronary sinus catheter (ECSC) in proper position as seen by fluoroscopy in an anteroposterior imaging plane. The transesophageal echocardiography probe is seen overlying the vertebral column at the top just to the left of the center of the photograph. (From the Heartport training video, Insertion of Endocoronary Sinus Catheter, Heartport, Inc., Redwood City, CA, with permission)

lieve that the EPV is not a very effective drain and that its use is not essential to successful PACS. Correct positioning is confirmed by a typical pulmonary artery pressure tracing or by TEE echocontrast injection.

Transesophageal echocardiography facilitates EVD placement. While the anesthesiologist monitors with TEE in the bicaval view, the surgeon advances the guidewire until it is located in the superior vena cava. The EVD should not be advanced if the guidewire is in either the right ventricle or the right atrial appendage, as cardiac perforation could occur. The EVD is advanced over the guidewire until the tip of the cannula is 1 to 2 cm above the junction of the right atrium and superior vena cava. This position generally achieves the best venous drainage.

Fluoroscopy and TEE aid placement of both the EARC and EAC. The aortic diameter at the sinotubular junction measured by TEE grossly indicates the balloon volume required for aortic occlusion. Before either of these cannulas is advanced, it is crucial to obtain TEE confirmation of the descending aortic intraluminal position of the guidewire. Any resistance to passing the guidewires or cannulas must be investigated before advancement is continued to prevent potential vascular damage. As visualized with TEE, the tip of the EAC should rest above the sinotubular ridge approximately 3 cm above the aortic valve (Fig. 35.9). Fluoroscopy and contrast dye injection through the aortic root vent can confirm the correct placement of the EAC either at this time or after EAC balloon inflation (Fig. 35.10).

Monitoring Considerations during Port-Access Cardiopulmonary Bypass

Venous Drainage

The adequacy of venous drainage is assessed by monitoring the AVD flow and pressure, central venous pressure, EPV

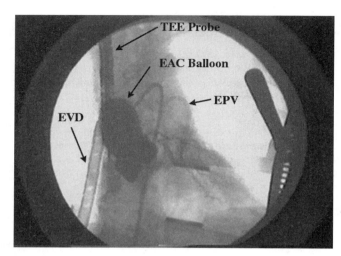

FIG. 35.10. A lateral-view fluoroscopic image (anterior is to the right) of the endoaortic clamp (*EAC*) in the correct position about 3 cm above the aortic valve. Note the flattened side walls of the balloon showing adequate contact with the aortic wall. Both the balloon and the aortic root are outlined by contrast, with the aortic valve located at the bottom of the torpedo-shaped contrast image. *TEE*, transesophageal echocardiography; *EVD*, endovenous drainage cannula; *EPV*, endopulmonary artery vent.

flow, arterial pressure waveform, cardiac chamber size, and oxygenator circuit reservoir volume. Inadequate venous return is determined by inadequate venous inflow (despite adequate negative inlet pressure), failure to reduce central venous pressure, an EPV flow above 100 mL/min, a pulsatile arterial pressure, failure to empty the cardiac chambers on TEE, direct inspection, or continued right or left ventricular ejection (30). The differential diagnosis of inadequate venous return includes malpositioned EVD, application of excessive negative pressure during AVD, and inadequate intravascular volume. Repositioning the EVD and adjusting the AVD siphon should improve venous blood return if intravascular volume is adequate.

Arterial Outflow

Arterial return is monitored in the same fashion as in traditional CPB (i.e,. measurement of flow and pressure on the arterial side of the circuit). When initiating Port-Access CPB, the perfusionist should pay particular attention to any unexpected increases in arterial infusion line pressure, which may indicate dissection. The anesthesiologist can observe the descending aorta via TEE at the time of initiating CPB for signs of vascular damage. A layering effect produced by the blood–pump prime interface when antegrade cardiac ejection meets retrograde aortic flow from the CPB circuit can be misinterpreted as aortic dissection (36).

Myocardial Decompression

Transesophageal echocardiographic imaging, measurement of central venous pressure, and determination of both EPV

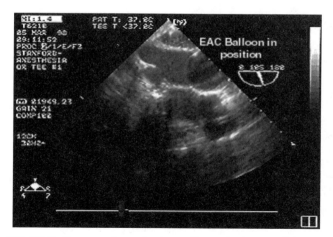

FIG. 35.9. Transesophageal echocardiography image of the endoaortic clamp (*EAC*) in the correct position in the ascending aorta approximately 3 to 4 cm beyond the aortic valve, which is seen in the top left portion of the image.

and EAC aortic root vent blood flow provide information about the adequacy of myocardial decompression. EPV flow should be less than 100 mL/min or less than 5% of the systemic flow. The pulmonary pressure should be zero or negative. Failure to satisfy either of these conditions may indicate a problem with venous drainage requiring repositioning of either the EPV or EVD. A reduction in EPV drainage may indicate obstruction of the lumen by malpositioning, kinking, failure to remove the guide cannula, reverse positioning of the negative pressure relief valve, or failure to turn the stopcock to the correct position. A small positive pressure (0 to 10 mm Hg) must be maintained in the aortic root to avoid EAC balloon migration. Excessive negative or positive pressure can result if the aortic wall abuts the tip of the catheter.

Cardioplegia

Antegrade or retrograde delivery of cardioplegia can be monitored via TEE because microbubbles will be present and can be visualized. With ECSC balloon inflation and initiation of retrograde cardioplegia, appropriate pressure (<40 mm Hg) should develop in the coronary sinus. Failure to generate the appropriate pressure may indicate that the ECSC has migrated out of the coronary sinus. ECSC migration can occur if the initial cardioplegia flow is too great, or if a rapid, transient pressure increase occurs. This emphasizes the need for slow changes in the cardioplegia flow rate. Overinflation of the ECSC balloon should be avoided because the coronary sinus can be damaged. High pressures in the coronary sinus may indicate distal migration or positioning in a small branch of the coronary sinus. In either case, TEE or fluoroscopy with contrast may delineate the problem. As with any operation in which cold cardioplegia is used, myocardial temperature and the electrocardiogram are used to monitor its efficacy.

Aortic Occlusion

When occluded by the endoaortic balloon, the systemic circulation is isolated from the aortic root. This allows a pressure differential to develop across the balloon. The gradient between the systemic arterial pressure and the aortic root pressure indicates satisfactory aortic occlusion. The aortic root pressure should vary with cardioplegia delivery and venting. If the endoaortic balloon is adequately inflated in the presence of full systemic blood flow delivered from the extracorporeal circuit, the aortic root pressure should fall below 10 mm Hg (except when antegrade cardioplegia is being delivered) and the endoaortic vent flow should be minimal (except when retrograde cardioplegia is being infused). To assess endoaortic balloon occlusion, one can also image the balloon contour with TEE, observe the aortic–systemic pressure difference, measure the endoaortic balloon inflation pressure, or note the presence of blood

in the operative field. Balloon rupture, proximal balloon migration into a wider portion (see below) of the aorta, a slow balloon leak, or improper connection of the catheter to the stopcock can result in a loss of aortic occlusion. The problem can be identified by TEE imaging of the balloon, fluoroscopy, direct inspection of the balloon connections, or aspiration of the balloon lumen. The presence of blood in the aspirate indicates balloon rupture. EAC balloon rupture can follow the placement of sutures in the mitral valve annulus if the balloon migrates too far toward the aortic valve. Loss of occlusion requires repositioning, reinflation of the EAC, replacement of the EAC (in the case of rupture), or conversion (when possible) to external cross-clamping of the ascending aorta under direct vision.

Migration of the Endoaortic Occlusion Clamp

Migration of the EAC is one of the major concerns in operating the system. During retrograde CPB, the flow tends to push the balloon toward the aortic valve. This can result in loss of occlusion, damage to the aortic valve, prolapse of the balloon into the left ventricle, and ineffective delivery of antegrade cardioplegia. Conversely, delivery of antegrade cardioplegia tends to push the balloon cephalad and occlude the innominate artery and possibly the left carotid artery (Fig. 35.11). Balloon migration can also damage the aortic wall or dislodge atheromatous debris or plaque. In most instances, TEE adequately monitors EAC position during CPB. However, cardiac manipulation, particularly during mitral valve procedures, can make observation by TEE difficult, and fluoroscopy should be used to assess balloon placement if TEE findings are inconclusive. Preventing proximal migration depends on removing excessive slack from the EAC catheter during placement, ensuring that balloon inflation pressures are adequate, avoiding excessive aortic root vent flow rates, and changing systemic arterial perfusion flows gradually.

Monitoring the systemic regional perfusion is important, as distal balloon migration can occlude the cerebral vessels. Monitoring of innominate artery and cerebral perfusion can be carried out by a number of methods. Table 35.4 describes these methods and their limitations. Arterial pressure should always be monitored in the right radial, brachial, or axillary artery because this pressure will fall if distal EAC migration partially or completely occludes the innominate artery. Simultaneous pressure monitoring in an artery supplied by the innominate artery and in one distal to (but not supplied by) the innominate artery (usually the left radial or femoral artery) will demonstrate balloon migration. The clinician should recognize that partial innominate artery occlusions may be difficult to detect, and that preexisting right-to-left or arm-to-leg pressure differences can complicate interpretation. Transcranial Doppler can also be used to detect distal migration and may identify partial occlusions more readily than does regional arterial pressure monitoring (37). How-

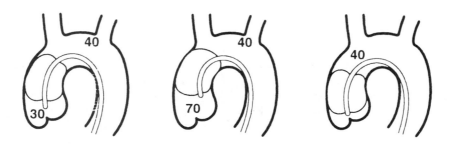

A,B A CLAMPING   B CARDIOPLEGIA   C VENTING   C

FIG. 35.11. Migration of the endoaortic clamp (*EAC*). **A:** Correct position of the EAC. **B:** Migration into the aortic arch tends to occur during antegrade cardioplegia and is driven by the changing pressure gradient across the balloon, illustrated by the hypothetical pressures on the diagram. **C:** Migration tends to occur toward the aortic valve during venting of the aortic root, again driven by the pressure gradient across the EAC balloon. Adequate balloon inflation, accurate initial positioning, minimization of the pressure differential across the balloon, and fixation of the catheter at the groin insertion site all decrease the tendency of the balloon to migrate. (From Peters WS, Siegel LC, Stevens JH, et al. Closed-chest cardiopulmonary bypass and cardioplegia: basis for less invasive cardiac surgery. *Ann Thorac Surg* 1997;63:1748–1754, with permission.)

TABLE 35.4. POTENTIAL STRATEGIES TO MONITOR CEREBRAL BLOOD FLOW DURING PORT-ACCESS CARDIOPULMONARY BYPASS

Monitor	Limitations	Observation with Cephalad Migration of Endoaortic Clamp[a]
Fluoroscopy	Must interrupt surgery to monitor	EAC occluding great vessels
TEE	May be difficult to visualize EAC position during surgery	EAC in area of great vessels
Carotid Doppler	1. Difficult to monitor signal continuously; dependent on index of suspicion 2. Difficult to obtain signal continuously with nonpulsatile blood flow	Sudden loss of blood flow signal
Transcranial Doppler	1. Difficult to monitor MCA blood flow continuously; dependent on index of suspicion 2. Difficult to insonate MCA during nonpulsatile blood flow 3. Poor sensitivity and specificity	1. Loss of MCA blood flow velocity signal 2. Change in ratio of right-to-left MCA flows 3. Possible reversal of flow direction in right MCA
Cerebral venous blood oximetry (right vs. left)	Sensitivity and specificity undefined	Decrease in cerebral venous blood oxygen saturation[b]
Transcranial oximetry	Sensitivity and specificity undefined	Right-sided decrease in oxygen saturation[b]
EEG	Hypothermia, anesthetics and roller pump artifacts limit interpretation	EEG slowing; change in right-vs.-left EEG signal
Right and left arm arterial pressures	1. Requires cannulation of both arteries in both arms 2. Left radial arterial free graft difficult (can cannulate radial artery stump)	Change in ratio of right MAP to left MAP
Right radial and femoral artery pressures	Femoral artery damage	Change in ratio of right arm MAP to femoral artery MAP

[a] Hypothetical observation; the sensitivity and specificity of these monitors in this clinical setting have not been evaluated.
[b] The rate and magnitude of the change depend on many factors, including the patient's cerebral temperature, magnitude of obstruction, and collateral blood flow. Right side theoretically more sensitive than left.
EAC, endoaortic clamp; EEG, electroencephalogram; MAP, mean arterial pressure; MCA, middle cerebral artery; TEE, transesophageal echocardiography.

ever, transcranial Doppler equipment is expensive, expertise is required for its placement and interpretation, and a signal cannot be obtained in 10% to 20% of patients even in the presence of pulsatile flow. Carotid or temporal artery pulse wave Doppler can also be used, but continuous monitoring is difficult to maintain for long periods. EEG monitoring theoretically should provide information about the adequacy of cerebral perfusion, but no data are available regarding its utility in this clinical setting. Similarly, bilateral cerebral transcranial oximetry may reflect acute changes in unilateral cerebral O_2 delivery following balloon occlusion of the innominate artery, but again no data are available.

The prevention of distal migration depends on adequate balloon inflation and avoidance of high aortic root pressures during antegrade cardioplegia delivery, so that a balance between the aortic root pressure and the systemic arterial pressure is maintained. If distal migration occurs, cessation of cardioplegia delivery may return the balloon to its correct position. In this case, the balloon inflation pressure should be increased. If the balloon does not return to the correct position, then it should be deflated, repositioned, and reinflated.

Cardiac De-airing

Transesophageal echocardiography monitors the adequacy of "de-airing." Air is found in the usual locations after the left side of the heart or coronary arteries are opened. Methods for de-airing the heart include patient positional changes, cardiac manipulation, discontinuation of the EPV, mechanical ventilation, rendering the mitral valve incompetent, venous drainage manipulations, vigorous aortic root venting, and retrograde cardioplegia. A recommended "de-airing" sequence is provided in Table 35.5. CO_2 gas can also be used to displace air from the operative field.

RESULTS AND COMPLICATIONS OF PORT-ACCESS CARDIAC SURGERY

Port-Access cardiac surgery does not eliminate some of the pathophysiologic consequences of CPB. However, certain complications may result from the unique technologic aspects of Port-Access CPB, such as vascular access via the femoral vessels, placement of a large balloon clamp in the ascending aorta, migration of the endoaortic balloon, and percutaneous cannulation and occlusion of the coronary sinus. The incidence of these complications is unknown at present. Much of the available data reside in the proprietary Port-Access International Registry sponsored by Heartport, Inc., which collects voluntary data from a number of centers performing PACS. Voluntary reporting risks underestimation of the complication rates. Table 35.6 lists the potential complications of PACS.

Local complications at the site of femoral cannulation

TABLE 35.5. DE-AIRING PROCEDURES AFTER PORT-ACCESS MITRAL VALVE SURGERY

A. During left atrial closure: EAC inflated
1. Trendelenburg position, 45° left lateral decubitus.
2. EPV off.
3. Catheter across mitral valve to make incompetent.
4. Fill left ventricle with physiologic saline solution.
5. As atrial closure progresses:
   a. Generous preload.
   b. Inflate and deflate lungs.
6. Shake patient and manipulate left ventricle to mobilize air.

B. Left atrium closed: EAC inflated
1. Aortic root venting with EAC.
2. Retrograde cardioplegia.
3. Massage heart.
4. Steep Trendelenburg position
5. Decrease systemic flow, slowly deflate EAC.

C. After EAC deflation
1. Continue aortic venting.
2. Decompress heart.
3. Place needle vent in aortic root if appropriate.

D. Monitor de-airing
1. Transesophageal echocardiography.
2. ECG.
3. Direct inspection of
   a. Atriotomy.
   b. Right coronary artery.
   c. Aortic root needle vent.

EAC, endoaortic occlusion clamp; ECG, electrocardiogram; EPV, endopulmonary artery vent.
Adapted from the *Heartport Training Manual,* Heartport, Inc., Redwood City, CA, with permission.

TABLE 35.6. POTENTIAL COMPLICATIONS OF PORT-ACCESS CARDIAC SURGERY

Vascular: local
Local dissection of iliofemoral system
Stenosis at cannulation site
Acute limb ischemia
Damage to venous drainage of the leg
Lymphocele
Vascular: systemic
Aortic dissection
Retrograde embolism (e.g., plaque)
Damage to aortic wall
Coronary sinus or right ventricular perforation
EAC balloon migration
Proximal
  Loss of occlusion
  Aortic valve damage
  Prolapse of EAC into left ventricle
Distal: occlusion of cerebral supply vessels
Dislodgment of atheromatous plaque
Other: infection
  Hemorrhage (particularly intercostal artery)

EAC, endoaortic occlusion clamp.

include vascular damage, stenosis of femoral artery or vein, acute limb ischemia, thrombosis, lymphocele, and local groin infection. Cannulation of the femoral vein can also lead to deep vein thrombosis and pulmonary embolism. Arterial dissection related to cannulation or the EAC is probably the most feared complication. This can result from a ruptured or traumatized atheromatous plaque or from vascular trauma related to the passage or inflation of the EAC. Early experience reported dissections in 11 of 600 (1.8%) cases (38). Mohr et al. (39) reported two dissections in 51 patients. Some dissections resulting from Port-Access CPB have been fatal. These high incidences prompted changes in the EAC catheter and guidewire design, a revision of recommendations about patient screening and cannulation techniques, and reemphasis on the importance of vigilant monitoring of the arterial line pressure at initiation of Port-Access CPB. The overall incidence of aortic dissection in a large series of patients was 0.75% (8 of 1,063) but fell to 0.18% (1 of 532) in the second part of the series. If this reporting mechanism has yielded accurate figures, then this latter incidence places the risk for aortic dissection in the range of that for conventional cardiac surgical approaches to CPB (40).

Some aspects of the Port-Access platform may affect cerebral physiology (or pathophysiology) during extracorporeal circulation. In particular, the endoaortic clamp (positioning and interface with the aortic endothelium), retrograde aortic blood flow, and limited access to the cardiac chambers for "de-airing" maneuvers may affect cerebral integrity during and after CPB. The incidence of adverse central nervous system outcomes resulting from unrecognized EAC migration remains unknown.

Because the majority of adverse central nervous system events associated with CPB are thought to be related to macroembolic and microembolic events, the effect of the EAC on these phenomena merits consideration (41). A substantial proportion of these events occur with placement and removal of occlusive or partially occlusive aortic cross-clamps (42). The endoaortic clamp eliminates the need for "crushing" the aorta; the inflation of a soft balloon may result in less fracturing of atheromatous plaque and a reduction in the amount of embolic debris. Alternatively, retrograde arterial blood flow, passage of the cannulas and catheters associated with Port-Access CPB, and the relatively large contact area of the EAC with the ascending aorta could dislodge mobile atheromas or disrupt atherosclerotic plaques. Retrograde aortic blood flow associated with femoral artery cannulation for CPB has long been recognized as a potential risk factor for adverse central nervous system outcomes, presumably because reversal of flow tends to disrupt atheromatous debris and direct it toward the brain. How the incidence of adverse central nervous system events associated with conventional CPB techniques compares with that associated with the Port-Access platform remains unknown.

Residual air in the cardiac chambers constitutes another important source of cerebral emboli in cardiac surgery (43). It is frequently challenging to "de-air" the heart during conventional bypass procedures; various maneuvers, including manual shaking of the chest ("rock and roll"), increasing pulmonary pressures by manual inflation of the lungs, and direct massage of the heart, fail to evacuate all the air from the TEE-visualized "targets." The limited access to the heart with minimally invasive approaches further complicates "de-airing" maneuvers.

In summary, the effect of Port-Access CPB on perioperative cerebral pathophysiology remains unclear. In some respects, it may decrease the likelihood of adverse central nervous system events by permitting "gentler" handling of the aortic root, especially in the patient with a diseased aorta. The best technique (or combination of techniques) to monitor cerebral perfusion remains unknown.

The long-term effects of balloon inflation to pressures up to 350 mm Hg in the ascending aorta have not been investigated. There were no reports of aortic rupture at the time of this writing. Other complications that may occur include damage to the coronary sinus or other cardiac structures during passage of the ECSC or EPV. This stresses the need for gentle manipulation and avoidance of prolonged attempts at catheter placement.

Few data are available regarding the long-term patency of coronary artery bypass grafts created with the Port-Access method. Patency is of great importance in both PACS and MIDCAB grafting without CPB, as the standard median sternotomy technique with CPB is associated with high patency rates and low complication rates. The acute graft patency rate was assessed in 31 patients undergoing PACS that included both single internal mammary grafts and multiple-vessel grafts (44). Of 27 patients studied before discharge, the internal mammary artery was patent in 100%, with an overall graft patency rate of 97.7%. However, the study provided no data on long-term graft patency. Another study looked at left anterior descending graft patency in PACS versus MIDCAB and showed a patency rate of 100% for PACS versus 92.3% for MIDCAB (45). Other studies have also indicated acceptable outcomes (35,46). The length of hospital stay in these studies varied from 2 to 5 days.

A number of studies have assessed the use of the PACS platform for mitral valve surgery. Galloway et al. (47) used the Port-Access system in 131 patients undergoing either mitral valve replacement or repair. Overall mortality was 1.1%. Glower et al. (48) retrospectively investigated the advantages and disadvantages of PACS versus conventional sternotomy in 41 consecutive patients undergoing mitral valve surgery. The groups were matched for age, ejection fraction, mitral valve pathology, and comorbidity. They found overall duration of the surgical procedure, including bypass time and cross-clamp times, to be greater for PACS than for median sternotomy. The overall complication rates were similar. There was a tendency for a shorter hospital

TABLE 35.7. SUMMARY OF PORT-ACCESS CARDIAC RESULTS (UP TO 30 DAYS POSTOPERATIVELY)

Percent	CABG (n = 583) (%)	Mitral Valve Repair (n = 137) (%)	Mitral Valve Replacement (n = 184) (%)
Death	1.0	1.5	3.3
Stroke	2.2	3.6	1.1
Myocardial infarction	1.0	0.0	0.0
Reoperation of primary procedure	0.0	0.7	0.0
Reexploration for bleeding	1.5	1.5	3.8
Renal failure	0.2	0.7	0.5
Multiple organ failure	0.0	0.0	0.5
New atrial fibrillation	5.0	7.3	7.1

Data taken from 121 Port-Access International Registry centers from 4/1/97 to 12/31/97. Demographics for CABG patients: mean age, 60.5 years; mean weight, 83.1 kg. Demographics for mitral valve patients: mean age, 57.5 years; mean weight, 72.8 kg. CABG, coronary artery bypass graft.
From Galloway AC, Shemin RJ, Glower DD, et al. First report of the Port-Access International Registry. *Ann Thorac Surg* 1999;67:51–56.

stay in the PACS group, although it did not reach statistical significance. The major difference between the groups was the time to return to normal activity, which was significantly less in the PACS group (4 ± 2 vs. 9 ± 1 weeks). In the study of Port-Access mitral valve surgery by Mohr et al. (39), the mortality rate was 9.8%, although only one death could be directly attributed to the technique (aortic dissection). This may demonstrate a learning curve, as their most recent 28 patients had a low incidence of morbidity and no mortality. Other complications in that series included a high incidence of postoperative confusion and aortic dissection. One unusual complication of Port-Access mitral valve surgery is the entrapment of the EPV by atriotomy closure sutures. To eliminate this complication, the anesthesiologist should check the mobility of the EPV immediately after atriotomy closure while the patient is still on CPB.

Only one study looks at the overall adverse outcome rates for PACS, and the results, taken from Port-Access International Registry data, are summarized in Table 35.7 (40). Operative mortality was 1% for coronary artery bypass graft, 3.3% for mitral valve replacement, and 1.5% for mitral valve repair. Ninety-four percent of procedures that began as PACS were completed with this technology. The incidence of complications, including neurologic complications, was similar to those reported by the Society for Thoracic Surgeons for patients managed with conventional CPB. However, new-onset atrial fibrillation occurs less frequently in Port-Access patients. This may be attributable to the avoidance of atriotomy and decreased atrial manipulation and favorably affects the postoperative period and overall morbidity. Unfortunately, no prospective clinical trials comparing the two techniques have been performed.

SUMMARY

Port-Access CPB provides an alternative to minimally invasive cardiac surgery. However, it is more complex than conventional CPB and is technically challenging for the surgeon, anesthesiologist, and perfusionist. At present, overall operative and bypass durations are greater than those associated with conventional procedures. This relates both to the surgical difficulty and to the increased "anesthesia preparatory time" associated with placement of the ECSC and EPV (34). With experience, these times may decrease (33,48). PACS requires special training, and the initial learning curve is steep. TEE expertise is essential, as TEE plays a major role in the overall management of PACS. The Port-Access approach is rich in unanswered questions about perioperative brain monitoring and well-being. Appropriate patient selection is critical to reducing the likelihood of vascular (particularly aortic dissection), neurologic, and other complications. Present clinical trials are limited by the fact that they are neither randomized nor prospective. Preliminary data suggest that this technique can be carried out safely with proper precautions and patient selection. Further study is needed to analyze the outcomes, long-term efficacy, recovery times, and cost-effectiveness of PACS.

KEY POINTS

- New approaches to cardiac surgery in which smaller incisions are used have recently developed; in some of these, CPB is avoided, whereas in others, new approaches to CPB are utilized. This chapter addresses an approach to minimally invasive CPB called *Port-Access CPB*.
- Port-Access CPB involves the use of *several percutaneous catheters developed to permit minimally invasive CPB*, including the following:
  - A *femoral arterial cannula* designed to permit passage of an *endoaortic balloon catheter* that occludes the ascending aorta, infuses antegrade cardioplegia, vents the aortic root, and monitors aortic root pressure.
  - A *multilumen venous drainage cannula* that advances into the right atrium via the femoral vein.
  - A percutaneous *coronary sinus cannula* for the delivery of retrograde cardioplegia.
  - A *pulmonary artery vent* catheter.
- *Perfusion management* for Port-Access CPB requires separate pumps for the pulmonary artery and aortic

root vents, a pump or use of vacuum applied to a hard-shell venous reservoir to assist venous drainage, a flowmeter for the pulmonary artery vent, and additional pressure monitoring for the coronary sinus, endoaortic balloon, and aortic root.

■ The need to position and inflate an occlusive balloon in the ascending aorta excludes patients with severe aortic or peripheral vascular disease, aortic aneurysm or Marfan's syndrome, and severe aortic valvular incompetence.

■ The cannulation and management of patients undergoing Port-Access CPB requires *specific training* of the surgical team, including the perfusionist, anesthesiologist, surgeon, and scrub technician or nurse. Specialized monitoring required during cannulation and CPB includes pressure and flow monitoring and imaging with TEE, fluoroscopy, or both.

■ *Migration of the endoaortic cannula* constitutes a particular hazard of Port-Access CPB because distal migration can compromise cerebral blood flow and proximal migration can compromise antegrade cardioplegia delivery and left ventricular decompression. Cardiac de-airing maneuvers also are more complex than with traditional CPB via median sternotomy.

■ Experience and results continue to accumulate, with some reports suggesting complication rates (e.g., aortic dissection, inadequate valvular repair) exceeding those for traditional CPB. The voluntary Port-Access International Registry database suggests results comparable with those for traditional CPB and a reduced incidence of postoperative atrial fibrillation. To date, no prospective, randomized trials have compared Port-Access with traditional CPB.

REFERENCES

1. Benetti F, Naselli G, Wood M, et al. Direct myocardial revascularization without extracorporeal circulation: experience in 700 patients. *Chest* 1991;100:312–316.
2. Buffolo E, de Andrade JCS, Branco JNR, et al. Coronary artery bypass grafting without cardiopulmonary bypass. *Ann Thorac Surg* 1996;61:63–66.
3. Gayes JM, Emery RW. The MIDCAB experience: a current look at evolving surgical and anesthetic approaches. *J Cardiothorac Vasc Anesth* 1997;5:625–628.
4. Zenati M, Domit TM, Saul MS, et al. Resource utilization for minimally invasive direct and standard coronary artery bypass grafting. *Ann Thorac Surg* 1997;63:S84–S87.
5. Peters WS. Minimally invasive cardiac surgery by cardioscopy. *Australas J Card Thorac Surg* 1993;2:152–154.
6. Toomasian JM, Peters, WS, Siegel LC, et al. Extracorporeal circulation for Port-Access cardiac surgery. *Perfusion* 1997;12:83–93.
7. Toomasian JM, Williams DL, Colvin SB, et al. Perfusion during coronary and mitral valve surgery utilizing minimally invasive Port-Access technology. *J Extra-Corp Technol* 1997;29:66–72.
8. Peters WS, Siegel LC, Stevens JH, et al. Closed chest cardiopulmonary bypass and cardioplegia: basis for less invasive cardiac surgery. *Ann Thorac Surg* 1997;63:1748–1754.
9. Stevens JH, Burdon TA, Siegel LC, et al. Port-Access coronary artery bypass with cardioplegic arrest: acute and chronic canine studies. *Ann Thorac Surg* 1996;62:435–441.
10. Schwartz D, Ribakove GH, Grossi EA, et al. Single and multiple vessel Port-Access coronary artery bypass grafting with cardiplegic arrest. Technique and reproducibility. *J Thorac Cardiovasc Surg* 1997;114:46–52.
11. Stevens JH, Burdon TA, Peters WS, et al. Port-Access coronary artery grafting: a proposed surgical method. *J Thorac Cardiovasc Surg* 1996;111:567–573.
12. Schwartz D, Ribakove GH, Grossi EA, et al. Minimally invasive mitral valve replacement: Port-Access technique, feasibilty and myocardial function preservation. *J Thorac Cardiovasc Surg* 1997; 113:1022–1031.
13. Pompili MF, Stevens JH. Port-Access mitral valve replacement in dogs. *J Thorac Cardiovasc Surg* 1996;112: 1268–1274.
14. Schwarz DS, Ribakove GH, Grossi EA, et al. Minimally invasive cardiopulmonary bypass with cardioplegia arrest: a closed chest technique with equivalent myocardial protection. *J Thorac Cardiovasc Surg* 1996;111:556–566.
15. Reitz BA, Stevens JH, Burdon TA, et al. Port-Access coronary artery bypass grafting: lessons learned in a phase 1 clinical trial. *Circulation* 1996;94:1294(abst).
16. Reichenspuner H, Gulielmos V, Daniel WG, et al. Minimally invasive coronary bypass surgery. *N Engl J Med* 1997;336:67–68.
17. Pompili MF, Yakub A, Siegel LC, et al. Port-Access mitral valve replacement: initial clinical experience. *Circulation* 1996;94:I-3122(abst).
18. Bartlett RH. Extracorporeal life support for cardiopulmonary failure. *Curr Probl Surg* 1990;27:623–705.
19. Hirschl RB, Bartlett RH. Extracorporeal membrane oxygenation support in cardiorespiratory failure. *Adv Surg* 1987;21:189–212.
20. Vogel RA, Shawl F, Tommaso C, et al. Initial report of the National Registry of Elective Cardiopulmonary Bypass-Supported Coronary Angioplasty. *J Am Coll Cardiol* 1990;15:23–29.
21. Hill JG, Bruhn PS, Cohen SE, et al. Emergent applications of cardiopulmonary support: a multi-institutional experience. *Ann Thorac Surg* 1992;54:699–704.
22. Chyatte D, Elefteriades J, Kim B. Profound hypothermia and circulatory arrest for aneurysm surgery: case report. *J Neurosurg* 1989;70:489–491.
23. Mongero LB, Sistino JJ, Beck J, et al. Current perfusion techniques for repair of giant cerebral aneurysms using deep hypothermia and circulatory arrest. *J Extra-Corp Technol* 1994;26:13–17.
24. Reichman TR, Joyo CI, Dembitsky WP, et al. Improved patient survival after cardiac arrest using a cardiopulmonary support system. *Ann Thorac Surg* 1990;49:101–105.
25. Raithel SC, Swartz MT, Braun PR, et al. Experience with an emergency resuscitation system. *ASAIO Trans* 1989;35:475–477.
26. Bartlett RH. Physiology of extracorporeal life support. In: Zwischenberger JB, Bartlett RH, eds. *ECMO, extracorporeal cardiopulmonary support in critical care*. Ann Arbor, MI: Extracorporeal Life Support Organization, 1995:38.
27. Toomasian JM, McCarthy JP. Total extrathoracic cardiopulmonary support with kinetic assisted venous drainage: experience in 50 patients. *Perfusion* 1998;13:137–143.
28. Pederson TH, Videm V, Svennevig JL, et al. Extracorporeal membrane oxygenation using a centrifugal pump and servo regulator to prevent negative inlet pressure. *Ann Thorac Surg* 1997; 63:1333–1339.
29. Toomasian JM, Conte JV, Reitz BA. Kinetic assisted venous drainage as an adjunct to multiple redo sternotomy. In: Toomasian JM, Kurusz M, Stafford TB, eds. *Case reports: clinical studies*

in extracorporeal circulation. Houston: PREF Press, 1996:1–10 (vol 2).

30. Siegel LC, St.Goar FG, Stevens JH, et al. Monitoring considerations for Port-Access cardiac surgery. *Circulation* 1997;96: 562–568.

31. Applebaum RM, Cutler W, Bhardwaj N, et al. Utility of transesophageal echocardiography during Port-Access cardiac surgery. *Am J Cardiol* 1998;82:183–188.

32. Clements F, Wright SJ, De Bruijn N. Coronary sinus catheterization made easy for Port-Access minimally invasive cardiac surgery. *J Cardiothorac Vasc Anesth* 1998;12:96–101.

33. Yen ES. Brown GA, Carlson JL, et al. Rapid cannulation of the coronary sinus during Port-Access cardiac surgery. *Anesthesiology* 1998;89:A307(abst).

34. Mora Mangano CT. Show me the money. (But first show me the data) [Editorial]. *J Cardiothorac Vasc Anesth* 1998;12:615–616.

35. Chaney MA, Nikolov MP, Tuchek M, et al. An institution initial experience with Port-Access minimally invasive cardiac surgery. *J Cardiothorac Vasc Anesth* 1998;12:617–619.

36. Watke CM, Clements F, Glower DD, et al. False-positive diagnosis of aortic dissection associated with femoral cardiopulmonary bypass. *Anesthesiology* 1998;88:119–121.

37. Grocott HP, Stafford Smith M, Glower DD, et al. Endovascular balloon clamp malposition during minimally invasive cardiac surgery: detection by transcranial Doppler. *Anesthesiology* 1998;88: 1396–1399.

38. Reitz B. Presentation at the World Congress of Minimally Invasive Cardiac Surgery, Paris, May 1997.

39. Mohr FW, Falk V, Diegler A, et al. Minimally invasive Port-Access mitral valve surgery. *J Thorac Cardiovasc Surg* 1998;115: 567–576.

40. Galloway AC, Glower DD, Shemin RJ, et al. First report of the Port-Access International Registry. *Ann Thorac Surg* 1999;67: 51–56.

41. Roach GW, Kanchuger M, Mora Mangano C, et al. Adverse cerebral outcomes after coronary artery bypass surgery. *N Engl J Med* 1996;335:1857–1863.

42. Mora CT, Murkin JM. The central nervous system response to cardiopulmonary bypass. In: Mora CT, ed. *Cardiopulmonary bypass: principles and techniques of extracorporeal circulation.* New York: Springer-Verlag, 1995:114–146.

43. Pugsley W, Klinger L, Paschalis C, et al. The impact of microemboli during cardiopulmonary bypass on neuropsychological functioning. *Stroke* 1994;25:1393–1399.

44. Ribakove GH, Miller JS, Anderson RV, et al. Minimally invasive Port-Access coronary artery bypass grafting with early angiographic follow-up: initial clinical experience. *J Thorac Cardiovasc Surg* 1998;115:1101–1110.

45. Galloway AC, Ribacove GH, Esposito JS, et al. Port-Access MID-CAB: clinical experience and follow-up. *J Am Coll Cardiol* 1998; 31:69A(abst).

46. Reichenspurner H, Guliemos V, Wunderlich J, et al. Port-Access coronary artery bypass grafting with the use of cardiopulmonary bypass and cardioplegic arrest. *Ann Thorac Surg* 1998;65: 413–419.

47. Galloway AC, Ribakove GH, Grossi EA, et al. Minimally invasive Port-Access valvular surgery: initial clinical experience. *Circulation* 1997;96 [Suppl 1]:2845 I-508.

48. Glower DD, Landolfo KP, Clements F, et al. Mitral valve operation via Port-Access versus median sternotomy. *Eur J Cardiothorac Surg* 1998;14[Suppl 1]:S143–S147.

Note: Page numbers followed by t and f denote tables and figures, respectively.